# Textbook of Sports and Exercise Cardiology

Axel Pressler • Josef Niebauer
Editors

# Textbook of Sports and Exercise Cardiology

Springer

*Editors*
Axel Pressler
Private Center for Sports and Exercise Cardiology
München
Bayern
Germany

Josef Niebauer
University Institute of Sports Medicine
Prevention and Rehabilitation
Paracelsus Medical University Salzburg
Salzburg
Austria

ISBN 978-3-030-35373-5 ISBN 978-3-030-35374-2 (eBook)
https://doi.org/10.1007/978-3-030-35374-2



This Springer imprint is published by the registered company Springer Nature Switzerland AG
The registered company address is: Gewerbestrasse 11, 6330 Cham, Switzerland

# Preface

Sports and exercise cardiology have been increasingly acknowledged in recent years as important components of diagnostic and treatment pathways in modern medicine. Originating historically from the evaluation of the impact of intensive exercise on cardiac morphology and function, they have developed over time into much broader subspecialties in covering all aspects of both positive and potentially negative associations of regular physical activity and exercise with the cardiovascular system. Given both the drastic increase in inactive, obese individuals at high risk for subsequent cardiometabolic diseases and, in turn, millions of leisure time athletes participating in strenuous exercise events, specialists are increasingly needed who have been appropriately educated and trained to enable both patients and athletes to safely benefit from participation in leisure time or competitive sports.

Regarding sports cardiology, besides competitive athletes in their adolescent and young adult years, also an increasing number of those who exercise not only do so leisurely but strive to participate in competitions. These leisure time athletes increasingly practice at volumes and intensities that come close to or even exceed that of full-fledged athletes. In both groups, adaptations of the cardiovascular system occur that are commonly summarized as athlete's heart and may mimic pathologies that are known to be associated with cardiovascular complications including sudden cardiac death. It is the aim of sports cardiology to protect the physically active from untoward effects of exercise training and therefore to identify physiologic cardiac adaptations secondary to an increased hemodynamic demand from overt pathologies.

Regarding exercise cardiology, physical activity and exercise training have become the mainstay of prevention and treatment of noncommunicable diseases. National and international recommendations and guidelines from leading professional organizations attest the highest level of evidence. Nonetheless, just like any other potent drug, exercise not only helps prevent disease but also has its side effects, and thus may trigger, among others, sudden cardiac death or disease progression. "Exercise is medicine" and must be applied as such. The choice of activity or sport as well as the "dosage" has to be tailored individually in order to maximize benefit and minimize risk.

Nonetheless, in both medical schools and specialist training, physical activity and exercise training do still not receive the attention they deserve and require, leaving the vast majority of colleagues rather oblivious to the benefits but also to the inherent risks. To overcome these educational limits, working groups on sports and exercise cardiology worldwide have proposed specific curricula enabling interested candidates to qualify themselves as specialists in sports and exercise cardiology by acquiring specific knowledge and skills beyond the traditional education pathways. In Germany, for example, sports cardiology can now be acquired as official subspecialty after following a specific curriculum endorsed by the German Cardiac Society.

This book is intended to support interested students and medical professionals in these undertakings by providing a comprehensive overview on all aspects of sports and exercise cardiology. In combining profound theoretical background with precise practical recommendations, it addresses a broad readership, ranging from inquisitive students who consider starting a career as sports and exercise cardiologists over clinicians searching for precise information readily transferable to everyday care up to experienced professionals who will find up-to-date reviews on scientific and clinical backgrounds. We are happy, grateful, and proud of having assembled the world's leading experts in the field of sports and exercise cardiology, sharing with readers their wealth of knowledge in order to serve as a support during—among others—the process of pre-participation screening, comprehensive but sport- and exercise-specific diagnostics, and athletes' and patients' counseling, which shall result in healthy as well as efficient and effective exercise training. We hope that this book will become a companion during daily practice, as it encompasses all major aspects a physician in the field of physical activity, exercise training, cardiac prevention and rehabilitation, and above all sports cardiology needs to know.

München, Bayern, Germany — Axel Pressler
Salzburg, Austria — Josef Niebauer

---

The original version of this book was revised. The correction to this book can be found at https://doi.org/10.1007/978-3-030-35374-2_52

# Contents

# Contributors

**Paolo Emilio Adami** Department of Health and Science, World Athletics, Monaco Monaco

Department of Health and Science, International Association of Athletics Federations—IAAF, Monte Carlo, Monaco

**Volker Adams** Heart Center Dresden, Laboratory for Molecular and Experimental Cardiology, TU Dresden, Dresden, Germany

**Ross Arena** Department of Physical Therapy, College of Applied Health Sciences, University of Illinois at Chicago, Chicago, IL, USA

**Aaron L. Baggish** Cardiovascular Performance Program, Division of Cardiology, Massachusetts General Hospital, Boston, MA, USA

**Martin Bahls** Department of Internal Medicine B, University Medicine Greifswald, Greifswald, Germany

**Cristina Basso** Cardiovascular Pathology, Department of Cardiac, Thoracic and Vascular Sciences and Public Health, University of Padua Medical School, Padua, Italy

**Susanne Berrisch-Rahmel** MVZ DaVita CardioCentrum Düsseldorf, Düsseldorf, Germany

**Alessandro Biffi** Institute of Sports Medicine & Science, Italian Olympic Committee, Rome, Italy

**Birna Bjarnason-Wehrens** Department of Preventive and Rehabilitative Sport and Exercise Medicine, Institute for Cardiology and Sports Medicine, German Sports University Cologne, Cologne, Germany

**Mats Börjesson** Neuroscience and Physiology & Center for Health and Performance, University of Gothenburg, Gothenburg, Sweden

Neuroscience and Physiology & Center for Health and Performance, University of Gothenburg and Sahlgrenska University Hospital/Ostra, Gothenburg, Sweden

Department of Neuroscience and Physiology, Sahlgrenska Academy and Center for Health and Perfoamce, Gothenburg University and Sahlgrenska University Hospital/ Ostra, Gothenburg, Sweden

**Maria Joan Brosnan** Department of Cardiology and Sports Cardiology, St Vincent's Hospital and Baker Institute, Melbourne, VIC, Australia

**Martin Burtscher** Department of Sports Sciences, University of Innsbruck, Innsbruck, Austria

**François Carré** Department of Sports Medicine, University Hospital of Rennes, Rennes1 University, Inserm, Rennes, France

**Stefano Caselli** Cardiovascular Center Zurich, Hirslanden Klinik im Park, Zurich, Switzerland

**Silvia Castelletti** Center for Cardiac Arrhythmias of Genetic Origin, Istituto Auxologico Italiano, IRCCS, Milan, Italy

**Elena Cavarretta** Department of Medical-Surgical Sciences and Biotechnologies, Sapienza University of Rome, Rome, Italy

Mediterranea Cardiocentro, Naples, Italy

**Jeffrey Wilcox Christle** Division of Cardiovascular Medicine, Department of Medicine, Falk Cardiovascular Research Center, Stanford Sports Cardiology, Stanford University, Stanford, CA, USA

**Guido Claessen** Department of Cardiovascular Medicine, University Hospital Leuven, Leuven, Belgium

Department of Sports Cardiology, Baker Heart and Diabetes Institute, Melbourne, VIC, Australia

**Sheri R. Colberg** Old Dominion University, Norfolk, VA, USA

**Véronique Cornelissen** Department of Rehabilitation Sciences, KU Leuven, Leuven, Belgium

**Domenico Corrado** Department of Cardiac, Thoracic and Vascular Sciences and Public Health, University of Padova, Padova, Italy

**Lia Crotti** Center for Cardiac Arrhythmias of Genetic Origin, Istituto Auxologico Italiano, IRCCS, Milan, Italy

Laboratory of Cardiovascular Genetics, Istituto Auxologico Italiano, IRCCS, Milan, Italy

Department of Cardiovascular, Neural and Metabolic Sciences, San Luca Hospital, Istituto Auxologico Italiano, IRCCS, Milan, Italy

Department of Medicine and Surgery, University of Milano-Bicocca, Milan, Italy

**Flavio D'Ascenzi** Division of Cardiology, Department of Medical Biotechnologies, University of Siena, Siena, Italy

School of Medicine, University of Pittsburgh, Pittsburgh, PAUSA

**María Sanz de la Garza** Cardiovascular Institute, Hospital Clinic, Barcelona, Spain

**Mikael Dellborg** Department of Molecular and Clinical Medicine, Institute of Medicine, Sahlgrenska Academy, University of Gothenburg and Sahlgrenska University Hospital/Ostra, Gothenburg, Sweden

**Marcus Dörr** Department of Internal Medicine B, University Medicine Greifswald, Greifswald, Germany

**Jonathan A. Drezner** Department of Family Medicine/Sports Medicine, UW Medicine Center for Sports Cardiology, University of Washington, Seattle, WA, USA

**Frank Edelmann** Department of Internal Medicine and Cardiology, Charité Universitätsmedizin Berlin, Campus Virchow Klinikum, Berlin, Germany

**Thijs M.H. Eijsvogels** Department of Physiology, Radboud Institute for Health Sciences, Radboud University Medical Center, Nijmegen, The Netherlands

**Andrew Elagizi** Department of Cardiovascular Diseases, John Ochsner Heart and Vascular Institute, New Orleans, LA, USA

**Gherardo Finocchiaro** Division of Cardiovascular Sciences, Department of Cardiology, Guy's and St. Thomas' Hospitals and King's College London, London, UK

**Carla Frescura** Cardiovascular Pathology, Department of Cardiac, Thoracic and Vascular Sciences and Public Health, University of Padua Medical School, Padua, Italy

**Sabiha Gati** Department of Cardiology/Cardiac MRI, Royal Brompton & Harefield NHS Trust & National Heart and Lung Institute, Imperial College, London, UK

**Keith Phillip George** Research Institute for Sport and Exercise Science, Liverpool John Moores University, Liverpool, UK

**Belinda Gray** Cardiology Clinical Academic Group, St George's, University of London, London, UK

**Eduard Guasch** Arrhythmia Unit, Cardiology Department, Hospital Clínic/IDIBAPS, Barcelona, Spain

**Martin Halle** Department of Prevention, Sports Medicine and Sports Cardiology, University hospital 'Klinikum rechts der Isar', Technical University of Munich, DZHK (German Center for Cardiovascular Research), Munich, Germany

**Dominique Hansen** Heart Centre Hasselt, Jessa Hospital, BIOMED (Biomedical Research Institute) and REVAL (Rehabilitation Research Centre), Hasselt University, Hasselt, Belgium

**Kimberly G. Harmon** Department of Family Medicine, University of Washington School of Medicine, Seattle, WA, USA

Department of Orthopaedics and Sports Medicine, University of Washington School of Medicine, Seattle, WA, USA

**Mark J. Haykowsky** University of Alberta, Edmonton, AB, Canada

**Hein Heidbuchel** Department of Cardiology, Antwerp University Hospital and Antwerp University, Antwerp, Belgium

**Verena Heinicke** Department of Prevention, Sports Medicine and Sports Cardiology, University hospital 'Klinikum rechts der Isar', Technical University of Munich, DZHK (German Center for Cardiovascular Research), Munich, Germany

**Xavier Jouven** Paris-Sudden Death Expertise Center (Paris-SDEC), Paris, France

Paris Descartes University, Paris, France

Cardiology Department, European Georges Pompidou Hospital, Paris, France

Paris-Cardiovascular Research Center (Inserm U970), Paris, France

**Sergey Kachur** Department of Cardiovascular Diseases, John Ochsner Heart and Vascular Institute, New Orleans, LA, USA

**Dalane W. Kitzman** Kermit Glenn Phillips II Chair in Cardiovascular Medicine, Cardiovascular Medicine Section, Department of Internal Medicine, Wake Forest School of Medicine, Winston-Salem, NC, USA

**Efraim Kramer** Department of Sports Medicine, University of Pretoria, Pretoria, South Africa

**Nicolle Kränkel** Department of Cardiology, Charité–Universitätsmedizin Berlin, Berlin, Germany

**André La Gerche** Department of Sports Cardiology, Baker Heart and Diabetes Institute, Melbourne, VIC, Australia

National Centre for Sports Cardiology, St. Vincent's Hospital Melbourne, Melbourne, VIC, Australia

**Rachel Lampert** Department of Internal Medicine/Cardiology, Yale School of Medicine, New Haven, CT, USA

**Roman Laszlo** Division of Sports and Rehabilitation Medicine, Center of Medicine, Ulm University Hospital, Ulm, Germany

**Carl J. Lavie** John Ochsner Heart and Vascular Institute, Ochsner Clinical School–The University of Queensland School of Medicine, New Orleans, LA, USA

**Christine E. Lawless** Sports Cardiology Consultants LLC, Chicago, IL, USA

**Mark S. Link** Division of Cardiology, Department of Medicine, UTSouthwestern Medical Center, Dallas, TX, USA

**Herbert Löllgen** University of Mainz, Private Practice, Sports Cardiology and Cardiology, Remscheid, Germany

**Aneil Malhotra** Consultant Cardiologist-Inherited Cardiac Conditions and Sports Cardiology, Manchester University Hospitals, University of Manchester, Manchester, London, UK

**Eloi Marijon** Paris-Sudden Death Expertise Center (Paris-SDEC), Paris, France

Paris Descartes University, Paris, France

Cardiology Department, European Georges Pompidou Hospital, Paris, France

Paris-Cardiovascular Research Center (Inserm U970), Paris, France

**Andrew Maxwell** Department of Pediatric Cardiology, Heart of the Valley Pediatric Cardiology, Pleasanton, CA, USA

**Klaus Peter Mellwig** Department of Cardiology, Heart Center Northrhine Westfalia, Bad Oeynhausen, Germany

**Hielko Miljoen** Department of Cardiology, Antwerp University Hospital, Antwerp, Belgium

**Stefan Möhlenkamp** Clinic of Cardiology and Intensive Care Medicine, Bethanien Hospital Moers, Moers, Germany

**Lluis Mont** Arrhythmia Unit, Cardiology Department, Hospital Clínic/IDIBAPS, Barcelona, Spain

**Jan Müller** Department of Preventive Pediatrics, Technical University of Munich, Munich, Germany

**Jonathan Myers** Cardiology Division, Veterans Affairs Palo Alto Health Care System and Stanford University, Stanford, CA, USA

**Kumar Narayanan** Paris-Sudden Death Expertise Center (Paris-SDEC), Paris, France

Cardiology Department, Medicover Hospitals, Hyderabad, India

Paris Cardiovascular Research Center, Inserm U970, Paris, France

**Josef Niebauer** Institute of Sports Medicine, Prevention and Rehabilitation, Paracelsus Medical University Salzburg, Salzburg, Austria

**David Niederseer** Department of Cardiology, University Heart Center Zurich, University of Zurich, Zurich, Switzerland

**Renate Oberhoffer** Department of Preventative Paediatrics, Faculty of Sports and Health Sciences, Technical University of Munich, Munich, Germany

**David Oxborough** Research Institute for Sports and Exercise Sciences, Liverpool John Moores University, Liverpool, UK

**Paolo Palatini** Department of Medicine, University of Padua, Padua, Italy

**Nicole M. Panhuyzen-Goedkoop** Department of Clinical and Experimental Cardiology, Amsterdam Cardiovascular Sciences, Amsterdam UMC, University of Amsterdam, Heart Center, Meibergdreef, Amsterdam, Germany

Department of Sports Cardiology, Sports Medical Centre Papendal Arnhem, The Netherlands

**Michael Papadakis** Cardiology Clinical Academic Group, St. George's, University of London, London, UK

**Antonio Pelliccia** Department of Medicine, Institute of Sports Medicine and Science, Rome, Italy

**Guido E. Pieles** Congenital Heart Unit, Bristol Heart Institute, Bristol, UK

**Axel Pressler** Private Center of Sports & Exercise Cardiology, Munich, Germany

**Jordan M. Prutkin** Division of Cardiology/Electrophysiology, UW Medicine Center for Sports Cardiology, University of Washington, Seattle, WA, USA

**Hanne K. Rasmusen** Department of Cardiology, Bispebjerg-Frederiksberg Hospital, Copenhagen, Denmark

**Nils Reiss** Institute for Cardiovascular Research, Schüchtermann-Klinik Bad Rothenfelde, Bad Rothenfelde, Germany

**Stefania Rizzo** Cardiovascular Pathology, Department of Cardiac, Thoracic and Vascular Sciences and Public Health, University of Padua Medical School, Padua, Italy

**Mahdi Sareban** University Institute of Sports Medicine, Prevention and Rehabilitation, Paracelsus Medical University, Salzburg, Austria

**Thomas Schmidt** Institute for Cardiovascular Research, Schüchtermann-Klinik Bad Rothenfelde, Bad Rothenfelde, Germany

**Christian M. Schmied** Department of Cardiology, University Heart Center, Zurich, Switzerland

Department of Cardiology, Interdisciplinary Centre for Sports & Exercise Medicine, Inselspital, University Hospital of Bern, Bern, Switzerland

**Frédéric Schnell** Department of Sports Medicine, University Hospital of Rennes, Rennes1 University, Inserm, Rennes, France

**Martin Schwellnus** Sport, Exercise Medicine and Lifestyle Institute (SEMLI), University of Pretoria, Pretoria, South Africa

**Catherine Sedgwick** Cardiology Clinical and Academic Group, St Georges, University of London, London, UK

**Luis Serratosa** Rehabilitation, Sports Medicine and Physiotherapy Department, Hospital Universitario Quironsalud Madrid, Madrid, Spain

Ripoll & De Prado Sport Clinic, FIFA Medical Centre of Excellence, Madrid, Spain

**Sanjay Sharma** Cardiology Clinical Academic Group, St. George's, University of London, London, UK

**Erik Ekker Solberg** Medical Department, Diakonhjemmet Hospital, Oslo, Norway

**Tim Takken** Department of Medical Physiology, Child Development & Exercise Center, University Medical Center Utrecht, Utrecht, The Netherlands

**Kay Tetzlaff** Department of Sports Medicine, University of Tübingen, Tübingen, Germany

**Gaetano Thiene** Department of Cardiac, Thoracic and Vascular Sciences and Public Health, University of Padova, Padova, Italy

Cardiovascular Pathology, Department of Cardiac, Thoracic and Vascular Sciences and Public Health, University of Padua Medical School, Padua, Italy

**Wesley J. Tucker** College of Nursing and Health Innovation, University of Texas, Arlington, TX, USA

**Bharathi Upadhya** Cardiovascular Medicine Section, Department of Internal Medicine, Wake Forest School of Medicine, Winston-Salem, NC, USA

**Frank van Buuren** Cardiology, Angiology and Intensive Care Medicine, Catholic Hospital Southwestfalia, St. Martinus, Olpe, Germany

**Emeline van Craenenbroeck** Department of Cardiology, Antwerp University Hospital, Antwerpen, Belgium

**Luc Vanhees** Department of Rehabilitation Sciences, Research group Rehabilitation for internal disorders, University of Leuven, Leuven, Belgium

**Matthias Wilhelm** Department of Cardiology, University Heart Center, Zurich, Switzerland

Department of Cardiology, Interdisciplinary Centre for Sports & Exercise Medicine, Inselspital, University Hospital of Bern, Bern, Switzerland

**Mathew G. Wilson** Aspetar Orthopaedic and Sports Medicine Hospital, Doha, Qatar

**Alessandro Zorzi** Department of Cardiac, Thoracic and Vascular Sciences and Public Health, University of Padova, Padova, Italy

# Part I

# Sports Cardiology in Young Competitive Athletes

# Definition of Athletes and Classification of Sports

**1**

María Sanz de la Garza and Paolo Emilio Adami

**Learning Objectives**

1. Understand the meaning of the term athlete.
2. Be able to provide a complete description of a population of athletes including level of commitment, exercise training parameters and epidemiological characteristics.
3. Understand both the clinical and scientific need and the value of classifying athletes into subgroups based on various exercise stimuli.
4. Be aware of the main objectives, characteristics and limitations of the most used classifications of sports.

## 1.1 Definition of Athletes

The term athlete comes from the Greek word "athlos", which means "achievement" [1]. Indeed, athletes are commonly considered individuals with superior physical and psychological conditions leading them to athletic excellence. Within medical research, the term has been used with completely different meanings and without consensus between international guidelines [2–4].

For the purpose of this chapter, an athlete is considered to be an individual who is engaged in physical activity and exercise on a regular basis. This definition is intentionally much wider than previous ones, as we believe it is the responsibility of the medical and scientific community to engage and include all those individuals regularly participating in some type of physical activity. They are the one that will likely benefit the most, in terms of health enhancement, from sport participation.

M. Sanz de la Garza
Cardiovascular Institute, Hospital Clinic, Barcelona, Spain

P. E. Adami (✉)
Department of Health and Science, World Athletics, Monaco, Monaco
e-mail: paoloemilio.adami@worldathletics.org





A. Pressler, J. Niebauer (eds.), *Textbook of Sports and Exercise Cardiology*,
https://doi.org/10.1007/978-3-030-35374-2_1

There is a need for a cultural change, and this can only be achieved through education and direct engagement. The objective is to bring sport back to the people at grass root level. Therefore, we need a much more inclusive definition of what an athlete is. The population of athletes is thus quite heterogeneous and as such, further descriptors should be included when describing an athlete. The following are necessary descriptors to define a population of athletes:

- Level of commitment:
  - Recreational athletes: individuals engaged in recreational or open sport.
  - Competitive athletes: individuals engaged in exercise and training on a regular basis and participating in official sports competition, at any level.
  - Elite and professional athletes: constitute a subgroup within competitive athletes who achieve athletic excellence and usually compete at an international level, earning a living out of their sport participation.
- Exercise training parameters:
  - Frequency (days/week): the number of days per week an individual exercises or performs physical activity.
  - Intensity: can be measured or estimated using different methods (see below).
  - Duration (time per session, per day, per week): the amount of exercise performed.
  - Type of activity: describes the type of activity performed based on the discipline's characteristics and cardiovascular main adaptations.
  - Volume (Metabolic equivalent of tasks (MET)-min/week, kcal/week): the product of frequency (days/week), intensity (based on, e.g., heart rate (HR), heart rate reserve (HRR), maximal oxygen uptake ($VO_2$max), oxygen reserve ($VO_2$R)), and duration (of each training session/day or /week).
  - Sport discipline and role/position within this discipline.
  - Global exercise training load: years of exercise training in the specified sport discipline.

Regarding exercise intensity, the preferred method is the direct measurement of physiological responses to exercise through an incremental cardiopulmonary exercise test (i.e. maximal HR—$HR_{max}$, $VO_2$max). For exercise prescription purposes the HRR, %$HR_{max}$ or %$VO_2$max can be adopted [5]. Other indirect methods of estimating exercise intensity use the predicted $HR_{max}$ formulas (e.g. $HR_{max} = 220 - \text{age}$; $HR_{max} = 208 - (0.7 \times \text{age})$) [6, 7]. These methods, although easier to use, can underestimate or overestimate measured $HR_{max}$. Measured or estimated values of absolute exercise intensity include caloric expenditure (kcal/min), absolute oxygen consumption (mL/min or L/min), and METs which is roughly the energy expended in resting conditions, set by convention at 3.5 mL of oxygen per kilogram body weight per minute, or 1 kcal/kg body mass per hour. Nevertheless, these methods do not take into consideration individual factors such as body mass, sex and fitness level and can cause misclassification of exercise intensities. For ease of reference and adoption of METs, activities have been listed and classified, according to the measured METs, in a compendium of physical activities [8–10].

Measures of perceived effort can also be used to modulate and indirectly estimate the exercise intensity. These measures of affective valence (i.e. pleasantness of exercise) include the Borg Rate of Perceived Exertion (RPE) Scales [11, 12] and the Talk Test [13]. The Talk Test is based on the concept that exercising at or above the lactate or ventilatory thresholds prevents a comfortable conversational speech and thus constitutes a valid and reliable method for estimating exercise intensities [14–19] (see also Chaps. 11 and 45).

Regarding exercise volume, it can be used to estimate the individual's energy expenditure [20]. The volume of exercise usually increases progressively with the level of competition from ≥500–1000 MET-min/week in recreational athletes to ≥10,000 MET-min/week in competitive and elite athletes. However, this is not always the case and may vary depending on the sport discipline requirements and even on individual motivation (Table 1.1).

- Epidemiological characteristics:
  - Gender
  - Age: young or adolescents (12–17), adult (18–35) and master athletes (above 35 years old).

Regarding age, the above-mentioned traditional classification may be subject to changes according to each sport rules and regulations [21]. The current division between adult and master athletes is mainly based on the fact that 35 years is the age at which ischemic cardiovascular events tend to become a greater cause of mortality

**Table 1.1** Energy expenditure induced by various sports (arbitrarily selected from [8–10])

| Activity/sports | Intensity/type | METs |
|---|---|---|
| Cycling | Leisure | 4.0 |
| | General | 7.5 |
| | Vigorous | 10.0 |
| | Mountain, uphill | 14.0 |
| Conditioning exercise | Cycling, stationary, general | 7.0 |
| | Calisthenics, moderate | 3.8 |
| | Resistance training, 8–15 repetitions | 3.5 |
| | Rowing, stationary, general | 6.0 |
| Running | Jogging, general | 7.0 |
| | Marathon | 13.0 |
| Basketball | General | 6.5 |
| Soccer | Competitive | 8.0 |
| Golf | General | 4.8 |
| Hockey, ice | General | 8.0 |
| Horseback riding | General | 5.5 |
| Martial arts | Different types, moderate | 10.3 |
| Rock climbing | Moderate difficulty | 5.8 |
| Tennis | General | 7.3 |
| Walking | Hiking, cross-country | 6.0 |
| Water activities | Swimming, breaststroke, recreational | 5.3 |
| Winter activities | Skiing, general | 7.0 |

in the athlete's population while the separation between young and adult athletes at 18 years is related with the age at which puberty is usually completed.

Recreational athletes and those individuals participating in physical activity for health purposes, in some cases, might as well reach exercise training volumes and intensities as competitive or even elite athletes. Therefore, they may develop similar structural and electrical cardiovascular adaptations in response to the exercise stimulus. Thus, when describing an athlete, exercise training parameters described previously become mandatory.

## 1.2 Classification of Sports

According to the objective of the classification, sport disciplines have been classified in various ways. Existing classifications consider different aspects of the sport such as:

- physical demands induced by different sports
- impact of different exercise stimuli on performance and body composition
- cardiovascular adaptations induced by different modalities and intensities of exercise
- the potential consequences of a syncope while exercising.

For the purpose of this chapter we will present the two mainly adopted and recent classifications of sports.

### 1.2.1 Mitchell Classification of Sports

One of the most referred-to classifications is the Mitchell classification of sports [22] that was developed with the objective of clarifying whether an athlete with a specific cardiovascular abnormality was eligible to participate in competitive sport. The Mitchell classification considers:

1. the type and intensity of the sport
2. the risks of injuries from body collision
3. the consequences of a syncope.

The main components of each sport considered are **static** and **dynamic**. These terms refer to the exercise activities characteristics and are based on the biomechanical action of the muscles involved. These features do not consider the metabolic pathway mostly used (aerobic or anaerobic). Dynamic exercises involve changes in muscle length and joint movement through rhythmic contractions that usually develop a relatively small force. Static exercises, on the other hand, are characterized by relatively large forces, with very little or no change in muscle length and joint movement.

Based on these two "opposite" components of exercise, the Mitchell classification characterizes different sports according to their percental proportion of static and dynamic exercise stimuli and summarizes disciplines with similar proportions into particular subgroups (Fig. 1.1). It was first developed with the objective of defining whether an athlete with a specific cardiovascular abnormality is eligible to participate in a competitive sport. It provides clinical support when deciding whether certain cardiovascular adaptations observed in an athlete are likely to be sufficiently explained by the type of sports he or she is performing.

Although comprehensive and including most sports, the Mitchell classification:

- does not take into consideration the extent to which the physical fitness components are trained in successful athletes,
- carries a risk of underestimating the real work intensity, and
- might not be so intuitive for the clinician with less experience in sports cardiology.

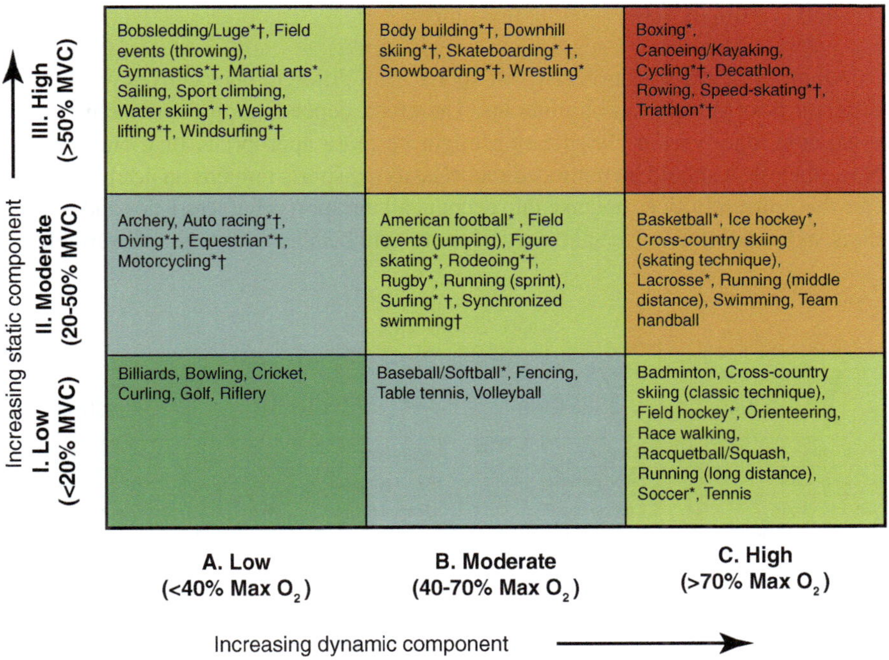


**Fig. 1.1** Classification of sports. This classification is based on peak static and dynamic components achieved during competition. It should be noted, however, that higher values may be reached during training. The increasing dynamic component is defined in terms of the estimated percent of maximal oxygen uptake ($VO_2$max) achieved, resulting in increasing cardiac output. The increasing static component is related to the estimated percent of maximal voluntary contraction (MVC) reached, resulting in an increasing blood pressure load. The lowest total cardiovascular demands (cardiac output and blood pressure) are shown in green and the highest in red. Blue, yellow and orange depict low moderate, moderate and high moderate total cardiovascular demands. (Modified from Mitchell and colleagues [22]). *Danger of body collision, †Increased risk if syncope occurs

### 1.2.2 Cardiovascular Classification of Sports

Another way in which sports have been also frequently classified is based on the **isotonic** and **isometric** exercise components and the resulting cardiovascular adaptations induced by exercise (Fig. 1.2 and [23]). Isotonic exercise mainly involves disciplines that are characterized by a predominant change in muscular length rather than tension, whereas isometric refers to the opposite. As such, this is rather similar to the Mitchell classification. However, apart from this, the classification also considers whether a particular discipline requires specific technical skills beyond muscular work to be performed successfully, such as the complex movement required to hit a golf ball or the concentration and reactivity to control a racing car.

Although comprehensive from a cardiovascular perspective, this type of classification

- does not take into consideration most of the physiological components defining different sports,
- relies mostly on imaging findings with the objective of facilitating the clinical sports cardiologists evaluating the athlete.

All types of classifications look at sports from different perspectives resulting in different positive sides and limitations. Therefore, depending on the objective of the evaluation, one type of classification might be more appropriate than another one. Nevertheless, it should be reminded that classifying sports remains an academic exercise that, currently, does not take into account all the sports characteristics and adaptations, at least until a universal theory of sports will be able to describe all variables.

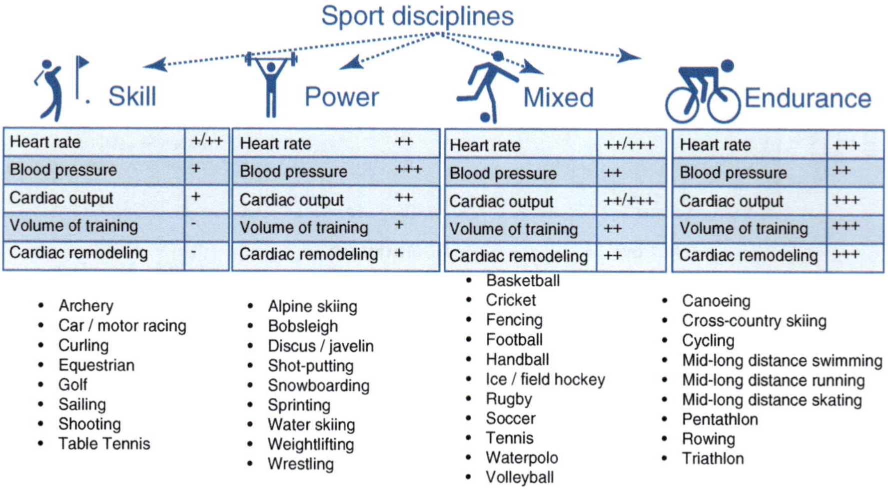


**Fig. 1.2** Simplified classification of the most common Olympic sport disciplines, according to the relative isometric and isotonic components of exercise and resulting cardiovascular adaptation. (Modified from Pelliccia and colleagues [23])

It should also be reminded that in many cases, training could be more demanding, from a cardiovascular perspective, than competition. Training regimens in most sports now include both static and dynamic components that might not be a specific part of that sport. The concept that training load could induce a greater cardiovascular load than competition must be considered also for non-competitive athletes who might reach large training volumes but do not compete.

**Clinical Pearls**

- An athlete is considered to be an individual who is engaged in physical activity and exercise on a regular basis. This definition is intentionally wide, to include all those individuals regularly participating in some type of physical activity.
- Variables to consider when describing exercise and athletic populations:
  - Level of commitment
  - Exercise training parameters
  - Epidemiological characteristics
- All types of classifications look at sports from different perspectives, have different positive sides and limitations. Therefore, depending on the objective of the evaluation, one type of classification might be more appropriate than another one.

## Review

## Questions

1. A 48-year old male triathlete reports an average training volume of 4–5 h per week. He used to perform a variety of sports during his adolescence without particular focus and with only occasional competitions. After a break over several years he started with more or less regular running roughly at the age of 36 with increasing frequency, added by cycling and swimming about 3–4 years later. This was also the time when training became more systematic, and he started to participate in his first short distance events. Over several years he then performed 3–4 Olympic distance triathlons per year and is now preparing for his first ironman distance. What would be your definition of this athlete in terms of level of commitment, exercise training parameters and, particularly, the potential impact of this training history on cardiovascular adaptation?
2. According to the Mitchell classification, how would you classify an athlete who is performing triathlon during summer and cross-country skiing (classic technique) during winter, taking part in long-distance competitions in both sports?
3. A 44-year old marathon runner presents with concentric left ventricular hypertrophy (12 mm). He started regular running at the age of 25 and finished his first marathon a few years thereafter. Since then he has participated in 1–2 marathons per year. How would you classify this athlete? Is the type of hypertrophy explained by your classification?

## Answers

1. A major issue in sports cardiology is to decide whether the presence of certain cardiovascular adaptations in athletes are adequately explained by their particular training histories. Regarding this, defining an athlete as either "recreational" or "competitive" and evaluating his exercise parameters and the accumulated training years is of clinical significance. Middle-aged athletes having started their regular training only during adulthood are particularly difficult to judge. In this borderline case, apart from taking part in competitions, the training volume is usually not sufficient to result in detectable clinical changes (although it cannot fully be excluded). In other words, in case of equivocal alterations, a more extensive diagnostic workup is reasonable. Since these athletes usually aim at goals during competition that may exceed realistic estimations, they should be regarded as competitive in order to carefully account for the excessive demands they tend to expose themselves to.
2. Many ambitious recreational or competitive athletes engage in more than one sports and can thus sometimes not be assigned to a particular subgroup. This indicates the limitations of these approaches. For clinical assessment or scientific purposes, it is reasonable to assign this athlete to Mitchell subgroup IB covering the best mixture between the different exercise stimuli he or she is exposed to.
3. This athlete perfectly suits into Mitchell subgroup IC, or into the "endurance" group according to the cardiovascular classification. These athletes may develop mild hypertrophy over time; thus, a value of 12 mm is at least possible. However, one would usually expect a more eccentric type of hypertrophy, with the left ventricular diameter also being markedly enlarged. If this is not the case, this athlete requires further evaluation, e.g. with respect to the presence of hypertension.

## References

1. Araujo CG, Scharhag J. Athlete: a working definition for medical and health sciences research. Scand J Med Sci Sports. 2016;26(1):4–7.
2. Maron BJ, Zipes DP, Kovacs RJ. Eligibility and disqualification recommendations for competitive athletes with cardiovascular abnormalities: preamble, principles, and general considerations: a scientific statement from the American Heart Association and American College of Cardiology. Circulation. 2015;132(22):e256–61.
3. Solberg EE, Borjesson M, Sharma S, Papadakis M, Wilhelm M, Drezner JA, et al. Sudden cardiac arrest in sports – need for uniform registration: a position paper from the Sport Cardiology Section of the European Association for Cardiovascular Prevention and Rehabilitation. Eur J Prev Cardiol. 2015;23(6):657–67.
4. Pelliccia A, Fagard R, Bjornstad HH, Anastassakis A, Arbustini E, Assanelli D, et al. Recommendations for competitive sports participation in athletes with cardiovascular disease: a consensus document from the Study Group of Sports Cardiology of the Working Group of Cardiac Rehabilitation and Exercise Physiology and the Working Group of Myocardial and Pericardial Diseases of the European Society of Cardiology. Eur Heart J. 2005;26(14):1422–45.

5. Mezzani A, Hamm LF, Jones AM, McBride PE, Moholdt T, Stone JA, et al. Aerobic exercise intensity assessment and prescription in cardiac rehabilitation: a joint position statement of the European Association for Cardiovascular Prevention and Rehabilitation, the American Association of Cardiovascular and Pulmonary Rehabilitation and the Canadian Association of Cardiac Rehabilitation. Eur J Prev Cardiol. 2013;20(3):442–67.
6. Fox SM III, Naughton JP, Haskell WL. Physical activity and the prevention of coronary heart disease. Ann Clin Res. 1971;3(6):404–32.
7. Tanaka H, Monahan KD, Seals DR. Age-predicted maximal heart rate revisited. J Am Coll Cardiol. 2001;37(1):153–6.
8. Ainsworth BE, Haskell WL, Leon AS, Jacobs DR Jr, Montoye HJ, Sallis JF, et al. Compendium of physical activities: classification of energy costs of human physical activities. Med Sci Sports Exerc. 1993;25(1):71–80.
9. Ainsworth BE, Haskell WL, Whitt MC, Irwin ML, Swartz AM, Strath SJ, et al. Compendium of physical activities: an update of activity codes and MET intensities. Med Sci Sports Exerc. 2000;32(9 Suppl):S498–504.
10. Ainsworth BE, Haskell WL, Herrmann SD, Meckes N, Bassett DR Jr, Tudor-Locke C, et al. 2011 Compendium of Physical Activities: a second update of codes and MET values. Med Sci Sports Exerc. 2011;43(8):1575–81.
11. Borg GA. Perceived exertion. Exerc Sport Sci Rev. 1974;2:131–53.
12. Noble BJ, Borg GA, Jacobs I, Ceci R, Kaiser P. A category-ratio perceived exertion scale: relationship to blood and muscle lactates and heart rate. Med Sci Sports Exerc. 1983;15(6):523–8.
13. Persinger R, Foster C, Gibson M, Fater DC, Porcari JP. Consistency of the talk test for exercise prescription. Med Sci Sports Exerc. 2004;36(9):1632–6.
14. Brawner CA, Vanzant MA, Ehrman JK, Foster C, Porcari JP, Kelso AJ, et al. Guiding exercise using the talk test among patients with coronary artery disease. J Cardpulm Rehabil. 2006;26(2):72–5; quiz 6–7.
15. Ballweg J, Foster C, Porcari J, Haible S, Aminaka N, Mikat RP. Reliability of the talk test as a surrogate of ventilatory and respiratory compensation thresholds. J Sports Sci Med. 2013;12(3):610–1.
16. Gillespie BD, McCormick JJ, Mermier CM, Gibson AL. Talk test as a practical method to estimate exercise intensity in highly trained competitive male cyclists. J Strength Cond Res. 2015;29(4):894–8.
17. Lyon E, Menke M, Foster C, Porcari JP, Gibson M, Bubbers T. Translation of incremental talk test responses to steady-state exercise training intensity. J Cardiopulm Rehabil Prev. 2014;34(4):271–5.
18. Rodriguez-Marroyo JA, Villa JG, Garcia-Lopez J, Foster C. Relationship between the talk test and ventilatory thresholds in well-trained cyclists. J Strength Cond Res. 2013;27(7):1942–9.
19. Woltmann ML, Foster C, Porcari JP, Camic CL, Dodge C, Haible S, et al. Evidence that the talk test can be used to regulate exercise intensity. J Strength Cond Res. 2015;29(5):1248–54.
20. Garber CE, Blissmer B, Deschenes MR, Franklin BA, Lamonte MJ, Lee IM, et al. American College of Sports Medicine position stand. Quantity and quality of exercise for developing and maintaining cardiorespiratory, musculoskeletal, and neuromotor fitness in apparently healthy adults: guidance for prescribing exercise. Med Sci Sports Exerc. 2011;43(7):1334–59.
21. Allen SV, Hopkins WG. Age of peak competitive performance of elite athletes: a systematic review. Sports Med. 2015;45(10):1431–41.
22. Mitchell JH, Haskell W, Snell P, Van Camp SP. Task Force 8: classification of sports. J Am Coll Cardiol. 2005;45(8):1364–7.
23. Pelliccia A, Adami PE, Quattrini F, Squeo MR, Caselli S, Verdile L, et al. Are Olympic athletes free from cardiovascular diseases? Systematic investigation in 2352 participants from Athens 2004 to Sochi 2014. Br J Sports Med. 2017;51(4):238–43.

# 2 The Cardiologist as Part of the Athlete Medical Team

Christine E. Lawless

**Learning Objectives**
1. Define the role of the cardiologist as part of the athlete care team.
2. Identify the core competencies necessary to practice sports cardiology.
3. Understand the significance of being familiar with the cardiovascular demands of different sports.
4. Provide a practical approach to the cardiovascular evaluation of the athlete.

## 2.1 Introduction

Participation on the athlete medical team can be one of the most rewarding aspects of a cardiologist's job. It is uplifting to associate with energetic goal-oriented individuals whose focus is on excellence, peak performance, and getting back in the game. Such work can serve to balance some of the more dreary aspects of our profession.

Here, I will discuss:

1. how a cardiologist gets started in caring for athletes (Sports Cardiology),
2. how to interact with team medical staff,
3. a brief history of sports cardiology, and
4. the knowledge base required to practice this discipline.

The emphasis will be on how this discipline is practiced in the United States, and how it differs from Europe.

C. E. Lawless (✉)
Sports Cardiology Consultants LLC, Chicago, IL, USA



A. Pressler, J. Niebauer (eds.), *Textbook of Sports and Exercise Cardiology*,
https://doi.org/10.1007/978-3-030-35374-2_2

## 2.2 How Does the Cardiologist Get Started in Caring for Athletes (Sports Cardiology)?

- While there are several Sports Cardiology Clinics scattered throughout the United States (US), there is currently no US Sports Cardiology board examination. So, the cardiologist typically "learns by doing."
- This will be the case until there are formal Sports Cardiology fellowships, leading to an American Board of Internal Medicine (ABIM) subspecialty board examination.

My own journey into the field serves as a good example as to how a cardiologist typically gets started. It all began with me being invited to assist with athlete ECG interpretation and consultations for a professional soccer team, and for National Collegiate Athletic Association (NCAA) athletes at the Ohio State University.

My cardiology background consisted of a sub-specialty in heart failure, cardiomyopathy, and heart transplantation. While this provided excellent preparation to understand the cardiac diseases that predispose to sudden cardiac death in athletes and to be able to recognize these diseases at an early stage, my practice provided little exposure to athletes. General cardiology with some knowledge of exercise physiology probably provides the best background for a sports cardiologist. However, electrophysiology, and cardiac imaging also provide an excellent foundation.

In 2002, I was asked to be a team doctor for United States Figure Skating (USFS) World Teams. Since I had significant sports medicine knowledge deficits, I decided to formally study Primary Care Sports Medicine. After doing the requisite fellowship, I sat for the Sports Medicine Board Exam (through ABIM) and passed in 2004. The knowledge allowed me to serve confidently as team physician, and chairperson of the USFS Sports Science and Medicine Committee. I do not recommend other US cardiologists take formal training in Sports Medicine, unless they aspire to a career as a team physician.

After completing Sports Medicine training, I began to see a need for Sports Cardiology in the US. In 2006, I offered a half day Sports Cardiology symposium at the Ohio State University in Columbus Ohio. The medical staff members of the Columbus Crew, an American professional soccer team, were in attendance, and asked me to serve as team cardiologist, primarily to interpret ECGs. Major League Soccer (MLS) was considering ECG screening in all US professional soccer athletes, since Fédération Internationale de Football Association (FIFA, soccer's global governing body), had already adopted ECG screening at the World Cup level in 2004. My work with the Columbus Crew and Ohio State University collegiate athletes led to 5 years of service as the MLS Consulting Cardiologist, where I served at the annual recruitment combine interpreting screening ECGs and echocardiograms, and wrote an extensive cardiac policy for the League.

- During my time with the Ohio State University and the MLS, I reached out to a small group of cardiologists with an interest in Sports Cardiology, and we began to meet informally.
- In 2009, with the help of a medical education company, I surveyed a group of general cardiologists as to their interaction with athlete-patients.

The survey revealed that while a significant number of cardiologists cleared ≥50 athlete-patients annually (Fig. 2.1a), only 11% consistently used the 36th Bethesda Guidelines (sports participation guidelines for those with heart disease), while 46% were either unaware of, or did not use, the guidelines (Fig. 2.1b). In addition, the surveyed cardiologists identified several important Sports Cardiology knowledge gaps: athletic adaptations, athlete ECG interpretation, commotio cordis, Marfan syndrome and aortic diseases, channelopathies, cardiac MRI, and the use of genetic testing.

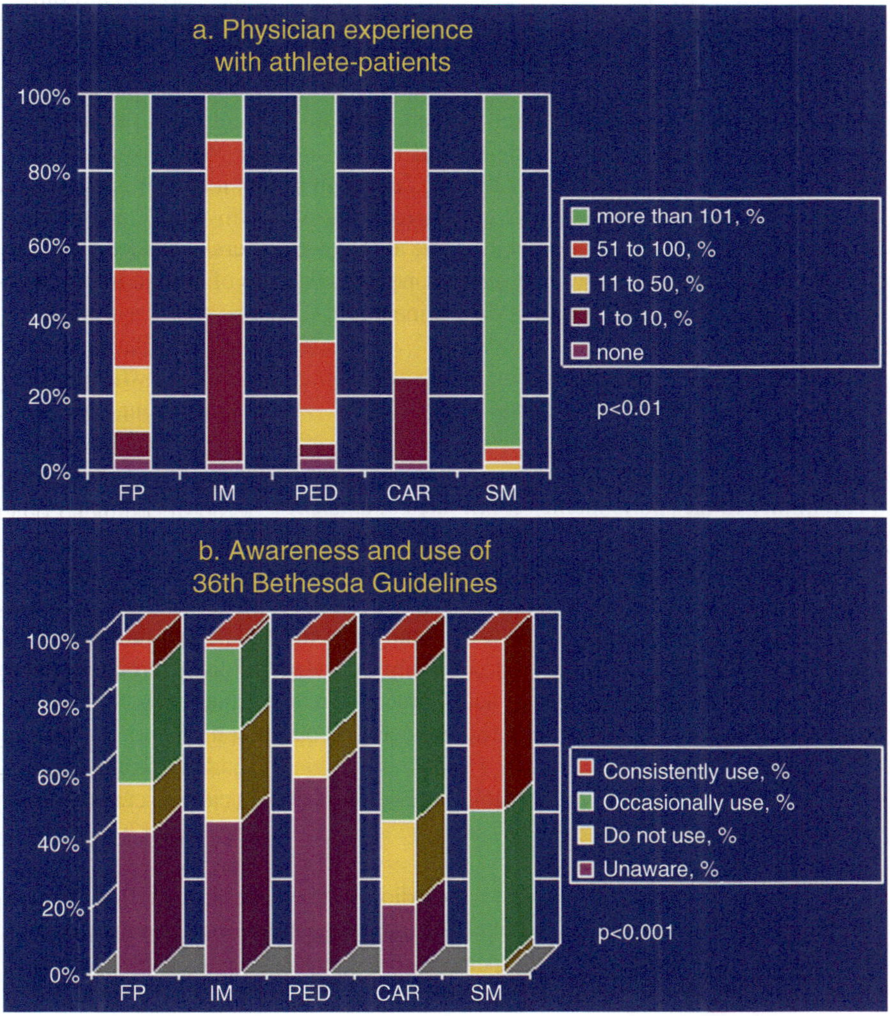


**Fig. 2.1** Sports cardiology needs assessment conducted in 2009 indicated 39% of cardiologists cleared ≥50 athlete-patients annually (**a**). Only 11% consistently used the 36th Bethesda Guidelines, while 46% were either unaware of, or did not use the guidelines (**b**) (reprinted with permission from [57]). *FP* family practice, *IM* internal medicine, *PED* pediatrics, *CAR* cardiologists, *SM* sports medicine

- Based on the survey results, in 2011, our informal US Sports Cardiology group petitioned the American College of Cardiology (ACC) to create the *ACC Sports and Exercise Cardiology Council and Section.*

Within just 1 year, our group grew from 150 members, to over 4000 [1]. We quickly held a think tank to discuss ECG screening in the United States [2] and wrote a white paper on the athlete as a unique cardiovascular patient [1]. The council and section continues to host annual symposia, and serves as a community for US Sports Cardiologists who work with athletes at all levels.

## 2.3 How to Interact with Team Medical Staff

Cardiologists are commonly recruited by the local team medical staff to either interpret athlete ECGs or see an athlete patient in consultation. When working with organized professional, university, Olympic, and high school teams, it is crucial to recognize that the cardiologist is merely a consultant in most instances, and that the athletic trainers and/or team physicians serve as the gatekeepers of athlete care. The cardiologist needs to be aware that *quality* and *efficiency* are of utmost importance to the team medical staff. *Quality* is determined by:

1. the cardiologist's reputation,
2. knowledge of subject matter, and
3. experience with athletes.

Proximity to the sports facility contributes to *efficiency*.

- Downtime is not healthy for an athlete, and deconditioning can occur quickly.

If the cardiologist states after ECG screening that the athlete can be seen in the office in 6 weeks, the cardiologist is not likely to get any future referrals, as team medical staff would not view this as acceptable athlete care. During those 6 weeks, the athlete would have to be kept out of practice, and out of competition.

- Thus, it is important that the cardiologist considers athlete cardiac evaluation an **urgent** priority.

This might be counter-intuitive to a cardiologist, whose priority is usually a patient who is the sickest, not a relatively healthy out-patient. But the consequences of deconditioning and its effect on performance are so grave, that timely cardiac evaluation is of utmost importance. Efficient work-ups will endear the cardiologist to the team medical staff.

My personal practice was to attend the pre-participation physicals, read the ECGs on-site, and have echocardiography on site, or nearby and ready to use. In this way, clearance to participate can be decided in a matter of minutes to hours. When performing cardiac consultations on symptomatic athletes, I would see the athlete immediately, and perform all necessary cardiac testing the same day, such as stress testing, echocardiography, and cardiac MRI. I worked carefully with colleagues to create and implement these protocols. We also designed "athlete specific" protocols. For example, visualization of the origin of the coronary arteries was part of the athlete echocardiogram, whereas this would not be performed on routine echocardiography. Gadolinium imaging was incorporated into the athlete cardiac MRI. Stress testing was tailored to meet the demands of the athlete's sport. Clearance decisions were made the same day if at all possible. Again, the emphasis is on the shortest downtime possible.

Some cardiologists in the United States have created stand-alone ECG screening programs. In this case, athletes and/or parents approach the screening program directly, and the team medical staff is not directly involved. But the same principles apply in that evaluations should be completed as quickly as possible.

## 2.4 Brief History of Sports Cardiology

Clinicians have long held a fascination for the interaction between the cardiovascular system and exercise.

- In the fifth century BC, Greek physicians promoted the health benefits of exercise [3, 4], while witnessing the first recorded episodes of exercise-related sudden cardiac death (SCD) in courier runners [5, 6].

It is now well known that SCD is more likely to occur during exercise than at rest [7–11], and while SCD risk is increased during athletic events, the long-term risk of SCD is actually decreased in athletic populations compared to the general population [12–14]. Furthermore, contemporary studies suggest that the risk of SCD in athletic populations is highly variable, dependent upon age, sex, ethnicity, level of play, and sport [15–19].

Association between regular exercise and cardiac enlargement has also intrigued clinicians, beginning in the late nineteenth century with Osler [20], and the Swedish physician Henschen. The latter first introduced the term "athlete's heart" in the literature in 1899 [21]. Later, when x-ray became available, researchers showed that cardiothoracic ratios $\geq 0.50$ were more common in athletes [22]. However, unable to distinguish between cardiomegaly due to pathology and that from athletic adaptation, concern surfaced that chronic training and competition actually resulted in pathology and could potentially shorten athletes' lifespans. In 1975, Morganroth first described the echocardiographic features of athletic adaptation [23] (see also Chap. 3). Italian researchers showed that athletic adaptation (by echocardiography) varied according to gender, size, age, and type of sport [24] (see Chaps. 3 and 4). Further details of the athlete's heart have emerged as imaging and technology have progressed [25–31].

No discussion of the history of Sports Cardiology would be complete without mentioning the importance of **ECG screening** to the development of this discipline. As beta blockers for heart failure began with the Swedes, ECG screening began with the Italians:

- In **1971**, Italy enacted legislation requiring National-caliber Italian athletes to undergo preparticipation examination (PPE) consisting of family and personal history, physical examination, resting 12 lead ECG, and limited exercise testing, with further cardiac testing performed on subjects who had positive findings at the initial evaluation.
- In **2006**, the Italians published longitudinal data indicating an 89% reduction in athlete SCD over a 25-year period [32], which they attributed directly to the use of ECG screening.
- Subsequent endorsement of ECG screening for all athletes prior to sports participation by the European Society of Cardiology (ESC), the International Olympic Committee (IOC), and the FIFA, have served to drive the adoption of ECG screening practices in many countries throughout the world.

The US experience has been unique, and not without controversy. Major US cardiology organizations have been reluctant to adopt mass or universal ECG screening for young people.

- In **2014**, the American Heart Association (AHA) and ACC concluded that "mandatory and universal mass screening with 12-lead ECGs in large general populations of young healthy people 12–25 years of age (including on a national basis in the United States) to identify genetic/congenital and other cardiovascular abnormalities is not recommended for athletes and non-athletes alike (Class III, no evidence of benefit; Level of Evidence C)" [33].
- However, US professional sports governing bodies such as the National Basketball Association (NBA), National Football League (NFL), and MLS uniformly embrace ECG screening in all athletes [34]. At the collegiate level in the US, it has been estimated about 50% of NCAA Division 1 member schools have adopted some degree of ECG screening [35].

The NCAA has not mandated the practice, primarily because there is no consensus as to the short- and long-term risk/benefit ratio of such an approach, and the knowledge base (to conduct and interpret athlete ECG) across the country is somewhat uneven [36]. For those schools that do perform athlete ECG screening, the NCAA recommends that certain protocols be followed (Table 2.1).

At the US high school level, screening ECG is not generally performed as part of the preparticipation physical examination (PPE), but some local screening organizations do offer ECG screening on either a volunteer basis, or for a fee.

Regardless how one feels about the merits of athlete ECG screening, it is evident that the global growth of ECG-based screening has served to drive the formal

**Table 2.1** NCAA inter-association task force recommendations for athlete ECG screening [36]

| |
|---|
| A. Pre-ECG screening planning and coordination: |
| • Before pre-participation physicals are conducted, team physicians, athletic trainers, and athletic administrators should meet to discuss the execution of ECG screening in student-athletes. A cardiovascular specialist with the requisite expertise to provide athlete ECG over-reading services and to coordinate any downstream testing dictated by ECG abnormalities should be identified. |
| • The implementation of ECG screening for all student-athletes versus targeted high-risk groups should be discussed and agreed upon. |
| • Student-athletes should be provided information regarding the rationale for utilizing ECG screening and the possible risk versus benefit of adding ECG screening. |
| • The standards for ECG interpretation should be reviewed and agreed upon, and avenues for prompt secondary cardiac testing of ECG abnormalities outlined. |
| B. Screening protocol: |
| • ECG screening should be implemented as part of an integrated cardiovascular screen using a standardized history and physical examination, such as the AHA 14-point recommendations or the PPE-4. |
| • The ECG should be obtained with equipment and by persons trained according to ACC/AHA/Heart Rhythm Society recommendations. |
| C. Interpretation and secondary testing: |
| • The ECG should be interpreted with modern standards that distinguish normal findings related to physiological cardiac remodeling in trained athletes from abnormalities suggestive of an underlying pathological cardiac condition. |
| • Consensus guidelines on ECG interpretation in athletes and a free online training course are available online at the BMJ learning web site (https://learning.bmj.com/learning/course-intro/.html?courseId=10042239). |
| • The institution should provide cardiology oversight and resources, either on-site or at a regional referral center, to interpret suspicious ECGs and guide and perform secondary testing that may be required for athletes whose ECG results call for further clarification. |
| D. Management of identified cardiac conditions associated with sudden cardiac death: |
| • In keeping with the NCAA's requirement that each member institution is responsible for protecting the health of and providing a safe environment for each student-athlete, the management of identified cardiac disorders and all sport eligibility decisions are ultimately the responsibility of the institutional primary athletics health care providers in consultation with subspecialty consultants, including a primary cardiology point person. |
| • The ACC/AHA provides recommendations for safe participation in athletes with cardiovascular conditions that can be used as an initial guideline. A model that utilizes a comprehensive evaluation, extensive patient/family counseling, and prudent medical management for risk reduction and informed decision-making that involves all key stakeholders in the oversight of the athlete (e.g. coaches, athletic trainers, team physicians, and athletic directors) provides a sensible strategy to structure difficult cardiac clearance decisions. |

*NCAA* National Collegiate Athletic Association, *AHA* American Heart Association, *PPE* Preparticipation Physical Evaluation, *ACC* American College of Cardiology

development of Sports Cardiology as a new discipline within cardiology, greatly advancing what we know about athletic adaptations, early identification of cardiomyopathies, distinguishing "normal" from pathologic conditions, and assessing risk of sports participation in those with cardiac disease.

## 2.5 Knowledge Base Required to Practice Sports Cardiology: Core Competencies

Beyond reading an athlete ECG, performing consultations, interpreting cardiac testing, and making sports participation decisions, Sports Cardiologists should have a well-defined set of competencies. There are two excellent references on this topic.

- In **2013**, the ESC proposed a 12-month training program in sports cardiology for both sports physicians and cardiologists, to include a sports cardiology core curriculum (Table 2.2 [37]).

In the US, although Sports Cardiology is developing at a rapid pace, an official core competency statement, such as those developed by the Core Cardiovascular Training Statement (COCATS) and endorsed by the ABIM, does not exist.

- However, in **2017**, in response to this unfulfilled need, the ACC Sports and Exercise Council defined the essential skills necessary to practice sports cardiology in the US [38].

Authors of this document took great care to format their recommendations to be consistent with ACC lifelong learning standards, to set the stage for incorporation of sports cardiology into existing cardiovascular training, and board processes. Core competencies are presented as skill sets in four domains (Fig. 2.2 [38]). As an example, the skill set for one domain (Essential skills for the Sports Cardiologist: Exercise Physiology and Exercise-induced Cardiovascular Remodeling) is illustrated in Table 2.3 [38].

While these references are quite comprehensive, in practice there are many more sports-specific nuances to the cardiovascular care of athletes. There can be significant cultural differences among sports governing bodies. As a cardiologist evaluates

**Table 2.2** Key issues of the core curriculum in Sports Cardiology as proposed by the European Society of Cardiology [37]

| |
|---|
| (a) Exercise anatomy, physiology, adaptation, and health benefits |
| (b) Cardiac evaluation in sports cardiology |
| (c) Sudden death in sports |
| (d) Prevention of sudden death by pre-participation screening |
| (e) Diagnostic conundrums |
| (f) Sports eligibility in individuals with cardiac disease |
| (g) Ethical and legal considerations of sports eligibility |
| (h) Cardiac rehabilitation and safe participation in sports |
| (i) Safety procedures in sports arenas (to include advanced life support certification) |
| (j) Substance abuse and doping |

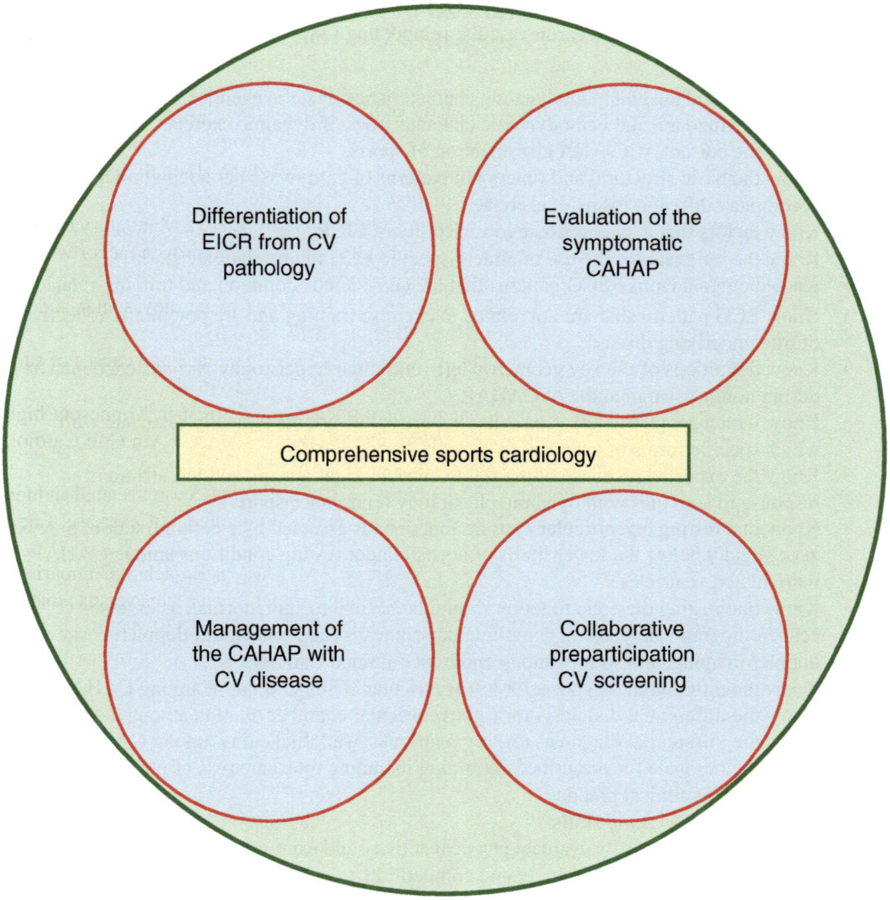


**Fig. 2.2** American College of Cardiology fundamental core competencies in Sports Cardiology. (Modified from [38]). *CAHAP* competitive athletes and highly active people, *CV* cardiovascular, *EICR* exercise-induced cardiac remodeling

a particular athlete patient, questions will arise as to how much remodeling is acceptable in a particular sport. For instance, left ventricular wall thickness of 1.5 cm might be normal for an African American basketball player, but would not be for an Olympic female Caucasian gymnast (see Chaps. 25 and 26).

When asked to participate on the athlete care team, I advise the cardiologist to find out as much as they can about that specific athlete population through interaction with team medical staff, and review of the published literature. Then, consider this five-step approach (using the professional soccer player to illustrate, adapted from [39]). This five-step approach to the cardiovascular care of an athlete can be adapted to fit any athlete, in any sport.

**Table 2.3** American College of Cardiology essential skills for the Sports Cardiologist: exercise physiology and exercise-induced cardiovascular remodeling [38]

| |
|---|
| A. Medical knowledge |
| • Know the fundamental hemodynamic characteristics of static exercise. |
| • Know the fundamental hemodynamic characteristics of dynamic exercise. |
| • Know the current ACC/AHA classification of sports. |
| • Know the basic structural and functional patterns of cardiovascular adaptation that accompany different forms of exercise. |
| • Know factors that may contribute to variability of EICR. |
| • Know the rationale for the use of athlete-specific ECG interpretation criteria. |
| • Know benign/adaptive ECG patterns that are considered "common and training-related." |
| • Know ECG patterns that are not related to exercise training and are potentially reflective of true underlying disease. |
| • Know definitions of the key geometric left ventricular hypertrophy variants encountered during noninvasive imaging of CAHAP. |
| • Know which geometric left ventricular hypertrophy variants typically associate with which specific forms of exercise. |
| • Know the expected response of the right ventricle, right atrium, and left atrium in response to activities with dynamic physiology (endurance sports). |
| • Know that resting biventricular systolic function, as assessed by ejection fraction, may be at or slightly below the lower limits of normal under resting conditions among CAHAP with dilated ventricles. |
| • Know that resting diastolic function should be normal to supranormal, as assessed echocardiographically, using complimentary indexes (i.e., transmitral doppler, tissue doppler imaging, and so on) among endurance-trained CAHAP. |
| • Know the differential diagnosis for left ventricular chamber dilation among CAHAP. |
| • Know the differential diagnosis for right ventricular chamber dilation among CAHAP. |
| • Know the differential diagnosis for left ventricular wall thickening among CAHAP. |
| • Know the rationale for prescribed detraining including relevant areas of physiological uncertainty in clinical practice. |
| B. Patient care and procedural skills |
| • Skill to comprehensively evaluate physical activity and exercise patterns, including type, duration, and intensity of training and competition, to determine expected patterns of underlying EICR. |
| • Skill to apply contemporary ECG interpretation criteria for CAHAP in varied clinical settings ranging from traditional clinical encounters to "in the field" pre-participation screening. |
| • Skill to interpret transthoracic echocardiographic data, in partnership with cardiovascular imaging experts, among CAHAP with emphasis on recognition of imaging data consistent with adaptive exercise-induced remodeling. |
| • Skill to prescribe physiological deconditioning in selected cases where multimodality diagnostic assessment fails to resolve "gray-zone" findings among CAHAP. |

*ACC* American College of Cardiology, *AHA* American Heart Association, *CAHAP* competitive athletes and highly active people, *EICR* exercise-induced cardiac remodeling

1. **Understand the sport, how it is governed, and define the role of the team doctor and cardiologist.**
   (a) With over 270 million active players (www.fifa.com), soccer is the world's most popular sport.
   (b) Soccer's governing body, FIFA, is comprised of 211 member associations.

(c) MLS (the American professional football association), is aligned with all of FIFA's policies and regulations.
(d) At the MLS player recruitment combine in Florida, local cardiologists partner with league medical staff to conduct and oversee athlete cardiovascular testing.
(e) Beyond the combine, each of the 24 MLS teams has engaged a local "team cardiologist," who is available to provide immediate athlete cardiac care, allowing for efficient evaluation.
(f) Most team cardiologists assist in the interpretation of baseline ECG, and/or echocardiograms, and evaluate symptomatic athletes.

2. **Define the cardiovascular demands of sport.**
   (a) Soccer is categorized as "IC" per the ACC/AHA sports participation guidelines [40] and is thus a highly dynamic sport (see Chap. 1).
   (b) During a 90-min soccer match, field players cover 10–12 km (6.2–7.5 mi) and goalkeepers about 4 km (2.5 mi); players also sprint 2–4 s every 90 s [41, 42].
   (c) During a soccer match, players average 80–90% of their heart rate maximum [42].
   (d) The highest maximal oxygen uptake recorded in soccer is about 80.9 ml/kg/min; most are in the 55–68 ml/kg/min range [43, 44].
3. **Consider the internal and external sports environment.**
   (a) During a 90-min soccer match, catecholamines and cortisol concentrations increase significantly compared to resting values [45, 46].
   (b) Similar to what has been observed in marathoners, troponin-I is elevated in 43% of soccer players after a match [47], and may remain elevated for up to 48 h [48].
   (c) Core temperature increases during play, starting at 20 min, and reaching 39 °C at the end of a match [49].
4. **Identify ranges of normal CV adaptations for this sport.**
   (a) Team doctors and cardiologists must develop proficiency in distinguishing normal soccer athletic adaptations from cardiac pathology.
   (b) Soccer poses a sustained volume load to the heart, resulting in four chamber enlargement and increased stroke volume at rest and exercise [50].
   (c) Soccer-induced electrophysiological adaptations appear on the ECG in the form of AV and interventricular blocks, ectopic beats, interval prolongations, increased voltage, and repolarization changes.
   (d) In 582 professional soccer players undergoing cardiac assessment at the 2006 FIFA World Cup, 4.8% were found to have a potentially "pathologic" ECG, most commonly due to T wave inversion [51].
   (e) Echocardiographic data in the same group suggests that ventricular enlargement is common. Thirty percent of players will demonstrate left ventricular end-diastolic dimension >55 mm, while 10% show right ventricular end-diastolic dimension >30 mm [51].

(f) Left ventricular ejection fraction ranges 45–85% in soccer players, while left atrial and aortic dimensions are 22–49 (mean 36 ± 4) and 19–43 (mean 31 ± 3) mm respectively [51].
(g) Three percent of players demonstrate left ventricular wall thickness >13 mm [51].
(h) In 558 professional soccer football players who completed ECG and echocardiographic screening in 2013 and 2014, 19 players (3.4%) presented with positive ECG findings [52].
(i) While MRI features of soccer have not been published, data on MRI in endurance athletes suggests that some normals may demonstrate late gadolinium enhancement [53]. The clinical significance of this is not known.

5. **Estimate cardiovascular risk, including that from performance enhancing agents.**
(a) Among 74.1% of FIFA member organizations surveyed, 107 cases of sudden cardiac arrest (SCA) or SCD were recalled over a 10-year period; mean age 24.9 years, with 20.5% overall survival [54].
(b) If an AED was placed on the pitch (field), survival was increased dramatically to 52.2% [54].
(c) Recently, it has been shown that the incidence of sudden cardiac death among previously screened adolescent soccer players is 1 per 14,794 person-years (6.8 per 100,000 athletes) [55].
(d) Similar to other endurance athletes, soccer players are prone to long term risk of atrial fibrillation [56].
(e) Professional soccer players have been known to test positive for performance enhancing agents and recreational drugs, primarily anabolic steroids, and stimulants (ephedrine, amphetamines, and cocaine).

**Clinical Pearls**

- In the United States, the cardiologist typically learns sports cardiology "by doing".
- Sports cardiologists must understand the cardiac diseases that cause sudden death in athletes and be able to recognize them at an early stage.
- Basic general cardiology with some knowledge of exercise physiology probably provides the best background for a sports cardiologist.
- Efficient work-ups will endear the cardiologist to the team medical staff.
- ECG screening has primarily driven the development of Sports Cardiology.
- Both the ESC and the ACC have published a set of core competencies in Sports Cardiology.
- A systematic approach to evaluation of athletes is recommended, taking into consideration sports specific cardiovascular demands, adaptations and their appearance on cardiac testing, any existing or potential interaction of the heart with the internal and external sports environment, cardiovascular risks, and prevalence of use of performance enhancing agents and rules for drug testing.

## Review

## Questions

1. The discipline of Sports Cardiology has been driven by:
   (a) ECG screening in Italy
   (b) Beliefs in health benefits of exercise
   (c) Observation that exercise triggers sudden cardiac death
   (d) Studies documenting cardiac enlargement in athletes
   (e) All of the above
2. If the cardiologist is asked to interpret ECGs and echocardiograms in basketball athletes:
   (a) Tests can be interpreted according to normal ranges in non-athletic populations
   (b) Tests are best interpreted according to published norms in basketball athletes
   (c) Should use the "International Recommendations for Electrocardiographic Interpretation in Athletes"
   (d) b and c are acceptable
   (e) None of the above
3. Core competencies for a Sports Cardiologist include:
   (a) Exercise physiology and adaptation
   (b) Cardiac evaluation
   (c) Substance abuse and doping
   (d) Sports eligibility in individuals with cardiac disease
   (e) All of the above

## Answers

1. **The correct answer is "e"**, as all of these observations and practices have contributed to the development of Sports Cardiology. The ancient Greek physician Herodicus promoted the health benefits of exercise to his patients. In fact, he recommended that his patients walk regularly from Athens to Megara, a distance of a little more than 20 miles. As mentor for Hippocrates, Herodicus passed these beliefs on to his famous student. Contemporary epidemiology has been able to demonstrate that the ancient Greeks were correct, and that regular exercise does, indeed, confer lower mortality and improved outcomes. The first episode of exercise related sudden cardiac death occurred in 490 BC, with sudden collapse of Athenian courier Pheidippides. But the abrupt unexpected death of young athletes continues to fascinate modern clinicians, prompting the creation and development of the Italian ECG based screening program. This practice has now "gone global", causing cardiologists who interpret cardiac testing in athletes to differentiate the nuances between athletic adaptation and early disease. As

echocardiography and advanced imaging have allowed more precise imaging of the heart, the normal limits of athletic adaptation have been defined.

2. **The correct answers are "b and c"**. An athlete's ECG cannot be interpreted as one would interpret an ECG in a non-athletic individual, as the athletic adaptations may result in a high incidence of false positives. One might use the "International Recommendations for Electrocardiographic Interpretation in Athletes" as a reference to interpret an athlete ECG; but the clinician is advised to dig deep into the published literature for normative data in a specific athletic population. In the case of the basketball athlete, excellent published references are available.
3. **The correct answer is "e"**, all of the above, as a sports cardiologist is required to have knowledge of all of these areas. See the ESC paper, and the ACC paper for details.

## References

1. Lawless CE, Olshansky B, Washington RL, Baggish AL, Daniels CJ, Lawrence SM, et al. Sports and exercise cardiology in the United States: cardiovascular specialists as members of the athlete healthcare team. J Am Coll Cardiol. 2014;63(15):1461–72.
2. Lawless CE, Asplund C, Asif IM, Courson R, Emery MS, Fuisz A, et al. Protecting the heart of the American athlete: proceedings of the American College of Cardiology Sports and Exercise Cardiology Think Tank October 18, 2012, Washington, DC. J Am Coll Cardiol. 2014;64(20):2146–71.
3. Georgoulis AD, Kiapidou IS, Velogianni L, Stergiou N, Boland A. Herodicus, the father of sports medicine. Knee Surg Sports Traumatol Arthrosc. 2007;15(3):315–8.
4. Park RJ. High-protein diets, "damaged hearts," and rowing men: antecedents of modern sports medicine and exercise science, 1867–1928. Exerc Sport Sci Rev. 1997;25:137–69.
5. Martin D, Benario H, Gynn R. Development of the marathon from Pheidippides to the present with statistics of significant races. Ann N Y Acad Sci. 1977;301:820–57.
6. Thompson PD. D. Bruce Dill Historical lecture. Historical concepts of the athlete's heart. Med Sci Sports Exerc. 2004;36(3):363–70.
7. Maron BJ, Roberts WC, McAllister HA, Rosing DR, Epstein SE. Sudden death in young athletes. Circulation. 1980;62(2):218–29.
8. Opie LH. Letter: Sudden death and sport. Lancet. 1975;1(7908):678.
9. Siscovick DS, Weiss NS, Fletcher RH, Lasky T. The incidence of primary cardiac arrest during vigorous exercise. N Engl J Med. 1984;311(14):874–7.
10. Thompson PD, Funk EJ, Carleton RA, Sturner WQ. Incidence of death during jogging in Rhode Island from 1975 through 1980. JAMA. 1982;247(18):2535–8.
11. Thompson PD, Stern MP, Williams P, Duncan K, Haskell WL, Wood PD. Death during jogging or running. A study of 18 cases. JAMA. 1979;242(12):1265–7.
12. Farahmand B, Hallmarker U, Brobert GP, Ahlbom A. Acute mortality during long-distance ski races (Vasaloppet). Scand J Med Sci Sports. 2007;17(4):356–61.
13. Farahmand BY, Ahlbom A, Ekblom O, Ekblom B, Hallmarker U, Aronson D, et al. Mortality amongst participants in Vasaloppet: a classical long-distance ski race in Sweden. J Intern Med. 2003;253(3):276–83.
14. Marijon E, Tafflet M, Antero-Jacquemin J, El Helou N, Berthelot G, Celermajer DS, et al. Mortality of French participants in the Tour de France (1947–2012). Eur Heart J. 2013;34(40):3145–50.
15. Harmon KG, Asif IM, Klossner D, Drezner JA. Incidence of sudden cardiac death in National Collegiate Athletic Association athletes. Circulation. 2011;123(15):1594–600.

16. Harris KM, Henry JT, Rohman E, Haas TS, Maron BJ. Sudden death during the triathlon. JAMA. 2010;303(13):1255–7.
17. Kim JH, Malhotra R, Chiampas G, d'Hemecourt P, Troyanos C, Cianca J, et al. Cardiac arrest during long-distance running races. N Engl J Med. 2012;366(2):130–40.
18. Maron BJ, Haas TS, Ahluwalia A, Rutten-Ramos SC. Incidence of cardiovascular sudden deaths in Minnesota high school athletes. Heart Rhythm. 2013;10(3):374–7.
19. Roberts WO, Stovitz SD. Incidence of sudden cardiac death in Minnesota high school athletes 1993–2012 screened with a standardized pre-participation evaluation. J Am Coll Cardiol. 2013;62(14):1298–301.
20. Osler W. The principles and practice of medicine. 1st ed. New York: Appleton; 1892.
21. Henschen S. Skilanglauf und Skiwettlauf: eine medizinische Sportstudie. Mitt Med Klin Upsala (Jena). 1899;2:15–8.
22. Gott PH, Roselle HA, Crampton RS. The athletic heart syndrome. Five-year cardiac evaluation of a champion athlete. Arch Intern Med. 1968;122(4):340–4.
23. Morganroth J, Maron BJ, Henry WL, Epstein SE. Comparative left ventricular dimensions in trained athletes. Ann Intern Med. 1975;82(4):521–4.
24. Pelliccia A, Maron BJ, Spataro A, Proschan MA, Spirito P. The upper limit of physiologic cardiac hypertrophy in highly trained elite athletes. N Engl J Med. 1991;324(5):295–301.
25. Basavarajaiah S, Boraita A, Whyte G, Wilson M, Carby L, Shah A, et al. Ethnic differences in left ventricular remodeling in highly-trained athletes relevance to differentiating physiologic left ventricular hypertrophy from hypertrophic cardiomyopathy. J Am Coll Cardiol. 2008;51(23):2256–62.
26. Di Paolo FM, Schmied C, Zerguini YA, Junge A, Quattrini F, Culasso F, et al. The athlete's heart in adolescent Africans. J Am Coll Cardiol. 2012;59(11):1029–36.
27. Galderisi M, Lomoriello VS, Santoro A, Esposito R, Olibet M, Raia R, et al. Differences of myocardial systolic deformation and correlates of diastolic function in competitive rowers and young hypertensives: a speckle-tracking echocardiography study. J Am Soc Echocardiogr. 2010;23(11):1190–8.
28. Kato TS, Noda A, Izawa H, Yamada A, Obata K, Nagata K, et al. Discrimination of nonobstructive hypertrophic cardiomyopathy from hypertensive left ventricular hypertrophy on the basis of strain rate imaging by tissue Doppler ultrasonography. Circulation. 2004;110(25):3808–14.
29. Magalski A, Maron BJ, Main ML, McCoy M, Florez A, Reid KJ, et al. Relation of race to electrocardiographic patterns in elite American football players. J Am Coll Cardiol. 2008;51(23):2250–5.
30. Pela G, Bruschi G, Montagna L, Manara M, Manca C. Left and right ventricular adaptation assessed by Doppler tissue echocardiography in athletes. J Am Soc Echocardiogr. 2004;17(3):205–11.
31. Zaidi A, Ghani S, Sharma R, Oxborough D, Panoulas VF, Sheikh N, et al. Physiological right ventricular adaptation in elite athletes of African and Afro-Caribbean origin. Circulation. 2013;127(17):1783–92.
32. Corrado D, Basso C, Pavei A, Michieli P, Schiavon M, Thiene G. Trends in sudden cardiovascular death in young competitive athletes after implementation of a preparticipation screening program. JAMA. 2006;296(13):1593–601.
33. Maron BJ, Friedman RA, Kligfield P, Levine BD, Viskin S, Chaitman BR, et al. Assessment of the 12-lead ECG as a screening test for detection of cardiovascular disease in healthy general populations of young people (12–25 years of age): a scientific statement from the American Heart Association and the American College of Cardiology. Circulation. 2014;130(15):1303–34.
34. Harris KM, Sponsel A, Hutter AM Jr, Maron BJ. Brief communication: cardiovascular screening practices of major North American professional sports teams. Ann Intern Med. 2006;145(7):507–11.
35. Asplund CA, Asif IM. Cardiovascular preparticipation screening practices of college team physicians. Clin J Sport Med. 2014;24(4):275–9.

36. Hainline B, Drezner JA, Baggish A, Harmon KG, Emery MS, Myerburg RJ, et al. Interassociation consensus statement on cardiovascular care of college student-athletes. J Am Coll Cardiol. 2016;67(25):2981–95.
37. Heidbuchel H, Papadakis M, Panhuyzen-Goedkoop N, Carre F, Dugmore D, Mellwig KP, et al. Position paper: proposal for a core curriculum for a European Sports Cardiology qualification. Eur J Prev Cardiol. 2013;20(5):889–903.
38. Baggish AL, Battle RW, Beckerman JG, Bove AA, Lampert RJ, Levine BD, et al. Sports cardiology: core curriculum for providing cardiovascular care to competitive athletes and highly active people. J Am Coll Cardiol. 2017;70(15):1902–18.
39. Lawless CE. How to practice sports cardiology: a cardiology perspective. Clin Sports Med. 2015;34:539–49.
40. Maron BJ, Zipes DP, Kovacs RJ. Eligibility and disqualification recommendations for competitive athletes with cardiovascular abnormalities: preamble, principles, and general considerations: a scientific statement from the American Heart Association and American College of Cardiology. J Am Coll Cardiol. 2015;66(21):2343–9.
41. Stolen T, Chamari K, Castagna C, Wisloff U. Physiology of soccer: an update. Sports Med. 2005;35(6):501–36.
42. Stroyer J, Hansen L, Klausen K. Physiological profile and activity pattern of young soccer players during match play. Med Sci Sports Exerc. 2004;36(1):168–74.
43. Hoff J. Training and testing physical capacities for elite soccer players. J Sports Sci. 2005;23(6):573–82.
44. Tumilty D. Physiological characteristics of elite soccer players. Sports Med. 1993;16(2):80–96.
45. Carli G, Bonifazi M, Lodi L, Lupo C, Martelli G, Viti A. Hormonal and metabolic effects following a football match. Int J Sports Med. 1986;7(1):36–8.
46. Haneishi K, Fry AC, Moore CA, Schilling BK, Li Y, Fry MD. Cortisol and stress responses during a game and practice in female collegiate soccer players. J Strength Cond Res. 2007;21(2):583–8.
47. Lowbeer C, Seeberger A, Gustafsson SA, Bouvier F, Hulting J. Serum cardiac troponin T, troponin I, plasma BNP and left ventricular mass index in professional football players. J Sci Med Sport. 2007;10(5):291–6.
48. Akyuz M. Changes in serum cardiac troponin T levels in professional football players before and after the game. Afr J Pharm Pharmacol. 2011;5:1365–8.
49. Ozgunen KT, Kurdak SS, Maughan RJ, Zeren C, Korkmaz S, Yazici Z, et al. Effect of hot environmental conditions on physical activity patterns and temperature response of football players. Scand J Med Sci Sports. 2010;20(Suppl 3):140–7.
50. Maron BJ, Pelliccia A. The heart of trained athletes: cardiac remodeling and the risks of sports, including sudden death. Circulation. 2006;114(15):1633–44.
51. Thunenkotter T, Schmied C, Dvorak J, Kindermann W. Benefits and limitations of cardiovascular pre-competition screening in international football. Clin Res Cardiol. 2010;99(1):29–35.
52. Bakken A, Targett S, Bere T, Adamuz MC, Tol JL, Whiteley R, et al. Health conditions detected in a comprehensive periodic health evaluation of 558 professional football players. Br J Sports Med. 2016;50(18):1142–50.
53. Breuckmann F, Mohlenkamp S, Nassenstein K, Lehmann N, Ladd S, Schmermund A, et al. Myocardial late gadolinium enhancement: prevalence, pattern, and prognostic relevance in marathon runners. Radiology. 2009;251(1):50–7.
54. Schmied C, Drezner J, Kramer E, Dvorak J. Cardiac events in football and strategies for first-responder treatment on the field. Br J Sports Med. 2013;47(18):1175–8.
55. Malhotra A, Dhutia H, Finocchiaro G, Gati S, Beasley I, Clift P, et al. Outcomes of cardiac screening in adolescent soccer players. N Engl J Med. 2018;379(6):524–34.
56. Abdulla J, Nielsen JR. Is the risk of atrial fibrillation higher in athletes than in the general population? A systematic review and meta-analysis. Europace. 2009;11(9):1156–9.
57. Lawless CE. Growth and development of sports and exercise cardiology in the US. In: Thompson PD, Fernandez AB, editors. Exercise and sports cardiology. 2nd ed. Singapore: World Scientific; 2018.

# Athlete's Heart: Basic Physiology and Adaptation to Exercise

3

Christian M. Schmied and Matthias Wilhelm

**Learning Objectives**

1. General knowledge of the structural and functional background of athlete's heart.
2. Historical perspective.
3. Acute response of the cardiovascular system to single bouts of exercise.
4. Electrical, structural, and functional cardiac adaptation to regular exercise training.

## 3.1 Historical Perspective

With the advent of modern medicine at the end of the nineteenth century, physicians became interested in exercise physiology. Sir William Osler observed in trained individuals "*a gradual increase in the capability of the heart*" and speculated that "*the large heart of athletes may be due to the prolonged use of their muscles, but no man becomes a great runner or oarsman who has not naturally a capable if not large heart*" [1]. The first systematic reports describing enlarged cardiac dimensions in athletes were based on physical examination, conducted in Sweden and the United States of America and published in 1899. Salomon Eberhard Henschen from the University of Uppsala performed chest percussion of Nordic skiers and sedentary individuals, concluding:

> Skiing causes an enlargement of the heart, and this enlarged heart can perform more work than a normal heart. [2]

---

C. M. Schmied (✉) · M. Wilhelm
Department of Cardiology, University Heart Center, Zurich, Switzerland

Department of Cardiology, Interdisciplinary Centre for Sports & Exercise Medicine, Inselspital, University Hospital of Bern, Bern, Switzerland
e-mail: christian.schmied@usz.ch; matthias.wilhelm@insel.ch



A. Pressler, J. Niebauer (eds.), *Textbook of Sports and Exercise Cardiology*,
https://doi.org/10.1007/978-3-030-35374-2_3

He thereby defined the "athlete's heart" for the first time, illustrating that exercise and athletic training may lead to a physiological enlargement of the heart with an enhanced function, in contrast to an enlargement of the heart due to a cardiomyopathy with a reduced function. Eugen Darling from Harvard University made a similar observation in Harvard rowers [3].

The introduction of radiological techniques made visualization of the athlete's heart possible and confirmed the findings from physical examination. The view of a beneficial adaptation to exercise was not universally accepted. In 1902, Fritz Moritz raised the concern that cardiac enlargement in athletes could be a form of overuse pathology, and that prolonged vigorous exercise could lead to premature cardiac failure [4]. In the next 60 years, chest x-ray contributed to a better understanding of exercise physiology and the athlete's heart, but did not solve the dilemma of discriminating physiology from pathology [5–11]:

- The size of the cardiac silhouette varies between sporting disciplines.
- Athletes engaged in high-intensity endurance sports have the largest hearts.
- A large cardiac silhouette is associated with a high aerobic capacity.
- Some cardiac silhouettes in athletes may mimic pictures of patients with valvular or congenital heart disease.

Alongside the advances in cardiac imaging, the development of the electrocardiogram (ECG) allowed the study of electrical activity of the athlete's heart and revealed distinct features of the athlete's ECG [11–14]:

- Sinus bradycardia and junctional rhythms
- PQ prolongation
- Increased QRS voltages fulfilling criteria for LV hypertrophy
- ST segment elevation
- Tall T waves

The introduction of transthoracic echocardiography substantially improved the understanding of structural and functional features of the athlete's heart. In 1975, Morganroth and colleagues were the first to publish a comparative cross-sectional study in predominantly endurance-trained (swimming and rowing) and strength-trained (wrestling and shot putting) athletes [15]. Based on M-mode echocardiography and reference values from sedentary controls, they demonstrated the following:

- Isotonic exercise was associated with an increased left ventricular (LV) mass and end-diastolic volume, but normal wall thickness.
- Isometric exercise was associated with an increased LV mass and wall thickness, but normal LV end-diastolic volume.

They concluded that isotonic exercise leads to an eccentric LV hypertrophy pattern similar to changes in chronic volume overload, whereas isometric exercise leads to a concentric LV hypertrophy pattern, similar to changes in chronic pressure overload [15]. The "Morganroth hypothesis" has been criticized because of relying on cross-sectional data and the paucity of supporting evidence from longitudinal exercise training studies [16, 17]. However, recent evidence from longitudinal studies supports the observation that long-term endurance exercise elicits eccentric LV hypertrophy [18]. Importantly, this study stimulated research on cardiac remodelling in athletes and opened the field of sports cardiology.

In 1991, Antonio Pelliccia, Barry Maron and colleagues published a seminal paper on upper limits of physiological cardiac hypertrophy in a large cohort of highly trained elite athletes from different sporting disciplines [19]. Eight years later, Pelliccia and colleagues reported on physiologic LV cavity dilatation in a cohort of Italian elite athletes [20]. The most important observations were

- LV wall thicknesses above normal limits (≥13 mm) were uncommon in elite Caucasian athletes (1.7%)
- Athletes from high dynamic and high static sports (see Chap. 1) like rowing or canoeing exhibited the thickest LV walls with values in the range of hypertrophic cardiomyopathy (up to 16 mm).
- Substantial LV cavity enlargement (LV end-diastolic diameter >60 mm), compatible with dilated cardiomyopathy, was more common in elite athletes (14%), most often in high dynamic sports such as cycling, cross-country skiing and canoeing, and in the absence of systolic dysfunction.

Although the problem of discriminating between physiology and pathology could not be solved by echography, this technique substantially led to a better understanding of the athlete's heart and subsequent studies investigated the impact of age, gender, ethnicity, type of sports and starting age of endurance sports [21–25].

Interestingly, for more than 25 years, sports cardiologists focused their interest on the LV. In 2003, Hein Heidbuchel and colleagues observed a high prevalence of right ventricular (RV) involvement in endurance athletes with ventricular arrhythmias [26]. Their hypothesis that endurance sport could be related to the development and/or progression of the underlying arrhythmogenic substrate stimulated research on function and structure of the RV. A recent study demonstrated that a significant percentage of Olympic athletes (namely 32% of included endurance athletes) exceed the RV reference dimensional limits proposed for the diagnosis of arrhythmogenic RV cardiomyopathy [27].

More than a century after the discovery of the athlete's heart by chest percussion, some controversies remain. Multimodal imaging has been proposed to better discriminate physiological adaptation in athletes from pathology. Computer tomography, nuclear imaging, two- and three dimensional echocardiography, and cardiac magnetic imaging have different potential for analysing perfusion, metabolism, morphology, function, and tissue characteristics, and will further improve our understanding of the consequences of exercise for the heart [28].

## 3.2 Cardiovascular Response to Exercise and Functional Changes in an Athlete's Heart

The ability to perform endurance exercise like running is a derived capability of the genus *Homo* and may have been instrumental in the evolution of human anatomy and physiology [29]. The acute response to a bout of exercise involves most organs of the body, in particular the autonomic nervous and cardiovascular system, and the respiratory and locomotor muscles. Chronic exercise leads to dose-dependent adaptations in form of a structural and functional remodelling of the involved organs [30]. Importantly, this includes a higher plasma and red blood cell volume for an improved oxygen and carbon dioxide transport [31–34].

Most of the cardiorespiratory effects of exercise are related to supplying adequate oxygen to the involved working muscles. During quiet sitting, the oxygen uptake is approximately 3.5 ml/min/kg (one metabolic equivalent, MET; see also Chap. 1) [35].

- In untrained individuals, maximum oxygen uptake can increase 10- to 12-fold from rest.
- In highly trained endurance athletes, maximum oxygen uptake can increase >20-fold from rest (to more than 6 l/min or 80 ml/min/kg) [36].

The Fick equation *"Cardiac output ($\dot{Q}_C$) is oxygen consumption ($\dot{V}_{O_2}$) divided by the difference in the oxygen content ($C_{O_2}$) of arterial and mixed venous blood ($a-\bar{v}$)"* illustrates the importance of cardiac output for the maximal oxygen uptake. Both heart rate (*HR*) and stroke volume (*SV*) contribute to the increase of the cardiac output:

- $\dot{Q}_C = \dfrac{\dot{V}_{O_2}}{C_{a-\bar{v}O_2}}$
- $\dot{V}_{O_2} = \dot{Q}_C \times C_{a-\bar{v}O_2}$
- $\dot{V}_{O_2} = SV \times HR \times C_{a-\bar{v}O_2}$

At rest, the cardiac output is approximately 5 l/min, both in athletes and in untrained individuals. Athletes have larger ventricular cavities and generate a larger SV, but their resting HR is lower (e.g. SV 120 ml and HR 40 beats per minute in an athlete, SV 70 ml and HR 70 beats per minute in an untrained person) [37–42].

- Heart rate increase is responsible for the majority of cardiac output augmentation during exercise.

The autonomic nervous system coordinates the transition from rest to exercise for a rapid matching between oxygen delivery and metabolic demand of the exercising muscles. A first phase of parasympathetic withdrawal is followed by sympathetic and neurohumoral activation. Maximal heart rate varies innately between individuals, decreases with age, and does not increase with exercise training. In contrast, stroke volume, both at rest and during exercise may increase significantly with prolonged exercise training [43]. However, the age dependant decrease of maximal heart rate can be decelerated by regular training [44, 45].

- LV end-diastolic filling and, to a lesser degree, sympathetically mediated reduction in LV end-systolic volume are responsible for stroke volume rise during exercise.

LV end-diastolic volume is determined by diastolic filling, a complex process that is affected by a variety of variables, including morphology, heart rate, intrinsic myocardial relaxation, ventricular compliance, ventricular filling pressures, atrial contraction, and extra cardiac mechanical factors such as pericardial and pulmonary constraints [43]. Newer inventions in cardiac imaging, such as echocardiographic tissue Doppler and strain imaging, improved the ability to understand diastolic mechanisms in athletes [46–48].

- Regular endurance training may lead to enhanced early diastolic LV filling [46, 49–51].

Furthermore, the ability of rapid relaxation of the left ventricle, particularly at maximal exercise with high heart rates, is an important mechanism in high-level endurance athletes. Systolic as well as diastolic LV function seem to be affected to a much lesser degree in strength athletes, although limited data is available for this population [52].

There is also only limited data regarding functional aspects of the right ventricle in athlete's heart, but the right ventricular systolic function at rest does not seem different between athletes and controls [53]. There is interesting data suggesting RV enlargement and diminished systolic function in high-level endurance athletes after highly intensive and/or repetitive exercise [54]. This phenomenon is commonly known as "right ventricular fatigue". However, whether these primarily temporary effects may result in chronic right ventricular failure is still a matter of debate [55].

- In untrained individuals, cardiac output can increase four- to fivefold from rest to 20–25 l/min.
- In highly trained endurance athletes, cardiac output can increase six- to eightfold from rest to 30–40 l/min [56].

Importantly, during intense whole-body exercise like cross-country skiing, the limiting factor of maximum oxygen uptake is the capacity of the heart to deliver oxygen, not the muscle to consume it.

- The capacity of the muscles to receive blood flow exceeds by a factor of 2–3 the capacity of the heart to supply the flow.

Vascular conductance and blood pressure are adjusted to match oxygen delivery with the local tissue oxygen demand [57, 58]. At high exercise intensities (>80% of peak work rate), where the metabolic acidosis has to be compensated by respiration, the circulatory system is unable to meet the demands of both locomotor and intercostal muscles. This leads to a reduced intercostal muscle blood flow and vascular conductance in favour of the locomotor muscles. This mismatch likely contributes to respiratory muscle fatigue [59].

The adaptations of the autonomic nervous and cardiovascular systems during an acute bout of exercise are illustrated in Fig. 3.1 in two individuals with different levels of exercise training.

## 3.3 Electrical Changes

The electrocardiogram classically depicts the electrical activity of the heart but, indirectly, it also allows conclusions on structural features. In athletes, the ECG represents a crucial tool in the screening to prevent adverse exercise-related cardiac events, as it may detect potentially harmful cardiac conditions with a very high accuracy. The current standard to assess an athlete's ECG are the so-called "International (Seattle) Criteria" that differentiate between pathologic, borderline and clearly physiologic changes [60, 61]. However, the ECG interpretation in athletes is challenging as it usually reflects the electrical and structural adaptions that may occur as a consequence of regular physical exercise. As many as 60% of (particularly endurance) athletes demonstrate physiologic ECG changes, such as sinus bradycardia or arrhythmia, ectopic atrial rhythm, low-degree atrioventricular (AV) block, early repolarisation, incomplete right bundle branch block (IRBBB) and voltage criteria for left or right ventricular hypertrophy (LVH/RVH) [62].

Distinguishing these frequent physiologic from pathologic findings is a big challenge for the sports physician, as not only false-positive but also potentially fatal false-negative interpretation may occur [63–65].

### 3.3.1 Physiologic Findings in Athletes

This section relies on the current recommendations for the interpretation of an athlete's ECG, where physiologic findings are particularly outlined [61] (see also Chap. 8). As highlighted before, the amount and intensity of regular exercise (minimum of 4 h/week) cannot be defined uniquely and depends on various denominators. However, the electrical manifestations reflect both increased vagal tone and enlarged cardiac chamber size. A typical athlete's ECG is shown in Fig. 3.2.

### 3.3.2 Increased QRS Voltage for LVH and/or RVH

There are various established criteria to define LVH and RVH [60, 61, 66]. Nevertheless, Sokolow-Lyon criteria are used most commonly. The Sokolow-Lyon

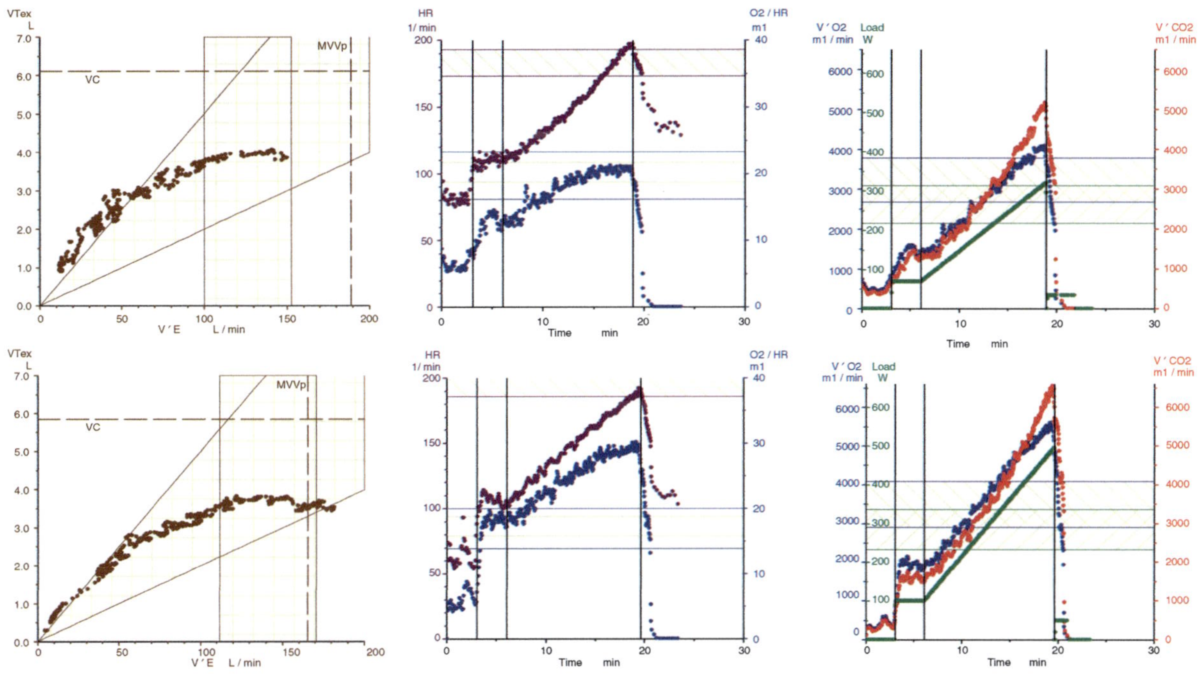


**Fig. 3.1** Comparison of cardiopulmonary exercise tests between a leisure-time sportsman (upper row) and a professional cyclist (lower row). Left panels: the athlete had a higher maximum ventilation (V′E), exceeding his predicted maximum voluntary ventilation (MVVp). Expiratory ventilatory tidal volume (VTex) was comparable between athlete and leisure-time sportsman until V′E 150 L/min. The athlete could further increase his breathing frequency (>50/min), but VTex slightly declined, possibly indicating respiratory muscle fatigue. Middle panels: the athlete had a lower resting heart rate (HR), and a higher HR recovery 1 min after peak exercise, indicating a higher contribution of the parasympathetic nervous system. Peak heart rate was comparable between the leisure-time sportsman and the athlete, but the difference of resting and peak HR was higher in the athlete. Oxygen pulse (O2/HR) increased both in the leisure-time sportsman and in the athlete and started to flatten at 70% of peak work load. Absolute O2/HR was higher in the athlete, indicating a higher stroke volume. Right panels: Oxygen uptake (V′O2) and $CO_2$ exhalation (V′CO2) in relation to incremental workload (W). Horizontal lines reflect 80% and 120% of predicted normal values. For a given work load, oxygen uptake was comparable between leisure-time sportsman and athlete. The athlete achieved a higher workload and oxygen uptake, indicating a higher delivery (cardiac output) and utilization (muscle) of oxygen

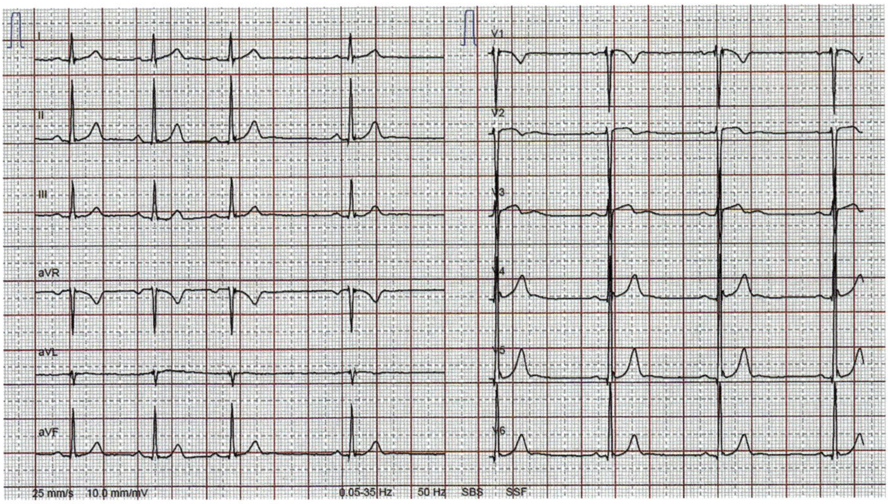


**Fig. 3.2** Typical ECG of a well-trained endurance athlete showing sinus bradycardia and sinus arrhythmia, high voltage criteria for LVH, as well as benign early repolarization

voltage criterion for LVH is defined as the sum of the S wave in V1 and the R wave in V5 or V6 (using the largest R wave) being >3.5 mV, using a standard amplification at 10 mm/1 mV speed [66].

Positive voltage criteria for RVH are a common finding in athletes with up to 13% of the athletes fulfilling the Sokolow–Lyon index [67, 68]. In isolation, positive criteria for RVH do not implicate underlying cardiac disease in athletes [68]. Positive voltage criterion for LVH is an even more frequent finding, in approximately 45% of male and 10% of female athletes, but can also be detected in 25% of young sedentary controls [22, 69–71]. Furthermore, it is relevantly more common in black Afro-Caribbean athletes and generally in children (see also Chaps. 24 and 26), where correlation with morphologic appearance (e.g. in the echocardiography or MRI) is poor [72, 73]. On the other hand, obesity, older age and pulmonary disease such as emphysema may cause lower voltage [73].

- An isolated electrical LVH (based on the QRS voltage criteria) is a normal finding in athletes and related to physiological increases in cardiac chamber size and/or wall thickness.

Further evaluation should only be considered in the presence of pathologic ECG findings as T wave inversion, ST segment depression or Q waves [61]. In the absence of additional pathologic ECG findings isolated QRS high voltage is extremely uncommon (2%) in patients with HCM [74].

### 3.3.3 Incomplete Right Bundle Branch Block

Generally, incomplete right bundle branch block (IRBBB) can be defined by a QRS duration <120 ms with a typical RBBB pattern resembling a terminal R wave in lead V1 (rsR′-pattern) and a wider terminal S wave in leads I and V6. While IRBBB is seen in up to 40% of well-trained endurance athletes, it is a much rarer finding in the general population (up to 10%) [71, 75, 76]. One common physiological correlate may be the increased cavity size of the RV due to athlete's heart with slightly increased conduction time, rather than an intrinsic delay within the conduction system itself [77].

- An IRBBB in an asymptomatic athlete with no additional pathologic findings does not prompt further evaluation.

However, an IRBBB may be confused with relevant ECG findings such as the Brugada ECG pattern or ARVC/D: Classical type I Brugada pattern is characterised by a high take-off and downsloping ST segment elevation followed by a negative T wave in ≥2 leads in V1–V3. Unlike the R′ wave in IRBBB, the 'J wave' seen in a Brugada-ECG pattern does not indicate delayed RV activation, but reflects early repolarisation with J point elevation and a high take-off with downsloping ST segment followed by a negative T wave [78]. IRBBB pattern may commonly be seen in patients with ARVC/D [79] but is only relevant if associated with other ECG abnormalities, such as T-wave inversion involving leads beyond V2, Epsilon waves, prolonged S wave upstroke, low limb-lead voltages and premature ventricular beats with a left bundle branch block appearance. Finally, IRBBB can be associated with an atrial septal defect which can also appear with a fixed splitting of the second heart sound during auscultation (see Chap. 7).

### 3.3.4 Early Repolarization and ST Segment Elevation

There is an ongoing debate regarding the definition of electrocardiographic early repolarisation. However, quite a unique characterisation is an ST segment elevation and/or J wave or "slur" on the downslope of the R wave [80]. Depending on the definition, early repolarisation is a very common finding in up to 45% of Caucasian athletes and 63–91% of black Afro-Caribbean athletes [67, 70–72, 81, 82] but considered a benign ECG pattern [81, 83]. It can appear in any lead but is most likely seen in the anterior leads [84–86].

- The typical early repolarisation pattern in athletes is defined as concave and ascending ST segment elevation [83, 86]. Interestingly, early repolarisation in athletes seems to underlie a dynamic process as it may appear more frequently at times of peak fitness [85].

Recently, some studies suggested that a specific pattern of late QRS slurring or notching with horizontal ST segment elevation in the inferolateral leads could be associated with an increased risk for sudden cardiac arrest due to ventricular arrhythmia [87, 88]. However, these data are controversial, particularly in athletic populations, and there is no evidence for an association between early repolarisation and SCD in athletes [87–90].

A special variant of a most apparently benign early repolarisation pattern in black Afro-Caribbean athletes is ST segment elevation followed by T-wave inversion V1–V4. Characteristically it is characterised with a convex "dome-shaped" ST-elevation followed by a negative T wave. More than two-thirds of black athletes exhibit ST segment elevation and up to 25% show T wave inversion [67, 72] (see Chap. 26). However, normal repolarisation changes in black Afro-Caribbean athletes do not extend beyond V4, and T wave inversion in the lateral leads (V5–V6 and I, aVL) is always considered an abnormal finding.

### 3.3.5 Sinus Bradycardia, Sinus Arrhythmia and Ectopic Atrial Rhythm

The classification of a true sinus rhythm is based on three criteria: (1) a P wave is preceding every QRS complex, (2) a QRS complex follows every P wave, and (3) the P wave must have a normal axis in the frontal plane (0–90°s). In healthy athletes, a normal heart rate is considered to range from 60 and 100 bpm, while sinus rhythm <60 bpm is labelled 'sinus bradycardia' and >100 bpm "sinus tachycardia".

- *Sinus bradycardia* at rest is one of the most common ECG findings in athletes, and is primarily due to increased vagal tone, but can also get a "structural" correlate by intrinsic adaptations within the sinus node [91, 92]. A typical hallmark of this benign finding is immediate increase of the heart rate during exercise.
- The physiologic adaptation of the heart rate to respiratory phases (increase during inspiration, decrease during expiration) is frequently exaggerated in children and in athletes (up to 55%), resulting in an irregular heart rhythm originating from the sinus node [69, 70]. Physiologic *sinus arrhythmia* should not be confused with sinus node dysfunction (e.g. in sick sinus syndrome).
- *Ectopic atrial rhythm* or *junctional escape rhythm* may occur due to a slowed resting sinus node activity prompting an ectopic focus within the atria to initiate cardiac conduction. A junctional or nodal rhythm appears with the QRS rate being faster than the resting P wave with a narrow QRS complex and a rate of typically less than 100 bpm (unless the baseline QRS complex is already enlarged). An ectopic atrial rhythm can be recognized if P waves are inverted in the inferior leads (II, III and aVF). Again, the atrial rate is typically less than 100 bpm.
- The appearance of two different morphologies of P waves in the resting ECG is called a wandering atrial pacemaker.

All these physiologic adaptions due to increased vagal tone change to a normal sinus rhythm as soon as heart rate increases during exercise.

### 3.3.6 Low Grade AV Block

PR interval prolongation (>200 ms) due to *AV block I* remains at the same duration on every beat, representing a delay in AV nodal conduction, particularly in endurance athletes, due to increased vagal activity (and additional intrinsic changes within the AV node). *In second degree AV block* (Mobitz type I/Wenckebach) the prolongation of the PR interval progressively increases from beat to beat, until a non-conducted P wave (not followed by a QRS complex) appears. Typically, the first PR interval after the dropped beat is shorter than the PR interval last conducted before. Similar to the adaptions of the sinus rhythm mentioned above, normal AV conduction immediately resumes during exercise [61].

### 3.3.7 Borderline and Pathologic ECG Findings in Athletes

Several ECG findings are not associated with the physiologic athlete's heart and are considered as being highly indicative of underlying cardiac disease [61]. These changes may suggest:

- *structural disease* (T wave inversion, ST segment depression, Q waves, complete Left Bundle Branch Block, Epsilon waves) or
- *electrical disease* (ventricular pre-excitation, QT prolongation, Brugada type I pattern, high degree AV block, atrial and ventricular tachyarrhythmia) [61].

T-wave inversions in V1–V3 are considered a normal finding in athletes up to the age of 16 [93, 94]. In addition, some changes have to be interpreted as "borderline" findings and may only warrant further investigation if they appear in combination with suspicious clinical findings or additional ECG alterations. These borderline changes include:

1. complete Right Bundle Branch Block
2. right or left axis deviation
3. signs of atrial enlargement [61, 94].

Complete RBBB is detected in approximately 1% of the general population but is a more common finding in athletes (0.5–2.5%) [95, 96]. In a recent study in U.S. collegiate athletes, RBBB was reported in 2.5%; compared with athletes with normal QRS complexes or incomplete RBBB, these athletes exhibited larger right ventricular dimensions and a lower right ventricular ejection fraction but none of them was found to have cardiac disease [97].

## 3.4 Structural Changes

### 3.4.1 General Aspects

The cardiovascular demand varies widely across sporting disciplines, experience of the athlete and level of competition (see Chap. 1). It can be characterized by different degrees of both isotonic (dynamic) and isometric (static) components [98, 99]:

- Isotonic (dynamic) exercise may substantially increase cardiac output and reduce peripheral vascular resistance, representing a transient volume challenge for the heart.
- Isometric (static) exercise increases peripheral vascular resistance with less increase in cardiac output, representing a transient pressure challenge for the heart.

Two classifications of sport disciplines have been proposed (see Chap. 1). The AHA/ACC classification is based on peak static and dynamic components achieved during competition [98], whereas the ESC classification groups the most common Olympic sport disciplines based on their main physiologic characteristics of exercise into skill, power, mixed and endurance disciplines [99].

Cardiac structural remodelling is most pronounced in professional endurance athletes in sports with an additional high isometric component, such as triathlon, cycling or rowing (Fig. 3.3; see also Chap. 4) [99]. Usually, athletes in these sports are involved in >10–15 h/week of intensive exercise training. Intense exercise places a disproportionate higher load on the RV, when compared with the LV [100]. Acutely after long-lasting competitions (8–11 h), a transient deterioration of the RV, but not of the LV function and an increase of the RV end-systolic volume and the RV/LV end-systolic volume ratio have been described [54]. Chronically, the combination of intense exercise training and competition leads to a balanced enlargement of all cardiac chambers.

- Compared to active controls (matched for body surface area), triathletes exhibited approximately 30% larger RV and LV cavities, and 30% higher RV and LV masses, resulting in comparable RV and LV mass-to-volume ratios [101].

In leisure-time athletes, endurance training protocols as low as 3 h/week may result in a measurable increase of cardiac mass, wall thickness and volume after 3 months [102]. However, long-term, non-elite endurance training and competition (<10 h/week) may have a more pronounced effect on the thin-walled atria, compared to the ventricles.

- Compared to non-marathon runners, regular marathon runners (>6 races) presented more often with right atrial (60% vs. 35%) and left atrial (74% vs. 24%) enlargement. There was a strong association between atrial and ventricular dimensions in the whole cohort, but RV and LV cavity dimensions did not differ between the groups, and exceeded normal limits in <3% of athletes [103].

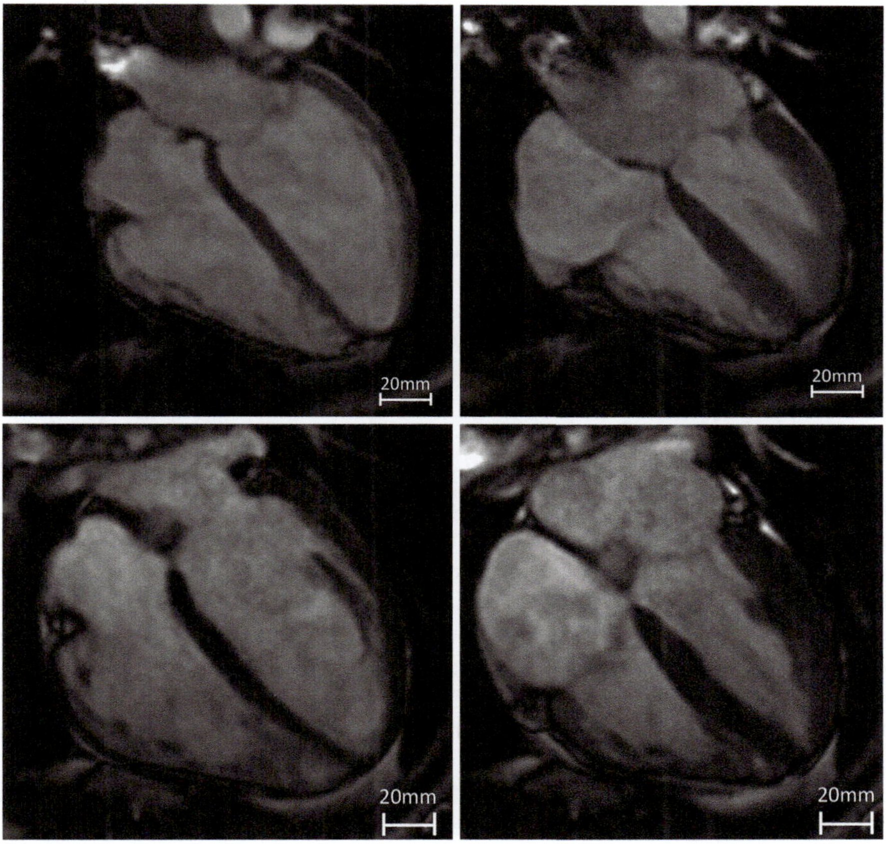


**Fig. 3.3** Comparison of cardiac magnetic resonance images between a non-athlete (upper row) and a triathlete (lower row, 10 h exercise training/week) (courtesy of Christoph Gräni, MD, PhD). Left panels: Four chamber view of the heart in diastole. Compared to the non-athlete, the triathlete showed an enlargement of the left and right ventricle and slightly thicker left ventricular walls, leading to eccentric left ventricular hypertrophy. Right panels: Four chamber view of the heart in systole. Compared to the non-athlete, the triathlete showed an enlargement of the left and right atria. Ventricular stroke volume is higher in the triathlete

### 3.4.2 Specific Aspects of Left Ventricular Remodelling

The LV geometry is characterized based on relative wall thickness (RWT) and left ventricular mass index (LVMI) [104].

- LV hypertrophy is defined as LVMI >95 g/m$^2$ in women, and >115 g/m$^2$ in men.
- Subjects with a normal LVMI can either have a normal geometry (RWT $\leq$ 0.42) or concentric remodeling (RWT > 0.42).
- Subjects with an abnormal LVMI can either have eccentric (RWT $\leq$ 0.42) or concentric (RWT > 0.42) hypertrophy.

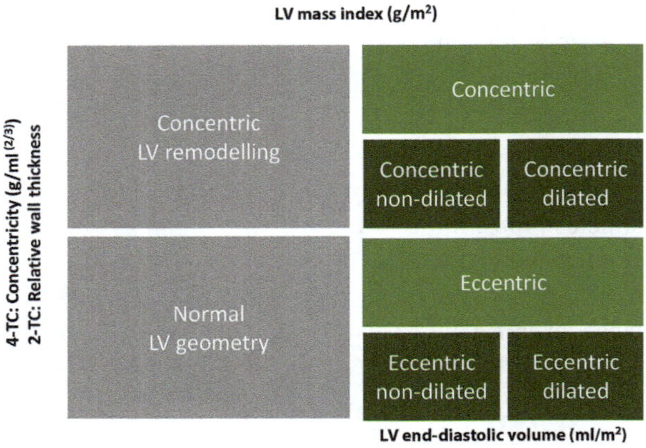


**Fig. 3.4** Two-tiered (2-TC, light green) and four-tiered (4-TC, dark green) classifications of left ventricular (LV) hypertrophy. Cut-of values for concentricity, LV mass index, and LV end-diastolic volume index depend on sex and imaging method (echocardiography or magnetic resonance imaging) [104, 105]

Compared to this 2-tiered classification of LV hypertrophy, a newer 4-tiered classification characterizes LV hypertrophy patterns based on LV concentricity ([LVM/LV end-diastolic volume]$^{2/3}$) and LV end-diastolic volume index, so that concentric and eccentric LV hypertrophy patterns are further stratified into a non-dilated and dilated category (Fig. 3.4) [105].

- In a cohort of normotensive endurance athletes, the 4-tiered classification demonstrated a superior discrimination of exercise-induced LV hypertrophy patterns, most likely because it takes three-dimensional information of the ventricular geometry into account [106].

Despite widespread acceptance of the Morganroth hypothesis on LV dimensions in athletes (see above), some investigators have questioned whether resistance exercise is exclusively a "pressure overload" stress, resulting in concentric LV hypertrophy, or whether endurance exercise is primarily a "volume overload" stimulus, resulting in eccentric LV hypertrophy [17].

Based on the Laplace's law, LV wall stress is a function of systolic arterial blood pressure and LV geometry:

- $LV\ wall\ stress = \dfrac{LV\ pressure\, x\, radius}{2x\, LV\ wall\ thickness}$

LV wall stress has been viewed as the most important determinant of concentric LV remodelling, since an increase in LV wall thickness contributes to a normalization of wall stress. However, to explain acute effects of resistance exercise on ventricular wall stress, heart-lung interactions have to be taken into account. When force production exceeds approximately 80% of maximum voluntary contraction, brief Valsalva manoeuvres are inevitable and affect the transmural pressure [17].

- Bilateral leg-press exercise at 80%, 95% and 100% of 1-repetition-maximum, performed with brief Valsalva manoeuvres, were not associated with an increase in LV end-systolic wall stress compared to rest in healthy young men [107].

This observation may explain why a large systematic review and meta-analysis (92 studies) found minimal support for concentric LV hypertrophy in resistance athletes [108]. Importantly, anabolic androgenic steroid abuse is not uncommon in strength-trained athletes. They may impair ventricular function and induce concentric LV remodelling, thereby confounding the association of LV geometry and resistance exercise [109]. Nevertheless, arterial hypertension is the most prevalent cardiovascular risk factor in athletes (see Chap. 13) [110, 111].

- Collegiate American-style football athletes have been shown to be at risk for the development of arterial hypertension and consecutive concentric LV hypertrophy during a season [112].

Acute effects of endurance exercise are associated with both a pressure and a volume load stress to the heart. LV transmural filling pressures increase during exercise.

- Compared to individuals with a high aerobic fitness ($VO_2$peak 60 ± 3 ml/min/kg), less fit subjects ($VO_2$peak 43 ± 6 ml/min/kg) demonstrated higher LV transmural filling pressures during exercise [113].

This finding may explain the different cardiac remodelling patterns of intensive endurance training observed in longitudinal studies of healthy subjects and elite athletes:

- In previously sedentary subjects (aged 29 ± 6 years, $VO_2$peak 40 ± 6 ml/min/kg), 1 year of endurance training with progressively increasing intensity led to an increase in LV mass and volume by 21% and 18%, respectively. During the first 6–9 months, LV mass-to-volume ratio increased, resulting in concentric LV remodelling. Thereafter, LV mass-to-volume ratio declined, ultimately leading to an eccentric LV hypertrophy pattern [102].
- In competitive young male rowers (aged 18.6 ± 0.5 years) with normal LV geometry at baseline, a 3-month augmentation phase of exercise training led to eccentric LV remodelling, with an increase of LV mass and volume of 14% and 11%, respectively. The following 36-months maintenance phase resulted in a further increase of LV mass and volume of 9% and 2%, respectively, leading to an eccentric LV hypertrophy pattern [114].

Despite the fact that exercise-induced LV remodelling has to be considered a phaseal phenomenon, long-term endurance exercise ultimately leads to an eccentric LV hypertrophy pattern, supporting the Morganroth hypothesis for isometric exercise [18]. Both pressure and volume load during athletic activities are transient

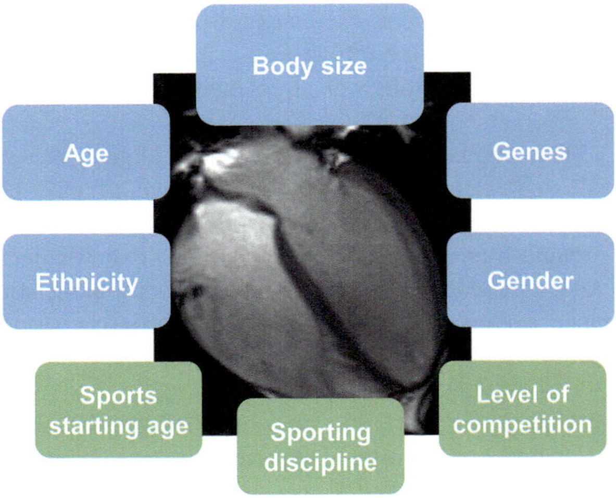


**Fig. 3.5** Important determinants of cardiac chamber size and geometry. Light blue determinants are individual characteristics of the athlete. Body size explains the largest proportion of overall variability in ventricular cavity size. Light green determinants are related to the athletes' sports behaviour

phenomena (in opposite to a cardiac pathology like hypertension, aortic stenosis or aortic regurgitation). However, long-term endurance exercise increases blood volume by up to 40%, compared to untrained individuals, placing an additional volume challenge on the heart [115].

Importantly, most data on exercise-induced LV remodelling are derived from young athletes. In middle-aged normotensive endurance athletes, both eccentric and concentric LV hypertrophy patterns have been reported.

- Early starting age of endurance training (<25 years) was associated with eccentric LV hypertrophy. In case of a mature starting age, endurance training led, contrary to what is commonly assumed, to concentric LV hypertrophy [25].

Besides differences in arterial vascular compliance, mechanisms on the cellular level may change with increasing age. At younger age, cardiomyocytes may have the ability to respond to a training stimulus with predominantly hyperplasia and an increase in length, whereas at an older age, cardiomyocytes may respond only with hypertrophy and an increase in width [116].

For a comprehensive evaluation of the athlete's heart, contributing factors such a sporting discipline, intensity of sports, body composition (see Chap. 4), age (see Chap. 24), gender (see Chap. 25), and ethnicity (see Chap. 26) must be considered (Fig. 3.5).

**Clinical Pearls**

- Regular exercise triggers structural, functional and electrical adaptations of the heart.
- Sporting discipline, starting age, intensity and duration of sports, body composition, age, sex, and ethnicity shape the phenotypic expression of the athlete's heart.
- Extreme expressions of the athlete's heart may overlap with cardiac diseases like hypertrophic cardiomyopathy.

## Review

### Questions

1. What are the major characteristics of the systolic function of an athlete's left ventricle?
2. What is the Morganroth hypothesis and what are the limitations of the hypothesis?
3. Occasionally, the right ventricle is named the "Achille's Heal" of the endurance athlete's heart. What are the reasons for that handle?

### Answers

1. Generally, the functional hallmark of an athlete's left ventricle is a rapid switch from parasympathetic to sympathetic activation during exercise, which enhances myocardial contractility as well as heart rate increase. Cardiac chamber enlargement enables a large stroke volume which leads to an increase of cardiac output. Left (and right) ventricular stroke volume rises as a direct consequence of an increased end-diastolic volume and a reduction of end-systolic volume.
2. The Morganroth hypothesis suggests that isotonic exercise leads to an eccentric LV hypertrophy pattern similar to changes in chronic volume overload, whereas isometric exercise leads to a concentric LV hypertrophy pattern, similar to changes in chronic pressure overload. It has been criticized because of relying on cross-sectional data and the paucity of supporting evidence from longitudinal exercise training studies.
3. The right ventricle is particularly susceptible to hemodynamic stress (especially to high volume loads). Although the right ventricular systolic function at rest does not seem different between athletes and controls, there is interesting data suggesting RV enlargement and diminished systolic function in high-level endurance athletes after highly intensive and/or repetitive exercise. This phenomenon is commonly known as "right ventricular fatigue". However, whether these primarily temporary effects may result in chronic right ventricular failure is still a matter of debate.

## References

1. Osler W. The principles and practice of medicine. New York: Appleton and Company; 1892.
2. Henschen S. Skilanglauf und Skiwettlauf: eine Medizinische Sportstudie. Mitt Med Klin Upsala (Jena). 1899;2:15–8.
3. Darling E. The effects of training: a study of the Harvard University crews. Boston Med Surg J. 1899;161:229–33.
4. Moritz F. Ueber orthodiagraphische Untersuchungen am Herzen. Muenchner Med Wochenschrift. 1902;49

5. Bulychev VV, Khmelevskii VA, Rutman IuV. [Roentgenological and instrumental examination of the heart in athletes]. Klin Med. 1965;43:108–114.
6. Buytendijk F, Snapper I. Ergebnisse sportaerztlichen Untersuchungen bei den IX. Olympischen Spielen in Amsterdam 1928. Berlin: Springer; 1929.
7. Deutsch F, Kauf E. Heart and athletics. St Louis: CV Mosby Company; 1927.
8. Der HW. Arbeits und Trainingseinfluss auf Kreislauf und Atmung. Darmstadt: Steinkopff; 1959.
9. Reindell H, Roskamm H, Steim H. [The heart and blood circulation in athletes]. Med Welt. 1960;31:1557–1563.
10. Roskamm H, Reindell H, Musshoff K, Koenig K. [Relations between heart size and physical efficiency in male and female athletes in comparison with normal male and female subjects. III]. Arch Kreislaufforsch. 1961;35:67–102.
11. Venerando A, Rulli V. Frequency morphology and meaning of the electrocardiographic anomalies found in Olympic marathon runners and walkers. J Sports Med Phys Fitness. 1964;4:135–41.
12. Van Ganse W, Versee L, Eylenbosch W, Vuylsteek K. The electrocardiogram of athletes. Comparison with untrained subjects. Br Heart J. 1970;32(2):160–4.
13. Smith WG, Cullen KJ, Thorburn IO. Electrocardiograms of marathon runners in 1962 Commonwealth Games. Br Heart J. 1964;26:469–76.
14. Beswick FW, Jordan RC. Cardiological observations at the Sixth British Empire and Commonwealth Games. Br Heart J. 1961;23(2):113–30.
15. Morganroth J, Maron BJ, Henry WL, Epstein SE. Comparative left ventricular dimensions in trained athletes. Ann Intern Med. 1975;82(4):521–4.
16. Naylor LH, George K, O'Driscoll G, Green DJ. The athlete's heart: a contemporary appraisal of the 'Morganroth hypothesis'. Sports Med. 2008;38(1):69–90.
17. Haykowsky MJ, Samuel TJ, Nelson MD, La Gerche A. Athlete's heart: is the Morganroth hypothesis obsolete? Heart Lung Circ. 2018;27(9):1037–41.
18. Lewis EJ, McKillop A, Banks L. The Morganroth hypothesis revisited: endurance exercise elicits eccentric hypertrophy of the heart. J Physiol. 2012;590(12):2833–4.
19. Pelliccia A, Maron BJ, Spataro A, Proschan MA, Spirito P. The upper limit of physiologic cardiac hypertrophy in highly trained elite athletes. N Engl J Med. 1991;324(5):295–301.
20. Pelliccia A, Culasso F, Di Paolo FM, Maron BJ. Physiologic left ventricular cavity dilatation in elite athletes. Ann Intern Med. 1999;130(1):23–31.
21. Pelliccia A, Maron BJ, Culasso F, Spataro A, Caselli G. Athlete's heart in women. Echocardiographic characterization of highly trained elite female athletes. JAMA. 1996;276(3):211–5.
22. Rawlins J, Carre F, Kervio G, Papadakis M, Chandra N, Edwards C, et al. Ethnic differences in physiological cardiac adaptation to intense physical exercise in highly trained female athletes. Circulation. 2010;121(9):1078–85.
23. Sharma S, Maron BJ, Whyte G, Firoozi S, Elliott PM, McKenna WJ. Physiologic limits of left ventricular hypertrophy in elite junior athletes: relevance to differential diagnosis of athlete's heart and hypertrophic cardiomyopathy. J Am Coll Cardiol. 2002;40(8):1431–6.
24. Basavarajaiah S, Boraita A, Whyte G, Wilson M, Carby L, Shah A, et al. Ethnic differences in left ventricular remodeling in highly-trained athletes relevance to differentiating physiologic left ventricular hypertrophy from hypertrophic cardiomyopathy. J Am Coll Cardiol. 2008;51(23):2256–62.
25. Ryffel CP, Eser P, Trachsel LD, Brugger N, Wilhelm M. Age at start of endurance training is associated with patterns of left ventricular hypertrophy in middle-aged runners. Int J Cardiol. 2018;267:133–8.
26. Heidbuchel H, Hoogsteen J, Fagard R, Vanhees L, Ector H, Willems R, et al. High prevalence of right ventricular involvement in endurance athletes with ventricular arrhythmias. Role of an electrophysiologic study in risk stratification. Eur Heart J. 2003;24(16):1473–80.
27. D'Ascenzi F, Pisicchio C, Caselli S, Di Paolo FM, Spataro A, Pelliccia A. RV remodeling in Olympic athletes. J Am Coll Cardiol Img. 2017;10(4):385–93.

28. La Gerche A, Taylor AJ, Prior DL. Athlete's heart: the potential for multimodality imaging to address the critical remaining questions. J Am Coll Cardiol Img. 2009;2(3):350–63.
29. Bramble DM, Lieberman DE. Endurance running and the evolution of Homo. Nature. 2004;432(7015):345–52.
30. Huonker M, Halle M, Keul J. Structural and functional adaptations of the cardiovascular system by training. Int J Sports Med. 1996;17(Suppl 3):S164–72.
31. Mairbaurl H. Red blood cells in sports: effects of exercise and training on oxygen supply by red blood cells. Front Physiol. 2013;4:332.
32. Faulkner JA, Heigenhauser GJ, Schork MA. The cardiac output–oxygen uptake relationship of men during graded bicycle ergometry. Med Sci Sports. 1977;9(3):148–54.
33. Lewis SF, Taylor WF, Graham RM, Pettinger WA, Schutte JE, Blomqvist CG. Cardiovascular responses to exercise as functions of absolute and relative work load. J Appl Physiol Respir Environ Exerc Physiol. 1983;54(5):1314–23.
34. Stringer WW, Hansen JE, Wasserman K. Cardiac output estimated noninvasively from oxygen uptake during exercise. J Appl Physiol (1985). 1997;82(3):908–12.
35. Ainsworth BE, Haskell WL, Whitt MC, Irwin ML, Swartz AM, Strath SJ, et al. Compendium of physical activities: an update of activity codes and MET intensities. Med Sci Sports Exerc. 2000;32(9 Suppl):S498–504.
36. Saltin B, Astrand PO. Maximal oxygen uptake in athletes. J Appl Physiol. 1967;23(3):353–8.
37. Bekaert I, Pannier JL, Van de Weghe C, Van Durme JP, Clement DL, Pannier R. Non-invasive evaluation of cardiac function in professional cyclists. Br Heart J. 1981;45(2):213–8.
38. Gilbert CA, Nutter DO, Felner JM, Perkins JV, Heymsfield SB, Schlant RC. Echocardiographic study of cardiac dimensions and function in the endurance-trained athlete. Am J Cardiol. 1977;40(4):528–33.
39. Fagard R, Van den Broeke C, Bielen E, Vanhees L, Amery A. Assessment of stiffness of the hypertrophied left ventricle of bicyclists using left ventricular inflow Doppler velocimetry. J Am Coll Cardiol. 1987;9(6):1250–4.
40. Abergel E, Chatellier G, Hagege AA, Oblak A, Linhart A, Ducardonnet A, et al. Serial left ventricular adaptations in world-class professional cyclists: implications for disease screening and follow-up. J Am Coll Cardiol. 2004;44(1):144–9.
41. Douglas PS, O'Toole ML, Hiller WD, Reichek N. Different effects of prolonged exercise on the right and left ventricles. J Am Coll Cardiol. 1990;15(1):64–9.
42. Pluim BM, Zwinderman AH, van der Laarse A, van der Wall EE. The athlete's heart. A meta-analysis of cardiac structure and function. Circulation. 2000;101(3):336–44.
43. Baggish AL, Wood MJ. Athlete's heart and cardiovascular care of the athlete: scientific and clinical update. Circulation. 2011;123(23):2723–35.
44. Jose AD, Stitt F, Collison D. The effects of exercise and changes in body temperature on the intrinsic heart rate in man. Am Heart J. 1970;79(4):488–98.
45. Uusitalo AL, Uusitalo AJ, Rusko HK. Exhaustive endurance training for 6–9 weeks did not induce changes in intrinsic heart rate and cardiac autonomic modulation in female athletes. Int J Sports Med. 1998;19(8):532–40.
46. Baggish AL, Yared K, Weiner RB, Wang F, Demes R, Picard MH, et al. Differences in cardiac parameters among elite rowers and subelite rowers. Med Sci Sports Exerc. 2010;42(6):1215–20.
47. Richand V, Lafitte S, Reant P, Serri K, Lafitte M, Brette S, et al. An ultrasound speckle tracking (two-dimensional strain) analysis of myocardial deformation in professional soccer players compared with healthy subjects and hypertrophic cardiomyopathy. Am J Cardiol. 2007;100(1):128–32.
48. Cardim N, Oliveira AG, Longo S, Ferreira T, Pereira A, Reis RP, et al. Doppler tissue imaging: regional myocardial function in hypertrophic cardiomyopathy and in athlete's heart. J Am Soc Echocardiogr. 2003;16(3):223–32.
49. Caso P, D'Andrea A, Galderisi M, Liccardo B, Severino S, De Simone L, et al. Pulsed Doppler tissue imaging in endurance athletes: relation between left ventricular preload and myocardial regional diastolic function. Am J Cardiol. 2000;85(9):1131–6.

50. Naylor LH, Arnolda LF, Deague JA, Playford D, Maurogiovanni A, O'Driscoll G, et al. Reduced ventricular flow propagation velocity in elite athletes is augmented with the resumption of exercise training. J Physiol. 2005;563(Pt 3):957–63.
51. Tumuklu MM, Ildizli M, Ceyhan K, Cinar CS. Alterations in left ventricular structure and diastolic function in professional football players: assessment by tissue Doppler imaging and left ventricular flow propagation velocity. Echocardiography (Mount Kisco, NY). 2007;24(2):140–8.
52. Baggish AL, Wang F, Weiner RB, Elinoff JM, Tournoux F, Boland A, et al. Training-specific changes in cardiac structure and function: a prospective and longitudinal assessment of competitive athletes. J Appl Physiol (1985). 2008;104(4):1121–8.
53. Scharhag J, Schneider G, Urhausen A, Rochette V, Kramann B, Kindermann W. Athlete's heart: right and left ventricular mass and function in male endurance athletes and untrained individuals determined by magnetic resonance imaging. J Am Coll Cardiol. 2002;40(10):1856–63.
54. La Gerche A, Burns AT, Mooney DJ, Inder WJ, Taylor AJ, Bogaert J, et al. Exercise-induced right ventricular dysfunction and structural remodelling in endurance athletes. Eur Heart J. 2012;33(8):998–1006.
55. La Gerche A, Robberecht C, Kuiperi C, Nuyens D, Willems R, de Ravel T, et al. Lower than expected desmosomal gene mutation prevalence in endurance athletes with complex ventricular arrhythmias of right ventricular origin. Heart. 2010;96(16):1268–74.
56. Ekblom B, Hermansen L. Cardiac output in athletes. J Appl Physiol. 1968;25(5):619–25.
57. Saltin B. Hemodynamic adaptations to exercise. Am J Cardiol. 1985;55(10):42D–7D.
58. Calbet JA, Jensen-Urstad M, van Hall G, Holmberg HC, Rosdahl H, Saltin B. Maximal muscular vascular conductances during whole body upright exercise in humans. J Physiol. 2004;558(Pt 1):319–31.
59. Vogiatzis I, Athanasopoulos D, Habazettl H, Kuebler WM, Wagner H, Roussos C, et al. Intercostal muscle blood flow limitation in athletes during maximal exercise. J Physiol. 2009;587(Pt 14):3665–77.
60. Drezner JA, Fischbach P, Froelicher V, Marek J, Pelliccia A, Prutkin JM, et al. Normal electrocardiographic findings: recognising physiological adaptations in athletes. Br J Sports Med. 2013;47(3):125–36.
61. Sharma S, Drezner JA, Baggish A, Papadakis M, Wilson MG, Prutkin JM, et al. International recommendations for electrocardiographic interpretation in athletes. Eur Heart J. 2018;39(16):1466–80.
62. Pelliccia A, Culasso F, Di Paolo FM, Accettura D, Cantore R, Castagna W, et al. Prevalence of abnormal electrocardiograms in a large, unselected population undergoing pre-participation cardiovascular screening. Eur Heart J. 2007;28(16):2006–10.
63. Papadakis M, Sharma S. Electrocardiographic screening in athletes: the time is now for universal screening. Br J Sports Med. 2009;43(9):663–8.
64. Drezner JA, Ackerman MJ, Cannon BC, Corrado D, Heidbuchel H, Prutkin JM, et al. Abnormal electrocardiographic findings in athletes: recognising changes suggestive of primary electrical disease. Br J Sports Med. 2013;47(3):153–67.
65. Drezner JA, Ashley E, Baggish AL, Borjesson M, Corrado D, Owens DS, et al. Abnormal electrocardiographic findings in athletes: recognising changes suggestive of cardiomyopathy. Br J Sports Med. 2013;47(3):137–52.
66. Weiner RB, Hutter AM, Wang F, Kim JH, Wood MJ, Wang TJ, et al. Performance of the 2010 European Society of Cardiology criteria for ECG interpretation in athletes. Heart. 2011;97(19):1573–7.
67. Papadakis M, Carre F, Kervio G, Rawlins J, Panoulas VF, Chandra N, et al. The prevalence, distribution, and clinical outcomes of electrocardiographic repolarization patterns in male athletes of African/Afro-Caribbean origin. Eur Heart J. 2011;32(18):2304–13.
68. Zaidi A, Ghani S, Sheikh N, Gati S, Bastiaenen R, Madden B, et al. Clinical significance of electrocardiographic right ventricular hypertrophy in athletes: comparison with arrhythmogenic right ventricular cardiomyopathy and pulmonary hypertension. Eur Heart J. 2013;34(47):3649–56.

69. Sharma S, Whyte G, Elliott P, Padula M, Kaushal R, Mahon N, et al. Electrocardiographic changes in 1000 highly trained junior elite athletes. Br J Sports Med. 1999;33(5):319–24.
70. Papadakis M, Basavarajaiah S, Rawlins J, Edwards C, Makan J, Firoozi S, et al. Prevalence and significance of T-wave inversions in predominantly Caucasian adolescent athletes. Eur Heart J. 2009;30(14):1728–35.
71. Pelliccia A, Maron BJ, Culasso F, Di Paolo FM, Spataro A, Biffi A, et al. Clinical significance of abnormal electrocardiographic patterns in trained athletes. Circulation. 2000;102(3):278–84.
72. Di Paolo FM, Schmied C, Zerguini YA, Junge A, Quattrini F, Culasso F, et al. The athlete's heart in adolescent Africans: an electrocardiographic and echocardiographic study. J Am Coll Cardiol. 2012;59(11):1029–36.
73. Hancock EW, Deal BJ, Mirvis DM, Okin P, Kligfield P, Gettes LS, et al. AHA/ACCF/HRS recommendations for the standardization and interpretation of the electrocardiogram: Part V: Electrocardiogram changes associated with cardiac chamber hypertrophy: a scientific statement from the American Heart Association Electrocardiography and Arrhythmias Committee, Council on Clinical Cardiology; the American College of Cardiology Foundation; and the Heart Rhythm Society. Endorsed by the International Society for Computerized Electrocardiology. J Am Coll Cardiol. 2009;53(11):992–1002.
74. Ryan MP, Cleland JG, French JA, Joshi J, Choudhury L, Chojnowska L, et al. The standard electrocardiogram as a screening test for hypertrophic cardiomyopathy. Am J Cardiol. 1995;76(10):689–94.
75. Moore EN, Boineau JP, Patterson DF. Incomplete right bundle-branch block. An electrocardiographic enigma and possible misnomer. Circulation. 1971;44(4):678–87.
76. Fagard R, Aubert A, Lysens R, Staessen J, Vanhees L, Amery A. Noninvasive assessment of seasonal variations in cardiac structure and function in cyclists. Circulation. 1983;67(4):896–901.
77. Langdeau JB, Blier L, Turcotte H, O'Hara G, Boulet LP. Electrocardiographic findings in athletes: the prevalence of left ventricular hypertrophy and conduction defects. Can J Cardiol. 2001;17(6):655–9.
78. Gussak I, Bjerregaard P, Egan TM, Chaitman BR. ECG phenomenon called the J wave. History, pathophysiology, and clinical significance. J Electrocardiol. 1995;28(1):49–58.
79. Corrado D, Basso C, Thiene G. Arrhythmogenic right ventricular cardiomyopathy: diagnosis, prognosis, and treatment. Heart. 2000;83(5):588–95.
80. Perez MV, Friday K, Froelicher V. Semantic confusion: the case of early repolarization and the J point. Am J Med. 2012;125(9):843–4.
81. Leo T, Uberoi A, Jain NA, Garza D, Chowdhury S, Freeman JV, et al. The impact of ST elevation on athletic screening. Clin J Sport Med. 2011;21(5):433–40.
82. Uberoi A, Jain NA, Perez M, Weinkopff A, Ashley E, Hadley D, et al. Early repolarization in an ambulatory clinical population. Circulation. 2011;124(20):2208–14.
83. Tanguturi VK, Noseworthy PA, Newton-Cheh C, Baggish AL. The electrocardiographic early repolarization pattern in athletes: normal variant or sudden death risk factor? Sports Med. 2012;42(5):359–66.
84. Junttila MJ, Sager SJ, Freiser M, McGonagle S, Castellanos A, Myerburg RJ. Inferolateral early repolarization in athletes. J Interv Cardiac Electrophysiol. 2011;31(1):33–8.
85. Noseworthy PA, Weiner R, Kim J, Keelara V, Wang F, Berkstresser B, et al. Early repolarization pattern in competitive athletes: clinical correlates and the effects of exercise training. Circ Arrhythm Electrophysiol. 2011;4(4):432–40.
86. Tikkanen JT, Junttila MJ, Anttonen O, Aro AL, Luttinen S, Kerola T, et al. Early repolarization: electrocardiographic phenotypes associated with favorable long-term outcome. Circulation. 2011;123(23):2666–73.
87. Haissaguerre M, Derval N, Sacher F, Jesel L, Deisenhofer I, de Roy L, et al. Sudden cardiac arrest associated with early repolarization. N Engl J Med. 2008;358(19):2016–23.
88. Tikkanen JT, Anttonen O, Junttila MJ, Aro AL, Kerola T, Rissanen HA, et al. Long-term outcome associated with early repolarization on electrocardiography. N Engl J Med. 2009;361(26):2529–37.

89. Quattrini FM, Pelliccia A, Assorgi R, DiPaolo FM, Squeo MR, Culasso F, et al. Benign clinical significance of J-wave pattern (early repolarization) in highly trained athletes. Heart Rhythm. 2014;11(11):1974–82.
90. Rosso R, Kogan E, Belhassen B, Rozovski U, Scheinman MM, Zeltser D, et al. J-point elevation in survivors of primary ventricular fibrillation and matched control subjects: incidence and clinical significance. J Am Coll Cardiol. 2008;52(15):1231–8.
91. Stein R, Medeiros CM, Rosito GA, Zimerman LI, Ribeiro JP. Intrinsic sinus and atrioventricular node electrophysiologic adaptations in endurance athletes. J Am Coll Cardiol. 2002;39(6):1033–8.
92. Stein R, Moraes RS, Cavalcanti AV, Ferlin EL, Zimerman LI, Ribeiro JP. Atrial automaticity and atrioventricular conduction in athletes: contribution of autonomic regulation. Eur J Appl Physiol. 2000;82(1–2):155–7.
93. Calo L, Sperandii F, Martino A, Guerra E, Cavarretta E, Quaranta F, et al. Echocardiographic findings in 2261 peri-pubertal athletes with or without inverted T waves at electrocardiogram. Heart. 2015;101(3):193–200.
94. Gati S, Sheikh N, Ghani S, Zaidi A, Wilson M, Raju H, et al. Should axis deviation or atrial enlargement be categorised as abnormal in young athletes? The athlete's electrocardiogram: time for re-appraisal of markers of pathology. Eur Heart J. 2013;34(47):3641–8.
95. Baggish AL, Hutter AM Jr, Wang F, Yared K, Weiner RB, Kupperman E, et al. Cardiovascular screening in college athletes with and without electrocardiography: a cross-sectional study. Ann Intern Med. 2010;152(5):269–75.
96. Fudge J, Harmon KG, Owens DS, Prutkin JM, Salerno JC, Asif IM, et al. Cardiovascular screening in adolescents and young adults: a prospective study comparing the pre-participation physical evaluation monograph 4th edition and ECG. Br J Sports Med. 2014;48(15):1172–8.
97. Kim JH, Noseworthy PA, McCarty D, Yared K, Weiner R, Wang F, et al. Significance of electrocardiographic right bundle branch block in trained athletes. Am J Cardiol. 2011;107(7):1083–9.
98. Levine BD, Baggish AL, Kovacs RJ, Link MS, Maron MS, Mitchell JH. Eligibility and disqualification recommendations for competitive athletes with cardiovascular abnormalities: Task Force 1: classification of sports: dynamic, static, and impact: a scientific statement from the American Heart Association and American College of Cardiology. J Am Coll Cardiol. 2015;66(21):2350–5.
99. Pelliccia A, Caselli S, Sharma S, Basso C, Bax JJ, Corrado D, et al. European Association of Preventive Cardiology (EAPC) and European Association of Cardiovascular Imaging (EACVI) joint position statement: recommendations for the indication and interpretation of cardiovascular imaging in the evaluation of the athlete's heart. Eur Heart J. 2018;39(21):1949–69.
100. La Gerche A, Heidbuchel H, Burns AT, Mooney DJ, Taylor AJ, Pfluger HB, et al. Disproportionate exercise load and remodeling of the athlete's right ventricle. Med Sci Sports Exerc. 2011;43(6):974–81.
101. Scharf M, Brem MH, Wilhelm M, Schoepf UJ, Uder M, Lell MM. Atrial and ventricular functional and structural adaptations of the heart in elite triathletes assessed with cardiac MR imaging. Radiology. 2010;257(1):71–9.
102. Arbab-Zadeh A, Perhonen M, Howden E, Peshock RM, Zhang R, Adams-Huet B, et al. Cardiac remodeling in response to 1 year of intensive endurance training. Circulation. 2014;130(24):2152–61.
103. Wilhelm M, Roten L, Tanner H, Schmid JP, Wilhelm I, Saner H. Long-term cardiac remodeling and arrhythmias in nonelite marathon runners. Am J Cardiol. 2012;110:129–35.
104. Lang RM, Badano LP, Mor-Avi V, Afilalo J, Armstrong A, Ernande L, et al. Recommendations for cardiac chamber quantification by echocardiography in adults: an update from the American Society of Echocardiography and the European Association of Cardiovascular Imaging. Eur Heart J Cardiovasc Imaging. 2015;16(3):233–70.
105. Khouri MG, Peshock RM, Ayers CR, de Lemos JA, Drazner MH. A 4-tiered classification of left ventricular hypertrophy based on left ventricular geometry: the Dallas heart study. Circ Cardiovasc Imaging. 2010;3(2):164–71.

106. Trachsel LD, Ryffel CP, De Marchi S, Seiler C, Brugger N, Eser P, et al. Exercise-induced cardiac remodeling in non-elite endurance athletes: comparison of 2-tiered and 4-tiered classification of left ventricular hypertrophy. PLoS One. 2018;13(2):e0193203.
107. Haykowsky M, Taylor D, Teo K, Quinney A, Humen D. Left ventricular wall stress during leg-press exercise performed with a brief Valsalva maneuver. Chest. 2001;119(1):150–4.
108. Utomi V, Oxborough D, Whyte GP, Somauroo J, Sharma S, Shave R, et al. Systematic review and meta-analysis of training mode, imaging modality and body size influences on the morphology and function of the male athlete's heart. Heart. 2013;99(23):1727–33.
109. Luijkx T, Velthuis BK, Backx FJ, Buckens CF, Prakken NH, Rienks R, et al. Anabolic androgenic steroid use is associated with ventricular dysfunction on cardiac MRI in strength trained athletes. Int J Cardiol. 2013;167(3):664–8.
110. De Matos LD, Caldeira Nde A, Perlingeiro Pde S, dos Santos IL, Negrao CE, Azevedo LF. Cardiovascular risk and clinical factors in athletes: 10 years of evaluation. Med Sci Sports Exerc. 2011;43(6):943–50.
111. Tucker AM, Vogel RA, Lincoln AE, Dunn RE, Ahrensfield DC, Allen TW, et al. Prevalence of cardiovascular disease risk factors among National Football League players. JAMA. 2009;301(20):2111–9.
112. Weiner RB, Wang F, Isaacs SK, Malhotra R, Berkstresser B, Kim JH, et al. Blood pressure and left ventricular hypertrophy during American-style football participation. Circulation. 2013;128(5):524–31.
113. Stickland MK, Welsh RC, Petersen SR, Tyberg JV, Anderson WD, Jones RL, et al. Does fitness level modulate the cardiovascular hemodynamic response to exercise? J Appl Physiol (1985). 2006;100(6):1895–901.
114. Weiner RB, DeLuca JR, Wang F, Lin J, Wasfy MM, Berkstresser B, et al. Exercise-induced left ventricular remodeling among competitive athletes: a phasic phenomenon. Circ Cardiovasc Imaging. 2015;8(12):e003651.
115. Heinicke K, Wolfarth B, Winchenbach P, Biermann B, Schmid A, Huber G, et al. Blood volume and hemoglobin mass in elite athletes of different disciplines. Int J Sports Med. 2001;22(7):504–12.
116. Caselli S, Pelliccia A. Interpretation of left ventricular geometry in athletes. Int J Cardiol. 2018;267:143–4.

# Impact of Sporting Disciplines and Body Size on the Athlete's Heart

4

Gherardo Finocchiaro and Keith Phillip George

**Learning Objectives**

1. To determine the impact of different athletic training regimes on the phenotypical presentation of the athlete's heart.
2. To evaluate how the presentation of the athlete's heart can influence the cardiac pre-participation screening process.
3. To understand that cardiac size is influenced by a wide range of factors, other than training status, including body size and composition.
4. To critically reflect on the different approaches and variables that can be used when scaling cardiac dimensions for individual differences in body size and composition.

## 4.1 Impact of Sporting Disciplines on the Athlete's Heart

The cardiovascular system supplies oxygen and nutrients to body tissues, removing carbon dioxide from the systemic circulation, both at rest and during exercise. The demands of the cardiovascular system during exercise may vary significantly according to the type of exercise [1]. For example the cardiovascular response to prolonged dynamic exercise is different from repetitive bouts of static exercise and may be influenced by many factors including exercise intensity, environmental conditions and training status [2]. Static exercise involves contraction of muscles in a stationary position, and the increase in blood flow which results in an increase in

G. Finocchiaro
Department of Cardiology and Division of Cardiovascular Sciences,
Guy's and St. Thomas' Hospitals and King's College London, London, UK

K. P. George (✉)
Research Institute for Sport and Exercise Science, Liverpool John Moores University,
Liverpool, UK
e-mail: k.george@ljmu.ac.uk





A. Pressler, J. Niebauer (eds.), *Textbook of Sports and Exercise Cardiology*,
https://doi.org/10.1007/978-3-030-35374-2_4

blood pressure is often accompanied by a minimal fall in peripheral vascular resistance; conversely in dynamic exercise the increase in blood flow parallels a significant fall in vascular resistance [2]. As a result, in static exercise the blood pressure response is disproportionate to the amount of work when compared to dynamic exercise. Moreover, while heart rate response is modest in static exercise it can be substantially larger in submaximal or maximal dynamic exercise. The terms dynamic and static exercise classify training activity on the basis of the mechanical action involved and are different from the terms aerobic and anaerobic exercise. These terms are used to differentiate sporting activity on the basis of the predominant type of metabolism. In general terms, static exercise is performed anaerobically, while highly dynamic exercise is predominantly supported by aerobic metabolism. Classification of sports, as per the Mitchell criteria [2], considers three categories (low, moderate, high) for both static and dynamic exercise (see Chap. 1).

Regular intensive exercise leads to a series of electrical, structural, and functional changes in the heart, collectively named as the "athlete's heart" [1, 3, 4]. These physiological changes are influenced by age, sex, sporting discipline, body size and ethnicity. A correct understanding of what is expected to be normal begins from taking into account all these variables in order to provide a "personalized assessment" of the athlete. As cardiac remodeling may be marked in some athletes resulting in significant overlap with potentially fatal cardiac disease such as cardiomyopathies [5], it is pivotal to differentiate between physiological and pathological changes with full knowledge of the impact of any moderating factors.

## 4.2 Historical Background (The "Morganroth Hypothesis")

In 1975 Morganroth et al. [6] hypothesized that physiological cardiac adaptation to exercise was highly dependent on the nature of the hemodynamic stimulus imposed on the heart. This hypothesis, based on a small number of athletes studied with echocardiography, postulated that dynamic exercise leads to eccentric hypertrophy with dilatation of the cardiac chambers, while static exercise results in concentric hypertrophy with an increase in wall thickness (Fig. 4.1).

- Although the "Morganroth hypothesis" was accepted in the scientific community for many years, its physiological basis has been recently questioned as several studies [7–9] suggested that the relationship between sporting discipline and cardiac adaptation is far more complex and cannot be reduced to a dichotomous approach.

The determinants of cardiac adaptation to exercise are not fully understood and although some sports have a clearly predominant static or dynamic component, most of sports are characterized by a mixture of the two components and particularly in these it is difficult to determine the exact nature of the hemodynamic load imposed by training to the left and right ventricle. Moreover, the "Morganroth hypothesis" was based on absolute cardiac dimensions, but we now understand that body size is a relevant determinant of cardiac dimensions in athletes.

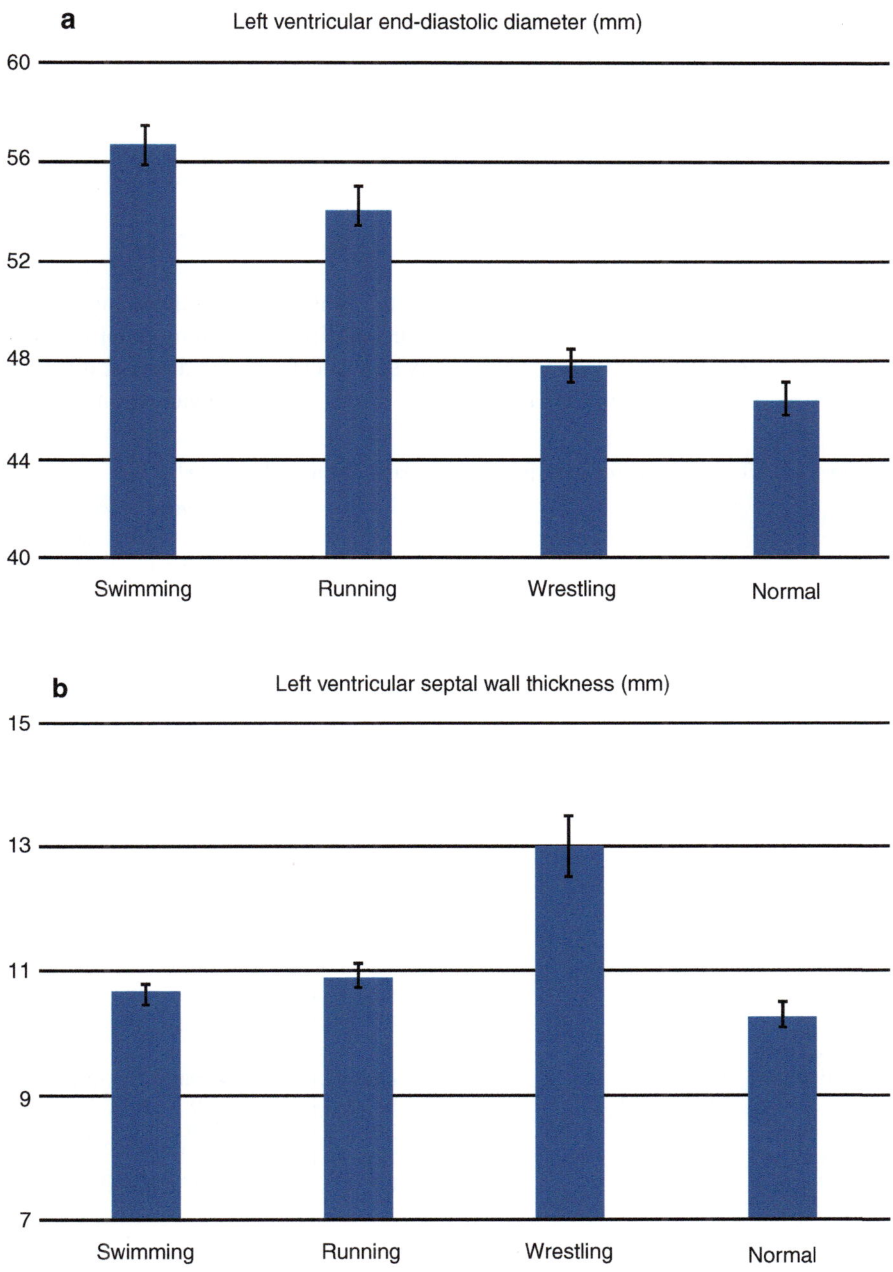


**Fig. 4.1** The Morganroth hypothesis. Athletes engaged in dynamic sports are expected to exhibit left ventricular dilatation (**a**) while athletes engaged in static sports are expected to show increased left ventricular wall thickness (**b**; modified from Morganroth et al. [6])

## 4.3 Impact on the Left Ventricle

The left ventricular (LV) physiological changes that can be observed in athletes include

1. an increase in size
2. an increase in wall thickness and
3. a decrease in ejection fraction.

According to the study by Pelliccia et al. [10] highly trained athletes engaging in different sports exhibit a wide range of significant differences in terms of LV size. Rowing was associated with the larger cavity size (mean LV end-diastolic diameter was 56 ± 3 mm) (Table 4.1). In the same study athletes engaging in rowing,

**Table 4.1** Left ventricular size and type of sport (adapted from Pelliccia et al. [10])

| | | | | | | Left ventricular measures | | |
|---|---|---|---|---|---|---|---|---|
| Sport | Athletes | Males | Females | Age (years) | BSA ($m^2$) | LVEDD (mm) | MWT (mm) | Mass index ($g/m^2$) |
| Rowing | 95 | 92 | 3 | 21 ± 4 | 2.04 ± 0.1 | 56.0 ± 3 | 11.3 ± 1.3 | 121 ± 22 |
| Track | 89 | 66 | 23 | 26 ± 4 | 1.79 ± 0.1 | 51.4 ± 4 | 9.8 ± 1.2 | 101 ± 24 |
| Cycling | 64 | 49 | 15 | 20 ± 3 | 1.86 ± 0.1 | 54.8 ± 5 | 10.4 ± 1.1 | 115 ± 23 |
| Soccer | 62 | 62 | 0 | 24 ± 4 | 1.95 ± 0.1 | 54.9 ± 4 | 9.9 ± 0.7 | 105 ± 17 |
| Canoeing | 60 | 52 | 8 | 20 ± 3 | 1.92 ± 0.1 | 54.5 ± 3 | 10.5 ± 1.5 | 110 ± 21 |
| Roller-skating | 58 | 32 | 26 | 19 ± 2 | 1.73 ± 0.1 | 49.0 ± 4 | 9.0 ± 1.0 | 85 ± 17 |
| Swimming | 54 | 26 | 28 | 19 ± 3 | 1.81 ± 0.1 | 53.0 ± 4 | 9.3 ± 1.2 | 98 ± 23 |
| Volleyball | 51 | 36 | 15 | 20 ± 4 | 2.08 ± 0.1 | 53.7 ± 3 | 9.4 ± 1.0 | 88 ± 14 |
| Pentathlon | 50 | 36 | 14 | 19 ± 4 | 1.77 ± 0.1 | 52.4 ± 4 | 9.2 ± 0.9 | 98 ± 18 |
| Tennis | 47 | 32 | 15 | 17 ± 2 | 1.76 ± 0.1 | 50.0 ± 3 | 9.1 ± 1.0 | 88 ± 16 |
| Fencing | 42 | 31 | 11 | 22 ± 3 | 1.85 ± 0.1 | 51.7 ± 5 | 9.2 ± 1.3 | 92 ± 23 |
| Alpine skiing | 32 | 24 | 8 | 21 + 2 | 1.89 ± 0.1 | 52.0 ± 3 | 8.9 ± 0.9 | 87 ± 15 |
| Cross-country skiing | 31 | 24 | 7 | 24 ± 4 | 1.77 ± 0.1 | 54.5 ± 4 | 9.6 ± 0.8 | 107 ± 19 |
| Equestrianism | 28 | 23 | 5 | 28 ± 6 | 1.78 ± 0.1 | 50.4 ± 3 | 9.0 ± 0.8 | 87 ± 14 |
| Team handball | 26 | 9 | 17 | 22 ± 2 | 1.86 ± 0.1 | 51.8 ± 4 | 8.5 ± 0.9 | 80 ± 13 |
| Yachting | 24 | 20 | 4 | 27 ± 4 | 1.88 ± 0.1 | 51.2 ± 4 | 9.0 ± 0.8 | 85 ± 15 |
| Roller hockey | 23 | 23 | 0 | 22 ± 2 | 1.92 ± 0.1 | 53.4 ± 3 | 9.7 ± 0.9 | 99 ± 17 |
| Water polo | 21 | 21 | 0 | 24 ± 2 | 2.03 ± 0.1 | 54.7 ± 3 | 10.7 ± 0.6 | 110 ± 15 |
| Tae kwon do | 17 | 14 | 3 | 21 ± 2 | 1.76 ± 0.1 | 50.6 ± 4 | 8.7 ± 1.2 | 85 ± 17 |
| Wrestling and judo | 16 | 14 | 2 | 24 ± 3 | 1.93 ± 0.2 | 52.6 ± 5 | 10.2 ± 0.9 | 100 ± 14 |
| Bobsledding | 16 | 16 | 0 | 26 ± 3 | 2.08 ± 0.1 | 55.1 ± 2 | 9.6 ± 0.5 | 96 ± 7 |
| Boxing | 14 | 14 | 0 | 22 ± 4 | 1.85 ± 0.2 | 52.5 ± 3 | 9.8 ± 1.0 | 101 ± 16 |
| Diving | 11 | 7 | 4 | 23 ± 3 | 1.71 ± 0.1 | 49.6 ± 3 | 8.7 ± 1.1 | 83 ± 15 |
| Field weight events | 9 | 8 | 1 | 24 ± 3 | 2.26 ± 0.1 | 55.5 ± 4 | 10.0 ± 0.5 | 91 ± 8 |
| Weightlifting | 7 | 7 | 0 | 24 ± 2 | 1.96 ± 0.1 | 53.2 ± 3 | 10.4 ± 0.7 | 100 ± 9 |

*BSA* body surface area, *LVEDD* left ventricular end-diastolic diameter, *MWT* maximal wall thickness

**Table 4.2** Left ventricular wall thickness and type of sport in single athletes (adapted from Pelliccia et al. [10])

| | | | | Left ventricular measures | | | | |
|---|---|---|---|---|---|---|---|---|
| Athlete No. | Age (years) | Sport | BSA ($m^2$) | LVEDD (mm) | MWT (mm) | Mass index ($g/m^2$) | Aortic root (mm) | Left atrium (mm) |
| 1 | 26 | Rowing | 2.14 | 59 | 13 | 158 | 39 | 41 |
| 2 | 18 | Rowing | 2.16 | 59 | 13 | 133 | 34 | 35 |
| 3 | 19 | Rowing | 2.18 | 61 | 13 | 156 | 34 | 42 |
| 4 | 19 | Rowing | 2.23 | 62 | 13 | 157 | 32 | 45 |
| 5 | 19 | Rowing | 2.22 | 58 | 13 | 141 | 33 | 39 |
| 6 | 20 | Cycling | 2.05 | 60 | 13 | 161 | 30 | 43 |
| 7 | 21 | Rowing | 2.24 | 58 | 13 | 147 | 37 | 43 |
| 8 | 23 | Rowing | 2.17 | 58 | 13 | 144 | 38 | 40 |
| 9 | 24 | Rowing | 2.14 | 62 | 13 | 163 | 34 | 30 |
| 10 | 25 | Rowing | 1.93 | 59 | 13 | 158 | 33 | 35 |
| 11 | 24 | Rowing | 2.21 | 59 | 15 | 162 | 34 | 37 |
| 12 | 20 | Canoeing | 2.17 | 55 | 15 | 140 | 32 | 34 |
| 13 | 24 | Canoeing | 2.08 | 63 | 15 | 172 | 31 | 37 |
| 14 | 26 | Rowing | 2.15 | 55 | 15 | 149 | 37 | 40 |
| 15 | 27 | Rowing | 1.94 | 60 | 15 | 171 | 33 | 40 |
| 16 | 25 | Canoeing | 2.02 | 57 | 16 | 176 | 38 | 38 |
| Mean | 22.5 | | 2.12 | 59.0 | 13.8 | 155 | 34.3 | 38.6 |
| SD | ±2.9 | | ±0.09 | ±2.2 | ±1.07 | ±12 | ±2.6 | ±3.7 |

*BSA* body surface area, *LVEDD* left ventricular end-diastolic diameter, *MWT* maximal wall thickness

canoeing and cycling exhibited the most marked increase in wall thickness (LV wall thickness >12 mm) (Table 4.2). A marked increase in wall thickness in athletes may result in a conundrum in the differential diagnosis with pathological forms of LV hypertrophy such as hypertrophic cardiomyopathy (HCM). Athletes characterized by marked increase in wall thickness, however, often exhibit also a proportional increase in LV cavity size, a feature that is rarely observed in HCM.

- LV geometry, which is often represented by the relationship between the LV cavity size and wall thickness, is usually **normal** in athletes.

Recently, Finocchiaro et al. [11] described the effect of sex and sport discipline on LV geometry in 1083 white elite athletes (41% female athletes). In the specific subgroup of athletes engaged in dynamic exercise, females showed eccentric hypertrophy more frequently than males, while more men than women had concentric remodeling/hypertrophy (Fig. 4.2), although these geometric presentations were less common than normal geometry. These findings underscore how the impact of sporting disciplines on the athlete's heart may be affected also by other variables such as gender (see Chap. 25).

- *Ejection fraction*: Highly trained athletes may be characterized not only by large LV cavity size, but also by a decrease in baseline **LV ejection fraction**. Abergel

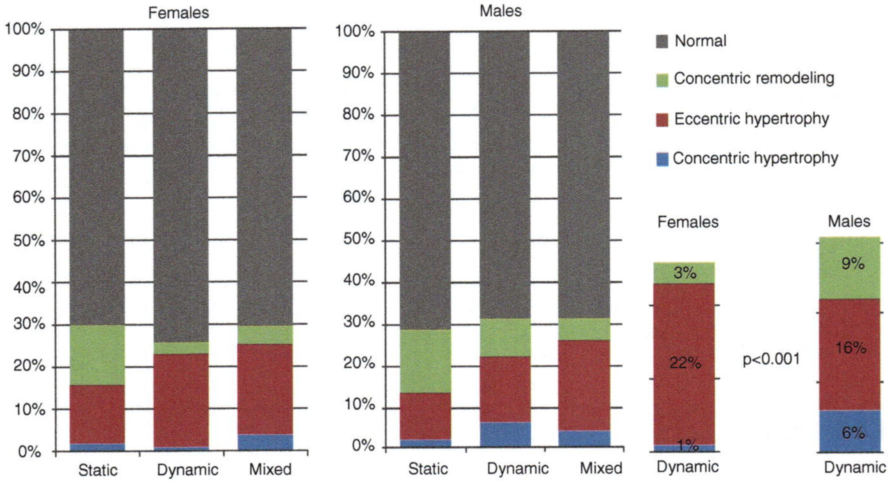


**Fig. 4.2** Left ventricular geometry in highly trained athletes. Normal geometry prevails regardless of sporting discipline. In the subgroup of athletes engaged in dynamic sports, female athletes most commonly show eccentric hypertrophy while males may exhibit concentric hypertrophy/remodelling. (Adapted from Finocchiaro et al. [11]; see also Chap. 3)

et al. [12] observed a LV ejection fraction of <52% in 17 out of 286 (6%) world-class professional cyclists; most individuals who exhibited a reduced LV ejection fraction were characterized by a significantly enlarged LV (LV end-diastolic diameter >60 mm). These findings appear to be limited to endurance athletes and have not been described in athletes engaging in other types of sport.

- Over the past decade, new echocardiographic techniques have been introduced to investigate cardiac function, such as deformation imaging by two-dimensional speckle-tracking echocardiography (STE). Caselli et al. [13] showed that athletes have similar distributions (and boundaries) for myocardial strain values as observed in untrained control subjects. No significant differences in **global longitudinal strain** (GLS) were found according to sport disciplines. Conversely, values of GLS are higher in athletes than in patients with pathologic LV hypertrophy, providing an additional tool for differential diagnosis [13].
- **Cardiovascular magnetic resonance** (CMR) has been increasingly used as a diagnostic tool in cardiology, due to its ability to accurately assess regional wall motion abnormalities, chamber volumes and possible myocardial fibrosis through late gadolinium enhancement. Although myocardial fibrosis is a final common pathway of several cardiac conditions, from hypertension to ischemia to cardiomyopathies, recent studies have shown that a non-negligible proportion of highly trained endurance athletes exhibit late gadolinium enhancement, suggestive of myocardial fibrosis at CMR [14]. Myocardial fibrosis has been described mostly in endurance athletes [15–17] with less data on other sporting disciplines. The underlying mechanisms of myocardial fibrosis in athletes as well as its clinical significance are largely unknown [14].

- **Diastolic filling** may also be affected as a result of cardiac adaptation to exercise. Invasive studies have shown that LV diastolic function plays a key role in the enhancement of stroke volume and is a major contributor to high levels of cardiorespiratory fitness and physical performance. However, a recent study [18] showed that most athletes reveal values within the normal range with less than one third of athletes exhibiting supernormal parameters of diastolic function. A significant relationship between septal velocities derived from Tissue Doppler Imaging (TDI) and LV cavity size was observed, and it is possible that reduced relaxation velocities just reflect that a large LV does not need to expand much to fill adequately in athletes. Interestingly, there were no significant sport-related differences in Doppler parameters of diastolic function.

## 4.4 Impact on the Right Ventricle

Although for many years the research on physiological adaptation to exercise has focused on the LV, recent studies showed that athletes often exhibit a significant right ventricle (RV) remodeling as a result of intense training [19, 20]. This is particularly relevant as RV structural changes may overlap with potentially fatal cardiac diseases as arrhythmogenic right ventricular cardiomyopathy (ARVC) [20–22] which may lead to sudden cardiac death during exercise [23]. Since in ARVC the RV often appears remodeled, it is pivotal to differentiate between physiological and pathological abnormalities to prevent possible tragedies (see Chap. 15).

- A large proportion of young athletes exhibit **increased RV dimensions** exceeding the reference values commonly used in clinical practice and the values proposed by the revised Task Force Criteria (TFC) for the diagnosis of ARVC [24]. Male sex and endurance sport are associated with the greatest extent of RV enlargement.
- The significant RV remodeling in endurance athletes is probably the expression of the hemodynamic overload with **increased pulmonary pressures** and bouts of RV systolic dysfunction that has been consistently observed immediately after high profile endurance events [25, 26]. Intriguingly, in a longitudinal model, Arbab-Zadeh et al. [27] showed that the left and right ventricle adapt differently to endurance training. In fact, while LV volumes did not change significantly after 6–9 months of training with initial concentric but not eccentric remodeling, RV volumes increased progressively with eccentric remodeling at all levels of training.
- The observed association between RV remodeling and endurance exercise led to the hypothesis that long-term intense exercise may result in pathological structural changes and a **pro-arrhythmic substrate**. La Gerche et al. [28] showed that a minority of athletes (13%) expressing a phenotype of ARVC showed desmosomal mutation (much less than in non-athletic ARVC cohorts), postulating the existence of an "exercise-induced right ventricular cardiomyopathy".

Although several studies described the RV remodeling occurring in endurance athletes, less data are available on athletes engaged in strength or mixed sports. D'Ascenzi et al. [29] used echocardiography to show a significant trend for an increasing enlargement of the RV chamber in athletes engaged in skill, strength, mixed, or endurance disciplines. Interestingly, when measuring the RV size in parasternal long axis, almost 60% of endurance athletes fulfilled a minor criterion and more than 20% a major criterion for the diagnosis of ARVC. Despite differences in morphological RV remodeling, RV systolic function was within the spectrum of normality as determined by fractional area change, even in endurance athletes, indicating a physiological process and providing insights for the differential diagnosis between athlete's heart and ARVC.

## 4.5 Impact on the Atria

Exercise-induced cardiac remodeling is not a prerogative of the left and the right ventricle. Atria often appear enlarged in highly trained athletes.

- Pelliccia et al. [30], in a cohort of 1777 competitive athletes, found that 18% of competitive athletes had mild increases of left atrial (LA) anteroposterior diameter (≥40 mm), while 2% exhibited marked LA enlargement (≥45 mm). Similar to the LA, the right atrium (RA) is able to adapt to the stimulus of training. Zaidi et al. [19] proposed reference values for right heart dimensions suggesting upper limits for RA area of 28 $cm^2$ in male athletes and 24 $cm^2$ in female athletes and upper limits for RA index of 14 $cm^2/m^2$ in male athletes and 13 $cm^2/m^2$ in female athletes.
- The extent of RA remodeling appears again more significant in endurance athletes, in comparison with strength athletes as shown by D'Andrea et al. [31] in a cohort of 650 highly trained athletes. In an elegant study, McClean et al. [32] compared biatrial size in high dynamic/high static and low dynamic/high static sporting disciplines and showed that biatrial enlargement was present in the first but not in the latter, suggesting that the dynamic component to training is the primary driver for both LA and RA adaptation.

## 4.6 Impact on the Aorta

Aortic-root dimensions in athletes are influenced by the same variables as in the general population but could be affected by exercise, given the hemodynamic stress on the aorta during exercise.

- Most studies examining aortic-root dimensions in athletes are cross-sectional often without appropriate matching for anthropometric parameters such as BSA.
- Systolic blood pressure rises during exercise increasing wall stress and, therefore, athletes with aortic disease may be at risk for an acute aortic event. This

concern is particularly relevant for athletes engaging in static exercise and specifically weightlifters, whose systolic blood pressure may rise above 300 mmHg during exercise.

- Only 17 (1.3%) of 1300 male and 10 (1.0%) of 1017 female Italian athletes had aortic-root diameters of more than 40 mm or more than 34 mm, respectively [33].
- Recently Engel et al. [34] showed the maximal aortic diameter was 42 mm in a cohort of basketball players with a mean BSA of 2.38 $m^2$. It appears that aortic root diameter might reach a plateau in those athletes with the uppermost biometric variables.

## 4.7 Body Size and the Need to "Normalise", "Index" or "Scale": Historical Background

Normalization, indexation or scaling (from here on we refer to this as scaling) of human and animal anatomical or physiological data is not unique to sports cardiology [35]. An example of a common functional parameter in human exercise physiology that is scaled for body size differences would be maximal oxygen uptake. In most scientific literature maximal oxygen uptake is often initially reported as an absolute value (ml/min) and then scaled to for individual differences in body mass (ml/kg/min).

As alluded to in earlier sections of this chapter and in the extant literature [36–39] body size is one of a number of factors that can mediate the phenotypical presentation of cardiac dimensions in any athlete. This is because the strong association between body size and cardiac dimensions has been demonstrated in a range of empirical research papers in normal adults as well as athletes [40–47].

When interpreting the cardiac dimensions in any athlete, it would make sense to study body-size independent or scaled cardiac data. By removing the influence of body size, you may unmask the independent impact of, for example, training load or a pathological disease process. Clearly, this could help facilitate any diagnostic process associated with cardiac screening in athletes. To derive a body size-independent cardiac index you must adopt a scaling process. Within sports cardiology this would be the case when interrogating, for example LV mass; firstly, you might analyze an absolute measure and then you would further your understanding by calculating and interpreting an LV mass index that takes into account the impact of body size.

One specific theory that is pertinent within scaling research generally, and sports cardiology specifically, is that of "geometric similarity" [35]. Briefly, this theory suggests that growth, change or development of any specific anatomic parameter is likely to occur in tandem with other parameters that have the same geometric status.

- Taken simply this would mean that change, growth and development of a linear cardiac dimension (e.g. aortic root dimension) would likely occur in tandem with a linear measure of body size (e.g. stature), as they are both one-dimensional variables.

This relationship would be similar if the cardiac dimension (LV mass) and body size variable (body mass) were both three-dimensional constructs. Scaling becomes problematic when geometric similarity is not clear; such as when a three-dimensional cardiac measure such as LV mass is scaled by body surface area (BSA), a two-dimensional parameter. This latter example is very common in sports cardiology literature and is often assumed to be best practice and supported by professional guidelines and published "normative data".

In the rest of this chapter we will; (1) illuminate the different scaling processes that have been used in sports cardiology research; (2) discuss the uses as well as pros and cons of using different measures of body size in any scaling process, and finally (3) provide some take home messages and guidance for future research.

## 4.8 Which Scaling Processes Have Been Used with "Athlete's Heart" Data?

Historically, body size has often been entirely ignored in sports cardiology literature. An early and important example was the cross-sectional study of Morganroth et al. [6] who reported absolute measures of LV chamber dimension and wall thickness in four groups (runners, swimmers, wrestlers and normal controls). Statistical comparison and thus data interpretation were made purely on absolute data (Fig. 4.1), despite the fact that it is highly likely that there were individual differences in body composition (as well as training status and background).

The lack of scaling for differences in body size is also evident in sports cardiology literature when absolute cut-offs for chamber dimension or wall thickness are used to aid differential diagnosis in athletes who may present, phenotypically, in the "grey zone" [39]. When sports cardiology studies have attempted to scale for individual differences in body size, this has most commonly been achieved through simple **ratiometric scaling**:

- Ratiometric scaling involves simply dividing Y (cardiac variable) by X (body size variable) to derive the index (Y/X). An example would be when LV mass is simply divided by the body surface variable (LV mass/BSA) (e.g. 47).

Ratiometric scaling is practically simple, widely adopted and has substantive norms-based literature associated with it [36]. This approach is theoretically problematic if the relationship between the two variables is not linear. Very few studies actually check if the "index" is in fact size-independent. You can do this by correlating the scaled variable to the body size variable. If a significant correlation is noted, body-size independence has not been achieved (Fig. 4.3a, b).

- We argue that this ratiometric scaling process may not always be theoretically or practically accurate, resulting in cardiac indices that are still body size-dependent. This only confuses clinical decision-making.

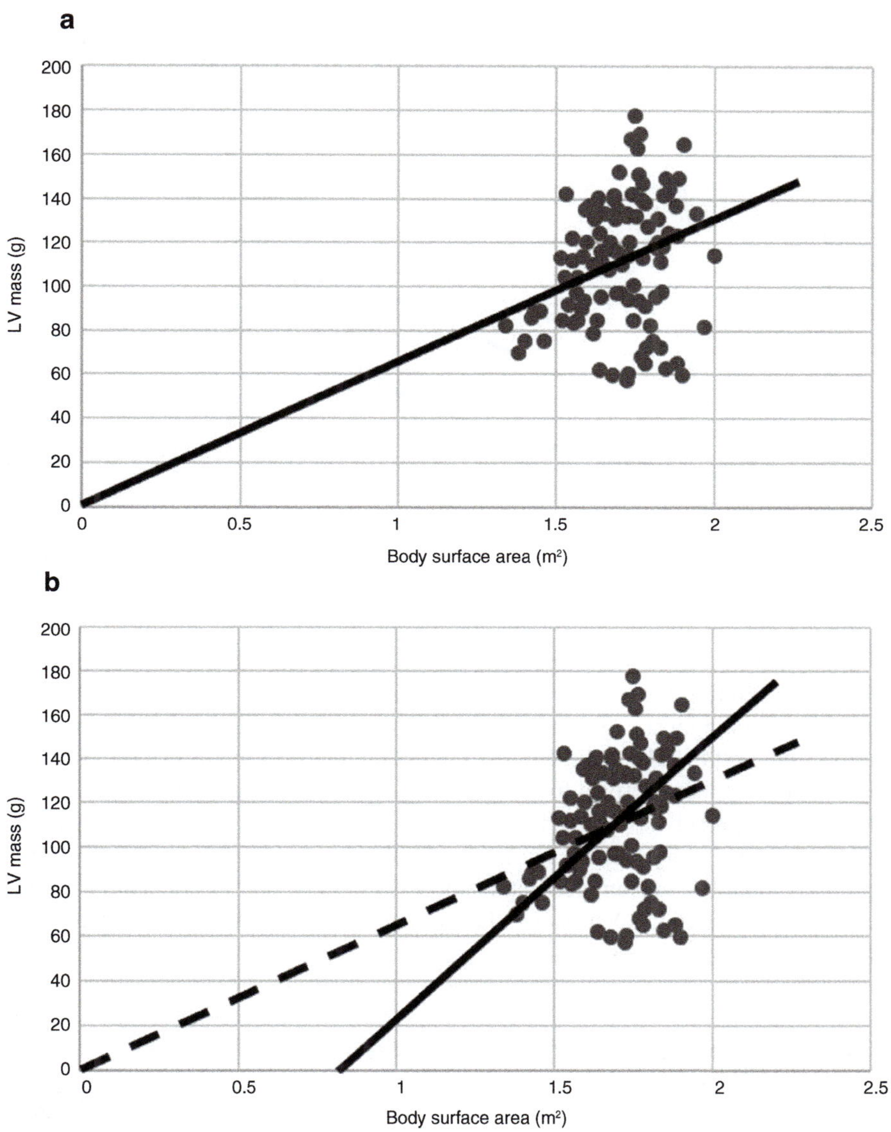


**Fig. 4.3** Scatterplot of LV mass against body surface area in female athletes and controls. In (**a**) the best fit line is constrained to the origin and the mean of both data sets and represents the ratiometric (y/X) approach to scaling. In (**b**) the same data has a linear best fit line that minimizes error but has a negative y-intercept which is biologically implausible. In (**c**) a curvilinear line of best fit is employed of the form $Y/X^b$ that minimizes error, passes through the origin and is likely to produce a size-independent cardiac index (unpublished data set from the author's lab)

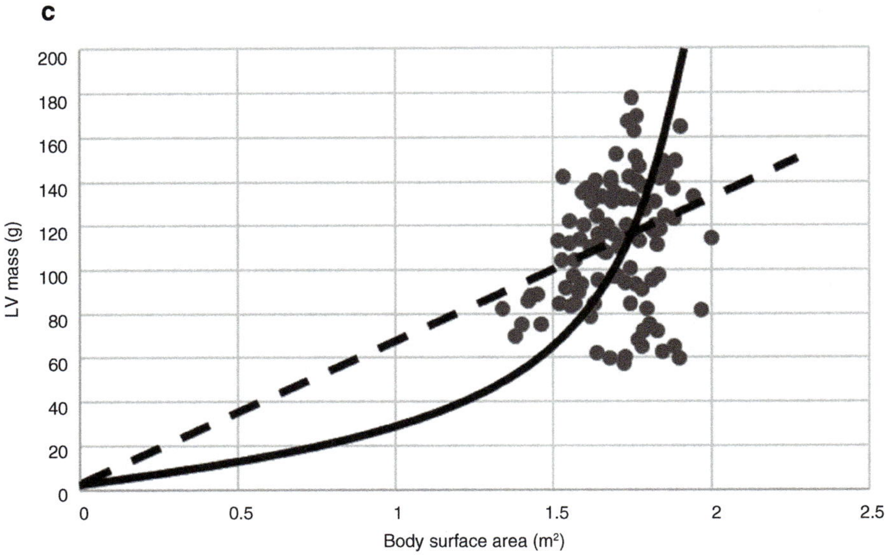


**Fig. 4.3** (continued)

Many cardiac dimensions and body size measures scale in a non-linear fashion (Fig. 4.3c) and thus the use of **"allometric" scaling** is useful [36, 39]. This is theoretically sound in most cases and practically tends to lead to body size-independent cardiac indices [43, 44]. Allometric scaling has an index of the form $Y/X^b$; where b is the slope exponent derived from simple log-log linear regression of the two variables. This approach has been adopted and shown to be more appropriate in various populations including healthy normal, clinical groups and athletes [40–47]. This approach should be encouraged within sports cardiology and its application to pre-participation screening. Dewey et al. [37] provide some simple but interesting clinical vignettes to support the allometric approach.

## 4.9 Which Scaling Variables Are Used with "Athlete's Heart" Data?

Body size is quite a broad term and has been used in a general sense to cover measurements such as

- height (stature)
- body mass, BSA (that mathematically combines both stature and mass in prediction equations)
- sub-components of overall body size such as fat mass, fat free mass and lean body mass.

Clearly different body size variables represent different anatomical components of any individual, are also measured in different units and reflect different dimensional constructs (1D, 2D and 3D). This can only complicate any scaling process, especially when there are multiple cardiac dimensions (or functional parameters) to be scaled.

- In sports cardiology literature the most common scaling variable used in an attempt to determine a size-independent index is **BSA** [36].

It is thought that BSA is a good "overall" surrogate of body size that can reflect changes or developments in fat mass and fat free mass [36]. This is despite the fact that BSA is estimated from prediction equations that are very rarely developed from the populations under investigation in sports cardiology research or screening.

Because of the issues associated with estimations of BSA and the desire to have highly accurate measures of body size a number of research studies have promoted the use of height (stature) as a scaling variable [40–42]. In most cases empirical data has supported the use of $height^{2.7}$ for scaling LV mass. This is not far from a geometrically consistent value of 3. Work specifically in athletes has questioned the use of height due to its limited variability in homogenous athlete groups [43, 44]. Despite this height does remain an option for scaling in athletes and other populations.

From a theoretical and evidence-based perspective, many authors [36, 37] have suggested that some estimate of the lean or muscle tissue component of body size in any individual would be a sensible option to reflect body size. Lean or muscle tissue represents the metabolic "sink" for blood flow and thus cardiovascular work requirements during exercise, and also likely reflects the component of body size that will differentiate most between individuals and groups (when compared to height, body mass or BSA); it has thus been employed in recent athletic heart studies [48, 49].

Recent research has extended scaling in sports cardiology research in a number of different directions:

- George et al. [50] investigated the application of scaling of cardiac dimensions in a longitudinal training study employing MRI to assess cardiac and body size variables.
- Riding et al. [49] specifically addressed the utility of scaling in athletes with an extreme body size. Other work has moved on from cardiac dimensions to more recent developments related to cardiac function, movement and mechanics.
- Batterham et al. [51] determined that basal septal wall peak tissue velocity in systole was highly dependent on LV length in athletes, suggesting some scaling adjustment.
- Conversely, Oxborough et al. [52] were able to demonstrate that longitudinal strain was independent of dimensional characteristics of the LV.

## 4.10 Take Home Messages and Guidance for Future Research

- Sporting disciplines have a significant impact on the type and the extent of physiological cardiac adaptation in athletes.
- While the "Morganroth hypothesis" interpreted the effect of sporting discipline on cardiac adaptation in a dichotomous way (static sports = concentric hypertrophy/remodelling, dynamic sports = eccentric hypertrophy), recent studies have shown that this relationship is far more complex.
- LV geometry, which is often represented by the relationship between the LV cavity size and wall thickness, is usually normal in athletes. In athletes engaged in dynamic exercise, females tend to show eccentric hypertrophy more frequently than males. Although occurring in only a small proportion of athletes, more men than women exhibit concentric remodeling/hypertrophy.
- Endurance athletes may exhibit a low normal or even mildly reduced LV ejection fraction, which is part of a physiological process of adaptation to exercise.
- With respect to scaling of cardiac dimensions (and in some cases cardiac function) we pose a number of simple questions.
  1. Why are you scaling?
  2. What do you need to scale?
  3. How are you going to scale (process and variable choice)?
  4. How are you going to demonstrate size-independence of your cardiac indices?
- It is prudent to develop an empirically supported and sample specific approach to scaling. Think about how you align your approach, theoretically and practically, to best practice and past literature.
- If it is difficult (sample size and variance) to provide sample specific scaling support, then you may have to resort to population specific and evidence-based approaches [35, 36].
- Future research should continue to advocate theoretically and practically valid scaling approaches to help accurately interpret cardiac dimensions in athletes. More work is needed in cardiac dimensions associated with the RV [26], the atria [32] and other cardiovascular structures.
- Further work should also address how cardiac and body dimensions relate to each other (and thus how scaling is performed) in a range of different athletic populations including
  - female athletes [48]
  - athletes with different ethnicity [50]
  - athletes of different age [53].
- All of this work, and that which has gone before, must contribute to the development of body-size-independent norms data for athletes to help differential diagnostic decisions in sports cardiology.

**Clinical Pearls**

- Eccentric hypertrophy of the LV is a common but not obligatory response to endurance-type training programs.
- Concentric hypertrophy of the LV is a rare finding in any athlete and should raise some suspicion at cardiac pre-participation screening.

- Balanced adaptions in the LV, RV and atria are the common form in most athletes undergoing long term training.
- Resting cardiac function is a poor clinical discriminator in most athletes and can even decline in some trained individuals.
- Big people have big hearts and smaller people tend to have smaller hearts.
- Choosing the right theoretical and mathematical approach to scaling your cardiac data, as opposed to the easiest, could be important in evaluating any given athletic heart accurately.

## Review

### Questions

1. What are the common forms of left ventricular geometry observed in highly trained athletes from different sporting disciplines?
2. Can you describe the impact of endurance sport on right ventricular adaptation to exercise?
3. Can you describe the nature of the relationship between a one-dimensional cardiac measure (e.g. septal wall thickness) with a three-dimensional body size variable (e.g. body mass)?
4. In the example above, can you describe possible different approaches to scaling, and how you would determine if the scaled index was, indeed, size-independent?

### Answers

1. Most athletes would exhibit a normal left ventricular geometry. Athletes may exhibit eccentric hypertrophy, concentric hypertrophy or concentric remodeling. A recent study [11] showed that in the specific subgroup of athletes engaged in dynamic exercise, females showed eccentric hypertrophy more frequently than males, while more men than women had concentric remodeling/hypertrophy, although these geometric presentations were less common than normal geometry.
2. A large proportion of young athletes exhibit increased RV dimensions exceeding the reference values commonly used in clinical practice and the values proposed by the revised Task Force Criteria (TFC) for the diagnosis of ARVC. Most available data are on endurance athletes, with less available data on athletes engaging in static sports.
3. Whilst the overall relationship will be positive (as body size increases so will septal wall thickness), careful analysis will likely reveal that over the range of data provided the relationship between septal wall thickness and body mass will be curvi-linear (i.e. non-linear) as it involves a one-dimensional cardiac measure and a three-dimensional body size parameter. The curvi-linear relationship is because of the lack of geometric similarity between the two variables.

4. Initially you would want to define your body size parameter to scale and in most cases this would likely be BSA or HT (in a clinical setting). Ratiometric approaches with BSA are likely to be problematic due to lack of geometric similarity in septal wall thickness and BSA. An allometric approach with the “b” exponent derived directly from the population to be studied would be optimal but an approach using 0.5 (1-D divided by 2-D) as the “b” exponent could be adopted. If HT was used, a ratiometric approach would likely be very similar to any allometric approach as both septal wall thickness and HT are one-dimensional parameters. To test for size independence all you would need to do is correlate the scaled index (wall thickness/BSA$^{0.5}$ or wall thickness/HT) to the body size measure (BSA or HT). Any significant residual correlation would suggest that size-independence of your index had NOT been achieved.

## References


1. Sharma S, Merghani A, Mont L. Exercise and the heart: the good, the bad, and the ugly. Eur Heart J. 2015;36:1445–53. https://doi.org/10.1093/eurheartj/ehv090.
2. Mitchell JH, Haskell WL, Raven PB. Classification of sports. J Am Coll Cardiol. 1994;24(4):864–6.
3. Spirito P, Pelliccia A, Proschan MA, et al. Morphology of the “athlete’s heart” assessed by echocardiography in 947 elite athletes representing 27 sports. Am J Cardiol. 1994;74(8):802–6.
4. Pelliccia A, Culasso F, Di Paolo FM, Maron BJ. Physiologic left ventricular cavity dilatation in elite athletes. Ann Intern Med. 1999;130(1):23–31.
5. Finocchiaro G, Sharma S. The safety of exercise in individuals with cardiomyopathy. Can J Cardiol. 2016;32(4):467–74. https://doi.org/10.1016/j.cjca.2015.12.005.
6. Morganroth J, Maron BJ, Henry WL, Epstein SE. Comparative left ventricular dimensions in trained athletes. Ann Intern Med. 1975;82(4):521–4.
7. Haykowsky MJ, Samuel TJ, Nelson MD, La Gerche A. Athlete’s heart: is the Morganroth hypothesis obsolete? Heart Lung Circ. 2018;27(9):1037–41. https://doi.org/10.1016/j.hlc.2018.04.289.
8. Kooreman Z, Giraldeau G, Finocchiaro G, et al. Athletic remodeling in female college athletes, the “Morganroth hypothesis” revisited. Clin J Sport Med. 2018;29:224–31. https://doi.org/10.1097/JSM.0000000000000501.
9. Naylor LH, George K, O’Driscoll G, Green DJ. The athlete’s heart: a contemporary appraisal of the “Morganroth hypothesis”. Sports Med. 2008;38(1):69–90. https://doi.org/10.2165/00007256-200838010-00006.
10. Pelliccia A, Maron BJ, Spataro A, Proschan MA, Spirito P. The upper limit of physiologic cardiac hypertrophy in highly trained elite athletes. N Engl J Med. 1991;324(5):295–301. https://doi.org/10.1056/NEJM199101313240504.
11. Finocchiaro G, Dhutia H, D’Silva A, et al. Effect of sex and sporting discipline on LV adaptation to exercise. JACC Cardiovasc Imaging. 2017;10(9):965–72. https://doi.org/10.1016/j.jcmg.2016.08.011.
12. Abergel E, Chatellier G, Hagege AA, et al. Serial left ventricular adaptations in world-class professional cyclists: implications for disease screening and follow-up. J Am Coll Cardiol. 2004;44(1):144–9. https://doi.org/10.1016/j.jacc.2004.02.057.
13. Caselli S, Montesanti D, Autore C, et al. Patterns of left ventricular longitudinal strain and strain rate in Olympic athletes. J Am Soc Echocardiogr. 2015;28(2):245–53. https://doi.org/10.1016/j.echo.2014.10.010.
14. van de Schoor FR, Aengevaeren VL, Hopman MTE, et al. Myocardial fibrosis in athletes. Mayo Clin Proc. 2016;91(11):1617–31. https://doi.org/10.1016/j.mayocp.2016.07.012.

15. La Gerche A, Claessen G, Dymarkowski S, et al. Exercise-induced right ventricular dysfunction is associated with ventricular arrhythmias in endurance athletes. Eur Heart J. 2015;36(30):1998–2010. https://doi.org/10.1093/eurheartj/ehv202.
16. Schnell F, Claessen G, La Gerche A, et al. Subepicardial delayed gadolinium enhancement in asymptomatic athletes: let sleeping dogs lie? Br J Sports Med. 2016;50(2):111–7. https://doi.org/10.1136/bjsports-2014-094546.
17. Tahir E, Starekova J, Muellerleile K, et al. Myocardial fibrosis in competitive triathletes detected by contrast-enhanced CMR correlates with exercise-induced hypertension and competition history. JACC Cardiovasc Imaging. 2018;11:1260–70. https://doi.org/10.1016/j.jcmg.2017.09.016.
18. Finocchiaro G, Dhutia H, D'Silva A, et al. Role of Doppler diastolic parameters in differentiating physiological left ventricular hypertrophy from hypertrophic cardiomyopathy. J Am Soc Echocardiogr. 2018;31:606–613.e1. https://doi.org/10.1016/j.echo.2017.11.022.
19. Zaidi A, Ghani S, Sharma R, et al. Physiological right ventricular adaptation in elite athletes of African and Afro-Caribbean origin. Circulation. 2013;127(17):1783–92. https://doi.org/10.1161/CIRCULATIONAHA.112.000270.
20. Zaidi A, Sheikh N, Jongman JK, et al. Clinical differentiation between physiological remodeling and arrhythmogenic right ventricular cardiomyopathy in athletes with marked electrocardiographic repolarization anomalies. J Am Coll Cardiol. 2015;65(25):2702–11. https://doi.org/10.1016/j.jacc.2015.04.035.
21. Sharma S, Zaidi A. Exercise-induced arrhythmogenic right ventricular cardiomyopathy: fact or fallacy? Eur Heart J. 2012;33(8):938–40. https://doi.org/10.1093/eurheartj/ehr436.
22. Corrado D, Basso C, Rizzoli G, Schiavon M, Thiene G. Does sports activity enhance the risk of sudden death in adolescents and young adults? J Am Coll Cardiol. 2003;42(11):1959–63.
23. Finocchiaro G, Papadakis M, Robertus J-L, et al. Etiology of sudden death in sports insights from a United Kingdom regional registry. J Am Coll Cardiol. 2016;67(18):2108–15. https://doi.org/10.1016/j.jacc.2016.02.062.
24. Marcus FI, McKenna WJ, Sherrill D, et al. Diagnosis of arrhythmogenic right ventricular cardiomyopathy/dysplasia: proposed modification of the task force criteria. Circulation. 2010;121(13):1533–41. https://doi.org/10.1161/CIRCULATIONAHA.108.840827.
25. Neilan TG, Januzzi JL, Lee-Lewandrowski E, et al. Myocardial injury and ventricular dysfunction related to training levels among nonelite participants in the Boston marathon. Circulation. 2006;114(22):2325–33. https://doi.org/10.1161/CIRCULATIONAHA.106.647461.
26. Oxborough D, Shave R, Warburton D, et al. Dilatation and dysfunction of the right ventricle immediately after ultraendurance exercise: exploratory insights from conventional two-dimensional and speckle tracking echocardiography. Circ Cardiovasc Imaging. 2011;4(3):253–63. https://doi.org/10.1161/CIRCIMAGING.110.961938.
27. Arbab-Zadeh A, Perhonen M, Howden E, et al. Cardiac remodeling in response to 1 year of intensive endurance training. Circulation. 2014;130(24):2152–61. https://doi.org/10.1161/CIRCULATIONAHA.114.010775.
28. La Gerche A, Robberecht C, Kuiperi C, et al. Lower than expected desmosomal gene mutation prevalence in endurance athletes with complex ventricular arrhythmias of right ventricular origin. Heart. 2010;96(16):1268–74. https://doi.org/10.1136/hrt.2009.189621.
29. D'Ascenzi F, Pisicchio C, Caselli S, Di Paolo FM, Spataro A, Pelliccia A. RV remodeling in Olympic athletes. JACC Cardiovasc Imaging. 2017;10(4):385–93. https://doi.org/10.1016/j.jcmg.2016.03.017.
30. Pelliccia A, Maron BJ, Di Paolo FM, et al. Prevalence and clinical significance of left atrial remodeling in competitive athletes. J Am Coll Cardiol. 2005;46(4):690–6. https://doi.org/10.1016/j.jacc.2005.04.052.
31. D'Andrea A, Riegler L, Golia E, et al. Range of right heart measurements in top-level athletes: the training impact. Int J Cardiol. 2013;164(1):48–57. https://doi.org/10.1016/j.ijcard.2011.06.058.
32. McClean G, George K, Lord R, et al. Chronic adaptation of atrial structure and function in elite male athletes. Eur Heart J Cardiovasc Imaging. 2015;16(4):417–22. https://doi.org/10.1093/ehjci/jeu215.

33. Pelliccia A, Di Paolo FM, De Blasiis E, et al. Prevalence and clinical significance of aortic root dilation in highly trained competitive athletes. Circulation. 2010;122(7):698–706, 3 pages following 706. https://doi.org/10.1161/CIRCULATIONAHA.109.901074.
34. Engel DJ, Schwartz A, Homma S. Athletic cardiac remodeling in US professional basketball players. JAMA Cardiol. 2016;1(1):80–7. https://doi.org/10.1001/jamacardio.2015.0252.
35. Schmidt-Nielsen K. Scaling: why is animal size so important? Melbourne: Cambridge University Press; 1984.
36. Batterham AM, George KP, Whyte G, Sharma S, McKenna W. Scaling cardiac structural data by body dimensions: a review of theory, practice, and problems. Int J Sports Med. 1999;20(8):495–502. https://doi.org/10.1055/s-1999-8844.
37. Dewey FE, Rosenthal D, Murphy DJ, Froelicher VF, Ashley EA. Does size matter? Clinical applications of scaling cardiac size and function for body size. Circulation. 2008;117(17):2279–87. https://doi.org/10.1161/CIRCULATIONAHA.107.736785.
38. Utomi V, Oxborough D, Ashley E, et al. Predominance of normal left ventricular geometry in the male "athlete's heart". Heart. 2014;100(16):1264–71. https://doi.org/10.1136/heartjnl-2014-305904.
39. Brown B, Somauroo J, Green DJ, et al. The complex phenotype of the athlete's heart: implications for preparticipation screening. Exerc Sport Sci Rev. 2017;45(2):96–104. https://doi.org/10.1249/JES.0000000000000102.
40. de Simone G, Daniels SR, Devereux RB, et al. Left ventricular mass and body size in normotensive children and adults: assessment of allometric relations and impact of overweight. J Am Coll Cardiol. 1992;20(5):1251–60.
41. Lauer MS, Anderson KM, Larson MG, Levy D. A new method for indexing left ventricular mass for differences in body size. Am J Cardiol. 1994;74(5):487–91.
42. Daniels SR, Kimball TR, Morrison JA, Khoury P, Witt S, Meyer RA. Effect of lean body mass, fat mass, blood pressure, and sexual maturation on left ventricular mass in children and adolescents. Statistical, biological, and clinical significance. Circulation. 1995;92(11):3249–54.
43. Batterham AM, George KP, Mullineaux DR. Allometric scaling of left ventricular mass by body dimensions in males and females. Med Sci Sports Exerc. 1997;29(2):181–6.
44. Batterham AM, George KP. Modeling the influence of body size and composition on M-mode echocardiographic dimensions. Am J Phys. 1998;274(2 Pt 2):H701–8.
45. George KP, Batterham AM, Jones B. Echocardiographic evidence of concentric left ventricular enlargement in female weight lifters. Eur J Appl Physiol Occup Physiol. 1998;79(1):88–92. https://doi.org/10.1007/s004210050478.
46. George KP, Batterham AM, Jones B. The impact of scalar variable and process on athlete-control comparisons of cardiac dimensions. Med Sci Sports Exerc. 1998;30(6):824–30.
47. George K, Sharma S, Batterham A, Whyte G, McKenna W. Allometric analysis of the association between cardiac dimensions and body size variables in 464 junior athletes. Clin Sci (Lond). 2001;100(1):47–54.
48. Giraldeau G, Kobayashi Y, Finocchiaro G, et al. Gender differences in ventricular remodeling and function in college athletes, insights from lean body mass scaling and deformation imaging. Am J Cardiol. 2015;116(10):1610–6. https://doi.org/10.1016/j.amjcard.2015.08.026.
49. Riding NR, Salah O, Sharma S, et al. Do big athletes have big hearts? Impact of extreme anthropometry upon cardiac hypertrophy in professional male athletes. Br J Sports Med. 2012;46(Suppl 1):i90–7. https://doi.org/10.1136/bjsports-2012-091258.
50. George KP, Birch KM, Pennell DJ, Myerson SG. Magnetic-resonance-imaging-derived indices for the normalization of left ventricular morphology by body size. Magn Reson Imaging. 2009;27(2):207–13. https://doi.org/10.1016/j.mri.2008.06.008.
51. Batterham A, Shave R, Oxborough D, Whyte G, George K. Longitudinal plane colour tissue-Doppler myocardial velocities and their association with left ventricular length, volume, and mass in humans. Eur J Echocardiogr. 2008;9(4):542–6. https://doi.org/10.1093/ejechocard/jen114.

52. Oxborough D, Batterham AM, Shave R, et al. Interpretation of two-dimensional and tissue Doppler-derived strain (epsilon) and strain rate data: is there a need to normalize for individual variability in left ventricular morphology? Eur J Echocardiogr. 2009;10(5):677–82. https://doi.org/10.1093/ejechocard/jep037.
53. McClean G, Riding NR, Ardern CL, et al. Electrical and structural adaptations of the paediatric athlete's heart: a systematic review with meta-analysis. Br J Sports Med. 2018;52(4):230. https://doi.org/10.1136/bjsports-2016-097052.

# 5 Sudden Cardiac Death in Athletes: Incidence, Causes and Prevention Strategies

Kimberly G. Harmon and Mathew G. Wilson

**Learning Objectives**

1. Understand the methodology behind incidence studies and be able to critically evaluate incidence studies with assessment of the accuracy of the numerators and denominators used to calculate risk of death.
2. Identify high risk populations at risk for sudden cardiac death.
3. Describe the causes of sudden cardiac death in young and older athletes and how they differ.
4. Discuss primary and secondary prevention strategies for sudden cardiac death.

## 5.1 Epidemiology

### 5.1.1 Prevalence

The prevalence of cardiovascular conditions that predispose to sudden cardiac arrest (SCA) and death (SCD) is about 1 in 300 individuals [1–4]. Not all those with cardiac conditions that predispose to SCA/D will die, however athletes with cardiac conditions

The original version of this chapter was revised. The correction to this chapter can be found at https://doi.org/10.1007/978-3-030-35374-2_52

K. G. Harmon (✉)
Department of Family Medicine, University of Washington School of Medicine, Seattle, WA, USA

Department of Orthopaedics and Sports Medicine, University of Washington School of Medicine, Seattle, WA, USA
e-mail: kharmon@uw.edu

M. G. Wilson
Aspetar Orthopaedic and Sports Medicine Hospital, Doha, Qatar
e-mail: Mathew.wilson@aspetar.com



A. Pressler, J. Niebauer (eds.), *Textbook of Sports and Exercise Cardiology*,
https://doi.org/10.1007/978-3-030-35374-2_5

are more likely to suffer SCA than non-athletes [5, 6]. The concept behind cardiovascular screening in athletes is to identify those with these conditions and to modify risk.

### 5.1.2 Incidence

SCD is the leading cause of medical death in young athletes [7]. The incidence of SCD in athletes has been reported between 1 in 3000 athlete-years (AY) to almost 1 in 1,000,000 AY [8, 9]. Much of the variability is related to study methodology, therefore it is important to have a granular understanding of methodology when evaluating any study on incidence. To arrive at an incidence calculation there must be an accurate numerator and denominator.

#### 5.1.2.1 Numerator

- How were the deaths recorded?
  - Mandatory reporting? Were the systems in place robust?
  - Death certificates?
  - Registry?

    Registries typically rely on next-of-kin reporting and are subject to ascertainment bias.
  - Media reports?

    Media reports will capture between 4% and 80% of deaths in given population depending on how high-profile the athlete is [7, 10–12].

    Media reports will also under-report SCD which occur while the athlete is sleeping or during activities of daily living.
- Is the numerator inclusive of death which occurs only during sports or death which occurs at any time?
  - Some studies only look at deaths which occur during sports which is appropriate if you are considering the type of medical coverage that is required for an event (i.e. AED placement).
  - When considering screening programs, the number of deaths which occur at any time is needed.
- How is "athlete" defined?
  - Some studies of SCD look at athletes while others look at young people or people participating in sporting activity (see also Chap. 1).
- What age-range is included?
  - Rates of SCD vary in age groups.
  - Rates of SCD in athletes >25 years of age increase because of increasing contribution of coronary artery disease [13].
  - Age range should ideally be inclusive of people with similar risk profiles.

#### 5.1.2.2 Denominator

- What unit is being used?
  - Most studies will use "athlete-years" or "person-years".
  - Other studies in sports injury epidemiology use "athlete-exposures" or "athlete-hours" but this is typically not used in studies of SCD.

- How was the denominator determined?
  - Actual numbers of athletes?
    Is there a breakdown into sub-populations that may be at higher risk (sex, race/ethnicity, sport)?
  - Estimated numbers of athletes
    Often with numbers reported by sporting associations, can lead to wide margins of error.
    Occasionally, reports on physical activity in a population are used to estimate the denominator. Depending on the methodology used, this can also lead to significant over or under-estimation of participation.

Table 5.1 includes studies on the incidence of sudden cardiac death in athletes with details about the study. In general, the overall incidence of SCD in athlete's aged between 18 and 24 is about 1 in 50,000 AY. However, studies have shown that males, Afro-American/Caribbean and Pacific Islanders have a higher risk of SCD. In addition, it appears that men's basketball, American football, and football (soccer) are higher risk sports [7, 14–16].

## 5.2 Conditions Associated with Sudden Cardiac Death

A variety of conditions are implicated in SCD with heterogeneous pathology based on age and other demographic factors. In addition, although the typical causes of SCD in athletes (listed below) are commonly reported, their percental proportion varies among different studies according to the characteristics of the particular athletic population evaluated (e.g. regional variations) (Fig. 5.1).

Causes of SCD in athletes vary from causes in a broader population. The prevalence of coronary artery disease in those with SCD increases precipitously after age 25 [13]. In those under 25 years old, congenital causes are more likely to predominate. More recent studies have seen an increasing prevalence of left ventricular hypertrophy (LVH) with fibrosis in cases of sudden death (Table 5.2) [17].

- Hypertrophic cardiomyopathy (HCM)
  - Prevalence in the general population of 1 in 500, in athletes 1 in 2000 [1].
  - Studies cite HCM as a cause of SCD in athletes in 2–36% of cases [7, 10, 12, 14, 17–22].
  - Characterized by asymmetric left ventricular hypertrophy (LVH).
  - Histologic analysis shows disorganized cellular architecture or myocyte disarray.
  - There is variable penetrance with some never developing phenotypic HCM. They are considered low risk for SCA.
  - Morphological features may appear in childhood but often develop in adolescence or young adulthood. Screening for HCM needs to continue into young adulthood to be effective [23].
  - The presenting symptoms of HCM is SCA 80% of the time. Exertional syncope or chest pain, light-headedness or dyspnea may also occur.

**Table 5.1** Incidence of sudden cardiac arrest and death in athletes

| Study | Study design and population | Case identification | Denominator | Sports-related SCD or all SCD? | SCD or all SCA/D? | Study years | Age range; number of cases | Annual incidence |
|---|---|---|---|---|---|---|---|---|
| Athletes | | | | | | | | |
| Van Camp [43] | Retrospective cohort; high school and college athletes | National Center for Catastrophic Sports Injury Research and media reports | Data from NCAA, NFHS, NAIA, and NJCAA, added together with conversion factor (1.9 for high school and 1.2 for college) used to account for multisport athletes "based on discussions with representatives from the national organizations" | Sports-related | SCD | 1983–1993 | 13–24; N = 160 | *College ± high school*<br>Overall 1:188,000<br>Male 1:134,000<br>Female 1:752,000<br>*High school*<br>Overall 1:213,000<br>Male 1:152,000<br>Female 1:861,000<br>*College*<br>Overall 1:94,000<br>Male 1:69,000<br>Female 1:356,000 |
| Maron [44] | Retrospective cohort; Minnesota high school athletes | Catastrophic insurance claims | Minnesota State High School League (estimated using conversion factor of 2.3 to account for multisport athletes) | Sports-related (school-sponsored only) | SCD | 1985–1997 | 16–17; N = 3 | *High school*<br>Overall 1:217,000<br>Male 1:129,000<br>Female 0 |
| Corrado [18] | Prospective cohort; athletes and non-athletes in the Veneto Region of Italy | Mandatory reporting of sudden death | Registered athletes in the Sports Medicine Database of the Veneto Region of Italy and the Italian Census Bureau | All | SCD | 1979–1999 | 12–35; N = 51<br>12–35; N = 208 | *Athletes*<br>Overall 1:47,000<br>Male 1:41,000<br>Female 1:93,000<br>*Non-athletes*<br>Overall 1:143,000 |

| | | | | | | | | |
|---|---|---|---|---|---|---|---|---|
| Drezner [45] | Retrospective survey; college athletes | Survey of NCAA Division I institutions (244/326 responded) | Reported number of athletes | All | SCD | – | N = 5 | _College_<br>Overall 1:67,000 |
| Corrado [4] | Prospective cohort; athletes and non-athletes in the Veneto Region of Italy | Mandatory reporting to the Registry on Juvenile Sudden Death | Registered athletes in the Sports Medicine Database of the Veneto Region of Italy and the Italian Census Bureau | All | SCD | 1979–2004 | 12–35; N = 55<br>12–35; N = 265 | _Athletes_<br>1:24,000 (pre-screen)<br>1:233,000 (post-screen)<br>_Non-athletes_<br>1:127,000 (unscreened) |
| Maron [20] | Retrospective cohort; amateur and competitive athletes | U.S. Registry for Sudden Death in Athletes | An estimated 10.7 million participants per year ≤39 years of age in all organized amateur and competitive sports | All | SCA + SCD | 1980–2006 | 8–39; N = 1046 | _Athletes_<br>1:164,000 |
| Drezner [46] | Cross-sectional survey; high school athletes | Survey of 1710 high schools with AEDs | Reported number of student athletes | All cases occurring on campus | SCA + SCD | 2006–2007 | 14–17; N = 14 | _High school_<br>1:23,000 (SCA + SCD)<br>1:64,000 (SCD) |
| Holst [10] | Retrospective cohort; athletes and general population in Denmark | Review of death certificates, Cause of Death Registry, and National Patient Registry in Denmark | Interview data of people age 16–35 years from the National Danish Health and Morbidity Study | Sports-related SCD in athletes versus all SCD in the general population | SCD | 2000–2006 | 12–35; N = 15<br>12–35; N = 428 | _Athletes_<br>1:83,000<br>_General population_<br>1:27,000 |

(continued)

**Table 5.1** (continued)

| Study | Study design and population | Case identification | Denominator | Sports-related SCD or all SCD? | SCD or all SCA/D? | Study years | Age range; number of cases | Annual incidence |
|---|---|---|---|---|---|---|---|---|
| Marijon [47] | Prospective cohort; general population in France | Data from emergency medical system | General population statistics, data from the Minister of Health and Sport to estimate young competitive athlete population | Sports-related SCA or SCD with moderate or vigorous exercise | SCA + SCD | 2005–2010 | 10–75; N = 820<br>10–35; N = 50 | *General population*<br>1:217,000<br>*Young competitive athlete*<br>1:102,000<br>*Young non-competitive athlete*<br>1:455,000 |
| Steinvil [48] | Retrospective cohort; athletes in Israel | Retrospective review of two Israeli newspapers | Competitive athletes registered in the Israel Sport Authority in 2009; extrapolated this data for prior 24 years based on the growth of the Israeli population (age 10–40) from the Central Bureau of Statistics; allowed for a presumed doubling of the sporting population over 24 years | All | SCD | 1985–2009 | 12–44; N = 24 | *Athletes*<br>1:38,000 |

| | | | | | | | | |
|---|---|---|---|---|---|---|---|---|
| Harmon [8] | Retrospective cohort; college athletes | Parent Heart Watch database, NCAA Resolutions list, catastrophic insurance claims | Participation data from the NCAA | All | SCD | 2004–2008 | 18–26 N = 37 | _College_<br>Overall 1:43,000<br>Male 1:33,000<br>Female 1:76,000<br>Black 1:17,000<br>White 1:58,000<br>Male, black 1:13,000<br>Male, basketball 1:7000<br>Male, Div. I basketball 1:3000 |
| Maron [49] | Retrospective cohort; Minnesota high school athletes | U.S. Registry for Sudden Death in Athletes | Minnesota State High School League statistics (estimated using conversion factor of 2.3 to account for multisport athletes) | All | SCD | 1986–2011 | 12–18; N = 13 | _High school_<br>Overall 1:150,000<br>Male 1:83,000<br>Female 0 |
| Roberts [9] | Retrospective cohort; Minnesota high school athletes | Catastrophic insurance claims | Minnesota State High School League statistics (Sum of unduplicated athletes 1993–1994 through 2011–2012 school years) | Sports-related (school-sponsored only) | SCD | 1993–2012 | 12–19; N = 4 | _High school_<br>1:417,000 (1993–2012)<br>1:909,000 (2003–2012)<br>Female 0 |
| Maron [50] | Retrospective cohort; college athletes | U.S. Registry for Sudden Death in Athletes and NCAA resolutions list | Participation data from the NCAA | All | SCD | 2002–2011 | 17–26; N = 64 | _College_<br>Overall 1:63,000<br>Male 1:56,000<br>Female 1:333,000<br>Black 1:26,000<br>White 1:143,000 |

(continued)

**Table 5.1** (continued)

| Study | Study design and population | Case identification | Denominator | Sports-related SCD or all SCD? | SCD or all SCA/D? | Study years | Age range; number of cases | Annual incidence |
|---|---|---|---|---|---|---|---|---|
| Toresdahl [5] | Prospective observational; high school students and student-athletes | 2149 high schools monitored for SCA events on school campus | Reported number of students and student-athletes | All cases occurring on school campus | SCA + SCD | 2009–2011 | 14–18; N = 44 | *Student-athlete*<br>Overall 1:88,000<br>Male 1:58,000<br>Female 1:323,000<br>*Student non-athlete*<br>Overall 1:326,000<br>Male 1:286,000<br>Female 1:357,000 |
| Drezner [51] | Retrospective cohort; Minnesota high school athletes | Public media reports | Minnesota State High School League statistics (sum of unduplicated athletes 2003–2004 through 2011–2012 school years) | All | SCA + SCD | 2003–2012 | 14–18; N = 13 | *High school*<br>Overall 1:71,000<br>Female 0<br>Male, basketball 1:21,000 |
| Harmon [14] | Retrospective cohort; high school athletes from 7 states in the U.S. | Public media reports | Participation data from the NFHS | All | SCA + SCD | 2007–2013 | 14–18; N = 109 | *High school*<br>Overall 1:67,000<br>Male 1:45,000<br>Female 1:238,000<br>Male, basketball 1:37,000 |
| Risgaard [11] | Retrospective cohort; competitive and non-competitive athletes in Denmark | Review of death certificates and the Danish National Patient Registry | Competitive and non-competitive athlete populations in Denmark estimated based on survey data from the Danish National Institute of Public Health | Sports-related SCD in competitive versus non-competitive athletes | SCD | 2007–2009 | 12–35; N = 44 | *Competitive athlete*<br>1:213,000<br>*Non-competitive athlete*<br>1:233,000 |

| | | | | | | | | |
|---|---|---|---|---|---|---|---|---|
| Harmon [7] | Retrospective cohort; college athletes | Parent Heart Watch database, NCAA Resolutions list, catastrophic insurance claims | Participation data from the NCAA | All | SCD | 2003–2013 | 17–26; N = 79 | _College_<br>Overall 1:53,000<br>Male 1:38,000<br>Female 1:122,000<br>Black 1:21,000<br>White 1:68,000<br>Football 1:36,000<br>Male, soccer 1:24,000<br>Male, black 1:16,000<br>Male, basketball 1:9000<br>Male, black, basketball 1:5300<br>Male, Div. I basketball 1:5200 |
| Bohm [12] | Prospective cohort; sports-related SCD in all persons in Germany | Voluntary reporting to German National Registry, web-based media search, regional institutes | Physical activity estimated from the German Health Update study and extrapolated to population data from the German Federal Statistical Office | Sports-related SCD | SCD | 2012–2014 | 10–79; N = 144 | _Sports participants_<br>1:1,200,000 |
| Grani [52] | Retrospective; sports-related SCD in all persons in German-speaking Switzerland | Forensic reports | Physical activity estimated from survey on sports participation by the Swiss Federal Office of Sports | Sports-related SCD | SCD | 1999–2010 | 10–39; N = 69 | _Sports participants_<br>Competitive: 1:90,000<br>Recreational: 1:192,000 |

(continued)

**Table 5.1** (continued)

| Study | Study design and population | Case identification | Denominator | Sports-related SCD or all SCD? | SCD or all SCA/D? | Study years | Age range; number of cases | Annual incidence |
|---|---|---|---|---|---|---|---|---|
| Maron [53] | Retrospective cohort | Records of the Medical Examiner | Data from the Minnesota Department of Education, National Center for Education Statistics, and the Minnesota State High School League for Hennepin County, Minnesota | All | SCD | 2000–2014 | 14–23; N = 27 | *Non-athlete* 1:39,000 *Athlete* 1:121,000 |
| Harmon [26] | Retrospective cohort, US high school athletes | Media reports | NFHS participation statistics | All | SCA/SCD | 2007–2013 | 14–18 N = 104 | *High school* Overall 1:67,000 Male 1:45,000 Female 1:237,000 Male, basketball 1:37,000 |
| Chatard [15] | Prospective, Pacific Island athletes who were screened | Prospectively followed | Defined cohort of 1450 athletes | | SCD | 2012–2015 | 10–40 N = 3 | *Pacific Island athletes* 1:2416 |
| Malhotra [16] | Prospective | Followed from time of screen to 2016 | Defined cohort of 11,168 elite soccer athletes | All | SCD | 1996–2016 | 15–17 N = 8 | *Elite male soccer athletes* 1:14,794 |

*SCD* sudden cardiac death, *SCA* sudden cardiac arrest, *NCAA* National Collegiate Athletic Association, *NFHS* National Federation of State High School Associations, *NAIA* National Association of Intercollegiate Athletics, *NJCAA* National Junior College Athletic Association, *U.S.* United States, *AED* automatic external defibrillator

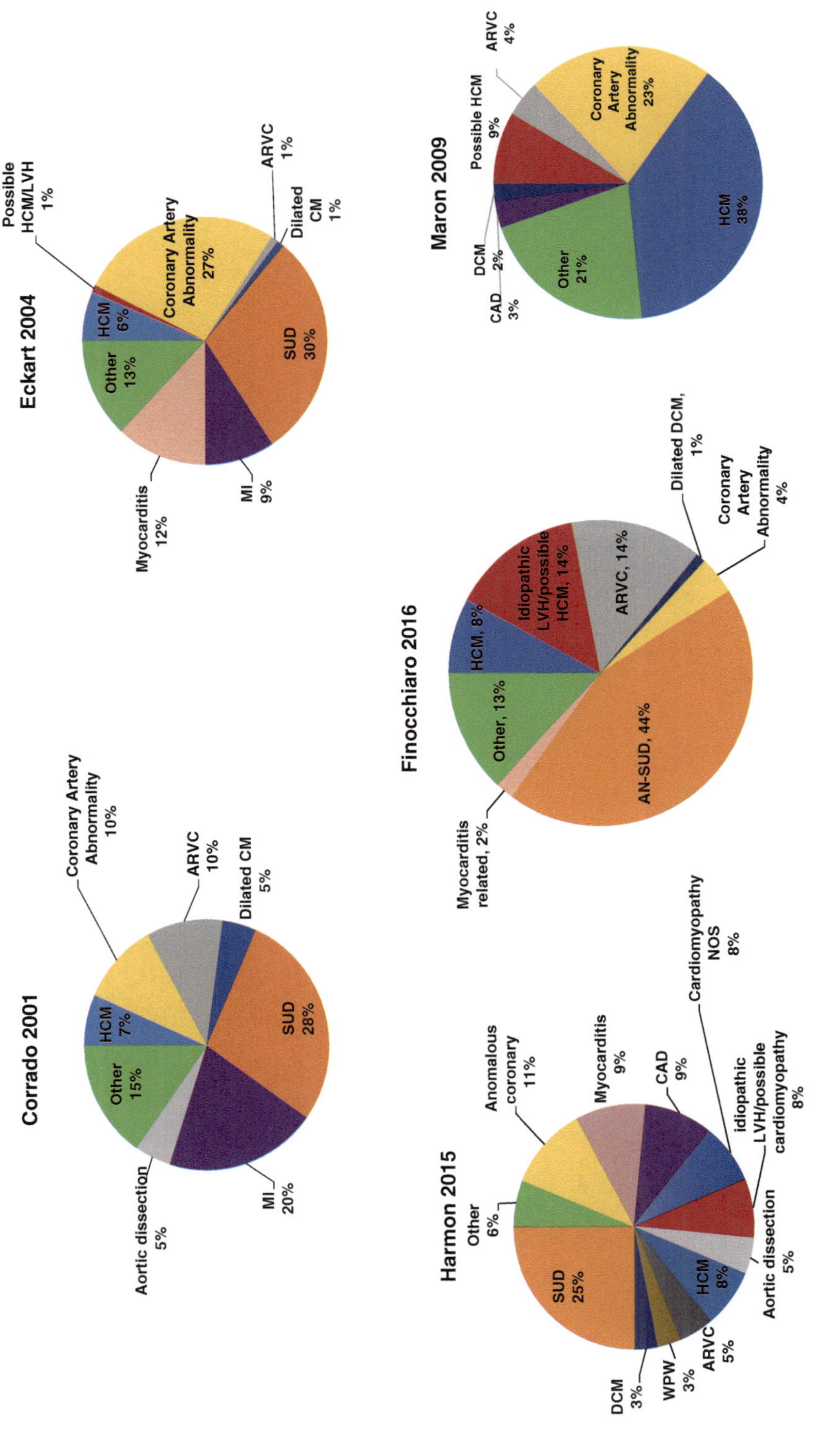


**Fig. 5.1** Graphic comparison of etiology of SCD in athletes. (Created from data reported in [7, 17, 18, 20])

**Table 5.2** Etiologies of sudden cardiac death in athletes

| Study | Years of study | Methods | Autopsy | Country | "Sports-related" or all deaths | Age range | Cases | HCM (%) | Idiopathic LVH/ fibrosis (%) | Coronary artery anomalies (%) | ARVC (%) | DCM (%) | SADS (%) | CAD (%) | Myocarditis related (%) | Aortic dissection (%) | LQTS (%) | WPW (%) | Other (%) |
|---|---|---|---|---|---|---|---|---|---|---|---|---|---|---|---|---|---|---|---|
| Corrado [18] | 1979–1999 | Prospective, mandatory reporting, all deaths in Veneto region | Standard procedure at referral center | Italy | All | 12–35 | 46 | 2 | 0 | 13 | 26 | 2 | 2 | 22 | 11 | 2 | 2 | 0 | 17 |
| De Noronha [19] | 1996–2008 | All cases SCD referred to CRY | Standard procedure at referral center | U.K. | All | 6–34 | 88 | 13 | 32 | 7 | 10 | 0 | 30 | 0 | 3 | 0 | 0 | 0 | 6 |
| Maron [20] | 1980–2006 | Retrospective, registry, media reports | Review of available autopsy, 359 had either pathologically normal heart or autopsy unavailable | U.S. | All—includes SCA | 8–39 | 1049 | 24 | 5 | 11 | 3 | 1 | 34 | 2 | 4 | 2 | 2 | 1 | 10 |
| Holst [10] | 2000–2006 | Retrospective, death certificates | Autopsy reports, hospital records | Denmark | Sports-related | 12–35 | 14 | 0 | 7 | 7 | 29 | 0 | 29 | 14 | 7 | 0 | 0 | 0 | 7 |
| Suarez-Mier [21] | 1995–2010 | All cases of SCD referred to National Institute of Forensic Sciences of Madrid | Standard procedure at referral center | Spain | Sports-related | 9–35 | 81 | 10 | 9 | 6 | 15 | 0 | 23 | 14 | 5 | 0 | 0 | 0 | 19 |
| Harmon [7] | 2003–2013 | Retrospective, media reports, NCAA database | Autopsy reports, ancillary reports | U.S. | All | 18–26 | 64 | 8 | 17 | 11 | 5 | 3 | 25 | 9 | 9 | 5 | 2 | 3 | 3 |
| Finochiaro [17] | 1994–2014 | All cases SCD referred to CRY | Standard procedure at referral center | U.K. | All | 18–35 | 179 | 8 | 14 | 4 | 14 | 1 | 44 | 0 | 2 | 0 | 0 | 0 | 13 |
| Bohm [12] | 2012–2014 | Retrospective | Media reports, registry | Germany | Sports-related | 10–34 | 29 | 7 | 3 | 10 | 3 | 3 | 17 | 21 | 31 | 0 | 0 | 0 | 3 |
| Harmon [26] | 2007–2013 | Retrospective, media reports | Autopsy reports | U.S. | All | 14–18 | 50 | 14 | 28 | 8 | 2 | 0 | 18 | 6 | 14 | 0 | 0 | 0 | 12 |
| Peterson [22] | 2014–2016 | Media reports, reports to NCCSIR | Autopsy reports | U.S. | All | 11–29 | 83 | 18 | 16 | 16 | 5 | 5 | 10 | 2 | 4 | 6 | 4 | 2 | 13 |
| Total | | | | | | | 1683 | 19 | 9 | 10 | 6 | 1 | 31 | 4 | 5 | 2 | 2 | 1 | 10 |

  - ECG will detect 93% of HCM [24] if suspected, a cardiac MRI is indicated as echocardiogram may miss apical hypertrophy, the most common variant in athletes [25].
  - Exercise increases the risk of ventricular tachycardia/fibrillation and is a modifiable risk factor. Shared-decision making for return-to-play is becoming more common, however, it should be noted that there are multiple cases of SCD after returning to play with HCM [15, 23]. An in-depth discussion of risks, including death, should be part of the decision-making process (see also Chap. 14).
- Idiopathic left ventricular hypertrophy/fibrosis (ILVH)
  - In studies examining the pathogenesis of SCD, there is an increasingly recognized category of ILVH or fibrosis, sometimes referred to as possible cardiomyopathy [7, 17, 26].
  - These hearts are sometimes larger than expected for age, weight and height but do not meet other pathologic criteria to be categorized as HCM, i.e. there is no myocyte disarray.
  - These hearts can also be normal sized with myocyte hypertrophy and fibrosis present.
  - It is unclear if this is an early expression of HCM, another entity or acquired response to exercise.
- Arrhythmogenic cardiomyopathy (AC)
  - Prevalence in population is 1 in 5000 [27].
  - Estimated to cause 3–29% of athlete SCDs [7, 10, 12, 14, 17–22].
  - Formerly characterized as arrhythmogenic right ventricular cardiomyopathy, there is increasing recognition as a biventricular entity [27].
  - AC is an inherited muscle disorder characterized by myocardial fibro-fatty replacement.
  - Exercise causes progression of disease and should be avoided after diagnosis (see Chap. 15) [28, 29].
- Dilated cardiomyopathy
  - Prevalence in population is 1 in 2500.
  - Dilated cardiomyopathy can be the end stage of other cardiomyopathies such as HCM or arrhythmogenic cardiomyopathy.
  - Less commonly diagnosed in athletes; 0–5% [7, 10, 12, 14, 17–22].
- Coronary artery anomalies
  - Causes 4–16% of SCD in athletes [7, 10, 12, 14, 17–22].
  - Abnormal origin of the left coronary artery arising from the right sinus of Valsalva is most common.
  - Other features that may contribute to ischemia during exercise include an acute angled take-off, hypoplastic ostium, or impingement of the anomalous artery as it traverses between the expanding great vessels during exercise.
  - May cause chest pain or exertional syncope.
  - Not detected with ECG. Transthoracic echocardiogram can visualize the coronary ostia in up to 98% of athletes [30].
  - Depending on abnormality, may be surgically repaired with successful return to play (see Chap. 22).
- Aortic rupture
  - Aortic rupture accounts for 0–6% of SCD in athletes and is usually associated with Marfan Syndrome [7, 10, 12, 14, 17–22].

  - Marfan Syndrome can cause progressive dilatation and weakness (cystic medial necrosis) of proximal aorta and myxomatous degeneration of mitral and aortic valves.
  - An echocardiogram to assess aortic diameter should be obtained in those with typical Marfanoid features (see also Chap. 7).
  - Return to play should be guided by a specialist familiar with aortic root pathology and is based on aortic dimensions and pathological features of the disease.
- Coronary artery disease (CAD)
  - Coronary heart disease is the leading cause of death in adults.
  - SCD due to CAD in athletes increases precipitously after age 25 and is the most frequent cause of cardiac disease in athletes after the age of 30 [13].
  - In general, exercise is protective from CAD, however exercise may be a stimulus for plaque disruption.
  - Recent studies of endurance athletes show a higher burden of coronary artery calcium than sedentary controls, however, the plaque appears predominantly calcific and more stable compared to mixed plaques which are prone to rupture (see also Chap. 32) [31].
- Myocarditis
  - Acute inflammatory process involving the myocardium. Coxsackie B virus is implicated in more than 50% of cases, but echovirus, adenovirus, influenza, and *Chlamydia pneumoniae* have also been associated with myocarditis.
  - Reported as the cause of death in 2–31% in studies of SCD in athletes [7, 10, 12, 14, 17–22].
  - Pathologic features include lymphocytic infiltrate of myocardium with necrosis or degeneration of adjacent myocytes.
  - Acute phase presents with flu-like illness, which may lead to dilated cardiomyopathy. SCD may occur in the presence of either active or healed myocarditis.
  - Characteristic symptoms include prodromal viral illness followed by progressive exercise intolerance and congestive symptoms of dyspnea, cough and orthopnea.
  - ECG may show diffuse low voltage, ST and T wave changes, heart block, or ventricular arrhythmias. Laboratory tests include leukocytosis, eosinophilia, elevated sedimentation rate or C-reactive protein, and increased myocardial enzymes. Echocardiography may show dilated LV, global hypokinesis, segmental wall abnormalities, and decreased LV ejection fraction.
  - Athletes with myocarditis should not exercise. Resolution is variable. Return to sports should not be considered until 3–6 months after onset of illness and ventricular systolic function has returned to normal, serum markers of myocardial injury have normalized, and clinically relevant arrhythmias are absent (see also Chap. 20).
- Sudden arrhythmic death syndrome (SADS)/Sudden unexplained death
  - A diagnosis of exclusion with a morphologically normal heart, normal histopathology, and negative toxicology screened. Presumed to be cardiac related to arrhythmia.

 - SADS in athletes is cited as a cause of death in 2–44% of cases [7, 10, 12, 14, 17–22].
 - Diagnoses that are represented in this category include channelopathies including Long QT Syndrome (LQTS) and Brugada Syndrome, and conduction abnormalities such as WPW (see also Chap. 21).
- LQTS
 - Most common channelopathy.
 - Characterized by prolongation of ventricular repolarization and QT interval corrected for heart rate.
 - Syncope or presyncope related to physical exertion or emotional stress may occur.
 - Family history of SADS, unexplained drowning or motor vehicle accident or sudden infant death should prompt further evaluation
 - In an asymptomatic athlete without a family history of SCD, current cutoffs for screening ECG are a $QT_c$ of 470 ms in males and 480 ms in females.
 - A prolonged $QT_c$ on an ECG does not equate to a diagnosis of LQTS. LQTS is a clinical diagnosed based on a number of criteria.
 - Return to play decisions should be guided by a heart rhythm specialist or genetic cardiologist experienced in the care of athletes. A shared decision making model should be used after the institution of treatment.
- Brugada Syndrome
 - A rare channelopathy more prevalent in males from Southeast Asia.
 - Caused by abnormalities in the sodium channels.
 - May present as syncope or sudden death while sleeping.
 - ECG shows a pattern of right bundle branch block and ST-segment elevation in leads $V_1$ to $V_3$.
 - Shared decision making for return to play should be implemented after appropriate treatment has been instituted.
- Catecholaminergic Polymorphic Ventricular Tachycardia (CPVT)
 - Inherited disorder characterized by stress-induced ventricular arrhythmias in children and young adults.
 - Caused by abnormalities in calcium channel function.
 - Syncope, sudden death, and polymorphic ventricular tachycardia can be precipitated by vigorous physical exertion or acute emotion.
 - Resting ECG is normal. Exertion or epinephrine challenge can induce ventricular tachycardia.
- Wolff-Parkinson-White Syndrome (WPW)
 - Most common abnormal finding on ECG in screening programs.
 - WPW is characterized by tachyarrhythmias caused by an accessory pathway (the Bundle of Kent) which directly connects the atria and ventricles and bypasses the AV node. The arrhythmia can be atrioventricular tachycardia (80%), atrial fibrillation (15–20%), or atrial flutter (5%).
 - Symptoms include palpitations, syncope and near-syncope.

- Once diagnosed, risk stratification can be performed.
- Symptomatic and high-risk pathways are candidates for ablation, with subsequent return to competition.

## 5.3 Prevention

Cardiovascular prevention strategies can be divided into two main categories:

1. primary prevention; identifying cardiac conditions that predispose to sudden cardiac arrest and attempting to mitigate risk or
2. secondary prevention; recognizing and treating SCA and preventing death.

### 5.3.1 Primary Prevention in Young Athletes

Some argue that the screening for conditions that predispose to sudden cardiac death in the young athletes is unnecessary, citing the relative infrequency of SCD and the resources required to screen, investigate and manage those with positive findings [11]. However, the incidence of SCD considered should be SCD in athletes occurring anytime, not sports-related sudden death (death occurring when participating in activity), as a substantial proportion of SCD in athletes occurs at rest or while sleeping [7, 17, 32]. There is broad agreement that the goal of cardiovascular screening in athletes is "to prospectively identify or raise suspicion of previously unrecognized and largely genetic congenital cardiovascular diseases known to cause SCA and sudden death in young people" [33–35].

- The American Heart Association and American College of Cardiology considers cardiovascular screening in athletes "justifiable and compelling, based on ethical, legal, and medical grounds" and recommends screening with a 14-point history and physical examination [33].

Others point out limited ability of screening with history and physical examination alone to effectively identify conditions that predispose to SCD or reduce SCD [36–38]. There is a high false positive rate to the screening questions [39].

- The European Society of Cardiology, the International Olympic Committee and most professional sports organizations recommend cardiovascular screening with history and physical as well as 12-lead electrocardiogram (ECG) [34, 40].
  - Previous concerns of a high false positive rate in screening ECGs are no longer valid with improved guidelines for interpreting ECGs in athletes, which account for the physiologic changes with training and have reduced the false positive rate to ~2% without affecting sensitivity [24, 25].

- Screening with ECG greatly improves the sensitivity and specificity of cardiovascular screening [1, 41].
- ECG will detect 2/3–3/4 of conditions that cause SCD.

Decisions on whether and how to screen for cardiovascular conditions that predispose to sudden cardiac death in young athletes should take into account regulations or requirements of sporting organizations, the risk of the population considered, the potential harms and benefits, and the available resources [37].

### 5.3.2 Primary Prevention in Older Athletes

- There is no debate that exercise improves physical health and well-being.
- CAD is the primary cause of death in athletes over 25.
- Screening strategies in older athletes in whom CAD is the primary concern should focus on risk factors for CAD.
- There is evidence that heavy exercisers have higher coronary artery calcium scores than sedentary controls. How this translates to risk is under investigation (see also Chap. 32) [31].

### 5.3.3 Secondary Prevention of SCD

Access to early cardiopulmonary resuscitation (CPR) and early defibrillation is the key to survival of SCA [42]. Recognition of SCA is first step to response.

- Anyone who collapses and is unresponsive should be presumed to have had a SCA.
- Over 50% of athletes with SCA will have tonic-clonic movement of the limbs which is often mistaken for a seizure causing critical delay.
- Agonal breaths or gasps should not be confused with respiration.
- Automated external defibrillators will not deliver shock unless indicated.

Every school or institution that sponsors athletic activities should have a written and structured Emergency Action Plan (EAP).

- The EAP should be developed in conjunction with local emergency medical services, school or venue safety officials, likely first responders, and administrators.
- The EAP should be specific to each venue and provide plans for:
  - A communication system should be in place to activate the emergency medical services (EMS) system, to alert local responders, and to expedite transfer of emergency equipment (AED) to the scene.
  - An identified team of targeted first responders (i.e. coaches, school health officials) should receive training in the recognition of SCA, CPR and AED use.

  - On-site AED programs are ideal and the best means of achieving early defibrillation.
  - Transportation routes for arriving EMS should be defined.
  - The EAP should be practiced at least annually by potential responders to SCA
  - The target time from collapse to first shock should be less than 3 min.

**Clinical Pearls**

- Reports on the incidence of SCD vary widely primarily due to differences in methodology and the population examined.
- Groups that are at higher risk for SCD include males, blacks, and men's basketball, American-style football, and football (soccer).
- The most common causes of SCD appear to be HCM/LVH with fibrosis and SADs. About 2/3 to 3/4 of cardiovascular conditions the cause SCD can be detected with ECG screening.
- No screening program will prevent all SCD, therefore an EAP should be developed and practiced at least annually at venues where sports are played.

## Review

### Questions

1. Which athlete statistically has the highest risk of sudden cardiac death?
   (a) Caucasian female volleyball athlete
   (b) Afro-American/Caribbean female basketball athlete
   (c) Caucasian male football (soccer) athlete
   (d) Afro-American/Caribbean basketball athlete
2. What is the most common cause of sudden cardiac death in athletes over the age of 25?
   (a) Hypertrophic cardiomyopathy
   (b) Sudden arrhythmic death syndrome
   (c) Coronary artery disease
   (d) Coronary artery abnormalities
3. Which primary prevention screening strategy has the highest likelihood of discovering conditions which predispose to SCD in a young athlete?
   (a) History including extensive personal and family history
   (b) ECG
   (c) Echocardiogram
   (d) Physical examination
4. The single most important factor in surviving SCA is
   (a) Early CRP
   (b) Early defibrillation

(c) Prompt arrival of emergency personnel
(d) The underlying cause of the arrest (i.e. hypertrophic cardiomyopathy, coronary artery anomaly, etc.)

## Answers

1. (**d**). The incidence of SCD is much higher in males, Afro-Americans/Caribbeans, and certain sports. Females are consistently demonstrated to be at lower risk for SCD. The highest risk sports include men's basketball, men's football (soccer) and American football. The highest demographic risk carries an Afro-American/Caribbean male basketball athlete.
2. (**c**). In athletes over 25 years, coronary artery disease is the primary cause of SCD. In athletes under 25 there are varying reports. More recent systematic reports suggest that SADS is the most common cause of death while earlier studies suggested HCM.
3. (**b**). Statistically ECG is much more likely to detect underlying cardiac conditions which predispose to SCD than history or physical examination. Although echocardiography has been suggested as a screening tool, it will not detect electrical causes of SCD, and will only detect some structural diseases often missing early or apical HCM.
4. (**b**). Early defibrillation is the primary determinant of survival from cardiac arrest, although early CPR also improves outcomes.

## References

1. Harmon KG, Zigman M, Drezner JA. The effectiveness of screening history, physical exam, and ECG to detect potentially lethal cardiac disorders in athletes: a systematic review/meta-analysis. J Electrocardiol. 2015;48(3):329–38.
2. Maron BJ, Thompson PD, Ackerman MJ, Balady G, Berger S, Cohen D, et al. Recommendations and considerations related to preparticipation screening for cardiovascular abnormalities in competitive athletes: 2007 update: a scientific statement from the American Heart Association Council on Nutrition, Physical Activity, and Metabolism: endorsed by the American College of Cardiology Foundation. Circulation. 2007;115(12):1643–455.
3. Drezner JA, Prutkin JM, Harmon KG, O'Kane JW, Pelto HF, Rao AL, et al. Cardiovascular screening in college athletes. J Am Coll Cardiol. 2015;65(21):2353–5.
4. Corrado D, Basso C, Pavei A, Michieli P, Schiavon M, Thiene G. Trends in sudden cardiovascular death in young competitive athletes after implementation of a preparticipation screening program. JAMA. 2006;296(13):1593–601.
5. Toresdahl BG, Rao AL, Harmon KG, Drezner JA. Incidence of sudden cardiac arrest in high school student athletes on school campus. Heart Rhythm. 2014;11(7):1190–4.
6. Corrado D, Migliore F, Basso C, Thiene G. Exercise and the risk of sudden cardiac death. Herz. 2006;31(6):553–8.
7. Harmon K, Asif IM, Maleszewski JJ, Owens DS, Prutkin JM, Salerno JC, et al. Incidence, cause, and comparative frequency of sudden cardiac death in National Collegiate Athletic Association athletes: a decade in review. Circulation. 2015;132(1):10–9.
8. Harmon KG, Asif IM, Klossner D, Drezner JA. Incidence of sudden cardiac death in National Collegiate Athletic Association athletes. Circulation. 2011;123(15):1594–600.

9. Roberts WO, Stovitz SD. Incidence of sudden cardiac death in Minnesota high school athletes 1993–2012 screened with a standardized pre-participation evaluation. J Am Coll Cardiol. 2013;62(14):1298–301.
10. Holst AG, Winkel BG, Theilade J, Kristensen IB, Thomsen JL, Ottesen GL, et al. Incidence and etiology of sports-related sudden cardiac death in Denmark—implications for preparticipation screening. Heart Rhythm. 2010;7(10):1365–71.
11. Risgaard B, Winkel BG, Jabbari R, Glinge C, Ingemann-Hansen O, Thomsen JL, et al. Sports-related sudden cardiac death in a competitive and a noncompetitive athlete population aged 12 to 49 years: data from an unselected nationwide study in Denmark. Heart Rhythm. 2014;11(10):1673–81.
12. Bohm P, Scharhag J, Meyer T. Data from a nationwide registry on sports-related sudden cardiac deaths in Germany. Eur J Prev Cardiol. 2016;23(6):649–56.
13. Winkel BG, Holst AG, Theilade J, Kristensen IB, Thomsen JL, Ottesen GL, et al. Nationwide study of sudden cardiac death in persons aged 1–35 years. Eur Heart J. 2011;32(8):983–90.
14. Harmon KG, Asif IM, Ellenbogen R, Drezner J. The incidence of sudden cardiac arrest in United States high school athletes. Br J Sports Med. 2014;48(7):605.
15. Chatard JC, Espinosa F, Donnadieu R, Grangeon JP, Sabot JM, Guivarch C, et al. Preparticipation cardiovascular evaluation in Pacific Island athletes. Int J Cardiol. 2019;278:273–9.
16. Malhotra A, Dhutia H, Finocchiaro G, Gati S, Beasley I, Clift P, et al. Outcomes of cardiac screening in adolescent soccer players. N Engl J Med. 2018;379(6):524–34.
17. Finocchiaro G, Papadakis M, Robertus JL, Dhutia H, Steriotis AK, Tome M, et al. Etiology of sudden death in sports: insights from a United Kingdom regional registry. J Am Coll Cardiol. 2016;67(18):2108–15.
18. Corrado D, Basso C, Rizzoli G, Schiavon M, Thiene G. Does sports activity enhance the risk of sudden death in adolescents and young adults? J Am Coll Cardiol. 2003;42(11):1959–63.
19. de Noronha SV, Sharma S, Papadakis M, Desai S, Whyte G, Sheppard MN. Aetiology of sudden cardiac death in athletes in the United Kingdom: a pathological study. Heart. 2009;95(17):1409–14.
20. Maron BJ, Doerer JJ, Haas TS, Tierney DM, Mueller FO. Sudden deaths in young competitive athletes. Analysis of 1866 deaths in the United States, 1980–2006. Circulation. 2009;119:1085–92.
21. Suarez-Mier MP, Aguilera B, Mosquera RM, Sanchez-de-Leon MS. Pathology of sudden death during recreational sports in Spain. Forensic Sci Int. 2013;226(1–3):188–96.
22. Peterson DF, Siebert DM, Kucera KL, Thomas LC, Maleszewski JJ, Lopez-Anderson M, et al. Etiology of sudden cardiac arrest and death in US competitive athletes: a 2-year prospective surveillance study. Clin J Sport Med. 2018; https://doi.org/10.1097/JSM.0000000000000598.
23. Malhotra R, West JJ, Dent J, Luna M, Kramer CM, Mounsey JP, et al. Cost and yield of adding electrocardiography to history and physical in screening Division I intercollegiate athletes: a 5-year experience. Heart Rhythm. 2011;8(5):721–7.
24. Zorzi A, Calore C, Vio R, Pelliccia A, Corrado D. Accuracy of the ECG for differential diagnosis between hypertrophic cardiomyopathy and athlete's heart: comparison between the European Society of Cardiology (2010) and International (2017) criteria. Br J Sports Med. 2018;52(10):667–73.
25. Drezner JA, Sharma S, Baggish A, Papadakis M, Wilson MG, Prutkin JM, et al. International criteria for electrocardiographic interpretation in athletes: consensus statement. Br J Sports Med. 2017;51(9):704–31.
26. Harmon KG, Asif IM, Maleszewski JJ, Owens DS, Prutkin JM, Salerno JC, et al. Incidence and etiology of sudden cardiac arrest and death in high school athletes in the United States. Mayo Clin Proc. 2016;91(11):1493–502.
27. Miles C, Finocchiaro G, Papadakis M, Gray B, Westaby J, Ensam B, et al. Sudden death and left ventricular involvement in arrhythmogenic cardiomyopathy. Circulation. 2019;139(15):1786–97.
28. James CA, Bhonsale A, Tichnell C, Murray B, Russell SD, Tandri H, et al. Exercise increases age-related penetrance and arrhythmic risk in arrhythmogenic right ventricular

dysplasia/cardiomyopathy-associated desmosomal mutation carriers. J Am Coll Cardiol. 2013;62(14):1290–7.
29. Sawant AC, Bhonsale A, te Riele AS, Tichnell C, Murray B, Russell SD, et al. Exercise has a disproportionate role in the pathogenesis of arrhythmogenic right ventricular dysplasia/cardiomyopathy in patients without desmosomal mutations. J Am Heart Assoc. 2014;3(6):e001471.
30. Hoyt WJ, Dean PN, Schneider DS, Conaway MR, Kramer CM, Battle RW. Coronary artery evaluation by screening echocardiogram in intercollegiate athletes. Med Sci Sports Exerc. 2017;49(5):863–9.
31. Merghani A, Maestrini V, Rosmini S, Cox AT, Dhutia H, Bastiaenan R, et al. Prevalence of subclinical coronary artery disease in masters endurance athletes with a low atherosclerotic risk profile. Circulation. 2017;136(2):126–37.
32. Johri AM, Poirier P, Dorian P, Fournier A, Goodman JM, McKinney J, et al. Canadian Cardiovascular Society/Canadian Heart Rhythm Society joint position statement on the cardiovascular screening of competitive athletes. Can J Cardiol. 2019;35(1):1–11.
33. Maron BJ, Friedman RA, Kligfield P, Levine BD, Viskin S, Chaitman BR, et al. Assessment of the 12-lead ECG as a screening test for detection of cardiovascular disease in healthy general populations of young people (12–25 years of age): a scientific statement from the American Heart Association and the American College of Cardiology. Circulation. 2014;130(15):1303–34.
34. Ljungqvist A, Jenoure P, Engebretsen L, Alonso JM, Bahr R, Clough A, et al. The International Olympic Committee (IOC) consensus statement on periodic health evaluation of elite athletes March 2009. Br J Sports Med. 2009;43(9):631–43.
35. American Academy of Family Physicians, American Academy of Pediatrics, American College of Sports Medicine, American Medical Society for Sports Medicine, American Orthopaedic Society for Sports Medicine, American Osteopathic Academy for Sports Medicine. PPE preparticipation physical evaluation. 4th ed. Elk Grove, IL: American Academy of Pediatrics; 2010.
36. Maron BJ, Shirani J, Poliac LC, Mathenge R, Roberts WC, Mueller FO. Sudden death in young competitive athletes. Clinical, demographic, and pathological profiles. JAMA. 1996;276(3):199–204.
37. Drezner JA, O'Connor FG, Harmon KG, Fields KB, Asplund CA, Asif IM, et al. AMSSM position statement on cardiovascular preparticipation screening in athletes: current evidence, knowledge gaps, recommendations and future directions. Br J Sports Med. 2016;26(5):347–61.
38. Hainline B, Drezner J, Baggish A, Harmon KG, Emery MS, Myerburg RJ, et al. Interassociation consensus statement on cardiovascular care of college student-athletes. Br J Sports Med. 2017;51(2):74–85.
39. Fudge J, Harmon KG, Owens DS, Prutkin JM, Salerno JC, Asif IM, et al. Cardiovascular screening in adolescents and young adults: a prospective study comparing the pre-participation physical evaluation monograph 4th edition and ECG. Br J Sports Med. 2014;48(15):1172–8.
40. Corrado D, Pelliccia A, Bjornstad HH, Vanhees L, Biffi A, Borjesson M, et al. Cardiovascular pre-participation screening of young competitive athletes for prevention of sudden death: proposal for a common European protocol. Consensus statement of the study Group of Sport Cardiology of the Working Group of Cardiac Rehabilitation and Exercise Physiology and the Working Group of Myocardial and Pericardial Diseases of the European Society of Cardiology. Eur Heart J. 2005;26(5):516–24.
41. Alattar A, Maffulli N. The validity of adding ECG to the preparticipation screening of athletes an evidence based literature review. Transl Med UniSa. 2015;11:2–13.
42. Larsen MP, Eisenberg MS, Cummins RO, Hallstrom AP. Predicting survival from out-of-hospital cardiac arrest: a graphic model. Ann Emerg Med. 1993;22(11):1652–8.
43. Van Camp SP, Bloor CM, Mueller FO, Cantu RC, Olson HG. Nontraumatic sports death in high school and college athletes. Med Sci Sports Exerc. 1995;27(5):641–7.
44. Maron BJ, Gohman TE, Aeppli D. Prevalence of sudden cardiac death during competitive sports activities in Minnesota high school athletes. J Am Coll Cardiol. 1998;32(7):1881–4.

45. Drezner JA, Rogers KJ, Zimmer RR, Sennett BJ. Use of automated external defibrillators at NCAA division I universities. Med Sci Sports Exerc. 2005;37(9):1487–92.
46. Drezner JA, Rao AL, Heistand J, Bloomingdale MK, Harmon KG. Effectiveness of emergency response planning for sudden cardiac arrest in United States high schools with automated external defibrillators. Circulation. 2009;120(6):518–25.
47. Marijon E, Tafflet M, Celermajer DS, Dumas F, Perier MC, Mustafic H, et al. Sports-related sudden death in the general population. Circulation. 2011;124(6):672–81.
48. Steinvil A, Chundadze T, Zeltser D, Rogowski O, Halkin A, Galily Y, et al. Mandatory electrocardiographic screening of athletes to reduce their risk for sudden death proven fact or wishful thinking? J Am Coll Cardiol. 2011;57(11):1291–6.
49. Maron BJ, Haas TS, Ahluwalia A, Rutten-Ramos SC. Incidence of cardiovascular sudden deaths in Minnesota high school athletes. Heart Rhythm. 2013;10(3):374–7.
50. Maron BJ, Haas TS, Murphy CJ, Ahluwalia A, Rutten-Ramos S. Incidence and causes of sudden death in U.S. college athletes. J Am Coll Cardiol. 2014;63(16):1636–43.
51. Drezner JA, Harmon KG, Marek JC. Incidence of sudden cardiac arrest in Minnesota high school student athletes: the limitations of catastrophic insurance claims. J Am Coll Cardiol. 2014;63(14):1455–6.
52. Grani C, Chappex N, Fracasso T, Vital C, Kellerhals C, Schmied C, et al. Sports-related sudden cardiac death in Switzerland classified by static and dynamic components of exercise. Eur J Prev Cardiol. 2016;23(11):1228–36.
53. Maron BJ, Haas TS, Duncanson ER, Garberich RF, Baker AM, Mackey-Bojack S. Comparison of the frequency of sudden cardiovascular deaths in young competitive athletes versus nonathletes: should we really screen only athletes? Am J Cardiol. 2016;117(8):1339–41.

# Medical Evaluation of Athletes: Medical History and Physical Examination

6

Hanne K. Rasmusen and Christian M. Schmied

**Learning Objectives**

1. To recognize "red flags" in an athlete's personal, systemic and family history.
2. To know the cornerstones of an accurate physical examination of athletes.
3. To understand and be able to classify the implications of specific clinical findings.
4. To recognize the limitations of the assessment of medical history and clinical examination in athletic populations.

## 6.1 Personal History/Symptoms

The clinical importance of personal, systemic and family medical history in athletic populations is apparent, but its accuracy very much depends on the particular circumstances. The yield of a questionnaire during pre-participation screening is sparse, with about two-thirds of the athletes indicating symptoms but with finally less than two percent leading to a cardiac diagnosis [1] (Fig. 6.1). This highlights the pivotal role of an experienced physician in classifying and clearing these subjective symptoms in order to prevent unnecessary anxiety and further examinations. On the other hand, athletes referred from their general practitioner because of particular cardiac symptoms have a high yield of 44% for having a cardiac diagnosis [2].

- Independent of the setting, the athlete's symptoms should always be evaluated in the context of personal and family history, as well as physical examination and the 12-lead ECG.

H. K. Rasmusen (✉)
Department of Cardiology, Bispebjerg-Frederiksberg Hospital, Copenhagen, Denmark
e-mail: hras0044@regionh.dk

C. M. Schmied
Department of Cardiology, University Heart Center Zurich, Zurich, Switzerland
e-mail: christian.schmied@usz.ch



A. Pressler, J. Niebauer (eds.), *Textbook of Sports and Exercise Cardiology*,
https://doi.org/10.1007/978-3-030-35374-2_6

| Physical Activity Readiness Questionnaire (PAR-Q) | | |
|---|---|---|
| Question | | Answer |
| 1. | Has your doctor ever said that you have a heart condition and that you should only do physical activity recommended by a doctor? | ☐ YES ☐ NO |
| 2. | Do you feel pain in your chest when you do physical activity? | ☐ YES ☐ NO |
| 3. | In the past month, have you had chest pain when you were not doing physical activity? | ☐ YES ☐ NO |
| 4. | Do you lose your balance because of dizziness or do you ever lose consciousness? | ☐ YES ☐ NO |
| 5. | Do you have a bone or joint problem (for example, back, knee or hip) that could be made worse by a change in your physical activity? | ☐ YES ☐ NO |
| 6. | Is your doctor currently prescribing drugs (for example, water pills) for your blood pressure or heart condition? | ☐ YES ☐ NO |
| 7. | Do you know of any other reason why you should not do physical activity? | ☐ YES ☐ NO |
| **YES** to one or more questions: medical examination reasonable before becoming much more physically active | | |

**Fig. 6.1** The Physical Activity Readiness Questionnaire (PAR-Q) as a classic example of a questionnaire designed to evaluate symptoms or conditions indicative of an increased risk during sports. This and similar, modified questionnaires are frequently recommended by various scientific or commercial sporting associations as a pre-participation screening tool (e.g. German Society of Sports Medicine, www.dgsp.de)

## 6.2 Syncope/Near-Syncope

The most alarming symptom among athletes is syncope. This is defined as

- "a sudden transient loss of consciousness and postural tone due to transient global cerebral hypoperfusion, characterized by rapid onset, short duration and spontaneous complete recovery" [3].

A syncope is not uncommon among athletes, as shown recently by Colivicchi and coworkers [4] on n = 7568 athletes undergoing pre-participation screening. A syncopal episode was reported in 6.2% within the preceding 5 years, but only 13.3% of these episodes were related to exercise (i.e. post-exertional in 12.0%, and during exercise in only 1.3%). At follow-up, those athletes with an exercise-unrelated syncope had a diagnosis of either vasovagal or situational syncope. Unlike post-exertional syncope, 50% of syncopal episodes occurring during exertion were cardiogenic, either due to structural heart disease or primary arrhythmia, and these causes are also associated with an increased risk of sudden cardiac death (SCD) [5].

- Exercise-related syncope is a red flag symptom that always warrants thorough and rapid evaluation.

Evaluation of an exercise-induced syncope should include obtaining a thorough history of circumstances related to its occurrence, including objective or subjective warning signs prior to the event (e.g. sweating, nausea, palpitations, chest pain), single or multiple appearance, duration, and state of mind at recovery. It should also be assessed whether the syncope had occurred during long-distance exercise with possible electrolyte derangement, during specific activities (e.g. swimming or sudden and loud noises as typically being associated with the long QT syndrome), during fever or after exercise in high temperature as observed in the Brugada syndrome, or after a blunt chest trauma as seen in commotio cordis. A syncope leading to an injury suggests cardiac, arrhythmogenic etiology.

Further issues that need to be evaluated within the diagnostic pathway are:

1. Use of medication and stimulants.
2. Familiar predisposition to early sudden unexplained death or cardiac disease.
3. Clinical examination with focus on cardiac murmurs (see below).
4. 12-lead ECG and, at least, 24 h of continuous Holter monitoring.
5. Basic clinical chemistry: hemoglobin, electrolytes, D-dimer and cardiac biomarkers.
6. Echocardiography including the detection of coronary ostia.
7. Exercise test if still uncertain or if symptoms have clearly been exercise-related, important to encourage to maximum exercise, preferably applying cardiopulmonary exercise testing (CPET)
8. Coronary computed (CT) angiography if coronary anomaly or coronary artery disease is suspected.
9. Cardiac magnetic resonance imaging (MRI) if possible and if structural disease is suspected, especially e.g. right heart disease as Arrhythmogenic Cardiomyopathy or apical Hypertrophic Cardiomyopathy (HCM; see Chaps. 14 and 15).
10. If still unclear: Loop recorder implantation.
11. Electrophysiologic examination for risk assessment (debatable).

## 6.3 Exertional Chest Pain/Discomfort

During lifetime, thoracic pain is experienced in 40–60% of adults in the general population and possibly similarly frequent in athletes [2, 6]. Fortunately, chest pain is most often benign and of non-cardiac origin, but in the acute setting the initial assessment is to rule-out potentially life-threatening causes. The most common cardiac cause of chest pain is ischemic heart disease (IHD) therefore the initial assessment includes assessment of risk factors for IHD:

- Age
- Gender
- Smoking history
- Plasma lipids
- Familiar predisposition
- Further cardiovascular risk factors

Other diagnostic considerations are pulmonary embolism, cardiomyopathies, peri-myocarditis, coronary anomaly, aortic stenosis (in young athletes often caused

**Table 6.1** Common causes of chest pain

| | |
|---|---|
| *Cardiac causes* | |
| Structural heart disease | • Ischemic heart disease<br>• Cardiomyopathy |
| Congenital | • Coronary artery anomaly<br>• Bicuspid aortic valve leading to premature aortic stenosis |
| Drug-induced | • Cocaine<br>• Other substances used for performance-enhancing purposes |
| Inherited | • Familial hypercholesterolemia leading to premature ischemic heart disease<br>• Marfan syndrome with aortic dissection |
| Infectious | • Perimyocarditis |
| Valvular | • Aortic stenosis |
| Traumatic | • Commotio cordis |
| Autoimmune | • Kawasaki disease (coronary aneurysms) |
| *Non-cardiac causes* | |
| Muscular-skeletal | • Costochondritis<br>• Intercostal/Serratus anterior strain<br>• Rib stress fracture |
| Gastrointestinal | • Gastroesophagal reflux<br>• Peptic ulcer<br>• Hiatal hernia |
| Respiratory | • Asthma (including exercise-induced)<br>• Pneumothorax (spontanously or traumatic)<br>• Pulmonary embolism<br>• Pleuritis<br>• Pneumonia |
| Miscellaneous | • Malignancy<br>• Herpes zoster<br>• Psychogenic (e.g. anxiety) |

prematurely by bicuspid aortic valve), mitral valve prolapse or aortic dissection (usually associated with systemic disease such as the Marfan syndrome). The main causes of acute chest pain in younger athletes origin from the muscular-skeletal system and the lungs [7], whereas in adults acute coronary syndrome, gastrointestinal disease, muscular-skeletal origin and (less common) pericarditis, pneumonia and pulmonary embolism should be suspected [8] (Table 6.1).

- In general, chest pain among athletes is often an unspecific symptom of non-cardiac origin such as gastroesophageal reflux, asthma or muscular-skeletal pain.
- Nonetheless, it should always be evaluated thoroughly to exclude any cardiac cause, given the significance of sudden cardiac arrest in this population.

## 6.4 Dyspnea and/or Reduced Exercise Capacity

Among athletes, exercise-induced shortness of breath is usually reported as reduced exercise capacity. If reported with concurrent symptoms as coughing and wheezing there is often a pulmonary cause such as exercise-induced asthma or vocal cord abnormalities [9].

- With a prevalence of 8%, asthma or airway hyperreagibility are the most common chronic medical conditions among Olympic athletes [10].

If a cardiac cause is suspected, cardiomyopathy should particularly be excluded in younger athletes whereas in older ones the prevalence of coronary artery disease poses the main risk factor for acute cardiac events during exercise (see Chap. 6). If a murmur appears, valvular heart disease (bicuspid aortic valve leading to premature aortic stenosis or regurgitation, or mitral valve prolapse), or innate cardiac disease (atrial or (less common) ventricular septal defects) should be suspected. Coarctatio aortae should particularly be considered if reduced exercise capacity is combined with blood pressure differences between upper and lower extremities and if additional symptoms such as abdominal angina and early fatigue of the legs during exercise are present. It also sometimes coincides with bicuspid aortic valve (see Chap. 24).

## 6.5 Palpitations

There is not a clear definition of palpitations but the symptom is often described by the athlete as an increased awareness of their own heartbeat [11]. Palpitations are common in athletes [2], and the symptom can represent the whole spectrum from benign ectopic beats to life-threatening ventricular tachycardia. To distinguish the different conditions it can often be helpful to ask the athlete to tap the rhythm of their palpitations or to choose from a range of rhythms tapped by the physician [12]. Palpitations followed by other cardiac symptoms such as lightheadedness or even syncope as well as shortness of breath most likely indicate a significant clinical arrhythmia. Correspondingly, it is important whether the palpitations are

- fast or slow
- regular or irregular
- start and terminate abruptly or gradually
- triggered by exercise or other external or internal factors.

Palpitations can be of *cardiac* or *non-cardiac* origin. The *cardiac* causes can either be secondary to structural heart disease or represent a primary cardiac arrhythmia. The structural conditions that can enhance cardiac irritability are most often due to cardiomyopathy (inherited as well as acquired), ischemic heart disease or valvular disease. The primary cardiac arrhythmias are of supraventricular and ventricular origin and include genetic channelopathies such as the Long QT syndrome, Brugada syndrome and Catecholaminergic Polymorphic Ventricular Tachycardia (CPVT; see Chap. 21). The *non-cardiac* causes of palpitations are often due to

- reactive sinus tachycardia caused by systemic disease (e.g. thyroid disease and anemia),
- psychosomatic disorders (e.g. anxiety, depression and panic attacks) and
- medication or drugs (e.g. alcohol, caffeine, performance-enhancing drugs/stimulants).

The most common cause of palpitations among athletes at rest are ectopic beats that decrease during exercise. Supraventricular arrhythmias are often influenced by vagal maneuvers, with a temporary reduction in heart rate or sudden interruption. In contrast, ventricular arrhythmias remain unaffected. Among middle-aged male master athletes, atrial fibrillation is up to five times more common than in age-matched non-athletes [13] (see Chap. 34). Athletes often suffer from irregular heart rhythm, associated weakness, fatigue and polyuria (as an effect of increased secretion of atrial natriuretic peptide).

Beyond medical history and physical examination, further clinical evaluation should always include ECG and echocardiography, and if no signs of structural heart disease are found, they should be followed by exercise testing and/or Holter monitoring. If the symptoms cannot be correlated to a specific finding during these tests, loop recorders or similar devices could be considered.

## 6.6 Family History

Obtaining a family history is of crucial importance as many of the causes of sudden cardiac arrest or death in young athletes are due to inherited cardiac disease. The goal of the investigation is to identify athletes at higher risk for inherited cardiovascular disorders. These include cardiomyopathies, valvular heart disease, channelopathies and other primary arrhythmic disturbances. Many of these diseases carry autosomal-dominant inheritance patterns; thus, a family history can specify the evaluation.

- If there is a positive family history of sudden unexplained death before the age of 50 years it is of utmost importance to obtain further information for risk assessment and stratification of the athlete.

This includes creating a pedigree to clarify the exact relation of the family member who died, getting an overview of who could be at risk and, if possible, clarifying the exact circumstances and cause of death from the deceased (e.g. autopsy). First degree relatives of SCD victims are at highest risk, as shown in a recent Danish study [14], and if genetic testing reveals positive findings it can be followed with family cascade screening.

## 6.7 Physical Examination

There is an ongoing debate about the ideal screening concept to prevent SCD in sport. The crux of the matter is the inclusion of an ECG, and most of the sports and cardiologic associations, like the European Society of Cardiology (ESC), the International Olympic Committee (IOC), the Federation Internationale de Football Association (FIFA), and various U.S. professional sporting organizations recommend a cardiac screening integrating an ECG.

However, the American Heart Association (AHA) still stands with a more traditional concept, using a 14-point personal and family history questionnaire (Fig. 6.2)

| The 14-Element AHA Recommendations | |
|---|---|
| Medical history* | |
| Personal history | |
| 1. | Chest pain/discomfort/tightness/pressure related to exertion |
| 2. | Unexplained syncope/near-syncope† |
| 3. | Excessive and unexplained dyspnea/fatigue or palpitations, associated with exercise |
| 4. | Prior recognition of a heart murmur |
| 5. | Elevated systemic blood pressure |
| 6. | Prior restriction from participation in sports |
| 7. | Prior testing for the heart, ordered by a physician |
| Family history | |
| 8. | Premature death (sudden and unexpected, or otherwise) before 50 years of age attributable to heart disease in ≥ 1 relative |
| 9. | Disability from heart disease in close relative < 50 years of age |
| 10. | Hypertrophic or dilated cardiomyopathy, long-QT syndrome, or other ion channelopathies, Marfan syndrome, or clinically significant arrhythmias; specific knowledge of genetic cardiac conditions in family members |
| Physical examination | |
| 11. | Heart murmur‡ |
| 12. | Femoral pulses to exclude aortic coarctation |
| 13. | Physical stigmata of Marfan syndrome |
| 14. | Brachial artery blood pressure (sitting position)§ |

•Parental verification is recommended for high school and middle school athletes. †Judged not to be of neurocardiogenic (vasovagal) origin: of particular concern when occurring during of after physical excertion. ‡Refers to heart murmurs judged likely to be organic and unlikely to be innocent: auscultation should be performed with the patient in both the supine and standing positions (or with valsalva maneuver), specifically to identify murmurs of dynamic left ventricular outflow tract obstruction. §Preferably taken in both arms.

**Fig. 6.2** The 14-Element AHA recommendations for preparticipation cardiovascular screening of competitive athletes (adapted from [17]) and a physical examination [15–19]. The questions focusing on medical history are mainly based on consensus expert opinion, and there are only few data regarding feasibility of these questions among various ethnic and socio-economic subgroups. The reliability of the questions is unclear, and existing data is ambiguous. With respect to the AHA-based history questions, prior to physician review, athletes reported positive rates in up to 35–60%, while other studies report positive history responses in only 1% of athletes [20, 21]. However, this once again highlights the importance of an accurate clinical assessment by a dedicated physician. Moreover,

- It should be kept in mind that in many athletes SCD occurs without suggestive preceding symptoms [22].

In a recent meta-analysis [23] physical examination even had a lower sensitivity than the athlete's history, but nevertheless, a relatively high specificity and negative likelihood ratio. However, despite all debates and limitations, a personal clinical evaluation is still the cornerstone of every medical assessment, including a population of competitive athletes. It may provide important information that relies on intuition and experience, not only regarding rather subjective questionnaires but also clinical findings during physical evaluation. Primary findings which may prompt further assessment of an athlete's heart and cardiovascular system are heart murmurs, clinical stigmata of connective tissue disease (e.g. Marfan syndrome) and high blood pressure [23].

The physical examination of an athlete should be focussed and clearly structured. As such, a standard approach, as in the assessment of other organs, would be as following:

1. Inspection
2. Palpation and percussion (incl. pulse and blood pressure measurement)
3. Auscultation

1. *Inspection.* Physical assessment of an athlete starts with an initial clinical impression. Complexion or obvious stigmata of an underlying disease should be noted. Particularly, clinical stigmata suggesting connective tissue disease are important to recognize, as affected athletes (e.g. in Marfan Syndrome) may develop aortic aneurysm with consecutive dissection. Table 6.2 provides an overview of the current criteria to assess an athlete regarding possible Marfan syndrome (revised Ghent nosology [24]).
2. *Palpation and percussion.* The examination of the heart should start with the classification of the *heart rhythm* as
   (a) regular
   (b) partly irregular (due to sinus arrhythmia or premature beats) or
   (c) absolutely irregular (due to atrial fibrillation).

   An accurate assessment of the athlete's *blood pressure* (BP) is crucial as it may gain false positive ("white coat hypertension") or false negative ("masked hypertension") results. The athlete should ideally be examined in a supine or sitting position with the arm supported at the level of the heart

**Table 6.2** Overview of the «Revised Ghent Nosology/Criteria» for the diagnosis of Marfan Syndrome (MFS) [24])

| | |
|---|---|
| *In the absence of family history* | |
| 1. Aortic root diameter (Z-score ≥ 2) and ectopia lentis | MFS[a] |
| 2. Aortic root diameter (Z-score ≥ 2) and causal FBN1 mutation | MFS |
| 3. Aortic root diameter (Z-score ≥ 2) and systemic score ≥ 7 points (see below) | MFS[a] |
| 4. Ectopia lentis and causal FBN1mutation with known aortic root dilatation | MFS |
| *In the presence of family history* | |
| 5. Ectopia lentis and family history of MFS (as defined above) | MFS |
| 6. Systemic score ≥ 7 points (see below) and family history of MFS (as defined above) | MFS[a] |
| 7. Aortic root diameter (Z-score ≥ 2 above 20 years old, ≥3 below 20 years) and family history of MFS (as defined above) | MFS[a] |
| *Scoring of systemic features of MFS* | *Score* |
| 1. Wrist AND thumb sign (alt.: wrist OR thumb sign) | 3 (1) |
| 2. Pectus carinatum deformity (pectus excavatum or chest asymmetry) | 2 (1) |
| 3. Hindfoot deformity (plain pes planus) | 2 (1) |
| 4. Pneumothorax | 2 |
| 5. Dural ectasia | 2 |
| 6. Protrusio acetabuli | 2 |
| 7. Reduced upper/lower body segment ratio AND increased arm/height AND no severe scoliosis | 1 |
| 8. Scoliosis or thoracolumbar kyphosis | 1 |
| 9. Reduced elbow extension | 1 |
| 10. Facial features (at least 3 out of the following 5: dolichocephaly, enophtalmos, downslanting palpebral fissures, malar hypoplasia, retrognathia) | 1 |
| 11. Skin striae | 1 |
| 12. Myopia >3 diopters | 1 |
| 13. Mitral valve prolapse (all types) | 1 |
| *Maximum Score* | 20 |
| *Indicative of systemic involvement* | ≥7 |

The Systemic score (lower part) refers to signs that can be detected by physical examination
[a]Caveat: without discriminating features of other forms of connective tissue syndromes AND certain genetic profiles (see [24] for details)

and after, at least, five minutes rest. Systolic pressure tends to be 2–3 mmHg higher and the diastolic pressure a similar degree lower in supine position. Mercury sphygmomanometers provide more accurate measurements than aneroid sphygmomanometers. Oscillometric BP measuring devices give readings that are typically lower than BP values obtained with the auscultatory method. A properly sized cuff use is essential, as an inappropriately small cuff provokes higher than intra-arterial pressure. As a rule of thumb, the length of the cuff bladder should be 80%, and the width at least 40% of the circumference of the upper arm. The cuff should be inflated to a pressure approximately 30 mmHg higher than the estimated systolic pressure (by pulse palpitation) and deflated slowly, at a rate of 2–3 mmHg per heartbeat.

Systolic pressure is equal to the pressure at which the pulse can first be detected by auscultation ("Korotkoff phase I") and the brachial/radial pulse can first be palpated again. As the cuff is further deflated, a brief period may follow during which the sounds soften (phase II) and then return to sharper

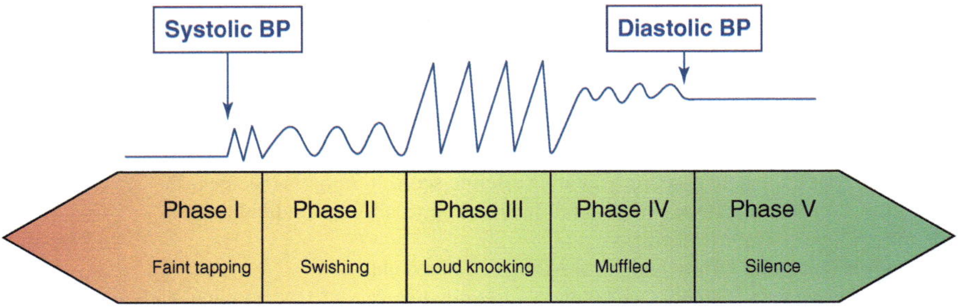


**Fig. 6.3** The five so-called Korotkoff phases that can be discriminated when measuring blood pressure by auscultation of the brachial artery

sounds again (phase III) before the pulse is first abruptly muffled (phase IV) and finally disappears (phase V), which generally equals the diastolic blood pressure (with the possible exception of high cardiac output in well trained athletes, where the pulse is continuously detectable) (Fig. 6.3).

(d) BP should at least once be measured on both arms to detect possible vascular perfusion deficits.

3. *Auscultation.* For more than a century, cardiac auscultation was the mainstay of cardiac examination. Despite all technical advances and possibilities to use cardiac imaging as a more accurate method to detect structural heart disease, a doctor's stethoscope has still the right to exist and clinical situations in which it should be used primarily, although the accuracy has been questioned repetitively [25, 26]. However, this cost-effective and highly available technique should be provided adequately to increase diagnostic accuracy and forego false positive findings. Examiner variability is a matter of fact; however, auscultation has a reported sensitivity of 70% and a specificity of 98% for the detection of valvular heart disease.

Cardiac auscultation is commonly performed with the athlete lying in a supine position in the end-expiratory phase. However, by changing the body position (e.g. left lateral position or prone) and varying respiratory phases (e.g. end-inspiratory, Valsalva manoeuvre, etc.) specific cardiac conditions can be provoked in case of clinical suspicion. The findings in auscultation can roughly be separated into *heart sounds* and *heart murmurs.*

## 6.8 Heart Sounds

*First heart sound (S1)*: The first heart sound (S1), normally best heard over the cardiac apex, consists of two high-frequency components: the first component is attributed to the dominant mitral valve closure while the second component refers to the closure of the tricuspid valve. The intensity of the valve closure sound is increased alongside an

- increased transvalvular gradient (e.g. in mitral stenosis)
- increased transvalvular flow (e.g. left-to-right shunt in ventricular septal defect or high output state)
- shortened diastole (tachycardia)
- short PR interval (pre-excitation syndrome).

Restricted valve mobility decreases the intensity of S1 (e.g. fibrosis or calcification of the mitral valve). Furthermore, S1 may also be diminished if the valve leaflets are already half-closed at the onset of systole, as it may occur in left ventricular systolic dysfunction. Abnormal splitting of S1 can result from delayed closure of the tricuspid valve (e.g. in patients with atrial septal defect). A widely split S1 can also occur in complete right bundle branch block (or after ectopic beats of LV origin).

*Second heart sound (S2)*: The second heart sound consists of two components: the aortic (A2) and pulmonary valve (P2) closure. P2 is best heard over the upper left sternal border, whereas A2 is widely transmitted to the right second interspace, along the sternal border and to the cardiac apex. Separation of A2 and P2 particularly occurs during inspiration, which allows comparison of the relative intensities of the two components and differentiation to a third heart sound (S3). This can best be heard over the left second interspace. Increased intensity of S2 occurs in

- systemic hypertension
- coarctation of the aorta
- ascending aortic aneurysm (mainly due to a louder A2)
- pulmonary hypertension (mainly due to a louder P2).

Decreased intensity of S2 is a rare finding in athletic screening but may occur in very low arterial diastolic pressure (e.g. in severe aortic regurgitation), immobilisation of the aortic valve due to calcification and severe aortic stenosis. Increased separation of A2 and P2 during inspiration may result from complete right bundle branch block (or premature beats or idioventricular rhythm of LV origin), the Wolff-Parkinson-White syndrome with LV pre-excitation and haemodynamic causes like pulmonary arterial hypertension of any aetiology. Fixed splitting of S2 is a relatively specific finding in case of interatrial communication (e.g. large atrial septal defect) or due to any condition with severe right ventricular failure. Paradoxical splitting (A2 following P2) may also be provoked during expiration, and is mostly seen with left bundle branch block, premature beats of RV origin or pre-excitation of the RV in Wolff-Parkinson-White syndrome.

*Third (S3) and fourth (S4) heart sounds*: S3 occurs at the very beginning of the passive filling phase of the ventricles and is a normal and common finding in healthy young athletes. However, beyond the age of 35–40 it may also suggest increased volume load due to a pathologic underlying condition.

In contrast, S4, which coincides with atrial systole, suggests increased LV pressure and is an unusual and suspicious finding in athletes. S3 as well as S4 are both low-frequency diastolic sounds and are thus best heard if the stethoscope is placed with slight pressure over the cardiac apex or over the lower left sternal border. Noise and murmurs of higher frequency will be eliminated like this and differentiation to components of S1 or S2, respectively, is easier.

So called aortic ejection sounds can occur in association with a geometrically deformed aortic valve (e.g. bicuspid aortic valve or aortic root dilatation). Another quite common finding is a mid-systolic click, suggesting mitral valve prolapse. The detection of a mitral-valve prolapse is important: Beside issues regarding valve function and training recommendations, this condition may be associated with concomitant cardiovascular anomalies such as cardiomyopathy, atrial septal defect, connective tissue disease (e.g. Marfan syndrome) or systemic lupus erythematosus.

Finally, a pericardial rub, that can be heard best during atrial systole, ventricular systole, and the rapid-filling phase of the ventricle ("three-component rub") is generated by friction of the two inflamed layers of the pericardium, suggesting peri(myo-)carditis.

## 6.9 Heart Murmurs

Heart murmurs are a common finding, particularly in young athletes, and are frequently of physiologic origin. However, an accurate characterisation of the murmur and thus detection of an eventual pathologic underlying condition is crucial. Heart murmurs can be characterised by five factors:

1. *Systolic versus diastolic murmurs* (including specification of whether the murmur is proto-, meso-, tele- or holosystolic or –diastolic, respectively).
2. *Localization* where the murmur can be heard loudest, according to the classical auscultation spots: Second intercostal space (ICS) parasternal right (aortic valve) and left (pulmonary valve), fifth ICS parasternal right (tricuspid valve), fifth ICS medio-clavicular left (mitral valve) and third ICS parasternal left (the so-called "Erb's point"). Transmission spots like the carotid arteries (aortic stenosis) or the left axilla (mitral valve pathology) should also be checked regularly (Fig. 6.4). Furthermore, the examiner should assess whether a murmur can be heard interscapular (aortic isthmus stenosis).
3. *Frequency* of a heart murmur (high or low frequency) can help differentiating between different conditions (e.g. the low frequent, harsh systolic murmur of an aortic stenosis versus the higher frequent systolic murmur of a mitral regurgitation).
4. The *shape* of a murmur is quite characteristic for certain pathologies and relies on the diagram of murmur intensity over time, as in a phonocardiogram:
   (a) Crescendo (increasing)
   (b) Decrescendo (diminishing)
   (c) Crescendo-decrescendo (increasing-decreasing or diamond/spindle shaped)
   (d) Plateau (unchanged in intensity)

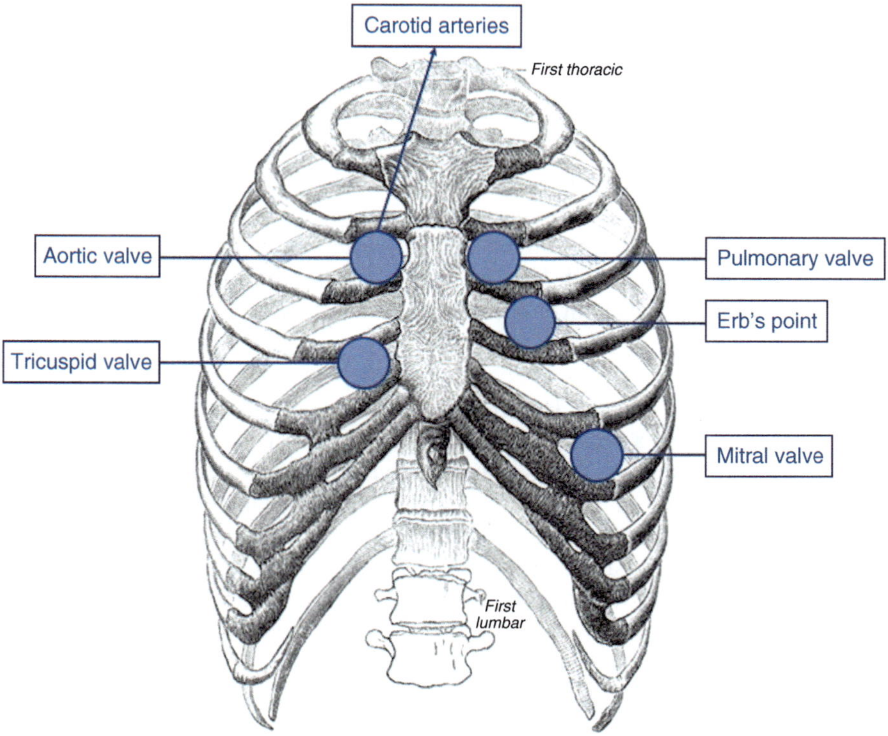


**Fig. 6.4** Overview of the most important cardiac auscultation points. It is important to note that murmurs implicating disorders of the aortic valve (i.e. aortic stenosis) typically can also be heard at the level of the carotid arteries

Assessing the shape of a murmur can, for example, help differentiating between the classic decrescendo shape of an aortic regurgitation and the spindle shaped murmur of aortic stenosis.

5. The *intensity* of a murmur may allow assessing the severity of a valve pathology:
   (a) Grade I (1/6) is the faintest murmur that can be heard (with difficulty)
   (b) Grade II (2/6) murmur is also a faint murmur but can be identified immediately
   (c) Grade III (3/6) murmur is moderately loud
   (d) Grade IV (4/6) murmur is loud (possibly associated with a palpable thrill)
   (e) Grade V (5/6) murmur is very loud (cannot be heard without the stethoscope)
   (f) Grade VI (6/6) murmur is the loudest (can be heard without the stethoscope)
      - A *systolic murmur* generally starts with or after S1 and terminates before or at S2 and is therefore recognised by identifying S1 and S2.
      - A diastolic *murmur* starts with or after S2 and ends at or before S1.

- Continuous *murmurs* continue through the whole systolic and diastolic phase, without interruption.
- *Mid*-systolic *murmurs* are most commonly benign flow murmurs due to physiologic flow, increased flow rate across a normal semilunar valve or due to aortic valve sclerosis. This kind of systolic murmur is present in up to 60% of athletes, however, in around 90% of these it is associated with a normal echocardiogram. Benign "flow" murmurs also occur when the relative flow volume across the semilunar valve is increased, as it occurs in high-level endurance athletes, during pregnancy but also in individuals with anaemia or thyrotoxicosis.

To distinguish between fixed valvular aortic stenosis (AS) and dynamic LV outflow obstruction (obstructive HCM) some clinical tests are established. With the patient changing from a squatting into a changing position, the intensity of the murmur in HCM increases, whereas the murmur of valvular aortic stenosis will decrease. In the straining phase of Valsalva manoeuvre, the murmur of HCM increases in intensity; both the intensity of the murmur and the carotid pulse volume decline with Valsalva in AS. It can be difficult to distinguish between a long mid-systolic murmur and a holosystolic regurgitant murmur in certain situations. Handgrip manoeuvre may help to distinguish between a mitral regurgitation murmur, where the intensity of the murmur increases (increased afterload effect), and an AS murmur, where intensity usually decreases.

- *Early systolic murmurs* most often result from mitral regurgitation (MR) and generally have a "plateau-configuration".
- *Late systolic murmurs* are most commonly caused by mitral valve prolapse. They are best heard with the diaphragm of the stethoscope and are usually preceded by single or multiple clicks.
- There are three classical causes of *holosystolic murmurs*—MR, tricuspid regurgitation and ventricular septal defect (VSD). The holosystolic murmur of MR is high pitched and is therefore best heard with the diaphragm of the stethoscope and the patient in the left lateral decubitus position [27].
- *Early diastolic murmurs* are most often due to aortic or pulmonary regurgitation and appear in decrescendo-shape with, in addition, a slight systolic murmur due to increased ventricular stroke volume.
- *Mid-diastolic murmurs* classically result from turbulent flow across the atrioventricular valves during the rapid filling phase because of mitral ("opening snap") or tricuspid valve stenosis. In mitral valve stenosis (MS) it can be stated that the longer the duration of the murmur, the more severe the MS might be.
- *Late diastolic or pre-systolic murmurs* usually have a crescendo configuration and result from increased flow across the mitral or tricuspid valve (e.g. in mitral or tricuspid stenosis, atrial fibrillation or left-to-right shunts).

**Clinical Pearls** An athlete's personal, systemic and particularly family history frequently detects "red flags" which lead to the diagnosis of a relevant underlying cardiovascular disease.

- Physical examination mainly targets connective tissue disease (with the potential for aortic dilation and dissection), as well as hypertensive blood pressure and cardiac murmurs.
- Blood pressure assessment needs to be performed correctly to differentiate physiologic findings (including "white coat hypertension") and pathologic findings (including "masked hypertension").
- Cardiac auscultation is challenging but, performed correctly, it may reliably detect underlying cardiac disease—particularly, valvular heart disease. It should follow a strict and standardized procedure (sounds vs. murmurs, systolic vs. diastolic, localization, shape, frequency, intensity, etc.).

## Review

## Questions

1. A 26-year old male leisure endurance athlete reports recurrent lightheadedness after brisk changing from a sitting to a standing position (i.e. after a meal). Two days ago, he experienced a syncope during his regular training (jogging of moderate intensity). The syncope appeared unheralded and the patient does not remember any warning symptoms and denied amnesia. However, due to his syncope he suffered from bruises on the knees, elbows and the forehead. What is your suspicion after knowledge of the patient's history?
2. You see a 19-year old asymptomatic male basketball player for routine pre-competition examination. During physical examination some clinical findings are suspicious. The skin on his back shows multiple slightly blue "scar-like" striae and during auscultation you can detect a mid-systolic click with a moderately loud tele-systolic murmur. What is your suspicion and what tests would you add?
3. A 54-year old marathon runner asks for consultation due to massive headaches, particularly during exercise, slowly decreasing vision and with a recent laboratory test which exhibited moderate renal failure. The patient's personal history is normal, and his family history only highlights systemic hypertension of his father. Physical examination shows normal findings with unsuspicious auscultation and normal blood pressure measurement (135/85 mmHg on both arms in supine position). In an additional exercise test the athlete performed well without abnormal ECG changes during exercise but headache and pronounced increase of blood pressure (up to 240/110 mmHg until exhaustion). What are your thoughts and what examination should be added to confirm your suspicion?

## Answers

1. The patient's history of the syncopal event is highly suspicious for cardiac/arrhythmic etiology. This is due to four classical points: The syncope occurred during exercise and without any prodromal symptoms. Amnesia has been denied but he suffered from (minor) injury (bruises) due to the syncope.
2. Skin striae are highly suspicious for connective tissue disease and are part of the so-called "Ghent Criteria" characterizing Marfan Syndrome. Thus, the next clinical step would be to complete these clinical criteria. The auscultatory findings are classical for mitral valve prolapse which is also part of the Ghent criteria and frequently seen in patients with connective tissue disease. To confirm this suspicion transthoracic echocardiography should be performed. It is also crucial, particularly in contact sports, to assess the diameter of the ascending aorta as aortic aneurysm (and possible dissection) may occur as another clinical finding in these patients.
3. The patient's history and physical examination raises suspicion for "masked hypertension". Systemic hypertension is genetically linked (positive family history) and may clinically appear with headaches. Ocular and renal damage can also be explained by longstanding hypertension. Although "office" blood pressure measurements were normal "masked hypertension" is most likely as up to 40% of athletes with exercise hypertension show underlying (often undetected and masked) hypertension. Thus, in a next diagnostic step ambulatory blood pressure monitoring (24-h automatic device or self-measurement at home) should urgently be recommended.

## References


1. Tischer SG, Mattsson N, Storgaard M, Hofsten DE, Host NB, Andersen LJ, et al. Results of voluntary cardiovascular examination of elite athletes in Denmark: proposal for Nordic collaboration. Scand J Med Sci Sports. 2016;26(1):64–73.
2. Kaiser-Nielsen LV, Tischer SG, Prescott EB, Rasmusen HK. Symptoms, diagnoses, and sporting consequences among athletes referred to a Danish sports cardiology clinic. Scand J Med Sci Sports. 2017;27(1):115–23.
3. Brignole M, Moya A, de Lange FJ, Deharo JC, Elliott PM, Fanciulli A, et al. 2018 ESC Guidelines for the diagnosis and management of syncope. Eur Heart J. 2018;39(21):1883–948.
4. Colivicchi F, Ammirati F, Santini M. Epidemiology and prognostic implications of syncope in young competing athletes. Eur Heart J. 2004;25(19):1749–53.
5. Vettor G, Zorzi A, Basso C, Thiene G, Corrado D. Syncope as a warning symptom of sudden cardiac death in athletes. Cardiol Clin. 2015;33(3):423–32.
6. Rogers E, Guerrero S, Kumar D, Soofi S, Fazal S, Martinez K, et al. Evaluation of the cost-effectiveness of the treatment of uncomplicated severe acute malnutrition by lady health workers as compared to an outpatient therapeutic feeding programme in Sindh Province, Pakistan. BMC Public Health. 2019;19(1):84.
7. Massin MM, Bourguignont A, Coremans C, Comte L, Lepage P, Gerard P. Chest pain in pediatric patients presenting to an emergency department or to a cardiac clinic. Clin Pediatr. 2004;43(3):231–8.
8. Fruergaard P, Launbjerg J, Hesse B, Jorgensen F, Petri A, Eiken P, et al. The diagnoses of patients admitted with acute chest pain but without myocardial infarction. Eur Heart J. 1996;17(7):1028–34.

9. Couto M, Moreira A. The athlete "out of breath". Eur Ann Allergy Clin Immunol. 2016;48(2):36–45.
10. Fitch KD. An overview of asthma and airway hyper-responsiveness in olympic athletes. Br J Sports Med. 2012;46(6):413–6.
11. Lawless CE, Briner W. Palpitations in athletes. Sports Med. 2008;38(8):687–702.
12. Abdelfattah RS, Froelicher VF. Palpitations in athletes. Curr Sports Med Rep. 2015;14(4):333–6.
13. Flannery MD, Kalman JM, Sanders P, La Gerche A. State of the art review: atrial fibrillation in athletes. Heart Lung Circ. 2017;26(9):983–9.
14. Ranthe MF, Winkel BG, Andersen EW, Risgaard B, Wohlfahrt J, Bundgaard H, et al. Risk of cardiovascular disease in family members of young sudden cardiac death victims. Eur Heart J. 2013;34(7):503–11.
15. Corrado D, Pelliccia A, Bjornstad HH, Vanhees L, Biffi A, Borjesson M, et al. Cardiovascular pre-participation screening of young competitive athletes for prevention of sudden death: proposal for a common European protocol. Consensus statement of the Study Group of Sport Cardiology of the Working Group of Cardiac Rehabilitation and Exercise Physiology and the Working Group of Myocardial and Pericardial Diseases of the European Society of Cardiology. Eur Heart J. 2005;26(5):516–24.
16. Bille K, Figueiras D, Schamasch P, Kappenberger L, Brenner JI, Meijboom FJ, et al. Sudden cardiac death in athletes: the Lausanne recommendations. Eur J Cardiovasc Prev Rehabil. 2006;13(6):859–75.
17. Maron BJ, Thompson PD, Ackerman MJ, Balady G, Berger S, Cohen D, et al. Recommendations and considerations related to preparticipation screening for cardiovascular abnormalities in competitive athletes: 2007 update: a scientific statement from the American Heart Association Council on Nutrition, Physical Activity, and Metabolism: endorsed by the American College of Cardiology Foundation. Circulation. 2007;115(12):1643–455.
18. Dvorak J, Grimm K, Schmied C, Junge A. Development and implementation of a standardized precompetition medical assessment of international elite football players--2006 FIFA World Cup Germany. Clin J Sport Med. 2009;19(4):316–21.
19. Drezner JA, Levine BD, Vetter VL. Reframing the debate: screening athletes to prevent sudden cardiac death. Heart Rhythm. 2013;10(3):454–5.
20. Zeltser I, Cannon B, Silvana L, Fenrich A, George J, Schleifer J, et al. Lessons learned from preparticipation cardiovascular screening in a state funded program. Am J Cardiol. 2012;110(6):902–8.
21. Hevia AC, Fernandez MM, Palacio JM, Martin EH, Castro MG, Reguero JJ. ECG as a part of the preparticipation screening programme: an old and still present international dilemma. Br J Sports Med. 2011;45(10):776–9.
22. Maron BJ, Shirani J, Poliac LC, Mathenge R, Roberts WC, Mueller FO. Sudden death in young competitive athletes. Clinical, demographic, and pathological profiles. JAMA. 1996;276(3):199–204.
23. Harmon KG, Zigman M, Drezner JA. The effectiveness of screening history, physical exam, and ECG to detect potentially lethal cardiac disorders in athletes: a systematic review/meta-analysis. J Electrocardiol. 2015;48(3):329–38.
24. Loeys BL, Dietz HC, Braverman AC, Callewaert BL, De Backer J, Devereux RB, et al. The revised Ghent nosology for the Marfan syndrome. J Med Genet. 2010;47(7):476–85.
25. Barron JT, Manrose DL, Liebson PR. Comparison of auscultation with two-dimensional and Doppler echocardiography in patients with suspected mitral valve prolapse. Clin Cardiol. 1988;11(6):401–6.
26. Guntheroth WG. Innocent murmurs: a suspect diagnosis in non-pregnant adults. Am J Cardiol. 2009;104(5):735–7.
27. Ishmail AA, et al. Interobserver agreement by auscultation in the presence of a third heart sound in patients with congestive heart failure. Chest. 1987;91(6):870–3.

# Medical Evaluation of Athletes: Electrocardiogram

7

Jordan M. Prutkin and Jonathan A. Drezner

**Learning Objectives**

1. Understand the most recent International Criteria for ECG interpretation in athletes.
2. Outline normal ECG findings in athletes related to physiologic cardiac adaptations from regular exercise training.
3. Recognize that two or more borderline ECG findings require further testing.
4. Define abnormal ECG findings in athletes which require further evaluation to exclude a pathologic cardiac disorder before participation in competitive sport.
5. Describe the minimum recommended evaluation for athletes with specific ECG abnormalities.

## 7.1 Introduction

While the American Heart Association and American College of Cardiology recommend that athletes undergo a preparticipation evaluation before competitive sports with a history and physical examination [1], many sporting organizations and the European Society of Cardiology (ESC) [2] recommend use of a screening electrocardiogram (ECG). The Canadian Cardiovascular Society recommends an ECG only if there is an abnormal history or physical examination [3], while the American

J. M. Prutkin
Division of Cardiology/Electrophysiology, UW Medicine Center for Sports Cardiology, University of Washington, Seattle, WA, USA
e-mail: jprutkin@cardiology.washington.edu

J. A. Drezner (✉)
Department of Family Medicine/Sports Medicine, UW Medicine Center for Sports Cardiology, University of Washington, Seattle, WA, USA
e-mail: jdrezner@uw.edu



A. Pressler, J. Niebauer (eds.), *Textbook of Sports and Exercise Cardiology*,
https://doi.org/10.1007/978-3-030-35374-2_7

Medical Society for Sports Medicine suggests an ECG should be considered in high risk athlete groups when adequate cardiology resources are available [3, 4]. Whether used for screening or diagnostic purposes, ECG interpretation is a fundamental skill for physicians responsible for the cardiovascular care of athletes.

An ECG increases the detection of disorders at increased risk of sudden cardiac death [5, 6], as most athletes who have a cardiac arrest are asymptomatic prior to their event [3] and the sensitivity and specificity of a screening history and physical examination are poor [6]. However, the ECG is not a perfect screening tool, and some disorders such as coronary artery anomalies or aortic dilatation do not demonstrate ECG abnormalities.

The distinction of ECG findings related to physiologic cardiac adaptations in trained athletes from ECG abnormalities suggesting the possibility of an underlying cardiac disorder is critical in the interpretation of an athlete's ECG. Certain ECG findings are considered normal in athletes that might be considered abnormal in non-athletes. For this reason, it is important to use athlete-specific ECG interpretation criteria. The first criteria from the ESC defined training-related and training-unrelated ECG findings [7] but there was a high rate of false positive ECG tests, especially in black athletes [8]. Other interpretation standards emerged, including the Seattle Criteria [9], that improved the specificity and reduced the false positive rate without compromising sensitivity [10–13]. Most recently, the International Criteria for ECG Interpretation in athletes were developed by an international panel of experts in sports medicine and cardiology which defines normal, borderline, and abnormal ECG findings and the secondary tests recommended for each ECG abnormality [14]. The International Criteria should be used for asymptomatic athletes with no concerning family history, and thus may need to be modified in the presence of clinical markers of concern. If there are symptoms suggestive of cardiac disease or a family history of sudden cardiac arrest, Marfan syndrome, cardiomyopathy, or channelopathy, then the athlete should be evaluated by a physician knowledgeable in these disorders.

Importantly, a normal ECG does not confirm a lifetime free of cardiac disease. ECG changes and phenotypic expression of a genetic disorder can occur over time, especially in pubertal age adolescents and young adults, where repeated screening is necessary to exclude the interval development of cardiomyopathies [15]. In addition, if an ECG is abnormal but the secondary testing is normal, serial evaluation is recommended to monitor for the later manifestation of phenotypic disease [16].

## 7.2 Normal ECG Findings

These findings do not require any further evaluation (Table 7.1; Fig. 7.1):

**Chamber Hypertrophy**

- Right and left ventricular hypertrophy are physiologic adaptations to regular exercise and can be manifested on the ECG as increased QRS voltage.

**Table 7.1** Definitions from the International Criteria for Electrocardiogram Interpretation in Athletes[14]

| | Definition |
|---|---|
| *Normal ECG finding* | |
| Increased QRS voltage | Isolated QRS voltage criteria for left (SV1 + RV5 or RV6 > 3.5 mV) or right ventricular hypertrophy (RV1 + SV5 or SV6 > 1.1 mV) |
| Incomplete RBBB | rSR′ pattern in lead V1 and a qRS pattern in lead V6 with QRS duration <120 ms |
| Early repolarization | J point elevation, ST elevation, J waves, or terminal QRS slurring in the inferior and/or lateral leads |
| Black athlete repolarization variant | J-point elevation and convex ("domed") ST segment elevation followed by T wave inversion in leads V1–V4 in black athletes |
| Juvenile T wave pattern | T wave inversion V1–V3 in athletes < age 16 |
| Sinus bradycardia | ≥30 bpm |
| Sinus arrhythmia | Heart rate variation with respiration: rate increases during inspiration and decreases during expiration |
| Ectopic atrial rhythm | P waves are a different morphology compared to the sinus P wave, such as negative P waves in the inferior leads ("low atrial rhythm") |
| Junctional escape rhythm | QRS rate is faster than the resting P wave or sinus rate and typically less than 100 beats/min with narrow QRS complex unless the baseline QRS is conducted with aberrancy |
| 1° AV block | PR interval 200–400 ms |
| Mobitz Type I (Wenckebach) 2° AV block | PR interval progressively lengthens until there is a non-conducted P wave with no QRS complex; the first PR interval after the dropped beat is shorter than the last conducted PR interval |
| *Borderline ECG Finding* | |
| Left axis deviation | −30° to −90° |
| Left atrial enlargement | Prolonged P wave duration of >120 ms in leads I or II with negative portion of the P wave ≥ 1 mm in depth and ≥40 ms in duration in lead V1 |
| Right axis deviation | >120° |
| Right atrial enlargement | P wave ≥ 2.5 mm in II, III, or aVF |
| Complete right bundle branch block | rSR′ pattern in lead V1 and a S wave wider than R wave in lead V6 with QRS duration ≥120 ms |
| *Abnormal ECG Finding* | |
| T wave inversion | ≥ 1 mm in depth in two or more contiguous leads; excludes leads aVR, III, and V1 |
| • Anterior | • V2-V4<br>– excludes: black athletes with J-point elevation and convex ST segment elevation followed by TWI in V2-V4; athletes < age 16 with TWI in V1-V3; and biphasic T waves in only V3 |
| • Lateral | • I and AVL, V5 <u>and/or</u> V6 (only one lead of TWI required in V5 or V6) |
| • Inferolateral | • II and aVF, V5-V6, I and AVL |
| • Inferior | • II and aVF |
| ST segment depression | ≥0.5 mm in depth in two or more contiguous leads |
| Pathologic Q waves | Q/R ratio ≥ 0.25 or Q wave ≥ 40 ms in duration in two or more leads (excluding III and aVR) |

(continued)

**Table 7.1** (continued)

| | Definition |
|---|---|
| Complete left bundle branch block | QRS ≥ 120 ms, predominantly negative QRS complex in lead V1 (QS or rS), and upright notched or slurred R wave in leads I and V6 |
| Profound nonspecific intra-ventricular conduction delay | Any QRS duration ≥140 ms |
| Epsilon wave | Distinct low amplitude signal (small positive deflection or notch) between the end of the QRS complex and onset of the T wave in leads V1–V3 |
| Ventricular pre-excitation | PR interval <120 ms with a delta wave (slurred upstroke in the QRS complex) and wide QRS (≥120 ms) |
| Prolonged QT interval (Bazett formula) | QTc ≥ 470 ms (male)<br>QTc ≥ 480 ms (female)<br>QTc ≥ 500 ms (marked QT prolongation) |
| Brugada Type 1 pattern | Coved pattern: initial ST elevation ≥2 mm (high take-off) with downsloping ST segment elevation followed by a negative symmetric T wave in ≥1 leads in V1–V3 |
| Profound sinus bradycardia | <30 beats/min or sinus pauses ≥3 s |
| Profound 1° AV block | ≥400 ms |
| Mobitz type II 2° AV block | Intermittently non-conducted P waves with a fixed PR interval |
| 3° AV block | Complete heart block |
| Atrial tachyarrhythmias | Supraventricular tachycardia, atrial fibrillation, atrial flutter |
| Premature ventricular contractions | ≥2 PVCs per 10 s tracing |
| Ventricular arrhythmias | Couplets, triplets, and non-sustained ventricular tachycardia |

*ECG* electrocardiogram, *PVCs* premature ventricular contractions, *RBBB* right bundle branch block, *TWI* T wave inversion

- Left ventricular hypertrophy (LVH) by Sokolow-Lyon criteria is seen in up to 45% of athletes in one study [17].
- While LVH may be present in those with hypertrophic cardiomyopathy (HCM), there are typically other ECG abnormalities such as ST depression, T wave inversions, or pathologic Q waves [16, 17].
- Right ventricular hypertrophy by voltage criteria is a normal finding seen in up to 12% of athletes [18, 19].
- Incomplete right bundle branch block usually with an rSR′ pattern and QRS duration <120 ms in lead V1 is also a common finding in trained athletes.

## Early Repolarization

- Early repolarization consists of J point elevation ≥0.1 mV, frequently with a notch called a J wave, and usually followed by ST segment elevation in a convex pattern [20].
- Early repolarization is often present in normal athletes [21], especially those who are young, male, or of African-Caribbean descent. It has been described in up to 45% of Caucasian [17] and 63% of Black athletes [18].
- This pattern is not associated with sudden death in young athletes and is considered normal.

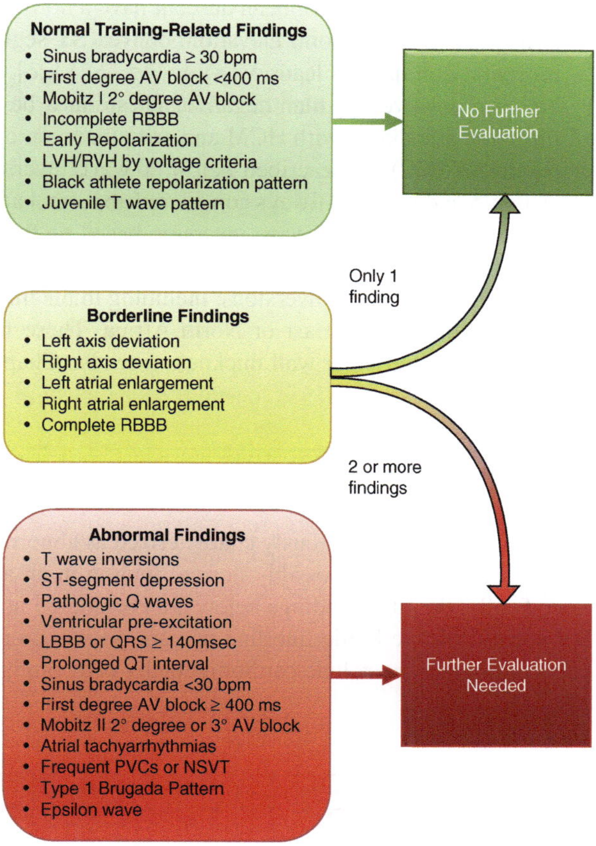


**Fig. 7.1** The International Criteria for ECG Interpretation in Athletes. *AV* atrioventricular, *LVH* left ventricular hypertrophy, *NSVT* non-sustained ventricular tachycardia, *PVCs* premature ventricular contractions, *RVH* right ventricular hypertrophy, *RBBB* right bundle branch block, *TWI* T wave inversion

### Bradycardia, First Degree Atrioventricular (AV) Block, and Second Degree Mobitz Type I AV Block (Wenckebach)

- Sinus bradycardia is commonly seen in elite athletes. This can also be manifested as an ectopic atrial rhythm or accelerated junctional rhythm.
- Sinus bradycardia is due to both enhanced vagal tone [22, 23] as well as changes in expression of the HCN4 and $I_f$ cardiac ion channels [24].
- First degree AV block between 200 and 400 ms and AV Wenckebach block are also considered normal.
- If there is any concern whether the findings are pathologic, a short burst of aerobic exercise should cause an increase in heart rate and normalization of AV conduction.

### Normal Patterns of T Wave Inversion

- There are several different normal T wave inversion patterns:
- An isolated negative T wave in V3.
- Persistent juvenile T wave pattern with T wave inversions in leads V1–V3 in athletes <16 years of age. T wave inversion extending beyond V2 is an uncommon finding in Caucasian athletes > age 16 [17, 25].

- Athletes of African-Caribbean descent have a normal T wave repolarization pattern consisting of J point elevation, convex ST segment elevation, and T wave inversion confined to leads V1–V4 (Fig. 7.2) [26]. Typically, the T waves are biphasic positive and then negative. These must be differentiated from T wave inversion associated with HCM and arrhythmogenic right ventricular cardiomyopathy (ARVC), as described below. T wave inversion extending to the lateral leads V5 and/or V6 is always considered abnormal and requires more evaluation. There is variation in T wave inversion based on the athlete's geographic origin even in normal individuals [27]. Those from Middle and West Africa have a higher rate of T wave inversions, including in the inferior and lateral leads, compared to those from East or North Africa. These findings are correlated with greater left ventricular wall thickness (see also Chap. 26).

## 7.3 Borderline ECG Findings

Some ECG findings previously characterized as abnormal have since been reclassified as a borderline or possibly normal finding in an athlete (Table 7.1; Fig. 7.1). Specifically, the ECG findings below are considered normal if present in isolation, but if two or more borderline findings are present then further evaluation with an echocardiogram to exclude cardiomyopathy is recommended [8].

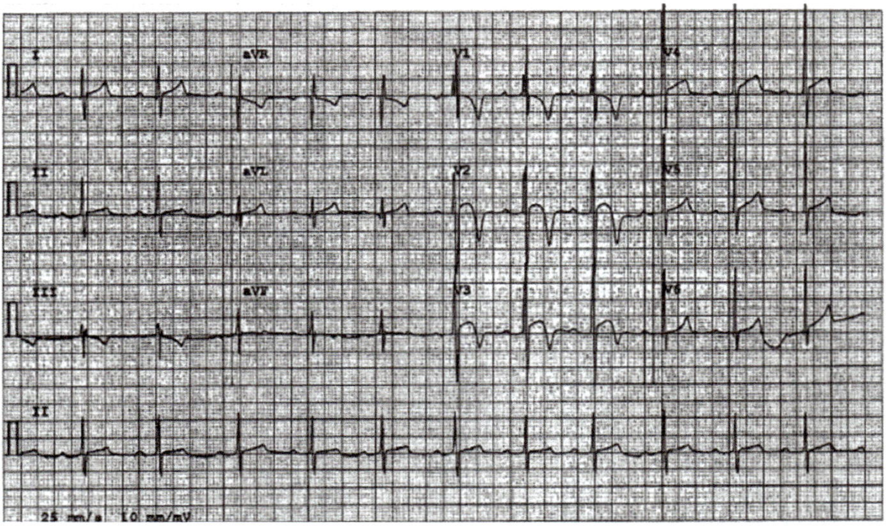


**Fig. 7.2** 19-year-old black male track athlete with ST-segment and J-point elevation followed by T wave inversion in leads V2–V3. This repolarization pattern represents a normal variant in black athletes

**Right Bundle Branch Block (RBBB)**

- While incomplete RBBB is common in athletes, complete RBBB (QRS duration ≥120 ms) is a less frequent finding in approximately 0.5–2.5% of athletes [28–30].
- Some highly trained athletes have physiologic right ventricular cardiac remodeling manifested as right ventricular dilatation, reduction in right ventricular systolic function at rest, and slight increase in the rate of right bundle branch block [31].
- While one study showed a slight increase in right ventricular size in those with RBBB, there were no pathologic abnormalities identified and no cardiac events occurred [30]. Other imaging studies have shown normal right ventricular size and function in those with RBBB [31].
- Complete RBBB when found in isolation without other borderline or abnormal ECG findings does not require additional investigation unless there are clinical markers of concern.

**Atrial Enlargement and Axis Deviation**

- Athletes are more likely to have left axis deviation or left atrial enlargement compared to non-athletes [32].
- There is no correlation, however, between axis deviation or atrial enlargement on ECG with abnormalities found on cardiac imaging.
- In patients with HCM, left axis deviation or left atrial enlargement in the absence of any other abnormality was not found to be more prevalent compared to normal athletes [25, 33, 34].
- Therefore, isolated right or left atrial enlargement or right or left axis deviation is considered a normal finding in the absence of any other ECG abnormality.

## 7.4 Abnormal ECG Findings

Abnormal ECG findings require further evaluation to exclude a pathologic cardiac disorder. The ECG abnormality alone does not necessarily imply a disease process, but rather indicates that more evaluation is needed. Temporary restriction from sport should be considered while the secondary evaluation is completed. Some ECG abnormalities may be the first manifestation of a cardiomyopathy before morphologic changes are present. Thus, serial evaluation is recommended on an annual basis for athletes with abnormal T wave inversion, ST segment depression, and/or pathologic Q waves.

**Pathologic T Wave Inversion**

- T wave inversions ≥1 mm in two or more contiguous leads are considered abnormal. T wave inversion in V5 or V6 alone satisfies the criteria (Fig. 7.3). Leads III, aVR, and V1 should be excluded from measurement.
- If a T wave is biphasic and the negative portion of the T wave is ≥1 mm in depth, then it is considered abnormal.

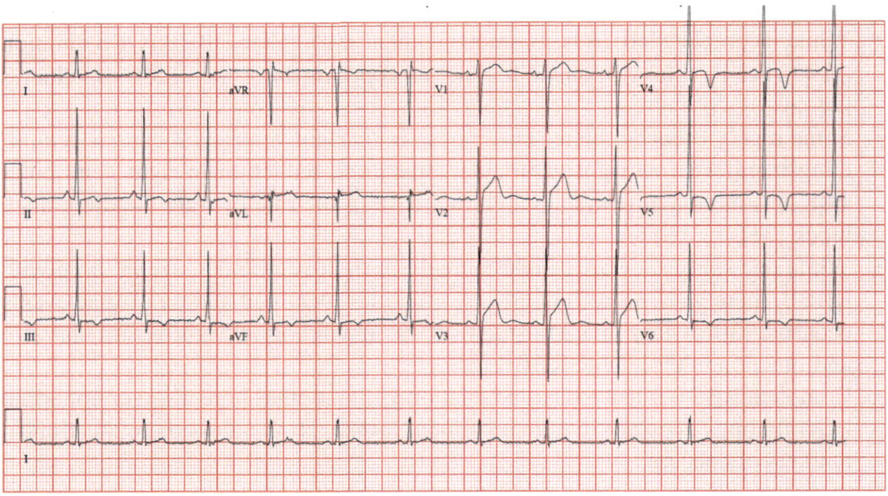

**Fig. 7.3** 19-year-old black baseball player with T wave inversion in V4–V6 and borderline in II and aVF. Lateral and inferolateral T wave inversion is an abnormal finding requiring investigation for cardiomyopathy. This athlete was later found to have hypertrophic cardiomyopathy

- T wave inversions should be described as anterior (V2–4), lateral (I, aVL, V5–V6), inferolateral (I, II, aVL, aVF, V5–6), or inferior (II, aVF) based on the leads involved. T wave inversions in the lateral leads are most concerning for cardiomyopathy.

T wave inversions may be an early finding for cardiomyopathy, often seen before the development of structural changes [8, 16, 35]. For instance, one study of 81 athletes with pathologic T wave inversions demonstrated that 6% later went on to manifest a cardiomyopathy, including two athletes who had a sudden cardiac arrest [16]. Another study demonstrated that 12.3% of athletes with lateral T wave inversions were found to be gene positive for a cardiac disease, most commonly for a mutation associated with HCM [36]. However, the specificity of this criterion is still imperfect, especially in black athletes with more prevalent T wave inversions [8, 18].

- There may be associated abnormalities to suggest a cardiomyopathy, including ST segment depression, pathologic Q waves, left bundle branch block, ventricular pre-excitation, or borderline ECG findings.
- The main disorders associated with T wave inversions include HCM, ARVC, dilated cardiomyopathy, left ventricular non-compaction cardiomyopathy, and myocarditis.

If T wave inversions are found in the lateral leads, an echocardiogram should be completed. In addition, a cardiac magnetic resonance imaging (MRI), which has better resolution for apical HCM, should be performed. Late gadolinium enhancement suggestive of myocardial fibrosis can be seen on MRI even when there is no significant hypertrophy. An exercise ECG test and ambulatory ECG monitoring should be considered if there is left ventricular hypertrophy which falls in the grey zone (13–15 mm wall thickness), where it is difficult to tell if the increased left ventricular hypertrophy is due to HCM or secondary to physiologic changes. If exercise-induced arrhythmias or non-sustained ventricular tachycardia are seen, it is more likely a cardiomyopathy is present.

T wave inversions in the inferior leads can also be seen in HCM though in a much smaller proportion and are usually associated with lateral T wave inversions if pathologic disease is present [18]. If T wave inversions are only present in the inferior leads, further evaluation with an echocardiogram should suffice [8].

Anterior T wave inversion may be related to ARVC, especially if there is an epsilon wave, premature ventricular contractions with a left bundle branch block morphology, prolonged S wave upstroke in leads V1–3, or low amplitude limb lead voltages. Evaluation should include an echocardiogram, cardiac MRI, Holter monitoring, exercise ECG test, and signal averaged ECG depending on clinical suspicion. Examination of the J point and T wave inversions can help distinguish between normal patterns and pathologic findings. If there is J point elevation ≥1 mm and T wave inversions in leads V1–V4, one study demonstrated 100% negative predictive value for cardiomyopathy [37]. However if there is no J point elevation, a flat or depressed ST segment, or additional T wave inversions in the inferior or lateral leads, then cardiomyopathy is more likely to be present.

**ST-Segment Depression**

- ST-segment depression is defined as ≥0.05 mV, or 0.5 mm in standard gain, in two or more contiguous leads.
- ST-segment depression is more commonly associated with cardiomyopathy. Approximately 50% of patients with HCM will have ST-segment depression though it is usually associated with other ECG abnormalities such as pathologic Q waves or T wave inversions [8, 18].
- Evaluation should include an echocardiogram if seen in isolation. However, if there are other ECG abnormalities, a cardiac MRI should be considered.

**Pathologic Q Waves**

- The current definition for a pathologic Q wave is a Q/R ratio ≥ 0.25 or a Q wave duration ≥40 ms in two or more contiguous leads, excluding leads III and aVR [14]. This was one of the significant changes from the Seattle Criteria [9], which used an absolute depth of >3 mm or > 40 ms in duration. The absolute depth was removed from the International Criteria as there was a greater rate of false-positive results in thinner people and those with physiologic left ventricular hypertrophy, who have high precordial voltage but no pathologic abnormalities. This problem is corrected by using the Q/R ratio.
- It is important to note that placement of ECG leads in the improper position can also cause abnormal Q waves, such as with limb lead reversal or placement of leads V1 and V2 into higher intercostal spaces [38].

- Recent data suggest that a Q + S wave amplitude in lead III > 1.0 mV may offer additive value to suggest HCM [39].
- The Q/R ratio ≥ 0.25 or a Q wave duration ≥40 ms is still not perfect as 1–2% of athletes may still have pathologic Q waves but no abnormalities seen [8, 40]. False positives are higher in black and male athletes.
- Pathologic Q waves are seen in various cardiomyopathies, including HCM, ARVC, dilated cardiomyopathy, and prior myocardial infarction. In addition, the Wolff-Parkinson-White (WPW) pattern can demonstrate pathologic Q waves.
- If pathologic Q waves are seen, the QRS should be examined for evidence of pre-excitation to suggest WPW. If this is not found, the specific leads where the Q waves are present will dictate the next step. If it is in V1 and V2, the ECG should be repeated with careful attention to correct lead placement in the fourth intercostal space.
- If the Q waves are still present after repeat ECG, or the pathologic Q waves are found in two or more other leads, an echocardiogram should be completed to exclude cardiomyopathy, especially if there are ST-segment or T wave abnormalities. If there is a high suspicion of cardiomyopathy, a cardiac MRI should be considered.
- If the athlete is over 30 years old or there is a clinical suspicion or risk factors of ischemic heart disease, especially if there is a wall motion abnormality on echocardiogram, a stress test is indicated [14].

**Left Bundle Branch Block (LBBB)**

- LBBB is a rare finding in screening studies of athletes and deserves a comprehensive evaluation to exclude myocardial disease if found [5, 41–43].
- A LBBB usually has other significant ST-segment and T wave changes which would be flagged by the screening criteria [29, 44, 45].
- There is a high rate of cardiomyopathy in patients with LBBB. One study comparing athletes and patients with HCM showed that 5.9% of patients with HCM had LBBB, but no athlete with normal cardiac imaging had LBBB [46].
- Athletes with LBBB require an echocardiogram and cardiac MRI with consideration for a stress perfusion study. Alternatively, a CT coronary angiogram or stress testing with imaging may be considered when ischemic heart disease is suspected.

**Widened QRS ≥ 140 ms**

- It is unclear whether a QRS duration ≥140 ms in a non-LBBB pattern represents pathologic disease in an athlete population [47].
- Increased myocardial mass and left ventricular hypertrophy in athletes, or alternatively, neurally-mediated conduction system slowing [48], can increase the QRS duration.
- Various cardiomyopathies can also have QRS widening.
- Until there is more data, however, it is prudent to perform further evaluation on those with a widened QRS complex ≥140 ms.
- An echocardiogram should be completed, and depending on these findings and clinical suspicion, further testing may be indicated.

**Wolff-Parkinson-White (WPW) Pattern**

- WPW (ventricular pre-excitation) is present in about 0.1–0.3% of people [49]. More than half of adolescents with WPW pattern are asymptomatic [49].
- The WPW pattern consists of a short PR interval <120 ms, widened QRS duration, and delta wave (slurred QRS upstroke).
- It is important to differentiate WPW from Lown-Ganong-Levine pattern or enhanced AV nodal conduction, which also have a PR interval <120 ms but no delta wave and a normal QRS duration, as these findings are not associated with sudden cardiac arrest (SCA).
- The most worrisome aspect of WPW is the associated risk of syncope or SCA. Syncope may be due to rapid supraventricular tachycardia from AV reciprocating tachycardia, rapid atrial fibrillation or flutter, or ventricular fibrillation.
- An echocardiogram should be completed on all patients with WPW as there is an association with Ebstein anomaly, L-transposition of the great arteries, and left ventricular hypertrophy due to LAMP2 or PRKAG2 mutations.

There is debate regarding the best method for risk stratification of patients with asymptomatic WPW to determine the risk of SCA. The most important feature is determining the refractory period of the bypass pathway, where faster pathway conduction is associated with an increased risk of SCA [50]. Intermittent pre-excitation on the resting ECG suggests a lower risk pathway. An exercise test should be performed looking for *abrupt* loss of bypass pathway conduction (Fig. 7.4). If present, this suggests a low risk pathway and in the absence of symptoms, no treatment is necessary. If there are symptoms, if the bypass pathway does not abruptly stop at

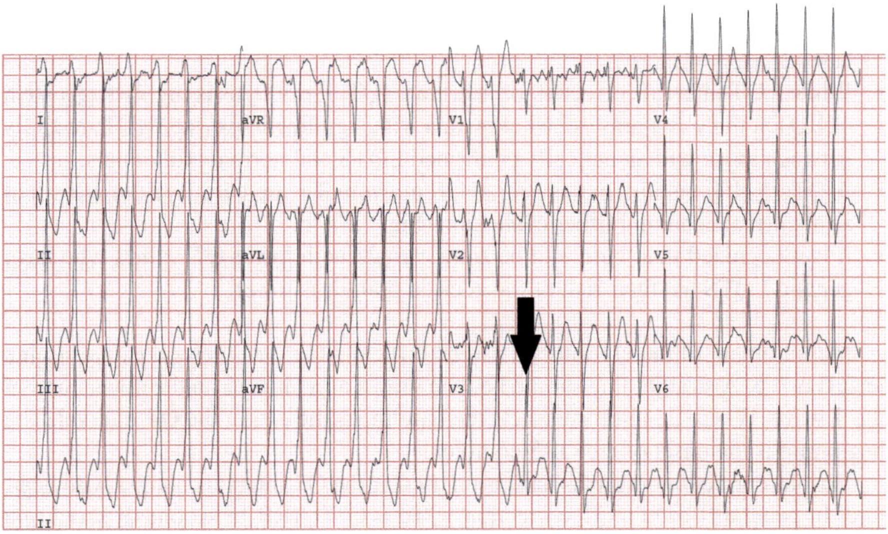


**Fig. 7.4** 18-year-old female basketball player with abrupt loss of pre-excitation (arrow) at 176 beats/minute on a treadmill test which suggests a bypass pathway at lower risk for causing sudden death

higher heart rates, or if the patient does not desire an exercise test, an electrophysiology (EP) study should be performed. The best predictor of SCA is a shortest pre-excited RR interval (SPERRI) in atrial fibrillation of ≤250 ms. In these patients, ablation is then performed if the pathway location is felt to be low risk for heart block or other complication. While this has a high sensitivity, this cutoff has a low specificity, meaning most patients with a low SPERRI will never have SCA [51].

A recent systematic review of 9 studies assessed the risk of SCA and method of risk stratification [52]. There was only one randomized controlled trial, however, on how to manage asymptomatic WPW. In addition, the age range of studies was from 19 to 50 years old so results may not be applicable to adolescents. Overall, malignant atrial fibrillation with an accessory pathway SPERRI ≤250 ms or ventricular fibrillation occurred in 9% and 1.5%, respectively. It is notable that there was no correlation of these outcomes with prior symptoms. Complication rates of EP study with ablation are low at 0.09% to 1% [53].

An autopsy study of 19 persons who died of SCA with an antemortem diagnosis of WPW showed that most events occurred at rest [54]. Four of these had a prior successful ablation. About half of these had other cardiac disease, including HCM, cardiac sarcoid, or idiopathic left ventricular hypertrophy. This argues that WPW can be implicated in SCA and that evaluation with echocardiography should be performed in all patients with WPW, with consideration for MRI if there is a suspicion for a cardiomyopathy.

**Prolonged QT Interval**

- Long QT syndrome (LQTS), a genetic disorder due to mutations in cardiac ion channels, is associated with torsade de pointes and SCA.
- The most common forms are LQT1, LQT2, and LQT3 due to mutations in KCNQ1, KCNH2, and SCN5A, respectively, which make up about 80% of cases.
- While a QT interval corrected for heart rate (QTc) ≥ 500 ms is highly suggestive of LQTS, there is a gray zone below this with significant overlap in QT intervals between those with genetically confirmed LQTS and normal individuals.
- A QTc ≥ 480 ms in females and ≥ 470 ms in males are cutoff values classified as abnormal needing further evaluation (Fig. 7.5).
- It is recognized that there will be some people with lower QT values who have genetic LQTS but their risk of torsades de pointes is lower.

Measurement of the QT interval can be difficult. The best method is to examine lead II or V5. A straight line should be then drawn as a tangent on the downslope of the T wave. Where this line intersects the baseline is the end of the QT interval. The beginning is the onset of the QRS complex.

Various correction formulas have been used as the QT interval changes with heart rate. In general, Bazett's QT correction [QTc = QT/√(RR in seconds)] should be used, noting that the accuracy is limited at heart rates below 50 or greater than 90. In these individuals, the athlete should be encouraged to do a small amount of exercise to increase the heart rate if the heart rate is low, or to give additional time for

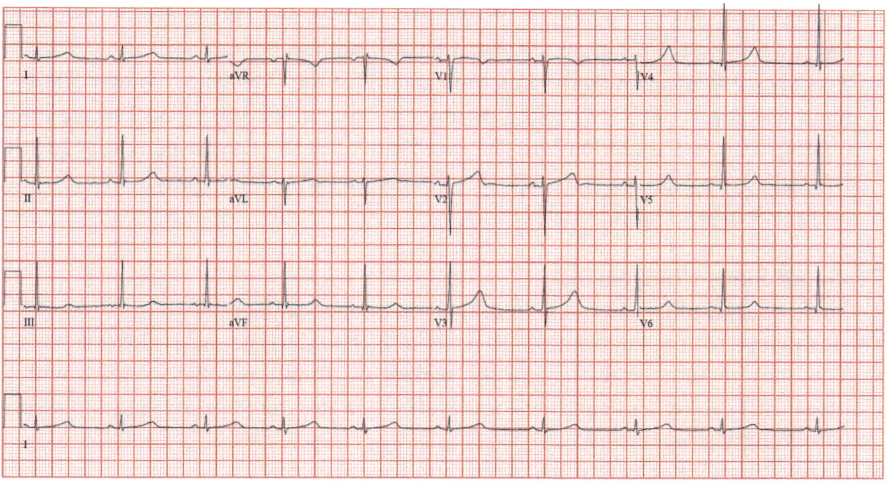


**Fig. 7.5** 18-year-old female soccer player with a prolonged QT interval measuring 508 ms, and a QTc using the Bazett formula of 494 ms. Genetic testing confirmed LQT1

relaxation for the heart rate to decrease. If there is an irregular heart rate due to sinus arrhythmia, an average of multiple beats of both the QT and RR should be used.

- There is variability in QT measurements even amongst experienced ECG readers [55]. The computer interpretation of the QT interval is about 90 to 95% accurate [14].
- T wave morphology may also suggest LQTS. Notching of the T wave in the lateral precordial leads, especially if the second part of the notch is greater than the first part of the notch, may suggest LQT2 even if the QT interval is normal [56].

Importantly, a single abnormal ECG with a prolonged QTc does not give a definitive diagnosis of LQTS. If a prolonged QT interval is found, a repeat ECG on a different day should be completed. ECGs of family members and a thorough family history of SCA, seizures, or unexplained deaths can be instructive. QT prolonging medications should be assessed (http://www.crediblemeds.org). In addition, an exercise stress test to assess for exercise-induced arrhythmias and whether the QTc is ≥ 470 ms at 2–5 min of recovery can be used [57]. Genetic testing and the Schwartz score also may be helpful (see also Chap. 21) [58].

**Brugada Pattern**

- The Type 1 Brugada pattern is defined as a coved rsR', ST elevation ≥ 2 mm with downsloping ST-segment, and symmetric T wave inversions in leads V1–V3.
- The Brugada Type 1 pattern is associated with syncope or SCA usually during rest or sleep.
- The Corrado index examines the height at the start of the ST-segment/J-point versus 80 ms later [59]. If this ratio is greater than one, the ST-segment is

downsloping and is concerning for the Brugada pattern. If the ratio is less than one, then there is upsloping ST elevation and is normal.
- The Type 2 Brugada pattern has a high takeoff of the r′ ≥ 2 mm, convex ST segment elevation ≥ 0.5 mm, and a positive T wave in V2 [60]. The T wave morphology can be variable in V1. The event rate of SCA or syncope is very low in Brugada Type 2 and for the purposes of screening would not warrant more evaluation (see also Chap. 21) [61].

**Profound Sinus Bradycardia**
- Sinus bradycardia is a typical finding in endurance athletes.
- However, a resting heart rate ≤ 30 beats/min should trigger an evaluation.
- This may include either having the patient do simple aerobic exercise with a repeat ECG at higher heart rates or performing a structured exercise test to assess chronotropic competence.
- If these are normal, no further evaluation is necessary.

**Profound First-Degree AV Block**
- First degree AV block is common in well-conditioned athletes.
- However, a PR interval ≥ 400 ms may represent conduction system disease.
- Limited aerobic exercise or a formalized stress test can be completed to assess for shortening of the PR interval with activity.
- If there is higher degree AV block with exercise, then further evaluation should be completed which may include an echocardiogram and/or ambulatory ECG monitor.

**Mobitz II and Complete AV Block**
- Mobitz II, second degree heart block and complete AV block are rare findings on screening ECG but would suggest significant conduction system disease. Rarely, congenital complete heart block will be found.
- It is important to differentiate Mobitz Type I versus Type II second degree AV block as Type I is a normal finding and much more common. Similarly, AV dissociation may be due to complete AV block or to sinus bradycardia with accelerated junctional or ventricular rhythms. More P waves than QRS complexes is consistent with complete AV block whereas more QRS complexes than P waves is consistent with accelerated rhythms.

**Frequent Premature Ventricular Contractions (PVCs) and Nonsustained Ventricular Tachycardia (NSVT)**
- PVCs have been associated with cardiomyopathy though they may also be seen in normal individuals. Specifically, ARVC, dilated cardiomyopathy, HCM, or myocarditis may have PVCs.
- On a standard ECG, two or more PVCs would suggest a high burden over a 24-h period and is considered abnormal. It is recognized that there is variability throughout the day or day-to-day in PVC burden and a single ECG may not necessarily pick up frequent PVCs.

An Italian study of 120 competitive athletes with no personal or family history of cardiomyopathy with a median of 3760 premature ventricular beats in 24 h showed that even in those who continued playing sport in the absence of treatment, the number of PVCs significantly decreased to 1240 beats per 24 h [62]. Another study with 5011 athletes undergoing exercise testing showed that 367 athletes had exercise-induced PVCs and demonstrated a reduction on repeat exercise testing even if allowed to continue playing sports [63]. While some have suggested that detraining may be necessary to show a reduction in PVC burden [64], it may simply be regression to the mean with or without detraining to explain why PVC burden decreases.

- NSVT is rarely seen and requires further evaluation.
- PVC morphology may have a role in identifying individuals with cardiac disease.
  - In normal individuals, PVCs with a LBBB morphology and an inferiorly directed axis with a variable precordial transition come from the right or left ventricular outflow tracts. PVCs with a RBBB morphology and superior axis frequently may be originating from one of the left bundle fascicles or the left ventricular papillary muscles.
  - If a PVC has a LBBB morphology with a superiorly directed axis, this might be indicative of ARVC as it suggests it is coming from the non-outflow tract portion of the right ventricle.

There has been concern for a form of ARVC induced by extreme endurance exercise [65–67]. Studies of some high-level endurance athletes with SCA showed findings of ARVC but a lower than expected rate of positive genetic testing and no family history of ARVC. This proposed type of exercise-induced ARVC may be manifest on ECG by frequent PVCs and in those with a history of intense endurance exercise.

Two or more PVCs on a 10 s ECG requires further evaluation including an echocardiogram, 24-h ambulatory monitor to assess the PVC burden, and additional investigation with exercise stress testing or cardiac MRI as indicated.

**Epsilon Wave**

- An epsilon wave is seen in the setting of ARVC (Fig. 7.6).
- It is a low amplitude, high frequency signal (small deflections and/or notches) between the end of the QRS complex and onset of the T wave in leads V1–V3 [68].
- It is rarely present on a screening ECG in the absence of other abnormalities such as T wave inversions in the anterior precordial leads.

**Atrial Tachyarrhythmias**

- The most common tachycardia on screening ECG is sinus tachycardia, especially if the athlete is anxious. A repeat ECG should be done a few minutes later if the heart rate is >120 bpm after the athlete has been given time to relax.

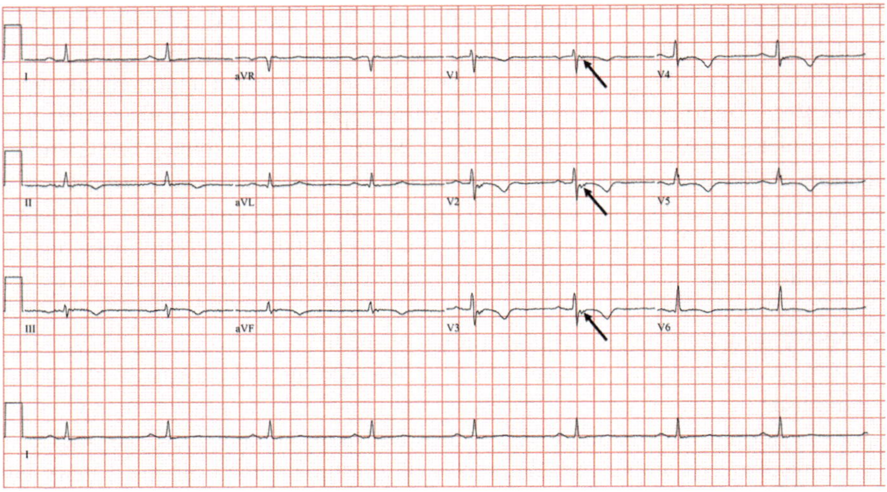


**Fig. 7.6** A 32-year-old male cyclist with an epsilon wave (arrows), defined as a low-amplitude high frequency signal between the QRS complex and T wave, present in leads V1–3. T wave inversions in V1–6, II, and aVF are also present

- Supraventricular tachycardia, atrial fibrillation and atrial flutter are rarely seen in athletes. If these are present, it may suggest the possibility of a cardiomyopathy or channelopathy.

## 7.5 Accuracy of Current Testing

Several studies have shown relatively good inter-observer agreement with ECG screening [69–71]. Even limited training can increase reader accuracy [72]. Open access to ECG training modules based on the International Criteria are available at: https://uwsportscardiology.org/e-academy/.

While ECG screening by experienced clinicians using athlete-specific standards typically produces false-positive rates <3–5%, some athlete groups may have a higher rate of ECG abnormalities. A study in athletes from the National Basketball Association showed that the new International Criteria were better than the Seattle Criteria, but 15.8% of African-American players and 11.5% of Caucasian players still had an abnormal ECG, with no disease based on echocardiogram findings [73]. However, cardiac MRI was not routinely performed in athletes with lateral or inferolateral T wave inversions.

Other studies demonstrate lower false-positive rates when applying the International Criteria [11, 12]. A study of 5000 athletes showed a 50% reduction in false positive results and all cases of true disease identified by the International Criteria [74].

**Clinical Pearls**

- ECG interpretation in athletes should be completed using athlete-specific standards, the most up-to-date of which is the International Criteria for ECG interpretation in athletes [14].
- Normal findings or one borderline finding do not require further testing, while two or more borderline findings and any abnormal finding requires further testing.
- The most frequent abnormal findings include T wave inversions, ST-segment depression, pathologic Q waves, and ventricular pre-excitation/WPW pattern.
- ECG abnormalities alone do not represent a disease in most cases, but should trigger additional evaluation to exclude pathologic cardiac disease.

## Review

### Questions

1. A 19-year-old male ice hockey player has a screening ECG that demonstrates 2 mm T wave inversion in V5–6 with no other abnormal findings. A follow-up transthoracic echocardiogram is normal. Which of the following is the most appropriate next step?
    1. 24-h Holter
    2. Cardiac magnetic resonance imaging
    3. Exercise treadmill test
    4. No further testing
    5. Signal averaged ECG
2. An 18-year-old black male football player undergoes a preparticipation evaluation with an ECG showing J point and ST-segment elevation and biphasic T wave inversion in leads V1–4. There is Sokolow-Lyon voltage criteria for left ventricular hypertrophy. Which of the following is the most appropriate diagnostic evaluation?
    1. 24-h Holter
    2. Cardiac magnetic resonance imaging
    3. No testing
    4. Signal averaged ECG
    5. Transthoracic echocardiogram
3. A 17-year-old female tennis player presents to the emergency room with abrupt onset of palpitations which terminate with the Valsalva maneuver. 12-lead ECG demonstrates a PR interval of 100 ms and QRS of 140 ms with a slurred upstroke. Which of the following is the most appropriate next test?
    1. 30-day event monitor
    2. Cardiac magnetic resonance imaging
    3. Electrophysiology study
    4. Exercise ECG treadmill test
    5. Observant management

## Answers

1. In an athlete with T wave inversion in V5–6, there is concern for apical hypertrophic cardiomyopathy. A transthoracic echocardiogram may not accurately image the apex of the left ventricle and a cardiac MRI should be completed.
2. The pattern of J point and ST-segment elevation with T wave inversion in leads V1–4 in a black athlete is a normal finding and does not require any further evaluation.
3. The 12-lead ECG demonstrates a Wolff-Parkinson-White pattern. In the presence of symptoms suggestive of an arrhythmia, an electrophysiology study should be completed to assess if atrioventricular reentrant tachycardia can be induced and to determine the shortest pre-excited RR interval in atrial fibrillation or the accessory pathway effective refractory period. In symptomatic patients an ablation should be considered depending on the safety and accessibility of the bypass pathway as determined by its location. An exercise treadmill test should only be used for asymptomatic patients. A 30-day event monitor could be considered if symptoms were not consistent with an arrhythmia. A transthoracic echocardiogram should be performed also to rule out structural heart disease, but a cardiac magnetic resonance imaging typically isn't needed.

## References

1. Maron BJ, Friedman RA, Kligfield P, Levine BD, Viskin S, Chaitman BR, et al. Assessment of the 12-lead electrocardiogram as a screening test for detection of cardiovascular disease in healthy general populations of young people (12–25 years of age): a scientific statement from the American Heart Association and the American College of Cardiology. J Am Coll Cardiol. 2014;64(14):1479–514.
2. Mont L, Pelliccia A, Sharma S, Biffi A, Borjesson M, Brugada Terradellas J, et al. Pre-participation cardiovascular evaluation for athletic participants to prevent sudden death: Position paper from the EHRA and the EACPR, branches of the ESC. Endorsed by APHRS, HRS, and SOLAECE. Eur J Prev Cardiol. 2017;24(1):41–69.
3. Johri AM, Poirier P, Dorian P, Fournier A, Goodman JM, McKinney J, et al. Canadian Cardiovascular Society/Canadian Heart Rhythm Society Joint Position Statement on the Cardiovascular Screening of Competitive Athletes. Can J Cardiol. 2019;35(1):1–11.
4. Drezner JA, O'Connor FG, Harmon KG, Fields KB, Asplund CA, Asif IM, et al. Infographic: AMSSM position statement on cardiovascular preparticipation screening in athletes: current evidence, knowledge gaps, recommendations and future directions. Br J Sports Med. 2017;51(3):168.
5. Fudge J, Harmon KG, Owens DS, Prutkin JM, Salerno JC, Asif IM, et al. Cardiovascular screening in adolescents and young adults: a prospective study comparing the pre-participation Physical Evaluation Monograph 4th Edition and ECG. Br J Sports Med. 2014;48(15):1172–8.
6. Harmon KG, Zigman M, Drezner JA. The effectiveness of screening history, physical exam, and ECG to detect potentially lethal cardiac disorders in athletes: a systematic review/meta-analysis. J Electrocardiol. 2015;48(3):329–38.
7. Corrado D, Pelliccia A, Heidbuchel H, Sharma S, Link M, Basso C, et al. Recommendations for interpretation of 12-lead electrocardiogram in the athlete. Eur Heart J. 2010;31(2):243–59.
8. Sheikh N, Papadakis M, Ghani S, Zaidi A, Gati S, Adami PE, et al. Comparison of electrocardiographic criteria for the detection of cardiac abnormalities in elite black and white athletes. Circulation. 2014;129(16):1637–49.

9. Drezner JA, Ackerman MJ, Anderson J, Ashley E, Asplund CA, Baggish AL, et al. Electrocardiographic interpretation in athletes: the Seattle Criteria. Br J Sports Med. 2013;47(3):122–4.
10. Brosnan M, La Gerche A, Kalman J, Lo W, Fallon K, MacIsaac A, et al. The Seattle Criteria increase the specificity of preparticipation ECG screening among elite athletes. Br J Sports Med. 2014;48(15):1144–50.
11. Zorzi A, Calore C, Vio R, Pelliccia A, Corrado D. Accuracy of the ECG for differential diagnosis between hypertrophic cardiomyopathy and athlete's heart: comparison between the European Society of Cardiology (2010) and International (2017) criteria. Br J Sports Med. 2018;52(10):667–73.
12. McClean G, Riding NR, Pieles G, Watt V, Adamuz C, Sharma S, et al. Diagnostic accuracy and Bayesian analysis of new international ECG recommendations in paediatric athletes. Heart. 2019;105(2):152–9.
13. Pickham D, Zarafshar S, Sani D, Kumar N, Froelicher V. Comparison of three ECG criteria for athlete pre-participation screening. J Electrocardiol. 2014;47(6):769–74.
14. Sharma S, Drezner JA, Baggish A, Papadakis M, Wilson MG, Prutkin JM, et al. International recommendations for electrocardiographic interpretation in athletes. J Am Coll Cardiol. 2017;69(8):1057–75.
15. Malhotra A, Dhutia H, Finocchiaro G, Gati S, Beasley I, Clift P, et al. Outcomes of cardiac screening in adolescent soccer players. N Engl J Med. 2018;379(6):524–34.
16. Pelliccia A, Di Paolo FM, Quattrini FM, Basso C, Culasso F, Popoli G, et al. Outcomes in athletes with marked ECG repolarization abnormalities. N Engl J Med. 2008;358(2):152–61.
17. Papadakis M, Basavarajaiah S, Rawlins J, Edwards C, Makan J, Firoozi S, et al. Prevalence and significance of T-wave inversions in predominantly Caucasian adolescent athletes. Eur Heart J. 2009;30(14):1728–35.
18. Papadakis M, Carre F, Kervio G, Rawlins J, Panoulas VF, Chandra N, et al. The prevalence, distribution, and clinical outcomes of electrocardiographic repolarization patterns in male athletes of African/Afro-Caribbean origin. Eur Heart J. 2011;32(18):2304–13.
19. Zaidi A, Ghani S, Sheikh N, Gati S, Bastiaenen R, Madden B, et al. Clinical significance of electrocardiographic right ventricular hypertrophy in athletes: comparison with arrhythmogenic right ventricular cardiomyopathy and pulmonary hypertension. Eur Heart J. 2013;34(47):3649–56.
20. Patton KK, Ellinor PT, Ezekowitz M, Kowey P, Lubitz SA, Perez M, et al. Electrocardiographic early repolarization: a scientific statement From the American Heart Association. Circulation. 2016;133(15):1520–9.
21. Noseworthy PA, Weiner R, Kim J, Keelara V, Wang F, Berkstresser B, et al. Early repolarization pattern in competitive athletes: clinical correlates and the effects of exercise training. Circ Arrhythm Electrophysiol. 2011;4(4):432–40.
22. Gourine AV, Ackland GL. Cardiac vagus and exercise. Physiology (Bethesda). 2019;34(1):71–80.
23. Stein R, Medeiros CM, Rosito GA, Zimerman LI, Ribeiro JP. Intrinsic sinus and atrioventricular node electrophysiologic adaptations in endurance athletes. J Am Coll Cardiol. 2002;39(6):1033–8.
24. D'Souza A, Bucchi A, Johnsen AB, Logantha SJ, Monfredi O, Yanni J, et al. Exercise training reduces resting heart rate via downregulation of the funny channel HCN4. Nat Commun. 2014;5:3775.
25. Migliore F, Zorzi A, Michieli P, Perazzolo Marra M, Siciliano M, Rigato I, et al. Prevalence of cardiomyopathy in Italian asymptomatic children with electrocardiographic T-wave inversion at preparticipation screening. Circulation. 2012;125(3):529–38.
26. Hermelin MJ, Prutkin JM. Black athlete electrocardiographic repolarization pattern. J Electrocardiol. 2018;51(4):680–2.
27. Riding NR, Sharma S, McClean G, Adamuz C, Watt V, Wilson MG. Impact of geographical origin upon the electrical and structural manifestations of the black athlete's heart. Eur Heart J. 2019;40(1):50–8.

28. Pelliccia A, Culasso F, Di Paolo FM, Accettura D, Cantore R, Castagna W, et al. Prevalence of abnormal electrocardiograms in a large, unselected population undergoing pre-participation cardiovascular screening. Eur Heart J. 2007;28(16):2006–10.
29. Baggish AL, Hutter AM Jr, Wang F, Yared K, Weiner RB, Kupperman E, et al. Cardiovascular screening in college athletes with and without electrocardiography: a cross-sectional study. Ann Intern Med. 2010;152(5):269–75.
30. Kim JH, Noseworthy PA, McCarty D, Yared K, Weiner R, Wang F, et al. Significance of electrocardiographic right bundle branch block in trained athletes. Am J Cardiol. 2011;107(7):1083–9.
31. Kim JH, Baggish AL. Electrocardiographic right and left bundle branch block patterns in athletes: prevalence, pathology, and clinical significance. J Electrocardiol. 2015;48(3):380–4.
32. Gati S, Sheikh N, Ghani S, Zaidi A, Wilson M, Raju H, et al. Should axis deviation or atrial enlargement be categorised as abnormal in young athletes? The athlete's electrocardiogram: time for re-appraisal of markers of pathology. Eur Heart J. 2013;34(47):3641–8.
33. Corrado D, Calore C, Zorzi A, Migliore F. Improving the interpretation of the athlete's electrocardiogram. Eur Heart J. 2013;34(47):3606–9.
34. Calore C, Melacini P, Pelliccia A, Cianfrocca C, Schiavon M, Di Paolo FM, et al. Prevalence and clinical meaning of isolated increase of QRS voltages in hypertrophic cardiomyopathy versus athlete's heart: relevance to athletic screening. Int J Cardiol. 2013;168(4):4494–7.
35. Schnell F, Riding N, O'Hanlon R, Axel Lentz P, Donal E, Kervio G, et al. Recognition and significance of pathological T-wave inversions in athletes. Circulation. 2015;131(2):165–73.
36. Sheikh N, Papadakis M, Wilson M, Malhotra A, Adamuz C, Homfray T, et al. Diagnostic yield of genetic testing in young athletes with T-wave inversion. Circulation. 2018;138(12):1184–94.
37. Calore C, Zorzi A, Sheikh N, Nese A, Facci M, Malhotra A, et al. Electrocardiographic anterior T-wave inversion in athletes of different ethnicities: differential diagnosis between athlete's heart and cardiomyopathy. Eur Heart J. 2016;37(32):2515–27.
38. MacAlpin RN. Clinical significance of QS complexes in V1 and V2 without other electrocardiographic abnormality. Ann Noninvasive Electrocardiol. 2004;9(1):39–47.
39. Chen AS, Bent RE, Wheeler M, Knowles JW, Haddad F, Froelicher V, et al. Large Q and S waves in lead III on the electrocardiogram distinguish patients with hypertrophic cardiomyopathy from athletes. Heart. 2018;104(22):1871–7.
40. Bent RE, Wheeler MT, Hadley D, Froelicher V, Ashley E, Perez MV. Computerized Q wave dimensions in athletes and hypertrophic cardiomyopathy patients. J Electrocardiol. 2015;48(3):362–7.
41. Marek J, Bufalino V, Davis J, Marek K, Gami A, Stephan W, et al. Feasibility and findings of large-scale electrocardiographic screening in young adults: data from 32,561 subjects. Heart Rhythm. 2011;8(10):1555–9.
42. Drezner JA, Owens DS, Prutkin JM, Salerno JC, Harmon KG, Prosise S, et al. Electrocardiographic screening in National Collegiate Athletic Association Athletes. Am J Cardiol. 2016;118(5):754–9.
43. Drezner JA, Prutkin JM, Harmon KG, O'Kane JW, Pelto HF, Rao AL, et al. Cardiovascular screening in college athletes. J Am Coll Cardiol. 2015;65(21):2353–5.
44. Pelliccia A, Maron BJ, Culasso F, Di Paolo FM, Spataro A, Biffi A, et al. Clinical significance of abnormal electrocardiographic patterns in trained athletes. Circulation. 2000;102(3):278–84.
45. Wilson MG, Chatard JC, Carre F, Hamilton B, Whyte GP, Sharma S, et al. Prevalence of electrocardiographic abnormalities in West-Asian and African male athletes. Br J Sports Med. 2012;46(5):341–7.
46. Bent RE, Wheeler MT, Hadley D, Knowles JW, Pavlovic A, Finocchiaro G, et al. Systematic comparison of digital electrocardiograms from healthy athletes and patients with hypertrophic cardiomyopathy. J Am Coll Cardiol. 2015;65(22):2462–3.
47. Dunn T, Abdelfattah R, Aggarwal S, Pickham D, Hadley D, Froelicher V. Are the QRS duration and ST depression cut-points from the Seattle criteria too conservative? J Electrocardiol. 2015;48(3):395–8.

48. Xiao HB, Brecker SJ, Gibson DG. Relative effects of left ventricular mass and conduction disturbance on activation in patients with pathological left ventricular hypertrophy. Br Heart J. 1994;71(6):548–53.
49. Cohen MI, Triedman JK, Cannon BC, Davis AM, Drago F, Janousek J, et al. PACES/HRS expert consensus statement on the management of the asymptomatic young patient with a Wolff-Parkinson-White (WPW, ventricular preexcitation) electrocardiographic pattern. Heart Rhythm. 2012;9(6):1006–24.
50. Klein GJ, Bashore TM, Sellers TD, Pritchett EL, Smith WM, Gallagher JJ. Ventricular fibrillation in the Wolff-Parkinson-White syndrome. N Engl J Med. 1979;301(20):1080–5.
51. Obeyesekere MN, Klein GJ. Intermittent preexcitation and the risk of sudden death: the exception that proves the rule? J Cardiovasc Electrophysiol. 2013;24(3):367–9.
52. Al-Khatib SM, Arshad A, Balk EM, Das SR, Hsu JC, Joglar JA, et al. Risk stratification for arrhythmic events in patients with asymptomatic pre-excitation: a systematic review for the 2015 ACC/AHA/HRS Guideline for the Management of Adult Patients With Supraventricular Tachycardia: A Report of the American College of Cardiology/American Heart Association Task Force on Clinical Practice Guidelines and the Heart Rhythm Society. Circulation. 2016;133(14):e575–86.
53. Pappone C, Vicedomini G, Manguso F, Saviano M, Baldi M, Pappone A, et al. Wolff-Parkinson-White syndrome in the era of catheter ablation: insights from a registry study of 2169 patients. Circulation. 2014;130(10):811–9.
54. Finocchiaro G, Papadakis M, Behr ER, Sharma S, Sheppard M. Sudden cardiac death in pre-excitation and Wolff-Parkinson-White: demographic and clinical features. J Am Coll Cardiol. 2017;69(12):1644–5.
55. Viskin S, Rosovski U, Sands AJ, Chen E, Kistler PM, Kalman JM, et al. Inaccurate electrocardiographic interpretation of long QT: the majority of physicians cannot recognize a long QT when they see one. Heart Rhythm. 2005;2(6):569–74.
56. Malfatto G, Beria G, Sala S, Bonazzi O, Schwartz PJ. Quantitative-analysis of T-wave abnormalities and their prognostic implications in the idiopathic long QT-syndrome. J Am Coll Cardiol. 1994;23(2):296–301.
57. Horner JM, Horner MM, Ackerman MJ. The diagnostic utility of recovery phase QTc during treadmill exercise stress testing in the evaluation of long QT syndrome. Heart Rhythm. 2011;8(11):1698–704.
58. Schwartz PJ, Crotti L. QTc behavior during exercise and genetic testing for the long-QT syndrome. Circulation. 2011;124(20):2181–4.
59. Zorzi A, Leoni L, Di Paolo FM, Rigato I, Migliore F, Bauce B, et al. Differential diagnosis between early repolarization of athlete's heart and coved-type brugada electrocardiogram. Am J Cardiol. 2015;115(4):529–32.
60. Bayes de Luna A, Brugada J, Baranchuk A, Borggrefe M, Breithardt G, Goldwasser D, et al. Current electrocardiographic criteria for diagnosis of Brugada pattern: a consensus report. J Electrocardiol. 2012;45(5):433–42.
61. Zorzi A, Migliore F, Marras E, Marinelli A, Baritussio A, Allocca G, et al. Should all individuals with a nondiagnostic Brugada-electrocardiogram undergo sodium-channel blocker test? Heart Rhythm. 2012;9(6):909–16.
62. Delise P, Sitta N, Lanari E, Berton G, Centa M, Allocca G, et al. Long-term effect of continuing sports activity in competitive athletes with frequent ventricular premature complexes and apparently normal heart. Am J Cardiol. 2013;112(9):1396–402.
63. Verdile L, Maron BJ, Pelliccia A, Spataro A, Santini M, Biffi A. Clinical significance of exercise-induced ventricular tachyarrhythmias in trained athletes without cardiovascular abnormalities. Heart Rhythm. 2015;12(1):78–85.
64. Biffi A, Maron BJ, Verdile L, Fernando F, Spataro A, Marcello G, et al. Impact of physical deconditioning on ventricular tachyarrhythmias in trained athletes. J Am Coll Cardiol. 2004;44(5):1053–8.

65. La Gerche A, Claessen G, Dymarkowski S, Voigt JU, De Buck F, Vanhees L, et al. Exercise-induced right ventricular dysfunction is associated with ventricular arrhythmias in endurance athletes. Eur Heart J. 2015;36(30):1998–2010.
66. Heidbuchel H, Hoogsteen J, Fagard R, Vanhees L, Ector H, Willems R, et al. High prevalence of right ventricular involvement in endurance athletes with ventricular arrhythmias. Role of an electrophysiologic study in risk stratification. Eur Heart J. 2003;24(16):1473–80.
67. La Gerche A, Robberecht C, Kuiperi C, Nuyens D, Willems R, de Ravel T, et al. Lower than expected desmosomal gene mutation prevalence in endurance athletes with complex ventricular arrhythmias of right ventricular origin. Heart. 2010;96(16):1268–74.
68. Marcus FI, McKenna WJ, Sherrill D, Basso C, Bauce B, Bluemke DA, et al. Diagnosis of arrhythmogenic right ventricular cardiomyopathy/dysplasia: proposed modification of the task force criteria. Circulation. 2010;121(13):1533–41.
69. Dhutia H, Malhotra A, Yeo TJ, Ster IC, Gabus V, Steriotis A, et al. Inter-rater reliability and downstream financial implications of electrocardiography screening in young athletes. Circ Cardiovasc Qual Outcomes. 2017;10(8):e003306.
70. Schneiter S, Trachsel LD, Perrin T, Albrecht S, Pirrello T, Eser P, et al. Inter-observer agreement in athletes ECG interpretation using the recent international recommendations for ECG interpretation in athletes among observers with different levels of expertise. PLoS One. 2018;13(11):e0206072.
71. Prutkin JM, Drezner JA. Training and experience matter: improving athlete ECG screening, interpretation, and Reproducibility. Circ Cardiovasc Qual Outcomes. 2017;10(8):e003881.
72. Drezner JA, Asif IM, Owens DS, Prutkin JM, Salerno JC, Fean R, et al. Accuracy of ECG interpretation in competitive athletes: the impact of using standised ECG criteria. Br J Sports Med. 2012;46(5):335–40.
73. Waase MP, Mutharasan RK, Whang W, DiTullio MR, DiFiori JP, Callahan L, et al. Electrocardiographic findings in National Basketball Association Athletes. JAMA Cardiol. 2018;3(1):69–74.
74. Dhutia H, Malhotra A, Finocchiaro G, Merghani A, Papadakis M, Naci H, et al. Impact of the International recommendations for electrocardiographic interpretation on cardiovascular screening in young athletes. J Am Coll Cardiol. 2017;70(6):805–7.

# Medical Evaluation of Athletes: Echocardiography

8

Flavio D'Ascenzi and David Oxborough

**Learning Objectives**

1. Understand the role of echocardiography in the assessment of the athlete, including pre-participation screening and secondary care.
2. Discuss normal conventional 2-dimensional, Doppler and tissue Doppler echocardiographic findings associated with the multi-factorial nature of the athlete's heart.
3. Discuss the role of conventional 2-dimensional, Doppler and tissue Doppler echocardiography in differentiating athlete's heart from conditions that predispose to sudden cardiac death.
4. Discuss the role of advanced echocardiographic techniques including strain imaging, 3-dimensional and exercise techniques in the assessment of the athlete's heart.

## 8.1 Introduction

Echocardiography is utilized ubiquitously in the assessment of cardiac structure and function. It is non-invasive and has the ability to provide high temporal and spatial resolution, making it an important diagnostic tool in the assessment of the athlete's heart. Although pre-participation evaluation is based in Europe mainly on physical

F. D'Ascenzi (✉)
Division of Cardiology, Department of Medical Biotechnologies, University of Siena, Siena, Italy

School of Medicine, University of Pittsburgh, Pittsburgh, PA, USA
e-mail: flavio.dascenzi@unisi.it

D. Oxborough
Research Institute for Sports and Exercise Sciences, Liverpool John Moores University, Liverpool, UK
e-mail: d.l.oxborough@ljmu.ac.uk



A. Pressler, J. Niebauer (eds.), *Textbook of Sports and Exercise Cardiology*,
https://doi.org/10.1007/978-3-030-35374-2_8

examination and resting ECG, echocardiography is becoming essential as screening tool in some conditions such as aortic dilatation and/or as the first important imaging technique to be used for the differential diagnosis.

## 8.2 The Athlete's Heart

### 8.2.1 The Left Ventricle

Structural physiological adaptation of the left ventricle (LV) is a common manifestation of the athlete's heart. Although enlargement is often within the constraints of normal geometry [1] there is evidence to suggest

- that those athletes engaged in high training volumes are more likely to develop an **eccentric** hypertrophy (chamber enlargement with concomitant increase in wall thickness) [2].
- **Concentric** hypertrophy (increased wall thickness without chamber enlargement) is less common particularly in female athletes (see also Chaps. 3 and 4) [3].

LV adaptation has been observed in athletes

(a) from multiple disciplines [4],
(b) in adults and children [5] and
(c) across ethnic groups [6, 7]

with specific cut-offs being applied (Fig. 8.1; Table 8.1) [8]. The greatest chamber adaptation is seen in adult male athletes whilst increased concentricity has been reported in athletes of black African/Afro-Caribbean ethnicity. In addition to an increase in overall LV mass, there is evidence to suggest that chronic training and hence frequent exposure to elevated preload can induce excess trabeculation as part of the remodeling process and is more frequently seen in male athletes of black

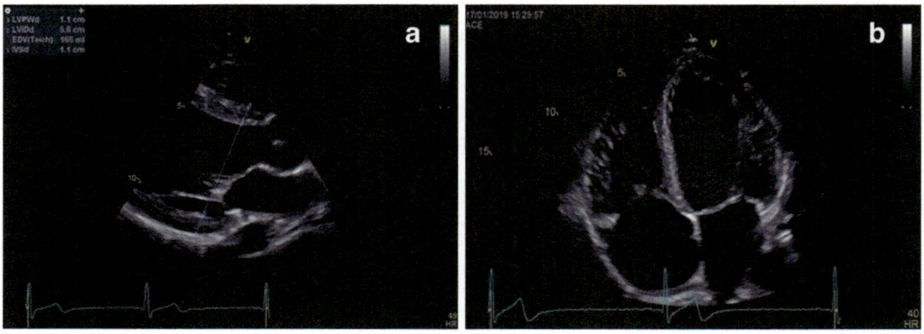


**Fig. 8.1** Physiological LV adaptation demonstrating balanced increases in wall thickness and cavity dimension in either the parasternal long axis (**a**) or the (**b**) apical 4-chamber view

**Table 8.1** Proposed cut-off values for LV and RV structure in athletes

| Parameter | Male athlete | Female athlete |
|---|---|---|
| LV dimension diastole (mm) | 64 | 57 |
| LV interventricular septal thickness (mm) | 13 | 11 |
| LV posterior wall thickness (mm) | 13 | 11 |
| LV mass (g) | 263 | 243 |
| $RVOT_1$ (short axis view, proximal; mm) | 43 | 40 |
| $RVOT_2$ (short axis view, distal; mm) | 32 | 29 |
| $RVD_1$ (apical view, basal; mm) | 55 | 49 |
| $RVD_2$ (apical view, middle-ventricle; mm) | 47 | 43 |
| $RVD_3$ (apical view, base-to-apex; mm) | 109 | 100 |

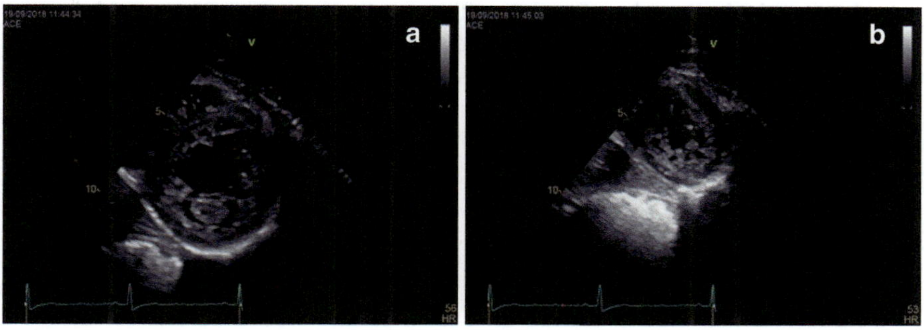


**Fig. 8.2** Examples of hypertrabeculation in athletes in a parasternal short axis view at the mid-level (**a**) and apex (**b**)

African/Afro-Caribbean ethnicity (see also Chap. 26) [9]. Careful attention should be made to ensure that normal myocardial function is present in the areas of hypertrabeculation to aid the differentiation from isolated LV non-compacted cardiomyopathy (Chap. 16) (Fig. 8.2) [10].

The impact of chronic training on LV function is less clear.

- In general, systolic function as determined by ejection fraction (EF) and tissue Doppler (TDI) is within normal limits.
- In a minority of athletes, specifically those with large chamber volumes, LV systolic function can be borderline low with ejection fraction falling below 50% [11]. This is likely a result of a large chamber requiring lower force to generate adequate stroke volumes at rest [12].
- In view of this, there is growing evidence to suggest that an exercise protocol should elicit a normal response with increases in EF consistent with cardiac reserve and may, therefore, serve as a useful indicator when differentiating from pathology (Chap. 10) [13].

The assessment of LV mechanics has shed further light into normal athletic adaptation. Previous studies have highlighted no significant differences in peak longitudinal strain between athletes and sedentary controls [14]. Although longitudinal function appears to be independent of training adaptation, circumferential and twist mechanics seem to change in tandem with physiological structural adaptation. Short axis function at the base and apex is mostly affected with apical rotation/twist demonstrating acute augmentation (i.e. increased twist during short training periods) followed by a reduction following longer periods of training exposure [15]. It has been suggested that the lower twist seen in the chronically adapted LV is driven by increased LV wall thickness [16]. The paradoxical nature and training load dependency of LV circumferential and twist mechanics exacerbates the grey area of differentiation from pathology and therefore these resting indices should be interpreted with caution.

Although some reports suggest diastolic function is supra-normal [17] this has not been evidenced across the literature and conventional values obtained from Doppler and tissue Doppler often fall within normal limits for the general population [18]. Reduced diastolic function is rarely seen in the athlete and specific cut-offs for TDI derived E' have been reported to aid differentiation from pathology.

### 8.2.2 The Right Ventricle

Dynamic exercise induces a disproportionate loading on the right ventricle (RV) [19] and hence RV structural adaptation is a frequent manifestation of the athlete's heart [20] (Table 8.1):

- There is proportional enlargement of the inflow and outflow and therefore the ratio between these is maintained (Fig. 8.3) [20].
- The magnitude of adaptation is reflective of training volumes with those athletes involved in dynamic activity demonstrating the greatest adaptation.
- In addition, age, body size and gender all seem to influence the degree of adaptation with male, older athletes having the largest dimensions [12].
- Unlike the LV, RV physiological adaptation appears to be similar across different ethnicity [21]. Although chamber enlargement is common, the thin wall of the RV is maintained and any evidence of an increased wall thickness (i.e. concentric hypertrophy) should be considered abnormal and is not reflective of physiological adaptation.

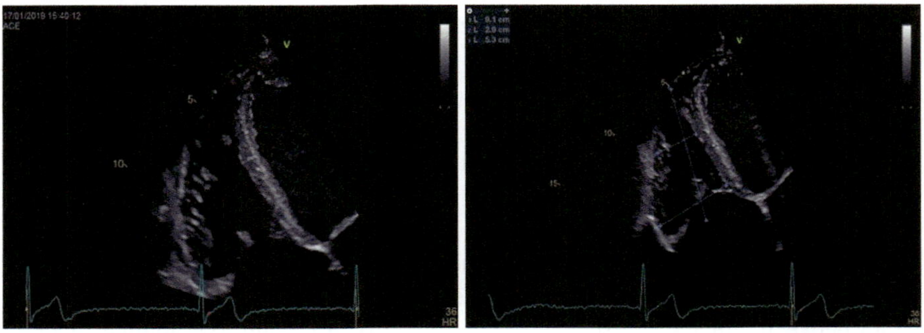

**Fig. 8.3** Modified RV inflow measurements demonstrating physiological enlargement

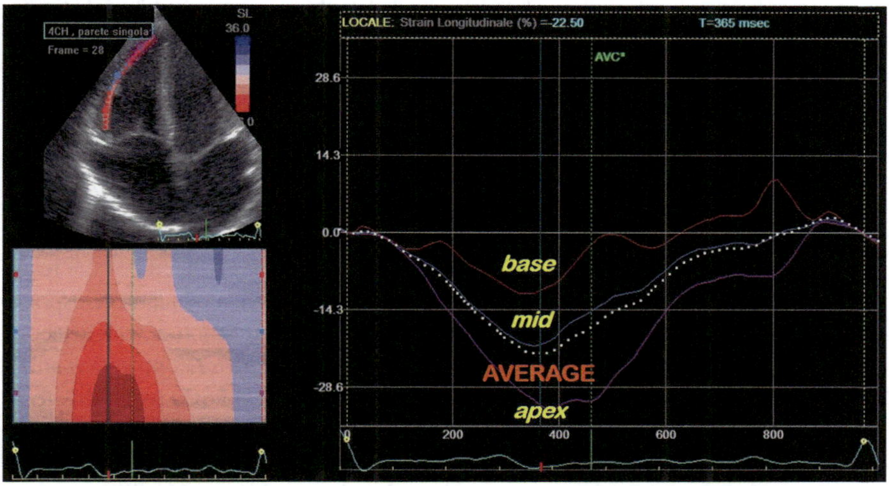


**Fig. 8.4** Speckle-tracking echocardiography applied to the right ventricle. Strain analysis is applied to the RV free wall, obtaining an average value of RV myocardial deformation

Global and conventional indices of RV function such as Fractional Area Change, Tricuspid Plane Systolic Excursion (TAPSE) and TDI are almost always normal [22]. Subtle assessment of longitudinal strain highlights regional variation related to segments of the RV free wall [23] which appear to be, in part, related to RV size (Fig. 8.4) [24]. Basal strain rate has been shown to be lower than non-athletic controls [25] whilst other studies have demonstrated lower apical function [24]. These regional variances appear to normalize during exercise, highlighting their physiological nature and providing a rationale for undertaking a stress protocol in the presence of low resting values [25]. That aside, global RV strain as determined as an average of the base, mid and apex is very rarely abnormal [26] and may aid the differentiation from pathology.

### 8.2.3 The Atria

Intensive training is associated with hemodynamic changes that typically induce an enlargement of cardiac chambers, involving not only the ventricles but also the atria.

- Indeed, typically competitive athletes have increased dimensions of left and right atria that have been interpreted as a physiologic adaptation to training both in males and females [27–31].
- Prospective studies have also found that exercise-induced atrial dilatation is dynamic in its nature and is reversible [32–34].
- Although most of the studies have been conducted in adults, biatrial remodeling has been confirmed also in children and adolescents practicing sport [35–37].

Although some authors have hypothesized that this increase in biatrial dimensions can be responsible for the higher incidence of supraventricular arrhythmias in athletes (and particularly in endurance athletes) as compared to controls [38, 39], echocardiographic studies assessing biatrial function in athletes have demonstrated that training-induced atrial remodeling is accompanied by a normal or even supranormal atrial function [17, 40]. Indeed, using echocardiography, and specifically by speckle-tracking echocardiography, it is possible to characterize atrial function and its specific phases. The application of speckle-tracking method to the atria allows the generation of a mean curve that presents a positive peak at the end of the reservoir phase, defined as *peak atrial longitudinal strain* (PALS), a plateau corresponding to the phase of diastasis and a measure of atrial reservoir function, and a second positive peak just before atrial contraction, defined as *peak atrial contraction strain* (PACS), a measure of atrial contractile function (Fig. 8.5). Studies using this technique have demonstrated that athlete's heart at rest is accompanied by supranormal atrial adaptation, with a normal reservoir function and a reduced atrial contractile function (compared to sedentary controls) related to a shift of LV filling toward early diastole [17, 40].

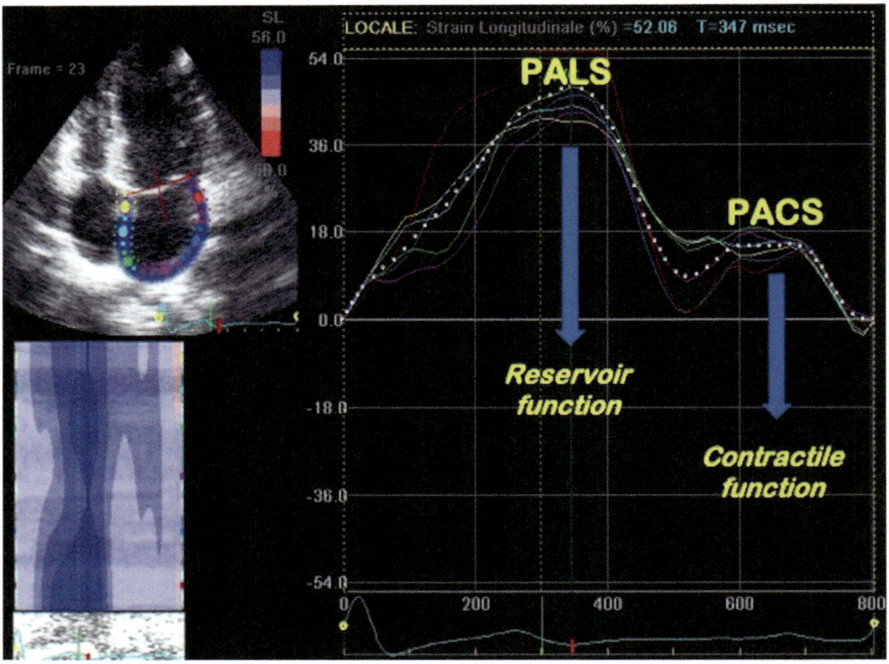


**Fig. 8.5** Application of speckle-tracking echocardiography to the left atrium of a control subject. Using this echocardiographic technique, two parameters of atrial function can be obtained: PALS, peak atrial longitudinal strain, a measure of atrial reservoir function, and PACS, peak atrial contraction strain, a measure of atrial contractile function

In other terms, the echocardiographic characterization of atrial function has demonstrated that atrial size is insufficient to provide mechanistic information about the atrium itself, and an increase in atrial size is not intrinsically an expression of atrial dysfunction. Furthermore, recent studies have found that characterization of atrial reservoir properties may be useful to differentiate physiologic remodeling induced by exercise from pathologic changes occurring in cardiac disorders in the early stages of these pathological conditions [41–43].

- Taken together, the current evidence suggests that atrial dilatation in athlete's heart can be regarded as a physiological rather than a pathological adaptation to sport and that the assessment of atrial function can be useful for distinguishing between a physiological vs. a pathological remodeling.

### 8.2.4 The Aortic Root

The aortic root is assessed as part of a standard echocardiographic examination and it is important to acknowledge normality in the athletic population (Fig. 8.6).

- There is evidence of mild adaptation with the athlete having a slight increase in aortic root dimensions compared to non-athletic controls [44].
- This adaptation is small and considered to be of little clinical relevance with the absolute dimensions at the Sinus of Valsalva unlikely to exceed 40 mm (0.3% prevalence) even in those individuals of extreme anthropometry [45].
- Recent evidence has highlighted the close linear relationship of aortic root to the height of the athlete and therefore a cut-off of 20 mm/m may aid interpretation [46].
- The morphology of the root is also important with the presence of normal effacement at the sino-tubular junction and proximal ascending aorta.
- Any evidence of enlargement or change in the aortic root morphology warrants further investigation.

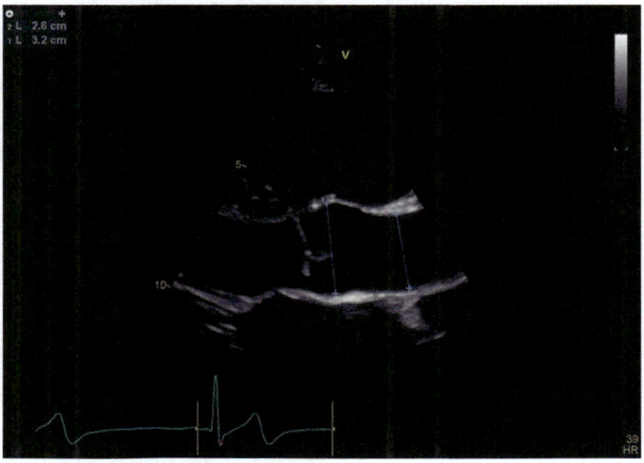


**Fig. 8.6** High parasternal long axis view demonstrating measurements at Sinus of Valsalva and proximal ascending aorta

## 8.3 Differentiation Between Physiological and Pathological Adaptations

### 8.3.1 Hypertrophic Cardiomyopathy

Hypertrophic cardiomyopathy (HCM) has an estimated prevalence of 1 in 500 [47] and has been suggested to account for 6–20% of all sudden cardiac deaths in the athletic population [48]. This inherited disease is characterized by myocardial disarray in the presence of variable phenotypes of LV hypertrophy (Fig. 8.7). The mild phenotypes pose a significant challenge when aiming to differentiate from physiological adaptation in that 14% of athletes with HCM have wall thicknesses between 13 and 16 mm [49]. Conventional echocardiographic criteria for HCM such as

(a) a small cavity,
(b) increased relative wall thickness,
(c) diastolic dysfunction and
(d) outflow obstruction

may be masked by the chronic adaptation to elevated preload during exercise and in this way, and athlete with HCM may present with eccentric hypertrophy and normal diastolic function with a preponderance to an apical phenotype [49]. This clearly exacerbates the differential diagnosis by increasing the potential of false negative findings and raises questions as to how best to utilize echocardiography in this setting.

- Finochiario et al. provided data from 1500 athletes and 58 patients with HCM in order to develop cut-offs to direct for further investigation [18].
  - In the presence of mild LVH, a combination of tissue Doppler and conventional trans-mitral Doppler should be utilized.
  - Reduced septal E′ < 10 cm/s and lateral E′ < 12 cm/s with elevated E/E′ > 7.9 are more consistent with a pathological phenotype.

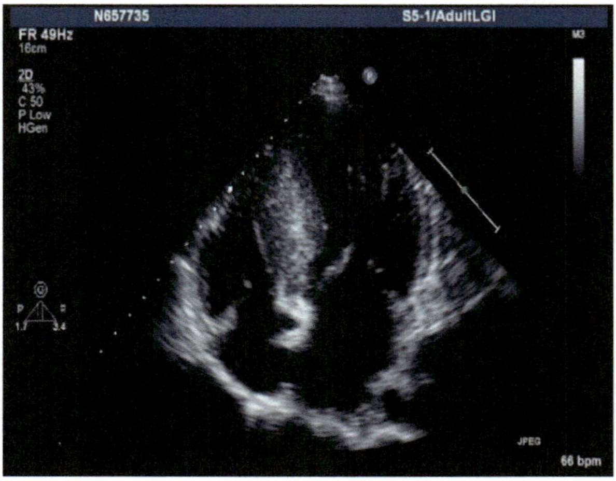


**Fig. 8.7** Apical 4-chamber view demonstrating asymmetric septal hypertrophy in an athlete with hypertrophic cardiomyopathy

It is important to note that these cut-offs have only reasonable sensitivity and specificity as other studies have highlighted low diastolic indices in a small minority of the athletic population [12, 16]. It is important in this setting to interpret the echocardiographic data within the clinical context and alongside the 12-lead ECG which is likely to be provide similar criteria between athletes and non-athletes with HCM [49].

In order to overcome some of the challenges of conventional echocardiography the use of longitudinal strain may provide additional diagnostic insight. Small studies have highlighted that, unlike the athlete's heart, global longitudinal strain (GLS) is often reduced in patients with HCM [50, 51]. These data inform current guidelines with recommendations that GLS > −16% should raise a suspicion of myocardial disease whilst > −12% is definitely abnormal [8].

### 8.3.2 Dilated Cardiomyopathy

Dilated cardiomyopathy (DCM) accounts for a small (<5%) proportion of athletes with SCD [48] either through an inherited form of the disease or secondary to myocarditis. LV dilatation is a common manifestation of the athlete's heart and in some cases, this structural adaptation may coexist with borderline low EF [11] and low longitudinal function/diastolic function. These findings can be compounded by the presence of RV and atrial dilatation. This raises a diagnostic dilemma and therefore careful assessment of the ventricle is required. Although often global, regional wall motion abnormalities may occur in DCM as the septum is under greater contractile stress than the free walls [52]. The normal structural and functional integrity of the athlete's heart dictate that regional abnormalities will not present and therefore the presence of any regional dysfunction serves to aid the diagnosis.

The important physiological phenomenon that is driving borderline/low function in an athlete underpins the concept of exercise reserve. When required, such as during bouts of exercise, the athlete's heart will improve in function in order to generate the higher stroke volumes. This mechanism serves as an important diagnostic criterion, in that a patient with DCM is less likely to be able to augment function when required:

- Although based on cardiac magnetic resonance imaging (CMR), Claessen et al. highlighted that EF improves in both athletes and DCM patients at low exercise workload but plateaus in the DCM patients with an inability to augment at higher exercise intensities [13].
  - An increase in EF of 11% at 75% $VO_2$max provides the ability to differentiate between the two groups.
- This 11% increase in EF has also been demonstrated with echocardiography during semi-recumbent exercise [53] and therefore highlights a role for stress echocardiography in these cases.

We are currently unaware of the magnitude of changes in TDI, diastolic indices and GLS in the same populations using the same methods and therefore further work in this area is warranted to provide additional discriminatory stress indices.

The rarer form of isolated left ventricular non-compaction (Chap. 16) is characterized by excess trabeculation and non-compacted layers of myocardium. The normal compacted layer of the myocardium is often thin and hypokinetic and results in ventricular dilatation and global dysfunction [10]. This form of DCM raises additional diagnostic challenges particularly in those athletes with physiological hypertrabeculation (Fig. 8.2) and low indices of systolic function [10]. It is recommended that regional dysfunction, myocardial thinning and gross excess non-compaction are not consistent with an athlete's heart and therefore careful assessment of ventricular structure and function is warranted in these cases.

As with other inherited conditions GLS may serve to provide additional diagnostic utility. GLS has been shown to be an early marker of DCM in the presence of normal EF [54] highlighted in those patients with intrinsic DCM or due to extrinsic factors such as cardiotoxicity [55]. Current guidelines recommend that GLS $> -16\%$ should raise a suspicion of myocardial disease whilst $>-12\%$ is definitely abnormal [8].

### 8.3.3 Arrhythmogenic Cardiomyopathy

Arrhythmogenic right ventricular cardiomyopathy (ARVC) is a rare genetic disease histologically characterized by replacement of myocardium with fibrous and fatty tissue, resulting in right ventricular (RV) dilation, dysfunction, and ventricular arrhythmia (Chap. 25) [56].

- ARVC is an important cause of sudden cardiac death (SCD) in youth and athletes [57].
- Diagnosis of ARVC is based on International Task Force Criteria, which combine family history and ECG, echocardiographic, CMR, and histological criteria [58].

Unfortunately, exercise-induced RV remodeling can mimic the pathological remodeling induced by ARVC and, as a consequence, athlete's heart may overlap some features of ARVC, especially in the early stages of the disease, and a relevant percentage of competitive athletes has been found to fulfill the dimensional criteria for the diagnosis of ARVC [21, 22]. Therefore, despite being crucial, the differential diagnosis between athlete's heart and ARVC can be very challenging. Indeed, RV is often dilated in competitive and top-level athletes: the greater the duration and intensity of exercise, the higher the cardiac output and, ultimately, the hemodynamic stimulus for the dimensional increase of the RV [22]. However, despite these similarities, ARVC patients usually exhibit a dilatation of the RV that is more evident at the level of RV outflow tract while RV enlargement in healthy athletes more often involves the RV main body.

In order to properly interpret RV remodeling,

(a) male gender,
(b) sports discipline,
(c) age, and
(d) years of training

should be taken into account. Indeed, RV enlargement is particularly evident in male athletes practicing endurance disciplines and in those who are engaged in sport activities for many years [21, 22, 59–61]. Notably, the impact of ethnicity is minimal, which obviates the need for race-specific RV reference values [21].

- According to the Task Force Criteria, diagnosis of ARVC by echocardiography requires a combination of regional RV wall motion abnormalities (WMAs) and global RV dilation and dysfunction. However, clinicians should be aware that physiological remodeling induced by exercise is not accompanied by the presence of RV WMAs, although WMAs are required for imaging diagnosis of ARVC in addition to RV dilation.
- Furthermore, despite a RV dilatation, RV function in competitive athletes is normal in most of the cases [22]. Therefore, the presence of RV dilatation and RV dysfunction should be regarded with high suspicion as it could be the early sign of a concealed cardiomyopathy potentially at risk of SCD.
- Finally, RV enlargement in athletes is usually accompanied by a concomitant remodeling of the LV, reflecting a global and symmetrical adaptation of the heart to the hemodynamic changes induced by training. Accordingly, a careful analysis of biventricular size and the estimation of RV/LV ratio can be useful in borderline cases in order to properly interpret RV enlargement [22].

In conclusion, although training-induced RV remodeling may mimic ARVC, some echocardiographic parameters can be very useful for the differential diagnosis between athlete's heart and ARVC. Table 8.2 summarizes the main echocardiographic parameters useful for the differential diagnosis.

**Table 8.2** Dimensional and functional parameters obtained by echocardiography in arrhythmogenic right ventricular cardiomyopathy vs. athlete's heart

| *Echocardiography and differential diagnosis between ARVC and athlete's heart* | | |
|---|---|---|
| ARVC | Findings | Athlete's heart |
| *Size* | | |
| + | Marked dilatation of RVOT | – |
| – | Moderate increase in RV main body with mild increase in RVOT | + |
| + | Disproportioned RV/LV ratio (<0.90) | – |
| – | Regression of RV dilatation after detraining | + |
| *Function* | | |
| + | RV wall motion abnormalities (bulging, akinesia, dyskinesia) | – |
| + | Reduced RV function (FAC <32%) | – |
| + | Reduced RV longitudinal strain (<20%) | – |
| + | Reduced RV s' velocity < 0.10 m/s | – |
| + | Reduced RV function by CMR | – |
| + | RV and/or LV tissue abnormalities (fat infiltration and LGE) at CMR | – |

*ARVC* arrhythmogenic right ventricular cardiomyopathy, *RVOT* right ventricular outflow tract, *RV* right ventricular, *LV* left ventricular, *FAC* fractional area change, *LGE* late gadolinium enhancement, *CMR* cardiac magnetic resonance

### 8.3.4 Coronary Artery Origin Anomalies

- Anomalous origin of coronary arteries is a rare congenital heart disease (prevalence between 0.17% and 1.3%).
- While it can be a benign finding, coronary artery anomalies have been recognized as major cause of SCD in competitive athletes, accounting for about 17% of such deaths in the USA and for 16% in Italy, particularly in case of an anomalous origin from the wrong sinus (Chap. 22) [62–65].
- The diagnosis can be suspected/defined non-invasively by transthoracic echocardiography as a first step [66, 67] and, according to their relevant clinical impact, a comprehensive echocardiographic examination in the athlete should include the visualization of coronary arteries ostia.

Figure 8.8 shows the normal and abnormal origin of coronary arteries identified by transthoracic echocardiography. However, we have to recognize that, although trans-thoracic echocardiography is a reliable noninvasive tool in detecting such anomalies, its sensitivity and specificity are influenced by the acoustic window and by expertise. The failure to demonstrate that a CA originates from its proper Valsalva

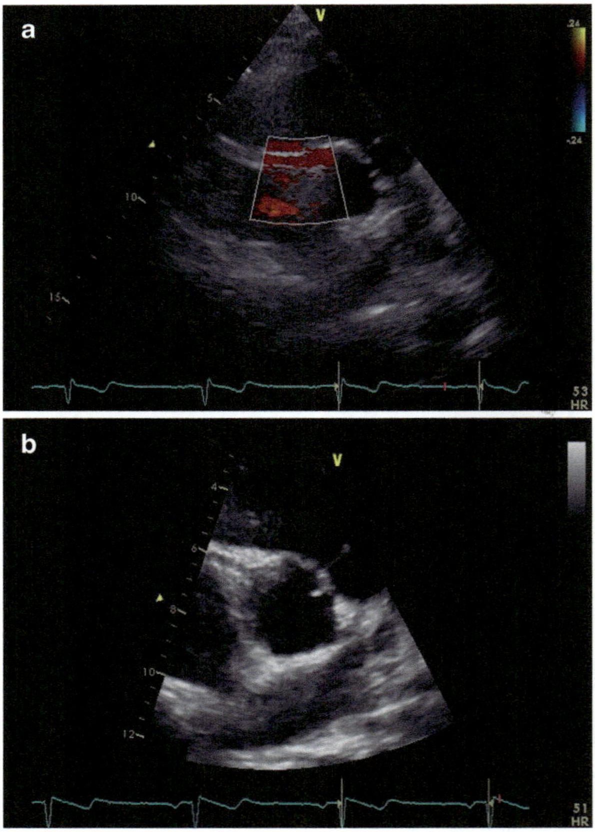


**Fig. 8.8** Origin of coronary arteries identified with colour Doppler (**a**) and without (**b**) by transthoracic echocardiography

sinus requires further anatomic confirmation with computed tomography (CT), CMR angiography or coronary angiography, as suggested [8]. In patients with a clinical suspicion of coronary artery anomalies, the European Society of Cardiology recommends CT and the American Heart Association either CT or CMR angiography, the latter preferred due to radiation concerns [68, 69].

Therefore, while a routine echocardiographic examination should include the visualization of coronary ostia, it should become mandatory in athletes with symptoms (e.g. chest pain/discomfort, presyncope or syncope, particularly if in relation with exercise) and/or with abnormal examinations (e.g. stress ECG testing).

**Clinical Pearls**

- For the differential diagnosis between athlete's heart and cardiomyopathies it is essential to evaluate the entire heart, taking into account whether ventricular or atrial dilatation occurs in the context of a harmonic and global remodeling, such as in athlete's heart
- The type of sports, gender, years of sports practice, weekly training volume and intensity, and training period should be taken into account to evaluate exercise-induced cardiac remodeling
- In the context of athlete's heart chamber dilatation is usually not accompanied by a reduction in cardiac function, as demonstrated by conventional and advanced echocardiographic techniques

## Review

### Questions

1. Are functional parameters useful for the differential diagnosis between athlete's heart and ARVC? If yes, which ones?
2. Is atrial dilatation always pathological?
3. Is it possible and useful to identify coronary arteries origin by transthoracic echocardiography?

### Answers

1. Yes, they are useful. Among the functional parameters, TAPSE, S′ velocity, RV-FAC and possibly RV strain should be analysed to help distinguishing between athlete's heart and ARVC.
2. No, it isn't. Indeed, usually atrial dilatation in competitive athletes is accompanied by normal atrial function, as demonstrated by speckle-tracking echocardiography.
3. Yes, it is possible in most of the cases and is useful in order to identify a potentially life-threatening condition.

## References


1. Utomi V, Oxborough D, Ashley E, Lord R, Fletcher S, Stembridge M, et al. Predominance of normal left ventricular geometry in the male athlete's heart. Heart. 2014;100(16):1264–71.
2. Beaudry R, Haykowsky MJ, Baggish A, La Gerche A. A modern definition of the athlete's heart-for research and the clinic. Cardiol Clin. 2016;34(4):507–14.
3. Finocchiaro G, Dhutia H, D'Silva A, Malhotra A, Steriotis A, Millar L, et al. Effect of sex and sporting discipline on LV adaptation to exercise. JACC Cardiovasc Imaging. 2017;10(9):965–72.
4. Utomi V, Oxborough D, Whyte GP, Somauroo J, Sharma S, Shave R, et al. Systematic review and meta-analysis of training mode, imaging modality and body size influences on the morphology and function of the male athlete's heart. Heart. 2013;99(23):1727–33.
5. Rowland T. Morphologic features of the Athlete's heart in children: a contemporary review. Pediatr Exerc Sci. 2016;28(3):345–52.
6. Rawlins J, Carre F, Kervio G, Papadakis M, Chandra N, Edwards C, et al. Ethnic differences in physiological cardiac adaptation to intense physical exercise in highly trained female athletes. Circulation. 2010;121(9):1078–85.
7. Sheikh N, Papadakis M, Ghani S, Zaidi A, Gati S, Adami PE, et al. Comparison of electrocardiographic criteria for the detection of cardiac abnormalities in elite black and white athletes. Circulation. 2014;129(16):1637–49.
8. Pelliccia A, Caselli S, Sharma S, Basso C, Bax JJ, Corrado D, et al. European Association of Preventive Cardiology (EAPC) and European Association of Cardiovascular Imaging (EACVI) joint position statement: recommendations for the indication and interpretation of cardiovascular imaging in the evaluation of the athlete's heart. Eur Heart J. 2018;39(21):1949–69.
9. Luijkx T, Velthuis BK, Prakken NH, Cox MG, Bots ML, Mali WP, et al. Impact of revised task force criteria: distinguishing the athlete's heart from ARVC/D using cardiac magnetic resonance imaging. Eur J Prev Cardiol. 2012;19(4):885–91.
10. Gati S, Chandra N, Bennett RL, Reed M, Kervio G, Panoulas VF, et al. Increased left ventricular trabeculation in highly trained athletes: do we need more stringent criteria for the diagnosis of left ventricular non-compaction in athletes? Heart. 2013;99(6):401–8.
11. Abergel E, Chatellier G, Hagege AA, Oblak A, Linhart A, Ducardonnet A, et al. Serial left ventricular adaptations in world-class professional cyclists: implications for disease screening and follow-up. J Am Coll Cardiol. 2004;44(1):144–9.
12. Brown B, Somauroo J, Green DJ, Wilson M, Drezner J, George K, et al. The complex phenotype of the Athlete's heart: implications for preparticipation screening. Exerc Sport Sci Rev. 2017;45(2):96–104.
13. Claessen G, Schnell F, Bogaert J, Claeys M, Pattyn N, De Buck F, et al. Exercise cardiac magnetic resonance to differentiate athlete's heart from structural heart disease. Eur Heart J Cardiovasc Imaging. 2018;19(9):1062–70.
14. Beaumont A, Grace F, Richards J, Hough J, Oxborough D, Sculthorpe N. Left ventricular speckle tracking-derived cardiac strain and cardiac twist mechanics in athletes: a systematic review and meta-analysis of controlled studies. Sports Med. 2017;47(6):1145–70.
15. Weiner RB, DeLuca JR, Wang F, Lin J, Wasfy MM, Berkstresser B, et al. Exercise-induced left ventricular remodeling among competitive athletes: a phasic phenomenon. Circ Cardiovasc Imaging. 2015;8(12):e003651.
16. Forsythe L, George K, Oxborough D. Speckle tracking echocardiography for the assessment of the Athlete's heart: is it ready for daily practice? Curr Treat Options Cardiovasc Med. 2018;20(10):83.
17. D'Ascenzi F, Cameli M, Zaca V, Lisi M, Santoro A, Causarano A, et al. Supernormal diastolic function and role of left atrial myocardial deformation analysis by 2D speckle tracking echocardiography in elite soccer players. Echocardiography. 2011;28(3):320–6.
18. Finocchiaro G, Dhutia H, D'Silva A, Malhotra A, Sheikh N, Narain R, et al. Role of doppler diastolic parameters in differentiating physiological left ventricular hypertrophy from hypertrophic cardiomyopathy. J Am Soc Echocardiogr. 2018;31(5):606–13. e1

19. La Gerche A, Heidbuchel H, Burns AT, Mooney DJ, Taylor AJ, Pfluger HB, et al. Disproportionate exercise load and remodeling of the athlete's right ventricle. Med Sci Sports Exerc. 2011;43(6):974–81.
20. Qasem M, George K, Somauroo J, Forsythe L, Brown B, Oxborough D. Influence of different dynamic sporting disciplines on right ventricular Structure and function in elite male athletes. Int J Cardiovasc Imaging. 2018;34(7):1067–74.
21. Zaidi A, Ghani S, Sharma R, Oxborough D, Panoulas VF, Sheikh N, et al. Physiological right ventricular adaptation in elite athletes of African and Afro-Caribbean origin. Circulation. 2013;127(17):1783–92.
22. D'Ascenzi F, Pisicchio C, Caselli S, Di Paolo FM, Spataro A, Pelliccia A. RV remodeling in olympic athletes. JACC Cardiovasc Imaging. 2017;10(4):385–93.
23. Forsythe L, Somauroo J, George K, Papadakis M, Brown B, Qasem M, et al. The right heart of the elite senior rugby football league athlete. Echocardiography. 2019;36(5):888–96.
24. Qasem M, George K, Somauroo J, Forsythe L, Brown B, Oxborough D. Right ventricular function in elite male athletes meeting the structural echocardiographic task force criteria for arrhythmogenic right ventricular cardiomyopathy. J Sports Sci. 2019;37(3):306–12.
25. La Gerche A, Burns AT, Mooney DJ, Inder WJ, Taylor AJ, Bogaert J, et al. Exercise-induced right ventricular dysfunction and structural remodelling in endurance athletes. Eur Heart J. 2012;33(8):998–1006.
26. D'Ascenzi F, Pelliccia A, Solari M, Piu P, Loiacono F, Anselmi F, et al. Normative reference values of right heart in competitive athletes: a systematic review and meta-analysis. J Am Soc Echocardiogr. 2017;30(9):845–58. e2
27. D'Andrea A, Riegler L, Cocchia R, Scarafile R, Salerno G, Gravino R, et al. Left atrial volume index in highly trained athletes. Am Heart J. 2010;159(6):1155–61.
28. Hauser AM, Dressendorfer RH, Vos M, Hashimoto T, Gordon S, Timmis GC. Symmetric cardiac enlargement in highly trained endurance athletes: a two-dimensional echocardiographic study. Am Heart J. 1985;109(5 Pt 1):1038–44.
29. Iskandar A, Mujtaba MT, Thompson PD. Left atrium size in elite athletes. JACC Cardiovasc Imaging. 2015;8(7):753–62.
30. Pelliccia A, Maron BJ, Di Paolo FM, Biffi A, Quattrini FM, Pisicchio C, et al. Prevalence and clinical significance of left atrial remodeling in competitive athletes. J Am Coll Cardiol. 2005;46(4):690–6.
31. Sanchis L, Sanz-de La Garza M, Bijnens B, Giraldeau G, Grazioli G, Marin J, et al. Gender influence on the adaptation of atrial performance to training. Eur J Sport Sci. 2017;17(6):720–6.
32. Baggish AL, Wang F, Weiner RB, Elinoff JM, Tournoux F, Boland A, et al. Training-specific changes in cardiac structure and function: a prospective and longitudinal assessment of competitive athletes. J Appl Physiol (1985). 2008;104(4):1121–8.
33. D'Ascenzi F, Pelliccia A, Natali BM, Cameli M, Lisi M, Focardi M, et al. Training-induced dynamic changes in left atrial reservoir, conduit, and active volumes in professional soccer players. Eur J Appl Physiol. 2015;115(8):1715–23.
34. D'Ascenzi F, Pelliccia A, Natali BM, Zaca V, Cameli M, Alvino F, et al. Morphological and functional adaptation of left and right atria induced by training in highly trained female athletes. Circ Cardiovasc Imaging. 2014;7(2):222–9.
35. D'Ascenzi F, Cameli M, Lisi M, Zaca V, Natali B, Malandrino A, et al. Left atrial remodelling in competitive adolescent soccer players. Int J Sports Med. 2012;33(10):795–801.
36. D'Ascenzi F, Solari M, Anselmi F, Maffei S, Focardi M, Bonifazi M, et al. Atrial chamber remodelling in healthy pre-adolescent athletes engaged in endurance sports: a study with a longitudinal design. The CHILD study. Int J Cardiol. 2016;223:325–30.
37. Zdravkovic M, Perunicic J, Krotin M, Ristic M, Vukomanovic V, Soldatovic I, et al. Echocardiographic study of early left ventricular remodeling in highly trained preadolescent footballers. J Sci Med Sport. 2010;13(6):602–6.
38. Gabrielli L, Bijnens BH, Butakoff C, Duchateau N, Montserrat S, Merino B, et al. Atrial functional and geometrical remodeling in highly trained male athletes: for better or worse? Eur J Appl Physiol. 2014;114(6):1143–52.

39. Oxborough D, Whyte G, Wilson M, O'Hanlon R, Birch K, Shave R, et al. A depression in left ventricular diastolic filling following prolonged strenuous exercise is associated with changes in left atrial mechanics. J Am Soc Echocardiogr. 2010;23(9):968–76.
40. D'Ascenzi F, Cameli M, Padeletti M, Lisi M, Zaca V, Natali B, et al. Characterization of right atrial function and dimension in top-level athletes: a speckle tracking study. Int J Cardiovasc Imaging. 2013;29(1):87–94.
41. D'Andrea A, De Corato G, Scarafile R, Romano S, Reigler L, Mita C, et al. Left atrial myocardial function in either physiological or pathological left ventricular hypertrophy: a two-dimensional speckle strain study. Br J Sports Med. 2008;42(8):696–702.
42. D'Ascenzi F, Anselmi F, Focardi M, Mondillo S. Atrial enlargement in the Athlete's heart: assessment of atrial function may help distinguish adaptive from pathologic remodeling. J Am Soc Echocardiogr. 2018;31(2):148–57.
43. Gabrielli L, Enriquez A, Cordova S, Yanez F, Godoy I, Corbalan R. Assessment of left atrial function in hypertrophic cardiomyopathy and athlete's heart: a left atrial myocardial deformation study. Echocardiography. 2012;29(8):943–9.
44. Boraita A, Heras ME, Morales F, Marina-Breysse M, Canda A, Rabadan M, et al. Reference values of aortic root in male and female white elite athletes according to sport. Circ Cardiovasc Imaging. 2016;9(10):e005292.
45. Gati S, Malhotra A, Sedgwick C, Papamichael N, Dhutia H, Sharma R, et al. Prevalence and progression of aortic root dilatation in highly trained young athletes. Heart. 2019;105(12):920–5.
46. Oates SA, Forsythe L, Somauroo JD, George KP, Papadakis M, Oxborough D. Scaling to produce size-independent indices of echocardiographic derived aortic root dimensions in elite Rugby Football League players. Ultrasound. 2019;27(2):94–100.
47. Maron BJ, Gardin JM, Flack JM, Gidding SS, Kurosaki TT, Bild DE. Prevalence of hypertrophic cardiomyopathy in a general population of young adults. Echocardiographic analysis of 4111 subjects in the CARDIA Study. Coronary artery risk development in (Young) adults. Circulation. 1995;92(4):785–9.
48. Finocchiaro G, Papadakis M, Robertus JL, Dhutia H, Steriotis AK, Tome M, et al. Etiology of sudden death in sports: insights from a United Kingdom Regional Registry. J Am Coll Cardiol. 2016;67(18):2108–15.
49. Sheikh N, Papadakis M, Schnell F, Panoulas V, Malhotra A, Wilson M, et al. Clinical profile of athletes with hypertrophic cardiomyopathy. Circ Cardiovasc Imaging. 2015;8(7):e003454.
50. Butz T, van Buuren F, Mellwig KP, Langer C, Plehn G, Meissner A, et al. Two-dimensional strain analysis of the global and regional myocardial function for the differentiation of pathologic and physiologic left ventricular hypertrophy: a study in athletes and in patients with hypertrophic cardiomyopathy. Int J Cardiovasc Imaging. 2011;27(1):91–100.
51. Kansal MM, Lester SJ, Surapaneni P, Sengupta PP, Appleton CP, Ommen SR, et al. Usefulness of two-dimensional and speckle tracking echocardiography in "Gray Zone" left ventricular hypertrophy to differentiate professional football player's heart from hypertrophic cardiomyopathy. Am J Cardiol. 2011;108(9):1322–6.
52. MacIver DH, Clark AL. Contractile dysfunction in sarcomeric hypertrophic cardiomyopathy. J Card Fail. 2016;22(9):731–7.
53. Millar L, Fernandez G, Dhutia H, Myott J, Malhotra A, Finocchiaro G, et al. Exercise echocardiography has a high sensitivity and specificity in differentiating athlete's heart from dilated cardiomyopathy. Circulation. 2016;134(suppl_1):A15662.
54. Okada M, Tanaka H, Matsumoto K, Ryo K, Kawai H, Hirata K. Subclinical myocardial dysfunction in patients with reverse-remodeled dilated cardiomyopathy. J Am Soc Echocardiogr. 2012;25(7):726–32.
55. Thavendiranathan P, Marwick TH. Reply: characteristic LV regional wall motion abnormality: sign of cardiotoxicity? J Am Coll Cardiol. 2015;65(7):758–9.
56. Basso C, Corrado D, Marcus FI, Nava A, Thiene G. Arrhythmogenic right ventricular cardiomyopathy. Lancet. 2009;373(9671):1289–300.
57. Corrado D, Thiene G, Nava A, Rossi L, Pennelli N. Sudden death in young competitive athletes: clinicopathologic correlations in 22 cases. Am J Med. 1990;89(5):588–96.

58. Marcus FI, McKenna WJ, Sherrill D, Basso C, Bauce B, Bluemke DA, et al. Diagnosis of arrhythmogenic right ventricular cardiomyopathy/dysplasia: proposed modification of the task force criteria. Eur Heart J. 2010;31(7):806–14.
59. D'Andrea A, Caso P, Sarubbi B, Limongelli G, Liccardo B, Cice G, et al. Right ventricular myocardial adaptation to different training protocols in top-level athletes. Echocardiography. 2003;20(4):329–36.
60. D'Andrea A, Caso P, Scarafile R, Salerno G, De Corato G, Mita C, et al. Biventricular myocardial adaptation to different training protocols in competitive master athletes. Int J Cardiol. 2007;115(3):342–9.
61. Pagourelias ED, Kouidi E, Efthimiadis GK, Deligiannis A, Geleris P, Vassilikos V. Right atrial and ventricular adaptations to training in male Caucasian athletes: an echocardiographic study. J Am Soc Echocardiogr. 2013;26(11):1344–52.
62. Angelini P. Coronary artery anomalies: an entity in search of an identity. Circulation. 2007;115(10):1296–305.
63. Basso C, Maron BJ, Corrado D, Thiene G. Clinical profile of congenital coronary artery anomalies with origin from the wrong aortic sinus leading to sudden death in young competitive athletes. J Am Coll Cardiol. 2000;35(6):1493–501.
64. Corrado D, Basso C, Rizzoli G, Schiavon M, Thiene G. Does sports activity enhance the risk of sudden death in adolescents and young adults? J Am Coll Cardiol. 2003;42(11):1959–63.
65. Maron BJ, Doerer JJ, Haas TS, Tierney DM, Mueller FO. Sudden deaths in young competitive athletes: analysis of 1866 deaths in the United States, 1980-2006. Circulation. 2009;119(8):1085–92.
66. Pelliccia A, Spataro A, Maron BJ. Prospective echocardiographic screening for coronary artery anomalies in 1,360 elite competitive athletes. Am J Cardiol. 1993;72(12):978–9.
67. Zeppilli P, dello Russo A, Santini C, Palmieri V, Natale L, Giordano A, et al. In vivo detection of coronary artery anomalies in asymptomatic athletes by echocardiographic screening. Chest. 1998;114(1):89–93.
68. Bluemke DA, Achenbach S, Budoff M, Gerber TC, Gersh B, Hillis LD, et al. Noninvasive coronary artery imaging: magnetic resonance angiography and multidetector computed tomography angiography: a scientific statement from the American heart association committee on cardiovascular imaging and intervention of the council on cardiovascular radiology and intervention, and the councils on clinical cardiology and cardiovascular disease in the young. Circulation. 2008;118(5):586–606.
69. Schroeder S, Achenbach S, Bengel F, Burgstahler C, Cademartiri F, de Feyter P, et al. Cardiac computed tomography: indications, applications, limitations, and training requirements: report of a Writing Group deployed by the Working Group Nuclear Cardiology and Cardiac CT of the European Society of Cardiology and the European Council of Nuclear Cardiology. Eur Heart J. 2008;29(4):531–56.

# Medical Evaluation of Athletes: Further Imaging Modalities—Stress Echo, CT and MRI

# 9

Guido Claessen and André La Gerche

**Learning Objectives**

1. Recognise the strength and weakness of different imaging modalities for the evaluation of athletes with symptoms.
2. Understand the utility of cardiac magnetic resonance imaging (CMR) in athletes in whom there is reasonable suspicion for underlying structural heart disease, even when an echocardiogram appears normal.
3. Resting biventricular systolic function, as assessed by ejection fraction, may be at or slightly below the lower limits of normal under resting conditions among athletes and highly trained individuals with dilated ventricles.
4. High levels of fitness are not mutually exclusive from cardiac pathology in athletes. It should not be assumed that an athlete is "too fit" to have a serious cardiac condition such as a cardiomyopathy.
5. Small patches of delayed gadolinium enhancement (DGE) are commonly seen in ostensibly healthy athletes and their presence should be interpreted in the appropriate clinical context. On the other hand, certain patterns of DGE may be a harbinger of significant pathology and risk of arrhythmias.

G. Claessen
Department of Cardiovascular Medicine, University Hospital Leuven, Leuven, Belgium

Department of Sports Cardiology, Baker Heart and Diabetes Institute, Melbourne, VIC, Australia
e-mail: guido.claessen@uzleuven.be

A. La Gerche (✉)
Department of Sports Cardiology, Baker Heart and Diabetes Institute, Melbourne, VIC, Australia

National Centre for Sports Cardiology, St. Vincent's Hospital Melbourne, Melbourne, VIC, Australia
e-mail: Andre.Lagerche@baker.edu.au



A. Pressler, J. Niebauer (eds.), *Textbook of Sports and Exercise Cardiology*,
https://doi.org/10.1007/978-3-030-35374-2_9

6. Understand that there are limitations to the implementation of cardiac imaging as a first-line screening modality including, but not limited to, the false positive findings associated with the significant overlap in appearance between healthy cardiac remodeling associated with the "athlete's heart" and cardiac pathology.

## 9.1 Introduction

Cardiac imaging techniques have become indispensable in identifying abnormalities that may be associated with symptoms such as chest pain, dyspnoea or palpitations but may also identify sub-clinical abnormalities associated with sudden cardiac death in athletes and highly active people. Although regular physical exercise is an effective means of reducing cardiovascular events, it does not confer complete immunity, and transiently increases the risk of events acutely, even in trained individuals with occult cardiovascular disease [1].

- Advanced cardiac imaging modalities such as stress echocardiography, computed tomography coronary angiography (CTCA) and cardiac magnetic resonance imaging (CMR) provide treating clinicians with a detailed evaluation of geometry, function and even tissue characterization of the heart and its blood supply.
- However, at the same time, the increased sensitivity of these advanced imaging methods may also paradoxically increase diagnostic uncertainty and false-positive results in athletes with little pre-test probability for disease [2].

As such, it is important to always interpret imaging findings in the context of symptoms and findings identified during clinical examination, the 12-lead electrocardiography and resting echocardiography. Furthermore, when evaluating athletic individuals, it is essential to have a thorough understanding of the structural and functional adaptations that accompany different forms of exercise.

In this chapter we will highlight state-of-the-art stress echocardiography, CTCA and CMR imaging techniques and propose a framework for the implementation of these techniques in the work-up of athletes with clinical suspicion of an underlying cardiovascular pathology raised by symptoms or abnormalities detected during screening evaluation. We will discuss findings that are frequently encountered in highly trained athletes and how to distinguish these from patients with underlying pathologies such as cardiomyopathies and coronary artery disease.

## 9.2 Advanced Cardiac Imaging in Athletes with Symptoms

In the following sections we aim to provide a framework for the work-up and interpretation imaging findings in highly active individuals with symptoms through several clinical scenarios. Using these scenarios, we will depict the use of advanced imaging methods in athletes with potential coronary artery disease, a suspected cardiomyopathy and/or an arrhythmogenic substrate. It stands to reason that the distinction into different sections is arbitrary, and overlap between these scenarios is to be anticipated in real-life clinical practice. For example, patients with ischemic heart disease can present with syncope whereas palpitations may be the first clinical manifestation of an athlete with a cardiomyopathy. Thus, the importance of flexible clinical decision making cannot be overestimated and epidemiological factors such as age and gender need to be incorporated into the diagnostic work-up of athletes.

### 9.2.1 The Athlete with Chest Pain

While a cardinal symptom of coronary artery pathology, (atypical) chest pain can occur in a number of clinical situations including

(a) musculoskeletal,
(b) gastro-intestinal and
(c) respiratory conditions [3].

Given its potential to induce life-threatening arrhythmias, particularly during vigorous exercise, it is important to exclude any underlying cardiac cause in highly active individuals presenting with chest pain. Despite the transiently increased risk of myocardial infarction and sudden cardiac death during each exercise bout, however, the clinical work-up of symptomatic athletes is essentially the same in non-athletes and includes an assessment of cardiovascular risk factors and epidemiological factors such as age.

- In highly active **young adults younger than 35 years**, congenital coronary artery anomalies represent the most prevalent cause of coronary artery pathology and have been reported to explain sudden cardiac death in up to 33% of cases [4].
- Therefore, in young athletes with suggestive symptoms (e.g. exertional chest pain or syncope) the origin and proximal course of the coronary arteries should be part of the work-up.

Although it has been argued that echocardiography may be a useful means of identifying coronary anomalies [5], we would contend that the sensitivity and specificity are insufficient for routine use in athletes presenting with symptoms. Examination using CTCA is preferred [6]. As an alternative, particularly for screening during less targeted evaluations, 3D CMR coronary angiography can be added to standard CMR imaging to enable assessment of the coronary ostia in more than 90% of patients [7]. This is not standard practice in most centres though and it cannot be assumed that coronary anomalies have been excluded in a CMR scan unless it has specifically been assessed and reported. On the other hand, CTCA is readily available and can be performed with high accuracy in the vast majority of patients.

Coronary arteries with an anomalous origin from the wrong aortic sinus, either an

- anomalous left coronary artery arising from the right sinus of Valsalva (ALCA) or
- an anomalous right coronary artery arising from the left sinus of Valsalva (ARCA),
- are considered of highest risk for sudden cardiac death and can be characterized by 1 of 5 course subtypes as
  1. inter-arterial,
  2. subpulmonic,
  3. pre-pulmonic,
  4. retro-aortic, or
  5. retrocardiac [8].

Of these subtypes, particularly an inter-arterial course between the aorta and the pulmonary artery has been linked with sudden cardiac death (see also Chap. 22). Despite the clear association between coronary anomalies and sudden death from autopsy series, management decisions regarding surgical or more conservative management strategies can be extremely difficult. Moreover, it is important to realize that data showing that any management strategy prevents sudden cardiac death are lacking. The mechanism of sudden cardiac death is presumed to be related to repetitive bursts of myocardial ischemia during exercise which may result in patchy areas of fibrosis [9, 10] serving as a substrate for life-threatening ventricular arrhythmias.

- Accordingly, surgical intervention is recommended for both (inter-arterial) ALCA and ARCA in patients with symptoms or evidence of ischemia (class I recommendation) [6].

Nevertheless, despite this clear rationale for stress testing, individuals with coronary anomalies rarely reveal features of inducible ischemia during exercise stress testing or pharmacological functional tests [9, 11]. Perfusion CMR sequences can be used to identify myocardial ischaemia whilst late enhancement images after gadolinium injection can be used to assess ischaemic scar in under-perfused regions [12]. However, the predictive value of these tests in the setting of congenital coronary artery disease remains to be established. Assessment with CTCA and/or CMR does provide essential information regarding anatomy of the coronary ostium and proximal coronary course (Fig. 9.1), which may facilitate guide individual risk assessment. Slit-like/fish-mouth-shaped orifice, acute angle take off, intramural course, inter-arterial course and hypoplasia of the proximal coronary artery have all been proposed as reasons for symptoms, ischemia and sudden cardiac death and should be taken into consideration [6, 8].

- In athletes **older than 35 years** the majority of cases of sudden cardiac death are related to atherosclerosis.
- Although chest pain (typical or atypical angina) constitutes the hallmark symptom of atherosclerotic heart disease, athletes may also present with dyspnoea, palpitations, light-headedness, syncope or even acute myocardial infarction or sudden cardiac death.

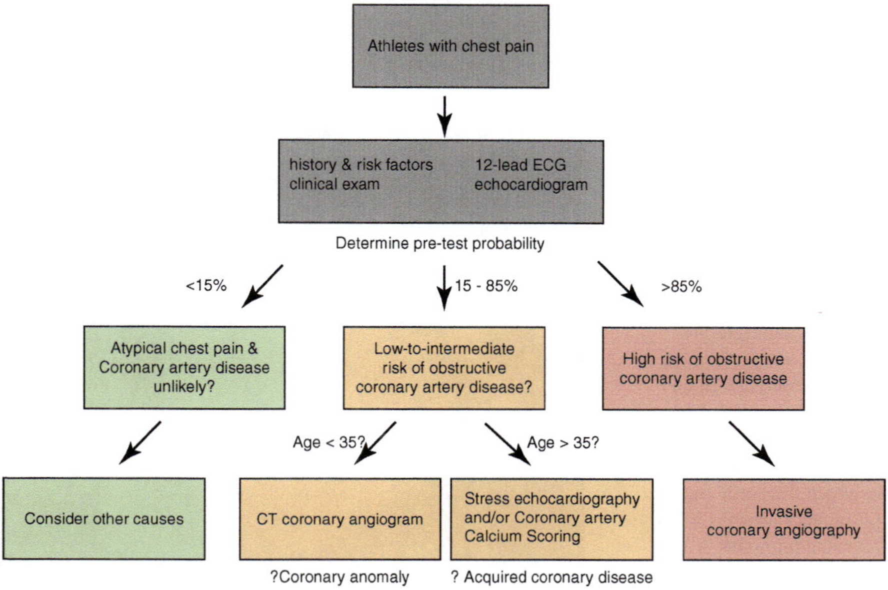


**Fig. 9.1** Initial diagnostic management of athletes with suspected angina pectoris. The process begins with clinical assessment of the pre-test probability that coronary artery disease is present. In athletes with a pretest probability <15% and atypical symptoms, no further testing is necessary and other causes should be considered. Both coronary calcium scoring and stress echocardiography can be used as first-line strategy in symptomatic athletes in whom there is a low-to-intermediate risk of acquired ischemic heart disease (15–85%), whereas invasive coronary angiography is reserved for athletes with high probability of coronary artery disease and typical angina symptoms

Over the last decades, the arsenal of diagnostic methods to examine patients with suspected coronary pathology has expanded enormously. These techniques can broadly be divided into those that assess the functional impact of myocardial lesions versus those that assess anatomy. Depending on the pre-test probability, a decision should be made as to which strategy is best suited for the athlete (Fig. 9.2). Although the common perception is that athletes are at very low risk of atherosclerotic heart disease, the effect of exercise in preventing coronary events is relative rather than absolute. It is critical that athletes understand that there are no "100% insurance policies" and that typical or atypical symptoms should be carefully evaluated.

- A recent Italian study highlighted the prevalence of sub-optimal primary prevention amongst some athletes in documenting an increased waist circumference in a substantial proportion (32% and 25%, respectively) of Olympic athletes (age range 15–45 years) [13].
- In addition, the exposure to cardiovascular risk factor in the past needs to be taken into account as illustrated by a study in recreational marathon runners (aged >50 years) showing a much higher than expected coronary artery calcification burden compared with age-matched controls [14]. Framingham risk was

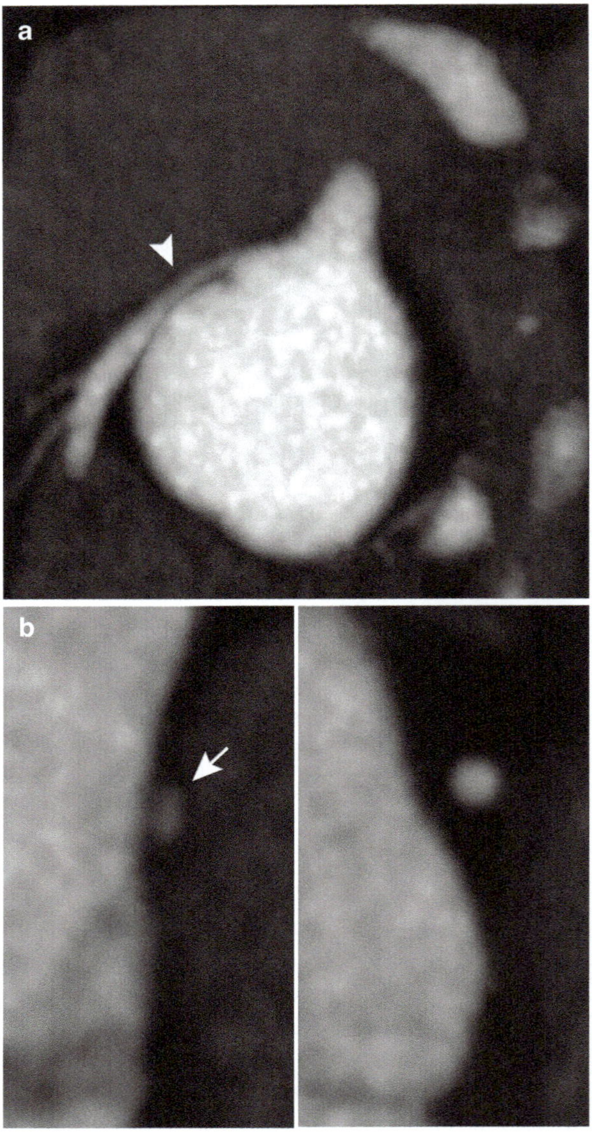


**Fig. 9.2** Anatomical high-risk features in an athlete with a congenital anomaly of the right coronary artery. Example of a 23-year-old recreational athlete who presented with abrupt syncope during high-intensity exercise. During diagnostic work-up, computed tomography coronary angiography (CTCA) was performed, which demonstrated an anomalous origin of the right coronary artery with inter-arterial course between the aorta and pulmonary artery. CTCA revealed high-risk anatomical features such as an acute take off angle (*arrowhead*) and proximal narrowing (*arrow*). Based on these findings, together with a convincing history (malignant syncope), the athlete was referred for cardiac surgery

only half of that in the controls, thereby presuming a healthy cardiovascular risk profile. However, up to 52% of the runners had smoked at some time during their lives and 4% were active smokers [14].

Although athletes are not immune to cardiovascular risk factors, only a minority has a high-risk profile and a substantial proportion does not have any risk factor [13]. In these subjects with low-to-intermediate risk profiles presenting with chest pain, further work-up should be pursued using non-invasive functional assessment (exercise ECG, stress echocardiography) or anatomic imaging (CTCA) (Fig. 9.2).

Although CMR is the ideal modality for investigating the possibility of previous infarction, it is not as good as CTCA for assessing the presence and burden of atherosclerosis and the risk of future ischemic damage. Stress perfusion CMR can be performed but in most centres other tests (exercise echocardiography or nuclear testing) are more routinely practiced.

Exercise ECG testing has long been the cornerstone of the initial assessment of suspected angina pectoris. The diagnostic accuracy of exercise ECG testing is, however, hindered by its low sensitivity, moderate specificity, and not infrequently equivocal results. As such, if local expertise and availability permit, exercise/pharmacological **stress echocardiography** may offer some advantages as the first-line test option in athletes with low-to-moderate risk:

- Stress echocardiography provides independent and incremental prognostic value for the prediction of cardiac events, over and above that of clinical, ECG, and stress ECG data by its capacity to accurately assess the extent and severity of the ischaemic burden of the myocardium (Fig. 9.3) [15].
  - Advantages include the lack of ionizing radiation exposure and high cost-effectiveness.
  - In addition, exercise echocardiography allows for the evaluation of filling pressures, valvular function and systolic/diastolic performance, which is useful in case of accompanying symptoms of dyspnoea or exercise intolerance.
  - However, like other imaging techniques, diagnostic accuracy is dependent on operator experience and requires sufficient annual activity to maintain competence with this technique.

An alternative approach to evaluate athletes with potential angina pectoris and low-to-intermediate risk profile is to assess the degree of coronary calcification (coronary calcium score) and, if abnormal, to directly visualize the coronary vasculature using **CTCA** in a non-invasive manner:

- Over the last years, important technological developments have led to a marked reduction in radiation, down to less than 1 mSv with the most recent dedicated CT scanners [16].
  - CTCA has a very high sensitivity for the detection of coronary stenoses considered significant by invasive arteriography [17].
  - Moreover, CTCA allows for a three-dimensional visualization of the coronary lumen and plaque volume, thereby providing insights into coronary plaque composition which may assist in the identification of unstable plaques.

The latter is important because acute coronary syndromes are most often the result of vulnerable atherosclerotic plaque events. Some CTCA-derived plaque characteristics have been associated with culprit lesions causing acute coronary syndromes. These features include

(a) a large necrotic core of lipid,
(b) a napkin rim of fibrous material,
(c) areas of plaque microcalcification, and
(d) a thin fibrous cap [18].

An important consideration in the use of CTCA is the potential for overestimation of the angiographic severity of coronary lesions because of the blooming artefact occurring near densely calcified plaques (Fig. 9.4) [19]. This may be particularly important in athletes given that recent studies reported a higher prevalence of atherosclerotic plaques compared with sedentary males (Chap. 32) [20, 21]. Furthermore, although the majority of athletes (60%) had a normal calcium score,

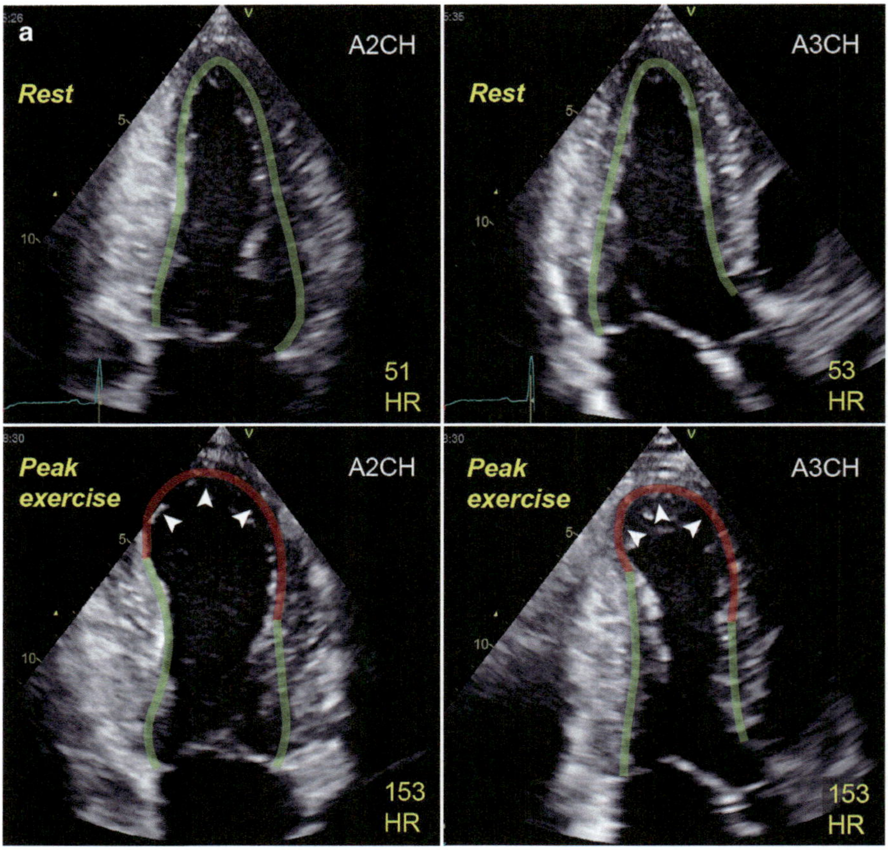


**Fig. 9.3** Example of exercise echocardiography in the work-up of an athlete with atypical chest complaints and dizziness during exercise. (Panel **a**) End-systolic image frames at rest demonstrate normal global and regional LV systolic function (green line denotes endocardial contour). At peak exercise, however, significant wall motion abnormalities (arrowheads and red line) appear with akinesia of the anteroapical left ventricular wall, suspicious of ischemia. (Panel **b**) Coronary angiogram confirms a tight stenosis in the proximal left anterior descending artery, consistent with the wall motion abnormalities observed during the stress echo. Bottom panels demonstrate the result after balloon angioplasty

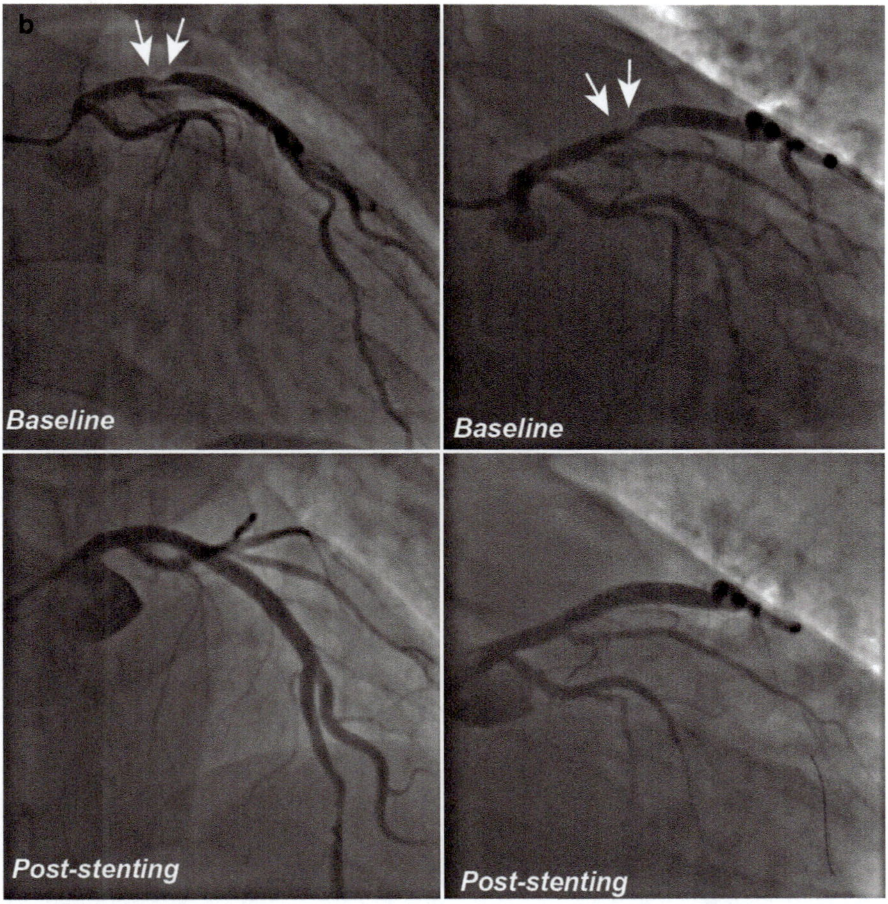


**Fig. 9.3** (continued)

moderate to severely elevated coronary calcium scores (≥300 AU) were exclusively observed in (11.3% of) athletes [21], which may increase the potential for further invasive investigations.

In athletes with a high risk probability of coronary artery disease and typical angina symptoms, **invasive coronary angiography** is the method of choice as interventional therapy may be performed during the same session.

- Moreover, invasive coronary angiography allows for additional assessment of the functional impact of epicardial coronary atherosclerosis and of any microvascular dysfunction, with the use of intracoronary pressure or/and Doppler guidewires at baseline and after pharmacological stimulation [22].
- Coronary angiography also remains the standard in diagnosing coronary artery dissection, which is an important cause of acute coronary syndrome, myocardial infarction, and sudden death, particularly among young women and individuals with few conventional atherosclerotic risk factors [23].

### 9.2.2 The Athlete with Exercise Intolerance and/or Breathlessness

Exertional breathlessness and/or intolerance are relatively common complaints in ostensibly healthy athletes and may be caused by numerous factors, ranging from poor aerobic fitness to serious, potentially fatal cardiac pathologies, such as

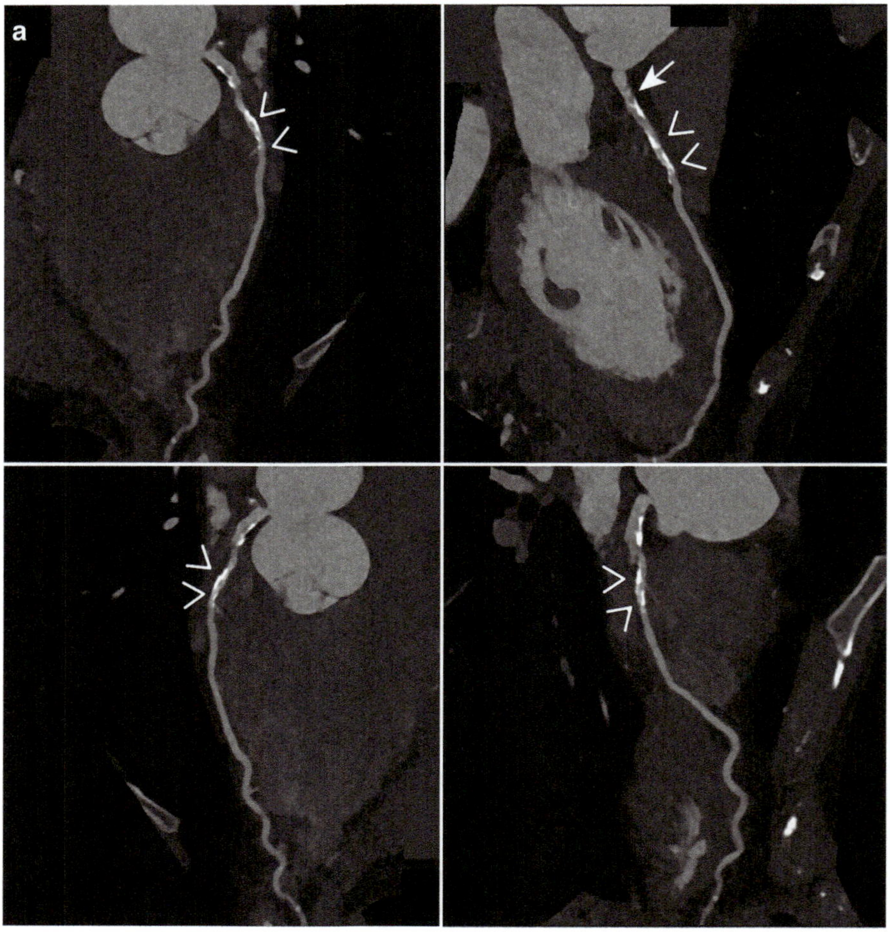


**Fig. 9.4** Illustration of the potential of coronary artery CT to overestimate luminal stenosis in an athlete with calcification in the coronary arteries. An asymptomatic 61-year-old endurance athlete underwent CTCA after coronary calcium score was elevated. (Panel **a**) CTCA suggested significant coronary artery disease with a mixed plaque of the left main coronary artery (arrow) and a calcified plaque with severe stenosis in the proximal left anterior descending artery (open arrowhead). (Panel **b**) Coronary angiography confirmed the presence of coronary lesions in the left main (arrow) and the proximal left descending aorta (arrowhead). However, neither of the lesions was flow-limiting (non-significant) and no intervention was performed

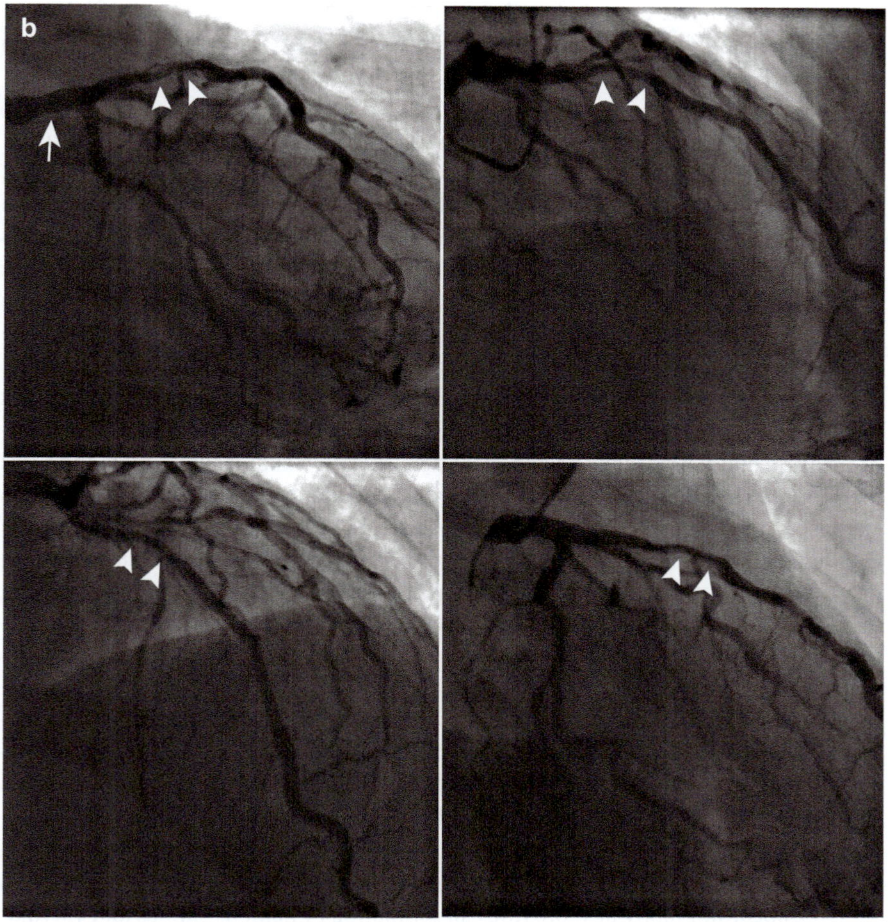


**Fig. 9.4** (continued)

hypertrophic cardiomyopathy (HCM) and dilated cardiomyopathy (DCM). It is important to realize, however, that cardiomyopathies may also be entirely asymptomatic and present with sudden cardiac death as first manifestation.

- Given the strong association between cardiac performance and aerobic exercise capacity, it stands to reason that the assessment of maximal oxygen consumption ($VO_2max$) has the potential to unmask athletes with structural heart disease.
  - However, the interpretation of $VO_2max$ values in the evaluation of athletes with a cardiomyopathy is a challenge because endurance-athletes, as well as those who engage in sprint-interval based sports, are expected to have high $VO_2max$ values.
  - A well trained athlete's $VO_2max$ may be well above average even in the presence of a dilated, hypertrophic or arrhythmogenic cardiomyopathy [24–26].

- It is reasonable to speculate that serial prospective measurements of $VO_2max$ may be more useful in identifying decreases in exercise capacity associated with a cardiomyopathic process but this is yet to be proven.

Another helpful point when interpreting $VO_2max$ values in athletic cardiovascular evaluation is the strong association between $VO_2max$ and cardiac size [27–29]. Extrapolating from these consistent findings, it may be reasonable to suspect a pathologic process when the cardiac dilation is excessive relative to the athlete's $VO_2max$ result. Conversely, it is not uncommon for athlete's to be referred after an imaging study and the question arises as to whether their cardiac dilation can be accounted for by their athletic history. In this context, a $VO_2max$ test may help establish the degree to which the physical conditioning accounts for the cardiac remodelling.

Substantial technical improvements in imaging modalities, such as **echocardiography** and **CMR**, have provided us with sensitive and accurate tools to assess the profound structural and functional cardiac adaptations underpinning the superb exercise capacity of highly trained athletes. However, at the same time, these exercise-induced changes overlap with those observed in patients with a cardiomyopathy, thereby creating diagnostic overlap. Therefore, imaging findings obtained in high-level athletes should be interpreted with caution and interpreted in the appropriate clinical context.

- Amongst different imaging techniques, we have many decades of experience in the evaluation of athletes with **echocardiography** and a clear description of normal reference values has evolved although it remains less complete for females and does not adequately encompass ethnic variability [30].
  - It is only with a clear definition of the normal athletic spectrum that we can start to accurately tease out pathological variants.
  - Echocardiography also provides an estimation of hemodynamics and valvular structures.
- On the other hand, **CMR** is more sensitive in identifying some abnormalities, particularly in potential echocardiographic 'blind-spots' such as the cardiac apex and right ventricle (RV), and should be included in the assessment of athletes in whom suspicion persists even if the echocardiogram fails to identify an abnormality.
- Finally, the combination of imaging during exercise testing (**exercise echocardiography or exercise CMR**) may provide additional valuable insights into functional reserve and prove to be a useful discriminator between physiological remodelling and pathology as well as provide an explanation for symptoms [25, 26] (Fig. 9.5).

Although athletes with **HCM** are often asymptomatic, exertional dyspnoea may occur because of several factors, including inefficient cardiac mechanics and/or dynamic obstruction of the left ventricular outflow tract.

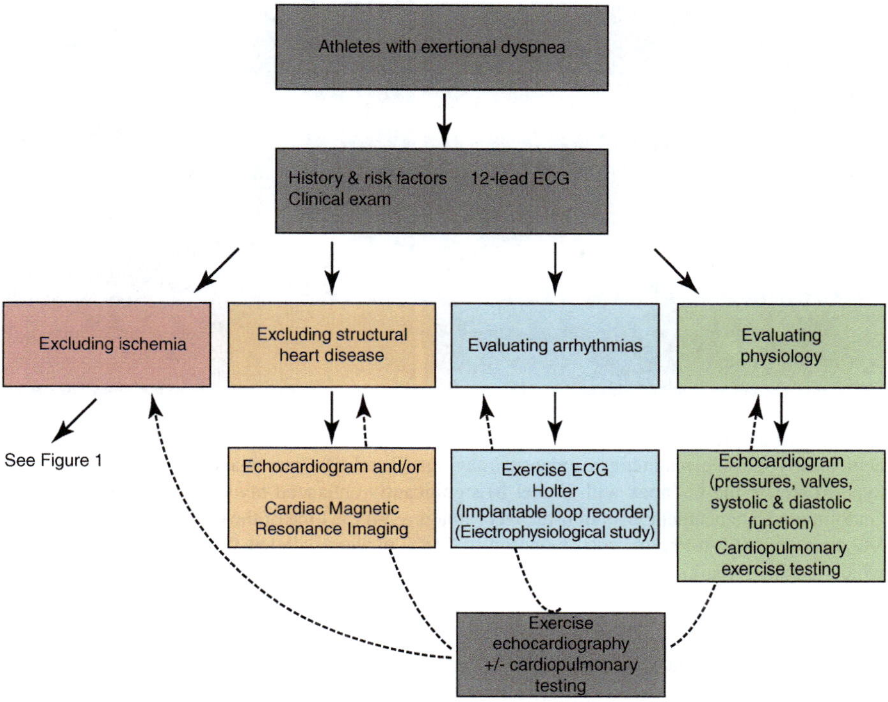


**Fig. 9.5** Evaluation of athletes presenting with dyspnea. The work-up can be divided into 4 parts. First, clinical appraisal of the pre-test probability of coronary artery disease should be performed and, when applicable, further diagnostic testing should be pursued. In addition, structural heart disease should be excluded and the presence of arrhythmias should be tested. The latter usually involves an exercise electrocardiogram (ECG) and/or Holter monitoring. Depending on the patients' individual circumstances, more advanced testing (including electrophysiological study and/or loop recording) may be required. Finally, it is also important to determine the mechanism of the athlete's symptoms and whether findings explain the exercise intolerance. In this regard, exercise echocardiography (ideally with simultaneous ergospirometry) represents a particularly useful technique as it provides information on different aspects of the patient's work-up at the same time

- Schnell and colleagues used exercise echocardiography to compare athletes with and without HCM versus non-athletic controls and non-athletic HCM patients [31].
  - Interestingly, athletes with HCM were far less likely to be dyspnoeic than non-athletes with HCM (8% versus 61%) and, expectedly, had superior exercise capacity, albeit lower than in healthy athletes.
  - The better functional status of athletes with HCM was associated with better systolic and diastolic function than the sedentary patients.
  - Furthermore, myocardial dispersion of longitudinal strain at rest (cut-off 40 ms) was the most robust and simple tool to differentiate athletes with HCM from healthy athletes, whereas exercise imaging did not provide any diagnostic benefit [31].

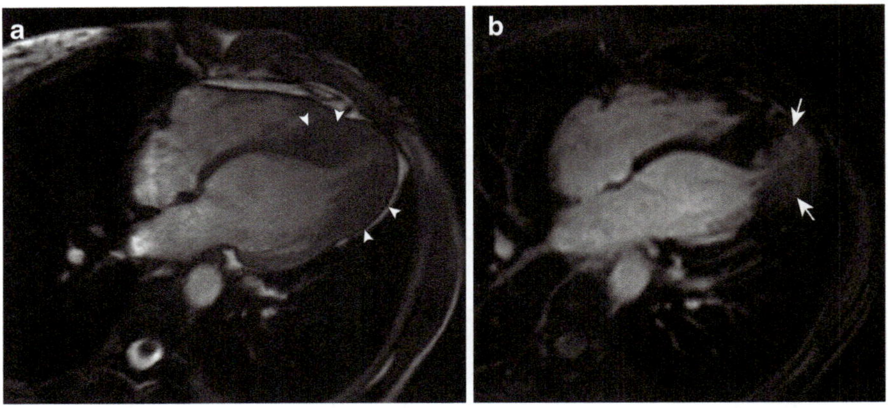


**Fig. 9.6** Example of a female former elite marathoner with hypertrophic cardiomyopathy as depicted by cardiac magnetic resonance imaging. (Panel **a**) Cine images depict asymmetrical hypertrophy of the LV apex with (Panel **b**) significantly enhanced myocardium during Delayed Gadolinium Enhancement inversion-recovery imaging. At the time of the CMR exam, the athlete's $VO_2max$ was 42.5 ml/kg/m$^2$ corresponding to 148% of the predicted value for age and gender, which is quite remarkable given the imaging findings. At the age of 29 her $VO_2max$ was 65.5 ml/kg/m$^2$

Beyond its diagnostic utility, however, exercise echocardiography can also provide insights into the mechanisms that explain symptoms or exercise intolerance, such as the demonstration of exercise-induced LV outflow tract obstruction (in approximately 28% of athletes with HCM) [31], mitral regurgitation or impaired diastolic functional reserve [32].

CMR has emerged as an important complementary technique to echocardiography for the diagnosis of HCM in athletes (Fig. 9.6), mainly because of superior visualization of specific areas of the LV, such as the apex and the anterolateral free wall.

- In a study of 6372 athletes referred for pre-participation screening, of which 155 presented with pathological T-wave inversion, CMR significantly provided incremental diagnostic value over echocardiography, as evidenced by the identification of a further 20 cases with HCM not diagnosed with echocardiography [33].

A second asset of CMR in the evaluation of athletes with suspected HCM is the ability to detect *fibrosis*.

- In the largest study of athletes with HCM (n = 106) to date, it was found that 33% had late gadolinium enhancement depicted by CMR [24].
- Although outcome data assessing the impact of DGE in athletic cohorts with HCM are unavailable, some studies in non-athletic HCM patients suggested that the presence of scar is a predictor of arrhythmias and is associated with cardiovascular death, heart failure death and all-cause mortality [34, 35].

- This remains contentious, however, as there is considerable overlap between scar burden and the presence of other prognostic markers such as the presence of non-sustained VT.

What is clear is that evidence of scar in HCM is common (one-third to half of patients) whilst cardiac arrest is uncommon and thus the presence of DGE should not be used as a sole criterion to determine suitability for defibrillator implantation. As the development of overt LV hypertrophy is preceded by a low-grade or more diffuse pro-fibrotic state without fibrosis visible with DGE imaging [36], CMR-based T1 mapping sequences are promising in identifying athletes with HCM in an earlier disease stage by demonstrating expansion of the extracellular matrix, with the two most common measures being native T1 and extracellular volume (ECV) fraction. As compared to athletic and non-athletic individuals, non-athletes with HCM have an increase of ECV and native T1, indicating extracellular matrix expansion, with both variables showing good diagnostic accuracy to depict HCM [37]. Further studies are required to validate these findings in athletes with HCM as it is known that athletic training significantly alters native T1 and ECV values [38].

In the context of a dilated ventricle and/or a reduced LV ejection fraction, exertional intolerance and/or dyspnoea in an athlete can also be the first manifestation of a **dilated cardiomyopathy** (most commonly idiopathic/inherited or after acute myocarditis). Again, it is important to point out that up to 10% of ostensibly healthy (particularly endurance) athletes may present with a mildly reduced ejection fraction (<52%) [39], which reinforces the need to integrate all clinical information when evaluating imaging findings in athletes. As for other types of structural heart disease, athletes with underlying LV damage constitute a different phenotype compared to sedentary individuals with DCM and may actually display superb exercise capacity [25]. As discussed earlier, it is possible that the onset of a cardiomyopathic process may be associated with a decline in $VO_2$max compared to pre-symptomatic values but, unfortunately, serial assessments of aerobic performance are often lacking, and clinicians have to rely on the test results at hand. Exercise imaging may be useful in this setting, both for the purpose of gaining insights into the pathophysiology of symptoms as well as for diagnostic reasons.

- Traditionally, it has been postulated that athletes with LV myocardial damage could be depicted by demonstrating a lack of increase in LVEF during exercise, as opposed to healthy athletes in whom LVEF is expected to increase [40].
  - Recent studies, however, showed that some athletes with LV pathology may actually demonstrate some LVEF reserve during exercise, but that the degree of augmentation is attenuated as compared to healthy athletes with borderline resting LVEF (<52% at rest by CMR) [25].
  - Using exercise CMR to assess LV contractile reserve, a cut-off of 11% was found to be most accurate in differentiating physiological from pathological remodelling [25].

- Using exercise echocardiography, the same cut-off value has been reported to yield superb accuracy for depicting athletes with DCM [41], which is important for clinical practice given the ubiquity of exercise echocardiography as opposed to exercise CMR.

An important asset of CMR is its ability to visualize tissue changes including

(a) oedema,
(b) hyperaemia and capillary leak (myocardial early gadolinium enhancement), and
(c) myocardial fibrosis (DGE) [42].

In patients with acute myocarditis, regional oedema can be visualized using T2-weighted images in up to 36% of patients with histologically active myocarditis [43]. In multiple conditions associated with LV myocardial damage, areas of late-gadolinium enhancement can be depicted, most typically involving the subepicardial regions of the LV with variable extension through the ventricular wall. Usually, this pattern can be distinguished from ischemic injury because the subendocardium is relatively less affected. However, identification of the underlying cause explaining LV dysfunction (e.g. DCM, myocarditis, LV-dominant ARVC or sarcoidosis) is more difficult.

Whilst DGE techniques are qualitative and able to detect irreversible replacement fibrosis, novel T1 mapping techniques allow quantitative CMR assessment of diffuse myocardial fibrosis, which is an earlier form of fibrosis that is potentially reversible. T1 mapping sequences have been used to compare athletes with early DCM patients. The native T1 times were similar for athletes and controls but both were significantly shorter than in the patients with cardiomyopathy [44]. Although very attractive in the work-up of athletes with symptoms suggestive of a cardiomyopathy, one consideration with these techniques is that, although they are capable of separating groups in research studies, there is significant overlap between groups which renders T1 mapping sequences currently unsuitable for use in diagnosing or excluding pathology in individual athletes.

### 9.2.3 The Athlete with Palpitations

Cardiac imaging plays an integral role in the evaluation of athletes with symptoms suggestive of arrhythmias (palpitations, syncope), both for determining the cause of symptoms as well as for risk stratification (Fig. 9.7).

- Evaluating the presence or absence of underlying structural heart disease is important as the overwhelming majority of arrhythmias in patients without structural heart disease carry an excellent prognosis [45].
  - For example, in athletes presenting with palpitations, the identification of ventricular dysfunction or myocardial scar may point towards an underlying cardiomyopathy, with implications for therapeutic decisions and sports restriction.

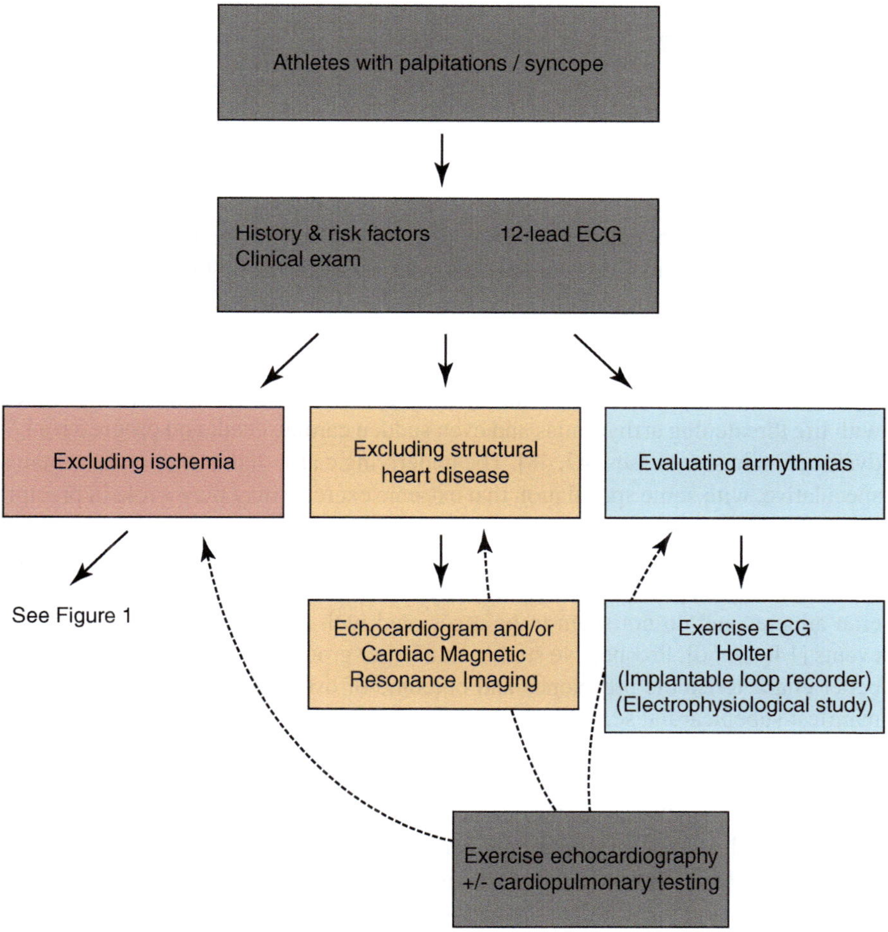


**Fig. 9.7** Evaluation of athletes presenting with palpitations. First, clinical assessment of the pre-test probability of coronary artery disease should be performed and, when applicable, further diagnostic testing should be pursued. Structural heart disease should be excluded, which requires echocardiography and/or cardiac magnetic resonance imaging. Third, the presence of arrhythmias should be evaluated, which generally starts by performing an exercise ECG and Holter monitoring. Depending on the clinical context, more advanced testing (including electrophysiological study and/or implantable loop recording) may be required. Exercise echocardiography can be particularly useful in the work-up of athletes with palpitations because of its ability to assess different aspects of the process at the same time

- On the other hand, in the absence of abnormalities of ventricular morphology or function, the demonstration of decreased atrial function may orient clinicians towards the diagnosis of atrial fibrillation as the explanation for symptoms [46].

In athletes presenting with ventricular arrhythmias as the explanation for palpitations, echocardiography and coronary angiography (particularly in athletes older than 35 years) represent the first-line diagnostic imaging modality, whereas CMR is indicated

1. to complement and clarify abnormalities identified on echocardiography and
2. as an additional evaluation even when the echocardiographic study appears normal but significant clinical suspicion persists.

In addition to its detailed assessment of cardiac morphology and function, CMR also enables detection of myocardial scar, which may be the first sign of an underlying cardiomyopathy. In recent years, two studies have reported on an association between ventricular arrhythmias and the presence of sub-epicardial DGE, in the absence of any other cardiomyopathic features. The delayed enhancement showed a predilection for the sub-epicardial layers of apical lateral wall and was associated with life threatening arrhythmias and even sudden cardiac death and progressive LV dysfunction in some cases [47, 48]. The underlying cause of this phenotype remains speculative, with some speculation that extreme exercise may play a role in precipitating this phenotype. It may be difficult to separate this sinister scar pattern from other patterns of scar in the athlete. Small patches of DGE, predominantly in the interventricular septum, have been reported in 12–50% of extensively trained veteran athletes and do not seem to be associated with a marked increase in clinical events [14, 49, 50]. Prospective studies in a larger group of athletes are underway to better characterise the prevalence and outcome of ostensibly healthy athletes with manifest subepicardial scar.

Amongst the different types of cardiomyopathies, **arrhythmogenic cardiomyopathy** (ACM) requires particular attention because it is associated with a high risk of ventricular arrhythmias and sudden cardiac death during competitive sports participation [51]. Data from a prospective multinational registry of athletes with ICDs identified ACM as the only diagnosis associated with appropriate shocks during competitive sport [52]. Cardiac imaging is part of the diagnostic criteria for making the diagnosis of ACM.

- However, it is important to realize that the current criteria are based on comparing ACM patients with normal controls, whereas 'athlete-specific' criteria are lacking, and are derived from cohorts with predominantly RV involvement.
- Few data are available comparing dimensions in normal athletes with (RV-dominant) ACM athletes, and those available have shown considerable overlap, especially when considering endurance athletes who have the largest RV [26, 53].
- Therefore, RV dimensions by itself are an unreliable criterion to distinguish physiologic from pathologic RV dilatation and currently there are no cut-offs to guide clinical practice [54].

As opposed to cardiac dimensions, functional measures are more useful for the diagnosis of ACM in athletes:

(a) RV ejection fraction ≤40–45%, as a measure of global RV dysfunction, has shown to be a reasonable discriminator between athlete's heart and RV-dominant ACM [53].
(b) Similarly, regional wall abnormalities limited to the RV are highly specific to the disease and occur in more than 50–94% of patients with ACM [53, 55], even in those with LV-dominant disease [56].

The utility of functional abnormalities may be limited to identify subjects with ACM who are engaged in endurance training. Hence, amongst endurance athletes presenting with complex ventricular arrhythmias of RV origin, functional abnormalities (both regional and global) are often relatively modest at rest and not distinguishable from athletic RV remodelling [26, 57]. Furthermore, patients with left-dominant ACM often have ventricular arrhythmias out of proportion to the mild degree of LV dilation/dysfunction, thereby causing overlap with physiological exercise-induced LV remodelling.

To overcome the challenges inherent to evaluating function in the rested state, demonstration of cardiac dysfunction during exercise (i.e. not at rest) using state-of-the-art CMR technology may facilitate the diagnosis of pathologic RV remodelling and contribute to risk stratification [26]. Similar diagnostic accuracy has been shown for exercise echocardiography [26], which is promising for the integration of functional cardiac reserve assessment into the diagnostic work-up of athletes presenting with symptoms suggesting ventricular arrhythmias (Fig. 9.7).

Although currently not included in the current Task Force Criteria, CMR tissue characterisation may be very useful in the evaluation of ACM.

- DGE has been observed in the RV in up to 88% of ACM patients [58, 59] and correlates with histopathology and inducibility of ventricular arrhythmias on electrophysiological studies (Fig. 9.8) [58].
- Furthermore, detection of DGE in the LV may provide important clues for the diagnosis of early and/or predominant LV involvement.
- This is important because fibrofatty infiltration, which can potentially be detected using DGE imaging, is isolated to the LV in 17% of sudden cardiac death cases due to ACM [60].

These data suggest that ventricular structural involvement may need to be included in future revision of Task Force diagnostic criteria.

## 9.3 Advanced Cardiac Imaging in Asymptomatic Athletes Following Screening

Although the efficacy of screening with electrocardiography has been the source of extensive debate, pre-participation screening has been advocated by the European Society of Cardiology (ESC) and has subsequently been implemented in multiple

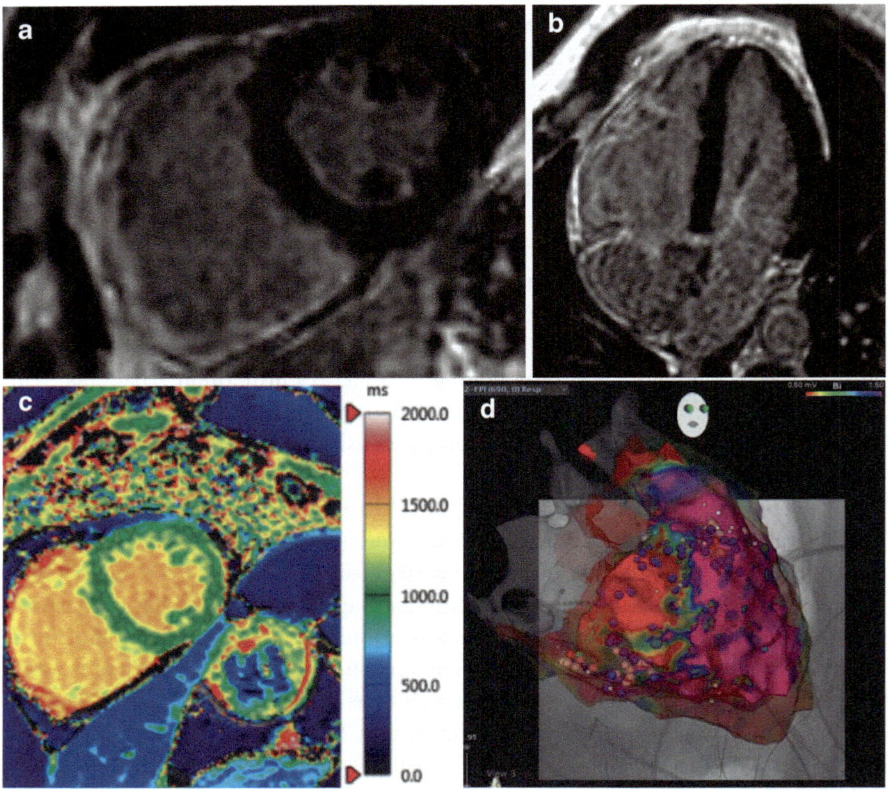


**Fig. 9.8** Example of delayed gadolinium enhancement in an athlete with arrhythmogenic cardiomyopathy. Example of a 50-year-old competitive cyclist presenting with exertional fatigue, chest discomfort and light headedness. (Panels **a**–**c**) During diagnostic work-up cardiac magnetic resonance (CMR) imaging is performed, which is highly suggestive of arrhythmogenic cardiomyopathy. CMR reveals significant Delayed Gadolinium Enhancement of the right ventricular (RV) free wall at the basal and midventricular level, with consistent abnormalities on T1 mapping. It is important to note though that the thin wall of the RV poses important challenges and makes T1 mapping more susceptible to partial volume effects. (**d**) In agreement with the CMR findings, electro-anatomical mapping during electrophysiological study reveals extensive scarring of the inferolateral RV free wall

sporting communities. Moreover, a number of sporting bodies also mandate the inclusion of exercise testing and echocardiography in screening protocols.

- Including imaging in screening protocols is based on the logic that some conditions, such as aortic dilation, would not be expected to be identified on ECG or clinical exam.
- However, it must also be recognised that the inclusion of imaging modalities such as echocardiography have potential to increase false-positive findings due to phenotypic overlap between athletes' heart and changes related to cardiac pathology and also to identify conditions such as bicuspid aortic valve that do not immediately represent a risk nor greatly alter clinical management.

At present, there is no evidence to support the inclusion of cardiac imaging tests as part of a pre-participation screening strategy in asymptomatic athletes. Because of the low pre-test probability of cardiac conditions related to sudden cardiac death in athletes, the predictive value of any imaging modality as a screening test is likely to be poor with a high rate of false positives [2, 61].

Most screening algorithms propose imaging as a "second-line" strategy reserved for any athlete with abnormal abnormalities on screening examination or ECG.

- In 2017, the international recommendations were revised by a group of American and European experts with the aim of unifying the recommendations for interpretation of the athlete's ECG [62].
  - In a single nationwide study of nearly 5000 young British athletes, the use of these criteria was associated with a reduction in the proportion of athletes requiring further investigation to 3% [63].
  - Although the exact specificity could not be calculated because the secondary investigation was limited to athletes with positive screening evaluations, it may be expected that the prevalence of underlying cardiac disease will be far greater among those 3% of athletes with significant abnormalities on ECG.

Thus, the predictive value of cardiac imaging is much improved when utilized as a second line strategy [2]. Further testing should be applied on a case-by-case basis and should focus on appraising the differential diagnoses arising from the clinical examination, history and ECG. The flowchart provided in Fig. 9.9 illustrates the manner in which a hierarchy of cardiac imaging modalities may enable differentiation of healthy athletes from those with conditions that require further management to minimize the risk of sudden cardiac death.

## 9.4 Conclusions

Advanced cardiac imaging modalities have become an essential part of the evaluation of athletes with symptoms, abnormalities on the ECG or a positive family history. The choice of imaging modality depends on the clinical appraisal and should be selected on a case-by-case basis. CTCA is the standard for anatomic evaluation of the coronary arteries and should be used when there is suspicion of a coronary anomaly. Both CT coronary angiography and stress echocardiography can be used as first-line strategy in symptomatic athletes in whom there is a low-to-intermediate risk of acquired ischemic heart disease, whereas invasive coronary angiography is reserved for athletes with high probability of coronary artery disease. Exercise echocardiography has the advantage of providing a physiological assessment of exercise hemodynamics and contractile reserve, which may be useful both for diagnostic purposes and the exploration of symptoms. CMR has superior sensitivity than other imaging modalities for identifying cardiomyopathies and myocarditis and thus should be included in the assessment of athletes in whom suspicion of a cardiomyopathy persists even if the echocardiogram fails to identify an abnormality or when further assessment, including scar imaging for risk stratification, is required.

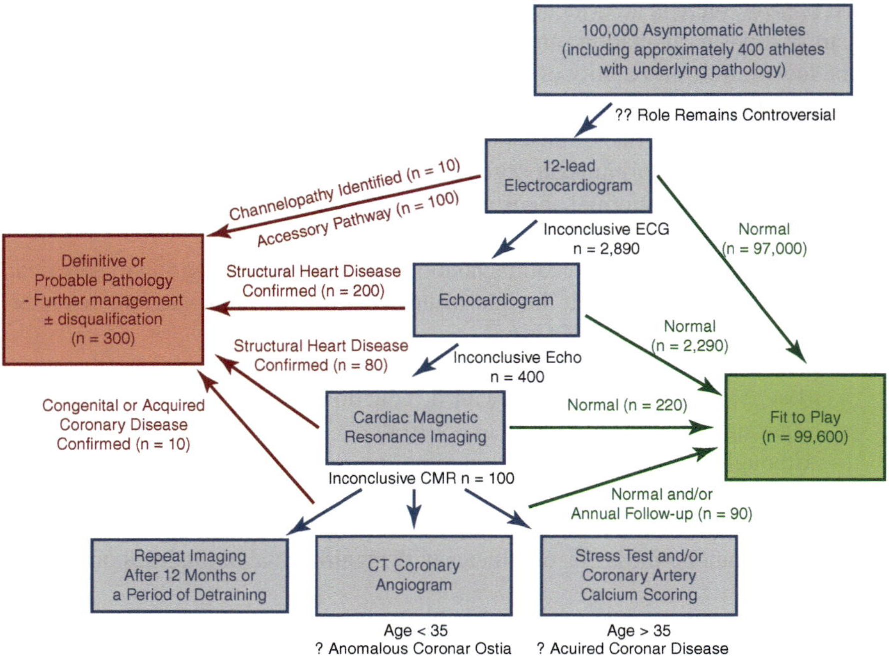


**Fig. 9.9** Screening asymptomatic athletes using a hierarchy of cardiac imaging modalities. This flowchart provides an algorithm whereby cardiac imaging may be employed as secondary screening modality following refinement of the "at-risk" population by means of electrocardiogram (ECG) screening. This flowchart represents an ideal scenario in which all potentially serious pathology is identified (100% sensitivity) and no healthy athletes are incorrectly diagnosed with pathology 100% specificity) following the cascade of tests. *CMR* cardiac magnetic resonance, *CT* computed tomography (reproduced with permission from [2])

Advanced imaging techniques are not appropriate for screening and also careful consideration should be given to findings that are unexpected or unrelated to the clinical question being addressed.

## Clinical Pearls

- Resting biventricular systolic function, as assessed by ejection fraction, may be at or slightly below the lower limits of normal under resting conditions among athletes and highly trained individuals with dilated ventricles. Evaluation of the response to exercise may be useful in case of borderline resting measurements.
- Both CT coronary angiography and stress echocardiography can be used as first-line strategy in symptomatic athletes in whom there is a low-to-intermediate risk of acquired ischemic heart disease
- Exercise echocardiography represents a particularly useful technique for the evaluation of athletes with symptoms as it provides information on different aspects (functional reserve, arrhythmias and hemodynamics) at the same time.
- Small patches of delayed gadolinium enhancement (DGE) are commonly seen in ostensibly healthy athletes and their presence should be interpreted in the

appropriate clinical context. On the other hand, certain patterns of DGE may be a harbinger of significant pathology and risk of arrhythmias.

## Review

## Questions

1. A 23-year old professional football player undergoes pre-participation screening. The club wants personal and family history, clinical examination, ECG as well as an echocardiography to be performed. The echo reveals an anomalous right coronary artery with inter-arterial course between the great vessels. All other investigations are negative. As part of further work-up an exercise echocardiogram is performed, which is unremarkable. What is the best management strategy for this athlete?
2. A 35-year old professional cyclist reports episodes of sudden fatigue and loss of power during high-intensity exercise. His medical history is unremarkable. The resting ECG shows features of athlete's heart, but no ST-segment abnormalities or T-wave inversion. He has no known cardiovascular risk factors and his family history is negative for cardiac diseases and/or sudden cardiac deaths. A resting echocardiogram is within the limits of normal for a highly trained athlete. Exercise testing reveals a superb exercise capacity with a $VO_2max$ of 76 ml/min/kg and runs of non-sustained ventricular tachycardia originating from the right ventricular apex. What is the next step in the work-up of this athlete?
3. A 16-year old competitive cyclist undergoes pre-participation screening, which includes an echocardiogram as mandated by the sports federation. The athlete is asymptomatic and his resting ECG is normal. The echocardiogram reveals profound hypertrabeculation of the midventricular-to-apical lateral LV wall with borderline LV systolic function (ejection fraction = 52%). Should the athlete be discouraged from competitive sport?

## Answers

1. Conservative strategy with annual follow-up. As the athlete is entirely asymptomatic and there are no signs of myocardial ischemia, coronary re-implantation is not indicated. Close follow-up is required to ensure timely detection of symptoms or inducible ischemia in the future.
2. Given the presence of exertional symptoms and documented non-sustained ventricular tachycardia, further work-up is mandatory and includes assessment of arrhythmias as well as excluding underlying structural heart disease. A stress echocardiogram was performed, which revealed impaired right ventricular (RV) as well as left ventricular (LV) reserve, but no regional wall motion abnormalities, which makes ischemia as the cause for the arrhythmias unlikely. Cardiac magnetic resonance imaging with delayed gadolinium sequences demonstrated

significant (>10% of LV mass) epicardial enhancement of the apical anterolateral LV wall as well as the RV free wall. Given the combination of ventricular arrhythmias, symptoms, significant myocardial fibrosis and impaired biventricular functional reserve, the athlete was referred for implantable cardioverter-defibrillator implantation.

3. Further evaluation should be considered, including stress echocardiography (cardiac reserve) and cardiac magnetic resonance imaging (to evaluate presence of myocardial scar and/or focal abnormalities). In this case, functional reserve of both ventricles was preserved (13% and 17% increase in ejection fraction from rest to peak exercise for LV and RV, respectively). As such, the observed hypertrabeculation is most likely explained by physiological adaptation to intensive endurance exercise. Annual follow-up is provided to ensure timely detection of potential maladaptive remodelling over time.

## References


1. Mittleman MA, Siscovick DS. Physical exertion as a trigger of myocardial infarction and sudden cardiac death. Cardiol Clin. 1996;14(2):263–70.
2. La Gerche A, Baggish AL, Knuuti J, Prior DL, Sharma S, Heidbuchel H, et al. Cardiac imaging and stress testing asymptomatic athletes to identify those at risk of sudden cardiac death. JACC Cardiovasc Imaging. 2013;6(9):993–1007.
3. Sik EC, Batt ME, Heslop LM. Atypical chest pain in athletes. Curr Sports Med Rep. 2009;8(2):52–8.
4. Eckart RE, Scoville SL, Campbell CL, Shry EA, Stajduhar KC, Potter RN, et al. Sudden death in young adults: a 25-year review of autopsies in military recruits. Ann Intern Med. 2004;141(11):829–34.
5. Maron BJ, Leon MB, Swain JA, Cannon RO 3rd, Pelliccia A. Prospective identification by two-dimensional echocardiography of anomalous origin of the left main coronary artery from the right sinus of Valsalva. Am J Cardiol. 1991;68(1):140–2.
6. Stout KK, Daniels CJ, Aboulhosn JA, Bozkurt B, Broberg CS, Colman JM, et al. 2018 AHA/ACC Guideline for the Management of Adults With Congenital Heart Disease: Executive Summary: A Report of the American College of Cardiology/American Heart Association Task Force on Clinical Practice Guidelines. J Am Coll Cardiol. 2019;73(12):1494–563.
7. Prakken NH, Cramer MJ, Olimulder MA, Agostoni P, Mali WP, Velthuis BK. Screening for proximal coronary artery anomalies with 3-dimensional MR coronary angiography. Int J Cardiovasc Imaging. 2010;26(6):701–10.
8. Cheezum MK, Liberthson RR, Shah NR, Villines TC, O'Gara PT, Landzberg MJ, et al. Anomalous aortic origin of a coronary artery from the inappropriate sinus of valsalva. J Am Coll Cardiol. 2017;69(12):1592–608.
9. Basso C, Maron BJ, Corrado D, Thiene G. Clinical profile of congenital coronary artery anomalies with origin from the wrong aortic sinus leading to sudden death in young competitive athletes. J Am Coll Cardiol. 2000;35(6):1493–501.
10. Finocchiaro G, Behr ER, Tanzarella G, Papadakis M, Malhotra A, Dhutia H, et al. Anomalous coronary artery origin and sudden cardiac death: clinical and pathological insights from a National Pathology Registry. JACC Clin Electrophysiol. 2019;5(4):516–22.
11. Brothers JA, McBride MG, Seliem MA, Marino BS, Tomlinson RS, Pampaloni MH, et al. Evaluation of myocardial ischemia after surgical repair of anomalous aortic origin of a coronary artery in a series of pediatric patients. J Am Coll Cardiol. 2007;50(21):2078–82.

12. Mavrogeni S, Spargias K, Karagiannis S, Kariofilis P, Cokkinos DD, Douskou M, et al. Anomalous origin of right coronary artery: magnetic resonance angiography and viability study. Int J Cardiol. 2006;109(2):195–200.
13. D'Ascenzi F, Caselli S, Alvino F, Digiacinto B, Lemme E, Piepoli M, et al. Cardiovascular risk profile in Olympic athletes: an unexpected and underestimated risk scenario. Br J Sports Med. 2019;53(1):37–42.
14. Mohlenkamp S, Lehmann N, Breuckmann F, Brocker-Preuss M, Nassenstein K, Halle M, et al. Running: the risk of coronary events: prevalence and prognostic relevance of coronary atherosclerosis in marathon runners. Eur Heart J. 2008;29(15):1903–10.
15. Chelliah R, Anantharam B, Burden L, Alhajiri A, Senior R. Independent and incremental value of stress echocardiography over clinical and stress electrocardiographic parameters for the prediction of hard cardiac events in new-onset suspected angina with no history of coronary artery disease. Eur J Echocardiogr. 2010;11(10):875–82.
16. Achenbach S, Marwan M, Ropers D, Schepis T, Pflederer T, Anders K, et al. Coronary computed tomography angiography with a consistent dose below 1 mSv using prospectively electrocardiogram-triggered high-pitch spiral acquisition. Eur Heart J. 2010;31(3):340–6.
17. Miller JM, Rochitte CE, Dewey M, Arbab-Zadeh A, Niinuma H, Gottlieb I, et al. Diagnostic performance of coronary angiography by 64-row CT. N Engl J Med. 2008;359(22):2324–36.
18. Small GR, Chow BJW. CT imaging of the vulnerable plaque. Curr Treat Options Cardiovasc Med. 2017;19(12):92.
19. Arbab-Zadeh A, Miller JM, Rochitte CE, Dewey M, Niinuma H, Gottlieb I, et al. Diagnostic accuracy of computed tomography coronary angiography according to pre-test probability of coronary artery disease and severity of coronary arterial calcification. The CORE-64 (coronary artery evaluation using 64-row multidetector computed tomography angiography) International Multicenter Study. J Am Coll Cardiol. 2012;59(4):379–87.
20. Aengevaeren VL, Mosterd A, Braber TL, Prakken NHJ, Doevendans PA, Grobbee DE, et al. Relationship between lifelong exercise volume and coronary atherosclerosis in athletes. Circulation. 2017;136(2):138–48.
21. Merghani A, Maestrini V, Rosmini S, Cox AT, Dhutia H, Bastiaenan R, et al. Prevalence of subclinical coronary artery disease in masters endurance athletes with a low atherosclerotic risk profile. Circulation. 2017;136(2):126–37.
22. Vrints CJM, Senior R, Crea F, Sechtem U. Assessing suspected angina: requiem for coronary computed tomography angiography or exercise electrocardiogram? Eur Heart J. 2017;38(23):1792–800.
23. Hayes SN, Kim ESH, Saw J, Adlam D, Arslanian-Engoren C, Economy KE, et al. Spontaneous coronary artery dissection: current state of the science: a scientific statement from the American Heart Association. Circulation. 2018;137(19):e523–e57.
24. Sheikh N, Papadakis M, Schnell F, Panoulas V, Malhotra A, Wilson M, et al. Clinical profile of athletes with hypertrophic cardiomyopathy. Circ Cardiovasc Imaging. 2015;8(7):e003454.
25. Claessen G, Schnell F, Bogaert J, Claeys M, Pattyn N, De Buck F, et al. Exercise cardiac magnetic resonance to differentiate athlete's heart from structural heart disease. Eur Heart J Cardiovasc Imaging. 2018;19(9):1062–70.
26. La Gerche A, Claessen G, Dymarkowski S, Voigt JU, De Buck F, Vanhees L, et al. Exercise-induced right ventricular dysfunction is associated with ventricular arrhythmias in endurance athletes. Eur Heart J. 2015;36(30):1998–2010.
27. La Gerche A, Burns AT, Taylor AJ, Macisaac AI, Heidbuchel H, Prior DL. Maximal oxygen consumption is best predicted by measures of cardiac size rather than function in healthy adults. Eur J Appl Physiol. 2012;112(6):2139–47.
28. Steding K, Engblom H, Buhre T, Carlsson M, Mosen H, Wohlfart B, et al. Relation between cardiac dimensions and peak oxygen uptake. J Cardiovasc Magn Reson. 2010;12(1):8.
29. Scharhag J, Schneider G, Urhausen A, Rochette V, Kramann B, Kindermann W. Athlete's heart: right and left ventricular mass and function in male endurance athletes and untrained individuals determined by magnetic resonance imaging. J Am Coll Cardiol. 2002;40(10):1856–63.

30. Prior DL, La Gerche A. The athlete's heart. Heart. 2012;98(12):947–55.
31. Schnell F, Matelot D, Daudin M, Kervio G, Mabo P, Carre F, et al. Mechanical dispersion by strain echocardiography: a novel tool to diagnose hypertrophic cardiomyopathy in athletes. J Am Soc Echocardiogr. 2017;30(3):251–61.
32. Mizukoshi K, Suzuki K, Yoneyama K, Kamijima R, Kou S, Takai M, et al. Early diastolic function during exertion influences exercise intolerance in patients with hypertrophic cardiomyopathy. J Echocardiogr. 2013;11(1):9–17.
33. Schnell F, Riding N, O'Hanlon R, Axel Lentz P, Donal E, Kervio G, et al. Recognition and significance of pathological T-wave inversions in athletes. Circulation. 2015;131(2):165–73.
34. Chan RH, Maron BJ, Olivotto I, Pencina MJ, Assenza GE, Haas T, et al. Prognostic value of quantitative contrast-enhanced cardiovascular magnetic resonance for the evaluation of sudden death risk in patients with hypertrophic cardiomyopathy. Circulation. 2014;130(6):484–95.
35. Green JJ, Berger JS, Kramer CM, Salerno M. Prognostic value of late gadolinium enhancement in clinical outcomes for hypertrophic cardiomyopathy. JACC Cardiovasc Imaging. 2012;5(4):370–7.
36. Ho CY, Lopez B, Coelho-Filho OR, Lakdawala NK, Cirino AL, Jarolim P, et al. Myocardial fibrosis as an early manifestation of hypertrophic cardiomyopathy. N Engl J Med. 2010;363(6):552–63.
37. Swoboda PP, McDiarmid AK, Erhayiem B, Broadbent DA, Dobson LE, Garg P, et al. Assessing myocardial extracellular volume by T1 mapping to distinguish hypertrophic cardiomyopathy from athlete's heart. J Am Coll Cardiol. 2016;67(18):2189–90.
38. McDiarmid AK, Swoboda PP, Erhayiem B, Lancaster RE, Lyall GK, Broadbent DA, et al. Athletic cardiac adaptation in males is a consequence of elevated myocyte mass. Circ Cardiovasc Imaging. 2016;9(4):e003579.
39. Abergel E, Chatellier G, Hagege AA, Oblak A, Linhart A, Ducardonnet A, et al. Serial left ventricular adaptations in world-class professional cyclists: implications for disease screening and follow-up. J Am Coll Cardiol. 2004;44(1):144–9.
40. Galderisi M, Cardim N, D'Andrea A, Bruder O, Cosyns B, Davin L, et al. The multi-modality cardiac imaging approach to the Athlete's heart: an expert consensus of the European Association of Cardiovascular Imaging. Eur Heart J Cardiovasc Imaging. 2015;16(4):353.
41. Millar L, Fernandez G, Dhutia H, Myott J, Malhotra A, Finocchiaro G, et al. Exercise echocardiography has a high sensitivity and specificity in differentiating athlete's heart from dilated cardiomyopathy. Circulation. 2016;134(suppl_1):A15662.
42. Friedrich MG, Sechtem U, Schulz-Menger J, Holmvang G, Alakija P, Cooper LT, et al. Cardiovascular magnetic resonance in myocarditis: A JACC White Paper. J Am Coll Cardiol. 2009;53(17):1475–87.
43. De Cobelli F, Pieroni M, Esposito A, Chimenti C, Belloni E, Mellone R, et al. Delayed gadolinium-enhanced cardiac magnetic resonance in patients with chronic myocarditis presenting with heart failure or recurrent arrhythmias. J Am Coll Cardiol. 2006;47(8):1649–54.
44. Mordi I, Carrick D, Bezerra H, Tzemos N. T1 and T2 mapping for early diagnosis of dilated non-ischaemic cardiomyopathy in middle-aged patients and differentiation from normal physiological adaptation. Eur Heart J Cardiovasc Imaging. 2016;17(7):797–803.
45. Al-Khatib SM, Stevenson WG, Ackerman MJ, Bryant WJ, Callans DJ, Curtis AB, et al. AHA/ACC/HRS Guideline for Management of Patients With Ventricular Arrhythmias and the Prevention of Sudden Cardiac Death: A Report of the American College of Cardiology/American Heart Association Task Force on Clinical Practice Guidelines and the Heart Rhythm Society. J Am Coll Cardiol. 2018;72(14):e91–e220.
46. Hubert A, Galand V, Donal E, Pavin D, Galli E, Martins RP, et al. Atrial function is altered in lone paroxysmal atrial fibrillation in male endurance veteran athletes. Eur Heart J Cardiovasc Imaging. 2018;19(2):145–53.
47. Schnell F, Claessen G, La Gerche A, Bogaert J, Lentz PA, Claus P, et al. Subepicardial delayed gadolinium enhancement in asymptomatic athletes: let sleeping dogs lie? Br J Sports Med. 2016;50(2):111–7.

48. Zorzi A, Perazzolo Marra M, Rigato I, De Lazzari M, Susana A, Niero A, et al. Nonischemic left ventricular scar as a substrate of life-threatening ventricular arrhythmias and sudden cardiac death in competitive athletes. Circ Arrhythm Electrophysiol. 2016;9(7):e004229.
49. La Gerche A, Burns AT, Mooney DJ, Inder WJ, Taylor AJ, Bogaert J, et al. Exercise-induced right ventricular dysfunction and structural remodelling in endurance athletes. Eur Heart J. 2012;33(8):998–1006.
50. Wilson M, O'Hanlon R, Prasad S, Deighan A, Macmillan P, Oxborough D, et al. Diverse patterns of myocardial fibrosis in lifelong, veteran endurance athletes. J Appl Physiol. 2011;110(6):1622–6.
51. Ruwald AC, Marcus F, Estes NA 3rd, Link M, McNitt S, Polonsky B, et al. Association of competitive and recreational sport participation with cardiac events in patients with arrhythmogenic right ventricular cardiomyopathy: results from the North American multidisciplinary study of arrhythmogenic right ventricular cardiomyopathy. Eur Heart J. 2015;36(27):1735–43.
52. Lampert R, Olshansky B, Heidbuchel H, Lawless C, Saarel E, Ackerman M, et al. Safety of sports for athletes with implantable cardioverter-defibrillators: long-term results of a prospective multinational registry. Circulation. 2017;135(23):2310–2.
53. Zaidi A, Sheikh N, Jongman JK, Gati S, Panoulas VF, Carr-White G, et al. Clinical differentiation between physiological remodeling and arrhythmogenic right ventricular cardiomyopathy in athletes with marked electrocardiographic repolarization anomalies. J Am Coll Cardiol. 2015;65(25):2702–11.
54. Luijkx T, Velthuis BK, Prakken NH, Cox MG, Bots ML, Mali WP, et al. Impact of revised task force criteria: distinguishing the athlete's heart from ARVC/D using cardiac magnetic resonance imaging. Eur J Prev Cardiol. 2012;19(4):885–91.
55. Te Riele AS, James CA, Philips B, Rastegar N, Bhonsale A, Groeneweg JA, et al. Mutation-positive arrhythmogenic right ventricular dysplasia/cardiomyopathy: the triangle of dysplasia displaced. J Cardiovasc Electrophysiol. 2013;24(12):1311–20.
56. Sen-Chowdhry S, Syrris P, Prasad SK, Hughes SE, Merrifield R, Ward D, et al. Left-dominant arrhythmogenic cardiomyopathy: an under-recognized clinical entity. J Am Coll Cardiol. 2008;52(25):2175–87.
57. Ector J, Ganame J, van der Merwe N, Adriaenssens B, Pison L, Willems R, et al. Reduced right ventricular ejection fraction in endurance athletes presenting with ventricular arrhythmias: a quantitative angiographic assessment. Eur Heart J. 2007;28(3):345–53.
58. Tandri H, Saranathan M, Rodriguez ER, Martinez C, Bomma C, Nasir K, et al. Noninvasive detection of myocardial fibrosis in arrhythmogenic right ventricular cardiomyopathy using delayed-enhancement magnetic resonance imaging. J Am Coll Cardiol. 2005;45(1):98–103.
59. Santangeli P, Pieroni M, Dello Russo A, Casella M, Pelargonio G, Macchione A, et al. Noninvasive diagnosis of electroanatomic abnormalities in arrhythmogenic right ventricular cardiomyopathy. Circ Arrhythm Electrophysiol. 2010;3(6):632–8.
60. Miles C, Finocchiaro G, Papadakis M, Gray B, Westaby J, Ensam B, et al. Sudden death and left ventricular involvement in arrhythmogenic cardiomyopathy. Circulation. 2019;139(15):1786–97.
61. Zeltser I, Cannon B, Silvana L, Fenrich A, George J, Schleifer J, et al. Lessons learned from preparticipation cardiovascular screening in a state funded program. Am J Cardiol. 2012;110(6):902–8.
62. Sharma S, Drezner JA, Baggish A, Papadakis M, Wilson MG, Prutkin JM, et al. International recommendations for electrocardiographic interpretation in athletes. J Am Coll Cardiol. 2017;69(8):1057–75.
63. Dhutia H, Malhotra A, Finocchiaro G, Merghani A, Papadakis M, Naci H, et al. Impact of the International recommendations for electrocardiographic interpretation on cardiovascular screening in young athletes. J Am Coll Cardiol. 2017;70(6):805–7.

# Medical Evaluation of Athletes: Exercise Testing

10

David Niederseer and Herbert Löllgen

**Learning Objectives**

1. Know the purpose, indications and contraindications of exercise testing in athletes.
2. Be able to interpret common findings during exercise testing in athletes.
3. Understand the role of exercise testing as part of pre-participation screening, clinical evaluation and performance assessment in athletes.
4. Understand the ECG findings during stress testing.
5. Know how to derive training recommendations from exercise testing.

## 10.1 Goals of Exercise Testing

Athletes are sportswomen and sportsmen who engage in regular (high) intensity training to improve her / his performance and competition results and who regularly participate in sports competitions. They devote several hours per day or week to training activities. Many of them are or want to become professionals specialized in single sport disciplines on an at least medium, preferably high level [1]. According to age, athletes can be classified into young (<18 years, mostly 12–17 years), adult (18–35 years) and master athletes (>35 years). Levels of performance range from regional over national to world class and Olympic level (see Chap. 1).

D. Niederseer
Department of Cardiology, University Heart Center Zurich, University of Zurich, Zurich, Switzerland
e-mail: david.niederseer@usz.ch

H. Löllgen (✉)
University of Mainz, Private Practice, Sports Cardiology and Cardiology, Remscheid, Germany
e-mail: herbert.loellgen@gmx.de



A. Pressler, J. Niebauer (eds.), *Textbook of Sports and Exercise Cardiology*,
https://doi.org/10.1007/978-3-030-35374-2_10

Exercise testing is used primarily to assess endurance fitness and progression during training or after training pauses e.g. due to diseases, or to measure the level of fitness during or after rehabilitation. However, exercise testing is also used to supplement clinical workup for known or suspected disease in athletes.

An abnormal exercise test is associated with cardiovascular events, total mortality, and sudden cardiac death (SCD) in asymptomatic adults [2–4]. The predominant factor that is associated with negative outcomes is a low fitness level. In a large-scale ($n > 30{,}000$, mean age 31, range 5–92 years) Italian evaluation of exercise stress testing in pre-participation screening (PPS) for competitive sports, abnormalities were found in 4.9%, leading to disqualification in 0.6% of an unselected population ranging from high level athletes to non-athletes, all of them seeking clearance to start exercising [5]. The efficacy of these disqualifications in preventing SCD remains unknown.

Exercise testing should be conducted with four main goals [6]:

1. To evaluate baseline fitness and prescribe an exercise program or training zones;
2. To evaluate continued progress after engaging in exercise training over a period of time;
3. To diagnose cardiopulmonary conditions affecting exercise performance; and
4. To provoke arrhythmias or evaluate hemodynamic response to exercise in an athlete with a known cardiovascular condition to determine whether it is safe to participate in competitive sports.

1. **Exercise testing for assessment of physical performance ability**, especially fitness or cardio-respiratory fitness (CRF) to evaluate the level of performance for forthcoming competitions.
   (a) Here, exercise testing is not primarily performed to search for disease but to measure performance.
   (b) However, also during exercise testing without medical intentions, pathological findings may be documented.
   (c) Further workup is then indicated as appropriate (Fig. 10.1).
   (d) Maximal exercise capacity itself represents an independent, important prognostic clinical finding in the general population associated with future morbidity and mortality. In athletes exercise capacity is usually significantly higher than in the general population; therefore, performing an exercise test to solely assess exercise capacity is generally not indicated.
2. **Exercise testing for monitoring** the level of performance and guiding training according to type and intensity before, during and after training cycles or sessions.
   (a) Repeated exercise testing to objectively measure the effect of training regimens.
   (b) Again, here medical issues are not the main reason to perform exercise testing.

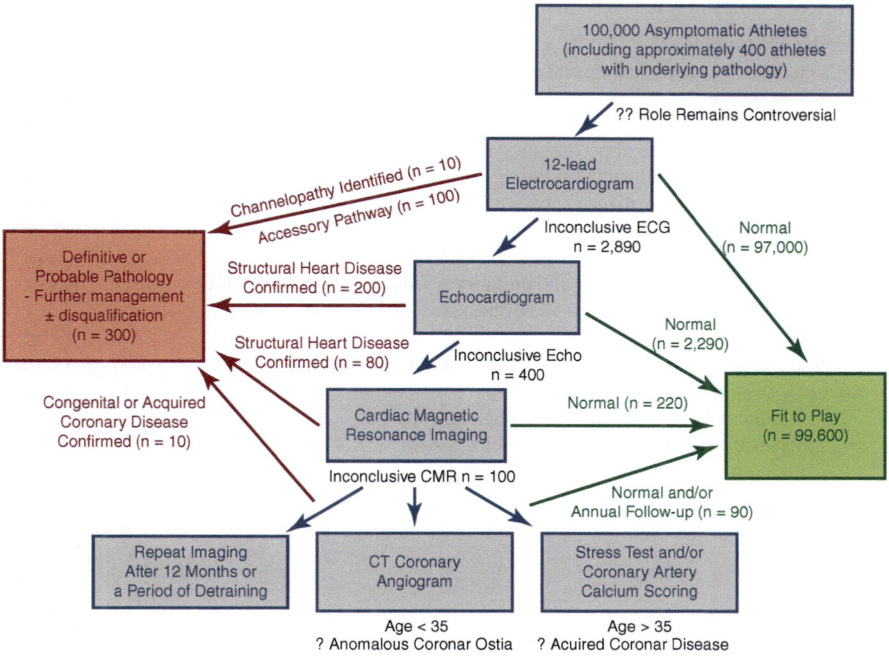


**Fig. 10.1** Diagnostic workflow in pre-participation screening in athletes with assumed incidences of pathological findings; Exercise testing is integrated in the diagnostic algorithm; however, it plays a minor role (adopted from [36])

   (c) However, if pathologic findings are documented they should be managed according to respective guidelines (e.g. Figure 10.1).
3. (3) and (4) can be summarized as: **Exercise testing for medical purposes/health examination.**
   (a) Exercise testing is not recommended to be included into routine PPS (see also Chap. 6).
   (b) In special situations, exercise testing may be included in the health examination of an athlete to exclude or detect congenital and/or acquired subclinical diseases (Table 10.1).
   (c) If physical examination, family and personal history and 12-lead ECG are normal, no further routine testing is needed to medically clear the athlete for sports participation.
   (d) If standard PPS reveals abnormalities, further workup is indicated that might include exercise testing.

A possible flowchart on PPS and the role of exercise testing is provided in Fig. 10.1. Possible diseases to look for in PPS are summarized in Table 10.2.

**Table 10.1** Indications for exercise testing in the medical assessment of athletes

| |
|---|
| *Asymptomatic individuals* |
| • Diagnosis of latent disease and of possible risks during sport |
| • Latent or occult conditions predisposing to exercise-induced arrhythmias or changes of ECG |
| • Assessment of physical performance ability and counselling before start of training |
| • Monitoring and guidance of training |
| • Assessment of performance capacity (e.g. cardio-respiratory fitness) and physical performance ability |
| *Athletes* with known disease who plan to return to play |
| • Diagnosis of cardiovascular and pulmonary function before start of training if applicable |
| • Evaluation of symptoms: dyspnea, chest pain, palpitations, dizziness, (syncope) |
| *Follow-up assessment during training* |
| • Recommendations for amount and intensity of training (FITT rule[a]) |
| *Diagnostic objectives* |
| • Assessment of performance, development, suitability, and structure of training/exercise |
| • Stress is measured by external parameters such as heart rate variability for autonomic cardiac function and effort by "internal" ones as a response of the subject's bodily organs to the exercise strain |

[a]*FITT* frequency of the training stage, **i**ntensity of training, type of training, time of the training session [12]

**Table 10.2** Occult cardiac diseases to be detected in athletes: Inherited and congenital diseases (frequently detected by resting ECG)

| |
|---|
| *Cardiomyopathies* |
| • Hypertrophic cardiomyopathy with and without outflow tract obstruction |
| • Dilated cardiomyopathy |
| • Arrhythmogenic (right ventricular) cardiomyopathy |
| • Non-compaction cardiomyopathy |
| *Congenital or inherited disorders* |
| • Marfan syndrome and other arteriopathies |
| • Coronary artery anomalies |
| *Channelopathies* |
| • Long or Short QT-syndrome |
| • Brugada syndrome |
| • Catecholaminergic Polymorphic Ventricular Tachycardia |
| • WPW and other pre-excitation syndromes |
| *Arrhythmias* |
| • Supraventricular tachycardia |
| • Premature ventricular contractions |
| • Ventricular tachycardia |
| • Bradycardic arrhythmias |

## 10.2 Mandatory Requirements and Pre-Exercise Screening

PPS in athletes is primarily indicated to protect the health of athletes and to enable safe sports participation. To recognise early possible risks during sports, history and clinical examinations are generally agreed upon to form the basis of PPS. It is now widely accepted that an ECG at rest should be a mandatory part of PPS.

PPS may detect cardiovascular diseases (Table 10.2) associated with a higher risk of sudden cardiac events in sports. It also serves to evaluate the proper sports eligibility. After PPS, training recommendations can be provided with regard to different types of sports. In addition, following diseases, PPS enables the sports physician to clear athletes to return to play. As indicated above, exercise testing is generally not included in PPS; however, certain societies or screening regimens recommend including exercise testing in PPS (e.g. Italian screening initiative mainly based in Veneto, German Society of Sports Medicine, German Olympic Sports Federation).

In the European Federation of Sports Medicine Associations (EFSMA) Statement on ECG for PPS [7], exercise testing (incl. ECG) is recommended in patients with diabetes (in males >40 years (yrs), females >50 yrs) and in asymptomatic subjects before engaging in vigorous sports (males >45 yrs., females >55 yrs), in line with the guidelines of the European Association of Cardiovascular Prevention and Rehabilitation (EAPCR [8] (now European Association of Preventive Cardiology)). Irrespective from these recommendations, top-level elite athletes may be required to undergo a more detailed examination (e.g. according to the International Olympic Committee (IOC) or the Fédération Internationale de Football Association (FIFA)) including exercise testing, spiroergometry (also termed cardiopulmonary exercise testing (CPET), see Chap. 45), and echocardiography, thus beyond of what is indicated according to standard cardiology guidelines. However, the scientific evidence for such broad screening investigations is questionable.

## 10.3 Methodological Approaches

The most common standard methods of exercise testing are bicycle ergometry (predominantly applied in Europe) and treadmill ergometry (predominantly applied in the USA) [9–11]. The Bruce testing protocol is the most widely used procedure in the USA. Other testing procedures, such as

- rowing ergometry
- the field step test
- Conconi-test
- rotational ergometry
- supine bicycle ergometry
- step-climbing
- six-minute walking test
- strength tests
- other sports-specific exercise tests

are used to measure performance in sport-specific testing modes and to answer specific clinical questions, sometimes even with mobile (spiroergometric) devices. These modalities of exercise testing will not be described in detail here.

| Stage | Bruce protocol | | | Balke protocol | | | Naughton protocol | | |
|---|---|---|---|---|---|---|---|---|---|
| | Speed | Incline | Duration | Speed | Incline | Duration | Speed | Incline | Duration |
| 1 | 2.7 | 0 | 3 | 5.3 | 0 | 1 | 3.2 | 0 | 3 |
| 2 | 2.7 | 5 | 3 | 5.3 | 2.5 | 1 | 3.2 | 3.5 | 3 |
| 3 | 2.7 | 10 | 3 | 5.3 | 5 | 1 | 3.2 | 7 | 3 |
| 4 | 4.0 | 12 | 3 | 5.3 | 7.5 | 1 | 3.2 | 10.5 | 3 |
| 5 | 5.4 | 14 | 3 | 5.3 | 10 | 1 | 3.2 | 14 | 3 |
| 6 | 6.7 | 16 | 3 | 5.3 | 12.5 | 1 | 3.2 | 17.5 | 3 |
| 7 | 8 | 18 | 3 | 5.3 | 15 | 1 | 4.8 | 12.5 | 3 |
| 8 | 8.8 | 20 | 3 | 5.3 | 17.5 | 1 | 4.8 | 15 | 3 |
| 9 | | | | 5.3 | 20 | 1 | 4.8 | 17.5 | 3 |
| 10 | | | | | | | 4.8 | 20 | 3 |
| 11 | | | | | | | 4.8 | 22.5 | 3 |
| 12 | | | | | | | 5.5 | 20 | 3 |

**Fig. 10.2** Overview of the most frequently applied treadmill protocols in athlete and patient populations

Treadmill testing is naturally more specific in runners or in sporting disciplines that at least partly include running elements. It might also be easier for some patients to perform at least walking protocols on a treadmill (Fig. 10.2). In addition, when performing CPET on a treadmill, usually a higher peak oxygen uptake ($VO_2$peak) is attained. In contrast, at least in European countries, the use of cycle ergometry is more common due to several advantages:

- Usually cheaper and easier to implement into laboratory settings (e.g. requires less space)
- Less ECG noise, thus easier to interpret, also blood pressure (BP) is much easier to measure during exercise
- If required, venous blood samples can much easier be obtained during exercise
- Can be combined with exercise echocardiography
- Usually less experience/training required compared with treadmill testing, thus safer procedure
- Direct power calculation possible
- Independent of weight
- Holding bars has no effect

Practical methodological tips include an adequate skin preparation for exact placement of ECG electrodes and reliable ECG tracings (such as an isoelectric PR and ST line). BP cuff should be tested prior to exercise and adjusted to the circumference of the upper arm. Athletes should receive clear and standardized instructions how to perform the test; they should be motivated to exercise until volitional exhaustion. ECG and BP should be documented at least at the end of each stage, otherwise every 1–2 min. Each test should be followed by a recovery phase of at least 3–5 min to assess vital signs, document heart rate recovery and ECG alterations during this phase.

## 10.4 Technical Prerequisites for Exercise Testing

Standardized conditions must be maintained in the exercise laboratory room (ambient temperature, humidity, etc.) [9, 12]. Continuous monitoring of heart rate (HR), BP, ECG and clinical signs are mandatory, in order to ensure that the stress test can be interrupted immediately in case of any complications. The response to emergency situations should be trained at regular intervals with the non-physician staff members. Requirements for exercise testing are summarized in Table 10.3.

## 10.5 When to Stop an Exercise Test

- Pathologic: athlete develops symptoms (relative, as sometimes exercise testing is performed to induce particular symptoms); ECG: ischemic changes and/or arrhythmias, drop in systolic BP (>20 mmHg), excessive increase in BP (>260/115 mmHg) (Table 10.4)
- Physiologic: maximal exhaustion [13, 14] (Table 10.5)

## 10.6 Desaturation

If assessed, a drop in oxygen saturation of more than 5% during exercise raises the suspicion of pulmonary disease causing exercise induced hypoxemia. However, in highly trained athletes changes of 5–10% may occur even in the absence of pathology!

**Table 10.3** Requirements for exercise testing

| |
|---|
| *Examination before starting the exercise test* |
| • History including current medications |
| • Physical examination including blood pressure at rest |
| • ECG at rest |
| *Test conditions* |
| • Room temperature 16–24 °C, humidity 30–60% |
| • Calibrated ergometer (certificate of conformity), control monitor, continuous digital ECG recording and storage |
| • Cadence 60–80 rpm (may be higher at maximal performance) |
| • Blood pressure measurement every 1–2 min (usually mid or end stage) |
| • Telephone number of emergency response team in sight |
| *Subject* |
| • Normal body temperature |
| • At least 1–2 h after last meal |
| • At least 12 h since last alcohol consumption or tobacco use |
| • Medication: adequate pause since last intake, if indicated |
| *Examiners* |
| • Presence of an experienced physician (up-to-date knowledge of resuscitation techniques) |
| • Appropriately trained personnel (trained in ECG monitoring, symptoms that may arise, first-aid measures, and cardiopulmonary resuscitation in case of an emergency) |

**Table 10.4** Criteria for the termination of ergometric testing

| |
|---|
| *Symptoms* |
| • Dizziness |
| • Incoordination |
| • Progressive chest pain |
| • Shortness of breath |
| *Objective signs* |
| • *ECG changes* |
| — progressively severe arrhythmias |
| — couplets, (non-)sustained ventricular tachycardia, increasing supraventricular extrasystoles, atrial tachycardias, atrial flutter, new-onset atrial fibrillation |
| — progressive intracardiac conduction disturbance |
| — increasing QRS widening |
| — appearance of a left bundle branch block |
| — progressive repolarization disorder |
| — ST depression: horizontal depression greater than 0.2 mV |
| — progressive ST elevation in the electrocardiogram (ECG) (>0.1 mV) |
| — ST elevation (obligatory termination of test) |
| • *Hemodynamic changes* |
| — progressive drop in blood pressure |
| — insufficient rise in blood pressure (less than 10 mmHg for each level of performance) |
| — excessive rise in blood pressure (either as unusually high values at low workloads (e.g. >200 mmHg at 100 W or excessive maximal response >240–260 mmHg) |

*Note:* A number of current guidelines and standard recommendations no longer distinguish between relative and absolute contraindications (see above) or criteria for test termination but refer to progressive changes instead

**Table 10.5** Criteria for peak word load and exhaustion (minimal values for adults)[a]

| Parameter | Criteria |
|---|---|
| Heart rate | Bicycle: >208–0.7 × age (years)<br>Treadmill: >209.3–0.72 × age 8 (years) |
| Perceived exertion | >17 (Borg scale 6–20) |
| Blood gas analysis | pH < 7.25<br>Base excess <9 mmol/l (healthy subjects), <5 mmol/l (patients) |
| Lactate | >9 mmol/L (healthy subjects), >5 mmol/L (patients) |
| Spiroergometry | $VO_2$peak > 35 ml/min/kg (males), >30 ml/min/kg (females)<br>Respiratory exchange ratio > 1.10 (patients) -1.15 (healthy subjects)<br>Ventilatory equivalent for $CO_2$ > 35 |

[a]Peak performance is assumed to have been achieved only when at least one of these values or more have been exceeded (according to [12]). Ergometric stress testing should not be terminated when one of these values has been reached; the person undergoing exercise testing should continue working up to the individual point of exhaustion. Ergometric testing should, however, be terminated if pathological changes arise

## 10.7 Interpretation of the Post-Exercise Phase

In the early recovery phase after ergometric stress testing, complications such as arrhythmias and circulatory collapse can arise, and therefore BP, HR and ECG should still be monitored. The HR response in this phase also provides further diagnostic information: the HR should fall by at least 12 beats/min in the first minute of the recovery period, indicating a good autonomic balance between sympathetic and parasympathetic function. Delayed HR renormalization may indicate disturbed neurohumoral function due to stress, hypertension, lack of training, or other factors. On the other hand, slow HR recovery kinetics and high HR in the recovery period are normal if the subject has performed physical work above the limit of sustainable performance. To avoid collapse, not an immediate stop of exercise, but a light workload is advisable. Monitoring is indicated until HR is <100/min and BP pressure has normalized [12].

## 10.8 Aspects to Particularly Pay Attention to During Exercise Testing in Athletes

- Apply suitable protocols for specific questions, e.g.:
  - Primary aim to provoke symptoms like angina, shortness of breath, palpitations, syncope
  - Primary aim to assess maximal exercise capacity
- ECG: ST-segment depression, arrhythmias, accessory pathways
- HR: chronotropic competence (e.g. recovery HR > 12 beats within 1 min after termination of exercise; achieving 80% of age-predicted maximum HR)
- BP response to exercise (unusual increase or drop; see also Chap. 13)

## 10.9 Ergometry vs. Cardiopulmonary Exercise Testing (CPET)

CPET is particularly useful to be additionally applied to athletes with medical issues such as exertional dyspnea, e.g. in case of suspected pulmonary disease like exercise-induced asthma. Moreover, it allows direct assessment of $VO_2$peak instead of calculating this parameter from maximal workload attained.

Important variables for interpretation of CPET in athletes (for a detailed description see Chap. 45 and [10])

- Peak or maximal oxygen uptake ($VO_2$max/$VO_2$peak)
- Ventilatory aerobic and anaerobic thresholds (VT1 and VT2)
- Oxygen pulse ($VO_2$/HR)
- Ventilatory reserve (Ratio of minute ventilation (VE) to maximal voluntary ventilation (MVV))
- Breathing frequency
- Ventilatory equivalents (VE/$VCO_2$ (slope, at VT2, at maximum), VE/$VO_2$)
- Dead space ventilation (VD/VT)
- Alveolar-arterial tension oxygen difference (P(A-a)$O_2$)

## 10.10 Challenges When Performing Exercise Tests in Athletes

Several issues deserve particular attention during exercise testing in athletes since they represent potential diagnostic conundrums due to either limited validity of this technique regarding specific scenarios, limited data or ongoing debates on the clinical consequences of particular findings. These include:

- False reassurance regarding coronary artery disease and negative exercise test for ischemia (limited sensitivity and specificity of exercise testing)
- Young athlete with exertional chest pain and syncope (difficult differential diagnosis)
- Accessory pathways that inconstantly conduct sinus tachycardia (to ablate or not to ablate?)
- Pseudo-Normalization of T-waves: negative T-waves at rest in supine and/or upright position that turn positive during exercise and return to be negative in the recovery phase (not clear if representing a normal or pathological variant such as ischemia or hypertrophic cardiomyopathy)
- Rapid hypertensive response to exercise vs. gradual increase and elevated blood pressure at peak exercise (to a certain degree normal in athletes or indication for medical treatment?)
- CPET: Desaturation and no residual breathing reserve at peak exercise (pulmonary limitation or high-level endurance athlete?)

## 10.11 Choosing the Right Protocol for Exercise Testing in Athletes

The protocol should be individualized to the assumed exercise capacity of the athlete, the specific medical question and the type of sport of the athlete. In general, exercise testing should be completed within 12–15 min to avoid early muscle exhaustion. A "one-size-fits-all" exercise testing protocol such as the Bruce protocol is not useful. Understanding the physiology involved in specific sports is important in assessing an athlete's performance. The ability to perform sport specific protocols is absolutely essential for evaluating athletes and will result in a much more informative test for both the athlete and sports cardiologist. Moreover, a profound understanding of the unique nature of an athlete's clinical event is essential to the design, interpretation, and counselling of an advanced exercise test. Thus, considerable thought needs to be given in the design of a sports specific protocol:

- For clinical assessment: when and how during the event do symptoms occur?
- Is the necessary testing equipment available to reproduce the type sport as close as possible?
- If not, can the metabolic demands of the particular sport sufficiently be reproduced with the equipment that is available or does the athlete have to be referred

**Table 10.6** Suggested nongraded exercise testing protocols for various sports (according to [6])

| Sport | Exercise protocol |
|---|---|
| Ice hockey | High intensity (>90–95% of maximal heart rate) intervals for 90 s with 90 s rest between bouts, repeated 6–10 times |
| American football | Very high intensity (>95% of maximal heart rate) intervals of 10 s with 30 s rest between bouts repeated 10–15 times |
| Soccer | Sustained moderate intensity effort (50–70% of maximal heart rate) for 2–3 min with 30–60 s of high-intensity effort (>90%of maximal heart rate) repeated 10–25 times |
| Basketball | Box jumps 3–5 times as quickly as possible followed by moderate level intensity (60–70% of maximal heart rate) intervals for 1 min repeated 10–15 times |
| Triathlon | Swimming (if available) 45 min, cycling 45 min, and running 45 min |

to another laboratory with more suitable devices (e.g. symptoms during running may not be observed during cycle ergometry)?

If the exercise test in the athlete is performed to assess symptoms during exercise, try to reproduce the symptoms during exercise testing by trying to closely mimic the exact condition during sports. Some examples are listed in Table 10.6.

Regarding the protocol, the following issues have to be considered:

- *Graded* (e.g. for lactate threshold assessment) vs. *non-graded* testing (e.g. for assessment of symptoms)
- A *ramp protocol* with intensities rising continuously may be preferred as an alternative (see Chap. 45). These protocols will more consistently achieve conditions comparable to other protocols, as they generate almost imperceptible increases in treadmill speed every few seconds and permit increases in external work in a continuous fashion. Ramp protocols offer the opportunity to individualize exercise testing through a wide range of athlete-patient capabilities [15, 16].
- *Bruce protocol*: the gradient and the speed of the treadmill are increased every 3 min in a predefined fashion [17]. Be aware that use of a formula rather than with direct measurements of oxygen consumption during the Bruce protocol leads to overestimated $VO_2$max in undertrained athletes and underestimated in well-trained athletes.
- *Balke protocol*: speed remains constant at 3.3 mph (=5.3 km/h) whereas the inclination is increased by 1% every minute [18]. This will take twice as much time to reach maximal state as Bruce protocol (Fig. 10.2).

Perhaps less common and restricted to special laboratories, but very important in specific athlete populations (e.g. the power athlete with efforts lasting 10–20 s) is **anaerobic exercise testing.** Usually, this has often turned out to be impractical for testing athletic teams or large groups because of the expense as well as the invasive (i.e. blood draw, muscle biopsies) nature of the activity [19], but tests have been developed over time that determine an athlete's anaerobic capacity quickly and easily. The Wingate Anaerobic Test is the most popular laboratory performance test

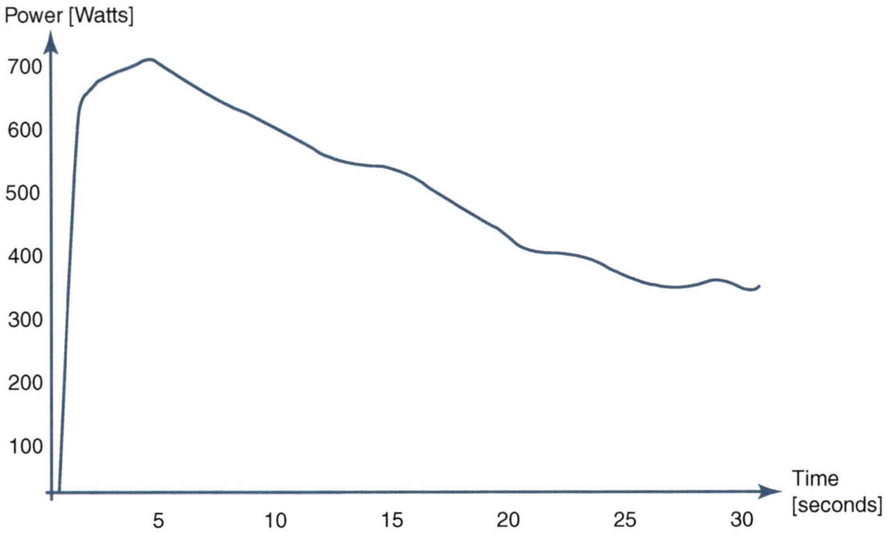


**Fig. 10.3** An example of a Wingate Anaerobic Test, showing the peak anerobic power attained during the initial phase of the test with a slow but steady decline during the further course

that evaluates anaerobic energy system power and provides a fatigue index based on the ability of the individual to sustain peak power [19]. It requires the subject to pedal a mechanically braked bicycle ergometer (an arm ergometer also can be used) for 30 s, at an "all out" pace [20]. The test provides values for peak power, relative peak power, anaerobic fatigue, and anaerobic capacity. These results can then be compared with previous testing to assess the progress of a specific anaerobic or power training regimen (Fig. 10.3).

## 10.12 Basic Principles of Exercise Prescription

Exercise prescription results in an individualized exercise program designed according to the particular conditions and demands of patients or athletes, similar to a prescription for medication. Each exercise prescription has four essential components: frequency, intensity, time (duration), and type of exercise (F.I.T.T). In addition, progression of training amount is another part of training recommendation. The ACSM recommends these F.I.T.T. guidelines for prescribing exercise [21] to achieve cardiovascular benefits. They recommend a frequency of 3–5 times per week, an intensity of 65–85% of maximal HR, and a duration of 20–60 min per session. Use of the F.I.T.T. guidelines is an easy way to prescribe exercise to the majority of people. With the addition of exercise testing, it is possible to provide a more individualized exercise prescription based on the current fitness level and the desired fitness goal.

There are several ways to calculate target HR to guide exercise intensity:

- Percentage of maximal HR (HRmax):
  - target heart rate (HR) = HRmax × % intensity
  - does not account for resting heart rate and assumes that the lower range of heart rate is zero
- Heart rate reserve (HRR):
  - target HR = (HRmax − resting HR) × % intensity + resting HR
  - a more accurate estimate of energy expenditure
  - considers the range of HR during exercise
  - This discrepancy between HRmax and HRR based on target heart rate calculations can result in a large difference when used for lower intensities; however, it becomes less apparent at near maximal intensity [22]
- Direct determination:
  - predominantly used in athletes
  - percentage of $VO_2$peak (if assessed) or percentage of ventilatory (or lactate) thresholds to set training zones
  - each zone carries its own benefits and purposes for a defined workout and can be used by athletes or coaches to achieve specific fitness gains

Lactate measurement during exercise can provide valuable information regarding the athlete's training status when preparing for a competition. Several established threshold models using lactate measurements are known, with no clear gold-standard. In German-speaking countries the workload at a fixed lactate value of 4 mmol/l representing the anaerobic threshold has traditionally been used, but nowadays threshold models calculated from the individual course during an exercise test are also established. Compared with $VO_2$max, athletic performance in endurance events of longer duration (such as marathon running) is often more closely correlated to performance at the lactate threshold [23], although such correlations largely depend on the duration of the particular sporting event. For example, lactate thresholds are particularly relevant to efforts lasting 2–3 h, whereas efforts lasting only 10–20 min are more closely linked to maximal parameters such as $VO_2$max. In contrast, efforts lasting less than 1–2 min largely depend on power output and lactate tolerance than on $VO_2$ and lactate thresholds [24].

## 10.13 Risk of Exercise Testing in Athletes

According to the Guidelines for Exercise Testing and Prescription from the American College of Sports Medicine (ACSM) [21] it should be recognized that

- clinical exercise testing is a part of the practice of medicine
- should always be conducted in consultation with a physician
- maximal exercise testing in healthy individuals, with adequate but simple pre-exercise screening, is an overall very safe procedure.

In an older study reporting the results of more than half a million clinical exercise tests in elderly individuals referred for evaluation of known or suspected cardiovascular or pulmonary disease [25], the rate of adverse events (including death, myocardial infarction and symptomatic hypotension) was only 0.04%, or about 1 event in 2500 tests. In a recent study on >5.000 multimorbid patients evaluated by CPET, the adverse event rate was also rather low (0.16%, that is 1 in 625 tests). It was concluded that CPET is a generally safe procedure, even in a high-risk population [26]. In young, healthy, physically active individuals or athletes [27], exercise tests were evaluated from 198 sites in 3 German-speaking countries; no deaths or life-threatening complications were reported among 353.638 tests.

Thus, apart from sudden cardiac death events in young athletes related to undiagnosed coronary artery disease or cardiomyopathies, the risk of undergoing exercise testing is insignificantly low. Furthermore, at least in athletes, the level of stress induced by laboratory testing is generally regarded to be much lower than the physical demands experienced in everyday living. Nonetheless, emergency equipment must be available in the exercise laboratory, including an external defibrillator device checked for functionality at regular intervals. The staff must be trained to react properly in cases of emergency, and a physician should be available to appear on-site within one minute [12].

## 10.14 The Role of Exercise Testing in Athletes with Specific Conditions

The following paragraphs provide a brief overview of the applicability and the potential additive value of exercise testing in cardiac conditions that may pose a particular risk. Please see the separate chapters on these conditions for more details.

**Hypertrophic Cardiomyopathy (HCM)**

- CPET may aid to distinguish athlete's heart from HCM; in athletes, $VO_2$peak is usually >50 ml/kg/min or >120% predicted as compared to HCM patients (can, however, be misleading in borderline cases) [28].
- CPET may be integrated into the holistic clinical differentiation between HCM and athlete's heart (Fig. 10.4).

**Arrhythmogenic (Right Ventricular) Cardiomyopathy (ARVC)**

- Exercise treadmill testing is considered to be safe in ARVC and does usually not induce sustained ventricular tachycardia (VT) (see Chap. 15).
- Exercise testing plays a limited role in diagnosis and does not help to discriminate between ARVC-associated and idiopathic VT.
- Frequent left bundle branch block and premature ventricular contractions with superior axis favor ARVC diagnosis.

| Hypertrophic Cardiomyopathy | "grey zone" LVWT 13-16 mm T-wave inversion | Athlete`s Heart |
|---|---|---|
| | **General information** | |
| • Female gender | | • Male gender |
| • Positive family history for HCM | | • Negative family history for HCM |
| | **ECG** | |
| • Additional ECG abnormalities such as ST-segment depression, deep T-wave inversion in inferolateral leads | | • Isolated Sokolow-Lyon criteria for LV hypertrophy, no ST-segment depression and/or T-wave inversion |
| | **Echocardiography** | |
| • LV cavity < 54 mm | | • LV cavity > 54 mm |
| • Bizarre patterns of LVH, LA > 50mm, LVOT obstruction | | • No or only mild LVH, LA < 50mm, no LVOT obstruction |
| • Impaired systolic or diastolic LV-function | | • Normal systolic and diastolic LV-function |
| | **Exercise testing and/or holter monitoring** | |
| • NSVT/VT during exercise testing or holter monitoring | | • No NSVT/VT during exercise testing or halter monitoring |
| • Abnormal BP response during exercise testing | | • Normal BP response during exercise testing |
| • Peak $VO_2$ < 50ml/kg/min or < 120% predicted | | • Peak $VO_2$ > 50 ml/kg/min or > 120% predicted |
| | **Cardiac magnetic resonance imaging** | |
| • Delayed gadolinium enhancement | | • No delayed gadolinium enhancement |

**Fig. 10.4** Integrative diagnostic assessment of hypertrophic cardiomyopathy vs. athlete's heart. *LVWT* left ventricular wall thickness, *HCM* hypertrophic cardiomyopathy, *ECG* electrocardiography, *LVH* left ventricular hypertrophy, *NSVT* non-sustained ventricular tachycardia, *VT* ventricular tachycardia, *LA* left atrium

- Decreased exercise capacity in ARVC predicts future development of symptomatic heart failure.
- Exercise testing exposes a latent electrical substrate in asymptomatic ARVC gene carriers that is shared by patients with ARVC with a history of ventricular arrhythmia.
- Exercise testing may be useful in guiding treatment decisions, exercise prescription, and prioritizing medical surveillance in asymptomatic ARVC gene carriers [29].

### Long-QT Syndrome

- The Schwartz score includes exercise testing to predict the probability of suffering from LQTS (Table 10.7) [30]. Risk classification: low probability ≤1, intermediate 1.5–3, high ≥3.5 (see also Chap. 21)
- Exercise testing may thus be integrated into the clinical assessment of patients with suspected LQTS.

### Catecholaminergic Polymorphic Ventricular Tachycardia (CPVT)

- Exercise testing is the primary diagnostic tool in CPVT; typical findings are bi-directional polymorphic ventricular arrhythmias increasing in frequency and complexity. Resting ECG is usually normal (Fig. 10.5 and Chap. 21)

**Table 10.7** The "Schwartz score" to calculate the probability for Long QT syndrome, **bold** indicates findings during exercise testing (according to [30])

| Findings | | | Points |
|---|---|---|---|
| ECG[a] | QTc[b] | ≥480 ms | 3 |
| | | =460–479 ms | 2 |
| | | =450–459 ms (in males) | 1 |
| | | **≥480 ms during fourth minute of recovery from exercise stress test** | 1 |
| | *Torsade de pointes*[c] | | 2 |
| | T wave alternans | | 1 |
| | Notched T wave in three leads | | 1 |
| | Low heart rate for age[d] | | 0.5 |
| Clinical history | **Syncope**[c] | **With stress** | 2 |
| | | Without stress | 1 |
| Family history | Family member(s) with definite LQTS[e] | | 1 |
| | Unexplained sudden cardiac death at age < 30 years in immediate family[e] | | 0.5 |
| **Total score** | | | X |

[a]In the absence of medications or disorders known to affect these electrocardiographic features
[b]QTc (corrected QT) calculated by Bazett's formula where $QTc = QT/\sqrt{RR}$
[c]Mutually exclusive
[d]Resting heart rate < 2nd %ile for age
[e]The same family member cannot be counted for both criteria

**Bradycardias**

- In athletes with AV block (see Chap. 8), exercise testing may aid to differentiate between a mostly benign supra-hisian and a usually pathological infra-hisian origin (Table 10.8).

**Post-Exertional Syncope**

- Exercise testing reveals the diagnosis: abrupt and massive blood pressure drop accompanied by symptoms immediately after cessation of exercise, following maximal exertion.
- Benign prognosis, symptomatic treatment with fluid management, compression garment.
- In part also caused due to augmented vagal tone in young athletes, thus increased parasympathetic release post exertion.
- Post-exercise peripheral vasodilation.
- However: Be aware of Brugada syndrome, as 10% of sudden cardiac deaths occur post-exertion.

**Brugada Syndrome**

- ST-segment elevation during the recovery phase of exercise testing predict cardiac events, as shown in a study on 93 Brugada patients (22 with documented ventricular fibrillation (VF), 35 with syncope; 36 asymptomatics; 102 healthy controls): 37% of Brugada patients but none of the controls exhibited ST elevation 1–4 min into recovery (≥0.05 mV in V1–V3). During 76 ± 38 months follow-up 44% with ST elevation vs. 17% without ST elevation exhibited VF ($p = 0.004$) [31].

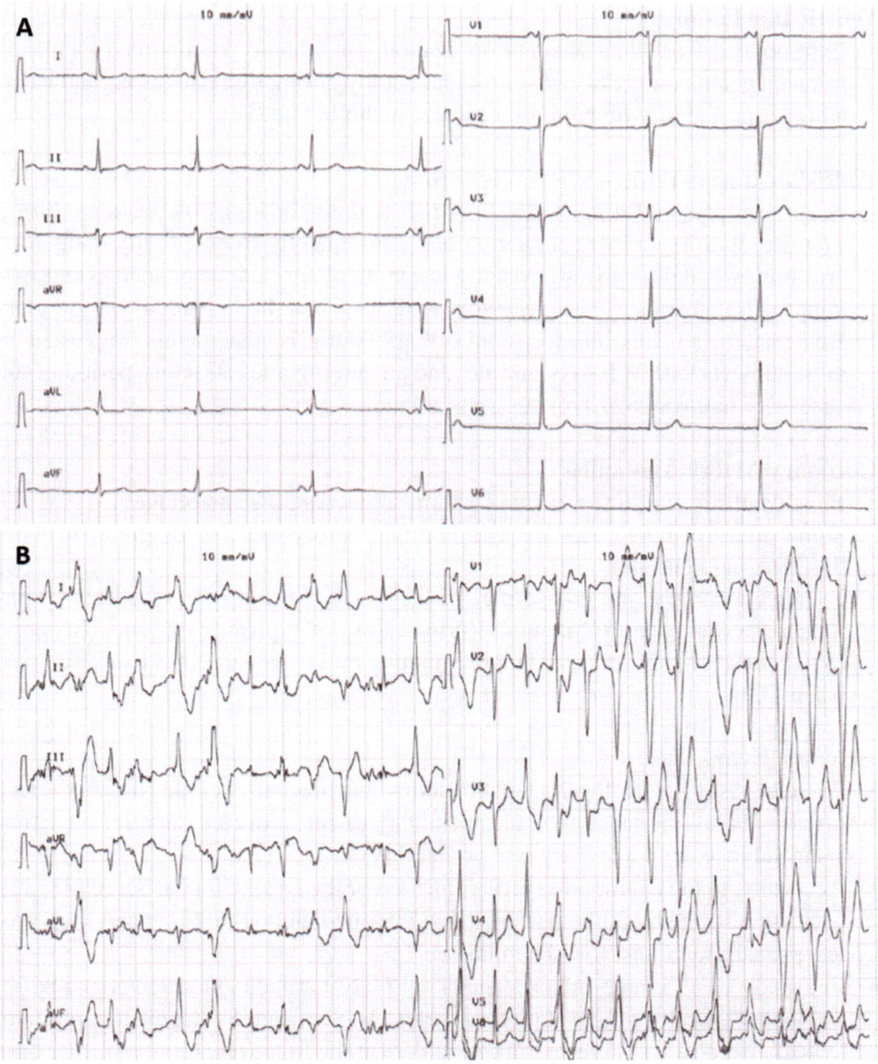


**Fig. 10.5** Example of a Catecholaminergic Polymorphic Ventricular Tachycardia (CPVT), typically showing a normal resting electrocardiogram (**a**) and polymorphic ventricular tachycardia induced by exercise (**b**)

**Table 10.8** Differential diagnosis of AV-block into supra-hisian (benign) and infra-hisian (pathological)

| Supra-hisian block | Infra-hisian block |
|---|---|
| Narrow QRS-complex | Wide QRS-complex |
| Normal QRS-axis | Abnormal QRS-axis |
| Bradycardia, first degree AV-Block, Mobitz Type 1 (Wenckebach) | Intrinsic, no extrinsic influence; second degree AV block, Mobitz Type 2; third degree AV-Block |
| Conduction ↑ with exercise | Conduction = or ↑ with exercise |
| Physiological | Pathological |
| Does usually not require treatment | Mostly needs treatment with a pacemaker |

**Ventricular Ectopy**

- Extrapolated from data obtained in general and athletic populations: Increased frequency and complexity of ventricular ectopy during exercise testing indicated a higher probability of exhibiting cardiac pathology [32].

**Wolff-Parkinson-White-(WPW)-Syndrome**

- Accessory pathway may exhibit low-risk features or high-risk features during exercise, with regard to conduction and consequently to potentially dangerous arrythmias. If delta-wave shows only intermittent appearance or sudden and sustained disappearance, the accessory pathway can be regarded as low-risk. However, in athletes an electrophysiologic study is nonetheless suggested in most subjects with WPW-syndrome, and an anterograde refractory period of the accessory pathway >270 ms suggests ablation.

**Coronary Artery Anomalies**

- Most deaths occur during exercise and in subjects <30 years of age
- Some affected individuals are symptomatic during exercise (angina, syncope, dyspnea, palpitations)
- Exercise testing as integrative part of diagnostic work-up for suspected symptomatic coronary artery anomaly (provocation of typical symptoms, ischemia (ST-depression) or drop in blood pressure during progressive exercise) (see Chap. 22)

**Ischemic Heart Disease**

- Exercise testing is not the diagnostic method of choice to exclude coronary artery disease due to low sensitivity and specificity to detect or rule out relevant stenosis in subjects with a low pre-test probability.
- According to the Diamond-Forrester method or the Duke Clinical Score [33, 34], exercise testing should be performed in intermediate, but not low and high pre-test probability to test for ischemia.
- In a study on 113 male subjects aged over 60 (79 trained; 34 sedentary), 88 (62; 26) were clinically followed up for 4 years. A significant ST segment depression at peak exercise was detected in one athlete at the first evaluation; a further case was seen during follow up in a previously "negative" athlete. Both were asymptomatic, and single photon emission tomography and/or stress echocardiography were negative for myocardial ischemia. The athletes remained symptom-free during the period of the study. One athlete died during follow up for coronary artery disease: he showed polymorphic ventricular tachycardia during both the exercise test and Holter monitoring, but no significant ST segment depression. The authors concluded, that the finding of false positive ST segment depression in elderly athletes, although still not fully understood, may be related to the physiological cardiac remodeling induced by regular training. Thus, athletes with exercise induced ST segment depression, with no associated symptoms and/or complex ventricular arrhythmias, and no adverse findings at second level cardiological testing, should be considered free from coronary disease and medically be cleared for continuation of athletic training [35].

**Clinical Pearls**

- Exercise testing in athletes is used to (a) evaluate baseline fitness and prescribe an exercise program or training zones, (b) evaluate continued progress after engaging in exercise training over a period of time, (c) diagnose cardiopulmonary conditions affecting exercise performance, and (d) provoke arrhythmias or evaluate hemodynamic response to exercise in an athlete with a known cardiovascular condition to determine whether it is safe to participate in competitive sports.
- Exercise testing is not part of routine pre-participation screening; however, it can supplement the clinical work-up in athletes with pathological findings and/or symptoms.

## Review

### Questions

1. A 29-year old Afro-Caribbean soccer player without symptoms and without any sudden cardiac deaths in his family is referred to you to be medically cleared before a transfer. The club wants personal and family history, clinical examination and ECG to be performed. These investigations are unremarkable. Other tests might be performed, however, only if you think they are clinically necessary. Do you perform an exercise test in this athlete?
2. A 53-year old high-level triathlete reports typical chest pain at exertion that disappears during recovery. His medical history is unremarkable. His resting ECG shows features of athlete's heart, but no ST-segment abnormalities. He has no known cardiovascular risk factors and his family history is unremarkable for cardiac diseases and/or sudden cardiac deaths. Do you perform an exercise test in this athlete to rule out coronary artery disease?
3. A 21-year old female ice-hockey player complains of exertional dyspnea and chest pain after maximal effort during competition, mostly in the third term. She never had these complaints during training. A cardiac work-up including ECG, echocardiography and standard exercise test (Bruce protocol) was unremarkable and revealed no condition that could explain the symptoms of the athlete. Besides other diagnostic work-up (e.g. pulmonary assessment of asthma, cardiac imaging, and laboratory workup): would another exercise test be of use?

### Answers

1. No. In asymptomatic young (<35 years) athletes with normal PPS including personal and family history, clinical examination and ECG, an exercise test is not useful and therefore not recommended.
2. In this athlete with typical angina but low risk profile an exercise test could be performed. If ST-segment depression would be seen, a further work-up including non-invasive ischemia testing and/or coronary angiography could be indicated. However,

if the exercise test would not show any sign of ischemia, this would not exclude relevant coronary artery disease. Therefore, exercise testing is not recommended to rule-out coronary artery disease. A coronary computed tomography would be the best choice to exclude significant coronary artery disease. Nevertheless, exercise testing may supplement the clinical picture in this athlete and could lead to additional clinically relevant information in the management of this athlete.

3. An exercise test that closely mimics the characteristics of ice hockey could help to shed light on the cause of the symptoms of this athlete. High intensity (>90–95% of maximal heart rate) intervals for 90 s with 90 s rest between bouts, repeated 6–10 times on a bicycle or treadmill ergometer including spiroergometric measurements would be our protocol of choice. Indeed, the symptoms of this athlete could be reproduced in the ninth interval, and ST-segment depression, drop in blood pressure and drop in oxygen pulse were noted. After cessation of exercise, the symptoms resolved, as were the abnormalities found during exercise testing. A coronary CT-scan revealed a coronary artery anomaly with interarterial course, and further management was planned.

## References


1. Araujo CG, Scharhag J. Athlete: a working definition for medical and health sciences research. Scand J Med Sci Sports. 2016;26(1):4–7.
2. Laukkanen JA, Makikallio TH, Rauramaa R, Kiviniemi V, Ronkainen K, Kurl S. Cardiorespiratory fitness is related to the risk of sudden cardiac death: a population-based follow-up study. J Am Coll Cardiol. 2010;56(18):1476–83.
3. Mora S, Redberg RF, Cui Y, Whiteman MK, Flaws JA, Sharrett AR, et al. Ability of exercise testing to predict cardiovascular and all-cause death in asymptomatic women: a 20-year follow-up of the lipid research clinics prevalence study. JAMA. 2003;290(12):1600–7.
4. Myers J, Prakash M, Froelicher V, Do D, Partington S, Atwood JE. Exercise capacity and mortality among men referred for exercise testing. N Engl J Med. 2002;346(11):793–801.
5. Sofi F, Capalbo A, Pucci N, Giuliattini J, Condino F, Alessandri F, et al. Cardiovascular evaluation, including resting and exercise electrocardiography, before participation in competitive sports: cross sectional study. BMJ. 2008;337:a346.
6. Sarma S, Levine BD. Beyond the Bruce protocol: advanced exercise testing for the sports cardiologist. Cardiol Clin. 2016;34(4):603–8.
7. Lollgen H, Borjesson M, Cummiskey J, Bachl N, Debruyne A. The pre-participation examination in sports: EFSMA statement on ECG for pre-participation examination. Dtsch Z Sportmed. 2015;66(6):151–5.
8. Borjesson M, Urhausen A, Kouidi E, Dugmore D, Sharma S, Halle M, et al. Cardiovascular evaluation of middle-aged/ senior individuals engaged in leisure-time sport activities: position stand from the sections of exercise physiology and sports cardiology of the European association of cardiovascular prevention and rehabilitation. Eur J Cardiovasc Prev Rehabil. 2011;18(3):446–58.
9. Fletcher GF, Ades PA, Kligfield P, Arena R, Balady GJ, Bittner VA, et al. Exercise standards for testing and training: a scientific statement from the American heart association. Circulation. 2013;128(8):873–934.
10. Guazzi M, Arena R, Halle M, Piepoli MF, Myers J, Lavie CJ. 2016 focused update: clinical recommendations for cardiopulmonary exercise testing data assessment in specific patient populations. Circulation. 2016;133(24):e694–711.
11. Meyer FJ, Borst MM, Buschmann HC, Claussen M, Dumitrescu D, Ewert R, et al. Exercise testing in respiratory medicine—DGP recommendations. Pneumologie. 2018;72(10):687–731.

12. Lollgen H, Leyk D. Exercise testing in sports medicine. Dtsch Arztebl Int. 2018;115(24):409–16.
13. Niebauer J. Call for truly maximal ergometries during clinical routine. Eur J Prev Cardiol. 2019;26(7):728–30.
14. Sirico F, Fernando F, Di Paolo F, Adami PE, Signorello MG, Sannino G, et al. Exercise stress test in apparently healthy individuals—where to place the finish line? The Ferrari corporate wellness programme experience. Eur J Prev Cardiol. 2019;26(7):731–8.
15. Myers J, Bellin D. Ramp exercise protocols for clinical and cardiopulmonary exercise testing. Sports Med. 2000;30(1):23–9.
16. Myers J, Buchanan N, Walsh D, Kraemer M, McAuley P, Hamilton-Wessler M, et al. Comparison of the ramp versus standard exercise protocols. J Am Coll Cardiol. 1991;17(6):1334–42.
17. Bruce RA, Kusumi F, Hosmer D. Maximal oxygen intake and nomographic assessment of functional aerobic impairment in cardiovascular disease. Am Heart J. 1973;85(4):546–62.
18. Balke B, Ware RW. An experimental study of physical fitness of air force personnel. U S Armed Forces Med J. 1959;10(6):675–88.
19. Vandewalle H, Peres G, Monod H. Standard anaerobic exercise tests. Sports Med. 1987;4(4):268–89.
20. Lockwood PA, Yoder JE, Deuster PA. Comparison and cross-validation of cycle ergometry estimates of VO2max. Med Sci Sports Exerc. 1997;29(11):1513–20.
21. Medicine ACoS. ACSM guidelines for exercise testing and prescription. Philadelphia: Lippincott Williams & Wilkins; 2000.
22. Forman DE, Myers J, Lavie CJ, Guazzi M, Celli B, Arena R. Cardiopulmonary exercise testing: relevant but underused. Postgrad Med. 2010;122(6):68–86.
23. Coyle EF, Coggan AR, Hopper MK, Walters TJ. Determinants of endurance in well-trained cyclists. J Appl Physiol (1985). 1988;64(6):2622–30.
24. Levine BD. VO2max: what do we know, and what do we still need to know? J Physiol. 2008;586(1):25–34.
25. Stuart RJ Jr, Ellestad MH. National survey of exercise stress testing facilities. Chest. 1980;77(1):94–7.
26. Skalski J, Allison TG, Miller TD. The safety of cardiopulmonary exercise testing in a population with high-risk cardiovascular diseases. Circulation. 2012;126(21):2465–72.
27. Kaltenbach M, Scherer D, Dowinsky S. Complications of exercise testing. A survey in three German-speaking countries. Eur Heart J. 1982;3(3):199–202.
28. Sharma S, Elliott P, Whyte G, Jones S, Mahon N, Whipp B, et al. Utility of cardiopulmonary exercise in the assessment of clinical determinants of functional capacity in hypertrophic cardiomyopathy. Am J Cardiol. 2000;86(2):162–8.
29. Perrin MJ, Angaran P, Laksman Z, Zhang H, Porepa LF, Rutberg J, et al. Exercise testing in asymptomatic gene carriers exposes a latent electrical substrate of arrhythmogenic right ventricular cardiomyopathy. J Am Coll Cardiol. 2013;62(19):1772–9.
30. Schwartz PJ, Crotti L. QTc behavior during exercise and genetic testing for the long-QT syndrome. Circulation. 2011;124(20):2181–4.
31. Makimoto H, Nakagawa E, Takaki H, Yamada Y, Okamura H, Noda T, et al. Augmented ST-segment elevation during recovery from exercise predicts cardiac events in patients with Brugada syndrome. J Am Coll Cardiol. 2010;56(19):1576–84.
32. Jouven X, Zureik M, Desnos M, Courbon D, Ducimetiere P. Long-term outcome in asymptomatic men with exercise-induced premature ventricular depolarizations. N Engl J Med. 2000;343(12):826–33.
33. Diamond GA, Forrester JS. Analysis of probability as an aid in the clinical diagnosis of coronary-artery disease. N Engl J Med. 1979;300(24):1350–8.
34. Pryor DB, Harrell FE Jr, Lee KL, Califf RM, Rosati RA. Estimating the likelihood of significant coronary artery disease. Am J Med. 1983;75(5):771–80.
35. Pigozzi F, Spataro A, Alabiso A, Parisi A, Rizzo M, Fagnani F, et al. Role of exercise stress test in master athletes. Br J Sports Med. 2005;39(8):527–31.
36. La Gerche A, Baggish AL, Knuuti J, Prior DL, Sharma S, Heidbuchel H, et al. Cardiac imaging and stress testing asymptomatic athletes to identify those at risk of sudden cardiac death. JACC Cardiovasc Imaging. 2013;6(9):993–1007.

# Medical Evaluation of Athletes: Genetic Testing

# 11

Belinda Gray and Michael Papadakis

**Learning Objectives**

1. Recognise the importance for pre- and post-test genetic counselling when offering athletes genetic testing.
2. Recognise the spectrum of genetic testing results and the challenges of determining pathogenicity and variant interpretation.
3. Appraise the indications for genetic testing in the evaluation of athletes with suspected cardiomyopathy or ion channelopathy.
4. Assess the implications of genetic testing in elite athletes, in terms of participation in competitive sports.
5. Explain the value of predictive testing in athletic individuals and their families.

## 11.1 Introduction

When evaluating athletes for conditions predisposing to sudden cardiac death (SCD), consideration must be given to the genetic basis of most of these conditions [1, 2]. This includes the cardiomyopathies such as hypertrophic cardiomyopathy [HCM], arrhythmogenic cardiomyopathy [ACM/ARVC], dilated cardiomyopathy [DCM] and left ventricular non-compaction [LVNC], and the channelopathies such as congenital long QT syndrome [LQTS], catecholaminergic polymorphic ventricular tachycardia [CPVT], Brugada syndrome [BrS], progressive cardiac conduction disease [PCCD] and short QT syndrome [SQTS] [1]. Genetic studies over the last 20–30 years have been integral in identifying the gene abnormalities that underpin these conditions, and technological advances have made genetic testing a readily available clinical tool.

B. Gray · M. Papadakis (✉)
Cardiology Clinical Academic Group, St George's, University of London, London, UK
e-mail: bgray@sgul.ac.uk; mipapada@sgul.ac.uk



A. Pressler, J. Niebauer (eds.), *Textbook of Sports and Exercise Cardiology*,
https://doi.org/10.1007/978-3-030-35374-2_11

- Genetic testing in an athlete can have diagnostic, therapeutic and prognostic value provided that the information is correctly assessed by a cardio-genetics expert [1].
- Genetic testing results are not binary but there is a probabilistic spectrum of pathogenicity using scoring criteria developed by the American College of Medical Genetics and Genomics (ACMG) [3, 4].
- The yield of genetic testing varies depending upon the condition assessed, from approximately 20% in dilated cardiomyopathy to 70% in long QT syndrome.

This chapter offers an overview of genetic testing and the technological advances that have made it readily available. The authors address the appropriate use of genetic testing in the assessment of athletes, using common clinical scenarios. For each scenario we outline the diagnostic, prognostic and therapeutic implications of genetic testing, including its impact on exercise recommendations.

## 11.2 Rationale for Genetic Testing in Athletes

- There are more than 40 cardiac diseases for which a genetic basis has been identified [5].
- Registries have consistently demonstrated that inherited cardiomyopathies and channelopathies account for the majority of SCDs in young (<35 years) athletes [6–9].
- To minimise such tragedies, preventive efforts have intensified and include targeted evaluation of high-risk individuals, such as athletes with symptoms or relevant family history, as well as wider cardiac screening of low risk individuals. Consequently, a large part of Sports Cardiology practice involves evaluation of athletes with symptoms or signs suggestive of an inherited cardiac condition (ICC).
- Genetic testing has primarily been used for familial cascade screening in athletes with clearly defined clinical phenotype of an inherited cardiac condition. Most ICCs are transmitted in an autosomal dominant pattern, meaning that first-degree family members have a 50% chance of carrying the causative genetic variant. Therefore, identification of the causative variant allows for predictive (cascade) testing in first-degree family members. Family members who are genotype-positive require surveillance, while those who are genotype-negative can be released from ongoing clinical evaluation [3, 5].
- Genetic testing may also be used for diagnostic, prognostic and therapeutic purposes, depending on the condition in question (Table 11.1, Fig. 11.1).
- The effects of exercise on the electrical and structural cardiac remodeling often pose significant challenges, and differentiation between "athlete's heart" and inherited cardiac diseases requires the use of several diagnostic tools.
- The yield varies from fairly limited, such as in dilated cardiomyopathy, approximately 20% compared with LQTS, approximately 70–80%. In addition, the identification of different genetic subtypes (LQT 1–3 particularly) can inform the risk of arrhythmic events, potential triggers to be avoided and targeted medical therapies [10].

**Table 11.1** Current utility of genetic testing in athletic individuals for the most commonly encountered cardiomyopathies and channelopathies (modified from [1])

| Disease under investigation in the athlete | Diagnostic utility | Prognostic utility | Therapeutic Implications (medical/device) | Impact on exercise recommendations |
|---|---|---|---|---|
| LQTS | +++ | +++ | +++ | +++ |
| CPVT | +++ | + | + | + |
| BrS | + | + | – | – |
| HCM | ++ | + | – | – |
| ACM | ++ | ++ | + | +++ |
| DCM | + | ++ | – | + |

– no utility, + limited utility, ++ utility in some athletes, +++ clear utility in most athletes
Impact on exercise recommendations derived from [12] and [59]

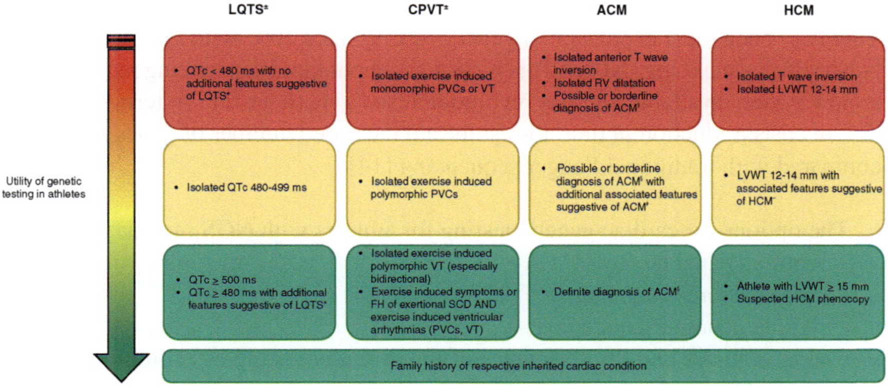


**Fig. 11.1** Utility of genetic testing in athletes suspected of an underlying inherited cardiac condition. The traffic light system is based on the pre-test probability of a positive yield and its use in terms of diagnosis, prognosis, treatment and exercise recommendation. Red: Not recommended, Orange: May be considered and Green: Should be considered. *LQTS* long QT syndrome, *CPVT* catecholaminergic polymorphic ventricular tachycardia, *ACM* arrhythmogenic cardiomyopathy, *HCM* hypertrophic cardiomyopathy, *QTc* corrected QT interval, *PVC* premature ventricular contractions, *VT* ventricular tachycardia, *LVWT* left ventricular wall thickness

±Structural heart disease, coronary artery disease and electrolyte abnormalities should be excluded

*Symptoms, documented polymorphic arrhythmias, paradoxical prolongation of the QT interval during exercise, T-wave alternans, T wave notching, congenital deafness, family history of unexplained SCD [41]

§According to the 2010 task force criteria, excluding genetic testing result [26]

#High propensity to ventricular arrhythmias, symptoms, family history of SCD in a first-degree relative under the age of 40 years, presence of scar on MRI (this list is not exhaustive)

~Symptoms, family history of SCD in a first-degree relative under the age of 40 years, ECG abnormalities, asymmetric hypertrophy, myocardial scar on cardiac MRI, blunted blood pressure response to exercise (this list is not exhaustive)

Genetic testing has been incorporated in contemporary exercise recommendations for elite and recreational athletes. The fact remains, however, that risk stratification and exercise prescription is predominantly dictated by the clinical phenotype. Although genetic testing has significant potential for individualized risk stratification, currently its role is limited to specific conditions.

- In ACM studies have shown that individuals carrying a pathogenic genetic variant have a greater chance of progression to overt disease, heart failure and life-threatening arrhythmias with high level athletic activity, even in the absence of any phenotypic evidence of disease, and therefore should be restricted from competitive sport [11, 12].
- It is important that prior to proceeding with genetic testing, the athlete has undergone appropriate genetic counselling relating to the potential implications, challenges and limitations of the testing [13]. Following the test, any variants identified should be conveyed to the athlete with appropriate post-test genetic counselling and support [5].

## 11.3 Approaches for Genetic Testing in Athletes

There has been rapid expansion of genetic testing since 2005 with the advent of next generation sequencing (NGS). This high-throughput rapid sequencing methodology is now widely available and has revolutionalised genetic testing in terms of reduction in costs, reduction in time-to-results and increased number of genes sequenced compared with traditional Sanger sequencing [14].

- The options for cardiac genetic testing for athletes with NGS include:
  - cardiac panel testing
  - whole exome sequencing
  - whole genome sequencing.
- The advantages and disadvantages of the different testing modalities are shown in Table 11.2.

**Table 11.2** Advantages and disadvantages of different genetic testing modalities (adapted from [14])

| Sequencing method | Advantages | Disadvantages |
|---|---|---|
| Sanger sequencing | Individual reads more accurate<br>Can sequence longer reads | Costly<br>Time-consuming<br>May miss large insertions or deletions |
| NGS cardiac panel testing | Quick<br>Multiple genes sequenced concurrently | Limited new gene discovery<br>Larger panels = more VUS |
| Whole exome sequencing | Quick<br>Less DNA required<br>High throughput<br>Acceptable cost | Only sequences exons (i.e. miss noncoding alleles)<br>May have inadequate coverage |
| Whole genome sequencing | Full genome sequenced<br>More even coverage than whole exome sequencing<br>Improved ability to assess large rearrangements | More costly<br>Requires more DNA than whole exome sequencing<br>Huge bioinformatic data set<br>High number VUS |

- Increased population databases such as the exome aggregation consortium (ExAC) and genome aggregation database (gnomAD, http://gnomad.broadinstitute.org) have highlighted an improved understanding of what is the true normal variation in the genome (so called "background noise").
- This is particularly true with cardiac channelopathy genes such as *SCN5A* which has been shown to have a background noise rate of 2% in caucasians and 4–5% in non-caucasians [15].
- This has also led to a significant increase in the number of variants classified as variants of uncertain significance (VUS), including variants previously considered as pathogenic, where the clinical utility is limited [14, 16, 17].
- The classification as a VUS means the variant cannot be used for predictive testing in family members, nor can it be ignored as unlikely to be implicated in disease (benign or likely benign). These variants remain in the "genetic purgatory" [17].

## 11.4 Determining Pathogenicity of Genetic Variants

- Genetic testing results are not binary but represent a spectrum of pathogenicity (Fig. 11.2).
- The basis for establishing pathogenicity is dependent upon a composite of criteria including rarity in the general population, whether the variant has been seen before in the disease phenotype under investigation, predicted effect on protein function and in silico computational prediction tools.
- These criteria have been published by the American College of Medical Genetics and Genomics (ACMG) [4].

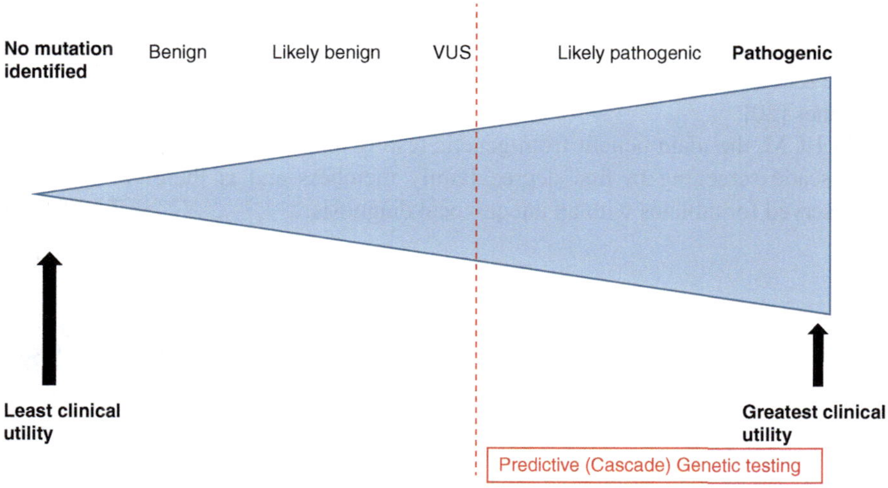


**Fig. 11.2** Spectrum of pathogenicity (modified from [14] and [60]). Only variants classified as likely pathogenic or pathogenic should be considered causative of the respective phenotype and used for predictive (cascade) genetic testing. *VUS* variant of uncertain significance

- Online databases such as ClinVar (www.ncbi.nlm.nih.gov/clinvar/) and ClinGen (https://clinicalgenome.org/) can be reviewed to identify previously reported unequivocally pathogenic variants in athletes with suspected inherited cardiac conditions.
- Online tools have been developed to help assess pathogenicity in genetic variants [18].
- Similar to all advanced cardiac investigations, in the absence of specific knowledge and experience, the sports cardiologist should liaise with a clinical geneticist when considering genetic testing to assist with appropriate use of the test and accurate interpretation.

## 11.5 Indications for Genetic Testing in Athletes

### 11.5.1 Cardiomyopathies

#### 11.5.1.1 Hypertrophic Cardiomyopathy

- Hypertrophic cardiomyopathy (HCM) has a prevalence of approximately 1 in 500 individuals and is characterised by left ventricular hypertrophy in the absence of loading conditions such as aortic stenosis or hypertension.
- HCM is inherited in an autosomal dominant manner and is associated with pathogenic variants in at least 11 genes, typically of cardiac sarcomeric proteins.
- The commonest genes causing HCM are myosin-binding protein C (*MYBPC3*) and beta-myosin heavy chain (*MYH7*).
- The full list of genes definitely involved in HCM is shown in Table 11.3.
- It has become apparent that increased gene panels beyond the core genes involved do not improve test yield or sensitivity but rather lead to increased numbers of variants of uncertain significance [19]. Therefore, large sequencing laboratories are recommending limiting genetic testing panels in HCM to a maximum of 11 genes [20].
- In HCM, the main benefit from genetic testing relates to an actionable result in cascade screening in first degree family members and is therefore typically reserved for athletes with an unequivocal diagnosis.

**Table 11.3** Common genes associated with cardiomyopathies and diagnostic yield

| Disease | Commonly associated genes | Overall yield (%) |
|---|---|---|
| HCM | *MYBPC3, MYH7, TTNT, TTNI, TPM1, MYL3, MYL2, ACTC, DES, PLN* | 40–60 |
| ACM | *PKP2, DSG2, DSP, DSC2, JUP, TMEM43, LMNA, DES, CTNNA3, CDH2, PLN* | 50–60 |
| DCM | *TTN, SCN5A, LMNA, FLNC, DSP, DES* | 20 |
| LVNC | *MYH7, MYBPC3, TNNT2, TPM1* | 9–15 (in association with cardiomyopathy)<br>~0% (in isolation) |

- Athletic individuals may develop LVH as part of physiological adaptation to exercise, but a wall thickness of ≥15 mm is likely to reflect a diagnosis of HCM and in these individuals genetic testing should be considered, especially in white athletes [12, 21].
- Genetic testing may also be considered in athletes with mild LVH (LVWT 12–14 mm), with additional features suggestive of HCM such as family history of HCM, ECG repolarisation anomalies, asymmetric patterns of LVH, relative apical hypertrophy and cavity obliteration out of keeping with athletic training, myocardial scar on cardiac MRI, the presence of non-sustained or sustained ventricular tachycardia, or a blunted blood pressure response to exercise (Fig. 11.1).
- The expected yield of genetic testing in individuals with a diagnosis of HCM is approximately 40–60% [22], however this may improve to as much as 70% in the context of a clear family history [23].
- Genetic testing may also help to identify HCM phenocopies; therefore comprehensive clinical evaluation is necessary to assess for features suggestive of Danon disease (*LAMP2*), Noonan Syndrome (*KRAS*, *SOS1*, *PTPN11*, *RAF1*) and Fabry's disease (*GLA*) [22].
- Genetic testing for *PRKAG2* should be considered in individuals with co-existent pre-excitation on the ECG [24].

#### 11.5.1.2 Arrhythmogenic Cardiomyopathy

- Arrhythmogenic cardiomyopathy has a prevalence of approximately 1:2000.
- ACM is characterised by fibro-fatty infiltration of the ventricular myocardium.
- ACM is inherited in an autosomal dominant pattern and genetic testing has a yield of approximately 50%, typically due to mutations in desmosomal protein genes, with the most commonly involved genes including *PKP2*, *DSC2*, *DSG*, *DSP*, and *JUP* (Table 11.3) [25].
- ACM is diagnosed through a composite scoring system which constitute the Task Force Criteria [26].
- Aside from familial cascade screening in individuals with a definite diagnosis of ACM, genetic testing may also be used for diagnostic and prognostic purposes. Identification of a pathogenic variant constitutes a major task force criterion, which may upgrade a case from a possible or borderline to a definite diagnosis [26].
- It should be emphasized that due to physiological adaptation a considerable proportion of elite athletes demonstrate anterior T wave inversion [27–29] or right ventricular dilatation in the spectrum of the echocardiographic and MRI criteria of the task force [30, 31] and their presence, in isolation, should not instigate genetic testing for ACM (Fig. 11.1).
- Genetic testing may, however, be considered in athletic individuals with high index of suspicion for ACM, such as athletes with anterior T wave inversion or right ventricular dilatation, who demonstrate high propensity to ventricular arrhythmias, or other red flags such as syncope, presence of scar on MRI or a family history of SCD (Fig. 11.1).
- Particular ACM genotypes such as *DSP* and *TMEM43* have a propensity for high arrhythmic burden which can pre-date the cardiomyopathy phenotype [25].

- ACM is an important cause of SCD in athletes due to ventricular arrhythmias provoked by exercise [32]. Sudden cardiac death due to ACM is up to 16 times more common in athletic individuals compared with non-athletes, often with no prior symptoms [6].
- Individuals with ACM who engage in competitive sport have a higher prevalence of ventricular arrhythmias and develop symptoms earlier, compared with those who are relatively sedentary [33].
- Participation in endurance exercise by gene carriers with no overt ACM phenotype (genotype-positive phenotype-negative individuals) is associated with higher penetrance of disease, worsening ventricular arrhythmias, more rapid progression to heart failure and earlier presentation of overt phenotype [11]. Therefore genetic testing is integral in first degree family members of a genotype positive ACM case to identify those individuals within the family who are genotype positive, in whom it is recommended to avoid competitive sports [12].

#### 11.5.1.3 Dilated Cardiomyopathy

- Dilated cardiomyopathy (DCM) is characterised by ventricular systolic dysfunction in association with chamber dilatation.
- The majority of cases of DCM are due to acquired causes such as ischaemia, toxins (e.g. viruses, alcohol), post-partum or metabolic disturbances. Approximately 20–30% of DCM is due to genetic mutations in sarcomere, cytoskeletal and nuclear envelope proteins [34]. The yield of genetic testing in DCM may increase up to 40% in the context of family history of the disease [35].
- Dilated cardiomyopathy is typically inherited in autosomal dominant pattern and there are over 50 genes implicated, with the commonest genes including *TTN*, *SCN5A*, *LMNA* and *DES* (Table 11.3) [36].
- In the context of the low yield, genetic testing in athletes presenting with a clear phenotype of DCM is recommended only in the context of a clear family history (clinical testing) or if there is a known familial variant (predictive testing).
- Genetic testing is also indicated in the context of other specific features such as a malignant family history, high burden of ventricular arrhythmias and coexisting conduction system disease. The presence of high burden of ventricular arrhythmias or family history of sudden death are more likely to be associated with mutations in *LMNA*, *DSP*, *RBM20*, *SCN5A* or *FLNC* [35].
- ECG evidence of conduction tissue disease provides a higher yield of *SCN5A* and *LMNA* pathogenic variants [1].
- Although unlikely in high-level athletes, DCM is also associated with skeletal myopathies such as Duchenne Muscular Dystrophy, myotonic dystrophy and Desmin-associated myopathies and therefore should be considered if there is coexisting skeletal muscle phenotype [1].

#### 11.5.1.4 Left Ventricular Non-compaction

- Left-ventricular non-compaction (LVNC) is characterised by increased trabeculations in the LV myocardium with associated deep recesses. LVNC is presumed to be due to failure of the developing heart to fully form and compact the myocardium during the later stage of cardiac development [1].

- Increased trabeculation can be seen in a significant proportion of athletes due to the physiological adaptation which is believed to be due to the increased pre-load [37].
- However, in some individuals, particularly in association with other features of cardiomyopathy such as depressed LV function or an abnormal ECG, the disease can be due to underlying genetic abnormalities [1].
- The yield of genetic testing in LVNC is 9–15%, however it is important to note that actionable gene results are almost 0% in individuals who fulfil diagnostic criteria for LVNC with no additional evidence of cardiomyopathy [38].
- Given the low yield and the significant phenotypic cross-over, genetic testing in athletes with an isolated LVNC phenotype is typically reserved for those with familial disease [1, 5].

### 11.5.2 Athletes with Isolated T Wave Inversion

- The presence of T-wave inversion on the ECG of an athletic individual can indicate underlying cardiomyopathy, particularly in white athletes.
- In these individuals comprehensive clinical evaluation provides a greater diagnostic utility than genetic testing (21% compared with 10%).
- The use of routine genetic testing in asymptomatic athletes with T-wave inversion is not recommended in the absence of a family history or other features suggestive of an inherited cardiac condition [39].

### 11.5.3 Inherited Arrhythmia Syndromes (Channelopathies)

#### 11.5.3.1 Long QT Syndrome

- Long QT syndrome (LQTS) is an inherited arrhythmia syndrome with a prevalence of approximately 1:2000 [40].
- LQTS is characterised by the presence of a prolonged QT interval (corrected for heart rate) in the absence of secondary causes for a prolonged QTc such as drugs or electrolyte disturbances [2].
- LQTS can also be diagnosed in the presence of an LQTS risk score (modified Schwartz score) $\geq$3.5 or in the presence of a pathogenic variant in a LQTS gene [2, 41].
- In LQTS genetic testing is an integral part of the diagnostic pathway.
- There are at least 15 genes described in the pathogenesis in LQTS (Table 11.4), however the top three genes account for >90% of genetically confirmed LQTS [2].
- The majority of LQTS is inherited in an autosomal dominant pattern, however a rare recessive form with associated sensorineural deafness (Jervell and Lange-Nielsen Syndrome) due to homozygous or compound heterozygous mutations also exists. This recessive form is highly lethal with early, severe onset and is unlikely to present in the adult athletic population.

**Table 11.4** Genes of autosomal dominant LQTS (modified from [14])

| LQTS type | Gene | Frequency |
|---|---|---|
| LQT1 | *KCNQ1* | 40–45% |
| LQT2 | *KCNH2* | 30–35% |
| LQT3 | *SCN5A* | 10% |
| LQT4 | *ANK2* | 1% |
| LQT5 | *KCNE1* | 1% |
| LQT6 | *KCNE2* | Rare |
| LQT7 | *KCNJ2* | Rare |
| LQT8 | *CACNA1C* | Rare |
| LQT9 | *CAV3* | Rare |
| LQT10 | *SCN4B* | Rare |
| LQT11 | *AKAP9* | Rare |
| LQT12 | *SNTA1* | Rare |
| LQT13 | *KCNJ5* | Rare |
| LQT14 | *CALM1* | Rare |
| LQT15 | *CALM2* | Rare |
| LQT16 | *CALM3* | Rare |
| LQT17 | *TRDN* | Rare |

- In an individual with a repeatedly prolonged QTc ≥ 480 ms and acquired causes for QT prolongation excluded, genetic testing should be considered, as this value represents the 99th percentile for the general population.
- Athletes tend to exhibit longer QT intervals compared to the general population and an isolated long QT interval in an athlete may represent the effect of increased vagal tone or delayed repolarization as a result of increased left ventricular mass [42]. In a study of 2000 elite athletes, athletes with a QTc in excess of 500 ms were more likely to exhibit additional features, including a pathogenic variant, suggestive of LQTS [43].
- Genetic testing in LQTS also provides therapeutic and prognostic utility.
  - There are known genotype associated triggers for arrhythmia including strenuous exercise and in particularly swimming and diving (LQT1), loud noise/alarm clocks (LQT2) and sleep (LQT3) [44].
  - These can guide lifestyle recommendations including exercise recommendations for genotype positive individuals.
  - Genotype directed therapies such as betablockers (particularly nadolol) in LQT1 or mexilitene in LQT3 can significantly reduce the life-threatening arrhythmic risk to the individual athlete [10, 45].
- Genetic testing assists in prognosis in LQTS as the individual's arrhythmic risk can be determined through a composite of the QTc value and the genotype. Individuals with a QTc < 460 ms and LQT1 genotype have an estimated 5-year risk of life-threatening arrhythmias <1%, even without betablocker therapy. On the contrary, individuals with QTc > 550 ms and a LQT2 or LQT3 genotype have an estimated 5-year risk of life-threatening arrhythmias in excess of 9% without therapy [10].

#### 11.5.3.2 Catecholaminergic Polymorphic Ventricular Tachycardia

- Catecholaminergic polymorphic ventricular tachycardia (CPVT) is an inherited arrhythmia syndrome characterised by adrenergically stimulated ventricular tachycardia, typically through physical exertion, in individuals with a structurally normal heart [2].
- CPVT is rare, with an estimated prevalence of 1:10,000.
- The pathophysiology of CPVT is due to abnormal intracellular calcium handling in ventricular myocytes, due to genetic mutations in calcium handling proteins [46].
- Individuals with CPVT have normal baseline ECG and echocardiogram, with the key diagnostic feature being the presence of exercise-induced ventricular arrhythmias, particularly bidirectional VT (Fig. 11.1).
- CPVT can be diagnosed in individuals who are found to be carriers of a clearly pathogenic genetic variant, as well as in family members of an index case who develop premature ventricular beats (PVBs) during exercise [2].
- The most common form of CPVT is due to autosomal dominant mutations in *RYR2* accounting for up to 60% of cases. There is a rarer recessive form due to mutations in *CASQ2* accounting for <5% of cases as well as a number of other very rare gene associations (Table 11.5). Recently, a family with autosomal dominant CPVT linked to a heterozygous *CASQ2* mutations has also been described [47].
- Any athlete with exercise induced syncope and a structurally normal heart should be assessed for CPVT and genetic testing should be considered if there is evidence of exercise induced ventricular tachycardia, particularly bi-directional tachycardia (Fig. 11.1).

#### 11.5.3.3 Brugada Syndrome

- Brugada syndrome (BrS) is diagnosed in individuals with a demonstrated type 1 Brugada pattern ECG (≥2 mm ST elevation with type 1 morphology in ≥1 right praecordial leads V1/V2 in the second, third or fourth intercostal space) either spontaneously, or after infusion of sodium-channel provocation testing in the presence of another feature such as documented ventricular arrhythmia, suspicious arrhythmic syncope or a family history of BrS or sudden unexplained death [48].
- High body temperature is known to be a trigger for arrhythmia in BrS and therefore in athletes, BrS may present in situations of hyperthermia, such as in or following an endurance race.

**Table 11.5** Genes associated with CPVT (modified from [14])

| Name | Gene | Frequency | Transmission |
|---|---|---|---|
| CPVT1 | *RYR2* | 50–60% | AD |
| CPVT2 | *CASQ2* | ~5% | AR (AD) |
| CPVT3 | Maps to chromosome 7 p14-p22 | Rare | AR |
| CPVT4 | *CALM1* | Rare | AR |
| CPVT5 | *TRDN* | Rare | AR |
| Possible LQT4 overlap | *ANK2* | Rare | AD |
| Possible LQT7 overlap | *KCNJ2* | Rare | AD |

*AD* autosomal dominant, *AR* autosomal recessive

- Our understanding of the genetic basis to BrS is evolving and therefore the utility of genetic testing is limited. Approximately 20% of BrS is due to autosomal dominant loss-of-function mutations in the gene encoding the cardiac sodium channel *SCN5A* [48]. This appears to be most evident in individuals with associated conduction disease.
- The remaining genetic basis underpinning BrS appears to be oligogenic based on data from genome wide association studies showing that multiple risk alleles confer an increased risk of disease [49].
- The prognostic utility of identification of a pathogenic *SCN5A* variant in an individual with BrS remains under debate. A single study has indicated *SCN5A* mutations may be associated with a worse prognosis in BrS, however this has not been seen in multiple prior similar studies [50].
- The indication for genetic testing in athletic individuals with BrS is limited to those who have demonstrated familial disease or with evidence of co-existing conduction disease.

#### 11.5.3.4 Progressive Cardiac Conduction Disease

- Progressive cardiac conduction system disease (PCCD) is diagnosed in young patients (<50 years) with ECG evidence of abnormal conduction in the absence of skeletal myopathies [2]. The majority of familial cases with a structurally normal heart are attributed to mutations in *SCN5A* and *TRPM4* [1].
- Athletes with premature advanced conduction disease, particularly those with evidence of familial disease, are recommended to proceed to genetic testing with the disease typically having an autosomal dominant inheritance [2].
- Cases due to *SCN5A* mutations can be associated with a BrS overlap syndrome [1, 51, 52].
- In individuals with abnormal LV function on echo, lamin A/C (*LMNA*) or desmin (*DES*) variants should be considered [1]. The presence of a *LMNA* mutation carries prognostic utility and may influence exercise prescription and recommendation for ICD implantation [2].

#### 11.5.3.5 Short QT Syndrome

- Short QT syndrome is a very rare inherited arrhythmia syndrome characterised by syncope or sudden cardiac death with a shortened QTc (QTc $\leq$ 330 ms, or $\leq$360 ms in the presence of symptoms or a family history).
- The disease is due to gain of function mutations in potassium channel proteins (*KCNH2*-SQT1, *KCNQ1*-SQT2, *KCNJ2*-SQT3) [2].
- Neither the genotype nor the duration of the QTc carries prognostic value in SQTS [53].
- There is limited evidence that quinidine may be more effective in prolonging the QTc in SQT1 and therefore genetic testing can help guide response to therapy [54]. Beyond this, the role of genetic testing is limited to benefiting first degree family members through predictive testing.
- Due to the very low prevalence of this disease, genetic testing in athletic individuals should be limited to those with high index of suspicion based on a combination of familial disease, symptoms and a QTc < 330 ms [1, 2].

## 11.6 Molecular Autopsy After Sudden Cardiac Death

- In some athletes, sudden cardiac death (SCD) is the first symptom or sign of an underlying inherited cardiac condition.
- In many cases the examining pathologist identifies structural abnormalities which establish the cause of death.
- Up to 40% of SCDs in athletes remain unexplained following specialised cardiac autopsy and toxicology screen [55, 56]. Such deaths are referred to as sudden arrhythmic death syndrome (SADS) or sudden unexplained death (SUD) and a significant proportion is thought to be due to inherited channelopathies.
- A diagnosis can be established through either clinical screening of first-degree family members or through post-mortem genetic testing ("molecular autopsy") in the deceased. Using a combined clinical and molecular autopsy approach can establish a diagnosis in approximately 40% of decedents [56].
- In cases of unexplained sudden cardiac death, the most recent guidelines for pathologists recommends retention of DNA-rich tissue for post mortem genetic analysis [57]. If an unequivocally pathogenic mutation is identified at molecular autopsy in the deceased, this result can be used for predictive testing in first-degree family members to identify those at risk [5].

## 11.7 Ethical and Medico-Legal Considerations and Genetic Counselling

- There are significant legal considerations for any athlete considering genetic testing.
  - The genetic result may have implications with regards to life insurance, whilst the particular club or sporting organization may have specific legal requirements.
- However, there are key diagnostic, prognostic and therapeutic benefits to genetic testing in some circumstances, including potentially initiating life-saving medication such as beta-blockers, which may also facilitate safe "return to play" [58].
- There are potential implications for first-degree family members of the athlete undergoing genetic testing which require consideration. Therefore, before any athlete proceeds with genetic testing pre- and post-test genetic counselling by an experienced cardiac genetic counsellor is essential [5, 13].

**Clinical Pearls**

- The clinical phenotype remains the cornerstone of the athlete's management.
- Appropriately considered genetic testing in athletes can help with diagnosis, prognosis, therapeutics and exercise recommendations.
- Genetic testing results fall on a probabilistic spectrum of pathogenicity. Variants of uncertain significance (VUS) have limited clinical utility, providing a challenge for the treating clinician.

- For LQTS and ACM genetic testing has a significant impact on exercise recommendations. For all other inherited cardiac conditions, recommendations are largely based on the clinical phenotype.
- Genetic testing is not recommended in athlete's who fall within the "grey zone" (isolated T wave inversion, cavity dilatation or LVH), in the absence of additional features suggestive of an inherited cardiac condition.

## Review

### Questions

1. An 18-year-old professional football player is identified to have a QTc of 490 ms on ECG screening. Which of the following statements is true regarding genetic testing?
   a. A variant of uncertain significance in *KCNQ1* (LQT1) is an indication to commence betablocker therapy
   b. Genetic testing in this athlete has no prognostic value as the QTc is <500 ms
   c. Genetic testing is not recommended as the diagnosis is not confirmed
   d. Genetic testing with a long QT panel may help to differentiate congenital long QT syndrome from athletic ECG adaptation
   e. The athlete should defer genetic testing to prevent disqualification from competitive football
2. A 45-year-old man presents following the unexplained sudden death of his younger brother on the football field, aged 35 years old. The deceased had undergone a negative postmortem and DNA was stored. Which of the following statements is true?
   a. Genetic testing for inherited arrhythmia syndromes can be considered in the deceased's DNA
   b. Genetic testing for inherited arrhythmia syndromes is indicated in the living 45-year-old brother
   c. Genetic testing should be performed in the brother and the deceased proband DNA concurrently
   d. Genetic testing should not be considered in the deceased's DNA as the postmortem is negative
   e. The DNA should be stored for research in the future, but no genetic testing should be performed at present
3. Which of the following statements regarding cascade family genetic testing is correct for an athlete with a diagnosis of HCM?
   a. All family members who undergo negative clinical screening based on ECG and echo should be referred for diagnostic genetic testing.
   b. First degree family members should be offered extensive genetic panel testing regardless of presence or absence of symptomatology
   c. First degree family members with cardiac symptoms or signs suggestive of HCM should be offered extensive genetic panel testing

d. If a likely pathogenic variant is found in the athlete, targeted (predictive) genetic testing of all first-degree family members is recommended
e. If a VUS is found in the athlete, genetic testing of all first-degree family members is recommended to determine its significance

## Answers

1. **D**: In an athlete with borderline QTc prolongation (480–500 ms), genetic testing for LQT 1–3 may assist in clarifying the diagnosis. In addition, by confirming the diagnosis in the athlete potentially lifesaving betablocker therapy can be initiated.

   A is not correct as variants of uncertain significance should not lead to an alteration in athlete's management [1].

   B is not correct, data shows the greater the QTc interval the higher the potential risk to the individual [10].

   C is not correct, genetic testing is indicated in this situation as it can assist in confirming the diagnosis [1].

   E is not correct, genetic testing can help facilitate appropriate therapy and return to play [58, 59].
2. **A**: HRS/EHRA guidelines state that an arrhythmia syndrome focused post mortem genetic testing "molecular autopsy" can be considered (Class IIa) [1].

   B is not correct, if DNA is stored on the deceased (the proband) then genetic testing should be initiated in them in the first instance. The brother should undergo clinical screening, and if there is evidence in him of an inherited cardiac condition then directed genetic testing can be ordered.

   C is not correct, usually the testing is initiated in the proband in the first instance (as above).

   D is not correct, a number of inherited cardiac conditions may present with sudden death as the first symptom, particularly channelopathies which are associated with a structurally normal heart [56].

   E is not correct, if DNA is stored then genetic testing for molecular autopsy should be initiated especially as the inherited cardiac conditions are autosomal dominant and therefore first degree family members have a 50% chance of having the same condition [1, 56].
3. **D**: Class I indication in EHRA/HRS guidelines with regards to genetic screening of first-degree relatives following a pathogenic variant being identified in an individual with hypertrophic cardiomyopathy.

   A/B/C are not correct as genetic testing should not be performed in family members in the first instance without a genetic diagnosis in the index case, independent of symptomatology. Clinical testing should be performed in all first-degree family members. The proband (i.e. the first person diagnosed in the family) is tested first whenever possible, and predictive testing is only offered to family members for likely pathogenic or pathogenic variants. Therefore, only the athlete should be tested genetically for known HCM genes in the first instance. If an actionable gene result is identified in the athlete this can then be used for predictive testing in the first-degree family members, independent of their clinical phenotyping.

E is not correct. A variant of uncertain significance is not an actionable genetic variant [4].

## References


1. Ackerman MJ, Priori SG, Willems S, Berul C, Brugada R, Calkins H, et al. HRS/EHRA expert consensus statement on the state of genetic testing for the channelopathies and cardiomyopathies this document was developed as a partnership between the Heart Rhythm Society (HRS) and the European Heart Rhythm Association (EHRA). Heart Rhythm. 2011;8(8):1308–39.
2. Priori SG, Wilde AA, Horie M, Cho Y, Behr ER, Berul C, et al. HRS/EHRA/APHRS expert consensus statement on the diagnosis and management of patients with inherited primary arrhythmia syndromes: document endorsed by HRS, EHRA, and APHRS in May 2013 and by ACCF, AHA, PACES, and AEPC in June 2013. Heart Rhythm. 2013;10(12):1932–63.
3. Semsarian C, Ingles J. Determining pathogenicity in cardiac genetic testing: filling in the blank spaces. Trends Cardiovasc Med. 2015;25(7):653–4.
4. Richards S, Aziz N, Bale S, Bick D, Das S, Gastier-Foster J, et al. Standards and guidelines for the interpretation of sequence variants: a joint consensus recommendation of the American College of Medical Genetics and Genomics and the Association for Molecular Pathology. Genet Med. 2015;17(5):405–24.
5. Ingles J, Semsarian C. The value of cardiac genetic testing. Trends Cardiovasc Med. 2014;24(6):217–24.
6. Miles C, Finocchiaro G, Papadakis M, Gray B, Westaby J, Ensam B, et al. Sudden death and left ventricular involvement in arrhythmogenic cardiomyopathy. Circulation. 2019;139:1786.
7. Maron BJ, Haas TS, Ahluwalia A, Murphy CJ, Garberich RF. Demographics and epidemiology of sudden deaths in young competitive athletes: from the United States National Registry. Am J Med. 2016;129(11):1170–7.
8. Harmon KG, Asif IM, Maleszewski JJ, Owens DS, Prutkin JM, Salerno JC, et al. Incidence and etiology of sudden cardiac arrest and death in high school athletes in the United States. Mayo Clin Proc. 2016;91(11):1493–502.
9. Finocchiaro G, Papadakis M, Robertus JL, Dhutia H, Steriotis AK, Tome M, et al. Etiology of sudden death in sports: insights from a united kingdom regional registry. J Am Coll Cardiol. 2016;67(18):2108–15.
10. Mazzanti A, Maragna R, Vacanti G, Monteforte N, Bloise R, Marino M, et al. Interplay between genetic substrate, QTc duration, and arrhythmia risk in patients with long QT syndrome. J Am Coll Cardiol. 2018;71(15):1663–71.
11. James CA, Bhonsale A, Tichnell C, Murray B, Russell SD, Tandri H, et al. Exercise increases age-related penetrance and arrhythmic risk in arrhythmogenic right ventricular dysplasia/cardiomyopathy-associated desmosomal mutation carriers. J Am Coll Cardiol. 2013;62(14):1290–7.
12. Pelliccia A, Solberg EE, Papadakis M, Adami PE, Biffi A, Caselli S, et al. Recommendations for participation in competitive and leisure time sport in athletes with cardiomyopathies, myocarditis, and pericarditis: position statement of the Sport Cardiology Section of the European Association of Preventive Cardiology (EAPC). Eur Heart J. 2019;40(1):19–33.
13. Ingles J, Yeates L, Semsarian C. The emerging role of the cardiac genetic counselor. Heart Rhythm. 2011;8(12):1958–62.
14. Gray B, Behr ER. New insights into the genetic basis of inherited arrhythmia syndromes. Circ Cardiovasc Genet. 2016;9(6):569–77.

15. Kapplinger JD, Giudicessi JR, Ye D, Tester DJ, Callis TE, Valdivia CR, et al. Enhanced classification of Brugada Syndrome-associated and long-QT syndrome-associated genetic variants in the SCN5A-encoded Na(v)1.5 cardiac sodium channel. Circ Cardiovasc Genet. 2015;8(4):582–95.
16. Rehm HL. Disease-targeted sequencing: a cornerstone in the clinic. Nat Rev Genet. 2013;14(4):295–300.
17. Ackerman MJ. Genetic purgatory and the cardiac channelopathies: exposing the variants of uncertain/unknown significance issue. Heart Rhythm. 2015;12(11):2325–31.
18. Patel RY, Shah N, Jackson AR, Ghosh R, Pawliczek P, Paithankar S, et al. ClinGen pathogenicity calculator: a configurable system for assessing pathogenicity of genetic variants. Genome Med. 2017;9(1):3.
19. Burns C, Bagnall RD, Lam L, Semsarian C, Ingles J. Multiple gene variants in hypertrophic cardiomyopathy in the era of next-generation sequencing. Circ Cardiovasc Genet. 2017;10(4):e001666.
20. Alfares AA, Kelly MA, McDermott G, Funke BH, Lebo MS, Baxter SB, et al. Results of clinical genetic testing of 2,912 probands with hypertrophic cardiomyopathy: expanded panels offer limited additional sensitivity. Genet Med. 2015;17(11):880–8.
21. Authors/Task Force m, Elliott PM, Anastasakis A, Borger MA, Borggrefe M, Cecchi F, et al. 2014 ESC Guidelines on diagnosis and management of hypertrophic cardiomyopathy: the Task Force for the Diagnosis and Management of Hypertrophic Cardiomyopathy of the European Society of Cardiology (ESC). Eur Heart J. 2014;35(39):2733–79.
22. Akhtar M, Elliott P. The genetics of hypertrophic cardiomyopathy. Glob Cardiol Sci Pract. 2018;2018(3):36.
23. Ingles J, Sarina T, Yeates L, Hunt L, Macciocca I, McCormack L, et al. Clinical predictors of genetic testing outcomes in hypertrophic cardiomyopathy. Genet Med. 2013;15(12):972–7.
24. Gollob MH, Green MS, Tang AS, Roberts R. PRKAG2 cardiac syndrome: familial ventricular preexcitation, conduction system disease, and cardiac hypertrophy. Curr Opin Cardiol. 2002;17(3):229–34.
25. Gandjbakhch E, Redheuil A, Pousset F, Charron P, Frank R. Clinical diagnosis, imaging, and genetics of arrhythmogenic right ventricular cardiomyopathy/dysplasia: JACC state-of-the-art review. J Am Coll Cardiol. 2018;72(7):784–804.
26. Marcus FI, McKenna WJ, Sherrill D, Basso C, Bauce B, Bluemke DA, et al. Diagnosis of arrhythmogenic right ventricular cardiomyopathy/dysplasia: proposed modification of the task force criteria. Circulation. 2010;121(13):1533–41.
27. Papadakis M, Carre F, Kervio G, Rawlins J, Panoulas VF, Chandra N, et al. The prevalence, distribution, and clinical outcomes of electrocardiographic repolarization patterns in male athletes of African/Afro-Caribbean origin. Eur Heart J. 2011;32(18):2304–13.
28. Brosnan MJ, Claessen G, Heidbuchel H, Prior DL, La Gerche A. Right precordial T-wave inversion in healthy endurance athletes can be explained by lateral displacement of the cardiac apex. JACC Clin Electrophysiol. 2015;1(1-2):84–91.
29. Malhotra A, Dhutia H, Gati S, Yeo TJ, Dores H, Bastiaenen R, et al. Anterior T-wave inversion in young white athletes and nonathletes: prevalence and significance. J Am Coll Cardiol. 2017;69(1):1–9.
30. Zaidi A, Ghani S, Sharma R, Oxborough D, Panoulas VF, Sheikh N, et al. Physiological right ventricular adaptation in elite athletes of African and Afro-Caribbean origin. Circulation. 2013;127(17):1783–92.
31. D'Ascenzi F, Anselmi F, Piu P, Fiorentini C, Carbone SF, Volterrani L, et al. Cardiac magnetic resonance normal reference values of biventricular size and function in male athlete's heart. JACC Cardiovasc Imaging. 2019;12:1755.
32. Corrado D, Link MS, Calkins H. Arrhythmogenic right ventricular cardiomyopathy. N Engl J Med. 2017;376(1):61–72.
33. Ruwald AC, Marcus F, Estes NA III, Link M, McNitt S, Polonsky B, et al. Association of competitive and recreational sport participation with cardiac events in patients with arrhythmogenic

right ventricular cardiomyopathy: results from the North American multidisciplinary study of arrhythmogenic right ventricular cardiomyopathy. Eur Heart J. 2015;36(27):1735–43.
34. Weintraub RG, Semsarian C, Macdonald P. Dilated cardiomyopathy. Lancet. 2017;390(10092):400–14.
35. Peters S, Kumar S, Elliott P, Kalman JM, Fatkin D. Arrhythmic genotypes in familial dilated cardiomyopathy: implications for genetic testing and clinical management. Heart Lung Circ. 2019;28(1):31–8.
36. Haas J, Frese KS, Peil B, Kloos W, Keller A, Nietsch R, et al. Atlas of the clinical genetics of human dilated cardiomyopathy. Eur Heart J. 2015;36(18):1123–35a.
37. Gati S, Papadakis M, Papamichael ND, Zaidi A, Sheikh N, Reed M, et al. Reversible de novo left ventricular trabeculations in pregnant women: implications for the diagnosis of left ventricular noncompaction in low-risk populations. Circulation. 2014;130(6):475–83.
38. Miller EM, Hinton RB, Czosek R, Lorts A, Parrott A, Shikany AR, et al. Genetic testing in pediatric left ventricular noncompaction. Circ Cardiovasc Genet. 2017;10(6):e001735.
39. Sheikh N, Papadakis M, Wilson M, Malhotra A, Adamuz C, Homfray T, et al. Diagnostic yield of genetic testing in young athletes with T-wave inversion. Circulation. 2018;138(12):1184–94.
40. Schwartz PJ, Stramba-Badiale M, Crotti L, Pedrazzini M, Besana A, Bosi G, et al. Prevalence of the congenital long-QT syndrome. Circulation. 2009;120(18):1761–7.
41. Schwartz PJ, Crotti L. QTc behavior during exercise and genetic testing for the long-QT syndrome. Circulation. 2011;124(20):2181–4.
42. Tanriverdi H, Kaftan HA, Evrengul H, Dursunoglu D, Turgut G, Kilic M. QT dispersion and left ventricular hypertrophy in athletes: relationship with angiotensin-converting enzyme I/D polymorphism. Acta Cardiol. 2005;60(4):387–93.
43. Basavarajaiah S, Wilson M, Whyte G, Shah A, Behr E, Sharma S. Prevalence and significance of an isolated long QT interval in elite athletes. Eur Heart J. 2007;28(23):2944–9.
44. Schwartz PJ, Ackerman MJ, George AL Jr, Wilde AAM. Impact of genetics on the clinical management of channelopathies. J Am Coll Cardiol. 2013;62(3):169–80.
45. Mazzanti A, Maragna R, Faragli A, Monteforte N, Bloise R, Memmi M, et al. Gene-specific therapy with mexiletine reduces arrhythmic events in patients with long QT syndrome type 3. J Am Coll Cardiol. 2016;67(9):1053–8.
46. Priori SG, Chen SR. Inherited dysfunction of sarcoplasmic reticulum Ca2+ handling and arrhythmogenesis. Circ Res. 2011;108(7):871–83.
47. Gray B, Bagnall RD, Lam L, Ingles J, Turner C, Haan E, et al. A novel heterozygous mutation in cardiac calsequestrin causes autosomal dominant catecholaminergic polymorphic ventricular tachycardia. Heart Rhythm. 2016;13(8):1652–60.
48. Antzelevitch C, Yan GX, Ackerman MJ, Borggrefe M, Corrado D, Guo J, et al. J-wave syndromes expert consensus conference report: emerging concepts and gaps in knowledge. Heart Rhythm. 2016;13(10):e295–324.
49. Bezzina CR, Barc J, Mizusawa Y, Remme CA, Gourraud JB, Simonet F, et al. Common variants at SCN5A-SCN10A and HEY2 are associated with Brugada syndrome, a rare disease with high risk of sudden cardiac death. Nat Genet. 2013;45(9):1044–9.
50. Yamagata K, Horie M, Aiba T, Ogawa S, Aizawa Y, Ohe T, et al. Genotype-phenotype correlation of SCN5A mutation for the clinical and electrocardiographic characteristics of probands with Brugada syndrome: a Japanese multicenter registry. Circulation. 2017;135(23):2255–70.
51. Bezzina C, Veldkamp MW, van Den Berg MP, Postma AV, Rook MB, Viersma JW, et al. A single Na(+) channel mutation causing both long-QT and Brugada syndromes. Circ Res. 1999;85(12):1206–13.
52. Makita N, Behr E, Shimizu W, Horie M, Sunami A, Crotti L, et al. The E1784K mutation in SCN5A is associated with mixed clinical phenotype of type 3 long QT syndrome. J Clin Invest. 2008;118(6):2219–29.
53. Mazzanti A, Kanthan A, Monteforte N, Memmi M, Bloise R, Novelli V, et al. Novel insight into the natural history of short QT syndrome. J Am Coll Cardiol. 2014;63(13):1300–8.
54. Giustetto C, Schimpf R, Mazzanti A, Scrocco C, Maury P, Anttonen O, et al. Long-term follow-up of patients with short QT syndrome. J Am Coll Cardiol. 2011;58(6):587–95.

55. Bagnall RD, Weintraub RG, Ingles J, Duflou J, Yeates L, Lam L, et al. A prospective study of sudden cardiac death among children and young adults. N Engl J Med. 2016;374(25):2441–52.
56. Lahrouchi N, Raju H, Lodder EM, Papatheodorou E, Ware JS, Papadakis M, et al. Utility of post-mortem genetic testing in cases of sudden arrhythmic death syndrome. J Am Coll Cardiol. 2017;69(17):2134–45.
57. Basso C, Aguilera B, Banner J, Cohle S, d'Amati G, de Gouveia RH, et al. Guidelines for autopsy investigation of sudden cardiac death: 2017 update from the Association for European Cardiovascular Pathology. Virchows Arch. 2017;471(6):691–705.
58. Turkowski KL, Bos JM, Ackerman NC, Rohatgi RK, Ackerman MJ. Return-to-play for athletes with genetic heart diseases. Circulation. 2018;137(10):1086–8.
59. Ackerman MJ, Zipes DP, Kovacs RJ, Maron BJ. Eligibility and disqualification recommendations for competitive athletes with cardiovascular abnormalities: task force 10: the cardiac channelopathies: a scientific statement from the American Heart Association and American College of Cardiology. J Am Coll Cardiol. 2015;66(21):2424–8.
60. Maron BJ, Maron MS, Semsarian C. Genetics of hypertrophic cardiomyopathy after 20 years: clinical perspectives. J Am Coll Cardiol. 2012;60(8):705–15.

# Specific Cardiovascular Diseases and Competitive Sports Participation: Arterial Hypertension

# 12

Stefano Caselli and Josef Niebauer

**Learning Objectives**

1. Recognize the definition of arterial hypertension and its classification.
2. Recognize risk factors of arterial hypertension and realize that blood pressure levels have to be within the normal range, regardless if one is an athlete or not—no exceptions.
3. Understand the safety even of competitive sports if blood pressure values are well controlled.
4. Understand the importance of target organ damage and associated clinical condition when making the decision regarding eligibility for competitive sports.
5. Appreciate that if indicated athletes have to be treated non-medically or medically just like any other patient, but that some drugs cannot be given because they are on the list of prohibited drugs, i.e. because of doping.
6. Recognize the beneficial effects of exercise training in everybody with arterial hypertension.

## 12.1 Introduction

Arterial hypertension is defined by the 2018 European Society of Cardiology Guidelines, as office systolic blood pressure (BP) values >140 mmHg and/or diastolic blood pressure values >90 mmHg [1]. These cut-off values are based on evidence from multiple randomized controlled trials having shown that treatment of patients with higher values is beneficial and outweighs potential side effects of this

S. Caselli
Cardiovascular Center Zurich, Hirslanden Klinik im Park, Zurich, Switzerland

J. Niebauer (✉)
University Institute of Sports Medicine, Prevention and Rehabilitation, Paracelsus Medical University, Salzburg, Austria
e-mail: j.niebauer@salk.at



A. Pressler, J. Niebauer (eds.), *Textbook of Sports and Exercise Cardiology*,
https://doi.org/10.1007/978-3-030-35374-2_12

treatment [1]. The same cut-off values are used in younger, middle-aged, and older people. Fewer data are available in children and adolescents; however, specific guidelines for the classification of blood pressure in boys and girls <16 years, have been published in 2016 by the European Society of Hypertension [2].

Due to the high prevalence of arterial hypertension in the general population, this condition is also one of the most common cardiovascular abnormalities reported in the setting of pre-participation screening of large athletic populations [3–5]. The common clinical scenarios in this context may include the middle-aged individual with cardiovascular risk factors including arterial hypertension, still aiming to participate in competitive sports; the middle-aged or even older individual with cardiovascular risk factors who aims to improve her/his cardiovascular risk profile by starting physical activity programs; the young individual with high blood pressure who engages in sport but follows an "unhealthy" diet and lifestyle.

Sport participation per se should not be considered as a risky undertaking, and as a matter of fact the ESC guidelines for cardiovascular disease prevention suggest at least 150 min of mild to moderate exercise activity per week [6]. However, hypertension as one of the most important cardiovascular risk factors may induce structural changes in target organs (Table 12.1) such as the kidneys, retina, brain and the heart that may be associated with increased morbidity and mortality in the long term. Arterial hypertension is also a risk factor for the occurrence of atherosclerotic plaques in peripheral vessels and in the coronary arteries [7, 8]. Furthermore, an acute increase in BP during effort may trigger atherosclerotic plaque rupture leading to acute myocardial infarction or cerebrovascular events [9–11].

A few other minor abnormalities have also been described in athletes with arterial hypertension. These athletes may achieve lower exercise performance on bicycle exercise and show lower cardiovascular fitness with an average 15% reduction in maximal oxygen consumption compared to non-hypertensive individuals [12]. Additionally, a study on vascular function in hypertensive athletes hypothesized that an early and subclinical vascular dysfunction (impaired reduction of peripheral vascular resistances) could be responsible for increased arterial stiffness and prevalence of elevated BP at effort, and this may be advocated to explain the reduced performance [13].

**Table 12.1** Signs of subclinical target organ damage and associated clinical conditions that may be helpful for risk stratification and sport eligibility in athletes with hypertension

| Target organ damage | Associated clinical conditions |
|---|---|
| LV hypertrophy induced by hypertension | Atrial fibrillation |
| LV diastolic dysfunction | Ischemic heart disease |
| Ultrasound evidence of arterial wall thickening or plaques | Heart Failure |
| Hypertensive eye fundus | Peripheral vascular disease |
| Increase in serum creatinine (men 1.3–1.5 mg/dl; women 1.2–1.4 mg/dl) | Renal impairment, proteinuria |
| Microalbuminuria | Advanced retinopathy |

In order to address the proper management of athletes with arterial hypertension, the Sports Cardiology Section of the European Association of Preventive Cardiology updated in 2018 the specific recommendations for participation in leisure-time and competitive sports [14]. This document, together with other important recent evidence, will be discussed in this chapter.

## 12.2 Prevalence

- Prevalence of arterial hypertension in the general population varies between countries.
- In Italy, a national cross-sectional study in 493 individuals aged 18–35 reported elevated BP values in 11% of young adults [15].
- In economically developed countries, the burden of hypertension in young adults has been reported as 14% and 21% in men aged 20–29 and 30–39, respectively and as 6% and 10% in women in the same age groups [16].
- The largest study on hypertension in athletes was recently published in Italy [3]. According to the ESC classification, optimal BP was found in 47%, normal BP in 38%, high-normal in 12% and a definite diagnosis of hypertension was made in 3%.
- Athletes with hypertension were in the large majority males (87%), and no differences were identified related to the sport discipline.
- Risk factors for hypertension were identified in family hypertension history and larger body size. Specifically, athletes with larger body size had also higher percentage of body fat, suggesting that overweight could be a determinant of hypertension.

## 12.3 Diagnosis

All athletes with a diagnosis of hypertension or suspected hypertension should undergo a complete cardiac evaluation including clinical history, physical examination, resting ECG, echocardiography and exercise testing [14]. Additional testing such as ambulatory BP measurements, specific laboratory tests or radiologic evaluation are not routinely performed and are warranted only in selected cases [1].

### 12.3.1 Medical History

Regarding clinical history, specific attention should be directed to the use of energy drinks, supplements (such as vitamins and minerals; see also Chap. 28) and herbal remedies, which are commonly used by athletes and are frequently not reported. Anti-inflammatory drugs including steroidal or non-steroidal agents are as well commonly used by athletes to reduce pain after injuries that are more frequent in contact sports such as boxing, soccer, rugby or American football.

Secondary hypertension may account for up to 8% of hypertension in young athletes and therefore should be always suspected and searched for [3, 17]. The **red flags** to suspect secondary hypertension are:

- age at onset younger than 40 years
- resistant hypertension at presentation
- absence of additional risk factors
- severe hypertension
- sudden increase in blood pressure
- obstructive sleep apnea syndrome.

Furthermore, the following combinations of symptoms should raise the suspicion of suffering from rare but clinically significant secondary causes of hypertension:

- anxiety, sweating, flushing, headache and paroxysmal hypertension may suggest *pheochromocytoma*
- palpitations, changes in body weight or fatigue may be indicative of *thyroid dysfunction*
- weight gain, fatigue, muscle weakness, hirsutism, skin atrophy and striae rubrae may be symptoms and signs of *Cushing's syndrome*
- fatigue, constipation, polyuria and muscle weakness may be caused by *primary hyperaldosteronism*
- abdominal bruits on physical examination are characteristic for *renal artery stenosis* [17].

### 12.3.2 Blood Pressure Measurement

According to the ESC guidelines the office BP measurement should be performed according to specific requirements [1]:

1. Patient should be seated comfortably in a quiet environment for 5 min before beginning BP pressure measurements.
2. 2 or 3 BP measurements should be recorded 1 or 2 min apart and additional measurements only if the first two readings differ by more than 10 mmHg. BP is recorded as the average of the last two blood pressure readings.
3. Additional measurements may have to be performed if BP values vary largely (e.g. due to arrhythmias).
4. Use correct size of cuff according to arm's circumference.
5. The cuff should be positioned at the level of the heart with the back and arm supported to avoid muscle contraction.
6. When using auscultatory methods use phase 1 and 5 (sudden reduction and disappearance) of Korotkoff sounds to identify systolic blood pressure and diastolic blood pressure respectively (see also Chap. 7).
7. During first visit, measure BP in both arms.

According to 2018 ESC guidelines blood pressure is classified [1]:

| | Systolic | | Diastolic |
|---|---|---|---|
| Optimal | <120 | and | <80 |
| Normal | 120–129 | and/or | 80–84 |
| High Normal | 130–139 | and/or | 85–89 |
| Grade 1 Hypertension | 140–159 | and/or | 90–99 |
| Grade 2 Hypertension | 160–179 | and/or | 100–109 |
| Grade 3 Hypertension | ≥180 | and/or | ≥110 |
| Isolated systolic hypertension | ≥140 | and | <90 |

In case of high or borderline office BP measurements or when a white coat hypertension or masked hypertension is suspected, home BP measurements with a well compiled diary of values, and/or ambulatory BP measurement could be considered for further evaluation. In the athletic population, ambulatory BP measurement is preferred, since it provides objective measurements also during the night and gives information about dipping. Home blood pressure measurements are useful for monitoring over longer time periods. However, information on self-measurements may not be precise and some athletes may provide false values fearing the potential consequences of high blood pressure on sport eligibility.

### 12.3.3 Blood Pressure Response During Exercise Testing

- Resting and exercise ECG should be performed in all individuals
- During ergometry BP needs to be documented. This may be more easily obtained during bicycle ergometry because the arm is more stable; during treadmill testing at higher velocities reliable measurements are more difficult to achieve [18].
- During maximal exercise, systolic BP increases by approximately 70 mmHg while diastolic BP usually remains unchanged.
- In a large cohort of Olympic athletes, the upper reference value (95th percentile) for systolic BP has been reported as 220 mmHg in males and 200 mmHg in females, and for diastolic BP 85 mmHg in male and 80 mmHg in female athletes [18, 19].
- These values were even exceeded in another large cohort of adolescent, professional and master athletes undergoing standardized exercise testing on bicycle ergometers. Only athletes fulfilling both subjective and objective criteria of complete exhaustion were selected for this study, and the upper normative value of systolic BP in male endurance athletes was 247 mmHg, whereas diastolic BP did also not change relevantly [20].

An exaggerated BP response to exercise testing may predict incident hypertension: In athletes with high blood pressure response (HBPR) to exercise, over 7-year follow-up no cardiac events occurred. However, the subsequent incidence of hypertension was higher in the HBPR group (13.5%) compared to controls (3.5%; $p = 0.009$). Baseline BP and HBPR were the strongest predictors of incident hypertension, being 3.6 times higher in these conditions compared to those with normal BP response during exercise [19]. Moreover, in a recent study on well-trained triathletes, HBPR was found to be associated with the presence of myocardial fibrosis detected by cardiac magnetic resonance imaging, but these preliminary observations require further evaluation in larger cohorts before definite conclusions on these potential deleterious effects are allowed [21].

- Overall, HBPR to exercise should not automatically raise concerns in terms of sport participation and should not be the reason for medical treatment. Nonetheless, these individuals should enter a periodical follow-up program.

### 12.3.4 Echocardiography

Echocardiography is particularly important to detect potential target organ damage. It has to be kept in mind, however, that left ventricular (LV) hypertrophy may both represent a physiologic cardiovascular adaptation to exercise or a pathological response to hypertension [12, 18]. Generally speaking, hypertrophy induced by hypertension can be suspected when the degree of hypertrophy is out of proportion in relation to the specific sport discipline.

- LV hypertrophy is defined as LV mass index >95 $g/m^2$ in women or >115 $g/m^2$ in men
- Geometry is described using the relative wall thickness (RWT = (interventricular septum + posterior wall)/(end-diastolic diameter)). The pattern of LV hypertrophy is defined concentric when associated with an RWT > 0.42 (see also Chap. 4).
- Diastolic dysfunction may be suspected by a trans-mitral E/A ratio <1 or by an e′ septal velocity on Tissue Doppler Imaging (TDI) <8 cm/s.
- Global longitudinal strain has been reported as an additional tool to detect subclinical left ventricular impairment and may help to identify athletes with pathological LV hypertrophy due to hypertension [22].

### 12.3.5 Further Evaluation

Further evaluation should be performed in order to rule out target organ damage. An ankle-brachial index <0.9 may suggest peripheral artery disease; carotid sonography may help identifying wall thickening or plaques; eye fundoscopy may reveal hypertensive retinopathy; lab tests are useful to detect impaired renal function through microalbuminuria, increased creatinine or reduced eGFR [1].

## 12.4 Management

Athletes should be treated according to the specific ESC guidelines. Management strategy is based on risk profile, specific risk scores, and presence or absence of target organ damage (Fig. 12.1).

Low, moderate, high, and very high risk correspond to absolute 10-year-risk of cardiovascular mortality of <1%, 1–4%, 5–10% and >10% respectively, according to the European score system as defined by the 2016 ESC prevention guidelines. Athletes with grade 1 hypertension and low risk profile could be treated with non-pharmacological measures:

| Other RFs, asymptomatic OD, or disease | Blood pressure (mmHg) | | | |
|---|---|---|---|---|
| | High normal SBP 130–139 or DBP 85–89 | Grade 1 HT SBP 140–159 or DBP 90–99 | Grade 2 HT SBP 160–179 or DBP 100–109 | Grade 3 HT SBP ≥180 or DBP ≥110 |
| No other RF | | Low risk | Moderate risk | High risk |
| 1–2 RF | Low risk | Moderate risk | Moderate to high risk | High risk |
| ≥3 RF | Low to moderate risk | Moderate to high risk | High risk | High risk |
| OD, CKD Stage 3, or diabetes | Moderate to high risk | High risk | High risk | High to very high risk |
| CVD, CKD stage ≥4, or diabetes with OD/RFs | Very high risk | Very high risk | Very high risk | Very high risk |

**Fig. 12.1** Stratification of total cardiovascular risk to quantify prognosis in patients with hypertension [14]. RF: blood pressure (high normal BP; Grades 1–3); gender, age (men > 55 years; women > 65 years); smoking; dyslipidaemia (total cholesterol > 190 mg/dL and/or LDL > 115 mg/dL and/or HDL < 40 mg/dL in men and <46 mg/dL in women); fasting plasma glucose 102–125 mg/dL; abnormal glucose tolerance test; body mass index >30 kg/m$^2$; abdominal obesity (men > 102 cm; women > 88 cm); First degree family history of premature cardiovascular disease (men < 55 years; women < 65 years). OD: hypertension-induced LV hypertrophy; carotid wall thickening or plaque; carotid-femoral pulse wave velocity >10 m/s; ankle-brachial index <0.9; CKD with eGFR 30–60 mL/min/1.73 m$^2$; presence of micro-albuminuria. Established cardiovascular or renal disease: cerebrovascular disease; coronary heart disease; heart failure; symptomatic peripheral artery disease; CKD: eGFR < 30 mL/min/1.73 m$^2$; proteinuria; and advanced retinopathy (haemorrhages; exudates; papilloedema). *CKD* chronic kidney disease, *CVD* cardiovascular disease, *DBP* diastolic blood pressure, *HT* hypertension, *OD* organ damage, *RF* risk factor, *SBP* systolic blood pressure

- salt restriction
- weight reduction
- alcohol restriction
- increased consumption of vegetables and fruits
- smoking cessation
- discontinuation of supplements, ergogenic and/or anti-inflammatory drugs
- aerobic exercise training

In most cases these measures are effective to control blood pressure. In case blood pressure remains elevated or in individuals with grade 2 hypertension or in those with higher risk profile, a pharmacological treatment should be taken into consideration. In any case, a periodical re-evaluation should be performed.

- The goal of antihypertensive therapy is to reduce blood pressure <140/90 and <140/85 mmHg in diabetic patients [14].

### 12.4.1 Pharmacologic Treatment

Choice of drugs has to be in keeping with the world anti-doping association regulation (www.wada-ama.org). First-choice treatment in athletes is an angiotensin converting enzyme inhibitor or an angiotensin II receptor blocker, since they do not affect exercise capacity and are not on the doping list. These are contraindicated, however, in female athletes because of potential adverse fatal neonatal effects. Alternatively, calcium channel blockers (nifedipine type) are a preferred choice. In case more than one drug is needed, combination drugs should be considered as they may improve compliance [14]. Beta blockers are usually not recommended due to their negative impact on aerobic exercise performance. Also, endurance athletes often present with significant bradycardia that may be further accentuated by this class of drugs. Beta blockers are also prohibited drugs in some specific sport disciplines in which the control of tremor is seeked such as archery and shooting. Diuretics should not be used; they are on the list of prohibited drugs since they may mask performance enhancing drugs. In selected cases, when a specific drug is considered mandatory to treat the athlete, a Therapeutic Use Exemption (TUE) can be requested at the national/international anti-doping associations.

## 12.5 Recommendations

- In competitive athletes, normal BP values similar to the general population have to be present or have to be attained, i.e. <140/90 and <140/85 mmHg in diabetic subjects. In case of higher values, temporary restriction may be advised, with possible exception for skill disciplines [14].
- Once blood pressure is well controlled, recommendations for appropriate sport disciplines are dependent upon the presence of target organ damage and associated clinical conditions (Fig. 12.2 and Table 12.2).

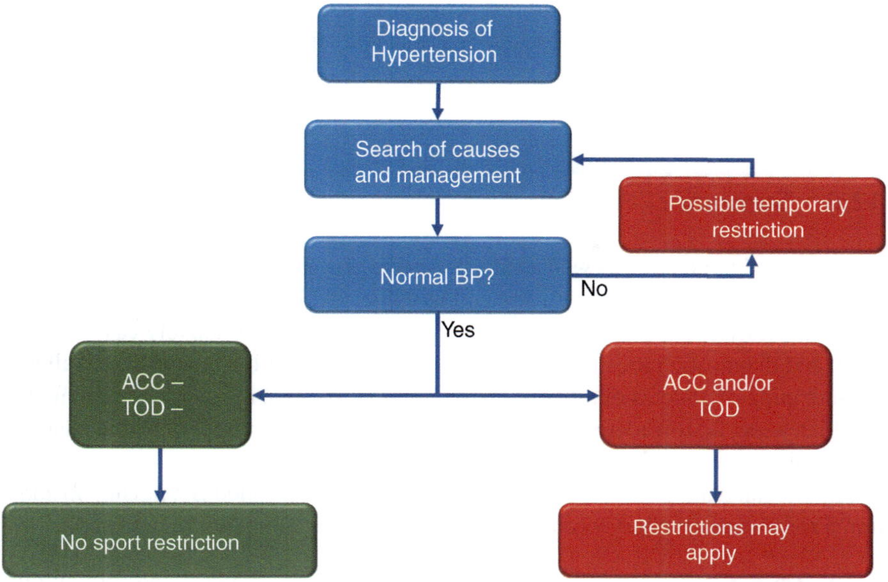


**Fig. 12.2** Recommended decision tree for clinical guidance of athletes with arterial hypertension. If blood pressure is well controlled, eligibility is dependent upon the presence of target organ damage and associated clinical conditions. (Modified from [14])

**Table 12.2** Criteria for risk stratification in athletes with hypertension (adapted from [14])

| Criteria for eligibility | Recommendations | Evaluation | Follow-up |
|---|---|---|---|
| BP well controlled<br>Further RF: none<br>TOD: none<br>ACC: none | All sports | History, PE, ECG, ET; echo[a] | Annually |
| BP well controlled<br>Further RF: well controlled<br>TOD: none<br>ACC: none | All sports | History, PE, ECG, ET; echo | 6–12 months |
| BP well controlled<br>Further RF: well controlled<br>TOD: present<br>ACC: none | All sports, except power sports known to severely increase BP | History, PE, ECG, ET; echo | 6 months |
| BP well controlled<br>Further RF: well controlled<br>TOD: none or present<br>ACC: present | All sports, except power sports known to severely increase BP[b] | History, PE, ECG, ET; echo | 6 months |

Individual recommendations need to also consider cardiovascular risk profile, target organ damage (TOD) and associated clinical conditions (ACC)

*BP* blood pressure, *ET* exercise testing, *PE* physical examination, including BP measurements, *RF* risk factors

[a]Echocardiography according to clinical condition, but once every 1–2 years

[b]Eligibility depending on type and severity of ACC and/or TOD

- Specifically, in the presence of target organ damage, power sport disciplines are not recommended. In the presence of associated clinical conditions (Table 12.2) the sport eligibility should be evaluated according to the severity of these conditions [14].

## 12.6 Summary

In the general population as well as in athletes the prevalence of arterial hypertension is relatively high, increases with age and is influenced by all negative effects of the Western lifestyle. On the other hand, arterial hypertension is relatively easy to diagnose, and diagnostic procedures are rather inexpensive and lend themselves suitable for screening of athletes of all ages. In case of confirmation of arterial hypertension, in athletes special considerations have to be taken into account regarding the pharmacological treatment. While eligibility for competitive sports may have to be restricted if target organ damage is present, an athlete with well-controlled BP, having no additional risk factor or target organ damage, is eligible for competition in all sports.

**Clinical Pearls**

- Definition of arterial hypertension is the same for athletes and non-athletes and defined by the 2018 European Society of Cardiology Guidelines as office systolic blood pressure values >140 mmHg and/or diastolic blood pressure values >90 mmHg.
- Sport participation per se should not be considered as a risky undertaking, and as a matter of fact, the ESC guidelines for cardiovascular prevention suggest at least 150 min of mild to moderate exercise activity per week.
- All athletes with a diagnosis of hypertension or suspected hypertension should undergo a complete cardiac evaluation including clinical history, physical examination, resting ECG, echocardiography and exercise testing.
- Regarding clinical history, ask for the use of energy drinks, supplements and herbal remedies as well as anti-inflammatory drugs to reduce pain, which are commonly used by athletes, frequently not reported, but may well result in increased blood pressure levels.
- Office blood pressure measurement should be performed according to guidelines [1].
- In the athletic population, ambulatory blood pressure measurement is preferred, since it provides objective measurements also during the night and gives information about dipping.
- During ergometry blood pressure needs to be recorded. This is easier during bicycle ergometry because the arm is more stable.
- In a large cohort of Olympic athletes, the upper reference value (95th percentile) for systolic blood pressure was 220 mmHg in male and 200 mmHg in females, and for diastolic blood pressure 85 mmHg in male and 80 mmHg in female athletes [18].
- Echocardiography is particularly important in hypertensive athletes to detect potential target organ damage.

- Recommendation for choice of competitive sports depends on the actual blood pressure values, target organ damage and associated clinical conditions.
- Athletes, just like any other patients, need to be regularly followed.

## Review

### Questions

1. Secondary hypertension may account for up to 8% of hypertension in young athletes and therefore should always be searched for. What are the red flags to suspect a secondary hypertension?
2. Both athletes and patients have to reach normal blood pressure values, if needed with the help of medical drugs. In athletes, generally speaking, what are the preferred types of drugs and which ones should usually not be prescribed?
3. Can athletes with well controlled blood pressure values participate in any competitive sport?

### Answers

1. Red flags to suspect secondary arterial hypertension are:
   (a) age at onset younger than 40 years
   (b) resistant hypertension at presentation
   (c) absence of additional risk factors
   (d) severe hypertension
   (e) sudden increase in blood pressure
   (f) obstructive sleep apnea syndrome.
2. First-choice treatment is an angiotensin converting enzyme inhibitor or an angiotensin II receptor blocker, which however is contraindicated in female athletes because of potential adverse neonatal effects. Alternatively, calcium channel blockers (nifedipine type) are a preferred choice. Beta blockers are not recommended due to their negative impact on aerobic exercise performance, frequent bradycardia and their presence on the list of prohibited drugs. The latter holds true for diuretics as well.
3. Generally speaking, decision about specific sports has to be made in the light of the individual cardiac risk and absence or presence of end organ damage and associated clinical conditions.

## References

1. Williams B, Mancia G, Spiering W, Agabiti Rosei E, Azizi M, Burnier M, et al. 2018 ESC/ESH Guidelines for the management of arterial hypertension. Eur Heart J. 2018;39(33):3021–104.

2. Lurbe E, Agabiti-Rosei E, Cruickshank JK, Dominiczak A, Erdine S, Hirth A, et al. 2016 European Society of Hypertension guidelines for the management of high blood pressure in children and adolescents. J Hypertens. 2016;34(10):1887–920.
3. Caselli S, Vaquer Sequi A, Lemme E, Quattrini F, Milan A, D'Ascenzi F, et al. Prevalence and management of systemic hypertension in athletes. Am J Cardiol. 2017;119(10):1616–22.
4. D'Ascenzi F, Caselli S, Alvino F, Digiacinto B, Lemme E, Piepoli M, et al. Cardiovascular risk profile in Olympic athletes: an unexpected and underestimated risk scenario. Br J Sports Med. 2019;53(1):37–42.
5. Karpinos AR, Roumie CL, Nian H, Diamond AB, Rothman RL. High prevalence of hypertension among collegiate football athletes. Circ Cardiovasc Qual Outcomes. 2013;6(6):716–23.
6. Authors/Task Force M, Piepoli MF, Hoes AW, Agewall S, Albus C, Brotons C, et al. 2016 European Guidelines on cardiovascular disease prevention in clinical practice: the Sixth Joint Task Force of the European Society of Cardiology and Other Societies on Cardiovascular Disease Prevention in Clinical Practice (constituted by representatives of 10 societies and by invited experts): developed with the special contribution of the European Association for Cardiovascular Prevention & Rehabilitation (EACPR). Eur J Prev Cardiol. 2016;23(11):NP1–NP96.
7. Mancia G, Fagard R, Narkiewicz K, Redon J, Zanchetti A, Bohm M, et al. 2013 ESH/ESC Guidelines for the management of arterial hypertension: the Task Force for the management of arterial hypertension of the European Society of Hypertension (ESH) and of the European Society of Cardiology (ESC). J Hypertens. 2013;31(7):1281–357.
8. Selden MA, Helzberg JH, Waeckerle JF. Early cardiovascular mortality in professional football players: fact or fiction? Am J Med. 2009;122(9):811–4.
9. Laukkanen JA, Jennings JR, Kauhanen J, Makikallio TH, Ronkainen K, Kurl S. Relation of systemic blood pressure to sudden cardiac death. Am J Cardiol. 2012;110(3):378–82.
10. Laukkanen JA, Khan H, Kurl S, Willeit P, Karppi J, Ronkainen K, et al. Left ventricular mass and the risk of sudden cardiac death: a population-based study. J Am Heart Assoc. 2014;3(6):e001285.
11. Laukkanen JA, Willeit P, Kurl S, Makikallio TH, Savonen K, Ronkainen K, et al. Elevated systolic blood pressure during recovery from exercise and the risk of sudden cardiac death. J Hypertens. 2014;32(3):659–66.
12. Mazic S, Suzic Lazic J, Dekleva M, Antic M, Soldatovic I, Djelic M, et al. The impact of elevated blood pressure on exercise capacity in elite athletes. Int J Cardiol. 2015;180:171–7.
13. Kim JH, Sher S, Wang F, Berkstresser B, Shoop JL, Galante A, et al. Impact of American-style football participation on vascular function. Am J Cardiol. 2015;115(2):262–7.
14. Niebauer J, Borjesson M, Carre F, Caselli S, Palatini P, Quattrini F, et al. Recommendations for participation in competitive sports of athletes with arterial hypertension: a position statement from the sports cardiology section of the European Association of Preventive Cardiology (EAPC). Eur Heart J. 2018;39(40):3664–71.
15. Bruno RM, Pucci G, Rosticci M, Guarino L, Guglielmo C, Agabiti Rosei C, et al. Association between lifestyle and systemic arterial hypertension in young adults: a national, survey-based, cross-sectional study. High Blood Press Cardiovasc Prev. 2016;23(1):31–40.
16. Kearney PM, Whelton M, Reynolds K, Muntner P, Whelton PK, He J. Global burden of hypertension: analysis of worldwide data. Lancet. 2005;365(9455):217–23.
17. Rimoldi SF, Scherrer U, Messerli FH. Secondary arterial hypertension: when, who, and how to screen? Eur Heart J. 2014;35(19):1245–54.
18. Caselli S, Vaquer Segui A, Quattrini F, Di Gacinto B, Milan A, Assorgi R, et al. Upper normal values of blood pressure response to exercise in Olympic athletes. Am Heart J. 2016;177:120–8.
19. Caselli S, Serdoz A, Mango F, Lemme E, Vaquer Segui A, Milan A, et al. High blood pressure response to exercise predicts future development of hypertension in young athletes. Eur Heart J. 2019;40(1):62–8.
20. Pressler A, Jahnig A, Halle M, Haller B. Blood pressure response to maximal dynamic exercise testing in an athletic population. J Hypertens. 2018;36(9):1803–9.

21. Tahir E, Starekova J, Muellerleile K, von Stritzky A, Munch J, Avanesov M, et al. Myocardial fibrosis in competitive triathletes detected by contrast-enhanced CMR correlates with exercise-induced hypertension and competition history. JACC Cardiovasc Imaging. 2018;11(9):1260–70.
22. Galderisi M, Lomoriello VS, Santoro A, Esposito R, Olibet M, Raia R, et al. Differences of myocardial systolic deformation and correlates of diastolic function in competitive rowers and young hypertensives: a speckle-tracking echocardiography study. J Am Soc Echocardiogr. 2010;23(11):1190–8.

# Specific Cardiovascular Diseases and Competitive Sports Participation: Hypertrophic Cardiomyopathy

13

Antonio Pelliccia and Stefano Caselli

**Learning Objectives**

1. Learn the abnormal ECG pattern not commonly seen in athletes which may suggest a structural heart disease.
2. Learn the clues on cardiovascular imaging to distinguish between physiological and pathological adaptation of the heart.
3. Understand the risk stratification for sudden cardiac death in athletes with hypertrophic cardiomyopathy (HCM).
4. Become familiar with the current recommendations for sport participation in individuals with HCM.

## 13.1 Introduction

Hypertrophic cardiomyopathy (HCM) is a relevant pathologic condition in athletes, because it represents one of the common causes of SCD [1–3]. The diagnosis of HCM relies on the presence of a hypertrophied left ventricle (LV; i.e. LV wall thickness >15 mm) in the absence of cardiac or systemic disease capable of producing the same magnitude of LV hypertrophy [4]. The diagnosis in young competitive athletes may be challenging when the extent of LV hypertrophy is mild and LV wall thickness is in the range of 13–15 mm, which identifies the 'gray zone' of overlap between the physiologic cardiac adaptation to intensive exercise training and mild phenotypic expression of the disease (Fig. 13.1) [5, 6].

A. Pelliccia (✉)
Department of Medicine, Institute of Sports Medicine and Science, Rome, Italy

S. Caselli
Cardiovascular Center Zurich, Hirslanden Klinik im Park, Zurich, Switzerland



A. Pressler, J. Niebauer (eds.), *Textbook of Sports and Exercise Cardiology*,
https://doi.org/10.1007/978-3-030-35374-2_13

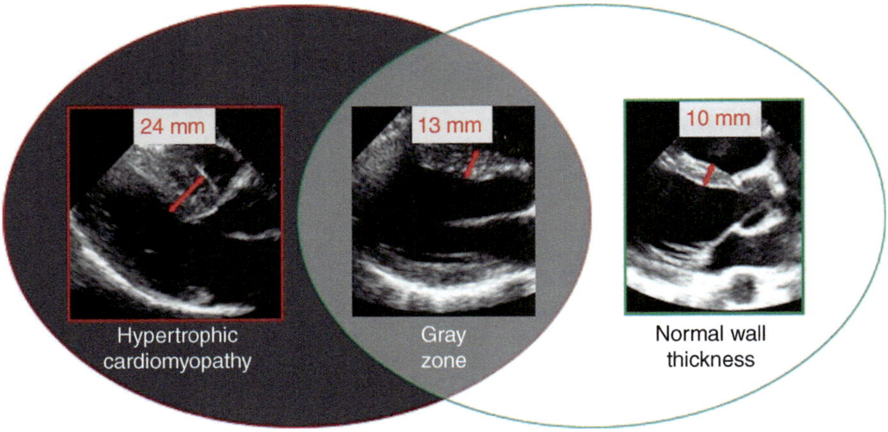


**Fig. 13.1** Schematic depiction of the so-called "gray zone" of athlete's heart. This zone indicates a certain range of mildly increased left ventricular wall thickness (usually 13–15 mm) that can either be explained by physiological adaptations to intensive sport or by an early expression of hypertrophic cardiomyopathy

## 13.2 Clinical Evaluation

Hypertrophic Cardiomyopathy may be difficult to identify during clinical evaluation of the athlete since the majority of young individuals are asymptomatic. However, the red flags that should rise a suspicion of a structural heart disease are represented by

- exercise induced *syncope and palpitations*; in these cases, extensive cardiac imaging should be warranted to rule out a cardiomyopathy.
- *Family history* should also be accurately investigated for the presence of cardiomyopathies and sudden cardiac death in young age.
- In a minority of subjects, especially those with more marked phenotypic expression, a *systolic murmur* which is accentuated in the sitting position, may suggest an obstructive form of hypertrophic cardiomyopathy.

## 13.3 The 12-lead ECG

The ECG is abnormal in over 95% of adult athletes with HCM [7, 8]. Large QRS voltages are common in all individuals with HCM, but this finding is also common in trained athletes. More relevant to the diagnosis are the repolarization abnormalities:

(a) T-wave inversion especially in inferior and lateral leads, and
(b) ST-segment depression,

which are unlikely to be present in case of physiologic LV hypertrophy (Fig. 13.2) (see also Chap. 8).

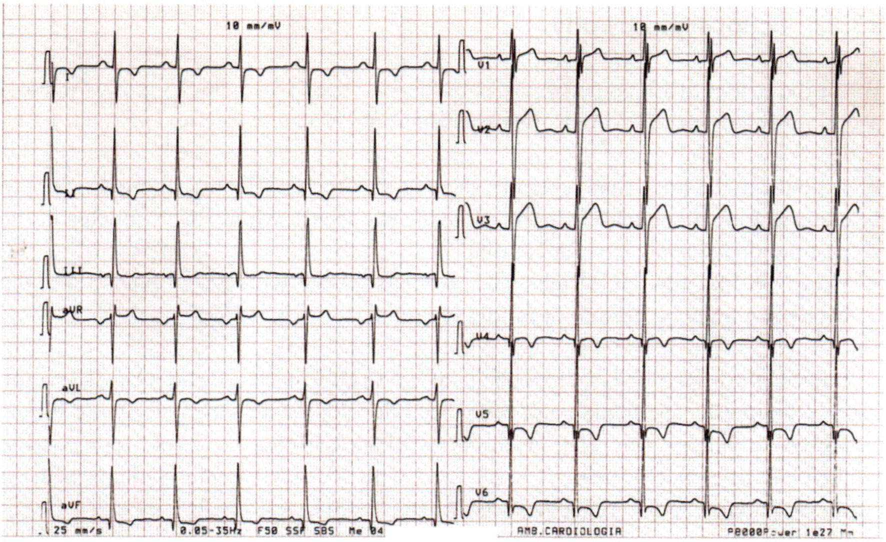


**Fig. 13.2** ECG of a 40-year-old asymptomatic marathon runner with family history of Hypertrophic Cardiomyopathy (HCM) and sudden cardiac death. ECG shows diffuse infero-lateral negative T Waves. Echocardiography showed concentric left ventricular hypertrophy suggestive of HCM

Cardiac MRI (see below) should be a standard component of the assessment for markedly abnormal ECGs suggestive of apical HCM, specifically ECGs with deep T-wave inversion and ST segment depression in the lateral or infero-lateral leads, in which echocardiography usually does not provide adequate assessment of the LV apex and inferior septum.

In addition, pathological Q waves, left atrial enlargement and left axis deviation are common abnormalities in HCM, and less frequent in trained hearts. To be noticed, lateral T-wave inversion has a 14% diagnostic yield for HCM, but is also detectable in 4% of normal black athletes [9] (see Chap. 26).

- Of relevance, the finding of abnormal repolarization patterns, particularly in adolescent and young athletes, may precede by several years the development of overt structural disease and require serial evaluation with imaging testing [10].
- Finally, a minority (5–10%) of young individuals with HCM may have a normal ECG, or just increased R/S wave voltage in isolation [11], which are overlapping the ECG findings common in young trained athletes.

## 13.4 Imaging Testing

Cardiac imaging offers several clues for diagnosis, having in mind that no single parameter may ultimately be diagnostic *per se*, but final decision should always consider all clinical information available. Diagnosis may be challenging when the extent of LV hypertrophy is mild (i.e., <15 mm), because detection of LV wall thickness, even segmentally above this value, is diagnostic for HCM.

### 13.4.1 Echocardiography

When the extent of LV hypertrophy is borderline (i.e., >12 but <15 mm), the most useful morphologic criterion is the assessment of LV cavity size and geometry.

- Athletes in the gray zone typically show an enlarged LV cavity (the cut off of LV end-diastolic diameter >54 mm has been suggested), while HCM athletes in the vast majority have a smaller cavity [12].
- However, in a few HCM athletes, especially those with apical phenotype, the cavity size may be normal or mildly enlarged (Fig. 13.3) [13].

Indeed, the shape of LV chamber is altered in most HCM patients, due to the usual asymmetric, segmental, and centripetal development of the pathologic hypertrophy. As a general rule, the development of physiologic LV hypertrophy in the context of the athlete's heart is associated with LV cavity enlargement, with an eccentric pattern, at difference from HCM [6, 13, 14].

The highest degree of LV hypertrophy in athletes is seen in male gender, with values up to 15 mm in white and 16 mm in Afro-American athletes [15, 16]. Less hypertrophy is found in female athletes, with values up to 11 mm in whites and 13 mm in Afro-Americans [17, 18] (regarding the latter see also Chap. 26). To be noticed that LV hypertrophy is typically found in individuals engaged in a combination of high volume and pressure overload, such as rowing, canoeing, cycling [5, 19, 20].

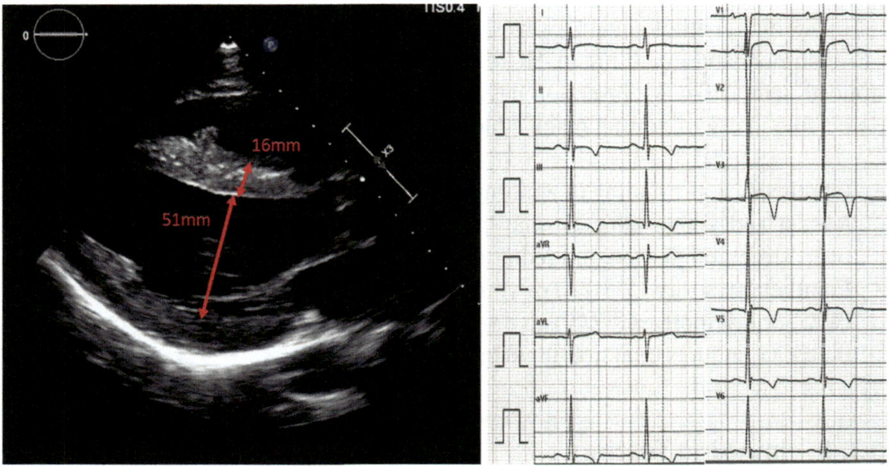


**Fig. 13.3** Echocardiographic findings in an 18-year-old black soccer player. LV wall thickness was 16 mm while cavity size in diastole was 51 mm, describing therefore a concentric hypertrophy. ECG on the right shows infero-lateral negative T waves. The overall clinical picture was suggestive of HCM

- Athletes usually show a homogeneous distribution of wall thickness with absolute differences of <2 mm between the thickest and the less thickened segments of the LV.
  - On the contrary, an asymmetric and heterogeneous pattern of LV hypertrophy represents a phenotypic expression of HCM.
- Athletes show a preserved LV chamber geometry with mitral valve normally located.
  - On the contrary, certain mitral abnormalities may be present in HCM athletes, such as elongation of mitral chordae, with systolic anterior motion and flow acceleration in the LV outflow tract [21, 22].

Additionally, while LV outflow obstruction may not be evident under resting conditions, it could be precipitated by exercise and thus be demonstrated on stress echocardiography in HCM patients [23].

LV systolic function is usually within the range of normality in both normal and HCM athletes. Only subtle differences in myocardial contraction can be detected by STE. Preliminary observations suggest that HCM with mild LV hypertrophy may already present a reduction in longitudinal endocardial strain, with a cut-off value <−15% able to identify pathologic hypertrophy with good accuracy (sensitivity 79%; specificity 67%). Therefore, values below this cut-off may be suggestive for pathologic LV hypertrophy [24, 25].

One of the most consistent features of the athlete's heart is the normal diastolic function, expression of preserved elastic, and recoil LV properties [26]. Conversely, in HCM, LV diastolic function may present impairment as an expression of myocyte alteration and interstitial fibrosis. Few individuals may show an inversion of the E/A ratio, but most frequently in HCM a subclinical impairment is associated with a reduction of the e′ velocity on TDI [26].

### 13.4.2 Cardiac Magnetic Resonance Imaging

Cardiac magnetic resonance imaging is indicated in all cases when echocardiographic images are not able to clearly identify all myocardial segments, in order to exclude segmental areas of hypertrophy (in particular, the apex and lateral wall).

- CMR should be performed in all cases with associated marked ECG abnormalities and/or arrhythmias.

The high-contrast of CMR images between endocardial surface and the blood pool allows a better definition and distribution of LV hypertrophy and areas of focal hypertrophy. Most importantly, the use of Late gadolinium enhancement techniques (LGE) enables tissue characterization and identification of focal areas of myocardial fibrosis [21]. The presence of LGE with a non-ischemic pattern in the hypertrophied segments is suggestive of myocardial fibrosis, and consistent with the diagnosis of HCM (see also Chap. 20).

| HCM | Findings | Athlete |
|---|---|---|
| + | Family history of SCD/A or HCM | - |
| + | Major ECG abnormalities (T wave inversions) | - |
| + | Normal or reduced LV cavity size (< 54 mm) | - |
| + | Abnormal LV geometry | - |
| + | LV outflow tract obstruction | - |
| + | Abnormal diastolic filling / relaxation | - |
| + | LGE on CMR | - |
| + | Unchanged LV wall thickness after detraining | - |

**Fig. 13.4** Criteria for the differential diagnosis of athlete's heart and HCM in the gray zone of 13–15 mm with cardiovascular imaging

It is worthy to mention that left atrial size may not be particularly helpful in this specific scenario. Left atrial enlargement has been described in athletes as an expression of global cardiac adaptation to training and is typically associated with increased LV size, at difference than in HCM where LV cavity is usually of normal size or even reduced, and LA appears disproportionately enlarged [6]. Additionally, while in older HCM patients LA enlargement is a common finding and is considered a reliable criterion for the diagnosis and risk stratification, in young and asymptomatic HCM patients with mild expression of the disease, this finding may not be present as well, with the apparent paradox that young athletes may have larger LA compared with young HCM patients (Fig. 13.4).

## 13.5 Genetic Testing

In the majority of cases, HCM is inherited as an autosomal dominant genetic trait with a 50% risk of transmission to offspring, but numbers of cases are due to *de novo* mutations. Indeed, apparently sporadic cases may be expression of incomplete penetrance and, less commonly, autosomal recessive inheritance.

In patients fulfilling HCM diagnostic criteria, sequencing of sarcomere protein genes identifies a disease-causing mutation in up to 60% of cases [4]. Therefore, at present time, genetic testing is not recommended as routine tool to make diagnosis of HCM, as the absence of a sarcomere mutation does not exclude familial HCM and variants of uncertain significance can be difficult to interpret [9].

- Genetic testing is advised only in patients already fulfilling the diagnostic criteria for HCM, to enable cascade genetic screening of their relatives.
- Therefore, in athletes with diagnosis of HCM, genetic testing should be advised by an experienced cardiologist after detailed clinical and family assessment (see also Chap. 12).

## 13.6 Exercise Testing and 24- to 48-h Holter Monitoring

The presence of non-sustained ventricular tachycardia (NSVT), or ST segment depression/T wave inversion during exercise, or flat blood pressure response (<20 mmHg rise in systolic pressure from baseline to peak exercise) and a low peak oxygen consumption (<84% predicted) are elements confirming the diagnosis of HCM and relevant for risk stratification of the individual patient [27].

In particular, detection of NSVT induced by exercise or an impaired blood pressure raise during effort are considered conveying a high-level of risk. However, it should also be reminded that absence of arrhythmias or normalization during exercise of T-wave inversion or ST-depression (present at rest) does not exclude the presence of HCM and does not necessarily imply a low-risk condition.

## 13.7 Detraining

Finally, when the differential diagnosis cannot be completely resolved with conventional tests, useful information may be gained from serial observation of the individual athletes after an adequate period of detraining. Serial echocardiographic studies (or even better, CMR images) demonstrating regression of LV hypertrophy after at least a 3-month period of complete deconditioning in a subject without family history of HCM are consistent with diagnosis of physiological LV hypertrophy [28, 29].

## 13.8 How to Stratify the Risk in Athletes with HCM

Risk stratification in athletes with HCM is challenging, due to the lack of prospective studies reporting the outcome of the disease in patients engaging in regular and intensive exercise programmes. The current ESC [4] and AHA [30] algorithms to assess the risk of sudden cardiac death/cardiac arrest (SCD/CA) in the HCM population cannot be extrapolated to individuals regularly exposed to the hemodynamic and metabolic stresses of an athletic lifestyle since they have not been validated in this particular population.

Circumstantial evidence has suggested that intensive exercise and sport participation itself may play a role in triggering SCD/CA [1]. This largely agreed belief is based on several considerations, as here summarized:

- Among young athletes in the US, HCM was reported in pathologic registries as one of the most common cause of exercise related SCD/CA (Chap. 6).
- Participation in high-intensity competitive sports has been considered as an independent risk for SCD/CA, even in the absence of the conventional risk markers, due to alterations in hydration, electrolyte and acid base status and surges in catecholamine levels that typically are induced by intensive exercise.

- The incidence of SCD/CA has been reported to be higher in highly-dynamic sport, such as basketball, football, swimming, particularly in athletes of Division I compared to Division II and III, suggesting that intensity of training schedule and level of athletic performance may have a causative role [31].
- Just recently, HCM has been reported as one of the most common causes of SCD/CA in adolescent athletes engaged in the English football championship [32].

However, over the years the concern for exercise and sport participation in patients with HCM has been softening, based on novel information. In fact, retrospective observations indicate that SCD/CA is rare in HCM, and less than 1% in high risk patients and likely much lower in the general HCM population. This assumption is supported by the observation that only a minority (i.e., <30%) of physically active HCM who die suddenly, do so during exercise [33], which suggests that most patients are not exposed to a significant additional risk being engaged in exercise programmes. Consistently, Lampert et al. reported that HCM patients implanted with ICD had similar rates of appropriate or inappropriate shocks during exercise or during resting condition [34].

Indeed, there has been accumulating scientific evidence to support the benefits of regular exercise programmes in patients with HCM:

- A recent randomized clinical trial demonstrated that patients with HCM may safely engage in moderate-intensity, regular exercise programmes [35].
  - Just after 16 weeks of an active lifestyle, a mild (+6%), statistically significant increase in $VO_2$max and exercise capacity was observed.
  - Of relevance, there were no episodes of sustained ventricular arrhythmia, cardiac arrest, or appropriate defibrillator shocks even in patients with a moderate or high-risk profile.
- Klempfner et al. reported similar results in symptomatic HCM patients enrolled in a supervised cardiac exercise program [36].
  - After a short-term period (average, 40 h exercise) the vast majority of patients (80%) reported subjective improvement in their clinical condition and the NYHA class improved from baseline by >1 grade.
  - Functional capacity, assessed by the change in maximally attained METs, improved by 46% and during the 12 months follow up period, none of the patients experienced clinical deterioration, significant adverse events or ICD discharges.
- Recently, Pelliccia et al. reported that in a small cohort of 35 HCM athletes, over a 9-year follow-up, there were no differences in the incidence of symptoms (syncope, palpitations, 2% per year), or major events between athletes who had become sedentary (n = 20) after diagnosis of HCM and athletes with the disease that continued to engage in competitive sport (n = 15).
  - In this cohort there was one cardiac arrest during the surveillance period, which was unrelated to exercise [37].

Overall, the scarce available literature indicates that, within the broad spectrum of the HCM, there are selected patients who are not exposed to a significant risk despite being engaged in exercise programmes for a long-time period.

It is indisputable, however, that absence of major risk factors does not convey immunity to SCD/CA, and even patients that are judged to be at low-risk (i.e., in the absence of major risk determinants) may die suddenly [38]. Therefore, when advising a patient with HCM regarding participation to intensive exercise programmes and competitive sport this consideration should be an integral part of discussion during the decision making.

Based on the evolving knowledge in this field, we believe:

1. that risk stratification should be individualized, taking into account symptoms, established risk factors for SCD/CA, natural history of the disease, age of the athlete and characteristics of the sport discipline.
2. that it is crucial to involve the athlete in the decision-making process, with the duty for the physician to inform comprehensively the patient of characteristics of the disease in the individual case, with special attention to the risk factors for SCD/CA. The physician should run an open discussion with the patient about the potential risks associated with on-going competitive sport and/or high-intensity exercise programmes.
3. that athletes should have full judgment and complete understanding of the physician explanation and should be free from patent conditions of misunderstanding, or obligation to sponsor, media or athletic team.

## 13.9 Advising Exercise and Sport Participation

It is reasonable that the actual risk associated with mild to moderate exercise programmes is less than previously anticipated and, therefore, the majority of patients with HCM should not be deprived of the many cardiovascular, metabolic and psychological benefits afforded by regular exercise. Regular exercise improves functional capacity and may reduce the impact of excessive body weight on symptom progression in HCM patients, in whom obesity promotes worsening of the disease [39].

Patients with HCM should be advised not to participate in exercise programmes that require pursuit of excellence or high pressure to excel against others and involves explosive bouts of intensive exercise. It is necessary for clinicians to individualize exercise prescription, balancing the clinical status of the patient with the type, intensity and frequency of the physical and/or sport activity deemed to be initiated.

Exercise prescription should be guided by exercise testing, aiming for a submaximal, well-tolerated level of exercise intensity. Exercise testing is useful not only to assess the individual response to exercise (i.e., induction of ischemic ECG changes, rise or drop in blood pressure, occurrence of arrhythmias and/or symptoms) but also to derive the heart rate range the individual patient should maintain during the exercise programme. The following issues should particularly be considered:

- Patients should be fully informed of the clinical peculiarities of the disease, including the modalities of clinical presentation, and warned about the incidence of potential symptoms that occur in association with exercise.
- Patients should be advised to start exercise sessions with a warm-up period, and at the end of the session an appropriate cool-down period is also recommended.
- Exercise programmes characterized by a progressive increase in intensity should be closely monitored by the physician (ideally in contact with the coach), in order to adapt the intensity, duration and frequency of training to the individual cardiac capabilities.
- As a general rule, patients should avoid exercising in adverse environments (high altitude, extreme climate conditions; see Chap. 35).
- In the choice of indoor activities, patients with HCM should be encouraged to exercise in environments equipped with automatic defibrillators and personnel trained in its use.
- Finally, patients should preferentially avoid high-intensity free weight lifting, to reduce the risk of injury in the event of a syncope.

### 13.9.1 Competitive Sport Activities

Participation in intensive exercise programmes and competitive sport should be considered on an individual basis, after full evaluation of the disease characteristics and risk determinants [40]. Specifically, conditions that reasonably represent absolute contraindications for sport participation include:

1. symptoms, particularly unheralded syncope
2. previous history of aborted SCD/CA
3. exercise induced ventricular tachycardia
4. documentation of a significant increase in LV outflow gradient (>50 mmHg)
5. abnormal blood pressure response to exercise
6. ESC 5-year risk score >4 [4].

Following comprehensive explanation of the disease characteristics, risk factors and potential outcomes, assuring that a reasonable understanding and agreement has been reached between the athlete and the physician, it seems reasonable that selected athletes, who respond to the previous criteria and present the following characteristics may be allowed to participate in all competitive sport (with exception of those at intrinsic risk):

1. adult age, with long-term previous experience of sport participation
2. mild clinical expressions of HCM
3. absence of exercise-induced tachyarrhythmias
4. low ESC risk profile (<4).

Such athletes should be reviewed annually to assess symptoms and changes in risk profile. This recommendation should be viewed in the context of the cultural and customary medical care in place and should not override the existing medical and legal boundaries existing in the different countries (Class IIb; Level of Evidence C).

**Clinical Pearls**

- ECG is abnormal in 95% of adult athletes with HCM. T-wave inversion especially in inferior and lateral leads, and ST-segment depression, are an unlikely expression of physiologic LV hypertrophy and should be investigated with extensive cardiovascular imaging.
- Physiologic LV hypertrophy is always associated with cavity enlargement in athletes, so that the chamber geometry is preserved.
- The highest degree of LV hypertrophy is usually detected in male athletes engaged in endurance or mixed disciplines. Females usually show a lower degree of hypertrophy.
- Routine genetic testing is not recommended as a diagnostic tool for HCM but is advised only in patients already fulfilling the diagnostic criteria for HCM, to enable cascade genetic screening of their relatives.
- All patients with HCM should be fully informed of the clinical peculiarities of the disease and warned about the risks associated with sport participation.
- As recommended by the current guidelines HCM individuals should be discouraged to participate in competitive sports.

## Review

### Questions

1. In the presence of infero-lateral T waves, is a normal echocardiography enough or should the athlete undergo cardiac magnetic resonance?
2. Is left atrial dilatation a marker of HCM?
3. Should HCM individuals avoid any sport activity?

### Answers

1. Infero-lateral negative T waves are uncommon in athletes and a likely expression of a structural cardiovascular disease and most common HCM. Therefore, it is advised that a CMR is performed in order to exclude small areas of focal hypertrophy or fibrosis.
2. No. Left atrial enlargement has been described in athletes as an expression of global cardiac adaptation to training and is typically associated with increased LV size. Therefore, dilated left atrium is not a specific sign of HCM.

3. Competitive sports are not recommended by the current guidelines. A tailored non-competitive exercise program may be recommended based on careful assessment of risk profile.

## References


1. Maron BJ, Doerer JJ, Haas TS, Tierney DM, Mueller FO. Sudden deaths in young competitive athletes: analysis of 1866 deaths in the United States, 1980-2006. Circulation. 2009;119(8):1085–92.
2. Maron BJ, Haas TS, Ahluwalia A, Rutten-Ramos SC. Incidence of cardiovascular sudden deaths in Minnesota high school athletes. Heart Rhythm. 2013;10(3):374–7.
3. Maron BJ, Haas TS, Murphy CJ, Ahluwalia A, Rutten-Ramos S. Incidence and causes of sudden death in U.S. college athletes. J Am Coll Cardiol. 2014;63(16):1636–43.
4. Elliott PM, Anastasakis A, Borger MA, Borggrefe M, Cecchi F, Charron P, et al. 2014 ESC Guidelines on diagnosis and management of hypertrophic cardiomyopathy: the Task Force for the Diagnosis and Management of Hypertrophic Cardiomyopathy of the European Society of Cardiology (ESC). Eur Heart J. 2014;35(39):2733–79.
5. Pelliccia A, Maron BJ, Spataro A, Proschan MA, Spirito P. The upper limit of physiologic cardiac hypertrophy in highly trained elite athletes. N Engl J Med. 1991;324(5):295–301.
6. Caselli S, Maron MS, Urbano-Moral JA, Pandian NG, Maron BJ, Pelliccia A. Differentiating left ventricular hypertrophy in athletes from that in patients with hypertrophic cardiomyopathy. Am J Cardiol. 2014;114(9):1383–9.
7. Calore C, Zorzi A, Sheikh N, Nese A, Facci M, Malhotra A, et al. Electrocardiographic anterior T-wave inversion in athletes of different ethnicities: differential diagnosis between athlete's heart and cardiomyopathy. Eur Heart J. 2016;37:2515.
8. Papadakis M, Carre F, Kervio G, Rawlins J, Panoulas VF, Chandra N, et al. The prevalence, distribution, and clinical outcomes of electrocardiographic repolarization patterns in male athletes of African/Afro-Caribbean origin. Eur Heart J. 2011;32(18):2304–13.
9. Sheikh N, Papadakis M, Wilson M, Malhotra A, Adamuz C, Homfray T, et al. Diagnostic yield of genetic testing in young athletes with T-wave inversion. Circulation. 2018;138(12):1184–94.
10. Pelliccia A, Di Paolo FM, Quattrini FM, Basso C, Culasso F, Popoli G, et al. Outcomes in athletes with marked ECG repolarization abnormalities. N Engl J Med. 2008;358(2):152–61.
11. Calore C, Zorzi A, Corrado D. Clinical meaning of isolated increase of QRS voltages in hypertrophic cardiomyopathy versus athlete's heart. J Electrocardiol. 2015;48(3):373–9.
12. Caselli S, Pelliccia A, Maron M, Santini D, Puccio D, Marcantonio A, et al. Differentiation of hypertrophic cardiomyopathy from other forms of left ventricular hypertrophy by means of three-dimensional echocardiography. Am J Cardiol. 2008;102(5):616–20.
13. Sheikh N, Papadakis M, Schnell F, Panoulas V, Malhotra A, Wilson M, et al. Clinical profile of athletes with hypertrophic cardiomyopathy. Circ Cardiovasc Imaging. 2015;8(7):e003454.
14. Finocchiaro G, Dhutia H, D'Silva A, Malhotra A, Steriotis A, Millar L, et al. Effect of sex and sporting discipline on LV adaptation to exercise. J Am Coll Cardiol Img. 2017;10:965.
15. Sharma S, Maron BJ, Whyte G, Firoozi S, Elliott PM, McKenna WJ. Physiologic limits of left ventricular hypertrophy in elite junior athletes: relevance to differential diagnosis of athlete's heart and hypertrophic cardiomyopathy. J Am Coll Cardiol. 2002;40(8):1431–6.
16. Basavarajaiah S, Boraita A, Whyte G, Wilson M, Carby L, Shah A, et al. Ethnic differences in left ventricular remodeling in highly-trained athletes relevance to differentiating physiologic left ventricular hypertrophy from hypertrophic cardiomyopathy. J Am Coll Cardiol. 2008;51(23):2256–62.
17. Pelliccia A, Maron BJ, Culasso F, Spataro A, Caselli G. Athlete's heart in women. Echocardiographic characterization of highly trained elite female athletes. JAMA. 1996;276(3):211–5.

18. Rawlins J, Carre F, Kervio G, Papadakis M, Chandra N, Edwards C, et al. Ethnic differences in physiological cardiac adaptation to intense physical exercise in highly trained female athletes. Circulation. 2010;121(9):1078–85.
19. Caselli S, Di Paolo FM, Pisicchio C, Di Pietro R, Quattrini FM, Di Giacinto B, et al. Three-dimensional echocardiographic characterization of left ventricular remodeling in Olympic athletes. Am J Cardiol. 2011;108(1):141–7.
20. Pelliccia A, Culasso F, Di Paolo FM, Maron BJ. Physiologic left ventricular cavity dilatation in elite athletes. Ann Intern Med. 1999;130(1):23–31.
21. Maron MS. Clinical utility of cardiovascular magnetic resonance in hypertrophic cardiomyopathy. J Cardiovasc Magn Reson. 2012;14:13.
22. Maron MS, Olivotto I, Harrigan C, Appelbaum E, Gibson CM, Lesser JR, et al. Mitral valve abnormalities identified by cardiovascular magnetic resonance represent a primary phenotypic expression of hypertrophic cardiomyopathy. Circulation. 2011;124(1):40–7.
23. Maron MS, Olivotto I, Zenovich AG, Link MS, Pandian NG, Kuvin JT, et al. Hypertrophic cardiomyopathy is predominantly a disease of left ventricular outflow tract obstruction. Circulation. 2006;114(21):2232–9.
24. Caselli S, Montesanti D, Autore C, Di Paolo FM, Pisicchio C, Squeo MR, et al. Patterns of left ventricular longitudinal strain and strain rate in Olympic athletes. J Am Soc Echocardiogr. 2015;28(2):245–53.
25. Kansal MM, Lester SJ, Surapaneni P, Sengupta PP, Appleton CP, Ommen SR, et al. Usefulness of two-dimensional and speckle tracking echocardiography in "Gray Zone" left ventricular hypertrophy to differentiate professional football player's heart from hypertrophic cardiomyopathy. Am J Cardiol. 2011;108(9):1322–6.
26. Caselli S, Di Paolo FM, Pisicchio C, Pandian NG, Pelliccia A. Patterns of left ventricular diastolic function in Olympic athletes. J Am Soc Echocardiogr. 2015;28(2):236–44.
27. Sharma S, Elliott PM, Whyte G, Mahon N, Virdee MS, Mist B, et al. Utility of metabolic exercise testing in distinguishing hypertrophic cardiomyopathy from physiologic left ventricular hypertrophy in athletes. J Am Coll Cardiol. 2000;36(3):864–70.
28. Weiner RB, Wang F, Berkstresser B, Kim J, Wang TJ, Lewis GD, et al. Regression of "gray zone" exercise-induced concentric left ventricular hypertrophy during prescribed detraining. J Am Coll Cardiol. 2012;59(22):1992–4.
29. Pelliccia A, Maron BJ, De Luca R, Di Paolo FM, Spataro A, Culasso F. Remodeling of left ventricular hypertrophy in elite athletes after long-term deconditioning. Circulation. 2002;105(8):944–9.
30. Gersh BJ, Maron BJ, Bonow RO, Dearani JA, Fifer MA, Link MS, et al. 2011 ACCF/AHA Guideline for the Diagnosis and Treatment of Hypertrophic Cardiomyopathy: a report of the American College of Cardiology Foundation/American Heart Association Task Force on Practice Guidelines. Developed in collaboration with the American Association for Thoracic Surgery, American Society of Echocardiography, American Society of Nuclear Cardiology, Heart Failure Society of America, Heart Rhythm Society, Society for Cardiovascular Angiography and Interventions, and Society of Thoracic Surgeons. J Am Coll Cardiol. 2011;58(25):e212–60.
31. Harmon KG, Drezner JA, Wilson MG, Sharma S. Incidence of sudden cardiac death in athletes: a state-of-the-art review. Heart. 2014;100(16):1227–34.
32. Malhotra A, Dhutia H, Finocchiaro G, Gati S, Beasley I, Clift P, et al. Outcomes of cardiac screening in adolescent soccer players. N Engl J Med. 2018;379(6):524–34.
33. Alpert C, Day SM, Saberi S. Sports and exercise in athletes with hypertrophic cardiomyopathy. Clin Sports Med. 2015;34(3):489–505.
34. Lampert R, Olshansky B, Heidbuchel H, Lawless C, Saarel E, Ackerman M, et al. Safety of sports for athletes with implantable cardioverter-defibrillators: long-term results of a prospective multinational registry. Circulation. 2017;135(23):2310–2.
35. Saberi S, Wheeler M, Bragg-Gresham J, Hornsby W, Agarwal PP, Attili A, et al. Effect of moderate-intensity exercise training on peak oxygen consumption in patients with hypertrophic cardiomyopathy: a randomized clinical trial. JAMA. 2017;317(13):1349–57.

36. Klempfner R, Kamerman T, Schwammenthal E, Nahshon A, Hay I, Goldenberg I, et al. Efficacy of exercise training in symptomatic patients with hypertrophic cardiomyopathy: results of a structured exercise training program in a cardiac rehabilitation center. Eur J Prev Cardiol. 2015;22(1):13–9.
37. Pelliccia A, Lemme E, Maestrini V, Di Paolo FM, Pisicchio C, Di Gioia G, et al. Does sport participation worsen the clinical course of hypertrophic cardiomyopathy? Clinical outcome of hypertrophic cardiomyopathy in athletes. Circulation. 2018;137(5):531–3.
38. Spirito P, Autore C, Formisano F, Assenza GE, Biagini E, Haas TS, et al. Risk of sudden death and outcome in patients with hypertrophic cardiomyopathy with benign presentation and without risk factors. Am J Cardiol. 2014;113(9):1550–5.
39. Sinagra G, Anzini M, Pereira NL, Bussani R, Finocchiaro G, Bartunek J, et al. Myocarditis in clinical practice. Mayo Clin Proc. 2016;91(9):1256–66.
40. Pelliccia A, Solberg EE, Papadakis M, Adami PE, Biffi A, Caselli S, et al. Recommendations for participation in competitive and leisure time sport in athletes with cardiomyopathies, myocarditis, and pericarditis: position statement of the Sport Cardiology Section of the European Association of Preventive Cardiology (EAPC). Eur Heart J. 2019;40(1):19–33.

# Specific Cardiovascular Diseases and Competitive Sports Participation: Arrhythmogenic Right Ventricular Cardiomyopathy

14

Domenico Corrado, Alessandro Zorzi, and Gaetano Thiene

**Learning Objectives**

1. Understand the pathophysiology of arrhythmogenic cardiomyopathy and its role as a cause of sudden death in the young.
2. Learn how to diagnose arrhythmogenic cardiomyopathy and to recognize the different phenotypes.
3. Differentiate arrhythmogenic cardiomyopathy from athlete's heart.
4. Become familiar with risk stratification and management of arrhythmogenic cardiomyopathy.
5. Be able to understand the implications for sports eligibility and exercise prescription of patients with arrhythmogenic cardiomyopathy.

## 14.1 Introduction

Arrhythmogenic cardiomyopathy (ACM) is an inherited heart muscle disease characterized pathologically by fibrofatty myocardial replacement and clinically by prominent ventricular arrhythmias and impairment of ventricular systolic function [1]. Although the original disease phenotype was characterized by predominant right ventricular (RV) involvement, with minor and late left ventricle (LV) disease, clinical variants characterized by early and greater LV involvement, which may parallel (i.e. biventricular ACM) or exceed (i.e. left-dominant ACM) the severity of RV involvement, have been increasingly reported. These findings have led over the past few years to the increasing use of the broader term of "arrhythmogenic cardiomyopathy," which encompasses all the phenotypic expressions [2].

D. Corrado (✉) · A. Zorzi · G. Thiene
Department of Cardiac, Thoracic and Vascular Sciences and Public Health, University of Padova, Padova, Italy
e-mail: domenico.corrado@unipd.it; gaetano.thiene@unipd.it





A. Pressler, J. Niebauer (eds.), *Textbook of Sports and Exercise Cardiology*,
https://doi.org/10.1007/978-3-030-35374-2_14

The fibro-fatty myocardial scar acts as a substrate of ventricular electrical instability which may lead to arrhythmic cardiac arrest, mostly in young people [3, 4]. Life-threatening ventricular arrhythmias are triggered by physical exercise, and participation in competitive athletics has been associated with an increased risk for sudden cardiac death (SCD) (Fig. 14.1) [5–7]. In addition, sport activity has been implicated as a factor promoting acceleration of disease progression [8–10]. This

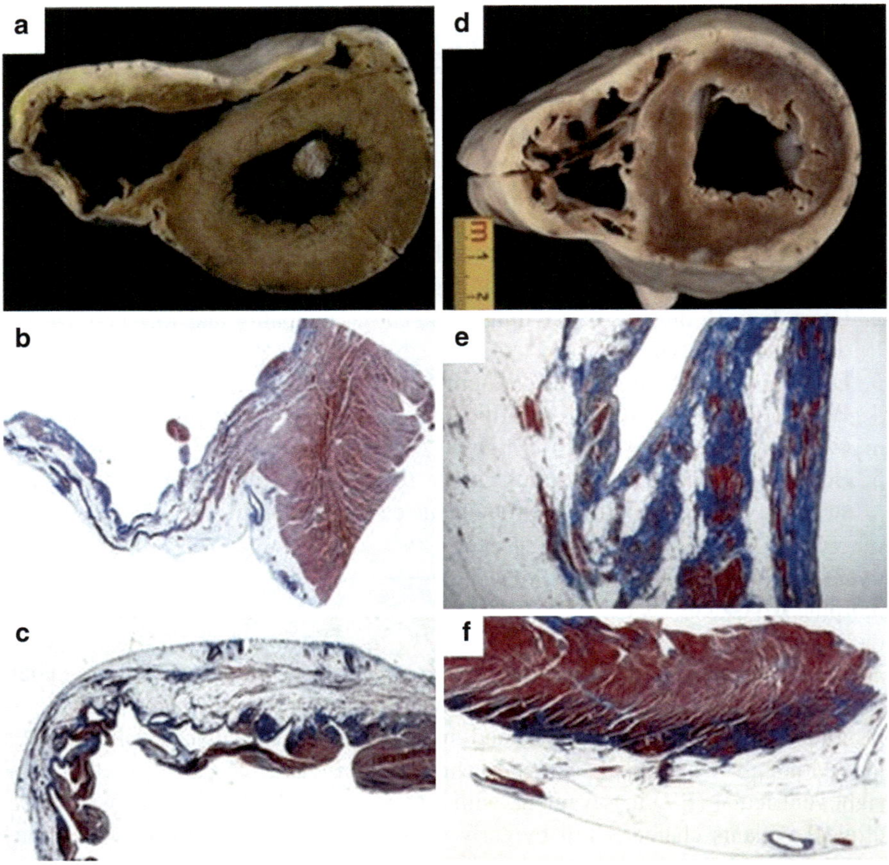


**Fig. 14.1** Pathologic features of arrhythmogenic cardiomyopathy. Classical right ventricular (RV) variant: (**a**) Gross transverse section of the heart that shows anterior and posterior RV wall thinning because of myocardial atrophy and a subtricuspidal aneurysm. Full-thickness histology of the posterior (**b**) and anterior (**c**) RV free wall that shows fibrofatty tissue replacement. There is thinning and residual myocardium confined to the endocardial trabeculae (trichrome stain). Biventricular variant: (**d**) Gross examination of a transverse section of the heart. Note the transmural RV free wall involvement as compared with the subepicardial midmural left ventricular (LV) free wall involvement. (**e**) Histology of the RV free wall confirms the transmural myocardial atrophy with fibrofatty replacement. (**f**) The histology of the LV free wall shows replacement-type fibrosis of the outer layer with preserved wall thickness (trichrome stain). (Reproduced with permission from Corrado D et al. [2])

chapter will examine the pathophysiology, natural history, diagnosis, prognosis and clinical management of ACM, with particular reference to the athletic population and relevance to risk of SCD during sports.

## 14.2 Disease Mechanism and Natural History

The prevalence of ACM is estimated to range from 1 case in 2000–5000 persons in the general population. Clinical presentation of ACM becomes clinically apparent between the second and fourth decades of life. The disease is more malignant in men and this has been in part ascribed to the sex-based differences in the amount or intensity of exercise [1, 2].

The disease process is characterized by

- the progressive loss of myocytes because of a genetically determined defect of the intercellular junction structures (desmosomes)
- subsequent fibrofatty replacement of the ventricular myocardium of both ventricles.

It has been postulated that the genetically-determined impairment of myocyte cell-to-cell adhesion may lead to tissue and organ fragility that is sufficient to promote myocyte death and subsequent fibrofatty repair, especially under conditions of mechanical stress such as those occurring during physical activity [4, 11]. The resulting alterations in the myocardial structure not only can impair the mechanical function of the ventricles but render affected individuals vulnerable to life-threatening ventricular arrhythmias. Patients may experience scar-related monomorphic ventricular tachycardia, which is caused by a re-entrant circuit related to the underlying fibrofatty ventricular scar [12]. Ventricular fibrillation and SCD may also occur in young patients during the so-called "hot phases" of the disease natural course, as a consequence of myocarditis-mediated bouts of acute myocyte death leading to acute electrical instability [4]. Loss of expression of desmosomal proteins might "per se" induce electrical myocardial instability by secondary sodium ion-channel dysfunction, and current reduction that predisposes to lethal ventricular arrhythmias even prior to the expression of an overt structural abnormality [13].

The natural history of the disease is typically characterized by four different phases:

1. "Concealed", characterised by the absence of subtle RV structural changes, with or without minor ventricular arrhythmias, during which SCD may occasionally be the first manifestation of the disease, mostly in young people during competitive sports or intense physical exercise.
2. "Overt electrical disorder" in which symptomatic RV arrhythmias possibly leading to sudden cardiac arrest are associated with overt RV functional and structural abnormalities.

3. "RV failure" caused by the progression and extension of RV muscle disease that provoke global RV dysfunction with relatively preserved LV function.
4. "Biventricular pump failure" caused by pronounced LV involvement. At this stage, ACM mimics biventricular dilated cardiomyopathy of other causes leading to congestive heart failure. A sizeable proportion of patients show early and severe LV involvement, which may either parallel ("biventricular") or exceed ("left dominant") the severity of RV disease [1, 2, 4, 11].

Exercise has been implicated as the most important environmental factor for promotion and progression of the ACM phenotypic expression: physical activity acutely increases the ventricular stress and accelerates the process of detachment, degeneration and death of genetically defective myocytes by disrupting intercellular junctions [4, 7, 11, 14]. In an animal model of plakoglobin-deficient mice, endurance training worsened the mechanical and electrical pathologic ventricular remodelling and induced RV dilatation, dysfunction and ventricular ectopy, supporting the concept that sport-related chronic ventricular overload might contribute to the development of the ACM phenotype in genetically susceptible individuals [15]. Studies in ACM-gene mutations carriers confirmed that endurance sports and sustained exercise increase age-related penetrance, risk of ventricular tachycardia/ventricular fibrillation and occurrence of heart failure. Moreover, in affected individuals physical activity is a strong pro-arrhythmic factor, because of adrenergic and mechanical stimulation of the diseased myocardium [7–10, 14].

It has been postulated that intense physical exertion may cause an ACM phenocopy characterized by dilatation and dysfunction of the RV in the absence of a pathological genetic substrate [16]. The theory, which has not been confirmed by other studies on large populations of highly trained athletes, was based on the study observations of a group of endurance athletes showing ventricular arrhythmias of RV origin and clinical features of underlying RV disease. However, the imaging features of the acquired phenocopy differed from those of desmosomal-gene related ACM, particularly due to the lack of RV wall motion abnormalities and fibrosis/late-gadolinium enhancement, which represent the distinctive pathologic abnormalities of ACM [17].

## 14.3 Diagnosis

The diagnosis is based on a series of criteria including

- histopathological manifestations
- alterations in cardiac structure and function
- electrocardiographic abnormalities
- arrhythmic manifestations
- identification of disease-causing genetic mutations (Figs. 14.2 and 14.3)

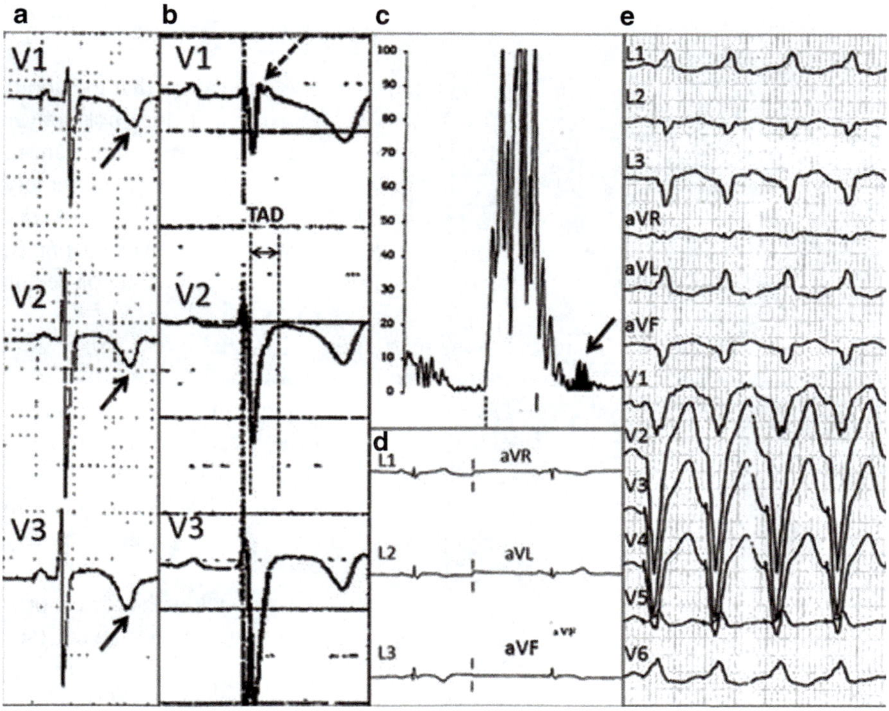


**Fig. 14.2** Electrocardiographic findings in arrhythmogenic cardiomyopathy. (**a**) Right precordial repolarization alterations characterized by negative T waves in leads $V_1$ through $V_3$ and (**b**) depolarization abnormalities consisting of epsilon waves (arrow) and prolongation of QRS complex because of delayed S-wave upstroke leading to a significant terminal activation delay (TAD). (**c**) Late potentials on signal-averaged ECG. (**d**) Low QRS voltages (<0.5 mV) in the limb leads. (**e**) Ventricular tachycardia with a left bundle brunch block and superior axis morphology. (Reproduced with permission from Corrado D et al. [2])

that were elaborated by an International Task Force of experts (Table 14.1) [18]. As no single criterion is accurate enough, the diagnosis requires a combination of criteria (classified as minor or major according to their specificity). Specifically, the diagnosis of "definite" disease is fulfilled in the presence of two major criteria, or, one major and two minor, or, four minor criteria from different categories. The diagnosis is considered "borderline" in the presence of one major and two minor criteria or three minor criteria, and "possible" when two minor criteria are met.

### 14.3.1 Classic Right Ventricular Phenotype

The classic phenotype is characterized by prevalent RV involvement with progressive fibro-fatty replacement of the ventricular myocardium, which is the histopathologic hallmark of the disease. Demonstration of fibrous or fibrofatty replacement on endomyocardial biopsy is the most specific diagnostic criteria [19].

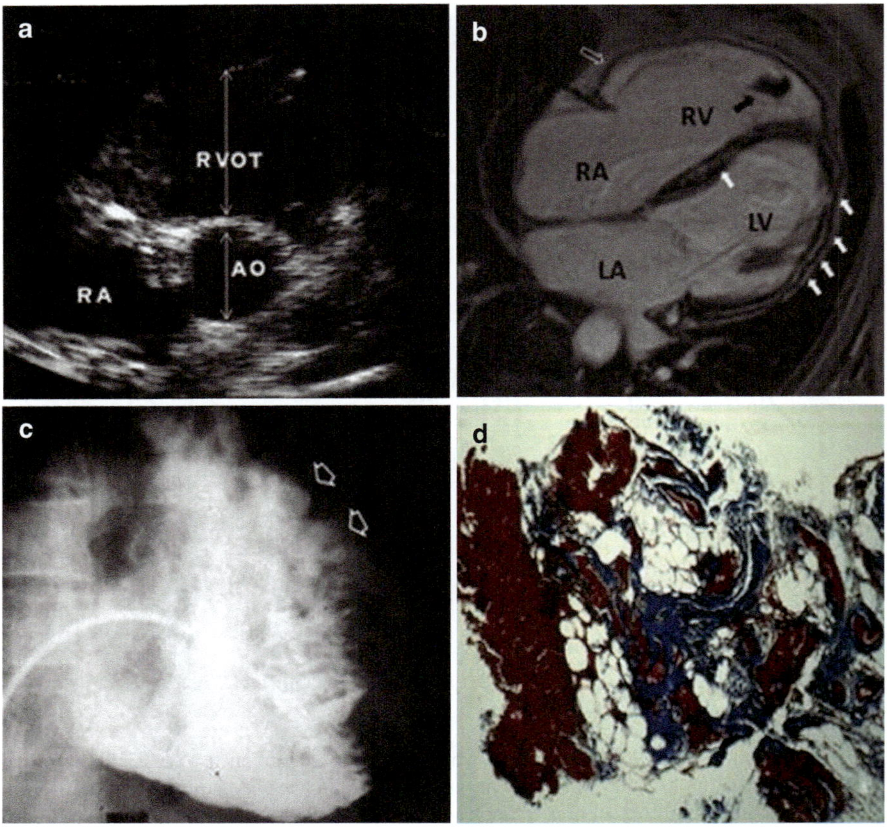


**Fig. 14.3** Imaging features of arrhythmogenic cardiomyopathy. Morphofunctional and histologic abnormalities on imaging and endomyocardial biopsy. (**a**) Two-dimensional echocardiogram (parasternal short-axis view), showing dilatation of the right ventricular outflow tract (PSAX-RVOT = 37 mm). (**b**) Diastolic frame of 4-chamber view on post-contrast sequences by cardiac magnetic resonance showing biventricular dilatation and wall thinning with evidence of a thrombus in the right ventricular (RV) apex (black arrow), diastolic bulging of the peritricuspid region (white empty arrow), and intramyocardial late gadolinium enhancement because of fibrofatty scar involving the left ventricular free wall (solid white arrows) and septum (solid white arrow). (**c**) Angiography showing RV dilatation with a bulging of the right ventricular outflow tract (arrows). (**d**) Endomyocardial biopsy revealing myocyte loss with fibrofatty replacement. Reproduced with permission from Corrado D et al. [2]. *AO* aorta, *LA* left atrial, *LV* left ventricle, *RA* right atrial

The process of progressive myocyte loss causes a gradual dilation and systolic dysfunction of the RV, initially at a regional level and, as the disease progresses, at a global level. The regional distribution of RV wall motion abnormalities (bulging, akinesis or diskinesis) is highly specific for ACM and allows differentiation from other RV conditions (e.g. congenital heart diseases, pulmonary hypertension, or athlete's heart), characterized by uniform dilation/dysfunction of the entire RV. Hence, imaging diagnosis of ACM requires demonstration of regional wall motion abnormalities [20].

**Table 14.1** International Task Force criteria for the diagnosis of arrhythmogenic cardiomyopathy

| |
|---|
| **1. Endomyocardial biopsy** |
| Major: |
| • *The total amount of the residual myocytes is less than 60% by morphometric analysis (or less than 50% if estimated), and the remaining of the free wall myocardium is replaced by fibrous tissue with or without fatty changes in more than one sample.* |
| Minor: |
| • *The total amount of the residual myocytes is 60% to 75% by morphometric analysis (or 50% to 65% if estimated), and the remaining of the free wall myocardium is replaced by fibrous tissue with or without fatty changes in more than one sample.* |
| **2. Right ventricular structural and functional abnormalities** |
| **A. Echocardiography** |
| Major:<br>• *Regional wall akinesis, diskinesis, or aneurismal dilatation of the RV*<br>plus one of the following:<br>*1. Right ventricular outflow tract more than 19 $mm/m^2$ in parasternal long axis view at the end diastole, or more than 21 $mm/m^2$ in parasternal short axis view at the end diastole*<br>*2. RV fractional area change <33%.* |
| Minor:<br>• *Regional wall akinesis or diskinesis*<br>plus one of the following:<br>*1. Right ventricular out flow tract of 16–19 $mm/m^2$ in parasternal short axis view at the end diastole or 18–21 $mm/m^2$ in parasternal short axis view at the end diastole*<br>*2. RV fractional area change 33–40%.* |
| **B. Cardiac magnetic resonance** |
| Major:<br>• *Regional wall akinesis or diskinesis or dyssynchronous contraction*<br>plus one of the following:<br>*1. Ejection fraction less than 40%,*<br>*2. End-diastolic volume t more than 110 $mL/m^2$ or more than 100 $mL/m^2$ in males and females, respectively.* |
| Minor:<br>• *Regional wall akinesis or diskinesis or dyssynchronous contraction*<br>plus one of the following:<br>*1. Ejection fraction less than 40%,*<br>*2. End-diastolic volume more than 110 $mL/m^2$ or more than 100 $mL/m^2$ in males and females, respectively.* |
| **B. Right ventricular angiography** |
| Major:<br>• *≥1 diskinetic, akinetic or aneurismatic right ventricular regions* |
| **3. Electrocardiographic repolarization abnormalities** |
| Major:<br>• *Inverted T waves in right precordial leads (V1, V2, and V3) or beyond in individuals >14 years of age (in the absence of complete right bundle-branch block QRS >120 ms).* |
| Minor:<br>• *Inverted T waves in leads V1 and V2 in individuals >14 years of age (in the absence of complete right bundle-branch block) or in V4, V5, or V6*<br>• *Inverted T waves in leads V1, V2, V3, and V4 in individuals >14 years of age in the presence of complete right bundle-branch block.* |

(continued)

**Table 14.1** (continued)

| |
|---|
| **4. Electrocardiographic depolarization abnormalities** |
| Major: |
| • *Epsilon wave (reproducible low-amplitude signals between end of QRS complex to onset of the T wave) in the right precordial leads (V1–V3).* |
| Minor: |
| • *Late potentials by Signal Averaged ECG in >1 of 3 parameters in the absence of a QRS duration of >110 ms on the standard ECG:* |
| 1. *Filtered QRS duration (fQRS) >114 ms.* |
| 2. *Duration of terminal QRS, 40 mV (low-amplitude signal duration) >38 ms* |
| 3. *Root-mean-square voltage of terminal 40 ms <20 mV* |
| • *Terminal activation duration of QRS > 55 ms measured from the nadir of the S wave to the end of the QRS, including R0, in V1, V2, or V3, in the absence of complete right bundle-branch block.* |
| **5. Arrhythmias** |
| Major: |
| • *Non-sustained or sustained ventricular tachycardia of left bundle-branch morphology with superior axis (negative or indeterminate QRS in leads II, III, and aVF and positive in lead aVL).* |
| Minor: |
| • *Non-sustained or sustained ventricular tachycardia of RV outflow configuration, left bundle-branch block morphology with inferior axis (positive QRS in leads II, III, and aVF and negative in lead aVL) or of unknown axis.* |
| • *>500 premature ventricular beats per 24 h (Holter).* |
| **6. Family history/genetics** |
| Major: |
| • *Positive family history of first-degree relative confirmed by current task force criteria.* |
| • *Pathological confirmation of the disease in first-degree relative either by autopsy or surgery.* |
| • *Discovering of a DNA pathogenic mutation that has been recognized to be associated or probably associated with ACM in the patient who has been evaluated for ACM.* |
| Minor: |
| • *Positive family history of first-degree relative in whom the diagnosis is not feasible to be confirmed by current Task Force criteria.* |
| • *Positive family history of young (<35 years) first degree relative with sudden death due to suspected ACM.* |
| • *Positive family history of disease in second degree relative who has been confirmed to have the disease either by current Task Force Criteria or pathologically.* |
| **Diagnosis** |
| ***Established*** |
| *At least two major criteria, one major criterion and three minor criteria, or four minor criteria from different categories* |
| ***Borderline*** |
| *One major criterion and two minor criteria, or three minor criteria from different categories* |
| ***Possible*** |
| *One major criterion or two minor criteria from different categories* |

Electrical abnormalities secondary to the fibro-fatty scarring process are also the basis for the typical ECG changes of ACM including depolarization (delayed intraventricular conduction with widening/slurring of the S wave in V1–V3, epsilon waves and late potentials) and/or repolarization (T wave inversion) abnormalities. Such features usually involve the right precordial leads (V1–V3/V4) [21].

Ventricular arrhythmias with a left-bundle branch block morphology (negative QRS complex in V1), suggestive of a RV origin, are another key feature of ACM [12]. However, arrhythmias originating from the RV outflow tract (negative QRS complex in V1 and inferior QRS axis in the limb leads) are less specific for ACM compared to those arising from other RV regions, because in the majority of cases are benign, non-familial and not related to an underlying cardiomyopathy ("idiopathic" RV outflow tract ventricular tachycardia) [22].

Finally, because of the genetic nature of the disease, a positive family history for SCD and/or ACM or the demonstration of a pathogenetic mutation in the genes encoding for desmosomal proteins represent a major diagnostic criterion.

### 14.3.2 Left-Dominant Phenotype

The classic ACM phenotype mostly involves the RV while morpho-functional abnormalities of the LV become evident only in the late stages of the disease. However, there are "left dominant" ACM variants characterized by early and predominant LV involvement, often because of specific genetic defects (i.e., mutations of genes encoding for desmoplakin, phospholamban, or filamin C) [1]. The phenotype is the counterpart of the classic variant, with

- T-wave inversion in the left precordial leads (V4–V6) and
- LV arrhythmias (right bundle branch block pattern, i.e. positive QRS complex in V1) [11].

A suggestive ECG finding is the presence of low QRS voltages (<0.5 mV) in the limb leads which reflects the reduction of the electrical activity of the LV wall due to fibro-fatty myocardial replacement. In contrast with the classic variant, the diagnostic power of echocardiography is limited because LV dilatation and systolic dysfunction, either regional or global, may be absent in patients with predominantly left-sided disease. The reason is that the fibro-fatty scarring process initially involves the sub-epicardial myocardial layers of the LV wall, which contribute marginally to the development of the contractile power and does not translate into prominent wall motion abnormalities or ejection fraction reduction. Therefore, the left-dominant ACM phenotype in isolation is difficult to diagnose and its incidence is probably underestimated. Contrast-enhanced cardiac magnetic resonance increases the diagnostic sensitivity because it allows identification of non-transmural LV scars (areas of late gadolinium enhancement) at a subepicardial and/or mid-mural level [23, 24].

### 14.3.3 Diagnosis in Athletes

The ultimate diagnosis of cardiomyopathy in a young competitive athlete may be problematic due to the presence of physiologic (and reversible) structural and electrical adaptations of the cardiovascular system to long-term athletic training.

This condition, known as "athlete's heart", is characterized by an increase in ventricular cavity dimension and wall thickness which may overlap with cardiomyopathies. In these circumstances, an accurate diagnosis is crucial because of the potentially adverse outcome associated with cardiomyopathy in an athlete and, conversely, the possibility of an erroneous diagnosis of a pathologic condition leading to unfair disqualifications from sport, with financial and psychological consequences. A sizable proportion of highly trained athletes have increased RV cavity dimensions which raises the question of ACM. Morphologic criteria in favour of a physiologic RV enlargement consist of preserved global and regional ventricular function, without evidence of wall motion abnormalities such as dyskinetic regions and/or diastolic bulging [25, 26]. During the last two decades, the advances in molecular genetics have allowed the identification of a growing number of defective desmosomal genes involved in the pathogenesis of ACM, and nowadays molecular genotyping is clinically available for differential diagnosis between desmosomal-gene related ACM and training-related physiologic RV changes. However, the presence of a large variety of polymorphisms and variants of uncertain significance of ACM-related genes makes it difficult to interpret the results of genetic testing (see also Chap. 12) [1, 27].

## 14.4 Prevention of Sudden Cardiac Death

Systematic monitoring and pathologic investigation of sudden death in young people and athletes of the Veneto Region of Italy showed that ACM is the most common pathologic substrate accounting for nearly a quarter of fatalities in young athletes and that the risk of sudden death from ACM is five times higher during competitive sports than during sedentary activity.

- The incidence of sudden death from ACM in athletes was estimated to be 0.5 per 100,000 persons per year. Sudden death victims with ACM were all males with a mean age of 22.6 ± 4 years [6].

Although ACM has been demonstrated to be the leading cause of SCD in athletes of the Veneto region of Italy, previous studies from other countries showed a higher prevalence of other pathologic substrates such as hypertrophic cardiomyopathy, anomalous coronary arteries and myocarditis [14, 28]. This discrepancy may be explained by several factors, including the experience of pathologists or coroners who perform post-mortem investigation of athletes who die suddenly. ACM is rarely associated with cardiomegaly and usually spares the LV, so that affected hearts may be erroneously diagnosed as normal hearts. Therefore, a number of SCDs in young people and athletes, in which the routine pathologic examination discloses a normal heart, may, in fact, be due to an unrecognised ACM. On the other hand, the high incidence of ACM in the Veneto region may be due to a genetic factor in the population of north-eastern Italy, although ACM can no longer be considered as peculiar

"Venetian disease" since there is growing evidence that it is ubiquitous and still largely underdiagnosed both clinically and at post-mortem investigation [29].

- The risk to die suddenly from ACM has been estimated to be 5.4 times greater during competitive sports than during sedentary activity and early identification of athletes with ACM plays a crucial role in the prevention of SCD during sport [6] (Fig. 14.4).

By reviewing clinical and ECG findings of 22 young competitive athletes who died suddenly from ACM proven at autopsy, it has been demonstrated that the majority of SCD victims exhibited ECG changes, ventricular arrhythmias, or both:

1. Right precordial T-waves inversion had been recorded in 88% of athletes.
2. Right precordial QRS duration >110 ms in 76%.
3. Ventricular arrhythmias with a left bundle branch block pattern in the form of isolated/coupled premature ventricular beats or non-sustained ventricular tachycardia in 76%.
4. Limited exercise testing induced ventricular arrhythmias in 50%.

Thus, the majority of young competitive athletes who died suddenly from ACM showed ECG abnormalities that could raise the suspicion of the underlying cardiovascular disease at preparticipation evaluation and could thus lead to further testing for a definitive diagnosis [11].

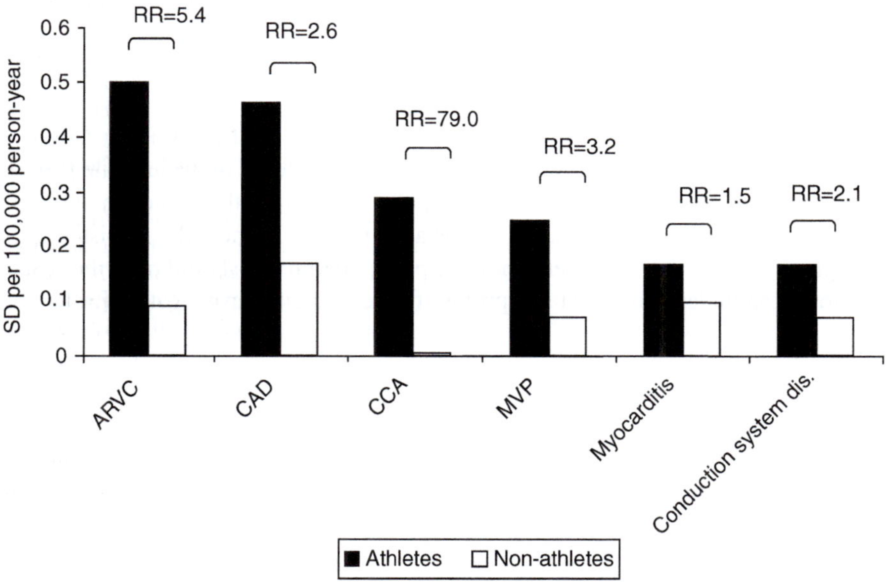


**Fig. 14.4** Incidence and relative risk (RR) of sudden death (SD) for specific cardiovascular causes among athletes and non-athletes. Reproduced with permission from Corrado D et al. [5]. *ARVC* arrhythmogenic right ventricular cardiomyopathy, *CAD* coronary artery disease, *CCA* congenital coronary artery anomaly, *MVP* mitral valve prolapse

For more than 20 years a systematic preparticipation screening, based on 12-lead ECG in addition to history and physical examination, has been the practice in Italy. A time-trend analysis of the incidence of SCD in young competitive athletes 12–35 year-old in the Veneto region of Italy between 1979 and 2004 has provided compelling evidence that ECG screening is a lifesaving strategy. The analysis demonstrated a 90% decrease of SCD in athletes after the introduction of the nationwide screening program. By comparison, the incidence of SCD in the unscreened nonathletic population of the same age did not change significantly over that time. Most of the mortality reduction was attributable to fewer deaths from hypertrophic cardiomyopathy and ACM. A parallel analysis of the causes of disqualifications from competitive sports at the Center for Sports Medicine in the Padua country area showed that the proportion of athletes identified and disqualified for cardiomyopathies doubled from the early- to the late-screening period. This indicates that mortality reduction was a reflection of a lower incidence of SCD from cardiomyopathies, as a result of increasing identification over time of affected athletes at ECG preparticipation screening [5].

## 14.5 Interpretation of Repolarization Abnormalities in Athletes

The 12-lead ECG is one of the most important tools for the disease diagnosis, follow-up and risk stratification. The inversion of the T-waves in the right precordial leads V1–V3/V4 and/or in the left infero-lateral leads is the most suggestive ECG sign. While inverted T-waves in the inferolateral leads are highly specific for a myocardial disease including left-dominant ACM, persistence of T-wave inversion in right precordial leads (known as persistence of the juvenile pattern of repolarization) may be occasionally observed in young athletes.

- It is noteworthy that the prevalence of a benign persistence of the juvenile pattern of repolarization declines sharply after puberty, whereas the clinical manifestations of cardiomyopathy usually occur after puberty. Hence, the persistence of right precordial T wave inversion in the post-pubertal age should raise the suspicion of an underlying ACM and prompt further imaging investigation [30].

Another cause of benign right precordial negative T waves in healthy athletes, especially of Afro-Caribbean descent, is an anterior early repolarization variant characterized by domed ST-segment elevation followed by negative T-wave in anterior leads V1–V4. The differential diagnosis requires careful analysis of the ST-segment morphology preceding the negative T-wave. Athletes exhibit J-point elevation (the hallmark of early repolarization), followed by an up-sloping ST-segment elevation with a domed morphology. On the other hand, ACM patients usually show no J-point elevation and no or minimal ST-segment elevation [31, 32] (Fig. 14.5).

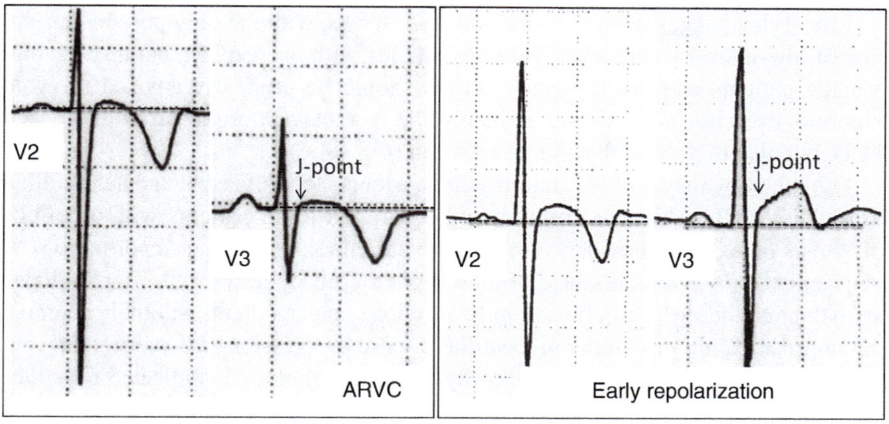


**Fig. 14.5** Differential diagnosis between cardiomyopathic negative T-waves and early repolarization of athlete's heart. Right-precordial leads V2–V3 of a patient with arrhythmogenic right ventricular cardiomyopathy (ACM) showing no J-point elevation and negative T-wave (**a**). Right-precordial leads V2–V3 of an Afro-Caribbean athlete showing an early repolarization pattern characterized by J-point elevation, dome ST-elevation and negative T-wave (**b**)

The clinical workup for differential diagnosis between pathological and non-pathological negative T waves traditionally includes electrocardiographic exercise testing. The current perception is that negative T waves usually revert to normal with exercise in healthy subjects whereas they persist in patients with structural heart muscle disease. However, the available data in favor of this concept are limited. In fact, by comparing ACM patients with healthy athletes with right precordial T wave inversion, the prevalence of complete or partial normalization of T wave polarity with exercise is observed in the majority of both groups [33].

## 14.6 Clinical Management

Patients with ACM should undergo lifelong clinical follow-up (every 6–24 months depending on the age, symptoms and disease severity) including echocardiography, 24-h Holter monitoring, and exercise testing to periodically evaluate new onset or worsening of symptoms, progression of morphological and/or functional ventricular abnormalities, and reassess the risk of SCD. Due to the age-related penetrance of ACM, healthy gene carriers and family members should also be offered repeat clinical assessment, mostly during adolescence and young adulthood. The four cornerstones of clinical management include:

1. Life-style changes
2. Drug therapy
3. Catheter ablation
4. ICD-Implantation

Life-style changes include restriction from sports, with the only possible exception of low-intensity activities. Not only patients with overt ACM, but also asymptomatic patients and healthy gene carriers should be prudently advised to avoid vigorous exercise, not only for reducing the risk of ventricular arrhythmias and SCD, but also to prevent disease progression (Fig. 14.6).

Drug therapy may include antiarrhythmic agents, beta-blockers, and heart failure drug therapy. Beta-blocker drugs should be offered to all patients with a definite diagnosis of ACM and evidence of morpho-structural ventricular abnormalities or ventricular arrhythmias because of their proven efficacy to prevent effort-induced arrhythmias, their proven efficacy in heart failure management, and their potential but unproven ability to hinder myocardial disease progression by lowering the ventricular wall stress. Adjunctive anti-arrhythmic drug therapy is indicated to reduce the arrhythmia burden in symptomatic patients with frequent premature ventricular

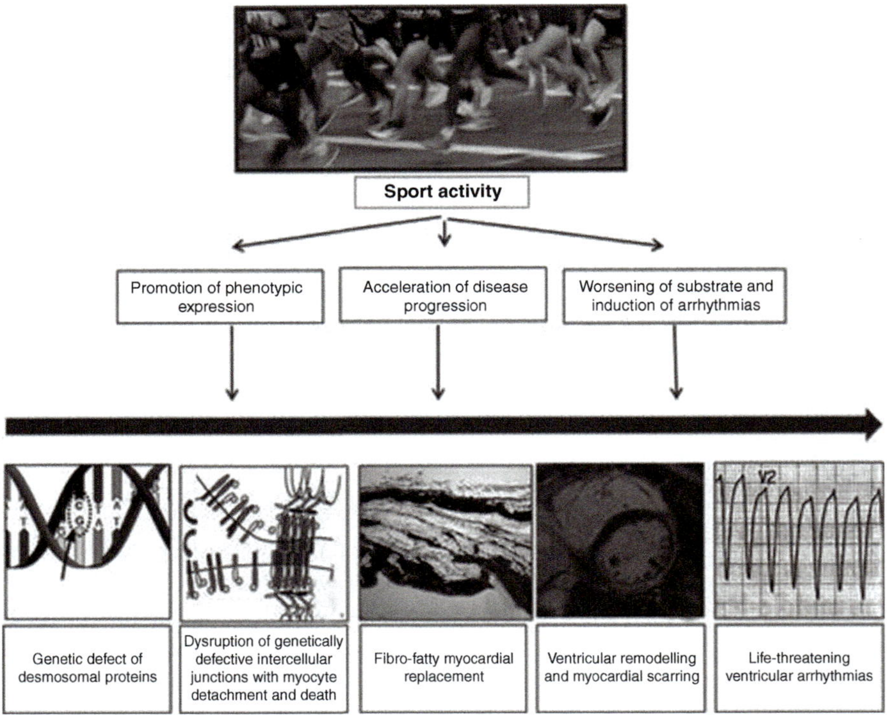


**Fig. 14.6** Impact of sports activity on arrhythmogenic cardiomyopathy. Schematic representation of natural history of arrhythmogenic cardiomyopathy from desmosomal gene mutation to phenotypic expression and life-threatening ventricular tachycardia. Sports activity may influence the disease course by promoting development of phenotypic expression, accelerating disease progression, and triggering malignant ventricular arrhythmias. (Reproduced with permission from Corrado D et al. [2])

beats and/or complex ventricular arrhythmia. For patients who developed heart failure, standard pharmacologic treatment with angiotensin-converting-enzyme inhibitors, angiotensin II receptor blockers, beta-blockers, and diuretics was prescribed as appropriate.

Catheter ablation is a therapeutic option for ACM patients who have recurrent ventricular tachycardia despite antiarrhythmic drug therapy. However, catheter ablation has not been proven to prevent SCD and should not be considered as an alternative to ICD therapy. Also, because of the progressive nature of the disease, repeated ablation procedures may be required to provide clinical control of ventricular arrhythmias.

Implantation of an implantable cardioverter defibrillator (ICD) is the most logical therapeutic strategy for patients with ACM, whose natural history is primarily characterised by the risk of arrhythmic cardiac arrest.

- There is general agreement that patients who survived an episode of ventricular fibrillation or sustained ventricular tachycardia most benefit from ICD implantation because of their high incidence of malignant arrhythmia recurrences.

Other risk factors identified by studies on ACM patients include

- unexplained syncope
- non-sustained VT on 24-h Holter monitoring
- systolic dysfunction of RV, LV, or both
- male gender
- compound and digenic heterozygosity of desmosomal-gene mutations
- young age at the time of diagnosis
- proband status
- inducibility at programmed ventricular stimulation
- amount of electroanatomic scar and electroanatomic scar-related fractionated electrograms
- extent of T-wave inversion across precordial and inferior leads
- low QRS amplitude and QRS fragmentation.

In patients with one of more of these risk factors, the decision to implant an ICD should be made on an individual basis, by assessing the overall clinical profile, the age, the strength of the risk factor identified, the level of SCD risk that is acceptable to the patient, and the potential risk of inappropriate interventions and complications. Finally, asymptomatic patients with no risk factors have a favourable long-term outcome regardless of familial history of SCD and electrophysiologic study findings. These results are particularly relevant for clinical management of the growing cohort of asymptomatic ACM patients or desmosomal gene mutation carriers [34] (Fig. 14.7).

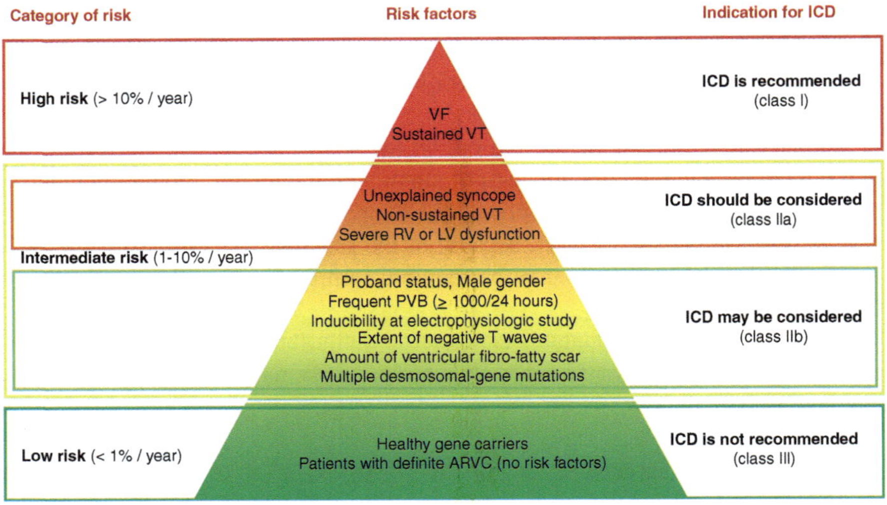


**Fig. 14.7** Pyramid of risk stratification in Arrhythmogenic Cardiomyopathy. Pyramid of risk and indications for implantable cardioverter defibrillator (ICD) therapy in arrhythmogenic cardiomyopathy. According to the available data on annual mortality rates associated to previous events and specific risk factors, the estimated risk of major arrhythmic events in the high-risk category (apex of pyramid) is >10% per year, in the intermediate-risk category (mid of pyramid) ranges from 1% to 10% per year and in the low-risk category (base of pyramid) is <1% per year. The recommendations for ICD implantation for different categories of arrhythmic risk are based on the 2015 International Task Force consensus document on treatment of arrhythmogenic right ventricular cardiomyopathy (ACM). Reproduced with permission from Corrado D et al. [2]. *LV* left ventricle, *PVB* premature ventricular beats, *RV* right ventricle, *VF* ventricular fibrillation, *VT* ventricular tachycardia

### 14.6.1 Eligibility to Sport Activity

According to current recommendations for sports eligibility, athletes with clinical diagnosis of ACM **should be excluded from all competitive sports** [34]. This recommendation is independent of age, gender, phenotype expression, symptoms, drug therapy, or interventions with surgery, catheter ablation, or implantable defibrillator. The presence of a free-standing automated external defibrillator at sporting events should not be considered absolute protection against sudden death, nor a justification for participation in competitive sports in athletes with ACM.

Patients with ACM may wish to participate in recreational and leisure-time exercise activity, given the recognized beneficial effects of a physically active lifestyle. It has been suggested that the absolute risk of ventricular tachyarrhythmias/death in patients practicing recreational sports does not significantly differ from that of physically inactive patients [10]. However, the conclusion that the recreational sports activity does not increase the risk of SCD or disease progression was not supported by adequate statistical power because of the small sample size.

- Thus, at the present time patients with a definitive diagnosis of ACM should be prudently restricted from participation in athletic activities, with the possible exception of recreational low intensity sports.

### 14.6.2 Implantable Cardioverter Defibrillator and Sports

The accurate prediction of the performance of ICD in athletes remains a challenging subject. Successful ICD therapy depends on a well-functioning device that is capable of both appropriate sensing of the malignant arrhythmia and delivering an adequate amount of energy to depolarize a critical myocardial mass to overcome the ongoing arrhythmic state. Sports may hinder the success of ICD therapy in many aspects:

1. Sinus tachycardia and other supraventricular tachyarrhythmias that are often present during sports activity represent an obstacle for appropriate differentiation of malignant ventricular arrhythmias.
2. Physical trauma whether due to direct or indirect contact may lead to device damage and malfunction.
3. Physiological changes associated with exertion such as high catecholamine levels, electrolyte imbalance, metabolic acidosis, and cardiac loading alterations can lead to persistent arrhythmogenic states in which defibrillation may not be successful (electrical storms) or—even worse—to SCD due to electromechanical dissociation where defibrillation will not be of any benefit [35].

The most compelling evidence on ICD efficacy and safety comes from a prospective, multinational Registry which recruited 372 athletes with an ICD from USA and Europe [36]. Over a median follow-up of 31 months, though ICD shocks occurred during and after sports participation, there were no arrhythmic deaths, resuscitated cardiac arrests, or shock-related injuries. The authors concluded that these data were similar to previously published data on non-athletic ICD patients and therefore do not support competitive sports restriction for all athletes with ICDs [36]. More recently, the same Authors confirmed these outcomes in the athletes enrolled in the same Registry over a long-term follow-up (44 months) [37]. The pro-arrhythmic effect of sports activity accounted for the occurrence of appropriate shocks respectively in 11% of participants during exercise and in 6% at rest. An underlying ARVC was the only variable associated with exercise-induced ICD shock.

Despite these reassuring data, it must be emphasized that the reasons for implementing restrictions from competition in sports in young athletes with ICD go beyond the increased risk of inappropriate interventions, injury to the patient, and damage of the system. Sports participation plays a major role in the disease progression, worsening of the substrate and adverse outcome. Although evidence has emerged in support of the safety of competitive sports in selected individuals carrying ICD, it is prudent to restrict competitive sports participation in ACM patients.

**Clinical Pearls**

- The natural history of arrhythmogenic cardiomyopathy progresses from a concealed phase to an overt disease characterized by ventricular arrhythmias and ventricular wall motion abnormalities. Exercise has been implicated as the most important environmental factor for progression of the disease.
- The diagnosis of arrhythmogenic cardiomyopathy is multiparametric and requires a combination of family history, electrocardiographic abnormalities, ventricular arrhythmias, regional right ventricular dilation/dysfunction associated with wall motion abnormalities and/or positive endomyocardial biopsy. No single criterion is accurate enough to support the diagnosis if present in isolation.
- The available scientific evidence suggests that patients with a definitive diagnosis of arrhythmogenic cardiomyopathy should be prudently restricted from participation in athletic activities, irrespective from ICD implantation, with the possible exception of recreational low intensity sports.

## Review

### Questions

1. A 19-year-old female dancer with a family history of arrhythmogenic cardiomyopathy was referred for frequent premature ventricular beats with a right-bundle-branch block morphology that increase in number and complexity with increasing workload during exercise testing. Resting electrocardiogram and echocardiography are unremarkable. Should other investigations be prescribed?
2. A 25-year-old black highly-trained competitive asymptomatic athlete shows T-wave inversion preceded by J-point and ST-segment elevation in V1–V3. Echocardiography shows a mildly dilated right ventricle in the absence of regional wall motion abnormalities. Is this pattern suggestive of arrhythmogenic cardiomyopathy?
3. A 36-year-old asymptomatic athlete has been diagnosed with definite arrhythmogenic cardiomyopathy. There is no family history of sudden death, only isolated premature ventricular beats are recorded during exercise test and 24-h Holter monitoring and echocardiography showed only a mild right ventricular dysfunction. Should he/she be allowed to engage in competitive non-professional soccer?

### Answers

1. The presence of premature ventricular beats with a right-bundle-branch block morphology, suggesting the origin from the left ventricular wall, in a young patient with a family history of arrhythmogenic cardiomyopathy may be the sign of an underlying left ventricular involvement. Echocardiography may not be

sensitive enough to detect segmental fibrofatty scarring of the left ventricle. Hence, prescription of a contrast-enhanced cardiac magnetic resonance is reasonable.

2. No, the presence of T-wave inversion preceded by J-point/ST-segment elevation is consistent with an early repolarization variant typical of black athletes. Moreover, a mildly dilated right ventricle without regional wall motion abnormalities is a usual finding in highly-trained athletes and does not support the diagnosis of arrhythmogenic cardiomyopathy.
3. There are two reasons for excluding patients with arrhythmogenic cardiomyopathy from all competitive sports. First, the risk of sudden death. Second, the fact that high-intensity exercise has been implicated as the most important environmental factor for progression of the disease.

## References

1. Corrado D, Link MS, Calkins H. Arrhythmogenic right ventricular cardiomyopathy. N Engl J Med. 2017;376(1):61–72.
2. Corrado D, Basso C, Judge DP. Arrhythmogenic cardiomyopathy. Circ Res. 2017;121(7):784–802.
3. Thiene G, Nava A, Corrado D, Rossi L, Pennelli N. Right ventricular cardiomyopathy and sudden death in young people. N Engl J Med. 1988;318(3):129–33.
4. Basso C, Bauce B, Corrado D, Thiene G. Pathophysiology of arrhythmogenic cardiomyopathy. Nat Rev Cardiol. 2012;9(4):223–33.
5. Corrado D, Basso C, Pavei A, Michieli P, Schiavon M, Thiene G. Trends in sudden cardiovascular death in young competitive athletes after implementation of a preparticipation screening program. JAMA. 2006;296(13):1593–601.
6. Corrado D, Basso C, Rizzoli G, Schiavon M, Thiene G. Does sports activity enhance the risk of sudden death in adolescents and young adults? J Am Coll Cardiol. 2003;42(11):1959–63.
7. Corrado D, Zorzi A. Arrhythmogenic right ventricular cardiomyopathy and sports activity. Eur Heart J. 2015;36(27):1708–10.
8. James CA, Bhonsale A, Tichnell C, Murray B, Russell SD, Tandri H, et al. Exercise increases age-related penetrance and arrhythmic risk in arrhythmogenic right ventricular dysplasia/cardiomyopathy-associated desmosomal mutation carriers. J Am Coll Cardiol. 2013;62(14):1290–7.
9. Saberniak J, Hasselberg NE, Borgquist R, Platonov PG, Sarvari SI, Smith HJ, et al. Vigorous physical activity impairs myocardial function in patients with arrhythmogenic right ventricular cardiomyopathy and in mutation positive family members. Eur J Heart Fail. 2014;16:1337.
10. Ruwald AC, Marcus F, Estes NA III, Link M, McNitt S, Polonsky B, et al. Association of competitive and recreational sport participation with cardiac events in patients with arrhythmogenic right ventricular cardiomyopathy: results from the North American multidisciplinary study of arrhythmogenic right ventricular cardiomyopathy. Eur Heart J. 2015;36:1735.
11. Basso C, Corrado D, Marcus F, Nava A, Thiene G. Arrhythmogenic right ventricular cardiomyopathy. Lancet. 2009;373:1289–300.
12. Lemola K, Brunckhorst C, Helfenstein U, Oechslin E, Jenni R, Duru F. Predictors of adverse outcome in patients with arrhythmogenic right ventricular dysplasia/cardiomyopathy: long term experience of a tertiary care centre. Heart. 2005;91(9):1167–72.
13. Cerrone M, Lin X, Zhang M, Agullo-Pascual E, Pfenniger A, Chkourko Gusky H, et al. Missense mutations in plakophilin-2 cause sodium current deficit and associate with a brugada syndrome phenotype. Circulation. 2014;129(10):1092–103.

14. Zorzi A, Pelliccia A, Corrado D. Inherited cardiomyopathies and sports participation. Neth Heart J. 2018;26(3):154–65.
15. Kirchhof P, Fabritz L, Zwiener M, Witt H, Schafers M, Zellerhoff S, et al. Age- and training-dependent development of arrhythmogenic right ventricular cardiomyopathy in heterozygous plakoglobin-deficient mice. Circulation. 2006;114(17):1799–806.
16. La Gerche A, Burns AT, Mooney DJ, Inder WJ, Taylor AJ, Bogaert J, et al. Exercise-induced right ventricular dysfunction and structural remodelling in endurance athletes. Eur Heart J. 2012;33(8):998–1006.
17. La Gerche A, Robberecht C, Kuiperi C, Nuyens D, Willems R, de Ravel T, et al. Lower than expected desmosomal gene mutation prevalence in endurance athletes with complex ventricular arrhythmias of right ventricular origin. Heart. 2010;96(16):1268–74.
18. Marcus FI, McKenna WJ, Sherrill D, Basso C, Bauce B, Bluemke DA, et al. Diagnosis of arrhythmogenic right ventricular cardiomyopathy/dysplasia: proposed modification of the task force criteria. Circulation. 2010;121(13):1533–41.
19. Basso C, Ronco F, Marcus F, Abudureheman A, Rizzo S, Frigo AC, et al. Quantitative assessment of endomyocardial biopsy in arrhythmogenic right ventricular cardiomyopathy/dysplasia: an in vitro validation of diagnostic criteria. Eur Heart J. 2008;29(22):2760–71.
20. Yoerger DM, Marcus F, Sherrill D, Calkins H, Towbin JA, Zareba W, et al. Echocardiographic findings in patients meeting task force criteria for arrhythmogenic right ventricular dysplasia: new insights from the multidisciplinary study of right ventricular dysplasia. J Am Coll Cardiol. 2005;45(6):860–5.
21. Steriotis AK, Bauce B, Daliento L, Rigato I, Mazzotti E, Folino AF, et al. Electrocardiographic pattern in arrhythmogenic right ventricular cardiomyopathy. Am J Cardiol. 2009;103(9):1302–8.
22. O'Donnell D, Cox D, Bourke J, Mitchell L, Furniss S. Clinical and electrophysiological differences between patients with arrhythmogenic right ventricular dysplasia and right ventricular outflow tract tachycardia. Eur Heart J. 2003;24(9):801–10.
23. Zorzi A, Perazzolo Marra M, Rigato I, De Lazzari M, Susana A, Niero A, et al. Nonischemic left ventricular scar as a substrate of life-threatening ventricular arrhythmias and sudden cardiac death in competitive athletes. Circ Arrhythm Electrophysiol. 2016;9(7):e004229.
24. Sen-Chowdhry S, Syrris P, Prasad SK, Hughes SE, Merrifield R, Ward D, et al. Left-dominant arrhythmogenic cardiomyopathy: an under-recognized clinical entity. J Am Coll Cardiol. 2008;52(25):2175–87.
25. Bauce B, Frigo G, Benini G, Michieli P, Basso C, Folino AF, et al. Differences and similarities between arrhythmogenic right ventricular cardiomyopathy and athlete's heart adaptations. Br J Sports Med. 2010;44(2):148–54.
26. D'Ascenzi F, Solari M, Corrado D, Zorzi A, Mondillo S. Diagnostic differentiation between arrhythmogenic cardiomyopathy and athlete's heart by using imaging. JACC Cardiovasc Imaging. 2018;11(9):1327–39.
27. Corrado D, Thiene G. Arrhythmogenic right ventricular cardiomyopathy/dysplasia: clinical impact of molecular genetic studies. Circulation. 2006;113(13):1634–7.
28. Maron BJ. Sudden death in young athletes. N Engl J Med. 2003;349(11):1064–75.
29. Elmaghawry M, Alhashemi M, Zorzi A, Yacoub MH. A global perspective of arrhythmogenic right ventricular cardiomyopathy. Glob Cardiol Sci Pract. 2012;2012(2):81–92.
30. Migliore F, Zorzi A, Michieli P, Perazzolo Marra M, Siciliano M, Rigato I, et al. Prevalence of cardiomyopathy in Italian asymptomatic children with electrocardiographic T-wave inversion at preparticipation screening. Circulation. 2012;125(3):529–38.
31. Corrado D, Pelliccia A, Heidbuchel H, Sharma S, Link M, Basso C, et al. Recommendations for interpretation of 12-lead electrocardiogram in the athlete. Eur Heart J. 2010;31(2):243–59.
32. Calore C, Zorzi A, Sheikh N, Nese A, Facci M, Malhotra A, et al. Electrocardiographic anterior T-wave inversion in athletes of different ethnicities: differential diagnosis between athlete's heart and cardiomyopathy. Eur Heart J. 2016;37(32):2515–27.
33. Zorzi A, ElMaghawry M, Rigato I, Cardoso Bianchini F, Crespi Ponta G, Michieli P, et al. Exercise-induced normalization of right precordial negative T waves in arrhythmogenic right ventricular cardiomyopathy. Am J Cardiol. 2013;112(3):411–5.

34. Corrado D, Wichter T, Link MS, Hauer RN, Marchlinski FE, Anastasakis A, et al. Treatment of arrhythmogenic right ventricular cardiomyopathy/dysplasia: an international task force consensus statement. Circulation. 2015;132(5):441–53.
35. Corrado D, Migliore F, Zorzi A. Sport activity in patients with implantable defibrillator: playing with death? Eur J Prev Cardiol. 2019;26:760.
36. Lampert R, Olshansky B, Heidbuchel H, Lawless C, Saarel E, Ackerman M, et al. Safety of sports for athletes with implantable cardioverter-defibrillators: results of a prospective, multinational registry. Circulation. 2013;127(20):2021–30.
37. Lampert R, Olshansky B, Heidbuchel H, Lawless C, Saarel E, Ackerman M, et al. Safety of sports for athletes with implantable cardioverter-defibrillators: long-term results of a prospective multinational registry. Circulation. 2017;135(23):2310–2.

# Specific Cardiovascular Diseases and Competitive Sports Participation: Left Ventricular Hypertrabeculation

15

Catherine Sedgwick and Sabiha Gati

**Learning Objectives**

1. Define Left Ventricular Non-Compaction (LVNC) and differentiate it from other cardiomyopathies.
2. Explain the likely pathogenesis of LVNC: abnormal myocardial morphogenesis or a sporadic, acquired phenomenon?
3. Understand the different criteria for diagnosing LVNC in both echocardiography and cardiac magnetic resonance imaging modalities.
4. Explain why pregnant women and athletes are more susceptible to LVNC.
5. Describe how an athlete exhibiting signs of LVNC should be investigated and managed.

## 15.1 Introduction

Left Ventricular Non-Compaction (LVNC) is a relatively rare cardiac condition which is characterised by prominent trabeculations and deep recesses in the myocardial tissue of the left ventricle. The precise stage of development of LVNC and the natural history of the disorder is poorly understood, however it can be congenital or acquired and is thought to be reversible [1]. LVNC features can be observed in healthy individuals with normal left ventricular function and dimensions [2–6]. There appears to be an association between LV hypertrabeculation and increased cardiac preload as observed in athletic cohorts and pregnant women [3, 4, 6].

C. Sedgwick
Cardiology Clinical and Academic Group, St Georges, University of London, London, UK
e-mail: catherine.sedgwick1@nhs.net

S. Gati (✉)
Department of Cardiology/Cardiac MRI, Royal Brompton & Harefield NHS Trust & National Heart and Lung Institute, Imperial College, London, UK
e-mail: sabiha.gati@nhs.net



A. Pressler, J. Niebauer (eds.), *Textbook of Sports and Exercise Cardiology*,
https://doi.org/10.1007/978-3-030-35374-2_15

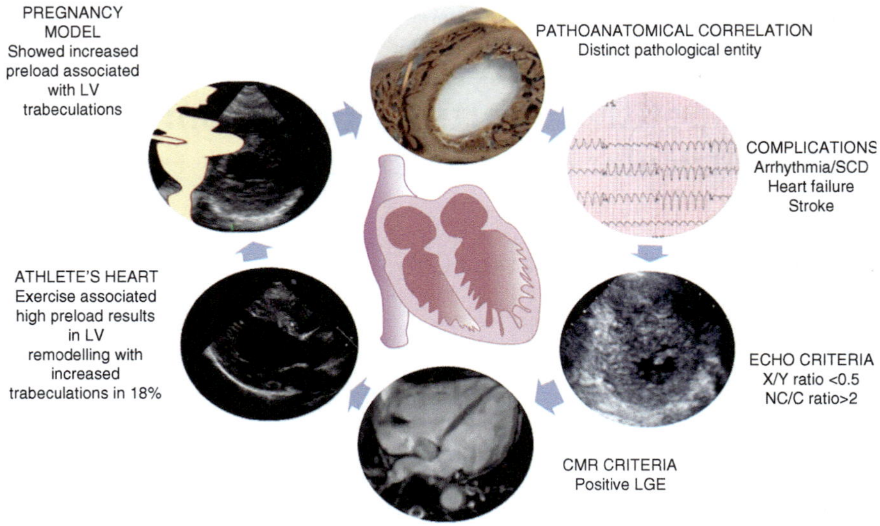


**Fig. 15.1** Central Illustration. Summary of the key features of left ventricular non-compaction. *LGE* late gadolinium enhancement, *LV* left ventricular, *SCD* sudden cardiac death

Athletic individuals are usually asymptomatic and are often diagnosed incidentally during routine preparticipation evaluation. Currently, there is no gold standard criteria for the diagnosis of LVNC, regardless of whether it is based on an echocardiographic definition or cardiac magnetic resonance imaging [1]. As a high proportion of athletes meet the criteria for a diagnosis of LVNC without exhibiting other clinical features of the disorder, it may be that increased left ventricular trabeculations are of limited significance in this group and simply form part of the 'athlete's heart' (Fig. 15.1: **central illustration**) [3]. Recent recommendations for athletes participating in competitive sport have been issued by the Sport Cardiology Section of the European Association of Preventive Cardiology (EAPC), offering guidance in the management of athletes with a suspected diagnosis of LVNC [7].

## 15.2 Definition

LVNC is characterised by conspicuous myocardial trabeculations and deep recesses that communicate with the left ventricular cavity [8]. On pathological specimens, a double-layered myocardium shows a compacted outer layer and an inner, non-compacted trabeculated layer [9, 10].

However, LVNC is not regarded as a distinct cardiomyopathy as it can be observed in healthy individuals with normal left ventricular function and dimensions, and is reversible [4]. LVNC still remains an unclassified cardiac condition because it is genetically heterogeneous and overlaps with other cardiomyopathies, cardiac conditions and even neuromuscular disease [1]. The precise stage of development of LVNC and the natural history of the disease is not yet fully understood.

There is some evidence to suggest that LVNC has a genetic basis although there is modest correlation between the genotypes and phenotypes of the disease [11, 12]. However, an alternative explanation of the features of LVNC may simply be attributed to increased cardiac preload, as demonstrated in the pregnancy model [4].

## 15.3 Epidemiology

### 15.3.1 Prevalence

The prevalence of LVNC is thought to be less than 0.3% of the population [13, 14].

## 15.4 Clinical Manifestations of LVNC

LVNC can manifest as a progressive LV dilatation, impairment in systolic function, predisposition to serious cardiac arrhythmias and systemic thromboembolism [15]. Athletic individuals are usually asymptomatic and are often diagnosed incidentally during routine testing when a conspicuous myocardial trabecular pattern is observed on cardiac imaging [3].

- *Systemic heart failure*
  A high prevalence of LV trabeculations has been observed in patients with heart failure, fulfilling the criteria for a diagnosis of LVNC, irrespective of the criterion used [16, 17].
- *Ventricular arrhythmias and sudden cardiac death*
  LVNC leads to a predisposition to ventricular tachyarrhythmias and sudden cardiac death [13].
- *Thromboembolic events*
  Individuals with LVNC are at a greater risk of thromboembolic events [13].

## 15.5 Pathogenesis of LVNC

There is a debate as to whether LVNC is a congenital abnormality or a sporadic, acquired phenomenon.

### 15.5.1 Abnormal Myocardial Morphogenesis In Utero

In early embryological development, the myocardium consists of a spongy network of recesses and trabeculations that interconnect with the left ventricular cavity [8]. Between weeks 5 and 8, the normal myocardium becomes compacted from base to apex and from the epicardial to endocardial layers. This compaction process causes involution of the trabeculations and converts the intertrabecular recess into capillaries, which later form the coronary vessels at 12–18 weeks [15].

However, in LVNC, it is postulated that this process of myocardial compaction is disrupted in some way, with the most severe cases occurring with an arrest of compaction in the earlier stages of development. In these cases, the relaxed appearance of the myocardium persists following delivery and results in the development of two discrete myocardial layers. LVNC may appear in isolation or may be linked with other congenital heart conditions associated with an increased cardiac preload.

### 15.5.2 Sporadic and Acquired

Alternatively, LVNC may be a sporadic, acquired disorder. Several case studies have demonstrated the development of new LV trabeculations during serial echocardiography. A study by Bleyl et al. [18] examined three infants with no evidence of LVNC on echocardiography who later went on to develop the disease.

- Possible explanations for LVNC as an acquired phenomenon could include:
  - A metabolic disorder or dysfunction of the microcirculation, resulting in myocardial ischaemia, producing a heightened trabecular response and clinical features of LVNC [1].
  - Myocarditis, causing midwall or subepicardial fibrosis and new LV trabeculations [1].
  - Chronic renal failure, sickle cell anaemia or heart valve disease, resulting in an increase in cardiac preload and afterload, and an increase in myocardial trabeculations (Fig. 15.2) [1, 4, 5, 19]. LVNC is observed in 30% of patients with valvular heart disease and 24% of patients with heart failure [20]. 8% of patients with sickle cell anaemia are observed to have the disease [5].
  - Ethnicity is a known factor as black individuals are found to have an 8% likelihood of displaying LVNC, although the aetiology remains unclear [3, 16].

In pregnancy, there is a 100% increase in circulating blood volume. In a study by Gati et al. [4], 102 pregnant women were observed to have normal echocardiograms at their booking visit. Participants were scanned in each trimester and 26 (25%) women were found to have myocardial trabeculations consistent with a diagnosis of LVNC by delivery. At 2 years follow up, 19 (73%) of participants had complete resolution of these trabeculations and six women had a marked reduction in the trabeculated layer of their myocardium. These observations support the assertion that a cardiomyopathy is not necessarily present in asymptomatic individuals who meet the diagnostic criteria for LVNC and, in the case of pregnant women, increased LV trabeculations are thought to be a benign, physiological response to increased cardiac preload.

Similarly, in a recent study of over 1000 asymptomatic athletic individuals, 18% were observed to have increased LV trabeculations, with 8% fulfilling the echocardiographic criteria for LVNC [3]. However, only 0.9% of those athletes diagnosed with LVNC had definitive electrocardiogram changes such as T-wave inversion.

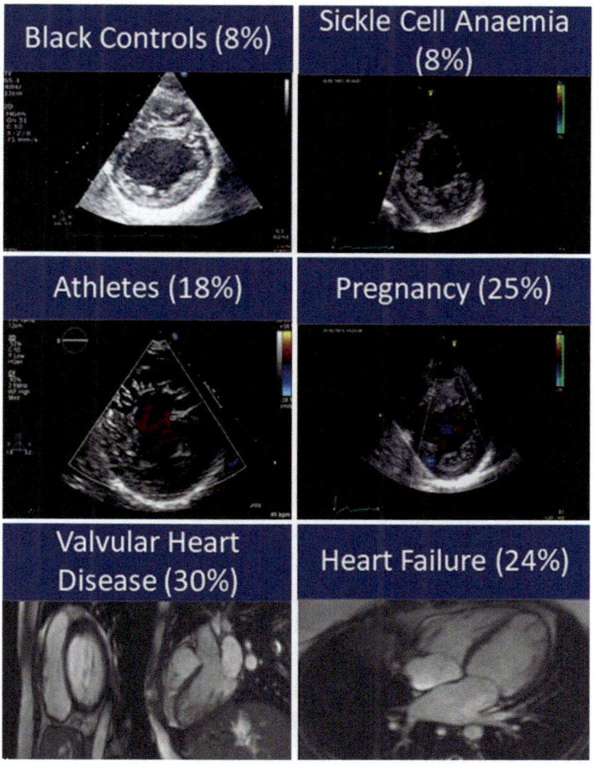


**Fig. 15.2** The estimated prevalence of increased left ventricular trabeculation in various cohorts including African/afro-Caribbean controls, healthy athletes, pregnancy and disease processes such as sickle cell anemia, heart failure and valvular heart disease

These results may suggest an incomplete expression of LVNC clinical features in predisposed athletes or they may simply represent a cardiac adaptation to exercise.

Increased myocardial trabeculations are likely to be a combination of genetic and acquired factors. An individual whose myocardium remodels as a result of increased cardiac preload or afterload is likely to have a genetic susceptibility to do so. It has also been postulated that myocardial non-compaction may be a compensatory mechanism in individuals with genetic myocardial contraction dysfunction.

## 15.6 Diagnosis of LVNC

There is no gold standard for the diagnosis of LVNC at present. Current diagnostic criteria is based on the ratio of compacted versus non-compacted left ventricular myocardium on echocardiography [14, 21, 22]. Cardiac magnetic resonance imaging modalities present with three different methods of LVNC assessment incorporating non-compacted to compacted ratio, LV trabecular mass and fractal analysis [23–25]. The presence of left ventricular systolic dysfunction, a thin epicardial layer and abnormal myocardial relaxation would support a pathological diagnosis. However, existing diagnostic criteria are based on a selection of small studies and there is a risk of overdiagnosing LVNC based on the current definitions [1].

## 15.7 Echocardiography

### 15.7.1 Echocardiography Criteria

Two-dimensional echocardiography is the current mainstay of diagnosis. There are three established echocardiography criteria for the diagnosis of LVNC, all of which describe increased trabeculations in the left ventricle and a double-layered myocardium—with an outer compacted layer and an inner non-compacted layer (Fig. 15.3). The exact area of compaction and non-compaction, and the timing of where in the cardiac cycle to measure these areas, differs between them. The most commonly used criteria in clinical practice is the Jenni et al. definition, outlined below.

- **Chin et al.**
  Chin et al. [22] offered the first echocardiographic criteria for the diagnosis of LVNC. Their study was based on eight paediatric cases and eight normal controls, validated by autopsy. They defined LVNC as $X/Y \leq 0.5$ (at end diastole), where: $X$ = the compacted later, i.e., the distance between the epicardial surface and the trough of the trabeculae; and $Y$ = the compacted layer plus the non-compacted layer, i.e., the distance between the epicardial surface and the highest point of the trabeculae. In patients with LVNC, a progressive decline in the X/Y ratio from the base to apex was noted. This was not observed in the control group. More recent studies suggest that a ratio of 0.5 would define LVNC, based on measurements from the parasternal short-axis view on echocardiography. The criteria proposed by Chin et al. [22] does not require a minimum number of trabeculae, the need to perfuse the intertrabecular recesses, nor a location for the non-compacted segments.
- **Jenni et al.**
  Jenni et al. [9] define LVNC as $NC/C \geq 2.0$ (at end-systole) on short-axis view, where NC = the non-compacted layer and C = the compacted layer, in addition

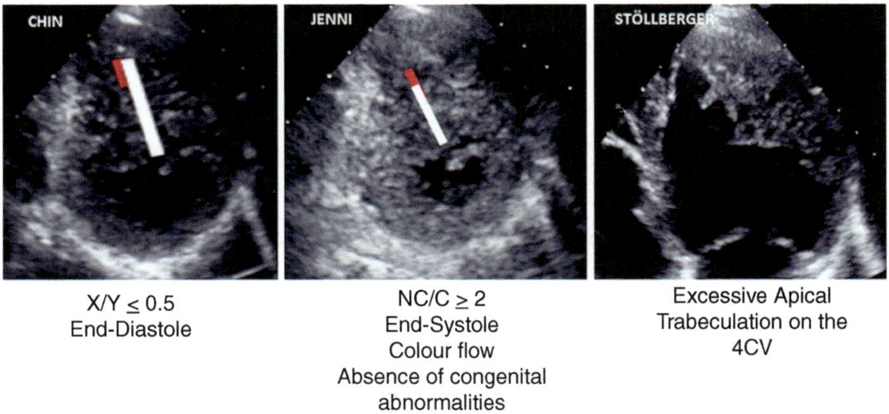


**Fig. 15.3** Echocardiographic criteria for left ventricular non-compaction. *C* compaction, *NC* non-compaction, *4CV* 4-chamber view, *X* compacted, *Y* compacted and non-compacted

to colour flow in the intra-trabecular pockets and an absence of congenital abnormalities. This is the most commonly used echocardiographic criteria to define LVNC. The Jenni et al. [9] study compared the hearts of 34 individuals with LVNC with nine patients with hypertensive cardiac disease, 10 patients with dilated cardiomyopathy and seven pathoanatomic specimens. They observed that the most common locations for non-compacted myocardial segments were the mid-lateral wall, the inferior wall and the apex. Whereas regional hypokinesia was originally included in the Jenni et al. [9] criteria, this was later removed as it was found to have a low specificity.

- **Stöllberger et al.**
  Stöllberger et al. [26] based their definition of LVNC on an analysis of 474 normal hearts that had been reviewed as part of a post-mortem study by Boyd et al. [10]. For a diagnosis of LVNC to exist, Stöllberger et al. proposed that more than three trabeculations, distal to the papillary muscle, must be present in any one axis plain. They refined their criteria further by suggesting that, at end diastole, there must also be a double-layered myocardium visible, with a ratio of non-compacted to compacted myocardium >2.0 [21, 27].

### 15.7.2 Advanced Echocardiographic Techniques

New echocardiographic techniques such as speckle tracking, tissue doppler imaging and strain rate imaging are being proposed as superior methods of assessing and diagnosing LVNC. Bellavia et al. [28] examined 20 patients with LVNC and compared these with 20 further individuals matched for age and sex. They demonstrated a reduction in systolic strain, rate of strain, displacement, rotation and torsion in those patients with LVNC, independent of ejection fraction. However, further studies have proved inconclusive with these findings. Three-dimensional echocardiography and contrast echocardiography may also offer useful evaluation tools in diagnosing LVNC, but both are user dependent and need further trials for validation.

### 15.7.3 Limitations of Echocardiographic Diagnosis of LVNC

Echocardiography is limited in that it is operator dependent and, occasionally, the apical segment of the heart may not be clearly visualised. Echocardiography may not visibly identify the double layers of the myocardium, critical for a diagnosis of LVNC. Occasionally, abnormal trabeculations can be mistaken for normal myocardial trabeculations however, in normal individuals, these are usually located in the left ventricular apex and are limited to fewer than three. A diagnosis of LVNC may get missed if abnormal trabeculations are confused with false tendons or aberrant bands, however these tend to cross the left ventricular cavity, so they can easily be identified. A left ventricular apical thrombus may be mistaken for abnormal trabeculations, but these can usually be differentiated by their altering echogenicity.

The current echocardiographic diagnostic criteria offered by Chin, Jenni and Stöllberger have its limitations. Their research is based on a small number of patients with LVNC, many of whom were paediatric (Chin et al. [22]) and few of whom were from different ethnic backgrounds. A study by Kohli et al. [16] demonstrated that, by using any one of the Chin, Jenni or Stöllberger criteria, 24% of patients with heart failure attending a general cardiology outpatient clinic were 'diagnosed' with LVNC, as were 8% of healthy black controls. This raises the question as to whether the current diagnostic echocardiographic criteria are appropriate for diagnosing LVNC in African and Afro-Caribbean individuals.

## 15.8 Cardiac MRI

Cardiac magnetic resonance (CMR) imaging is increasingly being used to confirm a diagnosis of LVNC. It is advantageous in diagnosing LVNC because of its superior image quality and better spatial resolution. CMR has an increased sensitivity for detecting myocardial trabeculations and can easily differentiate between endocardial trabeculations, apical hypertrophic cardiomyopathy and epicardial crypts, none of which can easily be seen on echocardiography. It can visualise the thin epicardial layer with ease and accurately assess left ventricular wall thickness and function (Fig. 15.4). It also allows one to appreciate the endocardial borders of the

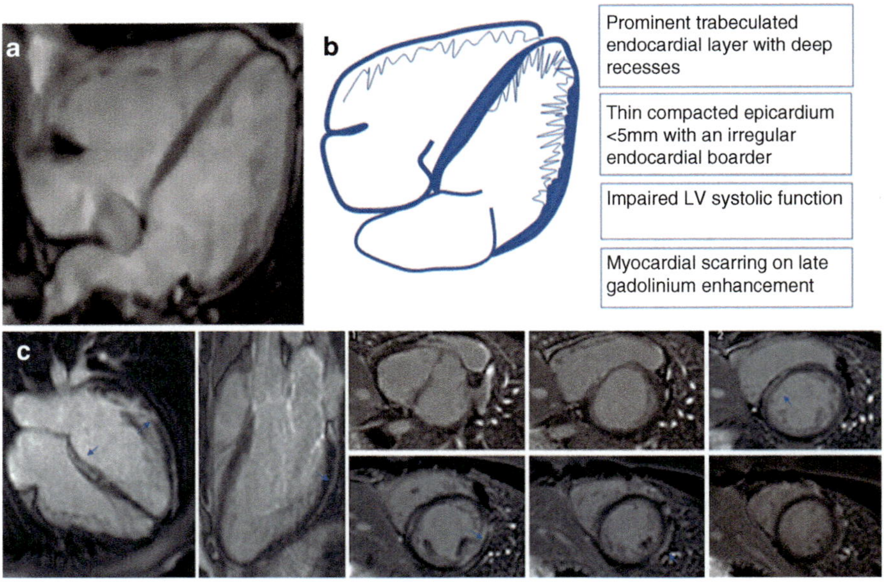


**Fig. 15.4** Further evaluation of left ventricular non-compaction on Cardiac Magnetic Resonance. (**a**) 4-chamber view demonstrating prominent LV trabeculations with a thinned compacted epicardial layer. (**b**) Schematic representation of features of left ventricular non-compaction on Cardiac Magnetic Resonance. (**c**) Presence of late gadolinium enhancement including mid-wall, subendocardial and subepicardial patterns (blue arrows)

compacted layer to identify the trabecular pockets. CMR calculates ejection fraction with precision by providing full coverage of the ventricles and having no inter-slice gap. It also enables the operator to view the heart in any plane and to identify the origins of the coronary vessels. CMR is more specific than echocardiography in detecting regional wall motion abnormalities and can also detect myocardial fibrosis via late gadolinium enhancement, often providing clarification when an athletic individual falls into the cardiomyopathy 'grey zone'.

### 15.8.1 CMR Late Gadolinium Enhancement

CMR late gadolinium enhancement software offers tissue characterisation and can identify myocardial fibrosis in up to 40% of patients with LVNC (Fig. 15.4). Nucifora et al. [29] identified 42 patients with confirmed LVNC and observed late gadolinium enhancement in 55% of these individuals. The strongest areas of enhancement occurred in the mid-myocardial regions of the left ventricle or at the point where the right ventricle inserted into the left ventricle. Enhancement was seen equally in compacted and non-compacted myocardial tissue. CMR late gadolinium enhancement can also identify endocardial fibrosis in paediatric patients, as well as mid-wall and epicardial fibrotic changes. However, the value of this advanced MRI technique has not been demonstrated in patients with LVNC experiencing concurrent ventricular arrhythmias nor has it been correlated to mortality.

### 15.8.2 Cardiac MRI criteria

There are three established Cardiac MRI criteria for the diagnosis of LVNC.

- **Petersen et al.:** In 2005, Petersen et al. [24] studied 177 individuals to determine whether CMR would accurately diagnose LVNC. They identified seven patients with LVNC using cine CMR images and compared them to the remaining control group of healthy volunteers, individuals with known athlete's heart, and patients with hypertrophic cardiomyopathy, dilated cardiomyopathy, hypertension and aortic stenosis. They identified a spectrum of non-compaction in the control group, most commonly located in the apex and lateral wall of the left ventricle, as opposed to the septal and basal areas of the left ventricle, commonly seen in LVNC.

  Petersen et al. defined LVNC as: $NC/C > 2.3$ (at end diastole, in long axis views), where $NC$ = the non-compacted layer, $C$ = the compacted layer. This criterion has a sensitivity of 86% and a specificity of 99%. However, the Multi-Ethnic Study of Atherosclerosis (MESA) [30] showed that 43% of 329 patients with no known heart disease met the diagnostic criteria for LVNC in at least one segment of the left ventricle, suggesting the Petersen et al. [24] criteria has low specificity in low risk individuals. It is further limited by difficulties in measuring in the long axis view because of the presence of the papillary muscle.

- **Jacquier et al.:** The Jacquier et al. [25] study compared 16 individuals with known (75%) or suspected (25%) LVNC versus patients with hypertrophic cardiomyopathy, dilated cardiomyopathy and healthy controls. They used steady-state free precession short-axis views to calculate the left ventricular trabecular mass. Jacquier et al. [25] defined LVNC as: Left ventricular trabecular mass > 20% of total mass. This criterion has a sensitivity of 91.6% and a specificity of 86.5%. However, the Jacquier et al. [25] study included the intratrabecular blood pool in its calculations which leads to an increased trabecular mass. Later evaluation in other published literature, criticises the Jacquier et al. [25] criteria for poor inter-observer variability.
- **Captur et al.:** Fractal analysis is a novel approach to assessing trabeculations that does not rely on the traditional comparison of compacted to non-compacted myocardial tissue. It is calculated using specialist software and involves superimposing a box grid onto 2D CMR images and counting the number of boxes that contain the data of interest. This method is repeated for four different box sizes in the short axis view. A line of best fit is applied across the points of the log-log plots of the box count, and the exponent of this gives the fractal dimension value.

  Captur et al. [23] examined 135 patients, 26% of whom had a known diagnosis of LVNC. A fractal dimension of 1.3 at end diastole gave the most accurate prediction of LVNC. This method is superior to the Petersen and Jacquier criteria in that there is less inter-observer variability because the machine is performing the measurements. However, specific software is required, and the scanner may struggle to differentiate between pooled blood and thinned myocardium, thus excluding apical segments. The extent to which contrast settings, blurring of motion artefacts, arrhythmogenic load or other technical aspects affect the performance of the fractal contour detection software remains unknown.

### 15.8.3 Advanced Cardiac MRI Techniques

- **T1 mapping and ECV:** The remaining 60% of patients with LVNC may be assisted by T1 mapping and ECV techniques. A study of 36 patients with LVNC versus healthy controls identified that the former had higher T1 values and expanded ECV, independent of left ventricular ejection fraction [31].

### 15.8.4 Limitations of Cardiac MRI Diagnosis of LVNC

Cardiac MRI is limited in that it is costly and access to scanners may prove problematic. Cardiac motion artefacts from patients with atrial fibrillation, or poor breath-holders, can result in blurred images. The current cardiac MRI diagnostic criteria is limited because:

(a) It is based on small cohorts
(b) It is not prospectively derived

(c) It is not validated
(d) Measurements are performed in different phases of the cardiac cycle
(e) The sites of measurements are variable
(f) It is oversensitive in certain populations such as black individuals
(g) It is non-specific in low risk populations

## 15.9 LVNC in Athletes

### 15.9.1 The Athlete's Heart

Competitive athletes regularly engage in intensive cardiovascular exercise, with many training more than 20 h per week. To perform at this level, cardiac output is increased by five to six times for prolonged periods (see Chap. 3). This leads to an increased cardiac preload and a series of structural, electrical and functional adaptations nominally termed the 'athlete's heart'. Changes include symmetrical enlargement of all four heart chambers with a 10–15% increase in cavity size of the left and right ventricles, compared to a healthy individual of the same age and size [32]. A 10–20% increase in left ventricular wall thickness may also be observed [32]. Athletes show greater filling in diastole, enhanced stroke volume and augmented oxidative capacity, resulting in improved oxygen consumption while training. While these cardiac adaptations to exercise are generally considered to be benign, it is important to differentiate them from the similar phenotype seen in cardiomyopathies, which remain the leading cause of sudden cardiac death in young athletes.

### 15.9.2 LVNC in Athletes

A study of 1146 athletes [3], 75 individuals with known LVNC and 415 controls found that 20% of athletes showed increased left ventricular trabeculations, with 8% of athletes fulfilling the echocardiography criteria for LVNC. These were predominantly black individuals, with T wave inversion on electrocardiogram and an ejection fraction of <50%. It has been postulated that the increased cardiac preload present in athletes unmasks pre-existing trabeculations, making them more apparent on imaging. As a high proportion of athletes meet the criteria for a diagnosis of LVNC without exhibiting other clinical features of the disorder, it may be that increased left ventricular trabeculations are of limited significance in this group and simply form part of the 'athlete's heart'. To reduce the risk of overdiagnosing LVNC in athletes, stricter diagnostic criteria may need to be applied to this cohort.

An Italian study by Caselli et al. [33] examined 2501 Olympic athletes with mean age 25 (range 15–45), 62% male and 99% Caucasian. Only 36 individuals exhibited prominent trabeculations following a physical examination, ECG, exercise test and echocardiography. LVNC was excluded in 24 of these athletes following further cardiac investigation with MRI scanning and genetic testing. Nine individuals were deemed unlikely to have LVNC and only three athletes with reduced ejection fraction and/or a positive family history, were labelled with the condition. Caselli et al. [33] concluded that, in a large athletic population, an LV trabecular pattern was only observed in 1.4% of individuals, with only a small subset of 0.1% of athletes demonstrating changes supporting a diagnosis of LVNC.

## 15.10 Investigating LVNC

- **History:** Individuals with LVNC may present with symptoms such as shortness of breath, palpitations, syncopal episodes, stroke, deep vein thrombosis, pulmonary embolism or sudden cardiac death [1]. However, many individuals remain asymptomatic and are diagnosed when LVNC is unmasked as an incidental finding on cardiac imaging or through family screening. Patients with a diagnosis of LVNC often express symptoms of left ventricular dysfunction but athletes are usually asymptomatic. It is important to clarify whether there is a family history of sudden cardiac death to help guide diagnosis (Fig. 15.5).
- **Electrocardiogram:** Common electrocardiogram (ECG) patterns seen in patients with LVNC are:
  - T-wave inversion in inferolateral leads
  - ST depression
  - Left bundle branch block (LBBB) or other ventricular conduction delay

  Athletic individuals may express similar ECG changes, but subtle differences may prevent overdiagnosis of LVNC in this cohort. Whilst LVNC patients have T-wave inversion in the inferolateral leads, athletes typically show T-wave inversion in V1–V3. LBBB is common in LVNC but is rarely seen in athletes [3].

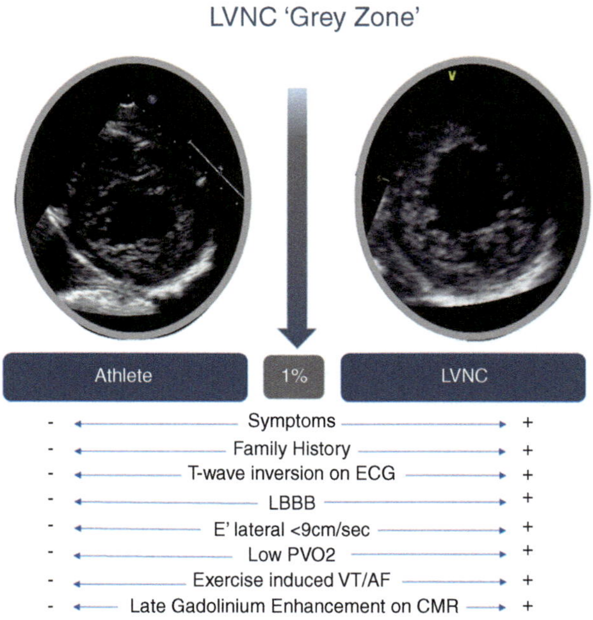


**Fig. 15.5** Differentiating physiological increased left ventricular trabeculation from pathological left ventricular non-compaction. *AF* atrial fibrillation, *CMR* cardiac magnetic resonance, *LBBB* left bundle branch block, *LV* left ventricular, *PVO2* peak oxygen uptake, *VT* ventricular tachycardia

- **Echocardiography and cardiac MRI:** Individuals with a diagnosis of LVNC often have impaired left ventricular filling (E' < 9 cm/s), an ejection fraction <45%, a left ventricular cavity of >64 mm in diameter and poor longitudinal left ventricular function (S′ < 9 cm/s). This differs from athletes presenting with a reduced ejection fraction and increased left ventricular trabeculations. In athletic individuals, the ejection fraction is typically 45–50% and their diastolic and longitudinal LV functions are usually within normal parameters [3, 7].
- **Further testing:** Further testing may be required to differentiate between the athlete's heart and pathological LVNC [1].
  - An **exercise stress test** may reveal a high peak $VO_2$ in athletes (>120% predicted for age and size) and a low peak $VO_2$ in LVNC patients. Identification of exercise induced ventricular arrhythmia particularly non-sustained ventricular tachycardia would support pathology [7].
  - A **peak exercise echocardiogram** is often considered for individuals with low LV ejection fraction to assess dynamic left ventricular contraction. In athletes, an increase in contractile reserve of >10% represents physiology [7].
- **Genetic testing**
  Genetic inheritance of LVNC is not yet fully understood and there is a poor correlation between genotype and LVNC phenotype [34]. However, a study by Waning et al. [12] examined the genetics and clinical features of children and adults with a diagnosis of LVNC. LVNC usually follows an autosomal dominant pattern of inheritance with variable penetration. Waning et al. [12] showed that nearly one-third of their LVNC patients had a mutation in a cardiomyopathy gene, 71% of which appeared in MYH7, MYBPC3 or TTN. They also noted that paediatric patients with confirmed LVNC genetic mutations were more likely to experience major adverse cardiovascular events than those with sporadic, acquired disease.

## 15.11 Management of LVNC

As observed in 1% of athletes [3], if there is a triad of:

1. Deep T-wave inversion on electrocardiogram
2. Reduced ejection fraction on echocardiography
3. Non-compaction features

then these individuals should remain under follow up to evaluate the natural history and progression of the disease process.

In the majority of athletes, isolated LV hypertrabeculation in the absence of symptoms and family history, is likely to be an epiphenomenon due to an increase in cardiac preload and does not require further follow up.

In the recent recommendations for participation in competitive and leisure time sport in athletes with cardiomyopathies, myocarditis, and pericarditis: position statement of the Sport Cardiology Section of the European Association of Preventive

Cardiology (EAPC) by Pelliccia et al. [35] guidance is given for athletic individuals with a suspected diagnosis of LVNC:

1. ***Athletes with incidental discovery of LV hypertrabeculation*** should not be diagnosed as LVNC in the absence of symptoms, positive family history, abnormal ECG patterns and, most importantly, impaired LV function. In such cases, no restriction for all competitive sports apply.
2. ***Athletes with unequivocal/reasonable diagnosis of LVNC but near-normal LV systolic function*** may participate in all competitive sports, with the exception of those where occurrence of syncope may cause serious harm or death, if they are:
   (a) asymptomatic,
   (b) without frequent and/or complex ventricular arrhythmias, or non-sustained VT on ambulatory monitoring and exercise ECG testing, and
   (c) no prior history of unexplained syncope
3. ***Athletes with an unequivocal diagnosis of LVNC*** and
   (a) impaired LV systolic function and/or
   (b) frequent and/or complex ventricular arrhythmias, or non-sustained VT on ambulatory monitoring or exercise testing should be advised to abstain from participation in competitive sports.

Athletes with an unequivocal diagnosis of LVNC should be advised to participate in leisure activities only and be closely monitored. Occasionally a period of detraining for 6–8 weeks may be required to aid diagnosis of LVNC.

## 15.12 Prognosis

Initial studies suggested that LVNC had a mortality rate of 35%, however, more recent research has found the mortality rate to be closer to 2–15% [36–39].

- A study by Stanton et al. [40] found that patients with LVNC had a similar mortality rate to patients with non-ischaemic dilated cardiomyopathy with a 3-year survival of 83–85%. Poor prognostic factors include increasing age, NYHA class III/IV, increased left ventricular filling pressures, an enlarged left atrium, concurrent ventricular arrhythmias, left ventricular dilatation, systolic dysfunction and cardiac complications. However, the prognosis of LVNC in low risk cohorts is good.
- A study by Oechslin et al. [13] examined 34 patients with known LVNC and found that those patients with complications such as low ejection fraction, atrial fibrillation and bundle branch block were found to be 'high risk' and as such had a poor prognosis. The authors suggest consideration of an implantable cardiac defibrillator or heart transplant in these patients.

## 15.13 Conclusion

In conclusion, LVNC may be genetic or acquired, however, the etiology of LVNC remains unclear. The identification of a high prevalence of hypertrabeculations in athletes and pregnant women suggests that, in low risk cohorts, LVNC may be an epiphenomenon associated with an increased cardiac preload. The echocardiographic and cardiac MRI diagnostic criteria for LVNC is based on small cohorts and is not ethnically diverse, risking overdiagnosis in some populations. Clearer diagnostic criteria, modified for ethnicity, is required. There is a poor genotype and phenotype correlation, so it is important to look at the overall clinical picture. However, prognosis of LVNC in low risk cohorts remains good.

**Clinical Pearls**

- LVNC is characterised by prominent myocardial trabeculations and deep recesses. The clinical spectrum of LVNC ranges from being completely asymptomatic to progressive LV systolic impairment
- The current imaging criteria for LVNC are non-specific in athletes and prone to erroneous diagnosis. The diagnosis of LVNC relies on multimodality imaging including echocardiography and cardiac MRI.
- Around 18% of asymptomatic athletes exhibit increased LV trabeculations and 8% fulfil echocardiographic criteria for LVNC suggesting that in most athletes, these findings represent an epiphenomenon in response to chronic increase in preload and afterload associated with exercise in the absence of a positive family history.
- A small minority of athletes (0.9%) fulfilling a triad of T-wave inversion, reduced resting indices of systolic function and LVNC imaging criteria may be supportive for a diagnosis of cardiomyopathy and require further evaluation and long-term follow-up.
- Cardiopulmonary exercise stress test followed by a peak exercise echocardiography is useful in differentiating athlete's heart from pathology. Athletes reveal a high peak VO2 (>120% predicted for age and size) and dynamic LV contraction, whereas patients with LVNC show low peak $VO_2$ and poor contractile reserve.

## Clinical Application

### Questions

1. A 17-year-old male, Caucasian, competitive rower is found to have features of LVNC on cardiac MRI, following a private health screening. He has no family history of cardiac disease or sudden cardiac death. His electrocardiogram is normal, and an echocardiogram shows an ejection fraction of 50% and normal LV function. What is the diagnosis, and can he continue to compete in his chosen sport?

2. A 23-year-old male, Afro-Caribbean, professional football player presents with syncopal episodes, shortness of breath on exertion and palpitations. His maternal Grandmother died aged 46 in unclear circumstances. His electrocardiogram shows deep inferolateral T-wave inversion. His echocardiogram shows an ejection fraction of 43% and normal LV function. A cardiac MRI shows features of mild myocardial non-compaction. What further tests would you order and how would you manage this patient?
3. A 34-year-old female, Caucasian, air race pilot has an annual health check as requested by her insurance company. She is asymptomatic apart from a recent bad cold. Her latest electrocardiogram shows ST depression. An echocardiogram shows an ejection fraction of 49% and normal LV dimensions and function. Cardiac MRI shows evidence of myocardial non-compaction. Ambulatory monitoring and an exercise electrocardiogram show no arrhythmias and no episodes of non-sustained VT. Can she compete in the air show this weekend?

## Answers

1. Although this young athlete has a feature of LVNC on imaging, in the absence of symptoms, positive family history, abnormal ECG patterns and, most importantly, impaired LV function, he has no restriction for any competitive sports.
2. This patient is symptomatic with concerning features on electrocardiogram and cardiac MRI. He should undergo further testing: an exercise stress test and peak exercise echocardiogram and should refrain from competitive sport until a diagnosis has been confirmed.
3. This air race pilot should not compete in the air show this weekend and should refrain from further air races. She is asymptomatic with no prior history of unexplained syncope and has no complex ventricular arrhythmias or episodes of non-sustained VT. She may compete in all competitive sports except those where occurrence of syncope may cause serious harm or death to herself or others. She should be encouraged to consider a ground sport if she wishes to continue competing.

## References

1. Gati S, Rajani R, Carr-White GS, Chambers JB. Adult left ventricular noncompaction: reappraisal of current diagnostic imaging modalities. JACC Cardiovasc Imaging. 2014;7(12):1266–75.
2. Gati S, Merghani A, Sharma S. Increased left ventricular trabeculation does not necessarily equate to left ventricular noncompaction in athletes left ventricular noncompaction in athletes letters. JAMA Intern Med. 2015;175(3):461–2.
3. Gati S, Chandra N, Bennett RL, et al. Increased left ventricular trabeculation in highly trained athletes: do we need more stringent criteria for the diagnosis of left ventricular non-compaction in athletes? Heart. 2013;99(6):401–8.

4. Gati S, Papadakis M, Papamichael ND, et al. Reversible de novo left ventricular trabeculations in pregnant women: Implications for the diagnosis of left ventricular noncompaction in low-risk populations. Circulation. 2014;130(6):475–83.
5. Gati S, Papadakis M, Van Niekerk N, Reed M, Yeghen T, Sharma S. Increased left ventricular trabeculation in individuals with sickle cell anaemia: physiology or pathology? Int J Cardiol. 2013;168(2)
6. Caselli S, Attenhofer Jost CH, Jenni R, Pelliccia A. Left ventricular noncompaction diagnosis and management relevant to pre-participation screening of athletes. Am J Cardiol. 2015;116(5):801–8.
7. Pelliccia A, Solberg EE, Papadakis M, et al. Recommendations for participation in competitive and leisure time sport in athletes with cardiomyopathies, myocarditis, and pericarditis: position statement of the sport cardiology section of the European Association of Preventive Cardiology (EAPC). Eur Heart J. 2018;40(1):19–33.
8. Sedmera D, Pexieder T, Vuillemin M, Thompson RP, Anderson RH. Developmental patterning of the myocardium. Anat Rec. 2000;258(4):319–37.
9. Jenni R, Oechslin E, Schneider J, Attenhofer Jost C, Kaufmann PA. Echocardiographic and pathoanatomical characteristics of isolated left ventricular non-compaction: a step towards classification as a distinct cardiomyopathy. Heart. 2001;86(6):666–71.
10. Boyd MT, Seward JB, Tajik AJ, Facc WDE. Morphologic studies frequency and location of prominent left ventricular trabeculations at autopsy in 474 normal human hearts: implications for evaluation of mural thrombi by two-dimensional echocardiography. J Am Coll Cardiol. 1987;9(2):323–6.
11. Arbustini E, Favalli V, Narula N, Serio A, Grasso M. Left ventricular noncompaction: a distinct genetic cardiomyopathy? J Am Coll Cardiol. 2016;68(9):949–66.
12. van Waning JI, Caliskan K, Hoedemaekers YM, et al. Genetics, clinical features, and long-term outcome of noncompaction cardiomyopathy. J Am Coll Cardiol. 2018;71(7):711 LP–722.
13. Oechslin EN, Jost CHA, Rojas JR, Kaufmann PA, Jenni R. Long-term follow-up of 34 adults with isolated left ventricular noncompaction: a distinct cardiomyopathy with poor prognosis. J Am Coll Cardiol. 2000;36(2):493–500.
14. Ritter M, Oechslin E, Sutsch G, Attenhofer C, Schneider J, Jenni R. Isolated noncompaction of the myocardium in adults. Mayo Clin Proc. 1997;72(1):26–31.
15. Oechslin E, Jenni R. Left ventricular non-compaction revisited: a distinct phenotype with genetic heterogeneity? Eur Heart J. 2011;32(12):1446–56.
16. Kohli SK, Pantazis AA, Shah JS, et al. Diagnosis of left-ventricular non-compaction in patients with left-ventricular systolic dysfunction: time for a reappraisal of diagnostic criteria? Eur Heart J. 2008;29(1):89–95.
17. Hutchins IM, Schaefer S. Progressive left ventricular noncompaction and systolic dysfunction. Exp Clin Cardiol. 2012;17(2):81–3.
18. Bleyl SB, Mumford BR, Brown-Harrison MC, et al. Xq28-linked noncompaction of the left ventricular myocardium: prenatal diagnosis and pathologic analysis of affected individuals. Am J Med Genet. 1997;72(3):257–65.
19. Frischknecht BS, Attenhofer Jost CH, Oechslin EN, et al. Validation of noncompaction criteria in dilated cardiomyopathy, and valvular and hypertensive heart disease. J Am Soc Echocardiogr. 2005;18(8):865–72.
20. Markovic NS, Dimkovic N, Damjanovic T, Loncar G, Dimkovic S. Isolated ventricular non-compaction in patients with chronic renal failure. Clin Nephrol. 2008;70(1):72–6.
21. Stollberger C, Gerecke B, Finsterer J, Engberding R. Refinement of echocardiographic criteria for left ventricular noncompaction. Int J Cardiol. 2013;165(3):463–7.
22. Chin TK, Perloff JK, Williams RG, Jue K, Mohrmann R. Isolated noncompaction of left ventricular myocardium. A study of eight cases. Circulation. 1990;82(2):507–13.
23. Captur G, Muthurangu V, Cook C, et al. Quantification of left ventricular trabeculae using fractal analysis. J Cardiovasc Magn Reson. 2013;15(1):36.
24. Petersen SE, Selvanayagam JB, Wiesmann F, et al. Left ventricular non-compaction insights from cardiovascular magnetic resonance imaging. J Am Coll Cardiol. 2005;46(1):101–5.

25. Jacquier A, Thuny F, Jop B, et al. Measurement of trabeculated left ventricular mass using cardiac magnetic resonance imaging in the diagnosis of left ventricular non-compaction. Eur Heart J. 2010;31(9):1098–104.
26. Stöllberger C, Finsterer J, Blazek G. Left ventricular hypertrabeculation/noncompaction and association with additional cardiac abnormalities and neuromuscular disorders. Am J Cardiol. 2002;90(8):899–902.
27. Stollberger C, Finsterer J. Left ventricular hypertrabeculation/noncompaction. J Am Soc Echocardiogr. 2004;17(1):91–100.
28. Bellavia D, Michelena HI, Martinez M, et al. Speckle myocardial imaging modalities for early detection of myocardial impairment in isolated left ventricular non-compaction. Heart. 2010;96(6):440–7.
29. Nucifora G, Aquaro GD, Pingitore A, Masci PG, Lombardi M. Myocardial fibrosis in isolated left ventricular non-compaction and its relation to disease severity. Eur J Heart Fail. 2011;13(2):170–6.
30. Kawel N, Nacif M, Arai AE, et al. Trabeculated (noncompacted) and compact myocardium in adults: the multi-ethnic study of atherosclerosis. Circ Cardiovasc Imaging. 2012;5(3):357–66.
31. Assuncao AN Jr, Nomura CH, Parga JR, et al. Myocardial T1 mapping and extracellular volume quantification in patients with left ventricular non-compaction cardiomyopathy. Eur Hear J Cardiovasc Imaging. 2018;19(8):888–95.
32. Sharma S, Merghani A, Mont L. Exercise and the heart: the good, the bad, and the ugly. Eur Heart J. 2015;36(23):1445–53.
33. Caselli S, Ferreira D, Kanawati E, et al. Prominent left ventricular trabeculations in competitive athletes: a proposal for risk stratification and management. Int J Cardiol. 2016;223:590–5.
34. Abela M, D'Silva A. Left ventricular trabeculations in athletes: epiphenomenon or phenotype of disease? Curr Treat Options Cardiovasc Med. 2018;20(12):100.
35. Pelliccia A. Differences in cardiac remodeling associated with race implications for preparticipation screening and the unfavorable situation of black athletes. J Am Coll Cardiol. 2008;51(23):2263–5.
36. Thavendiranathan P, Dahiya A, Phelan D, Desai MY, Tang WHW. Isolated left ventricular noncompaction controversies in diagnostic criteria, adverse outcomes and management. Heart. 2013;99(10):681–9.
37. Greutmann M, Mah ML, Silversides CK, et al. Predictors of adverse outcome in adolescents and adults with isolated left ventricular noncompaction. Am J Cardiol. 2012;109(2):276–81.
38. Lofiego C, Biagini E, Pasquale F, et al. Wide spectrum of presentation and variable outcomes of isolated left ventricular non-compaction. Heart. 2007;93(1):65–71.
39. Habib G, Charron P, Eicher J-C, et al. Isolated left ventricular non-compaction in adults: clinical and echocardiographic features in 105 patients. Results from a French registry. Eur J Heart Fail. 2011;13(2):177–85.
40. Stanton C, Bruce C, Connolly H, et al. Isolated left ventricular noncompaction syndrome. AJC. 2009;104(8):1135–8.

# Specific Cardiovascular Diseases and Competitive Sports Participation: Valvular Heart Disease

16

Frank van Buuren and Klaus Peter Mellwig

**Learning Objectives**
1. Learn how to diagnose different valve defects.
2. Learn which diagnostic tool is needed to find the adequate diagnosis.
3. Learn how sports activity influences the progression of VHD.
4. Learn how sports activity influences pulmonary pressure and ventricular function.
5. Learn which type of sports can be recommended in VHD individuals.

## 16.1 Introduction

The scope of this chapter is to provide an overview on the different types of VHD and to suggest a strategy how to diagnose them adequately. As the evaluation of the hemodynamic effects of competitive sport in individuals with VHD is challenging we describe the different consequences on cardiac function [1].

## 16.2 Aortic Valve Stenosis

The most common cause for aortic valve stenosis (AVS) is a rheumatic or congenital origin. Calcified degenerative stenosis is often associated with congenital abnormality of the aortic valve (e.g. bicuspid valve), especially when aortic stenosis is

F. van Buuren
Cardiology, Angiology and Intensive Care Medicine, Catholic Hospital Southwestfalia, St. Martinus, Olpe, Germany
e-mail: frank.van.buuren@onlinehome.de

K. P. Mellwig (✉)
Heart Center Northrhine Westfalia, Depart of Cardiology, Bad Oeynhausen, Germany



A. Pressler, J. Niebauer (eds.), *Textbook of Sports and Exercise Cardiology*,
https://doi.org/10.1007/978-3-030-35374-2_16

identified in young patients [2, 3]. Hemodynamic progression often shows marked individual variability and is not reflected by a single objective parameter.

Symptoms such as angina pectoris or dyspnea usually appear in a late stage of the disease. Occurrence of sudden cardiac death (SCD) is by far more probable if one of these symptoms is present. LA size can reflect hemodynamic burden in patients with asymptomatic severe aortic stenosis. Quantitative measurements of LA and diastolic function are helpful to evaluate left ventricular filling pressures with exercise and could be used to identify asymptomatic patients with increased hemodynamic burden [4].

- Congenital bicuspid aortic valve (BAV), one of the most common congenital heart diseases (0.9–2%), can lead to both AVS and aortic valve regurgitation (AVR; see below). In these individuals LV dimensions of athletes are often near the upper limits of normal.

*Evaluation.* AVS is frequently detected by auscultation. Determination of the gradient and valve opening area is initially carried out by Doppler-echocardiography (Table 16.1). Exercise testing is recommended in certain cases to assess LV function, development of ST segment depression, blood pressure behavior and possible arrhythmias [5, 6]. The role of exercise testing to clarify symptom status and the use of stress imaging (e.g. stress echocardiography) to evaluate the dynamic component of valvular abnormalities and to unmask subclinical myocardial dysfunction that could be missed at rest is of utmost importance. In patients with "low-flow, low-gradient AVS" (reduced systolic function, a valve opening area <1.0 cm$^2$ and a mean aortic valve gradient <40 mmHg) the use of stress echocardiography is often helpful when attempting to differentiate true severe aortic stenosis from pseudo-severe aortic stenosis, and it provides guidance for adequate therapy through evaluating the contractile reserve of the left ventricle.

**Table 16.1** Echocardiographic parameters indicative of the degree of severity of different valve lesions (adapted from [4])

| | Aortic valve stenosis | | |
|---|---|---|---|
| A | Low | Moderate | Severe |
| $V_{max}$ (m/s) | 2.6–2.9 | 3.0–4.0 | ≥4.0 |
| $\Delta p_{mean}$ (mmHg) | <30 | 30–40 | ≥40 |
| Valve orifice area (cm$^2$) | >1.5 | 1.0–1.5 | <1.0 |

| | Mitral valve stenosis | | |
|---|---|---|---|
| B | Low | Moderate | Severe |
| Valve orifice area (cm$^2$) | >1.5 | 1.0–1.5 | <1.0 |
| $\Delta p_{mean}$ (mmHg) | <5 | 5–10 | >10 |
| Pulmonary artery pressure (mmHg) | <30 | 30–50 | >50 |

| | Tricuspid valve stenosis |
|---|---|
| C | Clinical significant degree |
| $\Delta p_{mean}$ (mmHg) | >5 |

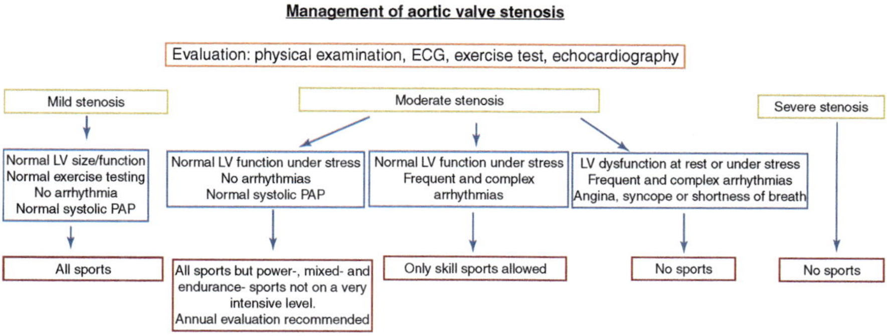


**Fig. 16.1** Decision tree on eligibility for different types and intensities of sport according to the clinical severity of aortic valve stenosis (see Chap. 1 for classification of sports). *ECG* electrocardiogram, *LV* left ventricular, *PAP* pulmonary artery pressure

The application of strain analysis during transthoracic echocardiography (TTE) allows a deeper physiological understanding of left ventricular (LV) contraction and its relationship with LV structure. Given that the severity of AVS is often progressive, periodical evaluation is necessary. Athletes with a BAV complicated by AVS are managed in the same fashion as athletes with a trileaflet valve.

*Classification.* Classification is based on the mean aortic valve gradient and aortic valve opening area (AVA):

1. Mild = mean gradient <20 mmHg (AVA > 1.5 $cm^2$).
2. Moderate = mean gradient between 21 and 49 mmHg (AVA 1.0–1.5 $cm^2$).
3. Severe = mean gradient ≥50 mmHg (AVA < 1.0 $cm^2$).

Recommendations for the allowed physical activity should be based on a distinguished strategy. Figure 16.1 shows an example for patients with AVS.

## 16.3 Aortic Valve Regurgitation

The commonest causes of AVR include BAV, rheumatic fever, infectious endocarditis, Marfan syndrome, aortic dissection, systemic arterial hypertension and rheumatoid spondylitis. AVR causes dilatation of the LV cavity with increases in LV diastolic and systolic volumes. Bradycardia can worsen the hemodynamic pattern, due to lengthening of the diastolic duration and increase of the regurgitant volume. AVR causes both pressure and volume loading of the left ventricle.

- Athletes involved in mainly isometric exercise can develop pressure overloads due to high systemic arterial pressure. Hence, the resulting chronically elevated aortic wall tension in strength-trained athletes can be associated with aortic dilatation and regurgitation.

- Athletes with AVR in the chronic compensated phase are often asymptomatic and can remain so far for many years.
- In patients with AVR, static exercise causes a reduction of preload resulting in a reduction in LV stroke volume and regurgitant volume.

AVR can be detected by auscultation and, of course, LV dilatation should be evaluated by echocardiography. Facing the fact that LV cavity dimension can also be increased in healthy athletes as a consequence of regular training, this should be considered when assessing LV size in the presence of AVR. As LV dysfunction proceeds, symptoms occur including dyspnea on exertion, arrhythmias and, in advanced cases, angina [7, 8].

People of Afro-Caribbean origin have a lower incidence of BAV. In athletes with BAV, aortic and LV dimensions increase significantly more than in athletes with tricuspid valves, but do not differ from those in the general, non-athlete BAV population. A normally functioning BAV usually does not represent a limit for competitive sport. However, progressive increase in the sizes of both aorta and LV in BAV athletes needs thorough and regular follow-up. Apart from echocardiographic evaluation also Cardiac Magnetic Resonance Imaging (MRI) is of good use. If LV dimensions and Doppler variables fall outside normal values, it may be necessary to interrupt or even stop competitive sport.

Exercise testing (or cardiopulmonary testing) can be helpful in the evaluation of exercise tolerance and blood pressure response. It should be carried out up to the level that is consistent with the particular sport in order to assess ventricular tolerance.

Because of possible progression of AVR over time, periodical evaluation is recommended.

*Classification.* The hemodynamic severity of AVR can be classified as follows:

1. Mild = absence of peripheral signs of AVR and normal LV and atrial size and function; small dimension of the diastolic flow signal on Doppler-echocardiography.
2. Moderate = peripheral signs of AVR, mild to moderate enlargement of the LV, normal systolic function, moderate dimension of the diastolic flow signal on Doppler-echocardiography.
3. Severe = peripheral signs of AVR, marked dilatation of the LV and/or evidence of LV dysfunction; enlarged atrial size and large dimension of the diastolic flow signal on Doppler-echocardiography.

## 16.4 Mitral Valve Stenosis

Mitral valve stenosis (MVS) in young individuals is generally of rheumatic origin. This disease can result in elevated left atrial (LA) pressure, leading to pulmonary hypertension. The increase in heart rate and cardiac output associated with intensive exercise can markedly increase the pulmonary arterial pressure and may eventually lead to acute pulmonary edema. In severe disease, left-sided cardiac output is compromised as a result of poor LV filling. However, exercise intolerance can also be influenced by restrictive lung function and chronotropic intolerance. Embolization by atrial thrombus represents a further complication, which usually occurs in the presence of atrial fibrillation and an enlarged left atrium. Long-term effects of repeated exertion-related increases in pulmonary artery wedge pressure on pulmonary circulation and on the right ventricle are still not well understood.

It still remains elusive to which extend chronic physical activity and especially competitive sports contribute in case of a negative course.

*Evaluation.* Presence of MVS can be detected by characteristic auscultation, and severity can be determined by non-invasive testing which includes

- ECG
- Echocardiography
- Chest x-ray
- Exercise testing.

TTE and transesophageal echocardiography (TOE) allow assessment of valve opening area, presence of calcification and papillary muscle function. The contribution of regurgitation should also be considered in the calculation of the valve opening area (Table 16.1). Pulmonary systolic arterial pressure can be assessed by Doppler-echocardiography in the presence of tricuspid regurgitation, even during or after exercise.

- Exercise testing (or cardiopulmonary testing) can add information regarding the hemodynamic behavior and occurrence of arrhythmias (particularly atrial fibrillation).
- Invasive testing, e.g. Swan Ganz catheterization, is indicated only in selected cases, when accurate assessment of pressure in the pulmonary circulation is needed for therapeutic or legal purposes.
- Stress echocardiography may provide additional objective information by assessing changes in mitral gradient and pulmonary artery pressure.

Athletes who develop a significant pulmonary artery systolic pressure during exercise are likely to develop severe adverse effects on RV function over time. Athletes/patients with MVS and atrial fibrillation must receive anticoagulation treatment to avoid systemic embolism. These individuals should avoid contact collision sport. Hemodynamic severity is best characterized by the planimetered mitral valve area and the calculated mitral valve area from the diastolic pressure half-time.

*Classification.* The severity of MVS can be categorized as follows:

1. Mild = mitral valve opening area 1.5–2.5 $cm^2$, with pulmonary systolic arterial pressure <35 mmHg, and mean gradient <7 mmHg.

2. Moderate = mitral valve opening area 1.0–1.5 $cm^2$, with resting pulmonary systolic arterial pressure between 35 and 50 mmHg, and a mean gradient between 8 and 15 mmHg.
3. Severe = mitral valve opening area <1.0 $cm^2$, with resting pulmonary systolic arterial pressure >50 mmHg, and a mean gradient >15 mmHg.

## 16.5 Mitral Valve Regurgitation

The most frequent cause of mitral valve regurgitation (MVR) is the prolapse of leaflets (mitral valve prolapse (MVP)). MVP can appear as a single or bileaflet protrusion and is of relevance in cases of a protrusion of at least 2 mm beyond the long-axis annular plane into the left atrium.

- It is worth to know that some trials showed that the prevalence of mitral valve prolapse syndrome is lower in black individuals.

  Other causes include

- post-rheumatic fever
- infectious endocarditis
- coronary heart disease (ischemic cardiomyopathy)
- connective tissue disease (e.g. Marfan syndrome)
- dilated cardiomyopathy.

MVR is responsible for regurgitated blood into the left atrium, which causes increased LV diastolic filling and subsequently raises left atrial pressure. Highly trained athletes presenting with mild mitral (and aortic) valve regurgitation are not disadvantaged regarding their cardiopulmonary capacity, but they have to be evaluated thoroughly.

MVR is clinically detected by dyspnea, exercise intolerance and auscultation. However, the majority of people with mild or moderate MVR remain asymptomatic. The severity of MVR can be assessed by Doppler-echocardiography. TTE is recommended as the first-line imaging modality, two-dimensional TOE is advocated when TTE is of non-diagnostic value or when further diagnostic refinement is required. Three-dimensional echo can provide additional information in patients with complex valve lesions. In assessing the severity of MVR, ECG and chest x-ray are also useful.

Since well-trained athletes often have an increased LV end-diastolic size due to their training history, this should be considered when a decision has to be made whether LV enlargement is caused by MVR or by a physiological adaptation to the years of training. MVR contributes to the unload of LV during systole which can lead to overestimation of true myocardial performance.

- In athletes, severity of MVR should be based on LV end-systolic volume, and a cut-off of 35 $mm/m^2$ in men (respectively 40 $mm/m^2$ in women) turned out to be useful to distinguish individuals with LV enlargement of clinical relevance.

Physical activity rarely leads to an increased regurgitation fraction due to the reduced systemic vascular resistance, but this effect can be diminished by elevated heart rate. The use of global longitudinal strain could be of potential interest for the detection of subclinical LV dysfunction.

The extent of LA enlargement should also be considered, because of the procliv-ity for atrial fibrillation. LA volume, systolic pulmonary artery pressure, tricuspid regurgitation, annular size and right ventricular (RV) function are important addi-tional parameters.

- A significant increase of pulmonary artery pressure with exercise of >60 mmHg has been reported to be of prognostic value.
- 24-h Holter monitoring is recommended when arrhythmias are evident or sus-pected, and when MVR is due to prolapse of the leaflets.

Athletes with atrial fibrillation must receive anticoagulation treatment, and they should avoid sports with risk of bodily collision. When MVR is due to an isolated MVP the prognosis is good and no sport restriction should be applied.

*Classification.* There are several methods to classify MVR. The widely accepted PISA-method uses the width of the jet and the velocity to assess the degree of regur-gitation, but also CW Doppler characteristics are helpful:

1. Mild = regurgitation width <0.3 cm (PISA), soft density and parabolic CW Doppler MR signal
2. Moderate = regurgitation width 0.3–0.6 cm (PISA).
3. Severe = regurgitation width >0.6 cm (PISA), dense and triangular CW Doppler MR jet, large central MR jet

## 16.6 Tricuspid Valve Stenosis

In most cases tricuspid valve stenosis (TVS) is caused by rheumatic fever and is associated with MVS. In the presence of MVS and TVS, patients should be assessed with reference to the MVS. An isolated TVS is very rare (Table 16.1).

- If the patient is asymptomatic (no dizziness, no dyspnea or peripheral edema), participation in competitive sports may be possible.

Thorough echocardiographic evaluation of the anatomy of the valve and its sub-valvular apparatus is important to evaluate the therapeutic strategy. There is no gen-erally accepted grading of TVS but a mean gradient ≥5 mmHg at normal heart rate is considered indicative of clinically significant TVS.

## 16.7 Tricuspid Valve Regurgitation

Tricuspid valve regurgitation (TVR) is often the consequence of RV dilatation. Rheumatic fever or infectious endocarditis are less common causes. Primary TVR leads to volume overload of the RV, increased venous pressure and congestive symptoms. The severity of TVR can be determined non-invasively by physical examination, chest x-ray and especially echocardiography. Dense and triangular early peaking regurgitant signal on colour flow, vena contracta flow, PISA radius and early diastolic filling velocity and RV outflow velocity are established echocardiographic parameters to assess the severity of TVR.

## 16.8 Multi-valvular Diseases

Multi-valvular diseases frequently occur in connection with rheumatic fever, myxomatous valvular diseases or infectious endocarditis. These conditions can be diagnosed by physical examination and assessed quantitatively by Doppler-echocardiography. If one valvular disease worsens, it might impact the other and result in unfavorable hemodynamic effects. Therefore, close follow-up is warranted in these athletes with regard to participation in competitive sports (see Table 16.1 for *recommendations*).

## 16.9 Postoperative Athletes with a (Bio)prosthetic Heart Valve

Although patients usually improve clinically after heart valve replacement, the long-term mortality can be higher than in a healthy control population. Furthermore, patients with normal hemodynamic patterns at rest may have abnormal values under physical stress.

- Exercise testing, preferably spiroergometry, should be carried out up to the intensity consistent with that of the sport the athlete wishes to pursue.

Noteworthy, patients with mechanical valves (or bioprosthetic valves in selected cases) need systematic anticoagulation treatment, which further limits their choice of competitive sports. Athletes with artificial valves should undergo periodic reevaluation. Athletes with a prosthetic or bioprosthetic valve who are receiving anticoagulation treatment should not participate in sports with a risk of bodily collision.

## 16.10 Athletes Post-valvuloplasty

Valvuloplasty is still performed in some patients with MVS, despite the probability of restenosis and no clear advantage when compared with valve replacement. Aortic valvuloplasty is performed extremely rare in young patients with AVS.

- In athletes after valvuloplasty, recommendations for sports participation are based on the residual degree of severity of stenosis and/or regurgitation.
- Exercise testing should be carried out up to the level consistent with the level reached in the sport in which the patient participates.

## 16.11 Mitral Valve Prolapse

Mitral valve prolapse (MVP) is mostly associated with myxomatous degeneration of the valve. It preferentially occurs in athletes of tall stature and shows a familial cluster. Ischemic cardiomyopathy and hypertrophic obstructive cardiomyopathy are potential secondary etiologies. Mitral valve prolapse is a disease of all connective tissues, including the tendinous chords; and so, the risk of chordal rupture remains after repair of the regurgitant valve.

- MVP is often associated with mitral regurgitation.
- Rhythm disorders (i.e. brady- or tachyarrhythmias), endocarditis, syncope or embolism can also occur.
- SCD in MVP patients is more common in women, occurs regardless of the degree of regurgitation, and is often associated with myocardial fibrosis in the papillary muscles on contrast-enhanced cardiac magnetic resonance imaging.

The typical auscultatory finding is a late-systolic click and a murmur due to late systolic or holosystolic regurgitation. Elongation and thickening of valve leaflets, degree of mitral regurgitation and LV dimension and function should be assessed by echocardiography. Evaluation should include exercise testing and/or Holter monitoring to assess the presence of arrhythmias. Frequent cardiological evaluation is recommended, because the regurgitation can get worse by progressive degeneration of the leaflets.

## 16.12 Transcatheter Interventions for Valvular Heart Disease

The recent development of devices for transcatheter aortic valve implantation (TAVI), mitral repair (mitral clipping), and closure of prosthetic paravalvular leaks has led to a greatly expanded armamentarium of catheter-based approaches to patients with regurgitant as well as stenotic valvular disease.

- The use of these new techniques is supposed to be rare in competitive athletes.
- However, athletes concerned should be judged according to the remaining cardiac defect and with respect to anticoagulation therapy.

In patients after TAVI, combined exercise training (endurance and resistance component) is safe and highly effective and often results in improved quality of life, muscular strength and exercise capacity. However, TAVI procedures are mainly used in elderly patients so far, showing corresponding comorbidities that make competitive sports in these individuals almost impossible. Latest trials on TAVI procedures showed also advantages in younger patients receiving this technique.

## 16.13 Prophylaxis for Endocarditis

Infective endocarditis (IE) is an endovascular, microbial infection of intracardiac structures facing the blood, including infections of the large intrathoracic vessels. The early lesion is a vegetation of variable size, although destruction, ulceration or abscess may follow. The increasing accuracy of echocardiography and therapeutic progress have contributed to the prognostic improvement in the last few years.

Patients with

- previous history of infective endocarditis
- prosthetic heart valves
- acquired valve disease

are considered high risk patients and should receive antibiotic prophylaxis when exposed to risk of bacteremia in accordance with the ESC recommendations.

- As a general rule, all sports activity should be avoided when active infection with fever is present. Resumption of sport activity can be considered when the inflammatory process is completely extinguished, and systematic maintenance of endocarditis prophylaxis must be observed strictly.

## 16.14 Aortopathies

The term aortopathies includes several aortic diseases that account for 1.6–5% of SCD in young athletes. Although Marfan syndrome (MFS) is the prototype for the aortopathies, maladaptive remodelling of the vascular extracellular matrix is not unique to MFS. Irrespective of etiology, altered vascular structure may lead to an increase propensity for aortic dilation, dissection, or rupture of aortic wall.

The evaluation of an athlete with suspected MFS includes

- family and personal medical history
- physical examination
- echocardiography
- genetic testing.

If transthoracic echocardiographic evaluation does not allow precise visualization of the aorta, computed tomography (CT) or MRI should be performed. Particular care should be paid in evaluating tall athletes engaged in certain sports such as basketball and volleyball which may exhibit most of the systemic features of the syndrome. The diagnosis of MFS relies on defined clinical criteria (Ghent nosology; see Chap. 7). Several factors influence aortic root dimensions, including body size, age, height, and gender, and they have to be taken into account [9].

- The abnormal range is an enlargement at the level of sinuses of Valsalva with a Z-score ≥2.
- Particular attention with close clinical surveillance should be paid when a rapid change in aortic dilatation is demonstrated (i.e. ≥0.5 cm/year) or when heart or valve function deteriorates.

Also, other rare connective tissue disorders may increase the risk of aortic dilatation/dissection in competitive athletes. These conditions may present a clinical overlap with MFS in the cardiovascular, ocular or skeletal systems.

Whether regular and intensive exercise has an impact on aortic root dimensions is still debated. However, a marked aortic root dilatation does not represent a physiological adaptation to exercise. Life expectancy in patients with aortopathies is largely determined by the risk of aortic dissection and lifestyle risk factors.

**Clinical Pearls**

- The majority of athletes with VHD are often asymptomatic for a long time and an abnormal ECG pattern raises a first suspicion on a potential valve defect. Possible symptoms are breathlessness that is disproportionate to the amount of exercise being performed, palpitation or syncope.
- TTE is the first line investigation to confirm the diagnosis of VHD and provides essential prognostic information in relation to severity of valve dysfunction, ventricular function and pulmonary artery pressure.
- Valve defects with a predominantly regurgitant component are often better tolerated than stenotic lesions.
- Recommendations for athletes with VHD need a detailed diagnostic approach and tailored guidance that respect not only the valve disease itself but also potential arrhythmia, pulmonary pressure, size and function of cardiac chambers.

## Review

### Questions

1. What is the most frequent cause of mitral valve regurgitation (MVR) and how can it be diagnosed adequately?
2. Are athletes with bicuspid aortic valve (BAV) allowed to perform sport on a higher level?
3. Which left ventricular size can be accepted in athletes with MVR?

### Answers

1. The prolapse of leaflets (mitral valve prolapse (MVP)) is the most frequent cause of MVR and can appear as a single or bileaflet protrusion. Typical symptoms are dyspnea, exercise intolerance and auscultation. Many individuals are

asymptomatic. MVR can be assessed by Doppler-echocardiography. Next to the valve function the extent of left atrial enlargement should also be evaluated, because of the proclivity for atrial fibrillation.
2. Congenital BAV is one of the most common congenital heart diseases appearing in up to every 50th individual and can lead to both AVS and aortic valve regurgitation. A normally functioning BAV usually does not represent a limit for competitive sport but these athletes need regular follow-up evaluation of both aorta and left ventricular size.
3. The relevance of MVR in athletes should also be based on LV end-systolic volume. A cut-off of 35 mm/m$^2$ in men (respectively 40 mm/m$^2$ in women) turned out to be useful to distinguish individuals with LV enlargement of clinical relevance.

## References

1. Pelliccia A, Fagard R, Bjornstad HH, Anastassakis A, Arbustini E, Assanelli D, et al. Recommendations for competitive sports participation in athletes with cardiovascular disease: a consensus document from the study group of sports cardiology of the working group of cardiac rehabilitation and exercise physiology and the working group of myocardial and pericardial diseases of the European society of cardiology. Eur Heart J. 2005;26(14):1422–45.
2. Gati S, Malhotra A, Sharma S. Exercise recommendations in patients with valvular heart disease. Heart. 2019;105(2):106–10.
3. Mellwig KP, van Buuren F, Gohlke-Baerwolf C, Bjornstad HH. Recommendations for the management of individuals with acquired valvular heart diseases who are involved in leisure-time physical activities or competitive sports. Eur J Cardiovasc Prev Rehabil. 2008;15(1):95–103.
4. Baumgartner H, Falk V, Bax JJ, De Bonis M, Hamm C, Holm PJ, et al. 2017 ESC/EACTS Guidelines for the management of valvular heart disease. Eur Heart J. 2017;38(36):2739–91.
5. Levine BD, Baggish AL, Kovacs RJ, Link MS, Maron MS, Mitchell JH, et al. Eligibility and disqualification recommendations for competitive athletes with cardiovascular abnormalities: task force 1: classification of sports: dynamic, static, and impact: a scientific statement from the American heart association and American college of cardiology. Circulation. 2015;132(22):e262–6.
6. Pelliccia A, Adami PE, Quattrini F, Squeo MR, Caselli S, Verdile L, et al. Are olympic athletes free from cardiovascular diseases? Systematic investigation in 2352 participants from Athens 2004 to Sochi 2014. Br J Sports Med. 2017;51(4):238–43.
7. Booher AM, Bach DS. Exercise hemodynamics in valvular heart disease. Curr Cardiol Rep. 2011;13(3):226–33.
8. Nishimura RA, Otto CM, Bonow RO, Carabello BA, Erwin JP 3rd, Guyton RA, et al. 2014 AHA/ACC guideline for the management of patients with valvular heart disease: executive summary: a report of the American college of cardiology/American heart association task force on practice guidelines. Circulation. 2014;129(23):2440–92.
9. Boraita A, Heras ME, Morales F, Marina-Breysse M, Canda A, Rabadan M, et al. Reference values of aortic root in male and female white elite athletes according to sport. Circ Cardiovasc Imaging. 2016;9(10):e005292.

# Specific Cardiovascular Diseases and Competitive Sports Participation: Arrhythmias

**17**

Alessandro Biffi, Alessandro Zorzi, and Domenico Corrado

**Learning Objectives**

1. Learn to distinguish those cardiac rhythm disorders which are the expression of physical training and do not have significant clinical impact (such as sinus bradycardia, low degree AV block etc.).
2. Give attention to the atrial and ventricular arrhythmias which may have a malignant consequence on athlete careers.
3. Set up a correct and appropriate diagnostic work up using modern and useful diagnostic tools.
4. Learn the decision-making protocols to grant sports eligibility and follow-up in athletes with arrhythmias.

## 17.1 Introduction

Arrhythmias represent a common finding in the evaluation of the athlete. They can be the expression of a benign phenomenon, such as bradyarrhythmias due to an increase of the vagal tone or raise the clinical suspect of an underlying heart disease, such as ventricular arrhythmias. In this chapter, we summarize the most frequent arrhythmias that can be encountered in athletes and the criteria for sports eligibility.

A. Biffi
Institute of Sports Medicine & Science, Italian Olympic Committee, Rome, Italy

A. Zorzi · D. Corrado (✉)
Department of Cardiac, Thoracic, Vascular and Public Health Sciences, University of Padova, Padova, Italy
e-mail: domenico.corrado@unipd.it

 
A. Pressler, J. Niebauer (eds.), *Textbook of Sports and Exercise Cardiology*,
https://doi.org/10.1007/978-3-030-35374-2_17

## 17.2 Sinus Bradycardia and Atrio-Ventricular Conduction Disturbances

### 17.2.1 Sinus Bradycardia, Sinus Arrhythmia and Sinus Pauses

Sinus bradycardia is a non-pathologic condition that represents a common feature of the athlete's heart as a consequence of the increased vagal tone [1]. Its prevalence varies widely among the populations oscillating from 4% to 8% in non-athletes, and from 40% to 90% in athletes according to the degree of training [1–5]. Sinus pauses > 2 s at 24-h ambulatory electrocardiogram (ECG) monitoring are also quite common and are observed in more than one third of athletes [6]. Sinus rates at rest in the 40–50 bpm range are common in endurance athletes [1–6].

- In highly trained athletes, even marked sinus bradycardia may be observed (<40 bpm), without pathological significance.
- Conversely, in athletes practicing sport at low cardiovascular intensity, a daytime resting heart rate (HR) <40 bpm is infrequent and potentially pathological.

With significant sinus bradycardia, a junctional or ventricular escape rhythm can compete with the sinus rhythm. Sinus arrhythmia and wandering atrial pacemaker are also more prevalent in athletes compared with the general population.

*Sports eligibility* can be granted in athletes without heart disease and without bradycardia-related symptoms (syncope, pre-syncope, dizziness, dyspnea, etc.).

- In cases of athletes with marked sinus bradycardia, exercise testing (ET) should show a normal chronotropic response (achievement of at least 85% of maximum theoretical heart rate for age) and 24-h ambulatory ECG monitoring should not record pauses >3 s.
- In athletes practicing aerobic sports, sinus pauses >3 s should not be considered as a sign of sinus node dysfunction, as long as they are not associated to symptoms or arrhythmias correlated with bradycardia.
- In selected case, 3–6 months of detraining can be very useful in documenting the significant reduction of the sinus arrhythmia or pauses, as expression of vagal tone.

### 17.2.2 Atrioventricular Block (AVB)

First-degree and second-degree type 1 AVB are not rare in athletes practicing aerobic sports and are also considered a major expression of adaptation to physical training, while Mobitz type II second-degree AVB and third-degree AVB are very rare and often pathological [7–11]. Second-degree type 1 AVB is frequently

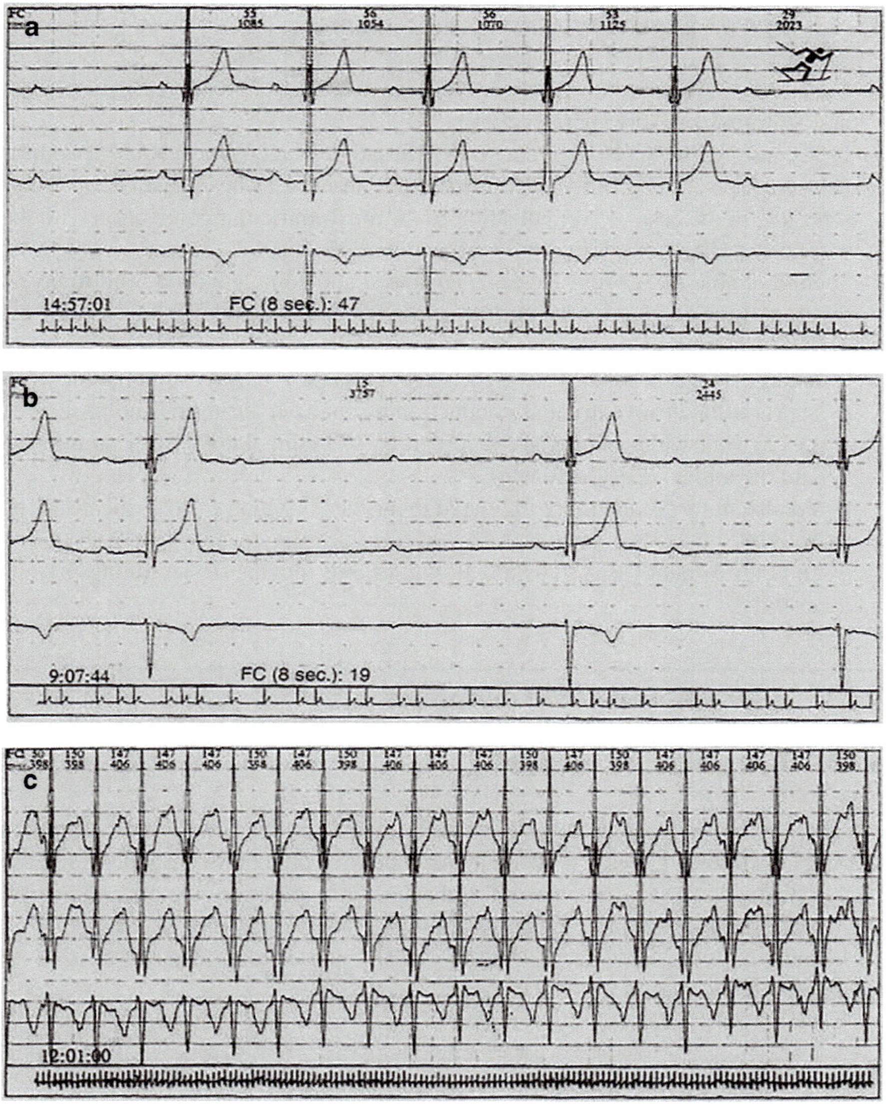


**Fig. 17.1** Cross-country skier, 28 years old, with asymptomatic resting/nocturnal Mobitz-1 atrio-ventricular block (**panel a**), occasionally advanced (3:1; **panel b**). The atrio-ventricular conduction disturbance is completely normalized by physical exercise (**panel c**)

observed during nighttime (i.e. when the vagal tone is highest) at 24-h ambulatory ECG monitoring, but it may rarely be observed at rest during daytime. Both first-degree and second-degree type 1 AVB should normalize during exercise or hyperpnoea (Fig. 17.1). On the other hand, appearance of an AVB during exercise is always pathological, suggesting an infra-hissian block (i.e. secondary to a disease of the conduction system).

### 17.2.3 Sports Eligibility

- First-degree AVB, which disappears during exercise or hyperventilation, does not contraindicate any sports activity.
- In second-degree AVB with narrow QRS and Luciani-Wenckebach periodism (Mobitz type-1), eligibility is granted in the absence of heart disease or symptoms and in the case of normalization of the atrioventricular conduction with the increase in HR during ET.
- Second-degree AVB Mobitz type-2, advanced and complete AVB require investigation of the conduction system by invasive electrophysiologic study [12].
  - If a disease of the cardiac conduction system is excluded and the AVB is considered to be secondary to hypervagotonia, they may be compatible with sports if the atrioventricular conduction normalizes during ET, no prolonged (>3 s) ventricular pauses are recorded at 24-h ambulatory ECG monitoring and the athlete is asymptomatic.
  - Persistent forms and those unrelated to physical training contraindicate sports activity.
  - In controversial cases, re-evaluation after 3–6 months of detraining may be useful.

## 17.3 Supraventricular Arrhythmias

### 17.3.1 Premature Atrial Beats

The presence of occasional premature atrial beats can be considered a common finding in healthy athletes. Frequent and/or repetitive premature atrial beats require further diagnostic testing, such as ET and echocardiography to rule out an underlying heart disease. Electrolytes and thyroid function should also be checked.

*Sports eligibility* may be granted in the absence of significant symptoms or underlying heart disease.

### 17.3.2 Paroxysmal Supraventricular Tachycardias (with No Overt Pre-Excitation)

Atrio-ventricular nodal re-entrant tachycardia (AVNRT) and orthodromic atrio-ventricular re-entrant tachycardia (ARVT) through a concealed accessory pathway are the two most common paroxysmal supraventricular tachycardias in young people [13]. Although benign, these arrhythmias may be poorly tolerated in athletes because they may occur during sports activity, and sympathetic stimulation increases their HR.

As a consequence, *sports eligibility* can be granted only if there is:

- no history of severe symptoms and the recurrences are rare and non-exercise related.

- In the other cases, catheter ablation is the best option, given the very high success rate (approximately 90% for AVRT and >95% for AVNRT) and the low risk of complications [14].
  - One month after successful ablation, in the absence of complications and recurrences, the athlete can resume competitions [15].

### 17.3.3 Wolff-Parkinson-White Syndrome

Wolff-Parkinson-White (WPW) syndrome is a congenital heart disease characterized by the abnormal persistence of a muscular bundle (accessory atrioventricular pathway) which provides an alternative way of electrical connection between atrial and ventricular myocardium, other than the normal atrioventricular node-His bundle axis [14, 15]. Typical ECG features of ventricular pre-excitation in the WPW syndrome include:

1. a PR interval less than 0.12 s
2. with a slurring of the initial segment of the QRS complex, known as a delta wave, and
3. a QRS complex widening with a total duration greater than 0.12 s.

The delta wave may be particularly evident in highly trained athletes who exhibit an increased vagal tone and prolonged atrioventricular node conduction time.

The WPW syndrome may be complicated by different types of arrhythmia, in particular:

(a) AVRT, either orthodromic or antidromic and
(b) pre-excited atrial fibrillation (AF) that can degenerate into lethal ventricular fibrillation in case of very rapid atrioventricular conduction through the accessory pathway.

Physical activity may increase the occurrence of arrhythmias in WPW syndrome [14, 15]. As the risk of sudden death is proportional to the ability of the accessory pathway to provide fast atrioventricular conduction in case of AF, evaluation of the accessory pathway refractoriness by transesophageal or endocavitary electrophysiological study is a prerequisite for sports eligibility. The study can be avoided in asymptomatic patients with intermittent delta wave and can be delayed in asymptomatic children aged <12 years who are at very low risk of sudden death [15].

*Sports eligibility* should be granted only in athletes

- with no history of supraventricular arrhythmias and
- if the electrophysiology study demonstrates a refractory period of the accessory pathway ≥250 ms at rest and ≥210 ms during exercise or isoproterenol infusion.

In case of previous symptoms or high-risk accessory pathway, the athlete should be referred for catheter ablation [15].

### 17.3.4 Atrial Fibrillation and Atrial Flutter

The association between sports activity and the risk of developing AF has been evaluated by several studies that have provided different results depending on the age, years of training, and type of sport of the study population [15–28]. Overall, these studies suggest that moderate intensity physical activity is associated with a lower incidence of AF, but high-intensity endurance sports increases the risk of AF in middle-aged athletes but not in younger individuals (see also Chaps. 34 and 51). The pathophysiological mechanisms responsible for the development of AF in athletes remain speculative and are mostly dependent on experimental data. Atrial enlargement and fibrosis, increased atrial ectopy, increased vagal tone and changes in electrolytes have been proposed as possible mechanisms [29].

Because AF in athletes usually occurs in the context of a structurally normal heart ("lone AF") and because anti-arrhythmic drugs may be poorly tolerated, pulmonary vein isolation by catheter ablation is been increasingly offered to athletes as a first line therapeutic option [30, 31]. Although observational studies suggest that the outcome of AF ablation in athletes is similar or better than in sedentary individuals, long-term arrhythmia-free survival after a single procedure ranges 50–70% and repeat ablations are required to achieve a 70–80% probability of freedom from AF [32–35]. Moreover, the rate of serious complications is not negligible (1–5%) and it has to be discussed with the patient before this strategy is chosen [36].

*Sports eligibility* in athletes with paroxysmal AF may be granted

- in the absence of structural heart disease,
- if the episodes are sporadic,
- not exercise-induced and
- not associated with severe symptoms.

Permanent AF usually contraindicates competitive sport at medium or high cardiovascular demand. In case of one of more risk factors for AF-related arterial thromboembolism (such as age > 65 years old, hypertension and diabetes) anticoagulation therapy should be considered and, if this is initiated, sports at-risk for trauma should be avoided because of the risk of bleeding.

Atrial tachycardia and atrial flutter are uncommon in athletes without heart disease and may cause elevated heart rates during exercise. Therefore, such arrhythmias are not usually compatible with athletic activity at medium-high cardiovascular intensity. Catheter ablation of the cavo-tricuspidal isthmus is a highly effective and safe therapy for the treatment of typical atrial flutter and should thus be considered as the treatment of choice [37].

## 17.4 Ventricular Arrhythmias

In the majority of cases, ventricular arrhythmias that may be encountered in athletes consists of simple premature ventricular beats (PVBs) resulting from the activity of a benign and idiopathic automatic focus that is usually suppressed by exercise, similarly to the sedentary population [38]. Only occasionally, idiopathic PVBs may increase in number and complexity during effort and cause non-sustained or sustained ventricular tachycardia that may be fast enough as to cause severe symptoms such as syncope [30, 31, 39], or be numerous enough as to cause PVBs-mediated left ventricular dysfunction [40]. Rarely, PVBs may represent the clinical manifestation of an underlying heart disease potentially at-risk of sudden cardiac death. Hence, the first objective in evaluating an athlete with ventricular arrhythmias is to exclude life-threatening cardiovascular diseases [41].

### 17.4.1 Features that may Suggest an Underlying Heart Disease

An increase in the arrhythmia at the beginning of exercise, disappearance at peak exercise, and reappearance during recovery usually suggest a benign process [38]. On the other hand, triggering or worsening of the arrhythmia during exercise may indicate an underlying cardiomyopathy or ion channel disease [42–49].

Careful assessment of the morphology of the arrhythmic QRS complex may help to identify the anatomic origin and the probability of an underlying disease:

- The most common benign PVBs of the athletes show a negative QRS complex in V1 (left-bundle-branch-block, LBBB pattern) and inferior axis in the limb leads (positive QRS complex in II, III and aVF), indicating origin from the ventricular outflow tract (either right or left).
  - Also, ventricular arrhythmias with a slightly prolonged QRS (0.12–0.13 s) and a morphology of the ectopic QRS resembling a typical right-bundle-branch-block (RBBB) in V1 suggests the origin from a fascicle of the left bundle and are usually benign.
- In contrast, arrhythmias with different configurations such as LBBB and intermediate/superior axis or RBBB with wide QRS are rarer in healthy athletes and may be the sign of an underlying structural heart disease [40–47] (Fig. 17.2).
  - In particular, PVBs with a RBBB configuration indicate a left ventricular origin and suggest possible left ventricular diseases such as
    dilated/inflammatory cardiomyopathy,
    hypertrophic cardiomyopathy,
    left ventricular non-compaction, or
    a predominantly left-sided arrhythmogenic cardiomyopathy (ARVC),

particularly if the arrhythmia increases in number and complexity with increasing workload during ET [39, 48].

The prevalence of concomitant repolarization/depolarization ECG abnormalities increases the probability of an associated disease. The association between PVBs with a LBBB pattern and repolarization abnormalities, such as T-wave inversion in the right precordial leads is highly suggestive of ARVC. The coexistence of a right ventricular conduction defect in the form of a prolonged QRS duration or a delayed S-wave upstroke in V1–V3 further increases the likelihood of ARVC [49].

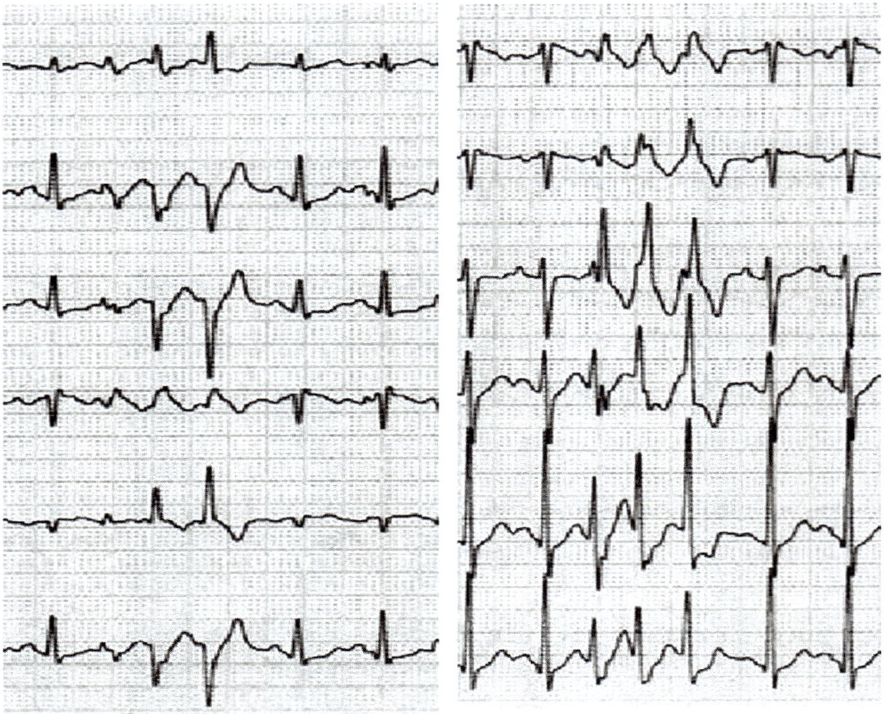

**Fig. 17.2** Swimmer, 26 years old, with a brief episode of exercise-induced non-sustained ventricular tachycardia. The ventricular arrhythmia has an uncommon morphology with wide right bundle branch block. Constrast enhanced cardiac magnetic resonance showed the presence of a subepicardial left ventricular scar

Finally, the induction of polymorphic VT during exercise always carries a bad prognosis. Polymorphic VT with alternating complexes ("bidirectional" pattern), induced during exercise, suggests the inherited ion channel disorder, catecholaminergic polymorphic ventricular tachycardia, which causes exercise-induced arrhythmic cardiac arrest in the absence of structural heart disease as discussed above [50].

### 17.4.2 Work-Up of Athletes with Ventricular Arrhythmias

The work-up of athletes with ventricular arrhythmias should always include

(a) echocardiography,
(b) 24-h ambulatory ECG monitoring and
(c) ET.

Ambulatory ECG monitoring should include a training session and, possibly, have a 12-lead configuration that allows to evaluate the PVBs morphology. Exercise tests should mimic the exercise/sport practiced by the patient, because a conventional ET may not replicate the specific clinical situation and the arrhythmogenic mechanisms produced by the sport. Echocardiography is the preferred imaging modality in the evaluation of athletes with ventricular arrhythmias in order to exclude an underlying a cardiomyopathy or a congenital heart disease. However, even if echocardiography is negative, contrast-enhanced cardiovascular magnetic resonance imaging may be particularly indicated in athletes with complex and/or exercise-induced PVBs with a RBBB configuration and wide-QRS, in order to exclude concealed left-ventricular scar tissue that may be a substrate for life-threatening ventricular arrhythmias and sudden cardiac death in the athlete [39, 48].

In selected athletes in whom non-invasive clinical and instrumental findings are inconclusive, other invasive tests such as

(a) electrophysiological study,
(b) coronary angiography (particularly in older athletes with coronary risk factors), and
(c) endomyocardial biopsy

may be required to achieve a definite diagnosis. Molecular genetic studies are increasingly available for the diagnosis of inherited arrhythmogenic heart muscle diseases, including channelopathies, and are particularly indicated if catecholaminergic polymorphic ventricular tachycardia is suspected (see Chap. 12). Work-up should also include a search for agents that may enhance electrical ventricular irritability, such as the use of excessive amount of alcohol, illicit drugs, or stimulants, particularly ephedrine and caffeine (see Chap. 28).

### 17.4.3 Sports Eligibility in Athletes with Premature Ventricular Beats

- The 2006 consensus document of the Working Group on Sports Cardiology of the European Society of Cardiology recommended to exclude from competitive sports activity athletes with >2000 PVBs/day, repetitive or exercise-induced PVBs even in the absence of an underlying structural heart disease, unless they disappear after 3–6 months of detraining [51].
  - However, these recommendations appear out-of-date considering the current perspective on the clinical meaning of PVBs based on more recent scientific data.
- The 2015 recommendations of the American Heart Association/American College of Cardiology suggest that athletes with PVBs and no underlying disease can participate in all competitive sports.
  - However, when PVBs increase in frequency during exercise or exercise testing and convert to repetitive forms, further evaluation by appropriate imaging or monitoring strategies is recommended before clearance for participation in high-intensity sports.
  - If exercise-induced arrhythmias cause symptoms, the athlete should be limited to exercise below the level at which arrhythmias occur.
  - Conversely, athletes with defined structural heart disease should be limited to low-intensity competitive sports.

- Finally, according to the 2017 recommendations of the Italian Society of Sports Cardiology, athletes with PVBs should be carefully assessed for an underlying heart disease.
  - The work-up should include cardiac magnetic resonance in case of PVBs with a left ventricular origin.
  - In case no disease is detected, the athlete is considered eligible to competitive sports activity in the absence of severe symptoms, complex arrhythmias (short-coupled PVBs or narrow couplets) or PVBs-induced left ventricular dysfunction [52].

### 17.4.4 Ventricular Tachycardia

Ventricular tachycardia (VT) can be either non-sustained (3 or more beats but lasting less than 30 s) or sustained (>30 s) and not leading to hemodynamic deterioration. Similar to PVBs, VT may be idiopathic and result from the activity of an ectopic focus or be secondary to a heart disease.

Benign idiopathic VTs include fascicular VT and ventricular outflow tract VT. These VTs are usually well tolerated but if they occur during exercise, they can show a high heart rate and lead to syncope [53, 54].

Consequently, *sports eligibility* can be granted only in cases there is

- no underlying heart disease (particularly arrhythmogenic cardiomyopathy),
- the athlete is asymptomatic, and
- the episodes are sporadic, of short duration, with low heart rate and unrelated to exercise.

In the other cases, catheter ablation is the preferred therapeutic option.

The occurrence of monomorphic sustained VT (>30 s) other than fascicular and infundibular, polymorphic VT, torsades de pointes, and/or cardiac arrest due to ventricular fibrillation, contraindicate both competitive and recreational sports activity. The only exceptions are VT arising in the context of acute and fully reversible disease with a low probability of recurrence, such as myocarditis, electrolyte disturbances and intake of drugs. In these cases, suspension of physical activity for 3–6 months and subsequent cardiovascular reassessment is recommended [51].

**Clinical Pearls**

- Due to an increased vagal tone, trained athletes commonly develop benign rhythm and conduction disturbances including sinus bradycardia, junctional rhythm, first-degree and second-degree Mobitz type-I atrioventricular block.
- These alterations usually disappear with adrenergic stimulation during exercise and do not preclude sports participation.
- Paroxysmal supraventricular tachycardia and atrial fibrillation usually occur in athletes with a structurally normal heart but may be incompatible with

competitive sports activity in case of severe symptoms or exercise-dependent episodes.

- Ventricular arrhythmias ranging from isolated premature ventricular beats to ventricular tachycardia require careful clinical investigation aiming to exclude an underlying structural heart disease potentially at risk of sudden cardiac death before the athlete can safely engage in high-intensity exercise.

## Review

### Questions

1. Top-level athlete, male, 28 years old, practicing soccer from 15 years, asymptomatic, without family and personal history for cardiovascular disease, presenting with a second-degree, type 1 atrio-ventricular block during resting 12-lead ECG. What examination may be useful to guarantee his sport eligibility?
2. Volleyball player, male, 27 years old, without clinical history of sudden death, asymptomatic, during pre-participation screening; occurrence of exercise-induced ventricular arrhythmias during an exercise stress test, sometimes as couplets, with RBBB morphology and wide QRS complex. What further examinations do you suggest?
3. 24 years old, male tennis player, presenting with paroxysmal palpitations and resting ECG showing a supraventricular tachycardia at HR 220 bpm, with narrow and regular QRS. The tachycardia has a spontaneous interruption after 10 min. When sinus rhythm is restored, ECG shows the presence of an overt ventricular pre-excitation. Can the athlete be considered eligible for competitive sports activity at this point?

### Answers

1. Exercise stress testing (EST) is the first exam to confirm the physiological, adaptive response of atrio-ventricular node to exercise training. EST usually normalizes the atrio-ventricular conduction during exercise and recovery phase. Also 24-h Holter ECG monitoring, including a training session, could be useful to verify the normalization of AV conduction during an exercise session and to show the maximal expression of AV disturbances during night sleeping.
2. The arrhythmia morphology (RBBB with wide QRS) is uncommon and could be associated with a concealed arrhythmogenic substrate, such as left ventricular scar. Therefore, beyond carrying out colour-doppler echocardiogram and 24-h Holter ECG monitoring, also contrast enhanced cardiac magnetic resonance, with tissue imaging typing, is requested.
3. No. Symptomatic WPW syndrome is not compatible with competitive sports activity. The athlete can be considered suitable for RF catheter ablation.

## References

1. Blake JB, Larrabee RC. Observations upon long distance runners. Boston Med Surg J. 1903;148:195.
2. Chapman JH. Profound sinus bradycardia in the athletic heart syndrome. J Sports Med Phys Fitness. 1982;22:45–8.
3. Hanne-Paparo N, Kellermann JJ. Long-term Holter ECG monitoring of athletes. Med Sci Sports Exerc. 1981;13:294–8.
4. Zehender M, Meinertz T, Keul J, et al. ECG variants and cardiac arrhythmia in athletes: clinical relevance and prognostic importance. Am Heart J. 1990;119:1378–91.
5. Huston TP, Puffer JC, Rodney WM. The athletic heart syndrome. N Engl J Med. 1985;313:24–32.
6. Viitasalo MT, Kala R, Eisalo A. Ambulatory electrocardiographic findings in young athletes between 14 and 16 years of age. Eur Heart J. 1984;5:2–6.
7. Palatini P, Maraglino G, Sperti G, et al. Prevalence and possible mechanisms of ventricular arrhythmias in athletes. Am Heart J. 1985;110:560–7.
8. Talan DA, Bauernfeind RA, Ashley WW, et al. Twentyfour hour continuous ECG recordings in longdistance runners. Chest. 1982;82:19–24.
9. Viitasalo M, Kala R, Eisalo A. Ambulatory electrocardiographic recording in endurance athletes. Br Heart J. 1982;47:213–20.
10. Meytes I, Kaplinsky E, Yahini JH. Wenckebach A-V block: a frequent feature following heavy physical training. Am Heart J. 1975;90:426–30.
11. Zeppilli P, Fenici R, Sassara M, et al. Wenckebach second-degree AV block in top-ranking athletes: an old problem revisited. Am Heart J. 1980;100:291–4.
12. Vidal A, Agorrody V, Abreu R, et al. Vagally third-degree AV block in a highly trained endurance athlete. Europace. 2017;19:1863.
13. Page RL, Joglar JA, Caldwell MA, et al. 2015 ACC/AHA/HRS guideline for the management of adult patients with supraventricular tachycardia: a report of the American college of cardiology/American heart association task force on clinical practice guidelines and the heart rhythm society. Heart Rhythm. 2016;13:e136–221.
14. Sarubbi B. The Wolff-Parkinson-White electrocardiogram pattern in athletes: how and when to evaluate the risk for dangerous arrhythmias. The opinion of the paediatric cardiologist. J Cardiovasc Med (Hagerstown). 2006;7:271–8.
15. Biffi A, Delise P, Zeppilli P, et al. Italian cardiological guidelines for sports eligibility in athletes with heart disease: part 1. J Cardiovasc Med. 2013;14:500–15.
16. Karjalainen J, Kujala UM, Kaprio J, et al. Lone atrial fibrillation in vigorously exercising middle aged men: case-control study. BMJ. 1998;316:1784–5.
17. Mont L, Sambola A, Brugada J, et al. Long-lasting sport practice and lone atrial fibrillation. Eur Heart J. 2002;23:477–82.
18. Elosua R, Arquer A, Mont L, et al. Sport practice and the risk of lone atrial fibrillation: a case-control study. Int J Cardiol. 2006;108:332–7.
19. Molina L, Mont L, Marrugat J, et al. Long-term endurance sport practice increases the incidence of lone atrial fibrillation in men: a follow-up study. Europace. 2008;10:618–23.
20. Masia R, Pena A, Marrugat J, et al. High prevalence of cardiovascular risk factors in Gerona, Spain, a province with low myocardial infarction incidence. REGICOR Investigators. J Epidemiol Community Health. 1998;52:707–15.
21. Mont L, Tamborero D, Elosua R, GIRAFA (Grup Integrat de Recerca en Fibril-lació Auricular) Investigators, et al. Physical activity, height, and left atrial size are independent risk factors for lone atrial fibrillation in middle-aged healthy individuals. Europace. 2008;10:15–20.
22. Myrstad M, Løchen ML, Graff-Iversen S, et al. Increased risk of atrial fibrillation among elderly Norwegian men with a history of long-term endurance sport practice. Scand J Med Sci Sports. 2014;24:e238–44.
23. Heidbuchel H, Anné W, Willems R, et al. Endurance sports is a risk factor for atrial fibrillation after ablation for atrial flutter. Int J Cardiol. 2006;107:67–72.

24. D'Ascenzi F, Cameli M, Ciccone MM, et al. The controversial relationship between exercise and atrial fibrillation: clinical studies and pathophysiological mechanisms. J Cardiovasc Med (Hagerstown). 2015;16:802–10.
25. Pelliccia A, Maron BJ, Di Paolo FM, et al. Prevalence and clinical significance of left atrial remodeling in competitive atheletes. J Am Coll Cardiol. 2005;46:690–5.
26. Woodward A, Tin Tin S, Doughty RN, Ameratunga S. Atrial fibrillation and cycling: six year follow-up of the Taupo bicycle study. BMC Public Health. 2015;15:23.
27. Kwok CS, Anderson SG, Myint PK, Mamas MA, Loke YK. Physical activity and incidence of atrial fibrillation: a systematic review and meta-analysis. Int J Cardiol. 2014;177:467–76.
28. Hoogsteen J, Schep G, Van Hemel NM, et al. Paroxysmal atrial fibrillation in male endurance athletes. A 9-year follow up. Europace. 2004;6:222–8.
29. Sarceviz Z, Tepavcecic A. Competitive endurance activities of middle-aged athletes as a risk factor for atrial fibrillation. Curr Sports Med Rep. 2018;17:391–5.
30. Zipes DP, Link MS, Ackerman MJ, Kovacs RJ, Myerburg RJ, Estes NA 3rd. Eligibility and disqualification recommendations for competitive athletes with cardiovascular abnormalities: task force 9: arrhythmias and conduction defects: a scientific statement from the American Heart Association and American College of Cardiology. Circulation. 2015;132:e315–25.
31. Lai E, Chung EH. Management of arrhythmias in athletes: atrial fibrillation, premature ventricular contractions, and ventricular tachycardia. Curr Treat Options Cardiovasc Med. 2017;19:86.
32. Kirchhof P, Benussi S, Kotecha D, et al. 2016 ESC guidelines for the management of atrial fibrillation developed in collaboration with EACTS. Europace. 2016;18:1609–78.
33. Furlanello F, Lupo P, Pittalis M, et al. Radiofrequency catheter ablation of atrial fibrillation in athletes referred for disabling symptoms preventing usual training schedule and sport competition. J Cardiovasc Electrophysiol. 2008;19:457–62.
34. Calvo N, Mont L, Tamborero D, Berruezo A, Viola G, Guasch E, Nadal M, Andreu D, Vidal B, Sitges M, Brugada J. Efficacy of circumferential pulmonary vein ablation of atrial fibrillation in endurance athletes. Europace. 2010;12:30–6.
35. Koopman P, Nuyens D, Garweg C, La Gerche A, De Buck S, Van Casteren L, Alzand B, Willems R, Heidbuchel H. Efficacy of radiofrequency catheter ablation in athletes with atrial fibrillation. Europace. 2011;13:1386–93.
36. Corrado D, Zorzi A. Risk of catheter ablation for atrial fibrillation. JACC Clin Electrophysiol. 2017;3:1434–6.
37. Schmieder S, Ndrepepa G, Dong J, Zrenner B, Schreieck J, Schneider MA, Karch MR, Schmitt C. Acute and long-term results of radiofrequency ablation of common atrial flutter and the influence of the right atrial isthmus ablation on the occurrence of atrial fibrillation. Eur Heart J. 2003;24:956–62.
38. Biffi A, Pelliccia A, Verdile L, et al. Long-term clinical significance of frequent and complex ventricular tachyarrhythmias in trained athletes. J Am Coll Cardiol. 2002;40:446–52.
39. Jacobson JT, Iwai S, Aronow W. Medical therapy to prevent recurrence of ventricular arrhythmia in normal and structural heart disease patients. Expert Rev Cardiovasc Ther. 2016;14:1251–62.
40. Delise P, Sitta N, Lanari E, et al. Long-term effect of continuing sports activity in competitive athletes with frequent ventricular premature complexes and apparently normal heart. Am J Cardiol. 2013;112:1396–402.
41. D'Ascenzi F, Zorzi A, Alvino F, et al. The prevalence of premature ventricular beats in the athlete. Scand J Med Sci Sports. 2017;27:140–51.
42. Steriotis AK, Nava A, Rigato I, et al. Noninvasive cardiac screening in young athletes with ventricular arrhythmias. Am J Cardiol. 2013;111:557–62.
43. Verdile L, Maron BJ, Pelliccia A, et al. Clinical significance of exercise-induced ventricular tachyarrhythmias in trained athletes without cardiovascular abnormalities. Heart Rhythm. 2015;12:78–85.
44. Rahilly GT, Prystowsky EN, Zipes DP, et al. Clinical and electrophysiologic findings in patients with repetitive monomorphic ventricular tachycardia and otherwise normal electrocardiogram. Am J Cardiol. 1982;50:459–68.

45. Buxton AE, Marchlinski FE, Doherty JU, et al. Repetitive, monomorphic ventricular tachycardia: clinical and electrophysiologic characteristics in patients with and patients without organic heart disease. Am J Cardiol. 1984;54:997–1002.
46. Zorzi A, De Lazzari M, Mastella G, Niero A, Trovato D, Cipriani A, et al. Ventricular arrhythmias in young competitive athletes: prevalence, determinants, and underlying substrate. J Am Heart Assoc. 2018;7(12):e009171.
47. Zorzi A, Mastella G, Cipriani A, Berton G, Del Monte A, Gusella B, et al. Burden of ventricular arrhythmias at 12-lead 24-hour ambulatory ECG monitoring in middle-aged endurance athletes versus sedentary controls. Eur J Prev Cardiol. 2018;25:2003–11.
48. Cipriani A, Zorzi A, Sarto P, Donini M, Rigato I, Bariani R, et al. Predictive value of exercise testing in athletes with ventricular ectopy evaluated by cardiac magnetic resonance. Heart Rhythm. 2019;16:239–48.
49. Zorzi A, Perazzolo Marra M, Rigato I, De Lazzari M, Susana A, Niero A, et al. Nonischemic left ventricular scar as a substrate of life-threatening ventricular arrhythmias and sudden cardiac death in competitive athletes. Circ Arrhythm Electrophysiol. 2016;9(7):e004229.
50. Priori SG, Napolitano C, Memmi M, Colombi B, Drago F, Gasparini M, et al. Clinical and molecular characterization of patients with catecholaminergic polymorphic ventricular tachycardia. Circulation. 2002;106(1):69–74.
51. Heidbuchel H, Corrado D, Biffi A, et al. Recommendations for participation in leisure-time physical activity and competitive sports of patients with arrhythmias and potentially arrhythmogenic conditions. Part II: ventricular arrhythmias, channelopathies and implantable defibrillators. Eur J Cardiovasc Prev Rehabil. 2006;13(5):676–86.
52. Comitato organizzativo cardiologico per l'idoneità allo sport (COCIS). Protocolli cardiologici per il giudizio di idoneità allo sport agonistico. Italy: C.E.S.I. ed. Roma; 2017.
53. John RM, Stevenson WG. Outflow tract premature ventricular contractions and ventricular tachycardia: the typical and the challenging. Card Electrophysiol Clin. 2016;8:545–54.
54. Sung R, Scheinman M. Spectrum of fascicular arrhythmias. Card Electrophysiol Clin. 2016;8(3):567–80.

# Specific Cardiovascular Diseases and Competitive Sports Participation: Pacemakers and ICD

18

Hielko Miljoen, Rachel Lampert, and Hein Heidbuchel

**Learning Objectives**

1. Understand the data on safety of sports for athletes with CIEDs, and the limitations of the data.
2. Obtain insight in available technologies and their place in the athletic population
3. Obtain knowledge of the scientific evidence concerning the rationale for choices regarding products and programming in the athletic population.
4. Obtain insight in the holistic approach of athletes with devices, including counseling, decision making and follow-up.

## 18.1 Athletes with Devices

- Before discussing or evaluating the CIED one should consider the underlying disease. If any cardiac condition such as congenital heart disease, cardiomyopathy or primary electrical disease (e.g. CPVT carries a higher risk for exercise induced arrhythmia) is present, the recommendations concerning management and sports eligibility for these specific conditions should be taken into account in

H. Miljoen
Department of Cardiology, Antwerp University Hospital, Antwerp, Belgium
e-mail: hielko.miljoen@uza.be

R. Lampert
Department of Internal Medicine/Cardiology, Yale School of Medicine, New Haven, CT, USA
e-mail: rachel.lampert@yale.edu

H. Heidbuchel (✉)
Department of Cardiology, Antwerp University Hospital and Antwerp University, Antwerp, Belgium
e-mail: hein.heidbuchel@uza.be





A. Pressler, J. Niebauer (eds.), *Textbook of Sports and Exercise Cardiology*,
https://doi.org/10.1007/978-3-030-35374-2_18

addition to the presence of the ICD [1–6]. These particular aspects are described in other chapters of the current book. The next paragraphs will cover the more specific issues concerning cardiac implantable devices in athletes.
- A second important message is that every patient is an autonomous individual. Physicians are counselors, not judges. If the safety of the environment and society are secured and the athlete/patient chooses to participate in sports despite a negative advice, our task is still to optimize his/her health and safety and not to leave the athlete without medical attention because of lack of compliance.

## 18.2 Pacemaker

### 18.2.1 General Considerations

- The vast majority of pacemakers are implanted in patients over 40 years of age [7, 8].
  - Very few professional athletes will be affected by this condition.
  - Exceptions are those with congenital complete AV-block or after congenital surgery.
  - However, pacemakers may be seen more commonly in master competitive athletes.
- Two main indication groups:
  - Sinus bradycardia with preserved AV-conduction.
  - AV-conduction disturbances, either permanent or intermittent.
- Recommendations for sports participation in the pacemaker population have changed considerably over the last decade:
  - Earlier recommendations were restricting pacemaker patients to sports with minor or moderate cardiovascular demand [4].
  - More recent guidelines are more liberal, generally allowing athletic participation in athletes with a pacemaker but without underlying structural heart disease [2].
  - A restriction is made for athletes participating in sports with risk of direct collision or impact to the device:

    Pacemaker dependent: cannot participate.

    Not pacemaker dependent: can participate, provided that adequate information of the potential risks and possible preventive measures is given.
  - Protective equipment must be considered for those participating in sports that are potentially hazardous to the device, although no prospective data have proven the effectiveness of such equipment.
  - Diving with a pacemaker is relatively contra-indicated. Outside pressure by the water can cause activity sensors to increase sensor indicated heart rate, and can even cause deformation of the can dependent on the depth [9]. As a general rule, diving must be restricted to depths of 20 m [10].

- Few data exist on sports participation in patients carrying a cardiac pacemaker.
  - Early Danish observation [11]: about half of the 72 patients that completed follow-up (aged 20–60 years) performed a type of leisure time sport in the 3 years following implantation, 83% of them felt improved or did not experience either psychological or physical hindrance from the pacemaker.
  - More recent Dutch study [12]: nine pacemaker patients were trained to successfully complete the Amsterdam (half) marathon without any evidence of pacemaker dysfunction or other complications during 2 years of follow-up.

### 18.2.2 Peri-Implant Management

- Side of implantation:
  - For some sports (e.g., riflery) direct impact on the side of implantation can lead to lead fracture and even complete detachment of the pacemaker header from the rest of the generator [13, 14]. Preferentially, implantation should be performed on the side least prone to such impacts.
  - Classification of sports according to their risk of impact can be found in the paper by Levine et al. [15].
  - Repetitive ipsilateral arm movements have the potential to result in lead failure [16, 17]. For these, the side of implantation should preferably be opposite to the dominant arm.
- Implantation technique:
  - Cephalic vein cutdown or, if not possible or sufficient, extra-thoracic axillary vein puncture is preferable to medial subclavian access, to reduce the risk of subclavian crush of the lead [18, 19].
  - The distance to the ipsilateral shoulder should be sufficient to allow for a full range of motion of this shoulder without hindrance by the device.
  - Subpectoral muscular implantation can be considered when the athlete performs a sport type that carries the risk of impact (for non-pacing-dependent athletes, or if a pacing-dependent athlete is not willing to follow the advice not to practice this sport at all). Only older ICD data are available comparing submuscular to subcutaneous placement. These data show no difference in pocket related complications between the two techniques [20]. However, replacement of the devices is more cumbersome. A randomized trial is ongoing [21].
- Material: one general concept should be kept in mind: the simpler the better.
  - Unipolar or bipolar lead design: while unipolar leads carry some advantages (lead design is less complex than in bipolar leads), and some evidence suggests an improved longevity [22], these benefits are outweighed by the possibility of unipolar oversensing of myopotentials [23]. This is of particular relevance in a more active population like athletes. Furthermore, clinical evidence demonstrates a considerable higher incidence of pacemaker malfunction (chest wall stimulation, myopotential oversensing) during unipolar as

compared to bipolar configuration [24, 25]. In the light of these findings we advocate use of bipolar leads.

- Passive or active fixation: conflicting evidence exists regarding complication rates in passive fixation leads as compared to active fixation models [8, 26–28]. Young (more active) people are prone to a higher long-term lead related complication rate than elderly (more sedentary) people [29]. This implies a higher probability of a future lead extraction. As this is less complicated in active fixation leads, we routinely use this lead type in the athletic population [30, 31].
- VVI, DDD or CRT: device related complications are linked to complexity, i.e. every additional lead implanted carries an increased risk of lead related complications [8]. The indication for more than an AAI or VVI device should therefore be carefully considered in light of available scientific evidence. The patient/athlete must be equipped with the least complex device possible.
- Lead position:

  Atrial:

    Some data point to less development of atrial fibrillation when the atrial lead is placed at Bachmann's bundle as compared to the right atrial appendage [32]. Because the available data are based on rather small groups, we feel that only in experienced hands lead placement in this position should be considered, since dislocation rates may be higher.

  Ventricular:

    RV apical pacing has potential deleterious effects, mainly new onset heart failure. The incidence of pacing-induced cardiomyopathy lies between 20 and 26% [33, 34]. In how far this is true in a younger athletic population with normal baseline LV function is unknown.

    Older data suggest that heart failure can occur with a cumulative ventricular pacing percentage of ≥40% [35]. More recent data suggest that this percentage may be even lower [33].

    CRT has shown to be of benefit when baseline ejection fraction is below 50% and a high pacing percentage is expected [36]. While some data do not suggest benefit in those with normal EF [37], data on young patients, who will be paced over decades, is not yet available.

    Permanent His bundle pacing might be an alternative in the athletic population to avoid development of heart failure when a high pacing percentage is expected. However, reported implant success rates are lower than for conventional pacing (average 92% when using catheter delivery) and chronic thresholds are higher (1.7 V) [38]. The pros and cons need to be discussed with the athlete.

  Lesion wave:

    During implantation special attention should be paid to obtaining a "sound" lesion wave (current of injury) on the signal, defined as at least 25% of the intrinsic atrial or ventricular amplitude. This is a marker of a good lead-tissue fixation [39].

  - Leadless pacing: recently the advent of leadless pacing provides one more option in this context, completely eliminating lead related issues [40, 41]. No data are available on athletes with such devices and real long-term data are not yet available. Although holding a certain promise for the future, we would not routinely advise implantation of such a system in young athletes since it is far from clear how patients needing many replacements in life will fare.
  - MRI conditionality: as various injuries in athletes are best imaged with MRI, we advise implantation of an MRI conditional device [42].
- Post implantation management:
  - Keep wounds dry until healed.
  - Avoid frequent or extreme ipsilateral arm movement until complete fixation of the leads (6 weeks).
  - Return to sports: this fully depends on the type of sports and should be discussed with the athlete, the trainer and the physician. A 6-week period of light training and abstinence from competition to allow fixation is recommended.

### 18.2.3 Device Programming

- Upper Tracking Rate (UTR)
  - In the absence of chronotropic incompetence, a maximum exercise test, or preferably Holter data or heart rate monitor data during a maximum training effort or competition, can be used to determine maximum heart rate. The UTR needs to be programmed accordingly.
  - If chronotropic incompetence is present, the maximum predicted heart rate for age must be employed as UTR. We routinely use 220 minus age in years for UTR programming.
  - Specific attention must be paid to allow tracking up to the desired UTR, taking the total atrial refractory period into account (TARP = AV interval + PVARP [post-ventricular atrial refractory period]). TARP (in ms) needs to be programmed below the upper tracking interval.

    In order to achieve this, rate dependent AV interval and PVARP may need to be programmed "ON".
- Minimize RV pacing
  - As RV pacing has the potential to provoke heart failure and algorithms to minimize ventricular pacing have demonstrated to be of benefit in patients with sinus node disease, we advise to program this algorithm "ON" in athletes with sinus node disease [43]. All manufacturers have such algorithms.
- Rate response
  - Guidelines state that rate response features should be activated for patients with chronotropic incompetence, especially if young and physically active (II A recommendation, level of evidence C) [44].
  - Attention must be payed to provide the athlete with a device with at rate response sensor that is compatible with the dominant type of sports performed by the athlete: a piezo-electric motion sensor will do less well in a cyclist who

does not generate excessive upper body movement during exercise. Horse riding would give the opposite result: here the horse generates the movement resulting in an increase in heart rate, while the rider does not necessarily perform the same heavy exercise [45].
- Minute ventilation sensors have been developed to overcome these limitations. They respond more proportionally but more slowly to exercise [46]. Currently they are most commonly used in dual sensor systems.
- Another option is closed loop stimulation where intracardiac impedance is measured on a beat-to-beat basis and compared to a reference curve.

  There is limited evidence that patients prefer this rate response method to an accelerometer [47].

  The largest body of evidence concerns patients with vasovagal syncope [48].

  No evidence in athletes is available.
- Dual sensor devices can be considered in selected cases. They have demonstrated to improve quality of life but not exercise capacity in a limited group of patients [49].
- Holter monitoring and exercise testing can be useful to optimize sensor response.

### 18.2.4 Follow-Up

- Training
  - Inform the athlete of possible sources of electromagnetic interference (starting gates, scoring equipment during fencing, also TENS during physical therapy). In case of doubt, a Holter or other heart rate monitor could be applied to evaluate device function under such circumstances.
  - Heart rate monitors:

    Measurement by heart rate monitors using a chest strap seems to be accurate when a bipolar but not always when a unipolar pacing mode is used [50].

    Limited data suggest that such heart rate monitors do not interfere with the pacemaker [51].

    There are no data on other means of heart rate monitoring in pacemaker patients (e.g. photoplethysmography). There should be no interference with unipolar and bipolar sensing, as there are no electromagnetic waves elicited by these systems. PPG-based monitors have demonstrated validity in measuring heart rate, also during exercise [52].
  - Ab stimulators, electronic body fat scales, and some other equipment producing electrical or electromagnetic signals have the potential to interfere with the pacemaker and need to be avoided. The following web-site lists sources of interference for devices: https://www.heart.org/en/health-topics/arrhythmia/prevention-treatment-of-arrhythmia/devices-that-may-interfere-with-icds-and-pacemakers

- CRT pacing will rarely be an issue in recreational or competitive athletes, by nature of its use in patients with severe LV systolic dysfunction, unless indicated prophylactically to prevent heart failure development in those with a high proportion of anticipated pacing.

  In this case His-bundle pacing can be considered (see above).

  If a CRT device is implanted, AV and VV optimization should be performed during exercise, as ventricular dyssynchrony can change during exercise [12, 53, 54].
- Remote monitoring is highly recommended: it allows for early detection of potential problems with the device or the leads, and also identifies arrhythmias that may impact sports participation.

## 18.3 ICD

### 18.3.1 General Considerations

- Patient population
  - In the general ICD population the median age for ICD-implantation is over 60 years old [55], with a limited number of younger patients (5.6% under 40 years of age) [56].
  - In a registry of 440 athletes continuing to compete with an ICD (the ICD Sports Safety registry) 61% of subjects were under 40 years of age. The average ejection fraction in this group was normal (60%) [57, 58].
  - As in the pacemaker population, CRT-patients (outside the above-mentioned prophylactic indication) will be rare. There were no CRT patients in the ICD Sports Registry.
- Existing recommendations
  - Older recommendations left no room for participation in sports more intensive than low dynamic, low static demand (IA (see Chap. 1), e.g., golf, bowling, and riflery) [6, 59, 60].
  - More recently, there has been a movement towards a more liberal approach to sports participation supported by reassuring findings from the ICD Sports Registry as described below [58, 61].
  - In this context the more recent (American) guidelines state [2]:

    Participation in IA sports is reasonable if more than 3 months free of device therapy (IIa, level of evidence C)

    Participation in more intensive sports may be considered if more than 3 months free of device therapy, after proper counseling is provided. (IIb, level of evidence C) The underlying cardiac condition should form the basis of sports eligibility, rather than the ICD itself.
  - The current European recommendations [5, 6] are in revision and will be published in 2019.

- Available scientific data
  - Even in the era of the more stringent 2005 guidelines, 71% of physicians reported to have ICD patients participating in numerous kinds of sports, even contact (15%) and high intensity (49%) sports (published 2006) [62].
  - Recently, the 4 year (median 44 months) follow-up data of the ICD Sports Safety Registry on 440 subjects (20% LQTS, 17% HCM, 13% ARVC/D, participating in mostly running, soccer, basketball, and for dangerous sport skiing) have been published [57].

    46% had a pre-ICD history of ventricular arrhythmia and/or cardiac arrest.

    No resuscitated sudden cardiac death or significant arrhythmia related injury occurred during follow-up (primary outcome).

    Two athletes died (one of worsening heart failure, the other at his desk after receiving multiple shocks). Neither death occurred during athletic participation.

    There were no generator malfunctions, and lead survival was similar to prior data in unselected populations (freedom of definite or possible lead failure 94% at 5 years, 85% at 10 years).

    10% of athletes received appropriate shocks during competition or practice, equaling 3/100 person-years.

    4% of athletes received multiple shocks for episode termination (0.5/100 person years)

    More participants received shocks during physical activity than while at rest (20% vs. 10%, $p < 0.0001$).

    The presence of ARVC/D was the only predictor of appropriate shocks during activity.

    A previous report from the same population reported that of those that received shocks, 27% stopped sports at least temporarily although most returned eventually [58].
  - A separate analysis was performed on 129 young (≤21 years) athletes with ICDs [63]:

    No resuscitated sudden cardiac death or significant arrhythmia related injury occurred over a median follow-up of 42 months.

    There were 20 varsity athletes, participating in soccer, baseball, basketball, tennis, triathlon, running, lacrosse and paintball.

    27% of athletes received at least one shock.

    Two athletes required more than one shock to convert an arrhythmia.

    Five athletes received inappropriate shocks during competition of practice.

    Freedom of lead malfunction was 92.3% at 5 years and 79.6% at 10 years.
  - An additional report compared 80 recreational athletes from Europe, Israel and Australia, who were engaged in intense physical activity on a regular basis (≥2×/week and/or ≥ 2 h/week, with the adults in the competitive cohort) [64, 65].

    Recreational athletes were older (median 44 vs. 37 years; $p = 0.0004$), more frequently men (79% vs. 68%; $p = 0.06$), with less idiopathic VF or

CPVT (1.3% vs. 15.4%), less congenital heart disease (1.3% vs. 6.9%) and more ARVC (23.8% vs. 13.6%) ($p < 0.001$).

They more often had a prophylactic ICD implant (51.4% vs. 26.9%; $p < 0.0001$) or were given a beta-blocker (95% vs. 65%; $p < 0.0001$).

Recreational athletes received fewer total (6.3% vs. 20.2%; $p = 0.003$), appropriate (3.8% vs. 11.4%; $p = 0.06$) and inappropriate (2.5% vs. 9.5%; $p = 0.04$) shocks during physical activity.

VT/VF storms during physical activity occurred in 0/80 recreational vs. 7/317 competitive athletes.

- Danger to patient
  - Unlike patients with an implanted pacemaker, ICD patients can experience unexpected loss of conscience at the time of occurrence of an arrhythmia or shock. Therefore, sports that carry risks when loss of conscience occurs, such as rock-climbing or open-water swimming, carry higher risk in this group. For patients choosing to participate in these sports, precautions (such as wearing a life-preserver when swimming in open water) should be taken.

### 18.3.2 Peri-Implant Management

Similar considerations as for pacemakers regarding the side of implantation, implantation technique and complexity of the device hold true for ICDs. Again the general rule is: the simpler the better [66]. The more ICD specific considerations will be discussed here.

- Implantation technique
  - Site of implantation of the can:

    Conventionally the left prepectoral position is used, because the field between the shock coil(s) and the active can covers a large area of the left ventricle.

    Alternative positions have been tested:

      Abdominal position: Historically the ICD can was placed abdominally. However, the risk of device infection increases about fourfold with an abdominal generator position [67] and dual-coil leads are necessary.

      Subcostal placement of the device in young patients has been reported [68]. In that series, the 2-year outcome was equivalent to prepectoral positioning. Longer follow-up is needed to know what happens with the long (100 cm) or epicardial leads used for subcostal placement.

      Right-sided implantation of the active can is an independent predictor of higher defibrillation thresholds [69, 70].

    For these reasons left-sided pectoral implantation still should be the technique of choice.

    Submuscular implantation may be considered in patients prone to direct impact on the can (see Sect. 18.2).

If the left side is not preferred or possible (e.g. for reasons of expected repeated left arm movements or other sports related issues) the right side is a valid alternative. In that case, however, Defibrillation Threshold Testing is mandatory [71].

- Specific points of attention during implantation:

  Signal amplitude: the R-wave signal needs to be large enough during implantation to reduce the risk of re-intervention for poor sensing or oversensing issues. Typically, one should strive for R-wave amplitudes of ≥7.0 mV.

  The presence of a lesion wave (current of injury) predicts a good lead stability, with few revisions for lead-dislocation. See Sect. 18.2.

  Ratio between T-wave amplitude and R-wave amplitude: the larger this ratio, the less risk of T-wave oversensing, understanding that the patient is supine and at rest during the procedure, so that no information can be gathered on this ratio when upright or exercise.

  Potential far-field signals. If atrial far field signal is present, repositioning is mandatory.

- Ventricular lead position:

  As a result of both the increased attention to the potential deleterious effects of apical pacing and the awareness that the RV apex is the thinnest region of the RV, which can lead to more complications during extraction, non-apical positions have been evaluated.

  A recent meta-analysis found non-inferiority of non-apical lead positions with regard to mortality, number of shocks (total, appropriate, inappropriate) and implant procedure time [72].

  A septal position is optimal, as the chance of a clinically significant perforation is lower. If no good sensing or stability can be obtained here, a switch to an apical position is defendable in athletes in whom the projected RV pacing percentage is low.

### 18.3.3 Material

- Integrated vs. true bipolar lead

  The potential advantage of integrated bipolar sensing is the lower lead complexity (obviating the additional ring electrode that is needed for true bipolar sensing)

  The limitation of using integrated bipolar leads is the impossibility of "electrical repositioning", switching the sensing from one mode to the other with the potential to have an increased R-wave sensing or better R-to-T-wave ratio.

  Taking those points into consideration we have no clear preference for either lead type.

- Single vs. dual coil lead

  The presence of an SVC coil increases the complexity of the lead design and lead extraction is more complex carrying a higher risk of complications when an SVC coil is present [73].

Recent data show similar defibrillation thresholds in dual and single coil leads [74, 75] and no difference in lead related complications was observed between the two lead types [76].

With these data in mind, we advocate the use of single coil leads for implantation of left prepectoral ICDs in most athletes. This is in line with reported trends [77, 78].

- Single vs. dual chamber ICD:

  Historically the majority of ICD implantations have been dual chamber devices [56].

  As with pacemaker therapy, patients with bradycardia indications should receive a dual chamber device (typically in 4–14% of the ICD population but probably lower in athletes) [71, 79].

  Dual chamber ICD can be considered in other specific conditions (e.g. LQTS3 with pause dependent arrhythmias, HCM with outflow tract gradient)

  Implantation of a dual chamber device for the sole purpose of tachycardia discrimination is not advocated (level of evidence IIa-NR) [71], due to the lack of firm evidence that dual chamber algorithms reduce the number of (in) appropriate shocks or improve mortality [79], including in the athlete population [80].

  As a general rule, unless DDD pacing is specifically indicated, we prefer implantation of single chamber devices in athletes, as an increased complexity carries an increased risk of complications [56, 81].

- S-ICD

  In patients without a pacing indication or need for ATP, the subcutaneous ICD has shown to be a valid alternative to the transvenous ICD (TV-ICD) with similar reported mortality rates in non-randomized trials [82], as well as similar shock success and fewer complication rates [77, 83, 84].

  With the currently optimal program settings for S-ICD the rate of inappropriate shocks is 4.3% in 1 year [85]. This must be compared with the PainFree-SST data, where optimal ICD programming resulted in a 1-year rate of inappropriate shocks of 2.5% in single chamber ICDs [86]. Real world data from the Altitude registry however show an inappropriate shock rate in TV-ICD of 6% at 1 year [87].

  There were no S-ICDs in the ICD Sports Registry, and no other data on S-ICDs in athletes. Theoretically, S-ICDs could be beneficial in sports with extensive arm-movement (swimming, rowing) in avoiding subclavian crush. For contact sports, whether the lead position outside of the protection of the thorax would increase likelihood of damage is unknown.

  In conclusion, the S-ICD is effective and as safe as the TV-ICD. The different location of the can and the probably lower lead related complication rates certainly hold a promise for athletes in the future. However, prospective data in athletes are not available. Moreover, the longevity of contemporary S-ICD is lower than that of TV-ICD. An open and honest discussion with the athlete on which system to implant is imperative in this context.

- Post implantation management
  - Instructions about (electromagnetic) interference:
    The athlete (and those in his environment) should be aware that the application of a magnet can switch off the device so that it does not deliver therapy (for the duration of the magnet application). This is important to avoid inadvertent inactivation in specific situations, although extremely rare.
    As for pacemakers, electromagnetic interference can cause oversensing. In ICDs, this can provoke inappropriate shocks [88]. This phenomenon seems to be declining over time [89].
  - Instruct the athlete about maximum heart rate:
    Inform the athlete of the programmed rate cut-offs.
    Performing an exercise test or Holter monitoring during training or competition can be of value to identify potential sensing of sinus tachycardia.
    Encourage the athlete to wear a heart-rate monitor during exercise.
    Some perform an exercise test while monitoring the ICD electrogram with the programmer to evaluate for T-wave oversensing. We do not routinely perform such a test.
    We usually advise the athlete to stay at least 10 bpm below the lowest programmed zone. This implies strategic programming of the device (see Sect. 18.3.4)
  - Instruct the athlete about what to do if a shock or syncope occurs [90]:
    One shock at rest, no symptoms: contact treating physician and discuss course of action
    One shock during exercise, no symptoms: stop the exercise, get home safely, contact treating physician and discuss further action.
    More than one shock over 24 h at rest or during exercise: immediate medical attention mandatory.
    Most often, physician consultation to determine any need for change in therapy or programming should be performed after one or more shocks during exercise, prior to resuming sports participation
    Remote monitoring can help to determine the actions that need to be taken.
  - Instruct those in the athlete's environment about possible shocks and actions that can be taken in case of the occurrence of shocks:
    Trainers, coaches, family members need to be aware of the presence of the ICD. Whether and how team members should be notified, should be discussed with the athlete, and the athlete should be encouraged to discuss team dynamics with his or her coach.
    Complete information about the possibility and consequences of a shock should be provided to these persons.
    We do not advocate specific extra measures while athletes with an ICD participate in sports, like having a resuscitation team on-site. Most sports venues now have AEDs available. In specific situations, it can be advisable that someone who knows how to perform CPR and use an AED is on-site while the athlete engages in sports.

- Driving restrictions:
  EHRA has issued recommendations concerning driving after ICD implantation or shocks [91]. Every country, however, has its own laws concerning this matter, which should be adhered to.
- Return to sports:
  No data are available on timing of return to sports. It seems reasonable to avoid vigorous arm movements or competition for at least 6 weeks after TV-ICD implantation
  After S-ICD implantation a similar period of time seems reasonable.
  The effective return to sports depends on the type of sports and needs to be the result of a clear communication between the physician, the athlete, and potentially other stakeholders (family, trainer, coaches, team).

### 18.3.4 Device Programming

- Allow for the necessary UTR/USR (see Sect. 18.2).
- Detection enhancements
  - No specific data for athletes is available. We recommend to use the settings proposed by the consensus document [71].
- Long detection times
  - The ICD programming consensus statement states that the tachyarrhythmia detection duration should be programmed to require the tachycardia to continue for at least 6–12 s or for 30 intervals before completing detection (class I A for primary and class II B-R for secondary prevention) [71].
  - In athletes programming detection times longer than factory settings reduces total and inappropriate shocks, with a trend toward reduction of "appropriate" shocks [80].
- VT zone programming:
  - The ICD programming consensus grants a class I level of evidence A indication to programming rate cut-offs for the VT zone of 185/min to 200/min in primary prevention [71].
  - The recommendation for zone programming in secondary prevention if VT cycle length is known is class IIa level of evidence C for VT rate minus 10/min [71].
  - Both recommendations state that rate cut-offs may be higher for young patients or those in whom SVT detection criteria cannot reliably distinguish SVT from VT [71].
  - Recent data in athletes show that programming higher rate cut-offs (≥200/min) did not increase the risk of syncope, and reduces total and inappropriate shocks, with a trend toward reduction in "appropriate" shocks [80].
  - This also allows for programming higher upper tracking and upper sensor rates (in most ICDs UTR and VT detection zones may not overlap).
- ATP and shock
  - Again, no specific data on athletes are available.

  - It seems logical, in the light of the PainFREE Rx II data, to program at least one sequence of ATP [92].
  - We routinely program all shocks at maximum output, the second to last one at reversed polarity if possible.
- S-ICD
  - Dual zone programming in S-ICD has the potential to reduce the rates of inappropriate shocks [93].
  - The Smart-Pass filter should be programmed "ON", as this halved the incidence of inappropriate shocks in a recent series [85].

### 18.3.5 Follow-Up

- One general point of attention in an ICD population is zone programming and change of medication: if e.g. betablocker or antiarrhythmic drug therapy is associated or increased, VT CL will likely decrease. Programming zones should be adapted accordingly.
- Exercise testing:
  - Exercise stress testing can be helpful to ensure that the slowest VT rate cut-off is above the maximum reached sinus rate.
  - In this context Holter monitoring "in the field" may even be more useful to identify maximum heart rate during competition, which in general can be higher than in lab settings.
  - Both in TV-ICD and S-ICD, exercise can provoke oversensing of T-waves (Fig. 18.1) or noise (Fig. 18.2) [94, 95].

    Unfortunately performing an exercise stress test with optimization of the device settings does not necessarily translate in less inappropriate shocks for this phenomenon [96, 97]. Therefore, we do not routinely perform exercise testing for this indication.
- Management of arrhythmias:
  - Supraventricular: endurance athletes have a higher risk of the development of atrial fibrillation [98]. This calls for aggressive treatment in ICD patients, including pulmonary vein isolation, to reduce the risk of inappropriate shocks as a result of fast conduction of AF. Also, other supraventricular arrhythmias should be treated aggressively and pro-actively to avoid inappropriate shocks.
  - Ventricular: if sustained VT or VF triggered by VPBs is the cause of appropriate therapy, VT ablation should be considered.
  - Sports participation should be deferred after device therapy of ventricular arrhythmias while evaluation and treatment are initiated.
- Remote monitoring:
  - Remote monitoring has shown to reduce mortality in the ICD population [99, 100].
  - It offers the possibility for early identification of arrhythmias and device related issues
  - All athletes should be monitored remotely.

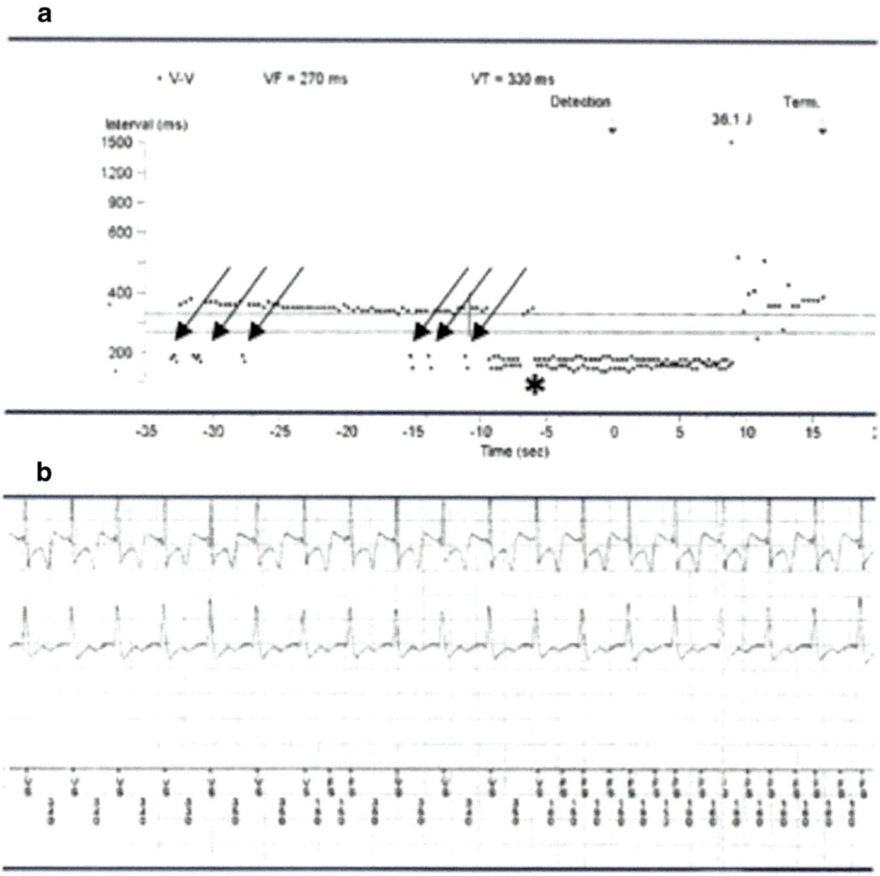


**Fig. 18.1** Exercise induced T-wave oversensing resulting in an inappropriate shock in a patient with Brugada Syndrome. Panel **a** shows the interval plot of the episode. One can appreciate a gradual increase in heart rate (exercise-related), with initially intermittent T-wave oversensing (arrows) and from the asterisk onwards sustained T-wave oversensing, giving rise to a typical "train-rail" aspect of the VV interval plot ending in an inappropriate shock. Panel **b** shows the EGM of the same episode. *VV* VV intervals, *VF* VF zone (faster than 270 ms), *VT* VT zone: between 330 ms and 270 ms, *VS* sense in the sinus rhythm zone, *FS* sense in the VF zone

### Clinical Pearls

- Clinical decisions in the context of sports participation in patients with cardiac electronic devices should be based on a process of shared decision making.
- Both the underlying disease and the device should be considered in this discussion.
- Recent scientific evidence can be helpful in supporting this process.

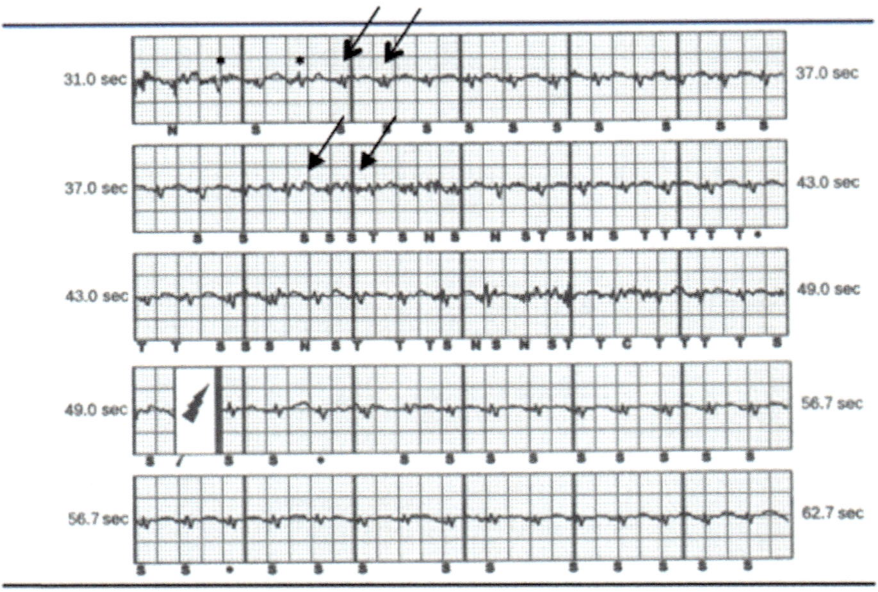


**Fig. 18.2** Exercise induced noise sensing in an S-ICD in a young patient with hypertrophic cardiomyopathy. As a result of the poor signal-to-noise ratio both undersensing (e.g. asterisk) appropriate sensing (open arrow) and inappropriate sensing (closed arrow) can be appreciated. *N* signal classified as noise, *S* signal classified as ventricular sensing in sinus rhythm zone, *T* signal classified as sensing in the VT zone, *C* tachycardia confirmation. Lightning Flash, shock. As a result of the poor signal-to-noise ratio both undersensing (e.g. asterisk) appropriate sensing (open arrow) and inappropriate sensing (closed arrow) can be appreciated

## Review

### Questions

1. A 33-year-old male athlete with ARVC presents to your office. He has received a VVI-ICD 2 years ago for sustained ventricular tachycardia (VT). After the implantation he underwent a radiofrequency ablation for recurrent VT. Since then no arrhythmias have occurred. He is taking Sotalol 80 mg bid. He wants to restart playing soccer. What would be your advice?
2. A 50-year-old male marathon runner has experienced three sudden, non-prodromal syncopes during the last year, not exercise-related. There is no indication of inducible ischemia and an echocardiography and cardiac MRI are normal. His Ajmaline test turns out positive. What would you discuss with this patient?
3. A 23-year-old female is planning to pick up her athletic career after a 2-year break. She was diagnosed with LQT syndrome and received an ICD for recurrence of syncope in spite of optimally titrated betablocker. She visits your consultation for cardiologic advice. What would be your standpoint?

## Answers

1. The discussion on participation in sports should start from the underlying heart disease. As ARVC can potentially worsen with exercise, high intense and/or endurance exercise should be discouraged, and hence, participation is not desirable from the perspective of the underlying disease state itself. If the athlete expresses a wish to participate regardless of your advice, he should be informed that there is a risk for collision during a match, with a potential harm to device and lead. Padding and protective garment should be explained. He must be aware of programmed rate cut-offs (that need to be programmed sufficiently high). Trainings and matches should preferably be conducted under heart rate monitoring and remote monitoring should be activated. His current medication should be continued unchanged. More frequent follow up of heart function should be performed.
2. The athlete has Brugada syndrome. There is a clear indication for an ICD given his recurrent syncope. There is no association between Brugada syndrome and exercise-induced arrhythmias. Based on the findings of the International ICD Sports Registry, there is no contra-indication for sports continuation. On the other hand, overheating and circumstances of hypervagotony could increase the propensity for arrhythmias, during sports or at rest. This is especially important in a long-distance runner. Moreover, there should be careful evaluation for supraventricular arrhythmias, as both Brugada syndrome and endurance exercise increase the risk of atrial fibrillation. The patient should also be evaluated for chronotropic incompetence to determine whether a dual chamber ICD is warranted. As he is still running marathons, this is unlikely. If a single chamber device suffices the option of transvenous or subcutaneous technology should be discussed, touching upon longevity, possibility of inappropriate shocks and the inability to pace with an S-ICD, and lead-related complications with a TV-ICD. After implantation, the patient must be instructed about the programmed rate cut-offs, the actions needed after experiencing a shock and sports participation. He can continue marathon running after a 6-week resting period, provided attention is payed to maintaining hydration and overheating. If shock recur at rest, hypervagotony induced by high-intensive endurance sports should be evaluated. Remote monitoring is highly recommended.
3. A first step, if not already performed, should be to perform genetic testing. If LQT1 is present, discuss the importance of exercise as trigger of events in this disease. As swimming has been shown to be important in this context, the patient should be advised to avoid swimming, especially when unsupervised. In LQT2 and LQT3 exercise as a trigger is less important but still can trigger events. As for sports participation and competition: if the athlete has been asymptomatic for at least 3 months and is fully evaluated, treated, and counseled by a LQT expert, participation can be considered, including competition. This can be placed in the context of the ICD Sports Safety Registry. Optimal betablocker therapy should be continued. The patient must be aware of a higher risk of shocks: this implies that those in the environment of the patient must be well-aware of the condition

and the presence of an ICD. Obviously, electrolyte disturbances (e.g. in the context of dehydration or overheating) and QT-prolonging drugs must be avoided. Again, remote follow-up is highly recommended.

## References


1. Budts W, Borjesson M, Chessa M, van Buuren F, Trigo Trindade P, Corrado D, et al. Physical activity in adolescents and adults with congenital heart defects: individualized exercise prescription. Eur Heart J. 2013;34(47):3669–74.
2. Zipes DP, Link MS, Ackerman MJ, Kovacs RJ, Myerburg RJ, Estes NA 3rd. Eligibility and disqualification recommendations for competitive athletes with cardiovascular abnormalities: task force 9: arrhythmias and conduction defects: a scientific statement from the American Heart Association and American College of Cardiology. Circulation. 2015;132(22):e315–25.
3. Maron BJ, Udelson JE, Bonow RO, Nishimura RA, Ackerman MJ, Estes NA 3rd, et al. Eligibility and disqualification recommendations for competitive athletes with cardiovascular abnormalities: task force 3: hypertrophic cardiomyopathy, arrhythmogenic right ventricular cardiomyopathy and other cardiomyopathies, and myocarditis: a scientific statement from the American Heart Association and American College of Cardiology. Circulation. 2015;132(22):e273–80.
4. Heidbuchel H, Panhuyzen-Goedkoop N, Corrado D, Hoffmann E, Biffi A, Delise P, et al. Recommendations for participation in leisure-time physical activity and competitive sports in patients with arrhythmias and potentially arrhythmogenic conditions. Part I: supraventricular arrhythmias and pacemakers. Eur J Cardiovasc Prev Rehabil. 2006;13(4):475–84.
5. Heidbuchel H, Corrado D, Biffi A, Hoffmann E, Panhuyzen-Goedkoop N, Hoogsteen J, et al. Recommendations for participation in leisure-time physical activity and competitive sports of patients with arrhythmias and potentially arrhythmogenic conditions. Part II: ventricular arrhythmias, channelopathies and implantable defibrillators. Eur J Cardiovasc Prev Rehabil. 2006;13(5):676–86.
6. Pelliccia A, Fagard R, Bjornstad HH, Anastassakis A, Arbustini E, Assanelli D, et al. Recommendations for competitive sports participation in athletes with cardiovascular disease: a consensus document from the Study Group of Sports Cardiology of the Working Group of Cardiac Rehabilitation and Exercise Physiology and the Working Group of Myocardial and Pericardial Diseases of the European Society of Cardiology. Eur Heart J. 2005;26(14):1422–45.
7. Proclemer A, Ghidina M, Gregori D, Facchin D, Rebellato L, Zakja E, et al. Trend of the main clinical characteristics and pacing modality in patients treated by pacemaker: data from the Italian Pacemaker Registry for the quinquennium 2003-07. Europace. 2010;12(2):202–9.
8. Kirkfeldt RE, Johansen JB, Nohr EA, Moller M, Arnsbo P, Nielsen JC. Risk factors for lead complications in cardiac pacing: a population-based cohort study of 28,860 Danish patients. Heart Rhythm. 2011;8(10):1622–8.
9. Lafay V, Trigano JA, Gardette B, Micoli C, Carre F. Effects of hyperbaric exposures on cardiac pacemakers. Br J Sports Med. 2008;42(3):212–6. discussion 6
10. Trigano A, Lafay V, Blandeau O, Levy S, Gardette B, Micoli C. Activity-based rate-adaptive pacemakers under hyperbaric conditions. J Interv Card Electrophysiol. 2006;15(3):179–83.
11. Mickley H, Petersen J. Leisure activities and sports in younger pacemaker patients. Ugeskr Laeger. 1989;151(42):2713–5.
12. Bennekers JH, van Mechelen R, Meijer A. Pacemaker safety and long-distance running. Neth Hear J. 2004;12(10):450–4.
13. Bohm A, Duray G, Kiss RG. Traumatic pacemaker lead fracture. Emerg Med J. 2013;30(8):686.
14. Chelu MG, Leahey EW. Fatigue attributable to broken pacemaker header by baseball. Circ Arrhythm Electrophysiol. 2013;6(5):e77.

15. Levine BD, Baggish AL, Kovacs RJ, Link MS, Maron MS, Mitchell JH. Eligibility and disqualification recommendations for competitive athletes with cardiovascular abnormalities: task force 1: classification of sports: dynamic, static, and impact: a scientific statement from the American Heart Association and American College of Cardiology. Circulation. 2015;132(22):e262–6.
16. Deering JA, Pederson DN. A case of pacemaker lead fracture associated with weightlifting. Pacing Clin Electrophysiol. 1992;15(9):1354–5.
17. Schuger CD, Mittleman R, Habbal B, Wagshal A, Huang SK. Ventricular lead transection and atrial lead damage in a young softball player shortly after the insertion of a permanent pacemaker. Pacing Clin Electrophysiol. 1992;15(9):1236–9.
18. Altun A, Erdogan O. Pacemaker lead failure suggestive of crush injury. Cardiol Rev. 2003;11(5):256.
19. Chan NY, Kwong NP, Cheong AP. Venous access and long-term pacemaker lead failure: comparing contrast-guided axillary vein puncture with subclavian puncture and cephalic cutdown. Europace. 2017;19(7):1193–7.
20. Gold MR, Peters RW, Johnson JW, Shorofsky SR. Complications associated with pectoral cardioverter-defibrillator implantation: comparison of subcutaneous and submuscular approaches. Worldwide Jewel Investigators. J Am Coll Cardiol. 1996;28(5):1278–82.
21. Magnusson P, Wennstrom L, Kastberg R, Liv P. Placement of cardiac PacemaKEr Trial (POCKET)—rationale and design: a randomized controlled trial. Heart Int. 2017;12(1):e8–e11.
22. Debski M, Ulman M, Zabek A, Boczar K, Haberka K, Kuniewicz M, et al. Lead-related complications after DDD pacemaker implantation. Kardiol Pol. 2018;76(8):1224–31.
23. Gialafos J, Maillis A, Kandilas J. Pacemaker inhibition by myopotentials associated with motion and exercise. Eur Heart J. 1987;8 Suppl D:149–54.
24. Wiegand UK, Bode F, Bonnemeier H, Tolg R, Peters W, Katus HA. Incidence and predictors of pacemaker dysfunction with unipolar ventricular lead configuration. Can we identify patients who benefit from bipolar electrodes? Pacing Clin Electrophysiol. 2001;24(9 Pt 1):1383–8.
25. Breivik K, Ohm OJ, Engedal H. Long-term comparison of unipolar and bipolar pacing and sensing, using a new multiprogrammable pacemaker system. Pacing Clin Electrophysiol. 1983;6(3 Pt 1):592–600.
26. Ellenbogen KA, Hellkamp AS, Wilkoff BL, Camunas JL, Love JC, Hadjis TA, et al. Complications arising after implantation of DDD pacemakers: the MOST experience. Am J Cardiol. 2003;92(6):740–1.
27. Hao Y, Li Y, Liao D, Yang L, Liu F. A comparative analysis of the effectiveness of active versus passive atrial lead fixation in Chinese patients with cardiac implantable electrical devices: a long term, retrospective, observational, single-center study. Curr Med Res Opin. 2017;33(3):573–8.
28. Wang Y, Hou W, Zhou C, Yin Y, Lu S, Liu G, et al. Meta-analysis of the incidence of lead dislodgement with conventional and leadless pacemaker systems. Pacing Clin Electrophysiol. 2018;41(10):1365–71.
29. Udo EO, Zuithoff NP, van Hemel NM, de Cock CC, Hendriks T, Doevendans PA, et al. Incidence and predictors of short- and long-term complications in pacemaker therapy: the FOLLOWPACE study. Heart Rhythm. 2012;9(5):728–35.
30. Hauser RG, Katsiyiannis WT, Gornick CC, Almquist AK, Kallinen LM. Deaths and cardiovascular injuries due to device-assisted implantable cardioverter-defibrillator and pacemaker lead extraction. Europace. 2010;12(3):395–401.
31. Henrikson CA, Zhang K, Brinker JA. A survey of the practice of lead extraction in the United States. Pacing Clin Electrophysiol. 2010;33(6):721–6.
32. Bailin SJ, Adler S, Giudici M. Prevention of chronic atrial fibrillation by pacing in the region of Bachmann's bundle: results of a multicenter randomized trial. J Cardiovasc Electrophysiol. 2001;12(8):912–7.

33. Khurshid S, Epstein AE, Verdino RJ, Lin D, Goldberg LR, Marchlinski FE, et al. Incidence and predictors of right ventricular pacing-induced cardiomyopathy. Heart Rhythm. 2014;11(9):1619–25.
34. Zhang XH, Chen H, Siu CW, Yiu KH, Chan WS, Lee KL, et al. New-onset heart failure after permanent right ventricular apical pacing in patients with acquired high-grade atrioventricular block and normal left ventricular function. J Cardiovasc Electrophysiol. 2008;19(2):136–41.
35. Sweeney MO, Hellkamp AS, Ellenbogen KA, Greenspon AJ, Freedman RA, Lee KL, et al. Adverse effect of ventricular pacing on heart failure and atrial fibrillation among patients with normal baseline QRS duration in a clinical trial of pacemaker therapy for sinus node dysfunction. Circulation. 2003;107(23):2932–7.
36. Curtis AB, Worley SJ, Adamson PB, Chung ES, Niazi I, Sherfesee L, et al. Biventricular pacing for atrioventricular block and systolic dysfunction. N Engl J Med. 2013;368(17):1585–93.
37. Stockburger M, Gomez-Doblas JJ, Lamas G, Alzueta J, Fernandez-Lozano I, Cobo E, et al. Preventing ventricular dysfunction in pacemaker patients without advanced heart failure: results from a multicentre international randomized trial (PREVENT-HF). Eur J Heart Fail. 2011;13(6):633–41.
38. Zanon F, Ellenbogen KA, Dandamudi G, Sharma PS, Huang W, Lustgarten DL, et al. Permanent His-bundle pacing: a systematic literature review and meta-analysis. Europace. 2018;20(11):1819–26.
39. Saxonhouse SJ, Conti JB, Curtis AB. Current of injury predicts adequate active lead fixation in permanent pacemaker/defibrillation leads. J Am Coll Cardiol. 2005;45(3):412–7.
40. El-Chami MF, Al-Samadi F, Clementy N, Garweg C, Martinez-Sande JL, Piccini JP, et al. Updated performance of the Micra transcatheter pacemaker in the real-world setting: a comparison to the investigational study and a transvenous historical control. Heart Rhythm. 2018;15(12):1800–7.
41. Tjong FVY, Knops RE, Neuzil P, Petru J, Sediva L, Wilde AAM, et al. Midterm safety and performance of a leadless cardiac pacemaker: 3-year follow-up to the LEADLESS trial (Nanostim Safety and Performance Trial for a Leadless Cardiac Pacemaker System). Circulation. 2018;137(6):633–5.
42. Indik JH, Gimbel JR, Abe H, Alkmim-Teixeira R, Birgersdotter-Green U, Clarke GD, et al. 2017 HRS expert consensus statement on magnetic resonance imaging and radiation exposure in patients with cardiovascular implantable electronic devices. Heart Rhythm. 2017;14(7):e97–e153.
43. Boriani G, Padeletti L. Management of atrial fibrillation in bradyarrhythmias. Nat Rev Cardiol. 2015;12(6):337–49.
44. Brignole M, Auricchio A, Baron-Esquivias G, Bordachar P, Boriani G, Breithardt OA, et al. 2013 ESC Guidelines on cardiac pacing and cardiac resynchronization therapy: the Task Force on cardiac pacing and resynchronization therapy of the European Society of Cardiology (ESC). Developed in collaboration with the European Heart Rhythm Association (EHRA). Eur Heart J. 2013;34(29):2281–329.
45. Lamas GA, Keefe JM. The effects of equitation (horseback riding) on a motion responsive DDDR pacemaker. Pacing Clin Electrophysiol. 1990;13(11 Pt 1):1371–3.
46. Israel CW, Hohnloser SH. Current status of dual-sensor pacemaker systems for correction of chronotropic incompetence. Am J Cardiol. 2000;86(9A):86K–94K.
47. Coenen M, Malinowski K, Spitzer W, Schuchert A, Schmitz D, Anelli-Monti M, et al. Closed loop stimulation and accelerometer-based rate adaptation: results of the PROVIDE study. Europace. 2008;10(3):327–33.
48. Rattanawong P, Riangwiwat T, Chongsathidkiet P, Vutthikraivit W, Limpruttidham N, Prasitlumkum N, et al. Closed-looped stimulation cardiac pacing for recurrent vasovagal syncope: a systematic review and meta-analysis. J Arrhythm. 2018;34(5):556–64.
49. Pilat E, Mlynarski R, Wlodyka A, Kargul W. Influence of DDD rate response pacing with integrated double sensors on physical efficiency and quality of life. Europace. 2008;10(10):1189–94.

50. Sudkamp M, Menzel C, Sindhu D, Savvidou-Zaroti P, La Rosee K, Hekmat K, et al. Is measuring by portable heart rate monitors (sport watches) dependable in patients with an implanted pacemaker? Dtsch Med Wochenschr. 2005;130(21):1307–10.
51. Joglar JA, Hamdan MH, Welch PJ, Page RL. Interaction of a commercial heart rate monitor with implanted pacemakers. Am J Cardiol. 1999;83(5):790–2. A10
52. Sartor F, Gelissen J, van Dinther R, Roovers D, Papini GB, Coppola G. Wrist-worn optical and chest strap heart rate comparison in a heterogeneous sample of healthy individuals and in coronary artery disease patients. BMC Sports Sci Med Rehabil. 2018;10:10.
53. Lafitte S, Bordachar P, Lafitte M, Garrigue S, Reuter S, Reant P, et al. Dynamic ventricular dyssynchrony: an exercise-echocardiography study. J Am Coll Cardiol. 2006;47(11):2253–9.
54. Valzania C, Eriksson MJ, Boriani G, Gadler F. Cardiac resynchronization therapy during rest and exercise: comparison of two optimization methods. Europace. 2008;10(10):1161–9.
55. Schmidt M, Pedersen SB, Farkas DK, Hjortshoj SP, Botker HE, Nielsen JC, et al. Thirteen-year nationwide trends in use of implantable cardioverter-defibrillators and subsequent long-term survival. Heart Rhythm. 2015;12(9):2018–27.
56. Hawkins NM, Grubisic M, Andrade JG, Huang F, Ding L, Gao M, et al. Long-term complications, reoperations and survival following cardioverter-defibrillator implant. Heart. 2018;104(3):237–43.
57. Lampert R, Olshansky B, Heidbuchel H, Lawless C, Saarel E, Ackerman M, et al. Safety of sports for athletes with implantable Cardioverter-Defibrillators: long-term results of a prospective multinational registry. Circulation. 2017;135(23):2310–2.
58. Lampert R, Olshansky B, Heidbuchel H, Lawless C, Saarel E, Ackerman M, et al. Safety of sports for athletes with implantable cardioverter-defibrillators: results of a prospective, multinational registry. Circulation. 2013;127(20):2021–30.
59. Zipes DP, Ackerman MJ, Estes NA 3rd, Grant AO, Myerburg RJ, Van Hare G. Task force 7: arrhythmias. J Am Coll Cardiol. 2005;45(8):1354–63.
60. Maron BJ, Chaitman BR, Ackerman MJ, Bayes de Luna A, Corrado D, Crosson JE, et al. Recommendations for physical activity and recreational sports participation for young patients with genetic cardiovascular diseases. Circulation. 2004;109(22):2807–16.
61. Heidbuchel H, Carre F. Exercise and competitive sports in patients with an implantable cardioverter-defibrillator. Eur Heart J. 2014;35(44):3097–102.
62. Lampert R, Cannom D, Olshansky B. Safety of sports participation in patients with implantable cardioverter defibrillators: a survey of heart rhythm society members. J Cardiovasc Electrophysiol. 2006;17(1):11–5.
63. Saarel EV, Law I, Berul CI, Ackerman MJ, Kanter RJ, Sanatani S, et al. Safety of sports for young patients with implantable cardioverter-defibrillators. Circ Arrhythm Electrophysiol. 2018;11(11):e006305.
64. Heidbuchel H, Olshansky B, Cannom D, Jordaens L, Willems R, Carre F, et al. Intensive recreational vs. competitive athletes in the prospective multinational ICD Sports Safety Registry: results from the European recreational cohort. Europace. 2017;19(Issue suppl_3):iii121.
65. Heidbuchel H, Willems R, Jordaens L, Olshansky B, Carre F, Lozano IF, et al. Intensive recreational athletes in the prospective multinational ICD Sports Safety Registry: results from the European cohort. Eur J Prev Cardiol. 2019;26(7):764–75.
66. Sweeney MO. The implantable cardioverter-defibrillator minimalist: an approach to patient follow-up and management of implantable defibrillators. Circulation. 2012;126(3):369–77.
67. Polyzos KA, Konstantelias AA, Falagas ME. Risk factors for cardiac implantable electronic device infection: a systematic review and meta-analysis. Europace. 2015;17(5):767–77.
68. Irfan G, Czapla J, Saitoh Y, Ciconte G, Mugnai G, Conte G, et al. Implantable cardioverter defibrillator therapy in young individuals: comparison of conventional and subcostal approaches-a single-centre experience. Europace. 2017;19(1):81–7.
69. Al-Atia B, Vandenberk B, Voros G, Garweg C, Ector J, Willems R. Predictors of a high defibrillation threshold test during routine ICD implantation. Acta Cardiol. 2018;73(3):267–73.

70. Ziegelhoeffer T, Siebel A, Markewitz A, Doll N, Barsch V, Reinartz M, et al. Intraoperative defibrillation testing should not be generally abandoned for all ICD procedures—a multicenter study on 4,572 consecutive patients. Thorac Cardiovasc Surg. 2016;64(8):679–87.
71. Wilkoff BL, Fauchier L, Stiles MK, Morillo CA, Al-Khatib SM, Almendral J, et al. 2015 HRS/EHRA/APHRS/SOLAECE expert consensus statement on optimal implantable cardioverter-defibrillator programming and testing. Heart Rhythm. 2016;13(2):e50–86.
72. Garg J, Chaudhary R, Shah N, Palaniswamy C, Bozorgnia B, Nazir T, et al. Right ventricular apical versus non-apical implantable cardioverter defibrillator lead: a systematic review and meta-analysis. J Electrocardiol. 2017;50(5):591–7.
73. Epstein LM, Love CJ, Wilkoff BL, Chung MK, Hackler JW, Bongiorni MG, et al. Superior vena cava defibrillator coils make transvenous lead extraction more challenging and riskier. J Am Coll Cardiol. 2013;61(9):987–9.
74. Aoukar PS, Poole JE, Johnson GW, Anderson J, Hellkamp AS, Mark DB, et al. No benefit of a dual coil over a single coil ICD lead: evidence from the sudden cardiac death in heart failure trial. Heart Rhythm. 2013;10(7):970–6.
75. Larsen JM, Heath FP, Riahi S, Holm K, Johansen MB, Hjortshoj SP, et al. Single and dual coil shock efficacy and predictors of shock failure in patients with modern implantable cardioverter defibrillators—a single-center paired randomized study. J Interv Card Electrophysiol. 2019;54(1):65–72.
76. Kutyifa V, Huth Ruwald AC, Aktas MK, Jons C, McNitt S, Polonsky B, et al. Clinical impact, safety, and efficacy of single- versus dual-coil ICD leads in MADIT-CRT. J Cardiovasc Electrophysiol. 2013;24(11):1246–52.
77. Hsu JC, Saxon LA, Jones PW, Wehrenberg S, Marcus GM. Utilization trends and clinical outcomes in patients implanted with a single- vs a dual-coil implantable cardioverter-defibrillator lead: insights from the ALTITUDE Study. Heart Rhythm. 2015;12(8):1770–5.
78. Leshem E, Suleiman M, Laish-Farkash A, Konstantino Y, Glikson M, Barsheshet A, et al. Contemporary rates and outcomes of single- vs. dual-coil implantable cardioverter defibrillator lead implantation: data from the Israeli ICD registry. Europace. 2017;19(9):1485–92.
79. Zeitler EP, Sanders GD, Singh K, Greenfield RA, Gillis AM, Wilkoff BL, et al. Single vs. dual chamber implantable cardioverter-defibrillators or programming of implantable cardioverter-defibrillators in patients without a bradycardia pacing indication: systematic review and meta-analysis. Europace. 2018;20(10):1621–9.
80. Olshansky B, Atteya G, Cannom D, Heidbuchel H, Saarel E, Anfinsen OG, et al. Competitive athletes with implantable cardioverter defibrillators—how to program? Data from the implantable cardioverter defibrillator sports registry. Heart Rhythm. 2019;16(4):581–7.
81. Lee DS, Krahn AD, Healey JS, Birnie D, Crystal E, Dorian P, et al. Evaluation of early complications related to De Novo cardioverter defibrillator implantation insights from the Ontario ICD database. J Am Coll Cardiol. 2010;55(8):774–82.
82. Basu-Ray I, Liu J, Jia X, Gold M, Ellenbogen K, DiNicolantonio J, et al. Subcutaneous versus transvenous implantable defibrillator therapy: a meta-analysis of case-control studies. JACC Clin Electrophysiol. 2017;3(13):1475–83.
83. Boersma LV, Barr CS, Burke MC, Leon AR, Theuns DA, Herre JM, et al. Performance of the subcutaneous implantable cardioverter-defibrillator in patients with a primary prevention indication with and without a reduced ejection fraction versus patients with a secondary prevention indication. Heart Rhythm. 2017;14(3):367–75.
84. Baalman SWE, Quast ABE, Brouwer TF, Knops RE. An overview of clinical outcomes in transvenous and subcutaneous ICD patients. Curr Cardiol Rep. 2018;20(9):72.
85. Theuns D, Brouwer TF, Jones PW, Allavatam V, Donnelley S, Auricchio A, et al. Prospective blinded evaluation of a novel sensing methodology designed to reduce inappropriate shocks by the subcutaneous implantable cardioverter-defibrillator. Heart Rhythm. 2018;15(10):1515–22.
86. Auricchio A, Schloss EJ, Kurita T, Meijer A, Gerritse B, Zweibel S, et al. Low inappropriate shock rates in patients with single- and dual/triple-chamber implantable

cardioverter-defibrillators using a novel suite of detection algorithms: PainFree SST trial primary results. Heart Rhythm. 2015;12(5):926–36.

87. Saxon LA, Hayes DL, Gilliam FR, Heidenreich PA, Day J, Seth M, et al. Long-term outcome after ICD and CRT implantation and influence of remote device follow-up: the ALTITUDE survival study. Circulation. 2010;122(23):2359–67.
88. Kolb C, Zrenner B, Schmitt C. Incidence of electromagnetic interference in implantable cardioverter defibrillators. Pacing Clin Electrophysiol. 2001;24(4 Pt 1):465–8.
89. von Olshausen G, Rondak IC, Lennerz C, Semmler V, Grebmer C, Reents T, et al. Electromagnetic interference in implantable cardioverter defibrillators: present but rare. Clin Res Cardiol. 2016;105(8):657–65.
90. Sears SF Jr, Shea JB, Conti JB. Cardiology patient page. How to respond to an implantable cardioverter-defibrillator shock. Circulation. 2005;111(23):e380–2.
91. Vijgen J, Botto G, Camm J, Hoijer CJ, Jung W, Le Heuzey JY, et al. Consensus statement of the European Heart Rhythm Association: updated recommendations for driving by patients with implantable cardioverter defibrillators. Europace. 2009;11(8):1097–107.
92. Wathen MS, DeGroot PJ, Sweeney MO, Stark AJ, Otterness MF, Adkisson WO, et al. Prospective randomized multicenter trial of empirical antitachycardia pacing versus shocks for spontaneous rapid ventricular tachycardia in patients with implantable cardioverter-defibrillators: Pacing Fast Ventricular Tachycardia Reduces Shock Therapies (PainFREE Rx II) trial results. Circulation. 2004;110(17):2591–6.
93. Gold MR, Weiss R, Theuns DA, Smith W, Leon A, Knight BP, et al. Use of a discrimination algorithm to reduce inappropriate shocks with a subcutaneous implantable cardioverter-defibrillator. Heart Rhythm. 2014;11(8):1352–8.
94. Srivathsan K, Scott LR, Altemose GT. T-wave oversensing and inappropriate shocks: a case report. Europace. 2008;10(5):552–5.
95. Ishibashi K, Noda T, Kamakura T, Wada M, Inoue Y, Okamura H, et al. Importance of exercise testing shortly after subcutaneous implantable cardioverter-defibrillator implantation in patients with Brugada syndrome—the first case of associated inappropriate shock in Japan. J Arrhythm. 2017;33(2):156–8.
96. Cohen MI, Shaffer J, Pedersen S, Sims JJ, Papez A. Limited utility of exercise-stress testing to prevent T-wave oversensing in pediatric internal cardioverter defibrillator recipients. Pacing Clin Electrophysiol. 2011;34(4):436–42.
97. Larbig R, Motloch LJ, Bettin M, Fischer A, Frommeyer G, Reinke F, et al. Postoperative ergometry-guided programming does not prevent T-wave oversensing and inappropriate shocks in S-ICD patients. Pacing Clin Electrophysiol. 2018;41(6):567–71.
98. Andersen K, Farahmand B, Ahlbom A, Held C, Ljunghall S, Michaelsson K, et al. Risk of arrhythmias in 52 755 long-distance cross-country skiers: a cohort study. Eur Heart J. 2013;34(47):3624–31.
99. Akar JG, Bao H, Jones PW, Wang Y, Varosy PD, Masoudi FA, et al. Use of remote monitoring is associated with lower risk of adverse outcomes among patients with implanted cardiac defibrillators. Circ Arrhythm Electrophysiol. 2015;8(5):1173–80.
100. Varma N, Piccini JP, Snell J, Fischer A, Dalal N, Mittal S. The relationship between level of adherence to automatic wireless remote monitoring and survival in pacemaker and defibrillator patients. J Am Coll Cardiol. 2015;65(24):2601–10.

# Specific Cardiovascular Diseases and Competitive Sports Participation: Myocarditis and Myocardial Fibrosis

19

Frédéric Schnell and François Carré

**Learning Objectives**

1. How to prevent myocarditis in athletes.
2. How to diagnose myocarditis in athletes.
3. How to treat myocarditis in athletes.
4. What are the current recommendations as regards to sport practice?

## 19.1 Introduction

Myocarditis is an inflammatory disease of the myocardium. There is a large heterogeneity in clinical presentation making myocarditis a very challenging diagnosis. In athletes, myocarditis is an underlying cause of sudden cardiac death (SCD), accounting for a rate of 5–24% of deaths in this population [1, 2]. Indeed, the impact of intense exercise on the occurrence of myocarditis in case of an infectious disease as well as its deleterious effect on ventricular remodelling and occurrence of ventricular arrhythmias in case of acute myocarditis has been demonstrated in animal models [3]. In this chapter, we will review the aetiology, diagnosis, treatment, and outcomes related to myocarditis in athletes. We will discuss the evidence of temporary restriction of sport practice. Lastly, we will also deal with the topic of non-myocardial scar without documented cardiomyopathy.

F. Schnell · F. Carré (✉)
Department of Sports Medicine, University Hospital of Rennes, Rennes1 University, Inserm, Rennes, France
e-mail: frederic.schnell@chu-rennes.fr; francois.carre@univ-rennes1.fr





A. Pressler, J. Niebauer (eds.), *Textbook of Sports and Exercise Cardiology*,
https://doi.org/10.1007/978-3-030-35374-2_19

## 19.2 Aetiology of Myocarditis

### 19.2.1 General Population

A large variety of infectious agents, systemic diseases, drugs and toxins can cause myocarditis (Table 19.1).

**Table 19.1** Causes of myocarditis and inflammatory cardiomyopathy

| | |
|---|---|
| **Infectious causes** | |
| Viral | *RNA viruses*: Coxsackieviruses A and B, echoviruses, polioviruses, influenza A and B viruses, respiratory syncytial virus, mumps virus, measles virus, rubella virus, hepatitis C virus, dengue virus, yellow fever virus, Chikungunya virus, Junin virus, Lassa fever virus, rabies virus, human immunodeficiency virus<br>*DNA viruses*: adenoviruses, parvovirus B19, cytomegalovirus, human herpes virus-6, Epstein-Barr virus, varicella-zoster virus, herpes simplex virus, variola virus, vaccinia virus |
| Bacterial | Chlamydia, Staphylococcus, Streptococcus, Pneumococcus, Meningococcus, Gonococcus, Salmonella, Corynebacterium diphtheriae, Haemophilus influenzae, Mycobacterium (tuberculosis), Mycoplasma pneumoniae, Brucella |
| Spirochaetal | Borrelia, Leptospira, Treponema pallidum |
| Fungal | Aspergillus, Actinomyces, Blastomyces, Candida, Coccidioides, Cryptococcus, Histoplasma, Mucormycoses, Nocardia, Sporothrix |
| Protozoal | Plasmodium falciparum, Trypanosoma cruzi, Toxoplasma gondii, Entamoeba, Leishmania |
| Parasitic | Trichinella spiralis, Echinococcus granulosus, Taenia solium |
| Rickettsial | Coxiella burnetii, R. rickettsii, R. tsutsugamushi |
| **Non-infectious causes** | |
| *Immune-mediated myocarditis* | |
| Allergens | Tetanus toxoid, vaccines, serum sickness<br>Drugs: penicillin, cefaclor, colchicine, furosemide, isoniazid, lidocaine, tetracycline, sulfonamides, phenytoin, phenylbutazone, methyldopa, thiazide diuretics, amitriptyline |
| Auto-antigens | Infection-negative lymphocytic, infection-negative giant cell<br>*Associated with autoimmune or immune-oriented disorders*: systemic lupus erythematosus, rheumatoid arthritis, Churg-Strauss syndrome, Kawasaki's disease, inflammatory bowel disease, scleroderma, polymyositis, myasthenia gravis, insulin-dependent diabetes mellitus, thyrotoxicosis, sarcoidosis, Wegener's granulomatosis, rheumatic heart disease (rheumatic fever) |
| Allo-antigens | Heart transplant rejection |
| *Toxic myocarditis* | |
| Drugs | Amphetamines, anthracyclines, cocaine, cyclophosphamide, ethanol, fluorouracil, lithium, catecholamines, hemetine, interleukin-2, trastuzumab, clozapine |
| Heavy metals | Copper, iron, lead |
| Miscellaneous | Scorpion sting, snake, and spider bites, bee and wasp stings, carbon monoxide, inhalants, phosphorus, arsenic, sodium azide |
| Hormones | Pheochromocytoma, vitamins: beri-beri |
| Physical agents | Radiation, electric shock |

- **Viral infections** are the most important causes of myocarditis in North America and Europe. The most common virus involves are
  - Enterovirus
  - Adenovirus
  - Influenza viruses
  - Human Herpes Virus 6
  - Epstein-Barr-virus
  - Cytomegalovirus
  - Hepatitis C virus
  - Parvovirus B19.

In human myocarditis, there is evidence for both viral and autoimmune mechanisms. The pathogenesis of myocarditis consists of three overlapping phases:

(a) Acute injury,
(b) The host innate and acquired immunologic response, and
(c) Recovery or a transition to scar and in few cases dilated cardiomyopathy (DCM).

Enteroviruses, for example, enter the host through the gastrointestinal or respiratory tract, reside in the reticuloendothelial system as an extra-cardiac reservoir, and attack the heart as a secondary target organ. There is a direct virus-related cytolysis of cardiomyocytes, but the antiviral immune response can also lead to acute myocardial injury [4]. Some other cardiotropic viruses such as human herpes virus 6 rather infect the vascular endothelium cells than directly the cardiomyocytes. This affects the myocardial contractility indirectly. Distinct viruses with different infection sites explain the heterogeneity of clinical presentation and prognosis. It is likely that there is a genetic predisposition in some cases of myocarditis, even if evidence is lacking in humans [5].

- **Auto-immune myocarditis** can occur with exclusive cardiac involvement or in the context of autoimmune disorders with extra-cardiac manifestations, most frequently in sarcoidosis, hypereosinophilic syndrome, scleroderma, and systemic lupus erythematosus. This underlines the importance of considering co-morbidities and extra cardiac symptoms.
- Myocarditis can also be caused by a great variety of **medical drugs or toxic causes** [6]. In the case of cocaine, drug-induced myocarditis is classified in dose-dependent hypersensitivity myocarditis and dose-dependent toxic myocarditis [7].

Nevertheless, the aetiology of myocarditis often remains undetermined. Indeed, although viral infections can cause symptoms, the majority of them are asymptomatic or oligosymptomatic; furthermore, due to a delayed onset of heart disease after the initial infection, these infections are frequently not recognized as the causes of myocarditis.

### 19.2.2 Distinctive Features in Athletes

In case of athletes, some specific features should be considered with respect to the aetiologies of myocarditis, in order to decrease their occurrence:

1. Avoidance of **recreational drugs** or **doping agents**: Recreational drugs or doping agents are responsible for myocarditis, for example anabolic androgenic steroids [8], amphetamines [9] or cocaine [7]. Unfortunately, the use doping agents appears not so rare among elite athletes [10], underlying the importance of a thorough lifestyle history in athletes (see Chap. 28). Of course, athletes may not always disclose the use of any performance enhancing substance to their caregiver. The risk of doping should be well explained to athletes, and this aetiology should be sought in order to prevent recurrences.
2. Prevention of **infectious diseases** and restriction of sport in case of infection: Athletes are **more susceptible to viral illness** than the untrained population [11]. Indeed, intensive sport can weaken immune function. Strenuous exercise has been shown to increase susceptibility to Coxsackie B3 infection in mice [12], and to upper respiratory tract infection in athletes [13]. A decrease in salivary IgA concentration was demonstrated in Nordic cross-country skiers [14]. This temporary antibody deficiency on the mucosal surface might lead to a susceptibility to acquiring viral and bacterial infections, especially during the interval immediately following strenuous exercise.

In case of viral infection, it has been demonstrated that intense exercising during an infectious illness may exacerbate symptoms, prolong the length of illness and increase the risk of potentially serious complications such as myocarditis [15]. Indeed, mice forced to exercise during the initial days of coxsackie B3 infections developed a replacement fibrous scar and had a poorer outcome (Fig. 19.1) [3]. In humans, 30 years ago, sudden cardiac deaths among young orienteers in Sweden were reduced after a recommendation not to train while infected [16], demonstrating that prevention can lead to a decrease of viral myocarditis in athletes.

### 19.2.3 When Should an Athlete Return to Play in Case of Infectious Disease?

This question is rather tricky, particularly at critical moments during an athlete's competitive season. In general, decisions about whether to continue exercising during an illness can be made using a **'neck check'** [17]. If symptoms are confined to above the neck, such as a runny nose, nasal congestion or sore throat, athletes may continue to participate as long as they feel able. If symptoms are below the neck (e.g., fever, malaise, severe cough, gastrointestinal symptoms), exercise should be delayed until all symptoms have resolved. If athletes have systemic symptoms, such as fever, myalgias, diarrhea or an elevated resting heart rate, they should refrain from exercising until symptoms have resolved for a period of 7–14 days. Indeed, in

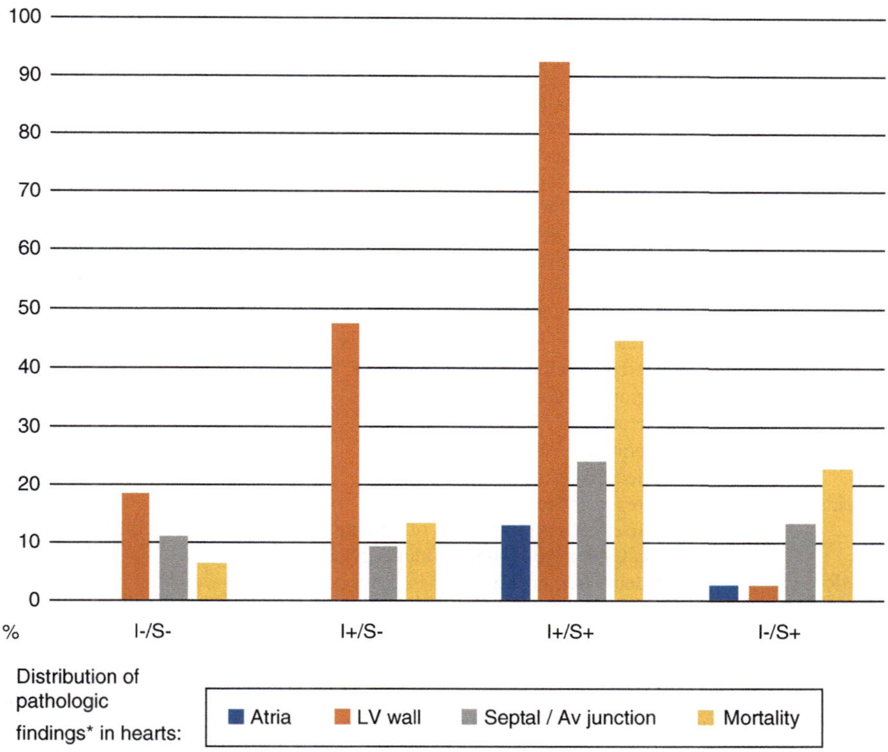


**Fig. 19.1** Externally induced myocarditis and outcome in a mouse model. Animals were either artificially infected with coxsackie B3 or not (I+ or I−) and were forced to swim or not (S+ or S−) and were followed up for a maximum of 15 months. Mice that were both infected and forced to swim showed the highest percental proportion of ∗pathological findings in their hearts (including fibrosis, mononuclear infiltrate, calcium deposition, and atrial thrombi) and also the highest mortality (created from data presented in [3]). *AV* atrioventricular, *LV* left ventricular

these circumstances, there is an increased risk of dehydration, prolonged illness or more serious complications [18].

Of course, when resuming training after recovering from an illness, athletes should start at a moderate pace and gradually increase his or her training intensity.

#### 19.2.3.1 Prevention of Myocarditis in Athletes

- *Restrict from training in case of infection and systemic symptoms (fever, myalgias, diarrhoea or an elevated resting heart rate).*
- *Education on the effect of doping agents and of recreational drugs.*

#### 19.2.3.2 Diagnosis of Myocarditis

As stated above, the diagnosis of myocarditis can sometimes be challenging due to its heterogenous clinical presentation and the lack of imaging finding being clearly diagnostic. The following paragraphs describe potential alterations suggestive of myocarditis, summarized in Table 19.2.

**Table 19.2** Diagnostic criteria of myocarditis

| | |
|---|---|
| Clinical presentation | Heterogeneous presentation<br>• Chest pain<br>• Symptoms related to arrhythmia (palpitations, dizziness, syncope)<br>• Symptoms related to heart failure (dyspnea, performance drop)<br>Context of infectious disease, drug intake or auto immune disease |
| ECG | • Arrhythmia (ventricular, supraventricular)<br>• PQ depression<br>• Conduction abnormalities (LBBB, AV block)<br>• Low QRS voltage<br>• Repolarization changes (ST-segment alterations, T-wave inversion) |
| Echocardiography | • LV dilation with thin myocardial walls<br>• Increase in myocardial wall thickness (myocardial *oedema*)<br>• Altered LV global systolic function<br>• Regional wall motion abnormalities<br>• Alteration of RV systolic function<br>• Alteration of diastolic function<br>• Pericardial effusion |
| Biomarkers | • Increase of Troponin<br>• Increase of serum markers of inflammation (erythrocyte sedimentation rate, C-reactive protein and leucocyte count) |
| CMR | • Oedema (regional increase in water content in T2-weighted images)<br>• Hyperaemia (increase in regional contrast-enhanced T1-weighted epicardial/midmyocardial signal within few minutes of gadolinium bolus)<br>• Myocardial fibrosis (epicardial/midmyocardial LGE) |

*LV* left ventricle, *RV* right ventricle, *LBBB* left bundle branch block, *AV* atrio-ventricular, *LGE* late gadolinium enhancement, *CMR* cardiac magnetic resonance imaging

### 19.2.4 Clinical Presentation

Myocarditis is a challenging clinical scenario, given its heterogeneous presentation. The suspicion of myocarditis may be raised when an athlete complains of chest pain simulating myocardial infarction, symptoms related to arrhythmia (palpitations, dizziness, syncope), or heart failure (dyspnoea or physical performance drop). The illness may be preceded by coryza or diarrhoea [19] or occur in the context of toxic drug intake or of auto immune disease.

### 19.2.5 12-Lead Electrocardiogram

ECG abnormalities are common in case of myocarditis; in a recent study ECG were abnormal in 42% of 670 patients with suspected myocarditis [20] (Fig. 19.2). These include repolarization changes such as ST-segment alterations and T-wave inversion, arrhythmias with frequent and/or complex ventricular and/or supraventricular arrhythmia, and occasionally conduction abnormalities with left bundle branch block or atrioventricular block [21]. Individuals may also present with low QRS voltages or PQ depression, particularly in the presence of an associated pericardial effusion.

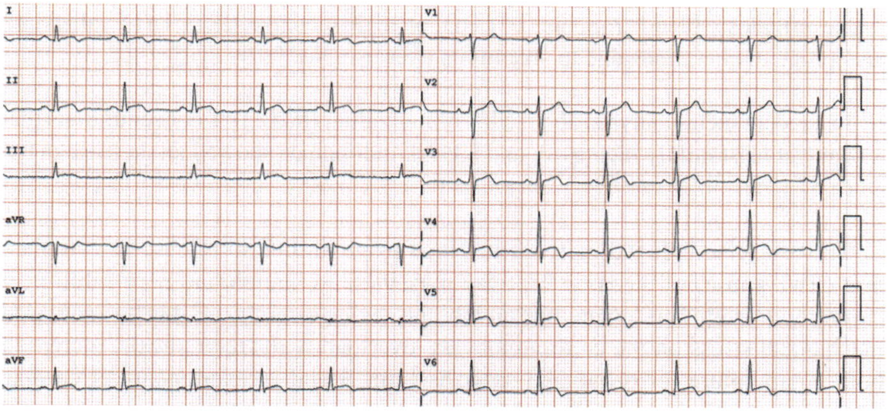


**Fig. 19.2** Example of an ECG in an athlete with acute myocarditis. Relative tachycardia for an athlete, infero-lateral ST elevation with T wave inversion, without reciprocal mirror ST-depression

### 19.2.6 Echocardiography

The left ventricle (LV) can be mildly dilated with thin myocardial walls, resembling a dilated cardiomyopathy, or there may be a non-dilated cavity with increased myocardial wall thickness due to myocardial oedema. Regional wall motion abnormalities can be present, and LV global systolic function can range from normal to severely altered. The right ventricle can also be altered, as well as diastolic function. Concomitant pericardial effusion suggests pericardial involvement [22].

### 19.2.7 Biomarkers

*Cardiovascular biomarkers.* Troponin is a hallmark for myocardial injury. It is not specific for inflammatory-mediated myocyte injury, but it will increase during the acute phase of myocarditis.

- Indeed, in patients aged less than 50 years, myocarditis is the second most cause of elevated troponins, after myocardial infarction [23].

Smith et al. demonstrated that among 53 patients with biopsy-proven myocarditis, 34% were found to have elevated cardiac troponin I (cTnI) values [24]. Of course, timing is a critical parameter for the efficacy of troponin measurement to detect myocarditis. cTnI is most likely to be elevated in patients with myocarditis early after the onset of symptoms (within 1 month). This finding is consistent with the hypothesis that the majority of myocyte injury and necrosis may occur early in the patient's clinical course [23].

Nevertheless, blood troponin T (cTnT or high-sensitive (hs)-cTnT) values are also prone to alterations due to **strenuous exercise**.

- In a recent meta-analysis, about 51% of individuals had cTnT concentrations that were at least mildly increased; and 83% of individuals showed an increase in hs-cTnT [25].

This exercise-induced increase in blood troponin due to release of cytoplasmic cTnT and cTnI, because exercise may increase membrane permeability of cardiomyocytes. This reversible membrane leakage might be due to increased mechanical stress on the cardiomyocytes, overload with free radicals, increased body temperature, or prolonged acidosis [26]. Serial measurements of cardiac troponin may help to differentiate between physiological and pathological changes of this parameter. Indeed, the troponin increase after strenuous exercise tends to be less prominent and monophasic rather than biphasic and resolves faster than in myocardial injury caused by myocarditis or acute coronary syndrome [26].

Hence, it is always necessary in athletes to take previous physical exercise into account when a cardiac emergency is suspected.

#### 19.2.7.1 Troponin Elevation After Exercise

- *Take previous physical exercise into account, as intense exercise can at least temporarily increase cardiovascular biomarkers.*

*Serum markers of inflammation.* Although non-specific as well, an elevation of several inflammatory biomarkers (erythrocyte sedimentation rate, C-reactive protein and leucocyte count) can be observed at the acute phase of myocarditis. The issue remains that these biomarkers can also be elevated in many other conditions.

*Viral serologies.* A previous study on the use of virus serology for patients with suspected myocarditis has shown limited utility [27]. Indeed, there was no correlation between virus serology and viral genome detected in the myocardium by endomyocardial biopsy. Circumstances in which serological testing might be helpful include suspected hepatitis C, rickettsia, Lyme disease in endemic areas, and HIV in high-risk patients [6].

### 19.2.8 Cardiac Magnetic Resonance Imaging (CMR)

CMR has evolved as the primary non-invasive diagnostic modality in suspected myocarditis cases. Indeed, beyond the assessment of wall motion and left ventricular ejection fraction, CMR is a non-invasive modality that allows tissue characterization with visualization of myocardial oedema and fibrosis (Fig. 19.3).

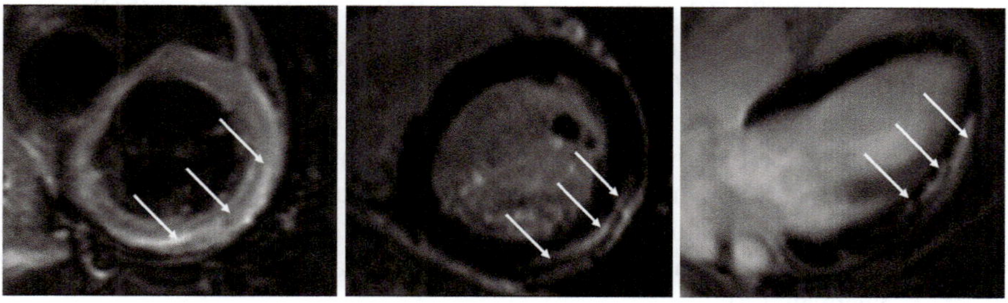


**Fig. 19.3** Example of CMR images in an athlete with acute myocarditis. On the T2 weighted images, the arrows indicate the regions with a regional increase in water content, which are related to intramyocardial oedema. On the LGE images, the arrows indicate the regions with sub-epicardial late gadolinium enhancement, which are related to focal fibrosis. *T2-w* T2 weighted imaging, *LGE* late gadolinium enhancement

According to the Lake Louise Criteria (LLC) [28], CMR features that may be used to diagnose probable myocarditis include:

1. a regional increase in water content visible on T2-weighted images,
2. an increase in regional contrast-enhanced T1-weighted epicardial or midmyocardial signal obtained within a few minutes of the gadolinium bolus ("hyperaemia" or "early-enhancement" sequences),
3. an epicardial or midmyocardial late gadolinium enhancement (LGE) indicating myocardial fibrosis as a residual finding after initial inflammation (i.e. non-ischemic pattern of LGE).

Regional and reversible increases in wall thickness might indicate myocardial oedema and are therefore a supportive finding of acute myocarditis. However, the sensitivity of CMR for the diagnosis of myocarditis also decreases a few weeks after the initial illness.

Some limitations of LGE have to be underlined. First of all, a certain number of patients with biopsy proven myocarditis do not show LGE [29, 30]. Indeed, active myocarditis may not always lead to regions with necrotic myocytes of sufficient size to be visually detectable with LGE-CMR. Secondly, myocardial fibrosis, the late sequelae of myocarditis, may be indistinguishable from active myocarditis on LGE sequences.

CMR may detect isolated myocarditis-like LGE on CMR in an athlete with non-acute symptoms (e.g. syncope, or palpitations without any clinical signs of acute myocarditis). Whether these findings represent an acute myocarditis, a myocarditis in a late stage without presence of myocardial oedema, a resolved myocarditis or another pathology can be challenging (we will discuss this question in the last paragraph of this chapter).

Furthermore, some clinical expressions of myocarditis do not fulfil the Lake Louise Criteria [28]. Therefore, LLC are now often complemented by novel CMR techniques such as T1/T2 mapping and extracellular volume fraction (ECV) measurement to provide a higher sensitivity and specificity [31, 32].

Nevertheless, even if LGE can fail to detect myocarditis, it seems to be a good prognostic marker in myocarditis. In fact, patients with suspected myocarditis with a large extent of LGE showed an increased risk for major adverse cardiovascular events (MACE) at follow-up [20]. Regarding location and pattern, septal, mid-wall, and patchy LGE demonstrated strong relations with MACE. On the contrary, a normal CMR study corresponded to low annual MACE and death rates of 0.8% and 0.3%, respectively [20].

***Lake Louise Consensus Criteria*** *should be used for CMR interpretation in suspected myocarditis. These criteria are based on:*

- *a regional increase in water content visible on T2-weighted images,*
- *an increase in regional contrast-enhanced T1-weighted epicardial or midmyocardial signal obtained within a few minutes of the gadolinium bolus ("hyperaemia" or "early-enhancement" sequences),*
- *an epicardial or midmyocardial late gadolinium enhancement (LGE) (i.e., non-ischemic LGE). Regional and reversible increase in wall thickness might indicate myocardial oedema and is therefore a supportive finding of acute myocarditis. The sensitivity of CMR for myocarditis decreases a few weeks after the initial illness.*

### 19.2.9 Invasive Endomyocardial Biopsy (EMB)

EMB is presented as the gold standard diagnostic tool for the diagnosis of myocarditis. Indeed, the World Health Organization/International Society and Federation of Cardiology definition of myocarditis is based on histology:

> An inflammatory disease of the myocardium diagnosed by established histological, immunological and immunohistochemical criteria.

According to the position statement on the diagnosis and management of myocarditis by the European Society of Cardiology Working Group on Myocardial and Pericardial Diseases "all patients with clinically suspected myocarditis should be considered for EMB" [6]. Nevertheless, they recognize that this is not done in routine practice. In a scientific statement from the American Heart Association, the American College of Cardiology, and the European Society of Cardiology, the role of EMB in the management of cardiovascular disease is recommended in more selective indications. Indeed, EMB should be performed in patients with severe clinical presentation in terms of recent heart failure or life-threatening arrhythmias, refractory to usual care [33].

EMB can differentiate between different types of inflammation (infectious, autoimmune, idiopathic) causative of myocarditis. Therefore, EMB might allow tailoring of therapy to the individual. However, EMB is an invasive diagnostic test, although with a rather low complication rate of <1% in experienced centres [34]. Hence, EMB should be performed for the in-depth evaluation of recent-onset high-risk major clinical syndromes not responding to standard optimized medical therapy in the short term [19].

One of the limitations of EMB is the rate of false negative results (sampling error) [35], the exact number of which is not known. To avoid focal sampling error, several precautions have to be undertaken. Preferably, EMB is performed soon after presentation, and at least three myocardial samples, each of sufficient size (1–2 mm), should be taken from the right or from the left ventricle [6]. Tissue obtained from EMB should be analysed using histology, immunohistochemistry and viral PCR (on heart tissue and blood sample).

- *EMB is the gold standard diagnostic tool for the diagnosis of myocarditis.*
- *EMB should be performed in of recent-onset high-risk major clinical syndromes not responding to conventional medical therapy.*

## 19.3 Therapy

In most of cases, myocarditis is a benign pathology which resolves favourably. To our knowledge, no controlled trial exists on the optimal therapy. Therefore, treatment is based on expert consensus [6], and is focused on optimal care of arrhythmias and heart failure. In all case of acute myocarditis, admission to hospital and clinical monitoring is mandatory.

- *Treatment of heart failure.* In patients with hemodynamic instability, a mechanical cardio-pulmonary assist device might be needed as bridge to recovery or to heart transplantation. As recovery may occur, cardiac transplantation should be deferred in the acute phase.
  In patients with hemodynamically stable heart failure, management should be in line with current guidelines on heart failure [36]. The decision for discontinuing heart failure therapy following recovery of ventricular function should be made on a case-by-case basis, as there is no defined consensus.
- *Treatment of arrhythmia.* Drug treatment of arrhythmia in patients with myocarditis does not differ from generally accepted clinical principles [37]. Pacemaker/ICD implantation should be deferred until resolution of the acute episode, as the conduction disorders may resolve spontaneously. Therefore, temporary pacing might be needed for complete atrio-ventricular block and bridging in-hospital monitoring with a wearable life-vest might be a transient solution.
- *Non-steroidal anti-inflammatory treatment* is recommended in acute pericarditis [38]; to date clinical data are inconclusive about their use in myocarditis.
- *Immunomodulatory anti-viral therapies* can be used in selected cases; the decision should be based on a shared consensus with an infectious disease specialist.

- *Immunosuppressive therapy* should be used in proven auto-immune forms of myocarditis (giant cell myocarditis, cardiac sarcoidosis, myocarditis with known extra-cardiac auto-immune disease).

***Treatment*** *is based on expert consensus and is focused on optimal care of arrhythmia and heart failure.*

- *Pacemaker/ICD implantation should be deferred until resolution of the acute phase of myocarditis*
- *Immunosuppressive therapy can be used in proven auto-immune forms of myocarditis*

### 19.3.1 Sport Restriction After Myocarditis

In the beginning of the chapter, we have already demonstrated that intense sport practice can favour infectious disease. Furthermore, it has been demonstrated in a murine model of coxsackie B3 myocarditis, that infected mice forced to swim developed more pronounced myocardial damage and had a higher mortality [39]. Furthermore, myocarditis is a leading cause of sudden cardiac death during strenuous physical exertion in young athletes or military recruits [1, 40].

- General consensus exists that athletes with a diagnosis of myocarditis should be *restricted from exercise programs for a period of 3–6 months* [41, 42], according to the clinical severity and duration of the illness, LV function at onset, and extent of inflammation on CMR. This time period is considered appropriate to ensure clinical and biological resolution of myocarditis.

After this period, the athletes should be tested thoughtfully before resuming training and competitive sport practice. They should undergo a resting echocardiogram, 24-h Holter monitoring (including a supervised training session), and an exercise test. Indeed, even if acute inflammation has resolved, these athletes may still be at risk for arrhythmias related to the resultant myocardial scar, or for heart failure related to negative ventricular remodeling.

Patients might be able to resume training and competition if:

1. asymptomatic
2. serum markers of myocardial injury, inflammation, and heart failure have normalized.
3. LV systolic function has returned to the normal range.
4. no significant arrhythmia occurs (such as frequent or complex repetitive forms of ventricular or supraventricular arrhythmias) on a 24-h ECG monitoring and during an exercise test.

Due to the risk of recurrence and silent progression of the disease, the ESC guidelines recommend a periodical re-assessment, particularly within the 2 first years.

The clinical significance of persistent LGE in an asymptomatic athlete with clinically healed myocarditis is unknown; however, myocardial scar is a potential source of ventricular tachyarrhythmias [43, 44]. At present, it seems reasonable for these athletes to resume training and participate in competitive sport if LV function is preserved and in the absence of frequent or complex repetitive forms of ventricular or supraventricular arrhythmias during maximal exercise and on 24-h ECG monitoring (including session of training/competition). Asymptomatic athletes with LGE, however, should remain under annual clinical surveillance [42].

- ***Athletes** with a diagnosis of myocarditis should be restricted from exercise programs for a period of 3–6 months*
- *Patients might be able to resume training and competition if:*
  - *asymptomatic*
  - *serum markers of myocardial injury, inflammation, and heart failure have normalized.*
  - *LV systolic function has returned to the normal range.*
  - *no significant arrhythmia occurs on a 24-h ECG monitoring and during an exercise test.*

#### 19.3.1.1 Focal Myocardial Fibrosis

Several studies have described an important prevalence of LGE in mostly asymptomatic middle-aged or veteran athletes, ranging from 12 to 50% [45–47]. According to the pattern of the LGE some aetiologies can be easily identified (Fig. 19.4).

- **Ischemic cardiomyopathy**: Sub-endocardial LGE is related to an ischemic cardiomyopathy. This pattern is the most frequently found in veteran athletes [45–47]. In the presence of such an ischemic scar the patients should be managed like every myocardial infarction patient to reduce their risk of an acute cardiac event. Indeed, ischemic LGE demonstrated the strongest association with major adverse cardiac events and cardiac mortality [48]. According to the latest recommendations for participation in leisure time or competitive sports in athletes-patients with coronary artery disease from the Sports Cardiology Section of the European Association of Preventive Cardiology (EAPC), a "high degree of myocardial scarring on CMR imaging "is related to a high probability for exercise-induced

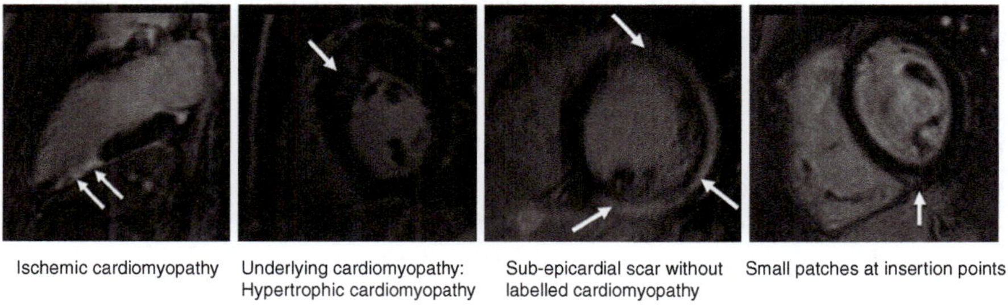


**Fig. 19.4** Examples of different patterns of Late Gadolinium Enhancement (LGE)

adverse cardiac events, and therefore this patients should be restricted from intense/competitive sport practice [49].

- LGE can also be related to an **underlying cardiomyopathy**. In hypertrophic cardiomyopathy (HCM), the presence of LGE can support the diagnosis in borderline cases, since this cannot be considered as physiological [41, 42, 50]. Some publications have underlined the relationship between LGE and cardiovascular mortality, heart failure death and all-cause death, as well as the occurrence of non-sustained ventricular tachycardia [51, 52]. Nevertheless, to date, there is no recommendation to adapt the management of these patients regarding to the presence/absence of myocardial scar; neither to adapt the recommendations with regard to their sport practice.
- In some cases, **sub-epicardial or mid-ventricular LGE is observed without underlying cardiomyopathy**. In two recent longitudinal series, which included athletes who had undergone CMR because of abnormal screening first line examination, a high rate of cardiac events during follow-up was reported in those with sub-epicardial LGE [53, 54]. This finding might be related to previous myocarditis, but this might also be related to a form of cardiomyopathy, for instance left dominant arrhythmogenic cardiomyopathy. Nevertheless, more data is needed in order to better characterize prevalence and outcome. For the moment, the same strategy might be applied as the one used in a scar resulting from previous myocarditis. This question has been addressed in the latest position statement of the Sport Cardiology Section of the EAPC on management with athletes with a myocarditis [42]. Although myocardial scar is a potential source of ventricular tachyarrhythmias, it seems reasonable for these athletes to resume training and participate in competitive sport if LV function is preserved and in the absence of frequent or complex repetitive forms of ventricular or supraventricular arrhythmias during maximal exercise and on 24-h ECG monitoring (including session of training/competition). Asymptomatic athletes with LGE, however, should remain under annual clinical surveillance.
- On the opposite of these pathological findings, **small patches of LGE at insertion points** are frequent in athletes, especially in the elite veterans [47]. As this is described in patients with more extensive history of training and greater cardiac dimensions it is hypothesized that this is related to stress bouts of intense exercise. Since the same pattern of scar is described in patients with pulmonary hypertension, it is supposed that this is due to increased interventricular wall stress due to chronic RV pressure overload [46]. A recent study has demonstrated a good prognosis in these athletes, even if associated with ventricular arrhythmias [54].

**Clinical Pearls**

- **Prevention of myocarditis in athletes**
  - Restrict from training in case of infection and systemic symptoms (fever, myalgias, diarrhea or an elevated resting heart rate).
  - Education on the effect of doping agents and of recreational drugs.

- **Sport restriction after myocarditis**
  - Athletes with diagnosis of myocarditis should be restricted from exercise programs for a period of 3–6 months
  - Patient might be able to resume training and competition if:
    asymptomatic
    serum markers of myocardial injury, inflammation, and heart failure have normalized.
    LV systolic function as returned to the normal range.
    no significant arrhythmia occurs on a 24-h ECG monitoring and exercise test.

## Review

### Questions

1. Regarding different diagnostic tools of myocarditis in athletes, which of the following statements is correct?
   (a) A slight increase of troponin after intense exercise is always pathological.
   (b) Pathological ECG changes are always present in myocarditis.
   (c) Regional wall motion abnormalities on imaging techniques are always present in myocarditis.
   (d) Late gadolinium enhancement is always present in myocarditis.
   (e) None of the answers is correct.
2. Which of the following statements are correct? Clearance of athletes regarding competitive sports practice after a myocarditis is possible:
   (a) If the athlete is asymptomatic.
   (b) If serum markers of myocardial injury, inflammation, and heart failure have normalized.
   (c) If LV systolic function has returned to the normal range.
   (d) If no significant arrhythmia occurs on a 24-h ECG monitoring and exercise test.
   (e) If there is no more LGE on control CMR.

### Answers

1. (e)
   The diagnosis of myocarditis is difficult. Indeed, except endomyocardial biopsy, none of the diagnostic tools that are at our disposal are specific nor sensitive.
   - Troponin can increase slightly after endurance exercise. Therefore, it is necessary to take previous physical exercise into account when a cardiac emergency is suspected.
   - ECG abnormalities are only present in less than 50% of patients with suspected myocarditis.

- Regional wall motion abnormalities can be present, and LV global systolic function can range from normal to severely altered, but this is also not always the case.
- A certain number of patients with biopsy proven myocarditis do not show LGE.

2. (a–d)
The clinical significance of persistent LGE in an asymptomatic athlete with clinically healed myocarditis is unknown, however, myocardial scar is a potential source of ventricular tachyarrhythmias. At present, it seems reasonable for these athletes to resume training and participate in competitive sport if LV function is preserved and in the absence of frequent or complex repetitive forms of ventricular or supraventricular arrhythmias during maximal exercise and on 24-h ECG monitoring (including a session of training or competition). Asymptomatic athletes with LGE, however, should remain under annual clinical surveillance.

## References

1. Bohm P, Scharhag J, Meyer T. Data from a nationwide registry on sports-related sudden cardiac deaths in Germany. Eur J Prev Cardiol. 2016;23(6):649–56.
2. Harmon KG, Asif IM, Maleszewski JJ, Owens DS, Prutkin JM, Salerno JC, et al. Incidence, cause, and comparative frequency of sudden cardiac death in National Collegiate Athletic Association Athletes: a decade in review. Circulation. 2015;132(1):10–9.
3. Reyes MP, Ho KL, Smith F, Lerner AM. A mouse model of dilated-type cardiomyopathy due to coxsackievirus B3. J Infect Dis. 1981;144(3):232–6.
4. Rose NR. Myocarditis: infection versus autoimmunity. J Clin Immunol. 2009;29(6):730–7.
5. Schultheiss HP, Kuhl U, Cooper LT. The management of myocarditis. Eur Heart J. 2011;32(21):2616–25.
6. Caforio AL, Pankuweit S, Arbustini E, Basso C, Gimeno-Blanes J, Felix SB, et al. Current state of knowledge on aetiology, diagnosis, management, and therapy of myocarditis: a position statement of the European Society of Cardiology Working Group on Myocardial and Pericardial Diseases. Eur Heart J. 2013;34(33):2636–48, 48a-48d
7. Rump AF, Theisohn M, Klaus W. The pathophysiology of cocaine cardiotoxicity. Forensic Sci Int. 1995;71(2):103–15.
8. Montisci M, El Mazloum R, Cecchetto G, Terranova C, Ferrara SD, Thiene G, et al. Anabolic androgenic steroids abuse and cardiac death in athletes: morphological and toxicological findings in four fatal cases. Forensic Sci Int. 2012;217(1-3):e13–8.
9. Schurer S, Klingel K, Sandri M, Majunke N, Besler C, Kandolf R, et al. Clinical characteristics, histopathological features, and clinical outcome of methamphetamine-associated cardiomyopathy. JACC Heart Fail. 2017;5(6):435–45.
10. Ulrich R, Pope HG Jr, Cleret L, Petroczi A, Nepusz T, Schaffer J, et al. Doping in two elite athletics competitions assessed by randomized-response surveys. Sports Med. 2018;48(1):211–9.
11. Roberts JA. Viral illnesses and sports performance. Sports Med. 1986;3(4):298–303.
12. Reyes MP, Lerner AM. Interferon and neutralizing antibody in sera of exercised mice with coxsackievirus B-3 myocarditis. Proc Soc Exp Biol Med. 1976;151(2):333–8.
13. Nieman DC. Is infection risk linked to exercise workload? Med Sci Sports Exerc. 2000;32(7 Suppl):S406–11.
14. Tomasi TB, Trudeau FB, Czerwinski D, Erredge S. Immune parameters in athletes before and after strenuous exercise. J Clin Immunol. 1982;2(3):173–8.
15. Primos WA Jr. Sports and exercise during acute illness. Phys Sportsmed. 1996;24(1):44–54.

16. Wesslen L, Pahlson C, Lindquist O, Hjelm E, Gnarpe J, Larsson E, et al. An increase in sudden unexpected cardiac deaths among young Swedish orienteers during 1979-1992. Eur Heart J. 1996;17(6):902–10.
17. Metz JP. Upper respiratory tract infections: who plays, who sits? Curr Sports Med Rep. 2003;2(2):84–90.
18. Exercise and febrile illnesses. Paediatr Child Health. 2007;12(10):885–92.
19. Sinagra G, Anzini M, Pereira NL, Bussani R, Finocchiaro G, Bartunek J, et al. Myocarditis in clinical practice. Mayo Clin Proc. 2016;91(9):1256–66.
20. Grani C, Eichhorn C, Biere L, Murthy VL, Agarwal V, Kaneko K, et al. Prognostic value of cardiac magnetic resonance tissue characterization in risk stratifying patients with suspected myocarditis. J Am Coll Cardiol. 2017;70(16):1964–76.
21. Morgera T, Di Lenarda A, Dreas L, Pinamonti B, Humar F, Bussani R, et al. Electrocardiography of myocarditis revisited: clinical and prognostic significance of electrocardiographic changes. Am Heart J. 1992;124(2):455–67.
22. Pinamonti B, Alberti E, Cigalotto A, Dreas L, Salvi A, Silvestri F, et al. Echocardiographic findings in myocarditis. Am J Cardiol. 1988;62(4):285–91.
23. Wu C, Singh A, Collins B, Fatima A, Qamar A, Gupta A, et al. Causes of troponin elevation and associated mortality in young patients. Am J Med. 2018;131(3):284–92. e1
24. Smith SC, Ladenson JH, Mason JW, Jaffe AS. Elevations of cardiac troponin I associated with myocarditis. Experimental and clinical correlates. Circulation. 1997;95(1):163–8.
25. Sedaghat-Hamedani F, Kayvanpour E, Frankenstein L, Mereles D, Amr A, Buss S, et al. Biomarker changes after strenuous exercise can mimic pulmonary embolism and cardiac injury—a metaanalysis of 45 studies. Clin Chem. 2015;61(10):1246–55.
26. Shave R, Baggish A, George K, Wood M, Scharhag J, Whyte G, et al. Exercise-induced cardiac troponin elevation: evidence, mechanisms, and implications. J Am Coll Cardiol. 2010;56(3):169–76.
27. Mahfoud F, Gartner B, Kindermann M, Ukena C, Gadomski K, Klingel K, et al. Virus serology in patients with suspected myocarditis: utility or futility? Eur Heart J. 2011;32(7):897–903.
28. Friedrich MG, Sechtem U, Schulz-Menger J, Holmvang G, Alakija P, Cooper LT, et al. Cardiovascular magnetic resonance in myocarditis: a JACC white paper. J Am Coll Cardiol. 2009;53(17):1475–87.
29. Grun S, Schumm J, Greulich S, Wagner A, Schneider S, Bruder O, et al. Long-term follow-up of biopsy-proven viral myocarditis: predictors of mortality and incomplete recovery. J Am Coll Cardiol. 2012;59(18):1604–15.
30. Yilmaz A, Kindermann I, Kindermann M, Mahfoud F, Ukena C, Athanasiadis A, et al. Comparative evaluation of left and right ventricular endomyocardial biopsy: differences in complication rate and diagnostic performance. Circulation. 2010;122(9):900–9.
31. Nadjiri J, Nieberler H, Hendrich E, Greiser A, Will A, Martinoff S, et al. Performance of native and contrast-enhanced T1 mapping to detect myocardial damage in patients with suspected myocarditis: a head-to-head comparison of different cardiovascular magnetic resonance techniques. Int J Cardiovasc Imaging. 2017;33(4):539–47.
32. Radunski UK, Lund GK, Saring D, Bohnen S, Stehning C, Schnackenburg B, et al. T1 and T2 mapping cardiovascular magnetic resonance imaging techniques reveal unapparent myocardial injury in patients with myocarditis. Clin Res Cardiol. 2017;106(1):10–7.
33. Cooper LT, Baughman KL, Feldman AM, Frustaci A, Jessup M, Kuhl U, et al. The role of endomyocardial biopsy in the management of cardiovascular disease: a scientific statement from the American Heart Association, the American College of Cardiology, and the European Society of Cardiology. Endorsed by the Heart Failure Society of America and the Heart Failure Association of the European Society of Cardiology. J Am Coll Cardiol. 2007;50(19):1914–31.
34. Holzmann M, Nicko A, Kuhl U, Noutsias M, Poller W, Hoffmann W, et al. Complication rate of right ventricular endomyocardial biopsy via the femoral approach: a retrospective and prospective study analyzing 3048 diagnostic procedures over an 11-year period. Circulation. 2008;118(17):1722–8.

35. Baughman KL. Diagnosis of myocarditis: death of Dallas criteria. Circulation. 2006;113(4):593–5.
36. Ponikowski P, Voors AA, Anker SD, Bueno H, Cleland JGF, Coats AJS, et al. 2016 ESC guidelines for the diagnosis and treatment of acute and chronic heart failure: The Task Force for the diagnosis and treatment of acute and chronic heart failure of the European Society of Cardiology (ESC)Developed with the special contribution of the Heart Failure Association (HFA) of the ESC. Eur Heart J. 2016;37(27):2129–200.
37. Priori SG, Blomstrom-Lundqvist C, Mazzanti A, Blom N, Borggrefe M, Camm J, et al. 2015 ESC guidelines for the management of patients with ventricular arrhythmias and the prevention of sudden cardiac death: The Task Force for the Management of Patients with Ventricular Arrhythmias and the Prevention of Sudden Cardiac Death of the European Society of Cardiology (ESC). Endorsed by: Association for European Paediatric and Congenital Cardiology (AEPC). Eur Heart J. 2015;36(41):2793–867.
38. Adler Y, Charron P, Imazio M, Badano L, Baron-Esquivias G, Bogaert J, et al. 2015 ESC Guidelines for the diagnosis and management of pericardial diseases: The Task Force for the Diagnosis and Management of Pericardial Diseases of the European Society of Cardiology (ESC)Endorsed by: The European Association for Cardio-Thoracic Surgery (EACTS). Eur Heart J. 2015;36(42):2921–64.
39. Kiel RJ, Smith FE, Chason J, Khatib R, Reyes MP. Coxsackievirus B3 myocarditis in C3H/HeJ mice: description of an inbred model and the effect of exercise on virulence. Eur J Epidemiol. 1989;5(3):348–50.
40. Phillips M, Robinowitz M, Higgins JR, Boran KJ, Reed T, Virmani R. Sudden cardiac death in Air Force recruits. A 20-year review. JAMA. 1986;256(19):2696–9.
41. Maron BJ, Udelson JE, Bonow RO, Nishimura RA, Ackerman MJ, Estes NAM 3rd, et al. Eligibility and disqualification recommendations for competitive athletes with cardiovascular abnormalities: task force 3: hypertrophic cardiomyopathy, arrhythmogenic right ventricular cardiomyopathy and other cardiomyopathies, and myocarditis: a scientific statement from the American Heart Association and American College of Cardiology. J Am Coll Cardiol. 2015;66(21):2362–71.
42. Pelliccia A, Solberg EE, Papadakis M, Adami PE, Biffi A, Caselli S, et al. Recommendations for participation in competitive and leisure time sport in athletes with cardiomyopathies, myocarditis, and pericarditis: position statement of the Sport Cardiology Section of the European Association of Preventive Cardiology (EAPC). Eur Heart J. 2019;40(1):19–33.
43. Mewton N, Dernis A, Bresson D, Zouaghi O, Croisille P, Flocard E, et al. Myocardial biomarkers and delayed enhanced cardiac magnetic resonance relationship in clinically suspected myocarditis and insight on clinical outcome. J Cardiovasc Med (Hagerstown). 2015;16(10):696–703.
44. van de Schoor FR, Aengevaeren VL, Hopman MT, Oxborough DL, George KP, Thompson PD, et al. Myocardial fibrosis in athletes. Mayo Clin Proc. 2016;91(11):1617–31.
45. Breuckmann F, Mohlenkamp S, Nassenstein K, Lehmann N, Ladd S, Schmermund A, et al. Myocardial late gadolinium enhancement: prevalence, pattern, and prognostic relevance in marathon runners. Radiology. 2009;251(1):50–7.
46. La Gerche A, Burns AT, Mooney DJ, Inder WJ, Taylor AJ, Bogaert J, et al. Exercise-induced right ventricular dysfunction and structural remodelling in endurance athletes. Eur Heart J. 2012;33(8):998–1006.
47. Wilson M, O'Hanlon R, Prasad S, Deighan A, Macmillan P, Oxborough D, et al. Diverse patterns of myocardial fibrosis in lifelong, veteran endurance athletes. J Appl Physiol (1985). 2011;110(6):1622–6.
48. Kwong RY, Chan AK, Brown KA, Chan CW, Reynolds HG, Tsang S, et al. Impact of unrecognized myocardial scar detected by cardiac magnetic resonance imaging on event-free survival in patients presenting with signs or symptoms of coronary artery disease. Circulation. 2006;113(23):2733–43.
49. Borjesson M, Dellborg M, Niebauer J, LaGerche A, Schmied C, Solberg EE, et al. Recommendations for participation in leisure time or competitive sports in athletes-patients

with coronary artery disease: a position statement from the Sports Cardiology Section of the European Association of Preventive Cardiology (EAPC). Eur Heart J. 2019;40(1):13–8.
50. Authors/Task Force members, Elliott PM, Anastasakis A, Borger MA, Borggrefe M, Cecchi F, et al. 2014 ESC Guidelines on diagnosis and management of hypertrophic cardiomyopathy: the Task Force for the Diagnosis and Management of Hypertrophic Cardiomyopathy of the European Society of Cardiology (ESC). Eur Heart J. 2014;35(39):2733–79.
51. Chan RH, Maron BJ, Olivotto I, Pencina MJ, Assenza GE, Haas T, et al. Prognostic value of quantitative contrast-enhanced cardiovascular magnetic resonance for the evaluation of sudden death risk in patients with hypertrophic cardiomyopathy. Circulation. 2014;130(6):484–95.
52. Rowin EJ, Maron MS. The role of cardiac MRI in the diagnosis and risk stratification of hypertrophic cardiomyopathy. Arrhythm Electrophysiol Rev. 2016;5(3):197–202.
53. Schnell F, Claessen G, La Gerche A, Bogaert J, Lentz PA, Claus P, et al. Subepicardial delayed gadolinium enhancement in asymptomatic athletes: let sleeping dogs lie? Br J Sports Med. 2016;50(2):111–7.
54. Zorzi A, Perazzolo Marra M, Rigato I, De Lazzari M, Susana A, Niero A, et al. Nonischemic left ventricular scar as a substrate of life-threatening ventricular arrhythmias and sudden cardiac death in competitive athletes. Circ Arrhythm Electrophysiol. 2016;9(7):e004229.

# Specific Cardiovascular Diseases and Competitive Sports Participation: Channelopathies

# 20

Silvia Castelletti and Lia Crotti

**Learning Objectives**

1. To learn the most important information about epidemiology, genetic background, clinical presentation, diagnosis, risk stratification and management of patients affected by cardiac channelopaties.
2. To learn when a cardiac channelopathy should be suspected.
3. To select the key diagnostic tools necessary to achieve the right diagnosis.
4. To learn the basis for correct treatment.

## 20.1 Long QT Syndrome

### 20.1.1 Definition and Prevalence

- The Long QT Syndrome is an inherited cardiac disorder characterized by QT prolongation on the ECG and increased risk of life-threatening arrhythmias, typically stress-induced Torsade-De-Point (TdP) [1, 2].

S. Castelletti
Center for Cardiac Arrhythmias of Genetic Origin, Istituto Auxologico Italiano, IRCCS, Milan, Italy
e-mail: s.castelletti@auxologico.it

L. Crotti (✉)
Center for Cardiac Arrhythmias of Genetic Origin, Istituto Auxologico Italiano, IRCCS, Milan, Italy

Laboratory of Cardiovascular Genetics, Istituto Auxologico Italiano, IRCCS, Milan, Italy

Department of Cardiovascular, Neural and Metabolic Sciences, San Luca Hospital, Istituto Auxologico Italiano, IRCCS, Milan, Italy

Department of Medicine and Surgery, University of Milano-Bicocca, Milan, Italy
e-mail: l.crotti@auxologico.it



A. Pressler, J. Niebauer (eds.), *Textbook of Sports and Exercise Cardiology*,
https://doi.org/10.1007/978-3-030-35374-2_20

- The QT corrected for heart rate (QTc) has traditionally been defined prolonged when it measures >440 ms in men and >460 ms in women after puberty [2]. Importantly, in athletes less stringent cut-off values are used to define a QTc as prolonged, based on expert consensus [3, 4]; specifically, a QTc > 470 ms in male athletes and a QTc > 480 ms in female athletes have been set as cut-off values (see Chap. 8).
- The prevalence of the disease is 1/2000 live births [5].
- Due to incomplete penetrance and phenotypic variability, affected individuals among family members may have a normal QT on ECG [6], and those are defined as "silent mutation carriers".
- Even though the risk of cardiac events in "silent mutation carriers" is lower than in patients with a prolonged QT, they have a 10% risk of experiencing a major cardiac event by age 40, with a 4% risk of cardiac arrest/sudden cardiac death [7]. Therefore, it is almost mandatory to perform a genetic testing in all family members, regardless of their QT interval, to identify all affected subjects [8].

### 20.1.2 Genetic Basis

Since the first genetic description, 17 genes have been linked to the disease. In the 1990s three genes have been associated with LQTS: *KCNQ1*, *KCNH2* and *SCN5A*. These genes are mutated in 75–80% of affected LQTS cases [9–12] and therefore are considered as the "major LQTS genes".

- *KCNQ1* encodes the α-subunit of the $K^+$ channel, generating $I_{Ks}$, which is essential for QT adaptation when heart rate increases. When $I_{Ks}$ is defective, the QT interval fails to shorten during tachycardia, thus creating a highly arrhythmogenic condition [12].
  - Heterozygous *KCNQ1* mutations cause the autosomal dominant Romano-Ward LQT1 syndrome [13–15].
  - Homozygous mutations in *KCNQ1*, or compound heterozygous mutations, cause the recessive Jervell and Lange-Nielsen Syndrome variant, characterized by deafness and aggressive cardiac phenotype [16, 17].
- *KCNH2* encodes the α-subunit of the $K^+$ channel conducting the rapid potassium rectifier current ($I_{Kr}$). Mutations in *KCNH2* cause a reduction in $I_{Kr}$ current and therefore a prolongation of action potential duration and QTc [10].
- *SCN5A* encodes the α-subunit of the cardiac sodium channel conducting the depolarizing sodium inward current. Mutations in this gene produce the LQTS phenotype by increasing the delayed $Na^+$ inward current and, therefore, prolonging the action potential duration [18].

Among the 14 "minor LQTS genes", those worth of note are the ones associated with specific or quite aggressive features:

- *KCNE1* and *KCNE2* encoding for the β-subunits of *KCNQ1* and *KCNH2* are responsible for LQT5 and LQT6 respectively. Mutations in *KCNE1* may cause either the dominant Romano Ward Syndrome or the recessive Jervell and Large-Nielsen Syndrome. Mutations in *KCNE2* are rare causes of LQTS while are more frequently implicated in acquired LQTS [19–24].

- *KCNJ2* is associated with a complex clinical disorder called "Andersen-Tawil Syndrome" (LQT7) in which the prolongation of the QT interval is modest and usually associated with prominent U waves. Additional clinical features, variably present, are ventricular arrhythmias, dysmorphic features and periodic paralysis [25].
- *CACNA1C*, encoding for the voltage-gated calcium channel, is the gene responsible for Timothy syndrome (TS; LQT8), a rare and syndromic disease, characterized by a malignant cardiac phenotype, with extracardiac findings ranging from syndactyly to cardiac developmental defects and autism [26].
- *CALM1*, *CALM2* and *CALM3* are genes encoding calmodulin, a $Ca^{2+}$-binding signal transducer messenger protein that influences the activity of ion channels. Mutations on these genes have been recently associated with aggressive forms (LQT14, LQT15, LQT16) characterized by extreme QTc prolongation and early-onset recurrent life-threatening arrhythmias [27–30].
- *TRDN* is the last gene identified. It encodes triadin, a major anchoring protein responsible for the structural integrity and crosstalk of sarcoplasmic reticulum $Ca^{2+}$-release channels, L-type $Ca^{2+}$ channels and $Ca^{2+}$-sensitive proteins. Homozygous or compound heterozygous mutations in this gene are responsible for another aggressive form of LQTS, the LQT17 [31, 32].

### 20.1.3 Clinical Presentation

- Syncopal episodes under emotional or physical stress are the main manifestations of the disease and are due to a typical polymorphic ventricular arrhythmia, i.e. TdP. This often degenerates into ventricular fibrillation accounting for a mortality rate of 5% per year among untreated symptomatic patients [33, 34].
- Due to incomplete penetrance and clinical heterogeneity, even in the presence of the same disease-causing mutation [35], clinical manifestation can range from no symptoms to sudden cardiac death [6, 35].
- Sudden death may represent the first clinical manifestation of the disease in 12% of untreated patients [6].
- Trigger for cardiac events is gene-specific [34, 36, 37]:
  - in LQT1 the main trigger is exercise or stress, with swimming being involved in 33% of cases [36];
  - LQT2 patients experience events during emotional stress, sudden auditory stimuli are responsible for 63% of cases. LQT2 women are particularly at risk also during hormonal changes like in the post-partum period and during menopause transition [36, 38];
  - in LQT3 patients, events occur typically while asleep or at rest [36].

### 20.1.4 Diagnostic Work-up

#### 20.1.4.1 ECG

Typical features on surface ECG are: QTc prolongation; peculiar T wave morphologies; T wave alternans; 2:1 functional atrio-ventricular blocks.

- QTc prolongation: an obvious QT prolongation is the main feature of the disease. QTc cut-offs are indicated above, and the most widely recognized formula to correct the QT is the Bazett's formula [1, 39–41]. Although in general, the longer the QT the greater is the risk for malignant arrhythmias, patients affected with normal QTc have a higher risk of cardiac events compared to normal subjects [6].
- T wave morphology: notched T waves in more than three precordial leads or diphasic T-waves are typical of the disease, and gene-specific ECG patterns (Fig. 20.1) exist [15, 29, 42]: LQT1 patients may present with broad based T waves, LQT2 patients have more frequently diphasic or notched T waves, while LQT3 patients, but also patients with Timothy Syndrome and CALM-LQTS, have late onset peaked T-waves [6, 29].

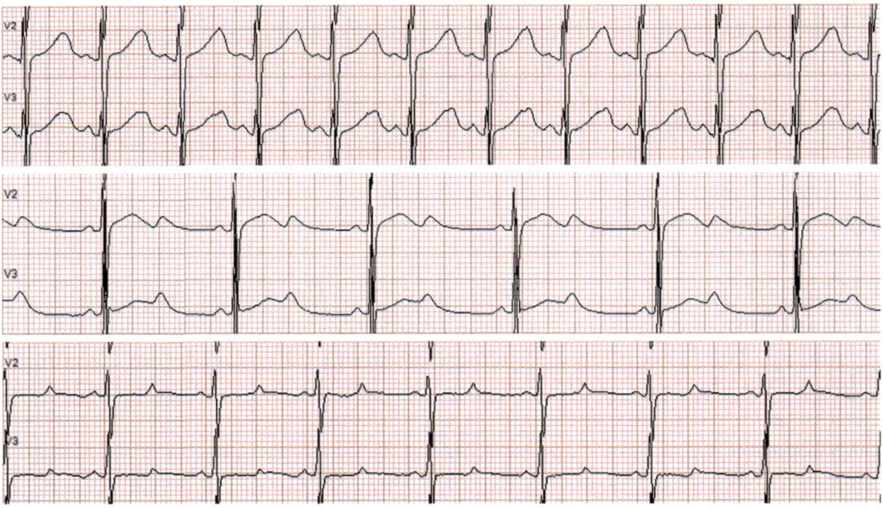


**Fig. 20.1** Electrocardiographic strips showing three LQTS ECG patterns: (1) LQT1 patient (upper panel): typical broad-based T waves, (2) LQT2 patient (middle panel): biphasic and notched T waves, and (3) LQT3 patient (lower panel): prolonged ST segment with sharpened T waves. Tracings are from a 24-h Holter recording. (Adapted from Crotti L, Kotta MC, Castelletti S. Long and Short QT Syndromes, *in* D. Thomas, C.A. Remme (eds.), *Channelopathies in Heart Disease*, Cardiac and Vascular Biology, p. 147–185, Springer International Publishing AG, part of Springer Nature 2018)

- T wave alternans: a beat-to-beat alternation of the polarity or amplitude of the T wave is a peculiar feature representing a sign of major electrical instability [43].
- 2:1 functional atrio-ventricular block, also called pseudo 2:1 AV block, occurs in very young patients with extreme QT prolongation: when sinus intervals are shorter than the ventricular refractory period, every two sinus beats one is not conducted because the ventricle is still in refractory period. This ECG feature represents a negative prognostic sign.

#### 20.1.4.2 Exercise Stress Test

- Exercise stress test is useful to check for QT adaptation during exercise that it is typically unpaired mainly in LQT1 patients, but also to a lesser extent in LQT2 patients [6].
- QT prolongation during the recovery phase of the exercise test is a typical feature of the disease and indeed a cut-off of QTc ≥ 480 ms at the fourth minute of recovery has been included among the last diagnostic criteria for the disease [44, 45]. In this phase, it is also possible to note the appearance of typical major repolarization changes [44]. Therefore, the exercise test should not be interrupted before the fourth minute after cessation of exercise.
- Heart rate reduction during the first minute of recovery could provide prognostic information in LQT1 patients [46].

#### 20.1.4.3 12-Lead 24-h Holter Monitoring

A 12-lead 24-h Holter recording is quite useful in the diagnostic process and for the follow-up [33, 47] as it allows the identification of:

- changes in QT duration during daytime and nighttime and the identification of the maximum QTc recorded;
- sudden sinus pauses;
- lower heart rate to modulate beta-blocker therapy;
- repolarization abnormalities, including T wave alternans.

### 20.1.5 Diagnosis

A score, the so-called "Schwartz score" (Table 20.1), has been developed to help the clinician in performing the diagnosis of LQTS [44] (see also Chap. 11). According to guidelines [2], clinical diagnosis can be performed:

- when the patient has a Schwartz score of ≥3.5 points;
- in presence of an unequivocally pathogenic mutation and/or in presence of a QTc ≥ 500 ms in repeated 12-lead ECGs.

**Table 20.1** Diagnostic criteria for Long QT Syndrome (adapted from [42])

| 11 Points | |
|---|---|
| Electrocardiographic findings[a] | |
| QTc[b] | |
| ≥480 ms | 3 |
| 460–479 ms | 2 |
| 450–459 ms (in males) | 1 |
| QTc fourth minute of recovery from exercise stress test ≥480 ms | 1 |
| Torsade de pointes[c] | 2 |
| T wave alternans | 1 |
| Notched T wave in three leads | 1 |
| Low heart rate for age[d] | 0.5 |
| Clinical history | |
| Syncope[c] | |
| With stress | 2 |
| Without stress | 1 |
| Congenital deafness | 0.5 |
| Family history | |
| Family members with definite LQTS[e] | 1 |
| Unexplained SCD below age 30 among immediate family members[e] | 0.5 |

SCORE: ≤1 point: low probability of LQTS; 1.5–3 points: intermediate probability of LQTS; ≥3.5 points high probability of LQTS

[a]In the absence of medications or disorders known to affect these electrocardiographic features

[b]QTc calculated by Bazett's formula

[c]Mutually exclusive

[d]Resting heart rate below the second percentile for age

[e]The same family member cannot be counted in both

### 20.1.6 Differential Diagnosis

A QT prolongation can be caused also by

1. Drugs: a list of medication causing QT prolongation in available on the website www.azcert.org;
2. Bradycardia;
3. Hypokalemia;
4. Hormonal changes.

It is therefore important to exclude secondary causes of QT prolongation that may lead to the so-called acquired Long QT Syndrome (aLQTS).

- A genetic predisposition is present in around one third of the subjects with aLQTS.
- A score, based on QTc, age and symptoms allow the identification of the aLQTS patients more likely to carry a predisposing mutation [48].

### 20.1.7 Risk Stratification

Risk stratification includes:

- gender, age, QTc and genotype [4];
- symptoms (patients with a previous syncopal episode are at higher risk for subsequent cardiac events if not correctly treated; clearly patients with a previous cardiac arrest are high-risk patients);
- Additional ECG features such as T-wave alternans, 2:1 functional AV block and sinus pauses, may increase the risk of events [46, 49, 50];
- Not only the gene, but also the type of mutation, the position of the mutation in the protein (i.e. pore region for KCNH2 or transmembrane region for KCNQ1) and sometimes the specific mutation can carry important prognostic information. Furthermore, common genetic variants, known as modifiers genes [51], may influence the arrhythmic risk [51, 52].

### 20.1.8 Therapy

The mainstay treatments for LQTS are beta-blockers and left cardiac sympathetic denervation (LCSD). ICD implantation is necessary only in a minority of the patients [2, 53]. Few gene-specific treatments are also available. All patients should be strongly advised to avoid QT-prolonging drugs (www.azcert.org) and to use potassium supplements whenever needed to keep adequate potassium levels.

- Betablockers: as the trigger for most of the events is a sudden increase in sympathetic activity, it is not surprising that the most effective therapy is represented by beta-blockers [53–56]. Not all of them, however, are equally effective: propranolol and nadolol are the wider used as they have been demonstrated to reduce the risk of recurrences of events more than metoprolol and bisoprolol [57].
- LCSD, a mini-invasive surgical approach consisting in the removal of the lower third of left stellate ganglion and the subsequent four thoracic ganglia [58], should be performed in patients symptomatic despite a full dose of beta-blockers or in those not tolerant to beta-blockers. The rationale for LCSD is largely based on its antifibrillatory effect and on the major reduction of norepinephrine release at ventricular level in the absence of post-denervation supersensitivity [53].
- The Implantable cardioverter defibrillator (ICD) is indicated in patients with a previous cardiac arrest and in patients with recurrences despite full antiadrenergic therapy possibly including LCSD [2].
- Gene-specific therapy and gene-specific recommendations:
  - LQT1 should avoid competitive sports activity, particularly swimming, as they are at higher risk during sympathetic activation [6, 59, 60];
  - LQT2 patients are at higher risk when aroused from sleep or rest by a sudden noise, therefore telephone and alarm clocks should be removed from the bedrooms. As they are also particularly sensitive to serum potassium levels, a

combination with potassium sparing agents should be considered in those patients with difficulties in maintaining reasonable levels of potassium [2, 36, 53]. Recently, in some specific *KCNH2*-mutations, Lumacaftor has been shown to correct the trafficking defect and shorten the QTc [61, 62].
  - LQT3 patients may benefit from mexiletine in addition to beta-blockers. As the effect of mexiletine is mutation-specific, its effectiveness should be tested by the acute oral drug test technique [63–65]. Recently, mexiletine showed to be effective also in some LQT2 patients [66].

## 20.2 Short QT Syndrome

### 20.2.1 Definition and Prevalence

- The Short QT syndrome (SQTS) is an arrhythmic cardiac disorder characterized by a short QT interval at the basal ECG and increased risk of life-threatening arrhythmias.
- SQTS is an autosomal dominant disease and it is expected to be equally prevalent in male and female patients; however, data from the European SQTS Registry suggest a higher prevalence of the disease among males with a mean age at diagnosis between 20 and 30 years [67].

### 20.2.2 Molecular Basis

- The genetic substrate is partially in common with Long QT Syndrome: while loss-of-function mutations in the *KCNQ1*, *KCNH2* and *KCNJ2* genes cause LQTS, gain-of-function mutations on the same genes cause SQTS [68–70]. On the contrary, loss-of-function mutations in genes encoding calcium channel subunits have been identified in patients with short QT, frequently associated with a Brugada ECG pattern [68–71].
- The first three are the main genes causing the disease [8, 72], with *KCNH2* being the most frequently involved.

### 20.2.3 Clinical Presentation

- The severity of symptoms and their age of onset are quite variable.
- The severity of symptoms ranges from asymptomatic (38%) [67] to sudden death, from atrial fibrillation to syncope [67, 72, 73].
  - Atrial fibrillation and flutter are probably due to short atrial refractory periods [67, 72, 73].
- The age of onset of clinical manifestations ranges from in utero to age 70 [67, 72, 73].
  - SQTS may manifest as sudden infant death syndrome (SIDS) [74];

   - the peak of occurrence of life-threatening arrhythmias seems to be the first year of life and then between age 14 and 40 [67, 72, 73]: more than 90% of males have cardiac arrest between 14 and 40 years of age; amongst females, the events are widely distributed across the years [67].

### 20.2.4 Diagnosis

- The diagnosis of SQTS is performed considering ECG data, symptoms and family history. Regarding the ECG, it is still debated how short the QTc should be to make a diagnosis of SQTS: SQTS patients reported so far have QTc in the range of 250–380 ms;
- In healthy populations (altogether >28,000 individuals) a QTc in the lowest 0.5 percentile of the normal distribution (≤330 ms) [75] or below 340 ms [76] and 320 ms [76, 77] was not associated with increased risk of SCD.
- Athletes have shorter QT intervals than non-athletes but athletic status does not predict short QT intervals [77].
- A diagnosis of SQTS should be performed, according to the 2015 ESC Guidelines for the prevention of SCD [65]:
   - in all patients with a QTc ≤ 340 ms;
   - in patients with a QTc between 340 and 360 ms, only in the presence of at least one additional criterion, such as either presence of a pathogenic mutation, family history of SQTS, family history of SCD below age 40 or survival of a VT/VF episode in the absence of heart disease.
- The HRS/EHRA/APHRS expert consensus statement on the diagnosis and management of patients with inherited primary arrhythmia syndromes [2] is more stringent, posing at 330 ms the cut off for the diagnosis of SQTS in the absence of additional criteria.
- Other ECG characteristics useful to suspect or diagnose the disease include (Fig. 20.2):

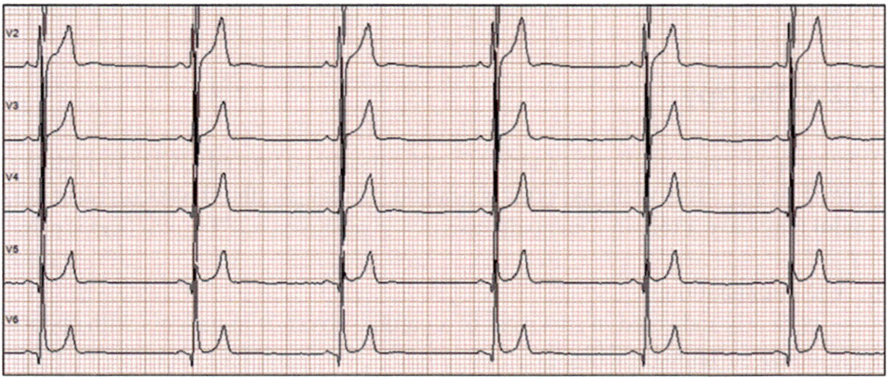


**Fig. 20.2** Electrocardiographic strip showing SQTS ECG typical features: tall, sharp, narrow and fine T waves with an early repolarization pattern and QTc 263 ms

- a short or absent ST segment, with the T wave initiating immediately from the S wave;
- SQT1 patients (those with a mutation in *KCNH2*) may have tall, sharp, narrow, fine and symmetrical T waves, especially in leads V2-V4, with a relatively prolonged $T_{peak}$-$T_{end}$ interval [78];
- SQT2 patients (those with a mutation in *KCNQ1*) show less narrow symmetrical T waves [79];
- SQT3 patients (those with a mutation in *KCNJ2*) present an asymmetrical pattern with a less steep ascending section of the T wave followed by a rapid descending terminal phase;
- Early repolarization has been described in 65% of SQTS patients and associated with arrhythmic events [80].

• Features that may help distinguishing healthy people from SQTS patients include:
  - a significantly shorter J point-T peak interval, a shorter $T_{peak} - T_{end}$/QT ratio [76, 80];
  - a less steep slope of the QT-RR relationship due to the lack of adequate QT shortening to heart rate increases during 24-h ECG recordings and exercise stress test [81];
  - presence of a PQ depression ≥0.05 mV, due to the heterogeneous abbreviation of atrial repolarization, rarely observed in healthy individuals [82].
• Reversible causes of short QTc should be excluded [78, 83, 84]:
  - hypercalcemia, hyperkalemia
  - digital toxicity
  - acidosis
  - hyperthermia
  - androgens use
  - increased vagal tone
• Genetic testing has a relatively low yield, ranging from 11 to 20% of cases [8, 72];
  - It may be considered for patients with a strong clinical suspicion [8];
  - it is recommended for the family members of a proband in whom a disease-causing mutation has already been identified [8].

### 20.2.5 Therapy

The therapy is quite challenging in SQTS patients and so far, only ICD implantation showed to be effective in preventing sudden cardiac death. Hydroquinidine and sotalol may have a role in some patients.

• ICD implantation:
  - is clearly indicated in survivors of a cardiac arrest or in patients with spontaneous sustained VT [2];
  - is quite controversial in asymptomatic patients for the high rate of inappropriate shocks due to T wave oversensing [85];

  - risk stratification remains challenging in asymptomatic patients as there are no data supporting the role of invasive electrophysiological study with programmed ventricular stimulation [2, 65].
- Hydroquinidine (HQ)
  - significantly increases QT interval and effective refractory period [67, 86] in SQT1 patients;
  - in patients without a mutation the effect appears weaker and quite variable [67, 86];
  - may represent an alternative option to ICD in those patients who would qualify for an ICD but present contraindications or refusal [65].
- Sotalol is considered a possible alternative to hydroquinidine [65]
- A pharmacological treatment may be considered also in asymptomatic patients with a family history of SCD and in those who already have an ICD to prevent the occurrence of multiple arrhythmic events [65].

## 20.3 Brugada Syndrome

### 20.3.1 Definition and Prevalence

- Brugada Syndrome (BrS) is a genetically transmitted heart disease characterized by coved-type ST elevation in the right precordial ECG leads and increased risk of sudden cardiac death (SCD).
- The diagnostic ECG pattern is not always present, even in affected subjects, therefore the prevalence of the disease is unclear and estimated to be between 5:10,000 and 1:2000 [87].
- It is considered responsible of 4–12% of all cases of SCD and 20% of those SCD with a structural normal heart [88], however a recent study evaluating relatives of SCD victims suggested that the prevalence may be even higher [89].

### 20.3.2 Molecular Basis

- BrS has always been considered a monogenetic disease with autosominal dominant pattern of inheritance; however, increasing evidences suggest that the BrS phenotype can be modulated by common genetic variants [90].
- *SCN5A*, encoding for the voltage-gated Nav1.5 sodium channel, is the major gene involved in the disease: mutations on this gene account for 20–30% of genotype positive patients [91].
- Other genes have been implicated in the disease [92–96]; however, they are responsible for a small number of cases.
- The emerging evidence of minor structural abnormalities in the right ventricular outflow has led to the identification of mutations also in genes responsible for the Arrhythmogenic Cardiomyopathy, of which BrS may be part of the spectrum [94, 97–99].

### 20.3.3 Clinical Presentation

- The clinical manifestation of the disease is quite heterogenous, ranging from no symptoms to syncope, from supraventricular arrhythmias to sudden cardiac death.
- Potentially lethal arrhythmias usually occur
  - at a mean age of 41 ± 15 years, eight times more frequently in males than females [100–102]. However, malignant forms responsible for SIDS or SCD in young children have been described [103, 104];
  - during fever [100, 105–107];
  - under vagal triggers [108–111]:
    
    at rest or while asleep, with a significant peak from midnight to 6 am, less frequently in the evening and during daytime [112, 113];
    
    after heavy meals and high alcohol intake [114, 115].
- Supraventricular arrhythmias have been reported in approximately 20% of patients [116–120], including
  - Atrial fibrillation
  - Atrioventricular nodal re-entrant tachycardia
  - Wolff-Parkinson-White syndrome
- Conduction delays have been reported in association with the syndrome, including:
  - prolonged sinus node recovery time and sinoatrial conduction time [121]
  - slowed atrial conduction and atrial standstill [122, 123]
  - prolonged atrio-ventricular conduction [96]
- Overlaps with Sick Sinus Syndrome and Lev-Lenègre syndrome (also called progressive cardiac conduction disease) have been reported, particularly in patients carrying mutations in *SCN5A* gene [124–128].

### 20.3.4 Diagnostic Work-up

#### 20.3.4.1 ECG

- Three ECG repolarization patterns in the right precordial leads have been associated with the disease (Figs. 20.3 and 20.4):
  - Type 1 ECG pattern ("coved-type") is characterized by incomplete right bundle brunch block and a coved ST-segment elevation ≥2 mm (0.2 mV) followed by a negative T wave in ≥1 right precordial lead (V1–V3).
  - Type 2 ECG pattern ("saddle-back type") is characterized by an ST-segment elevation ≥2 mm, in ≥1 right precordial lead (V1–V3), followed by a convex ST. The r′-wave may or may not overlap the J point, but it has a slow downward slope. The ST segment is followed by a positive T-wave in V2 and is of variable morphology in V1.
  - Type 3 ECG pattern has either a saddleback or coved appearance with an ST-segment elevation of <1 mm.

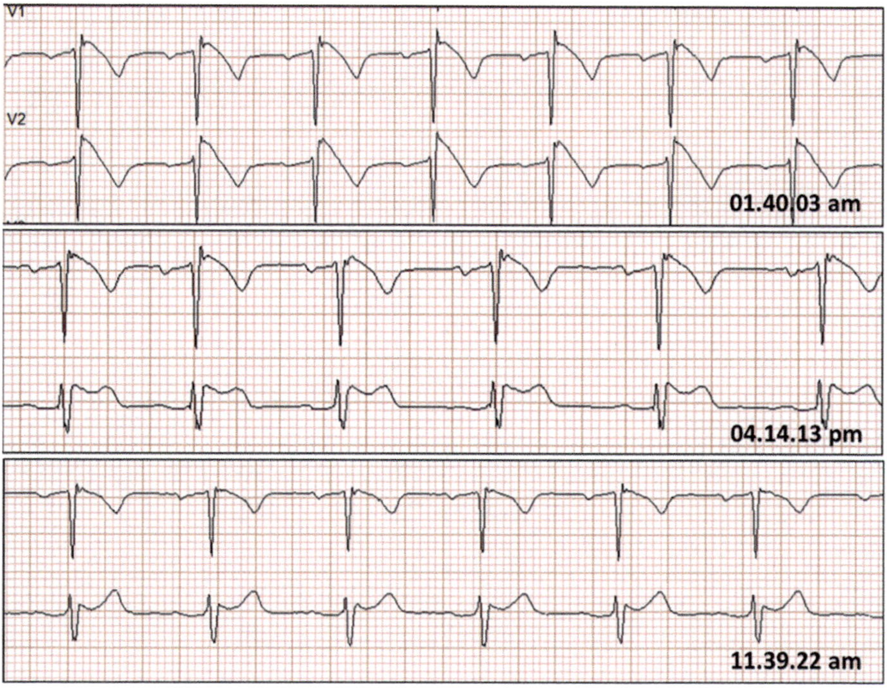


**Fig. 20.3** Electrocardiographic strips showing the three BrS ECG patterns: Type 1 ("coved-type" pattern) upper panel; type 2 ("saddle-back type") middle panel; Type 3 ECG lower panel. Only the type 1 ECG is diagnostic for the disease. Tracing are from a 24-h Holter recording of the same patient at different hours, reflecting the great fluctuation of the ECG pattern even in the single patient and the higher probability to see a diagnostic pattern during the night when there is an increased vagal-tone. The patient is a 59-year-old asymptomatic man referred for further investigations after an ECG performed for atypical chest pain showing a suspicious pattern

- The type 1 ECG pattern:
  - is the only one considered diagnostic for the disease [2];
  - may be absent on the surface ECG (concealed BrS);
  - can be unmasked by sodium channel blockers, during a febrile state or in vagotonic conditions [107, 108, 129, 130];
  - can be detected in the third or second intercostal spaces due to the variable anatomical correlation between the right ventricular outflow tract and V1–V2 in the standard position [131, 132]. The identification of a spontaneous or induced type 1 ECG in an high intercostal space is considered equal to its detection with a standard ECG in fourth intercostal space [133].
- The type 2 and type 3 ECG patterns are not diagnostic for the disease. Their detection should prompt further investigations [2].
- Conduction abnormalities are frequently observed [96, 124, 134]:
  - they include prolonged P wave, PR or QRS duration;
  - they are more common in patients carrying a mutation in SCN5A gene [96, 124];
  - PR prolongation is likely due to HV conduction delay [134].

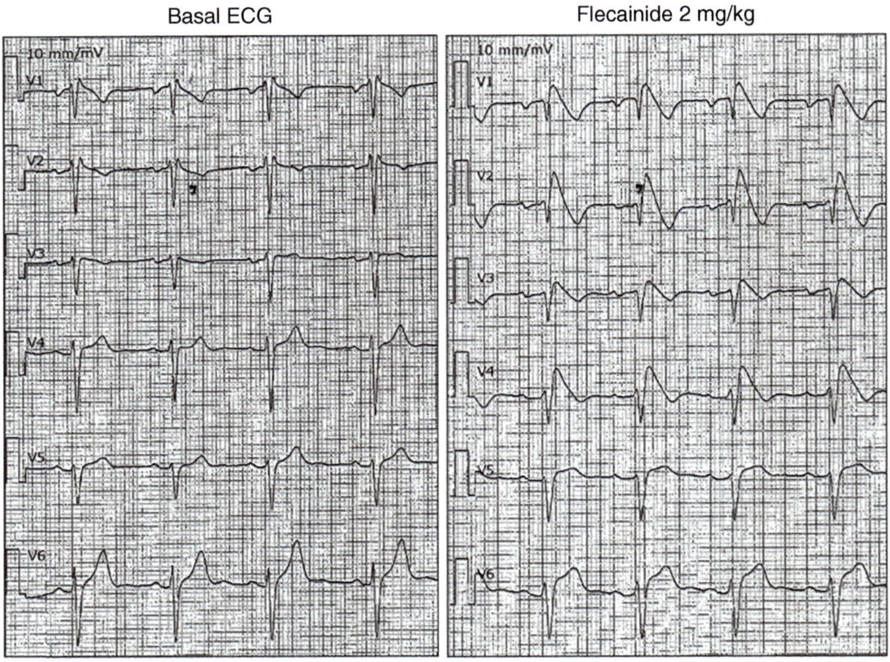


**Fig. 20.4** Induction of a Type 1 "coved-type" ECG by a flecainide drug challenge test. Lead V1 and V2 are placed in the second intercostal space, lead V3 and V4 are placed in the third intercostal space, lead V5 and V6 are placed in the fourth intercostal space. The type 1 ECG is clearly visible in the second and third intercostal space

- Depolarization and repolarization abnormalities in the inferior and lateral leads have been described and associated with a more severe phenotype [135–139].
- A slightly prolonged QTc can be occasionally observed [134, 140–142] and overlapping cases with LQTS have also been described [140, 143].

#### 20.3.4.2 12-Lead 24-h Holter Monitoring

- The fluctuation of the ECG pattern even in the single patient and the higher probability to see a diagnostic pattern during the night when there is an increased vagal tone justify the use of the 12-lead 24-h Holter monitoring (Fig. 20.3).
- Prolonged ECG monitoring has uncovered spontaneous intermittent type 1 ECG patterns in 20–34% of patients with only drug-induced type 1 ECG [113, 144].
- ECG recording should be performed placing the leads also in the higher intercostal spaces to increase the probability of identifying a diagnostic spontaneous Type 1 ECG pattern.

#### 20.3.4.3 Exercise Stress Testing

- Type 1 ECG pattern may be unmasked during the recovery phase of the exercise stress testing [111, 145, 146].
- The augmentation of ST-segment elevation during the recovery phase may identify patients with an higher risk profile [111, 146].

#### 20.3.4.4 Drug Challenge Test

- The detection of a type 2 or type 3 ECG pattern on surface ECG in absence of appearance of type 1 ECG during exercise testing and 12-lead 24-h Holter monitoring cannot exclude a concealed BrS (Fig. 20.3).
- Considering the greatness of ST-segment elevation fluctuation, when there is a clinical suspicious of the disease a drug challenge test with a sodium-channel blocking agent should be performed [2, 130].
- The drug challenge test (Fig. 20.4)
  - is considered positive when a type 1 ECG pattern appears [2];
  - is performed using a sodium-channel blocking agent such as ajmaline, flecainide, procainamide [147–150];
  - requires a continuous ECG monitoring because of its potential pro-arrhythmic risk: ECG monitoring should continue until the ECG reverts to the baseline condition [147];
  - should be interrupted before the end of the infusion when an excessive widening of the QRS is observed (>30% over the baseline value) or in the presence of frequent ventricular premature beats [147];
  - may result in false-negative in nearly 25% of cases [149];
    - flecainide and procainamide lead more often to false-negative results compared to ajmaline [131];
    - a repeated test using ajmaline should be considered in cases with a high probability of the disease;
- Drug-induced conversion of type 3 to type 2 ST-segment elevation is considered inconclusive for a diagnosis of Brugada syndrome [2].

#### 20.3.4.5 Genetic Testing

- According to the consensus statement on the state of genetic testing for the channelopathies and cardiomyopathies [8], genetic screening
  - is considered useful in all patients with a definitive diagnosis;
  - cannot be used to rule out BrS diagnosis in presence of an isolated type 2 or type 3 ECG pattern;
  - is recommended for family members following the identification of the BrS-causative mutation in the index case.

### 20.3.5 Diagnosis

- BrS is diagnosed when a type I ST-segment elevation is observed
  - either spontaneously or after intra-venous administration of a sodium channel blocking agent (ajmaline, flecainide or procainamide)
  - in at least one right precordial lead (V1 and V2), in a standard or a higher intercostal space (up to the second intercostal space) [2, 65].

### 20.3.6 Differential Diagnosis

- ST-segment elevation can be observed in several conditions (Brugada ECG phenocopies) [151] that should therefore be excluded before establishing a definite diagnosis. These conditions include:
  - Medical illness: RV ischemia, acute pulmonary embolism, acute pericarditis, acute myocardial ischemia or infarction, Prinzmetal angina, dissecting aortic aneurysm, Duchenne muscular dystrophy, various central and autonomic nervous system abnormalities [152–157];
  - Mechanical compression of RVOT: pectus excavatum, hemopericardium, mediastinal tumor [158, 159];
  - Cardiomyopathies: arrhythmogenic right ventricular cardiomyopathy, ventricular hypertrophy [160, 161];
  - Electrolyte imbalances: hyperkalaemia, hypercalcemia [162–165];
  - Hyperthermia and hypothermia [166, 167];
  - Other conditions: thiamin deficiency, elevated insulin level [168];
- The prominent differential diagnosis is with the ST-segment elevation observed in well-trained athletes, characterized by an upslope rather than a downslope. To help in the differentiation several criteria that use the triangle formed by the ascending and descending branch of the r′-wave have been suggested, such as:
  - The measurement of the β-angle [169];
  - The triangle base duration at the isoelectric line [170];
  - The relationship between the triangle base at the isoelectric line and its height [170];
  - Length of the base triangle of the r′-wave 5 mm below the maximum rise point [170];
  - The evolution of the β-angle during exercise testing [171];
  - The ratio between the measurement of the ST segment at the J point (STJ) and then 80 ms after the J point (ST80) [172].
- None of these additional criteria allow to definitely rule out the BrS diagnosis: a sodium-channel blocker test should be performed to exclude the diagnosis in athletes when there is a suspicious of BrS diagnosis.

### 20.3.7 Risk Stratification

- Clinical variables able to predict a worse outcome in patients with BrS include:
  - Presence of symptoms before diagnosis [102, 173–175];
  - Spontaneous type 1 ECG [102, 174–176];
  - Male gender [102, 174, 175, 177];
- Several additional clinical variables with prognostic significance have been proposed, however some of them derive from small observational studies and require validation. They include:
  - spontaneous atrial fibrillation [119];
  - presence of an SCN5A mutation, especially if in the pore region of the protein [178];
  - presence of QRS fragmentation [136];
  - augmentation of ST-segment elevation during recovery from exercise [146];
  - presence of late potentials [179];
  - early repolarization pattern in the inferior and/or lateral leads [180];
  - a prolonged $T_{peak}$–$T_{end}$ interval [181–183];
  - sinus node dysfunction [184];
  - prolonged QRS in V2 [184];
  - duration of the S-wave in DI [184];
  - prolonged QTc in V2 [184];
  - the "aVR sign" [184];
  - presence of the type 1 ECG pattern on limb leads [184];
  - presence of T-wave alternans [185, 186];
- The combined presence of a spontaneous type 1 ECG and the history of syncope identifies subjects at risk of cardiac arrest in which an ICD implantation should be considered [2, 65].
- The risk of life-threatening arrhythmias among asymptomatic patients without a spontaneous ECG pattern is below 0.5% a year. Only life-style changes are recommended [187].
- The risk of life-threatening arrhythmias among asymptomatic patients with a spontaneous type 1 ECG is not so high to require an ICD implantation, but it is higher than in those with only an induced ECG pattern [187]; there is not a consensus on what to do in this subgroup of patients, a possible option is the use of an electrophysiological study to evaluate inducibility of arrhythmic events. The current guidelines neither encourage nor discourage its use for BrS stratification [2, 65].

### 20.3.8 Therapy

Therapy include life-style changes in all patients and ICD and/or drugs in selected cases [8, 65].

- ICD implantation is
  - mandatory in patients with history of life-threatening arrhythmias;
  - can be useful in patients with a spontaneous diagnostic type I ECG who have a history of syncope suggestive of malignant arrhythmia origin;

  - may be considered in patients with a diagnosis of BrS who develop VF during programmed electrical stimulation;
  - is not indicated in asymptomatic patients with drug-induced type 1 ECG.
- Isoprotenerol has proved to be useful for the treatment of electrical storm in BrS.
- Quinidine, a Class Ia antiarrhythmic drug:
  - has shown to prevent the induction of VF and suppress spontaneous ventricular arrhythmias
  - can be useful in patients
    with BrS, carrying an ICD and experiencing arrhythmic storms;
    with a diagnosis of BrS who present a contra-indication to the ICD or refuse it;
    with supraventricular arrhythmias that require treatment.
  - may be considered in asymptomatic patients with a diagnosis of BrS with a spontaneous type I ECG.
- All patients should avoid
  - a list of drugs able to induce a type 1 ECG and VF, available on the website www.brugadadrugs.org;
  - prolonged febrile state at high temperatures (paracetamol should be promptly assumed);
  - electrolyte unbalance;
  - heavy meals in the evening;
  - excessive alcohol intake;
- Ablation of a fractionated electrogram in the epicardial RVOT may be considered in patients with a recurrent VF (Class IIb level C).

## 20.4 Catecholaminergic Polymorphic Ventricular Tachycardia

### 20.4.1 Definition and Prevalence

- Catecholaminergic Polymorphic Ventricular Tachycardia (CPVT) is a genetic cardiac disorder characterized by adrenergically-induced life-threatening arrhythmias.
- Basal ECG and echocardiogram are normal.
- The diagnosis is performed with exercise stress test that typically shows the occurrence of isolated ventricular beats at around 100–110 bpm; the complexity and frequency of arrhythmias progressively increase with the increase in workload, and the typical bidirectional ventricular tachycardia may occur. When the exercise is interrupted, arrhythmias generally disappear quickly.
- Prevalence is estimated to be 1:10,000, sudden cardiac death can be the first presentation, with a mortality rate in severely untreated patients up to 50% before age of 20 [2, 188].

### 20.4.2 Molecular Basis

All major genes causing the disease are involved in calcium handling. Mutations in these genes usually cause an excess calcium leak from the sarcoplasmic reticulum and electrical instability. The disease may be inherited with a:

- autosomal dominant trait, usually due to mutations in the following genes:
  - *RyR2*: is the gene responsible for the main form of the disease. It encodes the cardiac ryanodine receptor involved in the electromechanical coupling. Mutations in this gene are identified in approximately 60% of cases [189] and are responsible for the so-called CPVT type 1 form of the disease. They cause $Ca^{2+}$ "leakage" from the sarcoplasmic reticulum in conditions of sympathetic activation, creating an abnormal increase of the cytosolic free $Ca^{2+}$concentration leading to an electrically unstable substrate.
  - *KCNJ2*: mutations in this gene encoding the potassium inwardly rectifying channel, which usually is responsible for the Andersen-Tawil syndrome, are identified in less than 5% of cases and may be responsible for an atypical CPVT [190, 191].
  - *CALM1–3*: mutations in these genes causing a reduction of the calcium-binding affinity and an impaired calmodulin-ryanodine receptor interaction, may be responsible of a dominant form of the disease in less than 1% of cases [27, 29, 192].
- autosomal recessive trait, usually due to mutations in the following genes:
  - *CASQ2*: mutations in this gene encoding for cardiac calsequestrin, a calcium-buffering protein situated within the sarcoplasmic reticulum that also has inhibitory effects on RYR2 activity, underlie a malignant autosomal recessive form of the disease. Mutations in this gene have been identified in 5% of cases [193] and are responsible for the so-called CPVT type 2 form of the disease.
  - *TRDN*: mutations in triadin, a transmembrane sarcoplasmic reticulum protein functionally and physically related to RyR2, may affect the calcium release process leading to a calcium leak during diastole either though a reduction in CASQ2 protein levels or through an indirect destabilization of the RyR2 channel opening. Mutations in this gene are identified in 1% of cases [194].

### 20.4.3 Clinical Presentation

- Syncopal episodes triggered by exercise or acute emotion, due to ventricular tachycardia, are the typical manifestation of the disease.
- The first symptom usually occurs in childhood or early adolescence; less frequently later in life [188, 189, 195].
- Patients may also simply report palpitations or dizziness during exercise or emotion as the heart is structurally normal and therefore non-sustained ventricular arrhythmias can be tolerated.

- Sudden death may be the first manifestation of the disease [188].
- Supraventricular arrhythmias are part of the disease expression [120, 196, 197].
- Family history may be positive for juvenile sudden cardiac death or syncope under similar conditions.

### 20.4.4 Diagnostic Work-up

- Basal ECG and echocardiogram are normal.
- The exercise stress testing is the golden standard for diagnosis, as it allows to reproducibly induce ventricular arrhythmias.
- The pattern of arrhythmias onset is quite typical:
  - Ventricular arrhythmias are usually elicited when heart rate is >100–110 bpm.
  - The frequency and the complexity of arrhythmias increase with the increase in the workload: they start as isolated ventricular ectopic beats, then they increase in frequency becoming trigeminy and bigeminy, then couplets and runs of non-sustained ventricular tachycardia usually appear. If the exercise is not interrupted sustained ventricular tachycardia may occur.
  - Ventricular arrhythmias are typically polymorphic, with the bidirectional VT being the hallmark of the disease: there is an alternating QRS axis, with a rotation of 180 degrees, on a beat-to-beat basis (Fig. 20.5).
  - The QRS axis alternans may not be always present and patients may manifest an irregular polymorphic VT (Fig. 20.5).
  - Arrhythmias may originate from both the left and the right ventricle.
  - Isolated atrial ectopics, non-sustained supraventricular tachycardia and run of atrial fibrillation may occur during exercise with a pattern similar to the ventricular arrhythmias [196, 197].
- The arrhythmic pattern may be evoked also with isoprotenerol infusion in those patients who are unable to exercise. However, the sensitivity of this method is debated [198].
- A 12-lead 24-h Holter monitoring is useful in those patients with events during emotional stress. It is also very important in infants and younger children.
- The electrophysiological study has no diagnostic value as neither bidirectional nor polymorphic VT depends on re-entrant circuits [65, 115].

#### 20.4.4.1 Genetic Testing

- Molecular screening is recommended for any patient in whom a cardiologist has established a clinical index of suspicion for CPVT [2, 8].
- Mutation-specific genetic testing following the identification of the CPVT-causing mutation in the index-case, is recommended for all family members.

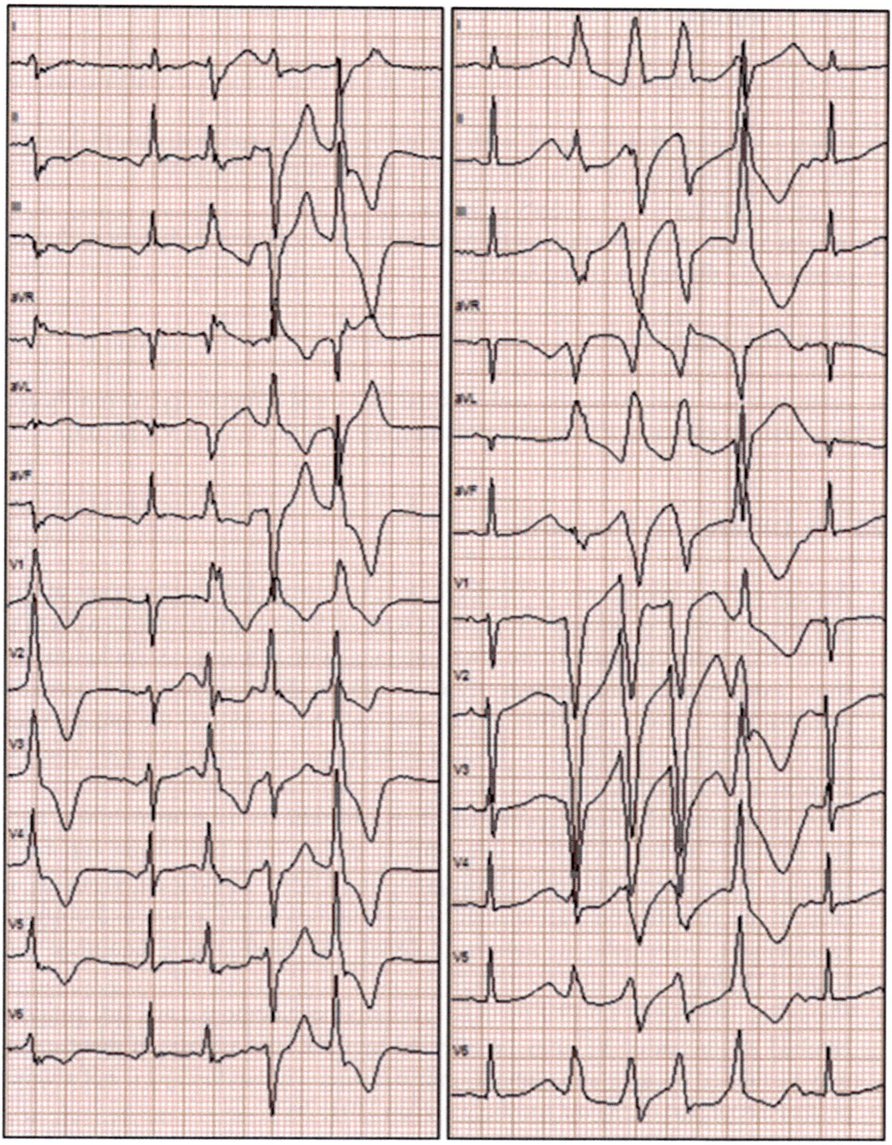

**Fig. 20.5** Electrocardiographic strips showing a bidirectional ventricular tachycardia (on the left) and a polymorphic ventricular tachycardia (on the right). There is an alternating QRS axis, with a rotation of 180°, on a beat-to-beat basis (on the left). The QRS complexes have a different morphology (on the right)

### 20.4.5 Diagnosis

Diagnosis is performed in:

- subjects younger than 40 years, with normal ECG and structurally normal heart, unexplained exercise or inducible polymorphic or bidirectional VT;
- subjects carrying a disease-causing mutation;
- in family members with premature ventricular beats or with bidirectional/polymorphic VT during exercise [2, 65];

CPVT can be diagnosed in

- subjects older than 40 years, with normal ECG and structurally normal heart, unexplained exercise or inducible polymorphic or bidirectional VT [2, 65].

### 20.4.6 Differential Diagnosis

- Andersen-Tawil Syndrome (ATS, LQT7): it is considered a phenocopy of the disease. However, unlike CPVT, patients with ATS have prominent U-waves on basal ECG, bidirectional VTs are often unrelated with adrenergic stimulation and show extracardiac abnormalities (typically facial dysmorphism and periodic paralysis). In those cases without extracardiac abnormalities, the presence of frequent ventricular ectopies on 12-lead 24-h Holter monitoring should raise the suspicion of ATS [191, 199].
- Arrhythmogenic Cardiomyopathy (AC): as AC patients have arrhythmias during exercise, and evidence of overlapping phenotypes have been reported, imaging assessment with echocardiogram and CMR should be performed in order to exclude the typical structure abnormalities of AC (such as fibrofatty replacement, ventricular dilatation, regional wall motion abnormalities; see Chap. 21) [200].
- Idiopathic ventricular fibrillation: it has recently been demonstrated that patients labelled as idiopathic VF may be affected by CPVT. Diagnosis in these cases may be missed because a maximal exercise testing without therapy is not always performed as part of the diagnostic work-up [201, 202].

### 20.4.7 Risk Stratification

There are no risk-scores available.

- The electrophysiological study is not indicated for risk stratification.
- Occurrence of cardiac arrest before diagnosis and/or the persistence of arrhythmias during exercise stress testing in patients on therapy are the two indicators of worse outcome [203, 204].

### 20.4.8 Therapy

Therapy includes: exercise restriction; beta-blockers; flecainide; left sympathetic cardiac denervation; ICD implantation [2, 65].

- Life-style changes: all patients are restricted from competitive sports and strenuous exercise and whenever possible they should also limit the exposure to stressful environments [2, 65].
- Beta-blockers: the adrenergic-mediated mechanism of the arrhythmias explains the high efficacy of the betablockers in the disease, acting through both a reduction in heart rate and a direct effect on calcium release from the sarcoplasmic reticulum.
  - Nadolol has been demonstrated to be the most effective [203].
  - Propranolol can be an alternative for those patients living in Countries where nadolol is not available.
  - Beta-blockers are recommended in all patients diagnosed with CPVT, and it is suggested also for patients with a disease-causing mutation even with a negative exercise stress testing [2, 65].
  - Exercise stress testing and 12-lead 24-h Holter monitoring should be periodically performed on therapy to assess the heart rate threshold of the arrhythmias onset.
- Flecainide: the addition of flecainide to beta-blockers has been shown to improve the arrhythmia control. This dual therapy should be considered in those patients with recurrence of syncope on beta-blocker therapy or complex arrhythmias during exercise [205].
- Left sympathetic cardiac denervation (LCSD): LCSD has been demonstrated to be able to provide an additional antiarrhythmic protection. It should be considered in symptomatic patients despite drug therapy and in those not tolerating beta-blockers [206].
- Implantable defibrillator: the implantation of an ICD should be the last choice therapy in CPVT due to its potential pro-fibrillatory effect. It is recommended in all symptomatic patients despite full medical therapy, plus LCSD [206] and in those with aborted sudden cardiac death, but always in conjunction with optimal medical therapy [2, 65].

**Clinical Pearls**

*Long QT Syndrome*

- Patients reporting syncopal events during exercise or awakening in the morning after the alarm clock sound should be checked for LQTS as they may be affected by LQT1 or LQT2 syndrome, respectively.
- As some patients may have a normal QTc on surface ECG, the LQTS diagnostic work-up should always include exercise stress test and 12-lead 24-h ECG recording.

- The QTc after cessation of exercise is a criterion for the LQTS diagnosis, therefore the ECG recording during exercise test should last at least until the fourth minute of the recovery phase.
- Genetic screening should be performed in all LQTS affected subjects because a gene-specific clinical management is available. Furthermore, if the disease-causing mutation is identified, it allows the identification of all affected family members in which preventive strategies should be employed.

*Short QT Syndrome*

- Although atrial fibrillation and a short QT can be observed in athletes, differential diagnosis with SQTS should be carefully performed considering: personal and family history, length of QTc, arrhythmic events, T-wave morphology, QT-RR relationship, PQ depression ≥0.05 mV and in some selected cases also molecular screening could be of some support;
- As the risk stratification of SQTS patients is challenging, a pharmacological treatment should be considered in asymptomatic patients with SQTS.

*Brugada Syndrome*

- An increased vagal tone may induce a spontaneous type 1 ECG diagnostic pattern. As athletes have an increased vagal tone and ST-segment elevation, it is important to correctly distinguish affected patients.
- Asymptomatic patients without a spontaneous type 1 ECG diagnostic pattern should only follow life-style changes.

*Catecholaminergic Polymorphic Ventricular Tachycardia*

- Whenever ventricular arrhythmias are evoked during exercise stress testing or syncope occurs during adrenergic stimulation, a diagnosis of CPVT should be taken in account.
- Life-style changes, including restriction from competitive sport and intensive exercise, and beta-blocker therapy are the first line treatments that should be recommended in all CPVT patients.

## Review

### Clinical Case 1

An 18-year-old girl has a syncope whilst swimming. Her physical examination is normal. She denies taking medications and any hormonal condition. On blood tests, potassium is 4.4 mEq/lt (normal values 3.5–5 mEq/lt). Also, glycemia is normal. Her ECG is shown below (Fig. 20.6). QTc is 460 ms.

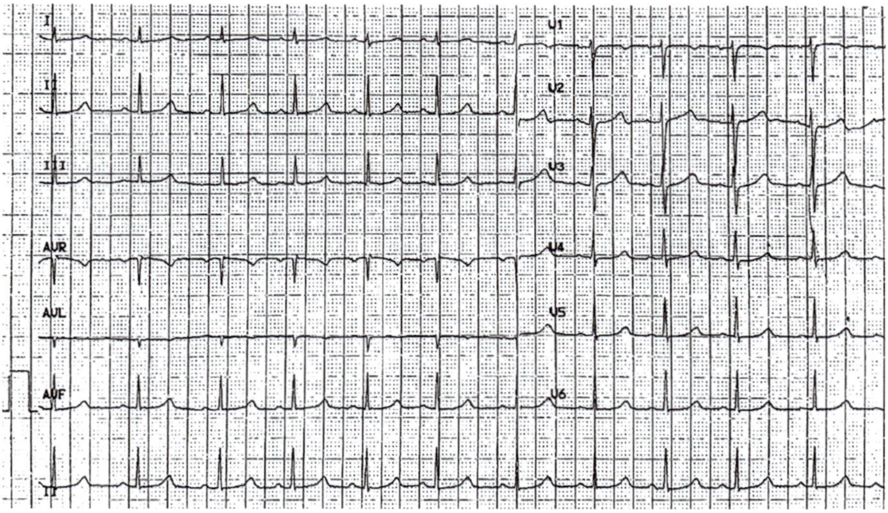


**Fig. 20.6** Clinical case 1. Basal ECG trace. It shows sinus rhythm, normal PR and QRS conduction, upper normal QTc (460 ms)

## Question 1

Would you perform further investigations?

(a) The QTc is upper normal, the syncope may be of vasovagal origin. A tilt-testing is the next step.
(b) Her ECG is normal. Electroencephalogram and head MRI should be performed to exclude an epilepsy.
(c) The QTc is upper normal, we cannot exclude a long QT syndrome based on this ECG: detailed personal and family history collection, exercise stress testing and 12-lead 24-h ECG monitoring should be performed.
(d) The QTc is upper normal, we cannot exclude a long QT syndrome based on this ECG: a genetic screening should be performed.

The patient reports a previous syncope when aged 16 whilst practicing sport at school. Her family history is positive for syncopal events: her mother reports loss-of-consciousness events in her teenage, all of them occurring during sport activity. Brain MRI and echocardiogram are normal. During exercise stress-testing, a QTc inability to shorten was observed. The ECG on the fourth minute of the recovery phase is shown below (Fig. 20.7). A 24-h 12-lead ECG monitoring was performed, and biphasic T-waves were observed during recording.

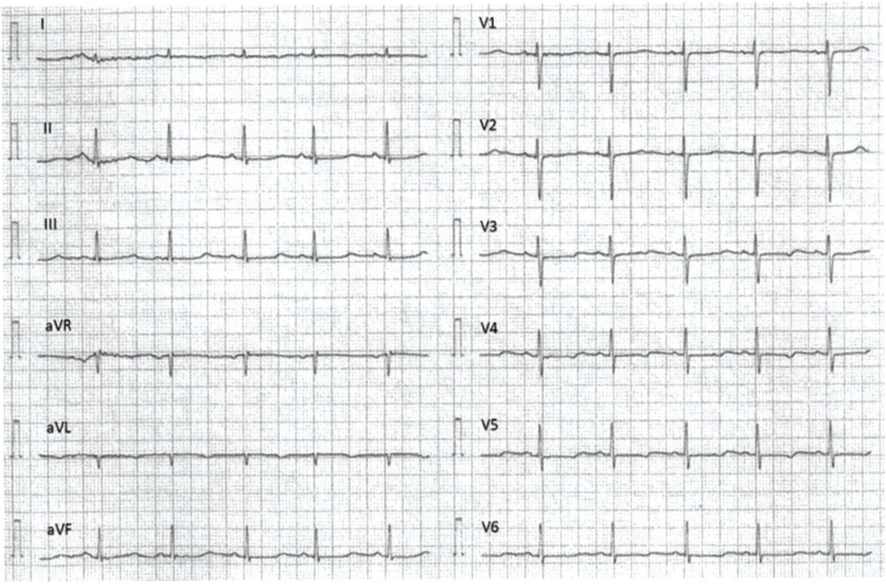


**Fig. 20.7** Clinical case 1. ECG trace on the fourth minute of the recovery phase of the exercise stress test. It shows marked prolonged QT interval (QTc 581 ms in lead II; QTc 589 in lead V1)

## Question 2

Based on the new information, what would you do next?

(a) According to the Schwartz score (=5), this patient has a high probability to be affected with long QT syndrome: a beta-blocker therapy with metoprolol should be started.
(b) According to the Schwartz score (=5), this patient has a high probability to be affected with long QT syndrome: a genetic testing should be performed. If positive, she will be started on betablocker therapy.
(c) According to the Schwartz score (=5), this patient has a high probability to be affected with long QT syndrome: a genetic testing should be performed, and the patient should be started on bisoprolol.
(d) According to the Schwartz score (=5), this patient has a high probability to be affected with long QT syndrome: a genetic testing should be performed and beta-booker therapy (propranolol or nadolol) should be prescribed. She should also be advised to avoid QT-prolonging drugs and to keep within a normal range potassium levels. Participation in competitive sports should be forbidden.

The patient was started on Propranolol 2 mg/kg/die. Genetic screening was performed and a *KCNQ1* mutation was identified. Cascade genetic screening was carried out and the mother was found to carry the same mutation. Since started on therapy, the patient has been asymptomatic.

### Question 3
**Which one of the following may be included among the ECG features of SQTS?**

(a) Biphasic T-waves
(b) Long QT segment
(c) tall, sharp, narrow, symmetrical T waves
(d) a long PQ interval

### Question 4
**Which one of the following may be responsible of a shorter QTc?**

(a) Hypokalaemia
(b) Androgens use
(c) Alkalosis
(d) Hydroquinidine toxicity

### Question 5
**Which one of the following is false? A diagnosis of BrS can be performed**

(a) in the presence of a type 1 ECG recorded at fourth intercostal space
(b) in the presence of a type 1 ECG recorded at third or second intercostal space
(c) when a type 2 to type 1 pattern conversion is observed after sodium channel blocker administration at fourth intercostal space
(d) when drug-induced conversion of type 3 to type 2 ST-segment elevation after sodium channel blocker administration is observed in fourth intercostal space

### Question 6
**Which one of the following is not responsible of BrS pattern?**

(a) Hyperkalaemia
(b) Fever
(c) Hypothermia
(d) Anti-allergic drugs

## Clinical Case 2

A 30-year-old swimmer with no family history for sudden death, syncope, or seizures started to report palpitations mainly during exercise and emotional stress. Basal ECG is shown below (Fig. 20.8).

### Question 7
**Based on the ECG, what is the most likely diagnosis?**

(a) Long QT Syndrome
(b) Short QT Syndrome

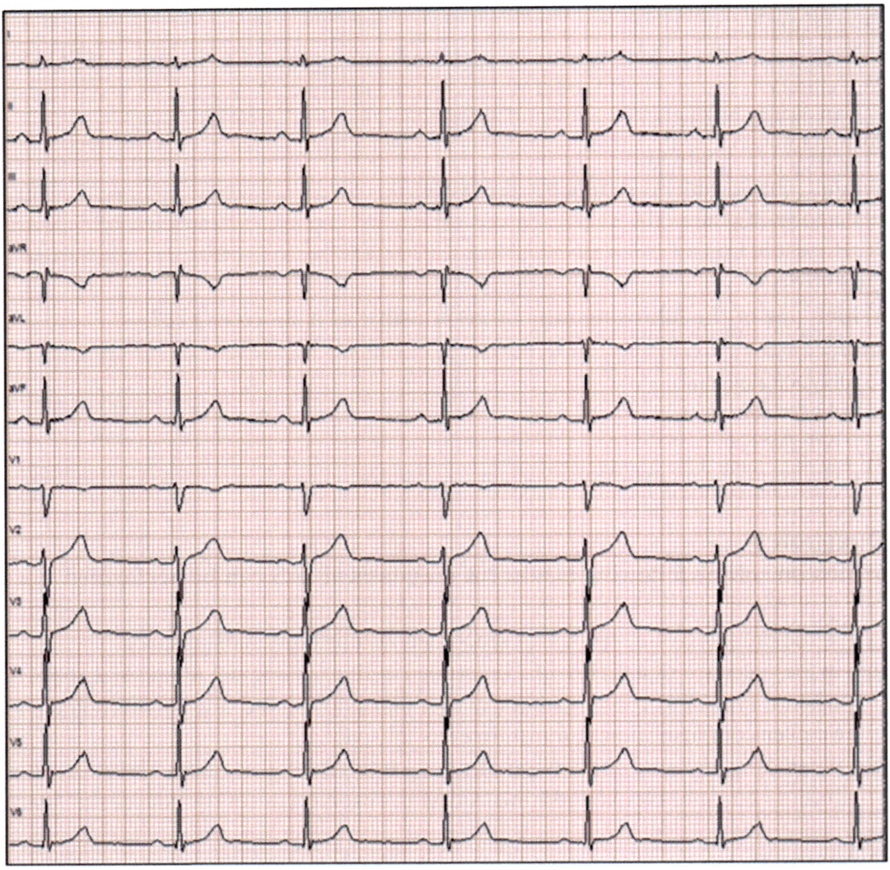

**Fig. 20.8** Basal ECG of clinical case 2

(c) Brugada Syndrome
(d) None of them

Echocardiogram was normal. A 12-leads 24-h Holter monitoring showed a run of non-sustained polymorphic ventricular tachycardia whilst exercising.

### Question 8
**What would be the most useful test to perform?**

(a) Exercise stress testing
(b) Cardiac Magnetic Resonance
(c) Flecainide drug challenging test
(d) Electrophysiological study

Exercise stress testing was performed (Bruce protocol). Isolated ventricular ectopic beats were noted when his heart rate was 113 bpm (Fig. 20.9a). A triplet and a couple appeared at 115 bpm (Fig. 20.9b) and a NSVT appeared at 123 bpm

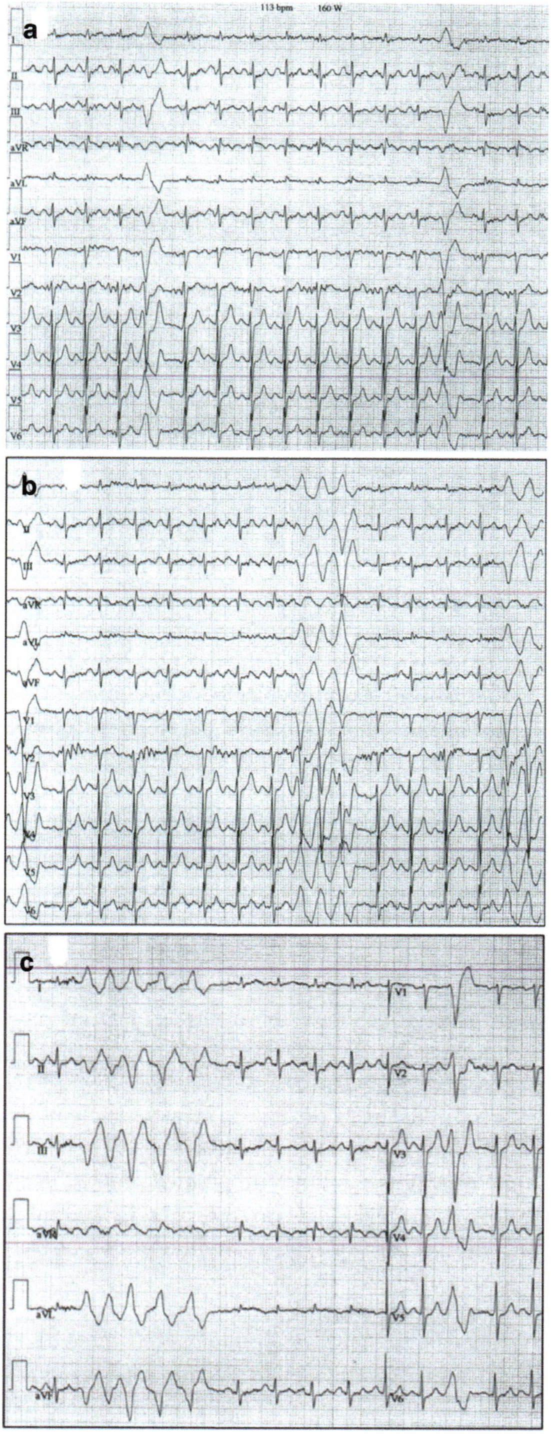


**Fig. 20.9** Electrocardiographic strips of the exercise stress test of clinical case 2. They show increasing frequency and complexity of ventricular arrhythmias with the increase in the workload

(Fig. 20.9c). The test was therefore interrupted, and arrhythmias disappeared as soon as he stopped cycling. The patient was started on Nadolol 2 mg/kg/die. Genetic analysis was performed on the major CPVT-related genes and a disease-causing mutation was identified on RyR2. The same mutation was then detected in the father.

## Answers

1. **Correct answer: (c).**
   Swimming is a well-known arrhythmic trigger in LQTS and the diagnosis cannot be excluded by a ECG [6]. Family history would elucidate her probability of being affected with a congenital Long QT Syndrome. The workup for clinical diagnosis includes exercise stress test and 12-lead 24-h ECG monitoring [2]. Genetic screening is recommended when there is an established strong clinical suspicious of LQTS [8].
2. **Correct answer: (d).**
   The Schwartz score of the patient is 5, this equals high probability of being affected with Long QT Syndrome (Table 20.1) [44, 53]. Therefore, betablocker therapy should be started [2]. Propranolol and nadolol are the two betablockers more effective in preventing arrhythmic events in patients with LQTS [57]. The trigger of the event and the morphology of the ECG are suggestive for LQT1 [6]. In this form, events typically occur upon exercise or stress, as the impairment of the $I_{Ks}$ current prevents the shortening of the QT during increases in heart rate [6]. Therefore patients are not allowed to participate in competitive sport activities [53]. Genetic screening is mandatory to confirm diagnosis: it would allow the genetic screening of family members and a genetic-specific therapy [8].
3. **Correct answer: (c).**
   Besides the short QTc, basal ECG of affected patients present with the T wave initiating immediately from the S wave, therefore with a short or absent ST segment [78]. T waves are tall, sharp, narrow, fine and symmetrical, especially in leads V2–V4, suggesting increased transmural dispersion of repolarization [78]. The heterogeneous abbreviation of atrial repolarization is responsible for the presence of a PQ depression $\geq$0.05 mV [82].
4. **Correct answer: (b).**
   Acquired causes of short QTc include electrolyte imbalance, such as hyperkalemia and hypercalcemia, acidosis, digitalis toxicity, increased vagal tone, and androgen use. A study in orchiectomized male rabbits showed that dihydrotestosterone (DHT) increased $I_{K1}$ and $I_{Kr}$ current densities and produced a left-shift in the V(1/2) for $I_{Kr}$ that could account, at least in part, for the observed differences in QTc between males and females [84].
5. **Correct answer: (d).**
   BrS is definitively diagnosed when a type I ST-segment elevation is observed
   (a) either spontaneously or after intra-venous administration of a sodium channel blocking agent (ajmaline, flecainide, pilsicainde or procainamide)

(b) in at least one right precordial lead (V1 and V2), which are placed in a standard or a superior position (up to the second intercostal space) [2, 65].

Drug-induced conversion of type 3 to type 2 ST-segment elevation is considered inconclusive for a diagnosis of Brugada syndrome.

6. **Correct answer: (d).**
   Several conditions may mimic a BrS, including medical illness [152–157], mechanical compression of RVOT [158, 159], cardiomyopathies [160, 161], electrolyte imbalances, hyperkalaemia, hypercalcemia [162–165], hyperthermia and hypothermia [166, 167], thiamin deficiency, elevated insulin level [168]. Anti-allergic drugs are not included. A list of drugs able to induce a type 1 ECG and VF is available on the website www.brugadadrugs.org.
7. **Correct answer: (d).**
   ECG shows sinus rhythm at 52 bpm, normal PR (160 ms) and QRS duration (90 ms), with a normal QTc. Therefore, LQTS and SQTS should be excluded. The repolarization is normal, therefore there are no criteria for a Brugada Syndrome diagnosis, even though this cannot be excluded, as the diagnostic ECG pattern is not always present.
8. **Correct answer: (a).**
   As echocardiogram is normal, an exercise stress testing should be performed to better evaluate the correlation with heart rate. Indeed, the ECG is normal. The absence of arrhythmias during the night-time on the 12-lead 24-h Holter monitoring and the correlation of the symptoms with exercise and emotional stress should arise the suspicious of CPVT diagnosis [65, 188, 189, 195].

## References


1. Merri M, Benhorin J, Alberti M, Locati E, Moss AJ. Electrocardiographic quantitation of ventricular repolarization. Circulation. 1989;80(5):1301–8.
2. Priori SG, Wilde AA, Horie M, Cho Y, Behr ER, Berul C, et al. HRS/EHRA/APHRS expert consensus statement on the diagnosis and management of patients with inherited primary arrhythmia syndromes. Heart Rhythm. 2013;10(12):1932–63.
3. Drezner JA, Sharma S, Baggish A, Papadakis M, Wilson MG, Prutkin JM, et al. International criteria for electrocardiographic interpretation in athletes: consensus statement. Br J Sports Med. 2017;51(9):704–31.
4. Sharma S, Drezner JA, Baggish A, Papadakis M, Wilson MG, Prutkin JM, et al. International recommendations for electrocardiographic interpretation in athletes. Eur Heart J. 2018;39(16):1466–80.
5. Schwartz PJ, Stramba-Badiale M, Crotti L, Pedrazzini M, Besana A, Bosi G, et al. Prevalence of the congenital long-QT syndrome. Circulation. 2009;120(18):1761–7.
6. Priori SG, Schwartz PJ, Napolitano C, Bloise R, Ronchetti E, Grillo M, et al. Risk stratification in the long-QT syndrome. N Engl J Med. 2003;348(19):1866–74.
7. Goldenberg I, Horr S, Moss AJ, Lopes CM, Barsheshet A, McNitt S, et al. Risk for life-threatening cardiac events in patients with genotype-confirmed long-QT syndrome and normal-range corrected QT intervals. J Am Coll Cardiol. 2011;57(1):51–9.
8. Ackerman MJ, Priori SG, Willems S, Berul C, Brugada R, Calkins H, et al. HRS/EHRA expert consensus statement on the state of genetic testing for the channelopathies and

cardiomyopathies: this document was developed as a partnership between the Heart Rhythm Society (HRS) and the European Heart Rhythm Association (EHRA). Europace. 2011;13(8):1077–109.
9. Attwell D. A cellular basis for the primary long Q-T syndromes. Lancet. 1988;331(8595):1136–9.
10. Curran ME, Splawski I, Timothy KW, Vincent GM, Green ED, Keating MT. A molecular basis for cardiac arrhythmia: HERG mutations cause long QT syndrome. Cell. 1995;80(5):795–803.
11. Wang Q, Shen J, Splawski I, Atkinson D, Li Z, Robinson JL, et al. SCN5A mutations associated with an inherited cardiac arrhythmia, long QT syndrome. Cell. 1995;80(5):805–11.
12. Wang Q, Curran ME, Splawski I, Burn TC, Millholland JM, VanRaay TJ, et al. Positional cloning of a novel potassium channel gene: KVLQT1 mutations cause cardiac arrhythmias. Nat Genet. 1996;12(1):17–23.
13. Romano C, Gemme G, Pongiglione R. Rare cardiac arrythmias of the pediatric age. II. Syncopal attacks due to paroxysmal ventricular fibrillation. (Presentation of 1st case in italian pediatric literature). Clin Pediatr (Bologna). 1963;45:656–83.
14. Ward OC. A new familial cardiac syndrome in children. J Irish Med Assoc. 1964;54:103–6.
15. Schwartz PJ, Crotti L, Insolia R. Long-QT syndrome: from genetics to management. Circ Arrhythm Electrophysiol. 2012;5(4):868–77.
16. Jervell A, Lange-Nielsen F. Congenital deaf-mutism, functional heart disease with prolongation of the Q-T interval, and sudden death. Am Heart J. 1957;54(1):59–68.
17. Schwartz PJ, Spazzolini C, Crotti L, Bathen J, Amlie JP, Timothy K, et al. The Jervell and Lange-Nielsen syndrome: natural history, molecular basis, and clinical outcome. Circulation. 2006;113(6):783–90.
18. Wang Q, Li Z, Shen J, Keating MT. Genomic organization of the human SCN5A gene encoding the cardiac sodium channel. Genomics. 1996;34(1):9–16.
19. Splawski I, Tristani-Firouzi M, Lehmann MH, Sanguinetti MC, Keating MT. Mutations in the hminK gene cause long QT syndrome and suppress lKs function. Nat Genet. 1997;17(3):338–40.
20. Barhanin J, Lesage F, Guillemare E, Fink M, Lazdunski M, Romey GK. (V)LQT1 and lsK (minK) proteins associate to form the I(Ks) cardiac potassium current. Nature. 1996;384(6604):78–80.
21. Sanguinetti MC, Curran ME, Zou A, Shen J, Spector PS, Atkinson DL, et al. Coassembly of K(V)LQT1 and minK (IsK) proteins to form cardiac I(Ks) potassium channel. Nature. 1996;384(6604):80–3.
22. Abbott GW, Sesti F, Splawski I, Buck ME, Lehmann MH, Timothy KW, et al. MiRP1 forms IKr potassium channels with HERG and is associated with cardiac arrhythmia. Cell. 1999;97(2):175–87.
23. Larsen LA, Fosdal I, Andersen PS, Kanters JK, Vuust J, Wettrell G, et al. Recessive Romano-Ward syndrome associated with compound heterozygosity for two mutations in the KVLQT1 gene. Eur J Hum Genet. 1999;7(6):724–8.
24. Westenskow P, Splawski I, Timothy KW, Keating MT, Sanguinetti MC. Compound mutations: a common cause of severe long-QT syndrome. Circulation. 2004;109(15):1834–41.
25. Nguyen H-L, Pieper GH, Wilders R. Andersen–Tawil syndrome: clinical and molecular aspects. Int J Cardiol. 2013;170(1):1–16.
26. Reichenbach H, Meister EM, Theile H. The heart-hand syndrome. A new variant of disorders of heart conduction and syndactylia including osseous changes in hands and feet. Kinderarztl Prax. 1992;60(2):54–6.
27. Crotti L, Johnson CN, Graf E, De Ferrari GM, Cuneo BF, Ovadia M, et al. Calmodulin mutations associated with recurrent cardiac arrest in infants. Circulation. 2013;127(9):1009–17.
28. Zühlke RD, Pitt GS, Deisseroth K, Tsien RW, Reuter H. Calmodulin supports both inactivation and facilitation of L-type calcium channels. Nature. 1999;399(6732):159–62.
29. Crotti L, et al. Calmodulin mutations and life-threatening cardiac arrhythmias: insights from the international calmodulinopathy registry. Eur Heart J. 2019;40(35):2964–75.

30. Boczek NJ, Gomez-Hurtado N, Ye D, Calvert ML, Tester DJ, Kryshtal D, et al. Spectrum and prevalence of CALM1-, CALM2-, and CALM3-encoded calmodulin variants in long QT syndrome and functional characterization of a novel long QT syndrome-associated calmodulin missense variant, E141G. Circ Cardiovasc Genet. 2016;9(2):136–46.
31. Altmann HM, Tester DJ, Will ML, Middha S, Evans JM, Eckloff BW, et al. Homozygous/compound heterozygous triadin mutations associated with autosomal-recessive long-QT syndrome and pediatric sudden cardiac arrest: elucidation of the triadin knockout syndrome. Circulation. 2015;131(23):2051–60.
32. Clemens DJ, Tester DJ, Giudicessi JR, Bos JM, Rohatgi RK, Abrams DJ, et al. International triadin knockout syndrome registry. Circ Genomic Precis Med. 2019;12(2):e002419.
33. Schwartz PJ, Periti M, Malliani A. The long Q-T syndrome. Am Heart J. 1975; 89(3):378–90.
34. Schwartz PJ, Zaza A, Locati E, Moss AJ. Stress and sudden death. The case of the long QT syndrome. Circulation. 1991;83(4 Suppl):II71–80.
35. Priori SG, Napolitano C, Schwartz PJ. Low penetrance in the long-QT syndrome: clinical impact. Circulation. 1999;99(4):529–33.
36. Schwartz PJ, Priori SG, Spazzolini C, Moss AJ, Vincent GM, Napolitano C, et al. Genotype-phenotype correlation in the long-QT syndrome: gene-specific triggers for life-threatening arrhythmias. Circulation. 2001;103(1):89–95.
37. Moss AJ, Robinson JL, Gessman L, Gillespie R, Zareba W, Schwartz PJ, et al. Comparison of clinical and genetic variables of cardiac events associated with loud noise versus swimming among subjects with the long QT syndrome. Am J Cardiol. 1999;84(8):876–9.
38. Buber J, Mathew J, Moss AJ, Hall WJ, Barsheshet A, McNitt S, et al. Risk of recurrent cardiac events after onset of menopause in women with congenital long-QT syndrome types 1 and 2. Circulation. 2011;123(24):2784–91.
39. Bazett HC. An analysis of the time-relations of electrocardiograms. Ann Noninvasive Electrocardiol. 1997;2(2):177–94.
40. Carnethon MR, Anthony MS, Cascio WE, Folsom AR, Rautaharju PM, Liao D, et al. A prospective evaluation of the risk of QT prolongation with hormone replacement therapy: the atherosclerosis risk in communities study. Ann Epidemiol. 2003;13(7):530–6.
41. Stramba-Badiale M, Spagnolo D, Bosi G, Schwartz PJ. Are gender differences in QTc present at birth? MISNES Investigators. Multicenter Italian Study on Neonatal Electrocardiography and Sudden Infant Death Syndrome. Am J Cardiol. 1995;75(17):1277–8.
42. Schwartz PJ. Idiopathic long QT syndrome: progress and questions. Am Heart J. 1985;109(2):399–411.
43. Schwartz PJ, Malliani A. Electrical alternation of the T-wave: clinical and experimental evidence of its relationship with the sympathetic nervous system and with the long Q-T syndrome. Am Heart J. 1975;89(1):45–50.
44. Schwartz PJ, Crotti L. QTc behavior during exercise and genetic testing for the long-QT syndrome. Circulation. 2011;124(20):2181–4.
45. Sy RW, van der Werf C, Chattha IS, Chockalingam P, Adler A, Healey JS, et al. Derivation and validation of a simple exercise-based algorithm for prediction of genetic testing in relatives of LQTS probands. Circulation. 2011;124(20):2187–94.
46. Crotti L, Spazzolini C, Porretta AP, Dagradi F, Taravelli E, Petracci B, et al. Vagal reflexes following an exercise stress test. J Am Coll Cardiol. 2012;60(24):2515–24.
47. Malfatto G, Beria G, Sala S, Bonazzi O, Schwartz PJ. Quantitative analysis of T wave abnormalities and their prognostic implications in the idiopathic long QT syndrome. J Am Coll Cardiol. 1994;23(2):296–301.
48. Itoh H, Crotti L, Aiba T, Spazzolini C, Denjoy I, Fressart V, et al. The genetics underlying acquired long QT syndrome: impact for genetic screening. Eur Heart J. 2016;37(18):1456–64.
49. Schwartz PJ, Vanoli E, Crotti L, Spazzolini C, Ferrandi C, Goosen A, et al. Neural control of heart rate is an arrhythmia risk modifier in long QT syndrome. J Am Coll Cardiol. 2008;51(9):920–9.

50. Brink PA, Crotti L, Corfield V, Goosen A, Durrheim G, Hedley P, et al. Phenotypic variability and unusual clinical severity of congenital long-QT syndrome in a founder population. Circulation. 2005;112(17):2602–10.
51. Schwartz PJ, Crotti L, George AL. Modifier genes for sudden cardiac death. Eur Heart J. 2018;39(44):3925–31. https://doi.org/10.1093/eurheartj/ehy502/5094987.
52. Schwartz PJ, Gentilini D. Can genetics predict risk for sudden cardiac death? The relentless search for the Holy Grail. Eur Heart J. 2018;39(44):3970–2.
53. Schwartz PJ, Ackerman MJ. The long QT syndrome: a transatlantic clinical approach to diagnosis and therapy. Eur Heart J. 2013;34(40):3109–16.
54. Vincent GM, Schwartz PJ, Denjoy I, Swan H, Bithell C, Spazzolini C, et al. High efficacy of beta-blockers in long-QT syndrome type 1: contribution of noncompliance and QT-prolonging drugs to the occurrence of beta-blocker treatment "failures". Circulation. 2009;119(2):215–21.
55. Priori SG, Napolitano C, Schwartz PJ, Grillo M, Bloise R, Ronchetti E, et al. Association of long QT syndrome loci and cardiac events among patients treated with beta-blockers. JAMA. 2004;292(11):1341–4.
56. Schwartz PJ, Spazzolini C, Crotti L. All LQT3 patients need an ICD: true or false? Heart Rhythm. 2009;6(1):113–20.
57. Chockalingam P, Crotti L, Girardengo G, Johnson JN, Harris KM, van der Heijden JF, et al. Not all beta-blockers are equal in the management of long QT syndrome types 1 and 2. J Am Coll Cardiol. 2012;60(20):2092–9.
58. Schwartz PJ, De Ferrari GM, Pugliese L. Cardiac sympathetic denervation 100 years later: Jonnesco would have never believed it. Int J Cardiol. 2017;237:25–8.
59. Johnson JN, Ackerman MJ. Competitive sports participation in athletes with congenital long QT syndrome. JAMA. 2012;308(8):764–5.
60. Choi G, Kopplin LJ, Tester DJ, Will ML, Haglund CM, Ackerman MJ. Spectrum and frequency of cardiac channel defects in swimming-triggered arrhythmia syndromes. Circulation. 2004;110(15):2119–24.
61. Schwartz PJ, Gnecchi M, Dagradi F, Castelletti S, Parati G, Spazzolini C, et al. From patient-specific induced pluripotent stem cells to clinical translation in long QT syndrome Type 2. Eur Heart J. 2019.
62. Mehta A, Ramachandra CJA, Singh P, Chitre A, Lua CH, Mura M, et al. Identification of a targeted and testable antiarrhythmic therapy for long-QT syndrome type 2 using a patient-specific cellular model. Eur Heart J. 2018;39(16):1446–55.
63. Schwartz PJ, Priori SG, Locati EH, Napolitano C, Cantu F, Towbin JA, et al. Long QT syndrome patients with mutations of the SCN5A and HERG genes have differential responses to Na+ channel blockade and to increases in heart rate: implications for gene-specific therapy. Circulation. 1995;92(12):3381–6.
64. Ruan Y, Liu N, Bloise R, Napolitano C, Priori SG. Gating properties of SCN5A mutations and the response to mexiletine in long-QT syndrome type 3 patients. Circulation. 2007;116(10):1137–44.
65. Priori SG, Blomström-Lundqvist C, Mazzanti A, Blom N, Borggrefe M, Camm J, et al. ESC Guidelines for the management of patients with ventricular arrhythmias and the prevention of sudden cardiac death: The Task Force for the Management of Patients with Ventricular Arrhythmias and the Prevention of Sudden Cardiac Death of the European Society of Cardiology (ESC)Endorsed by: Association for European Paediatric and Congenital Cardiology (AEPC). Eur Heart J. 2015;36(41):2793–867.
66. Bos JM, Crotti L, Rohatgi RK, Castelletti S, Dagradi F, Schwartz PJ, et al. Mexiletine shortens the QT interval in patients with potassium channel-mediated type 2 long QT syndrome. Circ Arrhythm Electrophysiol. 2019;12(5):e007280.
67. Giustetto C, Schimpf R, Mazzanti A, Scrocco C, Maury P, Anttonen O, et al. Long-term follow-up of patients with short QT syndrome. J Am Coll Cardiol. 2011;58(6):587–95.
68. Brugada R, Hong K, Dumaine R, Cordeiro J, Gaita F, Borggrefe M, et al. Sudden death associated with short-QT syndrome linked to mutations in HERG. Circulation. 2004;109(1):30–5.

69. Bellocq C, van Ginneken ACG, Bezzina CR, Alders M, Escande D, Mannens MMAM, et al. Mutation in the KCNQ1 gene leading to the short QT-interval syndrome. Circulation. 2004;109(20):2394–7.
70. Priori SG, Pandit SV, Rivolta I, Berenfeld O, Ronchetti E, Dhamoon A, et al. A novel form of short QT syndrome (SQT3) is caused by a mutation in the KCNJ2 gene. Circ Res. 2005;96(7):800–7.
71. Antzelevitch C, Pollevick GD, Cordeiro JM, Casis O, Sanguinetti MC, Aizawa Y, et al. Loss-of-function mutations in the cardiac calcium channel underlie a new clinical entity characterized by ST-segment elevation, short QT intervals, and sudden cardiac death. Circulation. 2007;115(4):442–9.
72. Mazzanti A, Kanthan A, Monteforte N, Memmi M, Bloise R, Novelli V, et al. Novel insight into the natural history of short QT syndrome. J Am Coll Cardiol. 2014;63(13):1300–8.
73. Gollob MH, Redpath CJ, Roberts JD. The short QT syndrome: proposed diagnostic criteria. J Am Coll Cardiol. 2011;57(7):802–12.
74. Arnestad M, Crotti L, Rognum TO, Insolia R, Pedrazzini M, Ferrandi C, et al. Prevalence of long-QT syndrome gene variants in sudden infant death syndrome. Circulation. 2007;115(3):361–7.
75. Gallagher MM, Magliano G, Yap YG, Padula M, Morgia V, Postorino C, et al. Distribution and prognostic significance of QT intervals in the lowest half centile in 12,012 apparently healthy persons. Am J Cardiol. 2006;98(7):933–5.
76. Anttonen O, Junttila MJ, Maury P, Schimpf R, Wolpert C, Borggrefe M, et al. Differences in twelve-lead electrocardiogram between symptomatic and asymptomatic subjects with short QT interval. Heart Rhythm. 2009;6(2):267–71.
77. Dhutia H, Malhotra A, Parpia S, Gabus V, Finocchiaro G, Mellor G, et al. The prevalence and significance of a short QT interval in 18,825 low-risk individuals including athletes. Br J Sports Med. 2016;50(2):124–9.
78. Schimpf R, Wolpert C, Gaita F, Giustetto C, Borggrefe M. Short QT syndrome. Cardiovasc Res. 2005;67(3):357–66.
79. Gaita F, Giustetto C, Bianchi F, Wolpert C, Schimpf R, Riccardi R, et al. Short QT syndrome: a familial cause of sudden death. Circulation. 2003;108(8):965–70.
80. Watanabe H, Makiyama T, Koyama T, Kannankeril PJ, Seto S, Okamura K, et al. High prevalence of early repolarization in short QT syndrome. Heart Rhythm. 2010;7(5):647–52.
81. Giustetto C, Scrocco C, Schimpf R, Maury P, Mazzanti A, Levetto M, et al. Usefulness of exercise test in the diagnosis of short QT syndrome. Eurpace. 2015;17(4):628–34.
82. Tülümen E, Giustetto C, Wolpert C, Maury P, Anttonen O, Probst V, et al. PQ segment depression in patients with short QT syndrome: a novel marker for diagnosing short QT syndrome? Heart Rhythm. 2014;11(6):1024–30.
83. Wolpert C, Schimpf R, Giustetto C, Antzelevitch C, Cordeiro J, Dumaine R, et al. Further insights into the effect of quinidine in short QT syndrome caused by a mutation in HERG. J Cardiovasc Electrophysiol. 2005;16(1):54–8.
84. Liu X-K, Katchman A, Whitfield BH, Wan G, Janowski EM, Woosley RL, et al. In vivo androgen treatment shortens the QT interval and increases the densities of inward and delayed rectifier potassium currents in orchiectomized male rabbits. Cardiovasc Res. 2003;57(1):28–36.
85. Schimpf R, Wolpert C, Bianchi F, Giustetto C, Gaita F, Bauersfeld U, et al. Congenital short QT syndrome and implantable cardioverter defibrillator treatment: inherent risk for inappropriate shock delivery. J Cardiovasc Electrophysiol. 2003;14(12):1273–7.
86. Gaita F, Giustetto C, Bianchi F, Schimpf R, Haissaguerre M, Calò L, et al. Short QT syndrome: pharmacological treatment. J Am Coll Cardiol. 2004;43(8):1494–9.
87. Antzelevitch C, et al. Brugada syndrome: report of the second consensus conference. Heart Rhythm. 2005;2(4):429–40.
88. Antzelevitch C. Brugada syndrome. Pacing Clin Electrophysiol. 2006;29(10):1130–59.
89. Papadakis M, Papatheodorou E, Mellor G, Raju H, Bastiaenen R, Wijeyeratne Y, et al. The diagnostic yield of Brugada syndrome after sudden death with normal autopsy. J Am Coll Cardiol. 2018;71(11):1204–14.

90. Bezzina CR, Barc J, Mizusawa Y, Remme CA, Gourraud J-B, Simonet F, et al. Common variants at SCN5A-SCN10A and HEY2 are associated with Brugada syndrome, a rare disease with high risk of sudden cardiac death. Nat Genet. 2013;45(9):1044–9.
91. Kapplinger JD, Tester DJ, Alders M, Benito B, Berthet M, Brugada J, et al. An international compendium of mutations in the SCN5A-encoded cardiac sodium channel in patients referred for Brugada syndrome genetic testing. Heart Rhythm. 2010;7(1):33–46.
92. Wilde AAM, Behr ER. Genetic testing for inherited cardiac disease. Nat Rev Cardiol. 2013;10(10):571–83.
93. Wang QI, Ohno S, Ding W-G, Fukuyama M, Miyamoto A, Itoh H, et al. Gain-of-function KCNH2 mutations in patients with Brugada syndrome. J Cardiovasc Electrophysiol. 2014;25(5):522–30.
94. Cerrone M, Lin X, Zhang M, Agullo-Pascual E, Pfenniger A, Chkourko Gusky H, et al. Missense mutations in plakophilin-2 cause sodium current deficit and associate with a Brugada syndrome phenotype. Circulation. 2014;129(10):1092–103.
95. Hennessey JA, Marcou CA, Wang C, Wei EQ, Wang C, Tester DJ, et al. FGF12 is a candidate Brugada syndrome locus. Heart Rhythm. 2013;10(12):1886–94.
96. Crotti L, Marcou CA, Tester DJ, Castelletti S, Giudicessi JR, Torchio M, et al. Spectrum and prevalence of mutations involving BrS1- through BrS12-susceptibility genes in a cohort of unrelated patients referred for Brugada syndrome genetic testing. J Am Coll Cardiol. 2012;60(15):1410–8.
97. Bastiaenen R, Cox AT, Castelletti S, Wijeyeratne YD, Colbeck N, Pakroo N, et al. Late gadolinium enhancement in Brugada syndrome: a marker for subtle underlying cardiomyopathy? Heart Rhythm. 2017;14(4):583–9.
98. Corrado D, Basso C, Thiene G, McKenna WJ, Davies MJ, Fontaliran F, et al. Spectrum of clinicopathologic manifestations of arrhythmogenic right ventricular cardiomyopathy/dysplasia: a multicenter study. J Am Coll Cardiol. 1997;30(6):1512–20.
99. Moncayo-Arlandi J, Brugada R. Unmasking the molecular link between arrhythmogenic cardiomyopathy and Brugada syndrome. Nat Rev Cardiol. 2017;14(12):744–56.
100. Brugada J, Brugada P, Brugada R. The syndrome of right bundle branch block ST segment elevation in V1 to V3 and sudden death—the Brugada syndrome. Eurpace. 1999;1(3):156–66.
101. Quan X-Q, Li S, Liu R, Zheng K, Wu X-F, Tang Q. A meta-analytic review of prevalence for Brugada ECG patterns and the risk for death. Medicine (Baltimore). 2016;95(50):e5643.
102. Gehi AK, Duong TD, Metz LD, Gomes JA, Mehta D. Risk stratification of individuals with the Brugada electrocardiogram: a meta-analysis. J Cardiovasc Electrophysiol. 2006;17(6):577–83.
103. Priori SG, Napolitano C, Giordano U, Collisani G, Memmi M. Brugada syndrome and sudden cardiac death in children. Lancet Lond Engl. 2000;355(9206):808–9.
104. Probst V, Denjoy I, Meregalli PG, Amirault J-C, Sacher F, Mansourati J, et al. Clinical aspects and prognosis of Brugada syndrome in children. Circulation. 2007;115(15):2042–8.
105. Mizusawa Y, Wilde AAM. Brugada syndrome. Circ Arrhythm Electrophysiol. 2012;5(3):606–16.
106. Chockalingam P, Rammeloo LA, Postema PG, Hruda J, Clur S-AB, Blom NA, et al. Fever-induced life-threatening arrhythmias in children harboring an SCN5A mutation. Pediatrics. 2011;127(1):e239–44.
107. Antzelevitch C, Brugada R. Fever and Brugada syndrome. Pacing Clin Electrophysiol. 2002;25(11):1537–9.
108. Miyazaki T, Mitamura H, Miyoshi S, Soejima K, Aizawa Y, Ogawa S. Autonomic and antiarrhythmic drug modulation of ST segment elevation in patients with Brugada syndrome. J Am Coll Cardiol. 1996;27(5):1061–70.
109. Kasanuki H, Ohnishi S, Ohtuka M, Matsuda N, Nirei T, Isogai R, et al. Idiopathic ventricular fibrillation induced with vagal activity in patients without obvious heart disease. Circulation. 1997;95(9):2277–85.

110. Agostini D, Scanu P, Loiselet P, Babatasi G, Darlas Y, Grollier G, et al. Iodine-123-metaiodobenzylguanidine SPECT of regional cardiac adrenergic denervation in Brugada syndrome. J Nucl Med. 1998;39(7):1129–32.
111. Makimoto H, Nakagawa E, Takaki H, Yamada Y, Okamura H, Noda T, et al. Augmented ST-segment elevation during recovery from exercise predicts cardiac events in patients with Brugada syndrome. J Am Coll Cardiol. 2010;56(19):1576–84.
112. Takigawa M, Noda T, Shimizu W, Miyamoto K, Okamura H, Satomi K, et al. Seasonal and circadian distributions of ventricular fibrillation in patients with Brugada syndrome. Heart Rhythm. 2008;5(11):1523–7.
113. Gray B, Kirby A, Kabunga P, Freedman SB, Yeates L, Kanthan A, et al. Twelve-lead ambulatory electrocardiographic monitoring in Brugada syndrome: potential diagnostic and prognostic implications. Heart Rhythm. 2017;14(6):866–74.
114. Ikeda T, Abe A, Yusu S, Nakamura K, Ishiguro H, Mera H, et al. The full stomach test as a novel diagnostic technique for identifying patients at risk of Brugada syndrome. J Cardiovasc Electrophysiol. 2006;17(6):602–7.
115. Nishizaki M, Sakurada H, Mizusawa Y, Niki S, Hayashi T, Tanaka Y, et al. Influence of meals on variations of ST segment elevation in patients with Brugada syndrome. J Cardiovasc Electrophysiol. 2008;19(1):62–8.
116. Morita H, Kusano-Fukushima K, Nagase S, Fujimoto Y, Hisamatsu K, Fujio H, et al. Atrial fibrillation and atrial vulnerability in patients with Brugada syndrome. J Am Coll Cardiol. 2002;40(8):1437–44.
117. Eckardt L, Kirchhof P, Johna R, Haverkamp W, Breithardt G, Borggrefe M. Wolff-Parkinson-White syndrome associated with Brugada syndrome. Pacing Clin Electrophysiol. 2001;24(9 Pt 1):1423–4.
118. Schimpf R, Giustetto C, Eckardt L, Veltmann C, Wolpert C, Gaita F, et al. Prevalence of supraventricular tachyarrhythmias in a cohort of 115 patients with Brugada syndrome. Ann Noninvasive Electrocardiol. 2008;13(3):266–9.
119. Kusano KF, Taniyama M, Nakamura K, Miura D, Banba K, Nagase S, et al. Atrial fibrillation in patients with Brugada syndrome relationships of gene mutation, electrophysiology, and clinical backgrounds. J Am Coll Cardiol. 2008;51(12):1169–75.
120. Olivotto I, Finocchiaro G, Maurizi N, Crotti L. Common presentation of rare cardiac diseases: arrhythmias. Int J Cardiol. 2018;257:351–7.
121. Morita H, Fukushima-Kusano K, Nagase S, Miyaji K, Hiramatsu S, Banba K, et al. Sinus node function in patients with Brugada-type ECG. Circ J. 2004;68(5):473–6.
122. Takehara N, Makita N, Kawabe J, Sato N, Kawamura Y, Kitabatake A, et al. A cardiac sodium channel mutation identified in Brugada syndrome associated with atrial standstill. J Intern Med. 2004;255(1):137–42.
123. Wang DW, Viswanathan PC, Balser JR, George AL, Benson DW. Clinical, genetic, and biophysical characterization of SCN5A mutations associated with atrioventricular conduction block. Circulation. 2002;105(3):341–6.
124. Smits JPP, Koopmann TT, Wilders R, Veldkamp MW, Opthof T, Bhuiyan ZA, et al. A mutation in the human cardiac sodium channel (E161K) contributes to sick sinus syndrome, conduction disease and Brugada syndrome in two families. J Mol Cell Cardiol. 2005;38(6):969–81.
125. Makiyama T, Akao M, Tsuji K, Doi T, Ohno S, Takenaka K, et al. High risk for bradyarrhythmic complications in patients with Brugada syndrome caused by SCN5A gene mutations. J Am Coll Cardiol. 2005;46(11):2100–6.
126. Watanabe H, Koopmann TT, Le Scouarnec S, Yang T, Ingram CR, Schott J-J, et al. Sodium channel β1 subunit mutations associated with Brugada syndrome and cardiac conduction disease in humans. J Clin Invest. 2008;118(6):2260–8.
127. Schott JJ, Alshinawi C, Kyndt F, Probst V, Hoorntje TM, Hulsbeek M, et al. Cardiac conduction defects associate with mutations in SCN5A. Nat Genet. 1999;23(1):20–1.
128. Benson DW, Wang DW, Dyment M, Knilans TK, Fish FA, Strieper MJ, et al. Congenital sick sinus syndrome caused by recessive mutations in the cardiac sodium channel gene (SCN5A). J Clin Invest. 2003;112(7):1019–28.

129. Brugada P, Brugada J, Brugada R. Arrhythmia induction by antiarrhythmic drugs. Pacing Clin Electrophysiol. 2000;23(3):291–2.
130. Brugada R, Brugada J, Antzelevitch C, Kirsch GE, Potenza D, Towbin JA, et al. Sodium channel blockers identify risk for sudden death in patients with ST-segment elevation and right bundle branch block but structurally normal hearts. Circulation. 2000;101(5):510–5.
131. Shimizu W, Matsuo K, Takagi M, Tanabe Y, Aiba T, Taguchi A, et al. Body surface distribution and response to drugs of ST segment elevation in Brugada syndrome: clinical implication of eighty-seven-lead body surface potential mapping and its application to twelve-lead electrocardiograms. J Cardiovasc Electrophysiol. 2000;11(4):396–404.
132. Nagase S, Kusano KF, Morita H, Nishii N, Banba K, Watanabe A, et al. Longer repolarization in the epicardium at the right ventricular outflow tract causes type 1 electrocardiogram in patients with Brugada syndrome. J Am Coll Cardiol. 2008;51(12):1154–61.
133. Miyamoto K, Yokokawa M, Tanaka K, Nagai T, Okamura H, Noda T, et al. Diagnostic and prognostic value of a type 1 Brugada electrocardiogram at higher (third or second) V1 to V2 recording in men with Brugada syndrome. Am J Cardiol. 2007;99(1):53–7.
134. Alings M, Wilde A. "Brugada" syndrome: clinical data and suggested pathophysiological mechanism. Circulation. 1999;99(5):666–73.
135. Crea P, Picciolo G, Luzza F, Oreto G. ST segment depression in the inferior leads in Brugada pattern: a new sign. Ann Noninvasive Electrocardiol. 2015;20(6):561–5.
136. Morita H, Watanabe A, Morimoto Y, Kawada S, Tachibana M, Nakagawa K, et al. Distribution and prognostic significance of fragmented QRS in patients with Brugada syndrome. Circ Arrhythm Electrophysiol. 2017;10(3).
137. Sarkozy A, Chierchia G-B, Paparella G, Boussy T, De Asmundis C, Roos M, et al. Inferior and lateral electrocardiographic repolarization abnormalities in Brugada syndrome. Circ Arrhythm Electrophysiol. 2009;2(2):154–61.
138. Potet F, Mabo P, Le Coq G, Probst V, Schott J-J, Airaud F, et al. Novel brugada SCN5A mutation leading to ST segment elevation in the inferior or the right precordial leads. J Cardiovasc Electrophysiol. 2003;14(2):200–3.
139. Kalla H, Yan GX, Marinchak R. Ventricular fibrillation in a patient with prominent J (Osborn) waves and ST segment elevation in the inferior electrocardiographic leads: a Brugada syndrome variant? J Cardiovasc Electrophysiol. 2000;11(1):95–8.
140. Bezzina C, Veldkamp MW, van Den Berg MP, Postma AV, Rook MB, Viersma JW, et al. A single Na(+) channel mutation causing both long-QT and Brugada syndromes. Circ Res. 1999;85(12):1206–13.
141. Priori SG, Napolitano C, Gasparini M, Pappone C, Della Bella P, Brignole M, et al. Clinical and genetic heterogeneity of right bundle branch block and ST-segment elevation syndrome: a prospective evaluation of 52 families. Circulation. 2000;102(20):2509–15.
142. Pitzalis MV, Anaclerio M, Iacoviello M, Forleo C, Guida P, Troccoli R, et al. QT-interval prolongation in right precordial leads: an additional electrocardiographic hallmark of Brugada syndrome. J Am Coll Cardiol. 2003;42(9):1632–7.
143. Makita N, Behr E, Shimizu W, Horie M, Sunami A, Crotti L, et al. The E1784K mutation in SCN5A is associated with mixed clinical phenotype of type 3 long QT syndrome. J Clin Invest. 2008;118(6):2219–29.
144. Cerrato N, Giustetto C, Gribaudo E, Richiardi E, Barbonaglia L, Scrocco C, et al. Prevalence of type 1 brugada electrocardiographic pattern evaluated by twelve-lead twenty-four-hour holter monitoring. Am J Cardiol. 2015;115(1):52–6.
145. García-Fuertes D, Villanueva-Fernández E, Crespín-Crespín M, Puchol A, Pachón M, Arias MA. Type 1 Brugada pattern unmasked during the recovery period of an exercise stress test. Arq Bras Cardiol. 2016;106(5):447–9.
146. Subramanian M, Prabhu MA, Harikrishnan MS, Shekhar SS, Pai PG, Natarajan K. The utility of exercise testing in risk stratification of asymptomatic patients with type 1 Brugada pattern. J Cardiovasc Electrophysiol. 2017;28(6):677–83.

147. Therasse D, Sacher F, Petit B, Babuty D, Mabo P, Martins R, et al. Sodium-channel blocker challenge in the familial screening of Brugada syndrome: safety and predictors of positivity. Heart Rhythm. 2017;14(10):1442–8.
148. Meregalli PG, Wilde AAM, Tan HL. Pathophysiological mechanisms of Brugada syndrome: depolarization disorder, repolarization disorder, or more? Cardiovasc Res. 2005;67(3):367–78.
149. Chauveau S, Le Vavasseur O, Chevalier P. Delayed diagnosis of Brugada syndrome in a patient with aborted sudden cardiac death and initial negative flecainide challenge. Clin Case Rep. 2017;5(12):2022–4.
150. Wolpert C, Echternach C, Veltmann C, Antzelevitch C, Thomas GP, Spehl S, et al. Intravenous drug challenge using flecainide and ajmaline in patients with Brugada syndrome. Heart Rhythm. 2005;2(3):254–60.
151. Baranchuk A, Nguyen T, Ryu MH, Femenía F, Zareba W, Wilde AAM, et al. Brugada phenocopy: new terminology and proposed classification. Ann Noninvasive Electrocardiol. 2012;17(4):299–314.
152. Wang K, Asinger RW, Marriott HJL. ST-segment elevation in conditions other than acute myocardial infarction. N Engl J Med. 2003;349(22):2128–35.
153. Myers GB. Other QRS-T patterns that may be mistaken for myocardial infarction; IV. alterations in blood potassium; myocardial ischemia; subepicardial myocarditis; distortion associated with arrhythmias. Circulation. 1950;2(1):75–93.
154. Abbott JA, Cheitlin MD. The nonspecific camel-hump sign. JAMA. 1976;235(4):413–4.
155. Hersch C. Electrocardiographic changes in subarachnoid haemorrhage, meningitis, and intracranial space-occupying lesions. Br Heart J. 1964;26:785–93.
156. Perloff JK, Henze E, Schelbert HR. Alterations in regional myocardial metabolism, perfusion, and wall motion in Duchenne muscular dystrophy studied by radionuclide imaging. Circulation. 1984;69(1):33–42.
157. Kataoka H. Electrocardiographic patterns of the Brugada syndrome in right ventricular infarction/ischemia. Am J Cardiol. 2000;86(9):1056.
158. Tarín N, Farré J, Rubio JM, Tuñón J, Castro-Dorticós J. Brugada-like electrocardiographic pattern in a patient with a mediastinal tumor. Pacing Clin Electrophysiol. 1999;22(8):1264–6.
159. Tomcsányi J, Simor T, Papp L. Images in cardiology. Haemopericardium and Brugada-like ECG pattern in rheumatoid arthritis. Heart. 2002;87(3):234.
160. Corrado D, Basso C, Buja G, Nava A, Rossi L, Thiene G. Right bundle branch block, right precordial st-segment elevation, and sudden death in young people. Circulation. 2001;103(5):710–7.
161. Corrado D, Nava A, Buja G, Martini B, Fasoli G, Oselladore L, et al. Familial cardiomyopathy underlies syndrome of right bundle branch block, ST segment elevation and sudden death. J Am Coll Cardiol. 1996;27(2):443–8.
162. Merrill JP, Levine HD, Somerville W, Smith S. Clinical recognition and treatment of acute potassium intoxication. Ann Intern Med. 1950;33(4):797–830.
163. Ortega-Carnicer J, Benezet J, Ruiz-Lorenzo F, Alcázar R. Transient Brugada-type electrocardiographic abnormalities in renal failure reversed by dialysis. Resuscitation. 2002;55(2):215–9.
164. Douglas PS, Carmichael KA, Palevsky PM. Extreme hypercalcemia and electrocardiographic changes. Am J Cardiol. 1984;54(6):674–5.
165. Sridharan MR, Horan LG. Electrocardiographic J wave of hypercalcemia. Am J Cardiol. 1984;54(6):672–3.
166. Osborn JJ. Experimental hypothermia; respiratory and blood pH changes in relation to cardiac function. Am J Phys. 1953;175(3):389–98.
167. Noda T, Shimizu W, Tanaka K, Chayama K. Prominent J wave and ST segment elevation: serial electrocardiographic changes in accidental hypothermia. J Cardiovasc Electrophysiol. 2003;14(2):223.
168. Read DH, Harrington DD. Experimentally induced thiamine deficiency in beagle dogs: clinical observations. Am J Vet Res. 1981;42(6):984–91.

169. Chevallier S, Forclaz A, Tenkorang J, Ahmad Y, Faouzi M, Graf D, et al. New electrocardiographic criteria for discriminating between Brugada types 2 and 3 patterns and incomplete right bundle branch block. J Am Coll Cardiol. 2011;58(22):2290–8.
170. Serra G, Baranchuk A, Bayés-De-Luna A, Brugada J, Goldwasser D, Capulzini L, et al. New electrocardiographic criteria to differentiate the Type-2 Brugada pattern from electrocardiogram of healthy athletes with r'-wave in leads V1/V2. Europace. 2014;16(11):1639–45.
171. Pospiech T, Jaussaud J, Sacher F, Hooks DA, Haïssaguerre M, Douard H. Characterization of repolarization in Brugada syndrome patients during exercise testing: dynamic angle evaluation. J Electrocardiol. 2015;48(5):879–86.
172. Zorzi A, Leoni L, Di Paolo FM, Rigato I, Migliore F, Bauce B, et al. Differential diagnosis between early repolarization of athlete's heart and coved-type Brugada electrocardiogram. Am J Cardiol. 2015;115(4):529–32.
173. Probst V, Veltmann C, Eckardt L, Meregalli PG, Gaita F, Tan HL, et al. Long-term prognosis of patients diagnosed with Brugada syndrome: results from the FINGER Brugada Syndrome Registry. Circulation. 2010;121(5):635–43.
174. Priori SG, Napolitano C, Gasparini M, Pappone C, Della Bella P, Giordano U, et al. Natural history of Brugada syndrome: insights for risk stratification and management. Circulation. 2002;105(11):1342–7.
175. Priori SG, Gasparini M, Napolitano C, Della Bella P, Ottonelli AG, Sassone B, et al. Risk stratification in Brugada syndrome: results of the PRELUDE (PRogrammed ELectrical stimUlation preDictive valuE) registry. J Am Coll Cardiol. 2012;59(1):37–45.
176. Brugada J, Brugada R, Brugada P. Right bundle-branch block and ST-segment elevation in leads V1 through V3: a marker for sudden death in patients without demonstrable structural heart disease. Circulation. 1998;97(5):457–60.
177. Benito B, Sarkozy A, Mont L, Henkens S, Berruezo A, Tamborero D, et al. Gender differences in clinical manifestations of Brugada syndrome. J Am Coll Cardiol. 2008;52(19):1567–73.
178. Yamagata K, Horie M, Aiba T, Ogawa S, Aizawa Y, Ohe T, et al. Genotype-phenotype correlation of SCN5A mutation for the clinical and electrocardiographic characteristics of probands with Brugada syndrome: a Japanese multicenter registry. Circulation. 2017;135(23):2255–70.
179. Huang Z, Patel C, Li W, Xie Q, Wu R, Zhang L, et al. Role of signal-averaged electrocardiograms in arrhythmic risk stratification of patients with Brugada syndrome: a prospective study. Heart Rhythm. 2009;6(8):1156–62.
180. Kawata H, Morita H, Yamada Y, Noda T, Satomi K, Aiba T, et al. Prognostic significance of early repolarization in inferolateral leads in Brugada patients with documented ventricular fibrillation: a novel risk factor for Brugada syndrome with ventricular fibrillation. Heart Rhythm. 2013;10(8):1161–8.
181. Maury P, Sacher F, Gourraud J-B, Pasquié J-L, Raczka F, Bongard V, et al. Increased Tpeak-Tend interval is highly and independently related to arrhythmic events in Brugada syndrome. Heart Rhythm. 2015;12(12):2469–76.
182. Zumhagen S, Zeidler EM, Stallmeyer B, Ernsting M, Eckardt L, Schulze-Bahr E. Tpeak-Tend interval and Tpeak-Tend/QT ratio in patients with Brugada syndrome. Eurpace. 2016;18(12):1866–72.
183. Tse G. (Tpeak - Tend)/QRS and (Tpeak - Tend)/(QT × QRS): novel markers for predicting arrhythmic risk in the Brugada syndrome. Eurpace. 2017;19(4):696.
184. Rollin A, Sacher F, Gourraud JB, Pasquié JL, Raczka F, Duparc A, et al. Prevalence, characteristics, and prognosis role of type 1 ST elevation in the peripheral ECG leads in patients with Brugada syndrome. Heart Rhythm. 2013;10(7):1012–8.
185. Fish JM, Antzelevitch C. Cellular mechanism and arrhythmogenic potential of T-wave alternans in the Brugada syndrome. J Cardiovasc Electrophysiol. 2008;19(3):301–8.
186. Tada T, Kusano KF, Nagase S, Banba K, Miura D, Nishii N, et al. Clinical significance of macroscopic T-wave alternans after sodium channel blocker administration in patients with Brugada syndrome. J Cardiovasc Electrophysiol. 2008;19(1):56–61.

187. Sroubek J, Probst V, Mazzanti A, Delise P, Hevia JC, Ohkubo K, et al. Programmed ventricular stimulation for risk stratification in the Brugada syndrome: a pooled analysis. Circulation. 2016;133(7):622–30.
188. Leenhardt A, Lucet V, Denjoy I, Grau F, Ngoc DD, Coumel P. Catecholaminergic polymorphic ventricular tachycardia in children. A 7-year follow-up of 21 patients. Circulation. 1995;91(5):1512–9.
189. Priori SG, Napolitano C, Memmi M, Colombi B, Drago F, Gasparini M, et al. Clinical and molecular characterization of patients with catecholaminergic polymorphic ventricular tachycardia. Circulation. 2002;106(1):69–74.
190. Plaster NM, Tawil R, Tristani-Firouzi M, Canún S, Bendahhou S, Tsunoda A, et al. Mutations in Kir2.1 cause the developmental and episodic electrical phenotypes of Andersen's syndrome. Cell. 2001;105(4):511–9.
191. Tester DJ, Arya P, Will M, Haglund CM, Farley AL, Makielski JC, et al. Genotypic heterogeneity and phenotypic mimicry among unrelated patients referred for catecholaminergic polymorphic ventricular tachycardia genetic testing. Heart Rhythm. 2006;3(7):800–5.
192. Nyegaard M, Overgaard MT, Søndergaard MT, Vranas M, Behr ER, Hildebrandt LL, et al. Mutations in calmodulin cause ventricular tachycardia and sudden cardiac death. Am J Hum Genet. 2012;91(4):703–12.
193. Lahat H, Pras E, Olender T, Avidan N, Ben-Asher E, Man O, et al. A missense mutation in a highly conserved region of CASQ2 is associated with autosomal recessive catecholamine-induced polymorphic ventricular tachycardia in Bedouin families from Israel. Am J Hum Genet. 2001;69(6):1378–84.
194. Roux-Buisson N, Cacheux M, Fourest-Lieuvin A, Fauconnier J, Brocard J, Denjoy I, et al. Absence of triadin, a protein of the calcium release complex, is responsible for cardiac arrhythmia with sudden death in human. Hum Mol Genet. 2012;21(12):2759–67.
195. Postma AV, Denjoy I, Kamblock J, Alders M, Lupoglazoff J-M, Vaksmann G, et al. Catecholaminergic polymorphic ventricular tachycardia: RYR2 mutations, bradycardia, and follow up of the patients. J Med Genet. 2005;42(11):863–70.
196. van der Werf C, Nederend I, Hofman N, van Geloven N, Ebink C, Frohn-Mulder IME, et al. Familial evaluation in catecholaminergic polymorphic ventricular tachycardia: disease penetrance and expression in cardiac ryanodine receptor mutation-carrying relatives. Circ Arrhythm Electrophysiol. 2012;5(4):748–56.
197. Fisher JD, Krikler D, Hallidie-Smith KA. Familial polymorphic ventricular arrhythmias: a quarter century of successful medical treatment based on serial exercise-pharmacologic testing. J Am Coll Cardiol. 1999;34(7):2015–22.
198. Marjamaa A, Hiippala A, Arrhenius B, Lahtinen AM, Kontula K, Toivonen L, et al. Intravenous epinephrine infusion test in diagnosis of catecholaminergic polymorphic ventricular tachycardia. J Cardiovasc Electrophysiol. 2012;23(2):194–9.
199. Kimura H, Zhou J, Kawamura M, Itoh H, Mizusawa Y, Ding W-G, et al. Phenotype variability in patients carrying KCNJ2 mutations. Circ Cardiovasc Genet. 2012;5(3):344–53.
200. Marcus FI, McKenna WJ, Sherrill D, Basso C, Bauce B, Bluemke DA, et al. Diagnosis of arrhythmogenic right ventricular cardiomyopathy/dysplasia: proposed modification of the Task Force Criteria. Eur Heart J. 2010;31(7):806–14.
201. Leinonen JT, Crotti L, Djupsjöbacka A, Castelletti S, Junna N, Ghidoni A, et al. The genetics underlying idiopathic ventricular fibrillation: a special role for catecholaminergic polymorphic ventricular tachycardia? Int J Cardiol. 2018;250:139–45.
202. Giudicessi JR, Ackerman MJ. Exercise testing oversights underlie missed and delayed diagnosis of catecholaminergic polymorphic ventricular tachycardia in young sudden cardiac arrest survivors. Heart Rhythm. 2019;16(8):1232–9.
203. Hayashi M, Denjoy I, Extramiana F, Maltret A, Buisson NR, Lupoglazoff J-M, et al. Incidence and risk factors of arrhythmic events in catecholaminergic polymorphic ventricular tachycardia. Circulation. 2009;119(18):2426–34.
204. Hayashi M, Denjoy I, Hayashi M, Extramiana F, Maltret A, Roux-Buisson N, et al. The role of stress test for predicting genetic mutations and future cardiac events in asymptomatic

relatives of catecholaminergic polymorphic ventricular tachycardia probands. Eurpace. 2012;14(9):1344–51.

205. Kannankeril PJ, Moore JP, Cerrone M, Priori SG, Kertesz NJ, Ro PS, et al. Efficacy of Flecainide in the treatment of catecholaminergic polymorphic ventricular tachycardia: a randomized clinical trial. JAMA Cardiol. 2017;2(7):759–66.

206. De Ferrari GM, Dusi V, Spazzolini C, Bos JM, Abrams DJ, Berul CI, et al. Clinical management of catecholaminergic polymorphic ventricular tachycardia: the role of left cardiac sympathetic denervation. Circulation. 2015;131(25):2185–93.

# Specific Cardiovascular Diseases and Competitive Sports Participation: Coronary Anomalies and Myocardial Bridging at Risk of Sudden Death

**21**

Gaetano Thiene, Stefania Rizzo, Carla Frescura, and Cristina Basso

**Learning Objectives**

1. Coronary artery anatomy.
2. Congenital coronary artery anomalies and risk of sudden death.
3. Prevalence of congenital coronary artery anomalies.
4. Identification in vivo of coronary artery anomalies.

## 21.1 Introduction

Coronary artery anomalies account for a significant rate of sudden cardiac deaths in the young [1–12] and particularly in athletes. Of 75 consecutive cases of sudden death in athletes, studied pathologically in the time interval 1981–2017 in the Veneto Region, Italy, 12 (16%) were ascribed to congenital malformations, either of origin or course, of coronary arteries as the sole cause of fatal outcome, the third major morbid entity, following arrhythmogenic right ventricular cardiomyopathy (27%) and coronary atherosclerosis (24%) (Fig. 21.1). Clearly, their detection at pre-participation screening for competitive sport eligibility plays a fundamental role for sudden death prevention. However, it represents a great challenge since it requires clinical imaging [13–24], because ECG (both 12 leads basal and stress test) has a scarce sensibility to raise suspicion. Classification of coronary artery anomalies is out of the scope of this chapter.

G. Thiene (✉) · S. Rizzo · C. Frescura · C. Basso
Cardiovascular Pathology, Department of Cardiac, Thoracic and Vascular Sciences and Public Health, University of Padua Medical School, Padua, Italy
e-mail: gaetano.thiene@unipd.it; cristina.basso@unipd.it



A. Pressler, J. Niebauer (eds.), *Textbook of Sports and Exercise Cardiology*,
https://doi.org/10.1007/978-3-030-35374-2_21

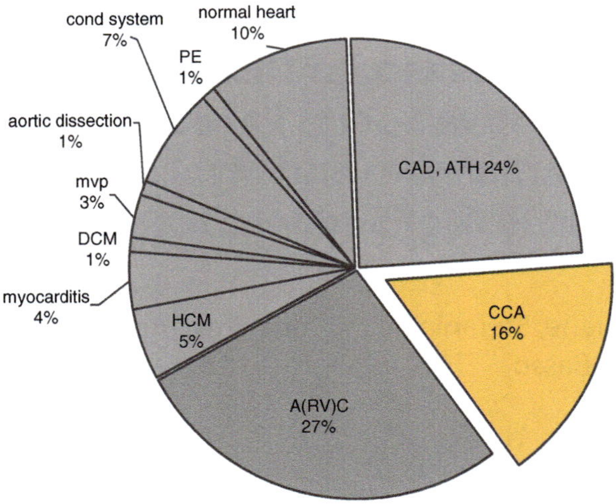


**Fig. 21.1** Causes of Sudden Cardiac Death in 75 athletes, Veneto Region Registry, Italy (1981–2014). Coronary artery anomalies accounted for 16% of cases. *A(RV)C* arrhythmogenic right ventricular cardiomyopathy, *CAD* coronary artery disease, *ATH* atherosclerosis, *CCA* congenital coronary anomalies, *DCM* dilated cardiomyopathy, *HCM* hypertrophic cardiomyopathy, *mpv* mitral valve prolapse, *PE* pulmonary embolism

## 21.2 Relevant Normal Anatomy

- The origin of the coronary arteries is extracardiac, in contrast to the venous drainage that occurs inside the right atrium through the coronary sinus.
- The coronary ostia are located at the aortic root, opposite to the sinuses of Valsalva facing the pulmonary artery, the right from the right anterior sinus and the left from the left sinus [25, 26]. The origin is perpendicular to the aorta and extraarterial, without the pulmonary trunk interfering with their proximal course (Fig. 21.2). Normally, the coronary ostia are round and located at the sino-tubular junction or up to 2.5 mm at maximum [27].
- In 75–90% of normal hearts, the coronary arterial circulation is right dominant, with the right coronary artery perfusing the postero-septal and sometimes even lateral walls of the left ventricle.
- Both the sino-atrial and atrioventricular (AV) node arteries originate from the right coronary artery in the right dominant pattern.

It was Banchi in 1903 [28] who first reported the various patterns of coronary circulation, introducing the concept of coronary arterial dominance. In 1965, Baroldi confirmed the variability by applying post-mortem injections with casts and published these in a book which is still considered a "bible" of coronary artery anatomy and pathology [29].

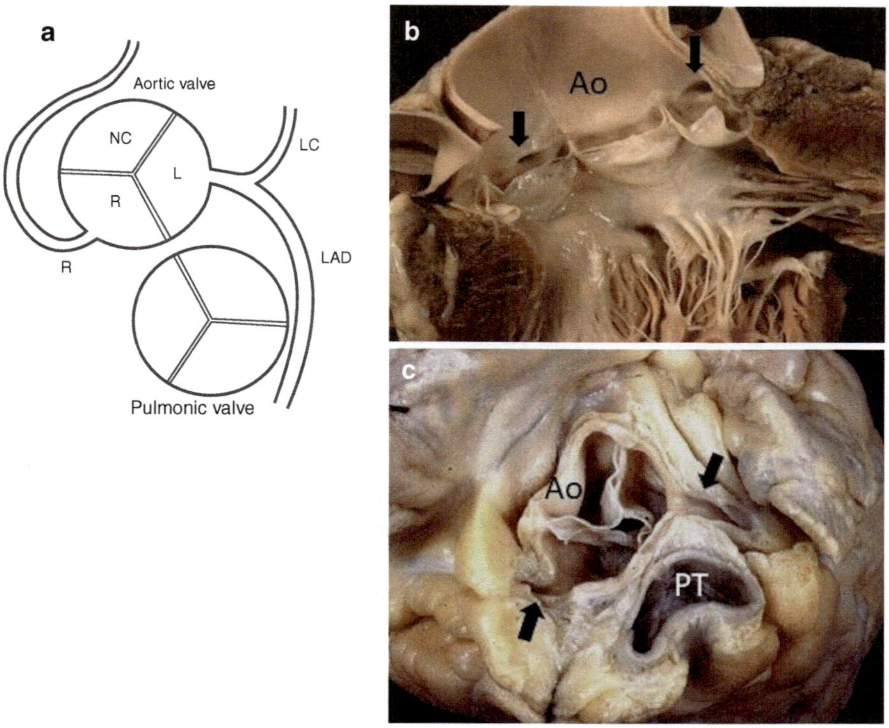


**Fig. 21.2** (**a**) Schematic representation of the origin of the coronary arteries. The coronary arteries normally arise perpendicularly from the aortic sinuses facing the pulmonary trunk, which does not interfere with their proximal course. (**b**) View of the left ventricle and aorta: note the origin of the right and left coronary artery (arrows) from the corresponding aortic sinus and the posterior non coronary aortic sinus in between. (**c**) Anatomical specimen corresponding to the diagram (**a**) with the relation of aorta and pulmonary trunk and the origin of the coronary arteries (arrows). *Ao* aorta, *L* left aortic coronary sinus, *LAD* left anterior descending artery, *LC* left circumflex artery, *NC* non-coronary aortic sinus, *PT* pulmonary, *R* right aortic sinus and right coronary artery

The left circumflex artery is a branch of the left main trunk or exceptionally originates separately from the left coronary sinus of Valsalva, a normal variant without pathological significance. Along its course overriding the anterior interventricular septum, in about 30% of normal hearts the left anterior descending coronary artery is covered by a thin (1–2 mm) layer of myocardium ("myocardial bridging") [30]. Intramural course of a major subepicardial coronary artery, mainly the left anterior descending artery, usually consists of such a thin layer of myocardium, overriding the coronary segment and considered as a benign variant. Floriano Caldani published the first beautiful drawing of this anomaly in Padua in 1810 [31].

## 21.3 Coronary Artery Anomalies Associated with Sudden Cardiac Death

The incidence of reported coronary artery anomalies is

- 0.17% in autopsy,
- 1.2% in coronary angiography, and
- 0.17% in echo series [32–34].

The true prevalence in general population is unknown, but presumably it is no more than 0.2%. In the Cardiac Registry with specimen collection of congenital heart diseases in our Institute (about 1700 hearts), isolated congenital anomalies of coronary arteries account for 3.5%.

Ogden [35] distinguished major, like origin from the pulmonary artery (Fig. 21.3) [36–38], and minor anomalies, such as high take off, single coronary artery, origin from a wrong coronary sinus [3, 8, 39–44]. However, this classification turned out to be untenable since Ogden "minor" anomalies may be life threatening as well.

Familial clustering of coronary artery anomalies has been sporadically reported [45]; however, it does not exceed the rate of recurrence in siblings and off-springs of other congenital heart diseases and, as such, they cannot be considered a mendelian disorder.

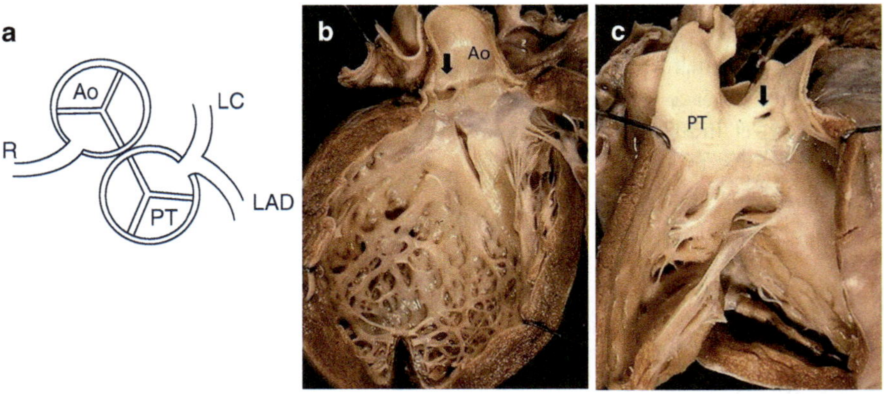


**Fig. 21.3** Origin of the left coronary artery from the pulmonary trunk. (**a**) Diagram of the origin of the left coronary artery from the pulmonary artery. (**b**) Left ventricle and aorta: only the orifice of the right coronary is present (arrow). (**c**) View of the right ventricular outflow and pulmonary artery: note the origin of the left coronary artery (arrow) from the pulmonary artery. *Ao* aorta, *LAD* left anterior descending artery, *LC* left circumflex artery, *PT* pulmonary trunk, *R* right coronary artery

## 21.4 Anomalous Origin of a Coronary Artery from the Opposite, Wrong Aortic Sinus

There are hearts in which both coronary ostia are located in one of the sinuses facing the pulmonary root: the right coronary artery from the left [46–48] (Fig. 21.4) or the left coronary artery from the right sinus [49–53] (Fig. 21.5).

- The proximal coronary artery originating from the opposite sinus displays a "flute bill" ostium and an inter-arterial course (Fig. 21.5), frequently within the aortic wall tunica media (intramural course) with a slit-like lumen (Fig. 21.6).
- Regarding the anomalous origin of left coronary artery from right aortic sinus, the intramural course corresponds to the left main trunk, which then bifurcates into left anterior descending and circumflex arteries (Fig. 21.7). When the aorta and the pulmonary artery dilate due to the increased cardiac output on effort, the lumen of the left main trunk is flattened. With this shape, the anomalous coronary artery is unable to compensate for the increased blood flow demand during exercise, thus resulting in an imbalance and mismatch between myocyte oxygen supply and request. A commissure is frequently located close to the anomalous coronary ostium (Fig. 21.7), thus interfering with the surgical repair.
- When the proximal course of the anomalous coronary artery lies anterior to the pulmonary outflow, the condition is not at risk of myocardial ischemia even during effort. Origin of a coronary artery from the posterior sinus is quite rare [49, 50, 54, 55].

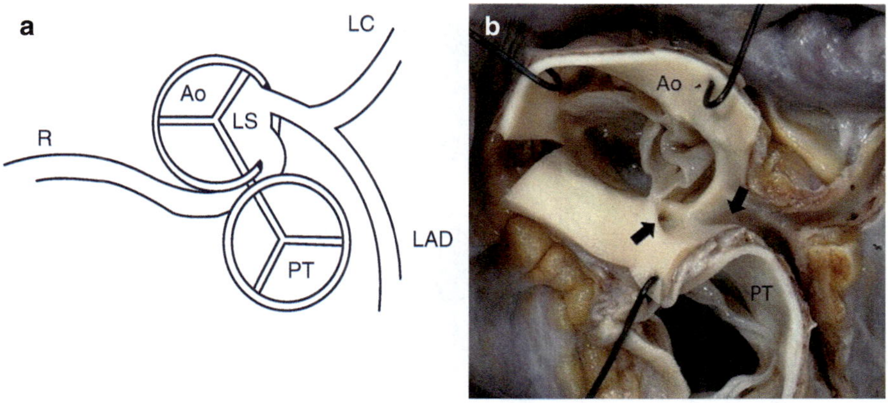


**Fig. 21.4** Origin of the right coronary artery from the left aortic sinus. (**a**) Diagram illustrating the anomalous origin of the right coronary artery from the opposite-wrong left sinus. (**b**) Anatomical specimen: the right coronary ostium is placed in the left aortic sinus, close to the left coronary ostium (arrows). The pathologist, while inspecting the right sinus, did not find a coronary ostium. *Ao* aorta, *LAD* left anterior descending artery, *LC* left circumflex artery, *LS* left aortic sinus, *PT* pulmonary trunk, *R* right coronary artery

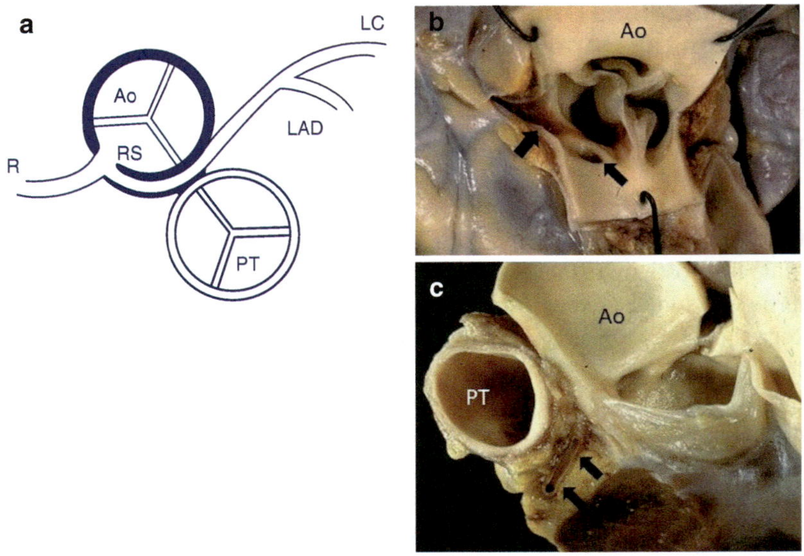


**Fig. 21.5** Origin of the left coronary artery from the right aortic sinus. (**a**) Schematic representation of the origin of the left coronary artery from the right anterior aortic sinus with a course between the aorta and the pulmonary trunk. (**b**) The left coronary ostium is located in the right aortic sinus close to the right coronary ostium (arrows). Note the "flute bill" shape with a slit-like lumen. (**c**) The left coronary artery courses between the aorta and the pulmonary trunk (arrows). *Ao* aorta, *LAD* left anterior descending artery, *LC* left circumflex artery, *RS* right aortic sinus, *PT* pulmonary trunk, *R* right coronary artery

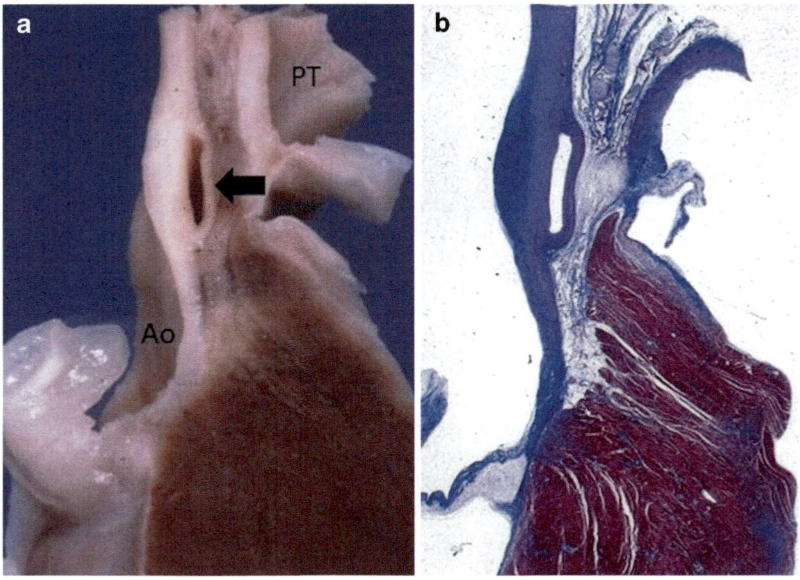


**Fig. 21.6** Anomalous origin of a coronary artery from the opposite wrong aortic sinus. Note the aortic intramural proximal course (arrow), at both gross (**a**) and microscopic (**b**) examination, (Heidenhain stain) with slit-like lumen. *Ao* aorta, *PT* pulmonary trunk

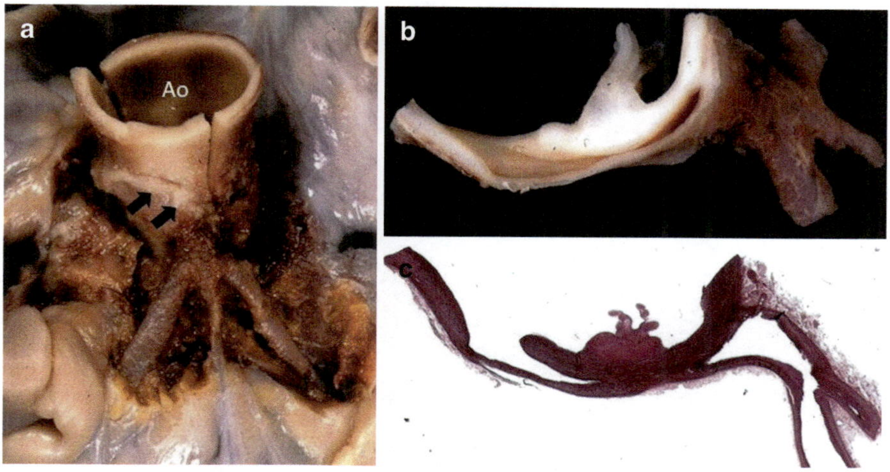


**Fig. 21.7** Origin of the left coronary artery from the right aortic sinus. Origin of the left coronary artery from the right wrong sinus, at gross anatomy (**a**, **b**) and histology (**c**). Note the intramural aortic course of the left main coronary trunk (arrows), reaching its normal position before bifurcating into descending and circumflex branches, and the position of the commissure. *Ao* aorta

Sudden cardiac death (SCD) occurs during strenuous exercise. Premonitory symptoms are present only in 30% of subjects (syncope, chest pain, palpitations on effort) and 12-lead ECG at rest or during exercise testing are normal [3], making clinical suspicion difficult and diagnosis almost impossible without imaging [13–24]. Moreover, in our experience, adverse cardiac events usually occur after long endurance performance (running, cycling, soccer in the second half), thus induced by an effort which is by far higher than that of exercise testing. This may explain the failure of the latter to unmask the underlying malformation. Beyond ECG end exercise testing, in the hands of experts and in case of good imaging quality 2-D echocardiography may be able to detect the anomaly [18, 19, 22, 24].

The mechanism of cardiac arrest is clearly arrhythmic in the form of ventricular fibrillation triggered by myocardial ischemia. Both acute myocardial injury following the last effort and chronic patchy fibrosis induced by previous strenuous episodes of exercise represent the structural substrates for life-threatening re-entry tachyarrhythmias (Fig. 21.8). The basic pathophysiological background is thus clearly ischemic. Acute take off, intramural aortic course and the "squeezing" effect of the inter-arterial course contribute to the myocardial blood flow mismatch, precipitating fatal tachyarrhythmias.

Of the two anomalous conditions, the most dangerous is the left from right, because of the greater proportion if involved myocardium at risk of ischemia. It can be regarded as an equivalent of left main coronary trunk disease (Fig. 21.7). In case of right from left, both sinus and AV node arteries are exposed to acute ischemia in a right dominant pattern, and cardiac arrest may occur with asystole due to sinoatrial or AV block.

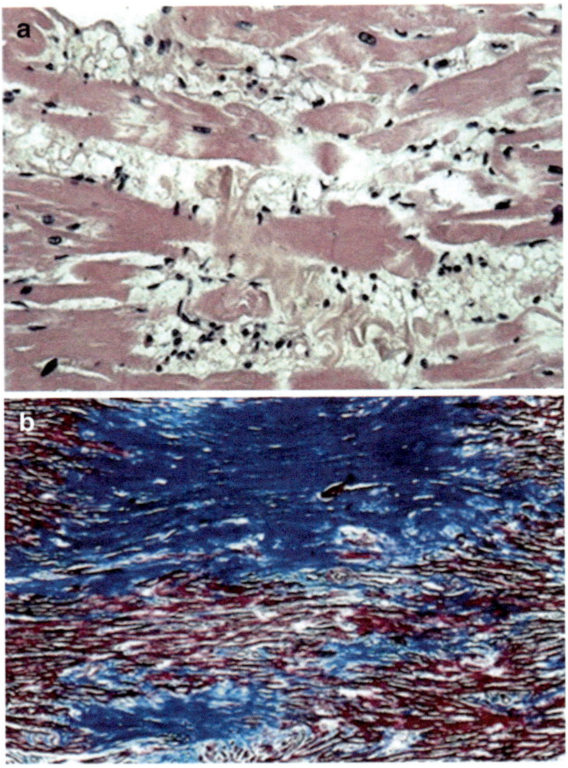


Fig. 21.8 Acute (cell death) (**a**) and chronic (fibrosis) (**b**) ischemic damage in the correspondence of left ventricular myocardium supplied by an anomalous coronary artery originating from wrong sinus. (**a**) Haematoxylin-Eosin stain, (**b**) Heidenhain stain

## 21.5 Anomalous Origin of the Left Circumflex Coronary Artery

- In this condition, the left circumflex artery, instead of originating from the left main stem, takes origin from the right coronary artery or from a separate ostium of the right sinus of Valsalva [56–58]. It runs behind the aortic root, reaches the left AV sulcus and, according to the type of coronary dominance, perfuses the lateral or even the posterior wall of the left ventricle (Fig. 21.9).
- During effort, the dilated aortic root may exert a squeezing effect with lumen stenosis.

The significance of this anomaly, whether a variant of normal or truly pathogenic, is still debated, despite being the only potential substrate in an otherwise normal heart. However, a case came to our attention (Fig. 21.10) presenting this abnormality with a patent lumen and posterolateral, subendocardial healed myocardial infarction, a clear-cut evidence for a pathogenic link.

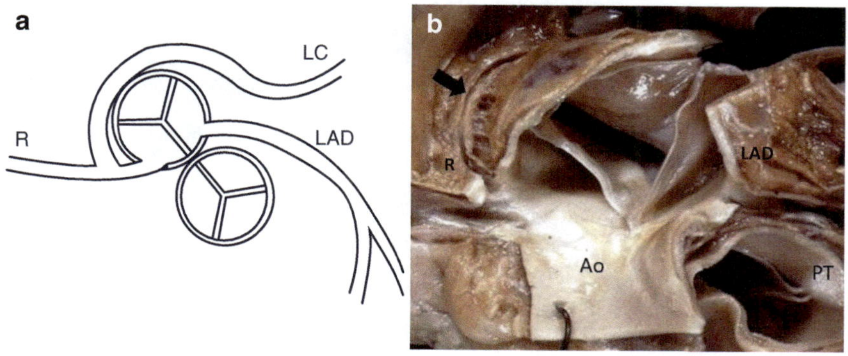


**Fig. 21.9** Origin of the left circumflex artery from the right coronary artery. (**a**) Diagram illustrating the anomalous origin of the left circumflex from the right coronary artery with a retro-aortic course. (**b**) Corresponding anatomical specimen. The arrow indicates the retro-aortic course of the circumflex artery. *Ao* aorta, *LAD* left anterior descending artery, *LC* left circumflex artery, *PT* pulmonary trunk, *R* right coronary artery

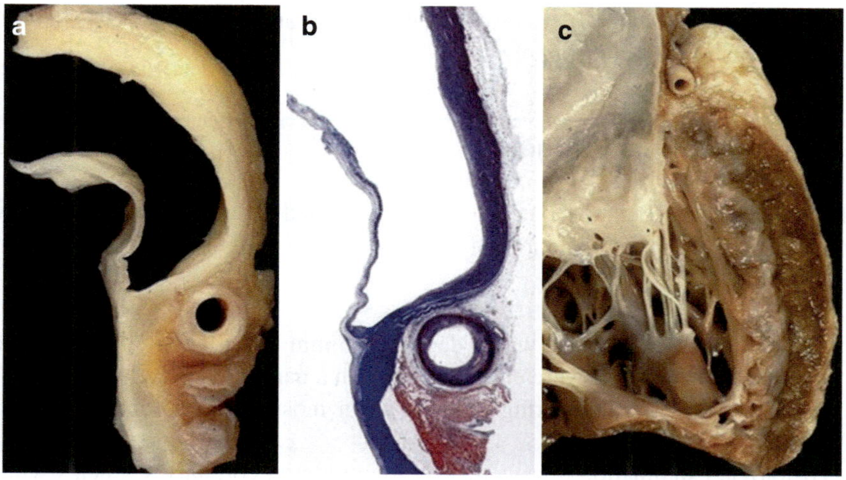


**Fig. 21.10** Origin of the circumflex artery from the right coronary artery. A case of sudden death with anomalous origin of the left circumflex coronary artery from the right aortic sinus, running behind the aorta (**a**, **b**). Note the presence subendocardial chronic myocardial infarction of the lateral wall of the left ventricle (**c**), in the absence of obstructive atherosclerosis in the infarct-related circumflex artery (**a**, **b**). (**b**) Heidenhain stain

## 21.6 High Take-off of a Main Coronary Artery

We observed cases of SCD in athletes, in whom at post-mortem evaluation the right coronary artery ostium was found to be located in the tubular part of the ascending aorta [59–61], well above the established normal upper limit of 2.5 mm [27]. The proximal course appeared vertical before reaching the right AV sulcus (Fig. 21.11).

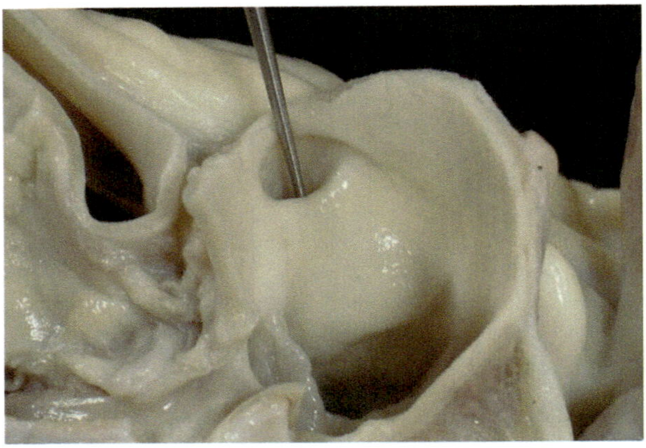

Fig. 21.11 High take off coronary artery. Sudden cardiac death in a patient with high take off of the right coronary artery (18 mm) and vertical proximal course

- Once again, intramural aortic course or squeezing during exercise-induced aortic dilatation may account for relevant lumen stenosis and imbalance between blood flow demand and actual supply.

## 21.7 Myocardial Bridging

This anomaly has been observed in athletes who died suddenly, in the absence of any other plausible explanation of the unexpected and abrupt fatal outcome (Fig. 21.12).

- An intramyocardial course with a depth of >5 mm and a length of >2.5 cm has been advocated to be severe enough to explain a narrow, flattened lumen during systole, also persisting during diastole when most of the coronary perfusion occurs [62–70].
- Histologic examination reveals that these intramural coronary segments with a flat lumen are surrounded by a muff of myocardium with disarray, in keeping with a sphincteric contraction that persists during diastole (Fig. 21.13).

It is interesting to observe that in the original paper by Morales et al. [69], who first drew the attention to mural left anterior descending coronary artery as a cause of sudden death during strenuous exercise, the accompanying picture of a heart discloses an asymmetric hypertrophy of the antero-lateral wall of the left ventricle, consistent with hypertrophic cardiomyopathy (HCM). In Fig. 21.14, we report a case of SCD in a boy with HCM and a massive infarction in a pronounced septal asymmetric hypertrophy, associated with long and deep intramural course of the left anterior descending coronary artery [71].

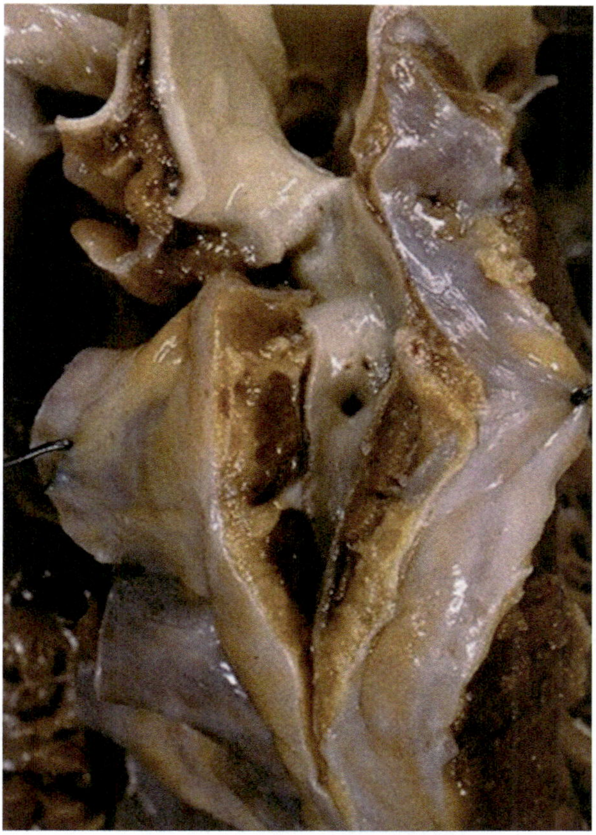

**Fig. 21.12** Intramyocardial course. Deep intramural course of the left anterior descending coronary artery segment, just over the first septal branch, in a patient having died suddenly

- A recent investigation of our group in a large cohort of HCM patients [72] revealed that the occurrence of "myocardial bridging" was much more frequent in this population as compared to healthy controls or to other causes of LV hypertrophy, suggesting that this phenomenon should be included in the spectrum of structural phenotypes of this cardiomyopathy.

The question is whether "myocardial bridging" plays a role in precipitating cardiac ischemic injury, which together with myocardial disarray may represent a morphological "cocktail" for triggering life-threatening arrhythmias and SCD as part of the natural history of HCM. Myocardial scars within asymmetric hypertrophy (but also elsewhere) are frequently observed in HCM patients dying suddenly, with (Fig. 21.15 left) or without (Fig. 21.15 middle) myocardial bridging, questioning the exclusive role of the latter in precipitating sudden death. Even intramural course without myocardial scarring was observed (Fig. 21.15 right).

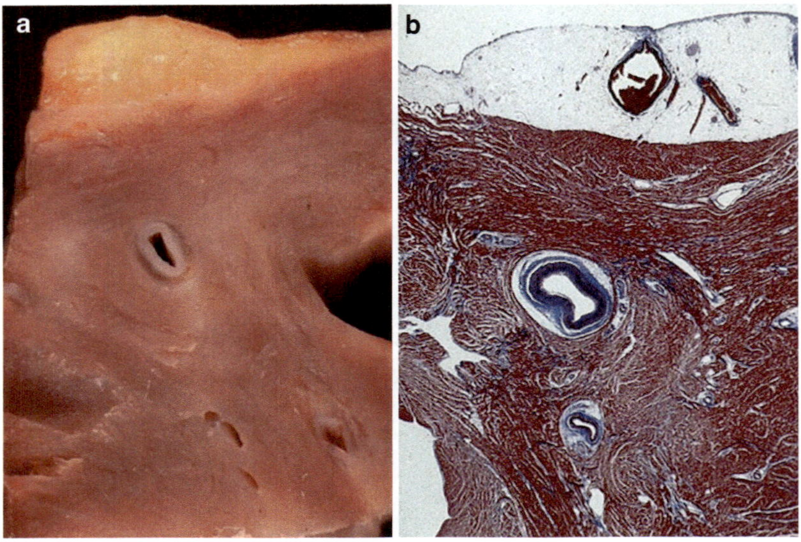


**Fig. 21.13** Intramural course of the left coronary artery. A segment of the left coronary artery runs deep in the myocardium and is surrounded by a muff of myocardium. Gross view of the heart (**a**) and histology (Heidenhain stain) (**b**)

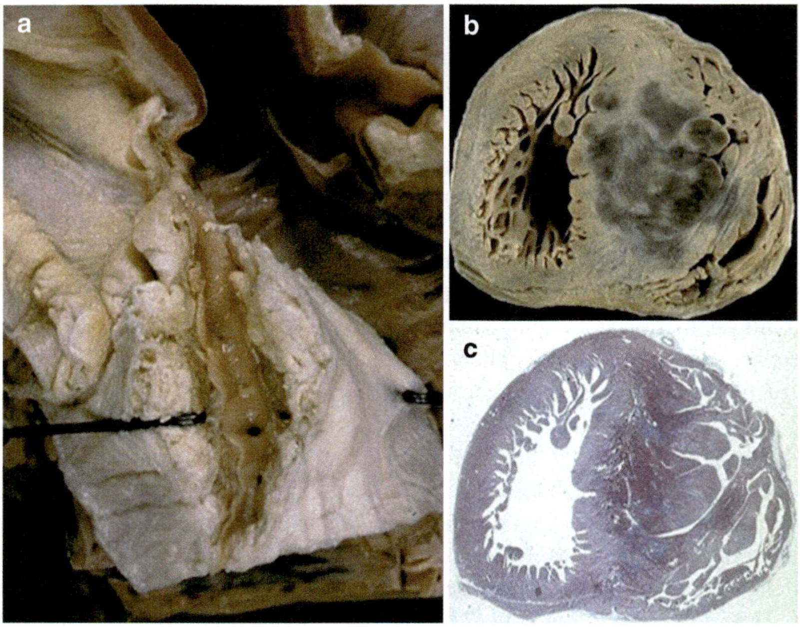


**Fig. 21.14** Intramural coronary course and hypertrophic cardiomyopathy. (**a**) Long and deep intramural course of the left anterior descending artery in a child with hypertrophic cardiomyopathy who died suddenly. (**b**) Anatomical specimen with massive acute myocardial infarction: note the huge asymmetric septal hypertrophy. (**c**) Corresponding histological view (Haematoxylin-Eosin stain)

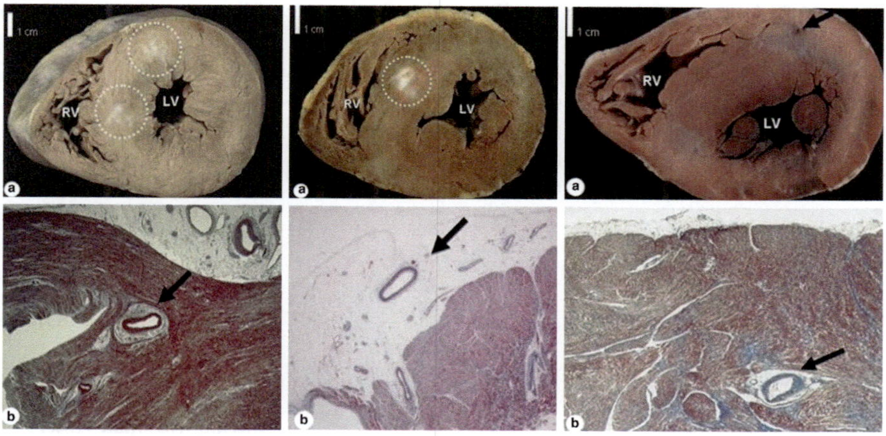


**Fig. 21.15** Hypertrophic cardiomyopathy. Three cases of hypertrophic cardiomyopathy and sudden death with scarring and intramural course (left panels), scarring and no intramural course (middle panels) and no scarring with intramural course (right panels) (**a**, gross view, **b**, histologic view)

## 21.8 Causal Relationship Between Coronary Artery Anomalies and SCD

According to the autopsy guidelines for the study of SCD cases of the Association for European Cardiovascular Pathology [73, 74] (Table 21.1), among coronary artery anomalies

1. an origin from the pulmonary trunk should be considered as a *certain* cause of SCD, in the absence of otherwise plausible explanations.
2. the origin of left coronary artery from the opposite right sinus of Valsalva has been classified as a *highly probable* cause of SCD
3. other forms (right from left, left circumflex from right and retro-aortic course, high take off and myocardial bridging) are classified as *uncertain* causes.

We believe that, if uncertain in the absence of other structural abnormalities, molecular genetic investigation together with family genetic study cascades should be carried out in search of pathogen mutations for channelopathies, to exclude a genetic origin.

**Clinical Pearls**

- Classically, coronary artery anomalies are divided in major, like those with origin from the pulmonary artery, and minor when originating from the aorta. This is not true since they are apparently minor anomalies that have been shown to cause arrhythmic sudden death.

**Table 21.1** Certainty of diagnosis in sudden cardiac death autopsies (issues referring to coronary artery anomalies are highlighted in bold; modified from [74])

| Certain | Highly probable | Uncertain |
|---|---|---|
| Massive pulmonary embolism | Stable atherosclerotic plaque with luminal stenosis >75% with or without healed myocardial infarction | **Minor anomalies of the coronary arteries from the aorta:**<br>**• RCA from the left sinus**<br>**• LCA from the right without inter-arterial course**<br>**• high take-off from the tubular portion**<br>**• LCx originating from the right sinus or RCA**<br>**• coronary ostia plication**<br>**• fibromuscular dysplasia**<br>**• intramural small vessel disease** |
| Haemopericard due to aortic or cardiac rupture | **Anomalous origin of the LCA from the right sinus and inter-arterial course** | Intra-myocardial course of a coronary artery (myocardial bridge) |
| Mitral valve papillary muscle or chordae tendineae rupture with acute mitral valve incompetence and pulmonary edema | Cardiomyopathies (hypertrophic, arrhythmogenic, dilated, others) | Focal myocarditis, hypertensive heart disease, idiopathic left ventricular hypertrophy |
| Acute coronary occlusion due to thrombosis, dissection or embolism | Myxoid degeneration of the mitral valve with prolapse, with atrial dilatation or left ventricular hypertrophy and intact chordae | Myxoid degeneration of the mitral valve with prolapse, without atrial dilatation or left ventricular hypertrophy and intact chordae |
| **Anomalous origin of the coronary artery from the pulmonary trunk** | Aortic stenosis with left ventricular hypertrophy | Dystrophic calcification of the membranous septum (± mitral annulus/aortic valve) |
| Neoplasm/thrombus obstructing the valve orifice | ECG documented ventricular pre-excitation (Wolff-Parkinson-White syndrome, Lown Ganong Levine syndrome) | Atrial septum lipoma |
| Thrombotic block of the valve prosthesis | ECG documented sinoatrial or AV block | AV node cystic tumor without ECG evidence of AV block, conducting system disease without ECG documentation |
| Laceration/dehiscence/poppet escape of the valve prosthesis with acute valve incompetence | Congenital heart diseases, operated | Congenital heart diseases, un-operated with or without Eisenmenger syndrome |
| Massive acute myocarditis | | |

- Among these, origin of the left coronary artery from the right aortic sinus has been proven a highly probable cause of sudden death during effort because not only the interarterial course, but also because mural running of the first tract into the tunica media. The mechanism is arrhythmic due to ischemic injury of the myocardium.

## Clinical Cases

### Questions

1. A 53-year-old man was admitted to the coronary care unit complaining of chest pain. ECG showed ST-segment elevation in leads II, III, aVF, V5 and V6 as well as a ST-segment depression in V1-V4. Echocardiogram showed posterolateral left ventricular wall akinesia with preserved ejection fraction. There was an increase of the serum level of troponin. The patient was found dead 1 month later. At autopsy, no signs of obstructive coronary atherosclerotic disease were found. The left circumflex coronary artery took off at an acute angle from the anterior right aortic sinus, separately from the right coronary ostium, and run behind the aorta to reach the left atrioventricular groove. Moreover, a myocardial infarction was detected in the posterolateral wall of the left ventricle. Which imaging testing do you perform in this man to rule out coronary artery disease? In the guidelines of autopsy of sudden death, is this anomaly considered as a certain, a probable or an uncertain cause of death?
2. A 3-month-old male baby was found dead in his crib. At autopsy, the origin of the dominant right coronary artery was found originating from above the left coronary sinus with an acute angle take-off, and the proximal segment coursed intramurally within the aortic tunica media, passing between the aorta and the pulmonary trunk before reaching the right atrioventricular groove. Could a fetal echocardiography provide the correct diagnosis of this condition?

### Answers

1. Coronary angiography is the gold standard method to provide an accurate study in vivo of coronary anatomy, to look at the origin and course of the proximal segments of right and left coronary artery, but also to rule out atherosclerotic coronary artery disease. Computed tomography angiography, due to its non-invasiveness and multiplanar reconstruction, is increasingly utilized for characterization of coronary artery origin anomalies. It provides a more accurate evaluation of the ostium as well as of the course and the presence of calcifications. Diagnostic methods such as computed tomographic angiography, nuclear magnetic resonance or coronarography are characterized by higher sensitivity and specificity as compared to echocardiography.
   The anomaly is considered an uncertain cause of sudden death; however, the subendocardial healed myocardial infarction in the setting of patently related coronary arteries strongly support a causal relationship.
2. Prenatal echocardiography does not allow visualization of the coronary artery origins in foetuses.

## References


1. Basso C, Corrado D, Thiene G. Congenital coronary artery anomalies as an important cause of sudden death in the young. Cardiol Rev. 2001;9(6):312–7.
2. Basso C, Corrado D, Thiene G. Coronary artery anomalies and sudden death. Card Electrophysiol Rev. 2002;6(1–2):107–11.
3. Basso C, Maron BJ, Corrado D, Thiene G. Clinical profile of congenital coronary artery anomalies with origin from the wrong aortic sinus leading to sudden death in young competitive athletes. J Am Coll Cardiol. 2000;35(6):1493–501.
4. Basso C, Perez-Pomares J, Thiene G, Houyel L. Coronary anomalies. In: Perez-Pomares J, Kelly R, editors. The ESC textbook of cardiovascular development. 1st ed. Oxford: OUP; 2018. p. 250–60.
5. Burke AP, Farb A, Virmani R, Goodin J, Smialek JE. Sports-related and non-sports-related sudden cardiac death in young adults. Am Heart J. 1991;121(2 Pt 1):568–75.
6. Cheitlin MD, MacGregor J. Congenital anomalies of coronary arteries: role in the pathogenesis of sudden cardiac death. Herz. 2009;34(4):268–79.
7. Corrado D, Thiene G, Cocco P, Frescura C. Non-atherosclerotic coronary artery disease and sudden death in the young. Br Heart J. 1992;68(6):601–7.
8. Frescura C, Basso C, Thiene G, Corrado D, Pennelli T, Angelini A, et al. Anomalous origin of coronary arteries and risk of sudden death: a study based on an autopsy population of congenital heart disease. Hum Pathol. 1998;29(7):689–95.
9. Maron BJ, Doerer JJ, Haas TS, Tierney DM, Mueller FO. Sudden deaths in young competitive athletes: analysis of 1866 deaths in the United States, 1980-2006. Circulation. 2009;119(8):1085–92.
10. Maron BJ, Haas TS, Doerer JJ, Thompson PD, Hodges JS. Comparison of U.S. and Italian experiences with sudden cardiac deaths in young competitive athletes and implications for preparticipation screening strategies. Am J Cardiol. 2009;104(2):276–80.
11. Maron BJ, Shirani J, Poliac LC, Mathenge R, Roberts WC, Mueller FO. Sudden death in young competitive athletes. Clinical, demographic, and pathological profiles. JAMA. 1996;276(3):199–204.
12. Taylor AJ, Rogan KM, Virmani R. Sudden cardiac death associated with isolated congenital coronary artery anomalies. J Am Coll Cardiol. 1992;20(3):640–7.
13. Angelini P, Cheong BY, Lenge De Rosen VV, Lopez A, Uribe C, Masso AH, et al. High-risk cardiovascular conditions in sports-related sudden death: prevalence in 5,169 schoolchildren screened via cardiac magnetic resonance. Tex Heart Inst J. 2018;45(4):205–13.
14. Cheng Z, Wang X, Duan Y, Wu L, Wu D, Liang C, et al. Detection of coronary artery anomalies by dual-source CT coronary angiography. Clin Radiol. 2010;65(10):815–22.
15. Duran C, Kantarci M, Durur Subasi I, Gulbaran M, Sevimli S, Bayram E, et al. Remarkable anatomic anomalies of coronary arteries and their clinical importance: a multidetector computed tomography angiographic study. J Comput Assist Tomogr. 2006;30(6):939–48.
16. Engel HJ, Torres C, Page HL Jr. Major variations in anatomical origin of the coronary arteries: angiographic observations in 4,250 patients without associated congenital heart disease. Catheter Cardiovasc Diagn. 1975;1(2):157–69.
17. Harikrishnan S, Jacob SP, Tharakan J, Titus T, Kumar VK, Bhat A, et al. Congenital coronary anomalies of origin and distribution in adults: a coronary arteriographic study. Indian Heart J. 2002;54(3):271–5.
18. Labombarda F, Coutance G, Pellissier A, Mery-Alexandre C, Roule V, Maragnes P, et al. Major congenital coronary artery anomalies in a paediatric and adult population: a prospective echocardiographic study. Eur Heart J Cardiovasc Imaging. 2014;15(7):761–8.
19. Maron BJ, Leon MB, Swain JA, Cannon RO 3rd, Pelliccia A. Prospective identification by two-dimensional echocardiography of anomalous origin of the left main coronary artery from the right sinus of Valsalva. Am J Cardiol. 1991;68(1):140–2.

20. Miller JA, Anavekar NS, El Yaman MM, Burkhart HM, Miller AJ, Julsrud PR. Computed tomographic angiography identification of intramural segments in anomalous coronary arteries with interarterial course. Int J Cardiovasc Imaging. 2012;28(6):1525–32.
21. Norgaard BL, Leipsic J, Gaur S, Seneviratne S, Ko BS, Ito H, et al. Diagnostic performance of noninvasive fractional flow reserve derived from coronary computed tomography angiography in suspected coronary artery disease: the NXT trial (Analysis of Coronary Blood Flow Using CT Angiography: Next Steps). J Am Coll Cardiol. 2014;63(12):1145–55.
22. Pelliccia A, Spataro A, Maron BJ. Prospective echocardiographic screening for coronary artery anomalies in 1,360 elite competitive athletes. Am J Cardiol. 1993;72(12):978–9.
23. Yamanaka O, Hobbs RE. Coronary artery anomalies in 126,595 patients undergoing coronary arteriography. Catheter Cardiovasc Diagn. 1990;21(1):28–40.
24. Zeppilli P, dello Russo A, Santini C, Palmieri V, Natale L, Giordano A, et al. In vivo detection of coronary artery anomalies in asymptomatic athletes by echocardiographic screening. Chest. 1998;114(1):89–93.
25. Angelini P. Normal and anomalous coronary arteries: definitions and classification. Am Heart J. 1989;117(2):418–34.
26. Angelini P, Villason S, Chan AJ, Diez J. Normal and anomalous coronary arteries in humans. In: Angelini P, editor. Coronary artery anomalies: a comprehensive approach. Philadelphia: Lippincott, Williams & Wilkins; 1999. p. 27–150.
27. Muriago M, Sheppard MN, Ho SY, Anderson RH. Location of the coronary arterial orifices in the normal heart. Clin Anat. 1997;10(5):297–302.
28. Banchi A. Le variazioni delle "arterie coronariae cordis" e la morfologia di questi vasi. Sperimentale. 1903;57:367–9.
29. Baroldi G, Scomazzoni G. Coronary circulation in the normal and the pathologic heart. Washington, DC: Armed Forces Institute of Pathology; 1965. p. 1–37.
30. Angelini P, Trivellato M, Donis J, Leachman RD. Myocardial bridges: a review. Prog Cardiovasc Dis. 1983;26(1):75–88.
31. Caldani L, Caldani F. Icones anatomicae ex optimis neotericum operibus summa diligentia depromtae et collectae. In: Picotti J, editor. Venetiis ex Calcographia; 1810.
32. Davis JA, Cecchin F, Jones TK, Portman MA. Major coronary artery anomalies in a pediatric population: incidence and clinical importance. J Am Coll Cardiol. 2001;37(2):593–7.
33. Kardos A, Babai L, Rudas L, Gaal T, Horvath T, Talosi L, et al. Epidemiology of congenital coronary artery anomalies: a coronary arteriography study on a central European population. Catheter Cardiovasc Diagn. 1997;42(3):270–5.
34. Yildiz A, Okcun B, Peker T, Arslan C, Olcay A, Bulent VM. Prevalence of coronary artery anomalies in 12,457 adult patients who underwent coronary angiography. Clin Cardiol. 2010;33(12):E60–4.
35. Ogden JA. Congenital anomalies of the coronary arteries. Am J Cardiol. 1970;25(4):474–9.
36. Bland E, White P, Garland J. Congenital anomalies of the coronary arteries: report of an unusual case associated with cardic hypertrophy. Am Heart J. 1933;8:787–801.
37. Dodge-Khatami A, Mavroudis C, Backer CL. Anomalous origin of the left coronary artery from the pulmonary artery: collective review of surgical therapy. Ann Thorac Surg. 2002;74(3):946–55.
38. Yau JM, Singh R, Halpern EJ, Fischman D. Anomalous origin of the left coronary artery from the pulmonary artery in adults: a comprehensive review of 151 adult cases and a new diagnosis in a 53-year-old woman. Clin Cardiol. 2011;34(4):204–10.
39. Chaitman BR, Lesperance J, Saltiel J, Bourassa MG. Clinical, angiographic, and hemodynamic findings in patients with anomalous origin of the coronary arteries. Circulation. 1976;53(1):122–31.
40. Elias MD, Meza J, McCrindle BW, Brothers JA, Paridon S, Cohen MS. Effects of exercise restriction on patients with anomalous aortic origin of a coronary artery. World J Pediatr Congenit Heart Surg. 2017;8(1):18–24.

41. Liberthson RR, Dinsmore RE, Fallon JT. Aberrant coronary artery origin from the aorta. Report of 18 patients, review of literature and delineation of natural history and management. Circulation. 1979;59(4):748–54.
42. Lim JC, Beale A, Ramcharitar S. Medscape. Anomalous origination of a coronary artery from the opposite sinus. Nat Rev Cardiol. 2011;8(12):706–19.
43. Lipsett J, Byard RW, Carpenter BF, Jimenez CL, Bourne AJ. Anomalous coronary arteries arising from the aorta associated with sudden death in infancy and early childhood. An autopsy series. Arch Pathol Lab Med. 1991;115(8):770–3.
44. Palmieri V, Gervasi S, Bianco M, Cogliani R, Poscolieri B, Cuccaro F, et al. Anomalous origin of coronary arteries from the "wrong" sinus in athletes: Diagnosis and management strategies. Int J Cardiol. 2018;252:13–20.
45. Youniss MA, Ghoshhajra B, Bernard S, Bhatt AB, Aranki SF, MacGillivray TE, et al. Familial anomalous origin of right coronary artery from the left coronary sinus. Am J Cardiol. 2018;122(10):1800–2.
46. Duran AC, Angelini A, Frescura C, Basso C, Thiene G. Anomalous origin of the right coronary artery from the left aortic sinus and sudden infant death. Int J Cardiol. 1994;45(2):147–9.
47. Munoz-Guijosa C, Permanyer E, Leta R. Anomalous origin of right coronary artery from the left coronary sinus: sudden death and successful surgical reimplantation. Eur Heart J. 2012;33(11):1308.
48. Roberts WC, Siegel RJ, Zipes DP. Origin of the right coronary artery from the left sinus of valsalva and its functional consequences: analysis of 10 necropsy patients. Am J Cardiol. 1982;49(4):863–8.
49. Angelini P, Uribe C. Anatomic spectrum of left coronary artery anomalies and associated mechanisms of coronary insufficiency. Catheter Cardiovasc Interv. 2018;92(2):313–21.
50. Arque JM, Thiene G, Cardo M, Franco D, Duran AC, Sans-Coma V. Anomalous origin of the left coronary artery from the nonfacing aortic sinus: a study in the Syrian hamster. Cardiovasc Pathol. 1993;2(1):35–9.
51. Barth CW 3rd, Roberts WC. Left main coronary artery originating from the right sinus of Valsalva and coursing between the aorta and pulmonary trunk. J Am Coll Cardiol. 1986;7(2):366–73.
52. Cheitlin MD, De Castro CM, McAllister HA. Sudden death as a complication of anomalous left coronary origin from the anterior sinus of Valsalva, A not-so-minor congenital anomaly. Circulation. 1974;50(4):780–7.
53. Murphy DA, Roy DL, Sohal M, Chandler BM. Anomalous origin of left main cononary artery from anterior sinus of Valsalva with myocardial infarction. J Thorac Cardiovasc Surg. 1978;75(2):282–5.
54. Adebo D, Jacobson Z, Harris MA. Anomalous origin of the right coronary artery from the posterior, non-coronary sinus of Valsalva diagnosed by cardiac magnetic resonance imaging. Cardiol Young. 2015;25(5):1006–8.
55. Padalino MA, Franchetti N, Hazekamp M, Sojak V, Carrel T, Frigiola A, et al. Surgery for anomalous aortic origin of coronary arteries: a multicentre study from the European Congenital Heart Surgeons Association dagger. Eur J Cardiothorac Surg. 2019;56(4):696–703.
56. Corrado D, Pennelli T, Piovesana P, Thiene G. Anomalous origin of the left circumflex coronary artery from the right aortic sinus of valsalva and sudden death. Cardiovasc Pathol. 1994;3(4):269–71.
57. Page HL Jr, Engel HJ, Campbell WB, Thomas CS Jr. Anomalous origin of the left circumflex coronary artery. Recognition, antiographic demonstration and clinical significance. Circulation. 1974;50(4):768–73.
58. Piovesana P, Corrado D, Contessotto F, Zampiero A, Camponeschi M, Lafisca N, et al. Echocardiographic identification of anomalous origin of the left circumflex coronary artery from the right sinus of Valsalva. Am Heart J. 1990;119(1):205–7.
59. Loukas M, Andall RG, Khan AZ, Patel K, Muresian H, Spicer DE, et al. The clinical anatomy of high take-off coronary arteries. Clin Anat. 2016;29(3):408–19.

60. Purvis J, Howe A, Morgan D. Aortic step: a clue to unusually high origin of right coronary artery. Heart. 2010;96(16):1334.
61. Virmani R, Chun PK, Goldstein RE, Robinowitz M, McAllister HA. Acute takeoffs of the coronary arteries along the aortic wall and congenital coronary ostial valve-like ridges: association with sudden death. J Am Coll Cardiol. 1984;3(3):766–71.
62. Alegria JR, Herrmann J, Holmes DR Jr, Lerman A, Rihal CS. Myocardial bridging. Eur Heart J. 2005;26(12):1159–68.
63. Bourassa MG, Butnaru A, Lesperance J, Tardif JC. Symptomatic myocardial bridges: overview of ischemic mechanisms and current diagnostic and treatment strategies. J Am Coll Cardiol. 2003;41(3):351–9.
64. Cheitlin MD. The intramural coronary artery: another cause for sudden death with exercise? Circulation. 1980;62(2):238–9.
65. Corban MT, Hung OY, Eshtehardi P, Rasoul-Arzrumly E, McDaniel M, Mekonnen G, et al. Myocardial bridging: contemporary understanding of pathophysiology with implications for diagnostic and therapeutic strategies. J Am Coll Cardiol. 2014;63(22):2346–55.
66. Faruqui AM, Maloy WC, Felner JM, Schlant RC, Logan WD, Symbas P. Symptomatic myocardial bridging of coronary artery. Am J Cardiol. 1978;41(7):1305–10.
67. Feldman AM, Baughman KL. Myocardial infarction associated with a myocardial bridge. Am Heart J. 1986;111(4):784–7.
68. Mohlenkamp S, Hort W, Ge J, Erbel R. Update on myocardial bridging. Circulation. 2002;106(20):2616–22.
69. Morales AR, Romanelli R, Boucek RJ. The mural left anterior descending coronary artery, strenuous exercise and sudden death. Circulation. 1980;62(2):230–7.
70. Schwarz ER, Gupta R, Haager PK, vom Dahl J, Klues HG, Minartz J, et al. Myocardial bridging in absence of coronary artery disease: proposal of a new classification based on clinical-angiographic data and long-term follow-up. Cardiology. 2009;112(1):13–21.
71. Gori F, Basso C, Thiene G. Myocardial infarction in a patient with hypertrophic cardiomyopathy. N Engl J Med. 2000;342(8):593–4.
72. Basso C, Thiene G, Mackey-Bojack S, Frigo AC, Corrado D, Maron BJ. Myocardial bridging, a frequent component of the hypertrophic cardiomyopathy phenotype, lacks systematic association with sudden cardiac death. Eur Heart J. 2009;30(13):1627–34.
73. Basso C, Aguilera B, Banner J, Cohle S, d'Amati G, de Gouveia RH, et al. Guidelines for autopsy investigation of sudden cardiac death: 2017 update from the Association for European Cardiovascular Pathology. Virchows Arch. 2017;471(6):691–705.
74. Basso C, Burke M, Fornes P, Gallagher PJ, de Gouveia RH, Sheppard M, et al. Guidelines for autopsy investigation of sudden cardiac death. Virchows Arch. 2008;452(1):11–8.

# Specific Cardiovascular Diseases and Competitive Sports Participation: Congenital Heart Disease

# 22

Tim Takken and Jan Müller

**Learning Objectives**

1. General importance of physical activity, recreational and competitive sport participation of patients with CHD.
2. Physical activity and exercise recommendations for patients with CHD.
3. General limitations to exercise in patients with CHD and physiological demands of competitive sports.
4. Actual situation of patients with CHD in competitive sports.
5. Necessity and content of a pre-participation screening before participation in competitive sports.
6. Exercise and training advices as well as specific recommendations for diagnostic subgroups.

## 22.1 Introduction

The importance of a physically active lifestyle to the health and wellbeing of children and adults with congenital heart defects (CHD) is undisputed [1–3]. Patients who are regularly participating in sports are generally more physically active, have a better exercise capacity and experience superior psychosocial outcomes. Moreover, in light of the improved life expectancy that has been observed in this cohort, sports participation is of particular relevance [4]. Adding to the consequences related to their type

T. Takken (✉)
Department of Medical Physiology, Child Development & Exercise Center, University Medical Center Utrecht, Utrecht, The Netherlands
e-mail: t.takken@umcutrecht.nl

J. Müller
Department of Preventive Pediatrics, Technical University of Munich, Munich, Germany
e-mail: j.mueller@tum.de





A. Pressler, J. Niebauer (eds.), *Textbook of Sports and Exercise Cardiology*,
https://doi.org/10.1007/978-3-030-35374-2_22

of CHD, patients are also affected by co-morbidities and risk factors that may favorably be influenced by regular PA and exercise [5]. These are in particular:

- Hypertension
- Overweight and Obesity
- Dyslipidemia
- Type 2 diabetes mellitus
- Cardiovascular events such as stroke and myocardial infarction
- Several types of cancer (e.g., colon and breast carcinoma)

Regular PA, exercise and sport participation do not only contribute to a favorable modification of the above-mentioned risk factors, they also improve:

- exercise capacity, the major predictor of morbidity and mortality in patients with CHD,
- health-related quality of life,
- self-confidence, and
- social relationships.

Several cardiac rehabilitation and exercise training studies [6–14] in patients with CHD have shown that exercise of moderate intensity is:

1. safe
2. improves exercise capacity
3. improves physical activity levels
4. improves health-related quality of life
5. beneficially contributes to psychosocial function.

## 22.2 Physical Activity Recommendations for Patients with CHD

Similar to their healthy counterparts children and adolescents with CHD should [15]:

- accumulate at least 60 min of moderate-to vigorous PA daily.
- Greater amounts than 60 min PA provide additional health benefits.
- Most of the daily physical activity should be aerobic.
- Vigorous-intensity activities should be incorporated, including those that strengthen muscles and bones (at least 3 times per week).

Likewise, the WHO recommendations for healthy adults can also be applied in adults with CHD. These patients should adhere to [15]:

- 150 min of moderate-intensity aerobic PA throughout the week or at least 75 min of vigorous-intensity aerobic physical activity throughout the week or an equivalent combination of moderate- and vigorous-intensity activities.

- Aerobic PA should be performed in bouts of at least 10 min duration.
- For additional health benefits, adults should increase their moderate-intensity aerobic physical activity to 300 min per week or engage in 150 min of vigorous-intensity aerobic physical activity per week, or an equivalent combination of moderate- and vigorous-intensity activity.
- Muscle-strengthening activities should be performed involving major muscle groups on 2 or more days per week.

## 22.3 Classification of Sports

To characterize whether a particular competitive sport is safe for an athlete with a specific cardiovascular abnormality, the Mitchell classification (Fig. 1.1) of sports is most widely used because it has been developed to specifically address this question [16]. It classifies an activity

1. on the basis of the mechanical action of the muscles and not on the metabolism.
2. according to two general types of exercise: dynamic (mainly involving endurance components) and static (mainly strength components).
3. by also recognizing those sports that pose significant risks due to bodily collision, or of hard impact between an object, projectile, or the ground.
4. on the degree of the risk of a sudden syncopal event.

For example, a sport with high static and high dynamic components will be classified as IIIC, whereas an exercise with low static and moderate dynamic components will be IB, and further on.

However, there are also some limitations to this classification that have to be taken into account:

- It does not consider the emotional stress and an increase in sympathetic drive, catecholamine concentrations and myocardial oxygen demand.
- Environmental exposure during athletic competition is not considered.
- In team sports, the classification is based on the highest cardiovascular demands.
- During training, stimuli might be higher than during the competition itself.

## 22.4 Exercise Limitations in CHD

Limitations to exercise in patients with CHD have been reported from the first studies on exercise testing until today. These impairments are prominent in all of the different diagnostic subgroups of patients with CHD, but the severity depends on complexity of the heart defect and the particular consequences [17]. Figure 22.1 characterizes the "Fick principle" where peak oxygen uptake ($VO_2$peak) is an estimate of cardiac output multiplied by the arteriovenous oxygen difference.

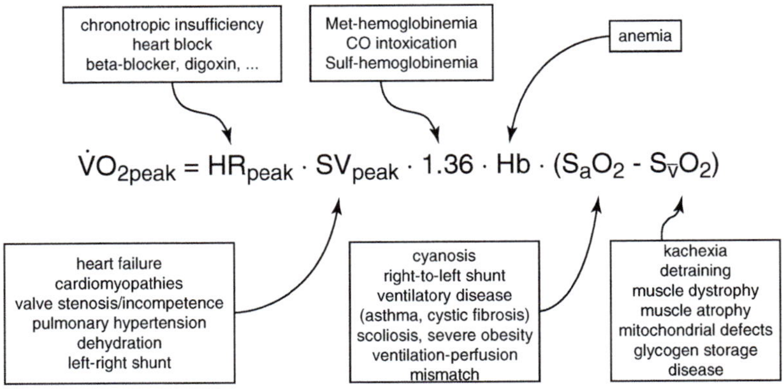


**Fig. 22.1** The classic Fick equation, calculating peak oxygen uptake ($VO_2$peak) as a function of arteriovenous oxygen difference (*S* saturation, *a* arterial, *v* venous), stroke volume (SV), hemoglobin concentration (Hb), and peak heart rate (HR). Each factor may be influenced and altered by particular conditions shown in the boxes, with impact on overall exercise capacity (used with permission from Müller and Hager [28])

Based on this principle the three following components are relevant:

1. Chronotropic insufficiency:
   (a) due to surgical scars around the right atria,
   (b) sinus node dysfunction, and
   (c) delayed electric conduction.
2. The inability to increase stroke volume under exercise:
   (a) Valvular stenosis limiting an adequate increase in stroke volume.
   (b) Right to left shunting where parts of the forward stroke volume shunt to the right heart side.
   (c) Systemic right ventricle that is morphologically not able to drive the systemic circulation.
   (d) Progressive heart failure due to systemic right ventricle.
3. Oxygen utilization:
   (a) Deconditioning or detraining leads to diminished oxygen utilization in the muscle.
   (b) Central cyanosis.
   (c) Comorbidities like respiratory diseases, asthma, obesity and scoliosis, leading to a ventilation-perfusion mismatch.

## 22.5 Physiological Demands of Competitive Sports

While in most exercise intervention studies on patients with CHD the chosen intensities are moderate and dynamic, the physiological demands of competitive sport are different to those applied in these interventions. Competitive athletes often perform higher dynamic intensities of both short and long nature, or have static components included as well as increased psychological pressure. However, there are only few studies that have implemented such demands as part of their interventions. The effect of aerobic training at higher exercise intensities has been evaluated in two studies:

1. *Novaković and colleagues* [12] randomized repaired Tetralogy of Fallot patients to either high-intensity interval, moderate intensity continuous training or usual care (no exercise) for 36 sessions of two to three times a week:
   (a) No adverse events occurred in none of the groups.
   (b) Both training groups improved in at least some parameters of cardiovascular health compared to no exercise.
   (c) Interval, but not continuous training improved $VO_2$peak.
   (d) Interval training appeared more effective in improving exercise capacity, vascular function, NT-proBNP and fibrinogen levels.
   (e) Continuous training was more effective in improving cardiac autonomic function and health-related quality of life.
2. *Sandberg and colleagues* [18] randomized 26 adults with complex CHD into 12 weeks of moderate-to-high intensity interval exercise training on a bicycle ergometer or to maintaining habitual physical activities as a control group:
   (a) Exercise time at a constant work rate cardiopulmonary exercise test increased in the intervention group compared to controls.
   (b) Peak workload at incremental cardiopulmonary exercise testing increased in the intervention group compared to controls.
   (c) At incremental cardiopulmonary exercise testing, $VO_2$peak increased 15% in relative terms in the intervention group, but this was not statistically different to the control group.

Currently there are a couple of randomized controlled trials underway, investigating the effect of high-intensity interval training in patients with CHD. Over the next few years, we will see what the actual requirements of competitive sports at CHD look like, how the body copes with these requirements and how physiological or pathological adaptive mechanisms work in these patients. Not to mention whether intensive and highly intensive exercise poses a safety risk in individual patients.

## 22.6 Competitive Sports Participation in CHD

Several competitive athletes with CHD have participated in the Olympic games. Examples are snowboarder and Olympic gold medal winner Shaun White or short track speed skater Yara van Kerkhof (silver medal winner). Beyond these single cases, there is not much data available on participation of CHD patients in sports in general or in competitive sports. Two studies have dealt with that issue so far. Both studies [19, 20] did not observe an increased incidence of adverse cardiac events in participants. On the other hand, both studies reported beneficial associations with exercise capacity and quality of life:

1. A survey of 177 adolescents and young adults with a mean age of 20 years that focused on physical activity, sports participation and sports restrictions, defining competitive sports as any sport with organized practices and competitions yielded the following findings [21]:
   (a) 52% of patients with CHD participated in competitive sports and 25% in recreational sports; 23% were inactive.
   (b) Male CHD patients were engaged more frequently in competitive sports (60%) than female patients (45%).
   (c) Patients participated in a wide range of competitive sports of different intensities and classifications.
   (d) Almost half of the patients with moderate or severe CHD participated in at least one competitive sport.
   (e) Almost a third of patients with severe CHD and almost half of the patients who had undergone a Fontan procedure participated in sports that would be restricted by the 36th Bethesda guidelines.
2. In adults with CHD a longitudinal study in patients with corrective surgery for atrial septal defect, ventricular septal defect, pulmonary stenosis, tetralogy of Fallot or transposition of the great arteries observed the following [19]:
   (a) Adults with CHD spent less hours in sports as compared with the general population.
   (b) More than half of the patients were involved in high-dynamic sports (Fig. 22.2).

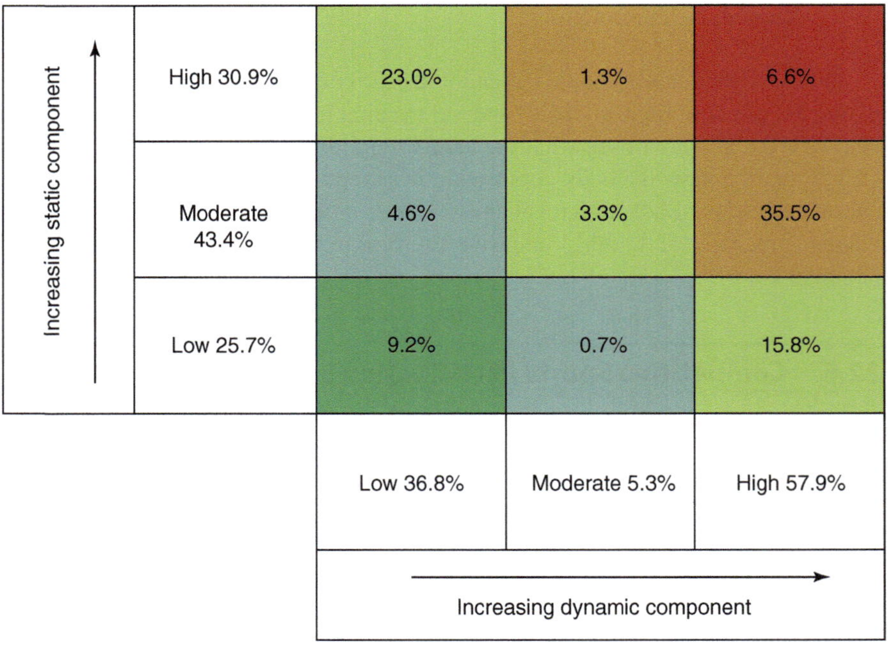


**Fig. 22.2** Distribution of sports participation in various disciplines among CHD patients, according to the Mitchell criteria (used with permission from Opic et al. [19])

(c) The rate of major cardiac events was similar in patients who participated or did not participate in sports.
(d) No relationship was found between practicing sports and the occurrence of sudden death.
(e) Patients who participated in sports showed better exercise capacity and systemic ventricular function.

## 22.7 Aspects of the Congenital Heart Defects

- Patients with CHD show on average a reduced exercise capacity [17, 22].
- The function of the respiratory, cardiovascular and musculoskeletal system are the most important contributing factors:
  - Pulmonary vascular disease with pulmonary hypertension and restrictive pulmonary function disorders can contribute to a reduced exercise capacity as well as a reduced ventilation-perfusion mismatch [23].
  - Cardiovascular factors such as volume and pressure load by the abnormality itself or by residual abnormalities, ventricular dysfunction, coronary anomaly, chronotropic incompetence and arrhythmias, pacing, intracardiac (rest) shunting and (relative) anemia, but also effects of medication may lead to reduction of the exercise capacity (Fig. 22.3).
  - Also, skeletal abnormalities (e.g. scoliosis) can give a limitation.
- Deconditioning is also an important factor in CHD, possibly because patients have often been subject to restrictions to PA in the past [24].

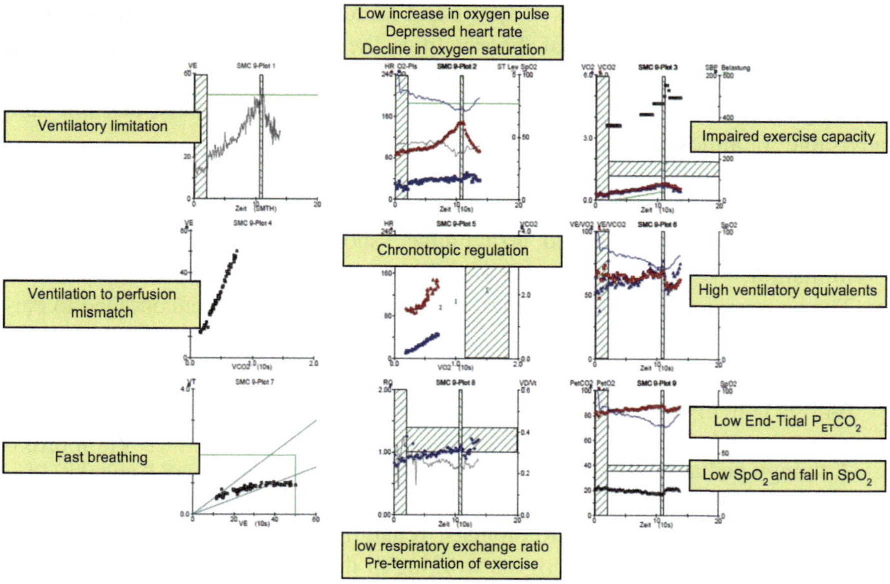


**Fig. 22.3** Special characteristics of a 9-panel-plot in a cardiopulmonary exercise test in a patient with Eisenmenger Syndrome

- Information is scarce on how many patients with CHD are actually engaged in recreational or competitive sport and on the type and intensities of sports they preferably are performing.

## 22.8 Pre-participation Screening

- A preparticipation screening following the Lausanne recommendations [25] including personal and medical history, physical examination, blood pressure and ECG is advised.
- Patients with positive personal history, family history of potentially inherited cardiac disease, or positive physical or ECG findings require further evaluation by cardiac specialist experienced with the particular age group to decide on medical clearance of the athlete for sports participation.
- Further evaluation may include transthoracic echocardiography, cardiac magnetic resonance imaging (MRI), cardiopulmonary exercise test (CPET), and 24-h ECG monitoring.
- Figure 22.4 outlines a thorough assessment in patients with CHD required prior to recommending exercise [14].

## 22.9 Exercise and Training Advices

A certain minimum amount of physical activity (150 min/week in adults; 60 min daily for children and adolescents) is required to achieve health effects. Hemodynamic balance in patients with CHD can vary considerably, also among patients with the same heart defect. Therefore, it is impossible to make recommendations that are applicable in all cases. The risk of sports and exercise participation depends on the specific heart defect and residual abnormalities, the tendency to arrhythmias and the type of sport. Recreational sports participation and exercise in daily life (cycling, walking, gardening, etc.), especially dynamic exercise, is usually possible and advisable for almost all patients with CHD [26].

- Only patients who may deteriorate hemodynamically as a result of exercise, or those with exercise-induced arrhythmias, should be subject to an exercise limitation;
- The large majority with a very low risk can be reassured and encouraged to participate in sporting activities;
- Competitive sports is generally not recommended for CHD patients if an interruption is not possible in case of complaints (logistically or socially).

Although pediatric and congenital cardiologists in general are not trained to provide detailed training advice, they are often confronted with individual requests regarding this issue. Sport cardiologists, rehabilitation specialists, sports physicians, but also exercise physiologists working in the sports medical advice centers

| | | |
|---|---|---|
| **Step 1:** | Assess current status | **A-Assessment of daily activities, including current exercise** (type, intensity, duration, frequency)<br>**B-Evaluation of the motivation for exercise training**<br>**C-Assessment of expectations regarding intended physical activities** (description, duration, enviorment) |
| **Step 2:** | Medical history | **A-Type of congenital heart disease, severity, physiological ramifications**<br>**B-Clinical history** (functional status, exercise intolerance, pre-syncope/syncope, chest pain, palpitations, hypoxia)<br>**C-Pharmacological history** (including anticoagulants and beta-blockers)<br>**D-Cardiac arrhythmia device** (pacemaker, defibrillator, cardiac resynchronization therapy)<br>**E-Associated comorbidities and cardiovascular risk factors** |
| **Step 3:** | Clinical exam | **A-Physical examination** [including a detailed cardiopulmonary exam, skeletal assessment (scoliosis, malformations), and neurologic exam (motor/sensory deficits)]<br>**B-Electrocardiogram** (rhythm, repolarization abnormalities, QRS duration, QTc)<br>**C-Oxygen saturation at rest** |
| **Step 4:** | Paraclinical investigations | **A-Recent assessment of systemic and subpulmonary ventricular function** [standard or stress echocardiography, magnetic resonance imaging (right ventricle), nuclear ventriculography]<br>**C-Assessment for pulmonary hypertension**<br>**D-Rule-out aortic dilation**<br>**B-Ambulatory ECG monitoring** (detection of asymptomatic arrhythmias)<br>**C-Blood tests** (anemia/relative anemia, iron deficiency) |
| **Step 5:** | CPET | **Peak oxygen consumption ($VO_{2max}$), peak oxygen pulse**<br>**$VE/VCO_2$ slope and $VE/VO_2$ slope**<br>**Anaerobic or lactate threshold**<br>**Oxygen saturation during exercise, exercise duration**<br>**Heart rate and blood pressure response** |

**Fig. 22.4** Preparticipation assessment scheme (used with permission from Chaix et al. [14])

can be consulted to give a formal training advice. The cardiologist will have an advisory role to adapt the advice to the specific CHD. Exercise is prescribed according to the **FITT** principle, indicating frequency, intensity, duration and type of sport (see also Chap. 11). A recommendation can be for example three times a week (**F**) at a moderate to intensive level (**I**) for 30–60 min (**T**) cycling (**T**) with the aim of aerobic endurance training. According to the same principle, the structure of interval training and strength training can be described. The results of a CPET are also useful to determine the extent and causes of potential limitations during physical effort.

- The scientific knowledge regarding the effects of training in CHD is limited. The studies that have been carried out show that patients basically benefit from a training program [10, 12] with respect to beneficial physical and psychosocial outcomes.
- An obstacle for implementing cardiac rehabilitation for patients with CHD is that, compared to standard cardiac rehabilitation, there are fewer patients who can participate in such a program and that reimbursement from insurance companies is not guaranteed in every case.
- In addition, the age of patients with CHD is much lower than the average participant in regular cardiac rehabilitation; CHD patients are thus underrepresented and do often not feel comfortable in these programs.

## 22.10 Specific Recommendations

The most recent eligibility and disqualification recommendations for competitive athletes with CHD have been published by the American Heart Association and the American College of Cardiology [27]. In this document, the level of sports participation recommended includes consideration of both the training and the competitive aspects of the activity; these must be individually tailored to the particular patient, taking into account the patient's functional status and a history of surgery.

### 22.10.1 Atrial Septal Defect (ASD)

- Small ASD with normal right ventricle (RV) and no pulmonary hypertension: Full participation (Class I, Level of evidence C)
- Large ASD and no pulmonary hypertension: Full participation (I, C)
- ASD and pulmonary hypertension: Allowed to participate in low intensity IA sports (Fig. 1.1) (I, C)
- ASD and pulmonary vascular disease, cyanosis, and right to left shunt: Restricted from all competitive sports, with the possible exception of IA (III, C)
- History of ASD repair or device and no pulmonary hypertension: Full participation (I, C)
- History of ASD repair or device and residual pulmonary hypertension, arrhythmias, or myocardial dysfunction: Allowed to participate in IA sports (IIb, C)

### 22.10.2 Ventricular Septal Defect (VSD)

- Small or restrictive VSD with normal RV size and no pulmonary hypertension: Full participation (I, C)
- Large, hemodynamically significant VSD and pulmonary hypertension: Allowed to participate in IA sports (IIb, C)
- History of VSD repair with no pulmonary hypertension, arrhythmias, or myocardial dysfunction: Full participation (I, C)

- History of VSD repair and residual pulmonary hypertension: Allowed to participate in IA sports (I, B)
- History of VSD repair with mild to moderate pulmonary hypertension or ventricular dysfunction: Restricted from all competitive sports, with the possible exception of IA (III, C)

### 22.10.3 Persistent Ductus Arteriosus (PDA)

- Small PDA with normal pulmonary artery pressures and normal left heart chambers: Full participation (I, C)
- Moderate to large PDA with persistent pulmonary hypertension: Only allowed to participate in IA sports (I, B)
- Moderate to large PDA with left ventricular enlargement: Full restrictions (III, C)
- History of surgical or catheter PDA closure and no evidence of pulmonary hypertension: Full participation (I, C)
- History of surgical or catheter PDA closure and residual pulmonary hypertension: Restricted from all competitive sports, with the possible exception of IA (I, B)

### 22.10.4 Pulmonary Valve Stenosis

- Mild pulmonary valve stenosis and normal RV function: Full participation (I, B)
- Moderate or severe pulmonary valve stenosis: Allowed to participate in IA and IB sports (IIb, B)
- History of pulmonary valve surgery or balloon valvuloplasty and gradient <40 mmHg: Full participation (I, B)
- Severe pulmonary insufficiency with marked RV enlargement: Allowed to participate in IA and IB sports (IIb, B)

### 22.10.5 Aortic Valve Stenosis

- Mild aortic valve stenosis: Full participation (I, B)
- Moderate aortic valve stenosis: Allowed to participate in IA, IB, IIA sports (IIb, B)
- Severe aortic valve stenosis: Allowed to participate in IA sports (I, B)
- Severe aortic valve stenosis: Restricted from all competitive sports, with the possible exception of IA (III, B)
- Residual aortic valve stenosis after surgical or catheter intervention: Considered for participation based on untreated recommendations (IIb, C)

### 22.10.6 Coarctation of the Aorta

- Untreated coarctation of the aorta without ascending aorta dilation and normal exercise test and <20 mmHg blood pressure gradient: Full participation (I, C)

- Untreated coarctation of the aorta and blood pressure gradient >20 mmHg or abnormal exercise stress test or significant ascending aorta dilation: Allowed to participate in IA sports (IIb, C)
- History of coarctation repair or stent and blood pressure gradient <20 mmHg, normal exercise test, no ascending aorta dilation, no aneurysm, and no concomitant aortic valve disease: Allowed to participate in IA, IB, IC, IIA, IIB, IIC sports (IIb, C)
- History of coarctation of the aorta repair or stent and significant aortic dilation or aneurysm: Allowed to participate in IA and IB sports (IIb, C)

### 22.10.7 Tetralogy of Fallot (ToF)

- History of ToF repair and no ventricular dysfunction, arrhythmias, or outflow tract obstruction and a normal exercise test: Full participation (IIb, B)
- History of ToF repair and severe ventricular dysfunction, severe outflow tract obstruction or recurrent or uncontrolled atrial or ventricular arrhythmias: Restricted from all competitive sports, with the possible exception of IA (III, B)

### 22.10.8 Ebstein Anomaly

- Mild to moderate Ebstein anomaly without cyanosis, normal RV size, less than moderate tricuspid valve regurgitation, and no arrhythmias: Full participation (IIb, C)
- Ebstein anomaly with severe tricuspid valve regurgitation but no arrhythmias: Allowed to participate in IA sports (IIb, C)

### 22.10.9 Transposition of the Great Arteries (d-TGA) After Atrial Switch (Senning or Mustard Procedure)

- History of Mustard or Senning procedure operation for d-TGA arteries if they have no arrhythmias or ventricular dysfunction: Allowed to participate in IA, IB, IIA, IIB sports (IIb, C)
- History of Mustard or Senning procedure operation for d-TGA and a history of arrhythmias, RV dysfunction, or severe RV outflow tract obstruction: Restricted from all competitive sports, with the possible exception of IA (III, C)

### 22.10.10 Transposition of the Great Arteries After Anatomical Correction (Arterial Switch Procedure)

- History of arterial switch procedure for d-TGA without symptoms, normal ventricular function and no tachyarrhythmias: Full participation (IIb, C)
- History of arterial switch procedure for d-TGA and more than mild hemodynamic abnormalities or ventricular dysfunction with normal exercise testing: Allowed to participate in IA, IB, IC and IIA (IIb, C)

- History of arterial switch procedure for d-TGA with evidence of ischemia: Restricted from all sports with possible exception of IA (III, C)

### 22.10.11 Congenital Corrected Transposition of the Great Arteries (CCTGA)

- CCTGA without arrhythmias, ventricular dysfunction, exercise intolerance, or exercise-induced ischemia: Participation in IA and IB sports and may be considered for IIA, IIB, IIIB and IIIB (IIb, C)
- CCTGA severe clinical systemic RV dysfunction, severe RV outflow tract obstruction, or recurrent or uncontrolled atrial or ventricular arrhythmias: Restricted from all competitive sports, with the possible exception of IA (III, C)

### 22.10.12 Univentricular Heart After any Kind of Fontan Procedure

- History of Fontan procedure with no symptoms and no hemodynamic abnormalities: Allowed to participate in IA sports (I, C)
- History of Fontan procedure without evidence of abnormalities on exercise stress test: Sports may be considered on individual basis (IIb, C)

### 22.10.13 Unrepaired or Palliated Cyanotic CHD

- Unrepaired cyanotic heart disease who are clinically stable and asymptomatic: Allowed to participate in IA sports (IIb, C)

**Clinical Pearls**

- Patients with CHD should adhere to an active lifestyle and participate in leisure sport activities. However, the boundaries between leisure time and competitive sport have already become blurred.
- Comprehensive pre-participation screening is essential for minimizing the risk of adverse events during sport participation.
- Recommendations for competitive sports but must be individualized to the particular patient, taking into account the patient's preferences, functional status and history of surgery.

## Review

## Questions

1. During preparticipation screening a 20-year old male soccer player with repaired coarctation of the Aorta develops slight ST segment depression during a cardiopulmonary exercise test. Would you initiate further examinations, or would you basically disqualify him from exercising, with this information in mind?
2. Why is chronotropic insufficiency often observed in patients with CHD?

3. Which factors play a role in the observed exercise intolerance of patients with CHD?

## Answers

1. Mild ST depressions can frequently be observed during physical stress in patients with coarctation of the Aorta; they do not require further diagnostics. Therefore, at this point there is no reason to prohibit exercise. However, this finding should nonetheless be monitored regularly.
2. Chronotropic incompetence is often caused by surgical scars around the right atria, sinus node dysfunction and/or delayed electric conduction.
3. The function of the respiratory, cardiovascular and musculoskeletal system are the most important factors. Musculoskeletal abnormalities can also play a role (e.g. scoliosis). Moreover, deconditioning is also an important factor contributing to reduced exercise capacity.

## References

1. Hirth A, Reybrouck T, Bjarnason-Wehrens B, Lawrenz W, Hoffmann A. Recommendations for participation in competitive and leisure sports in patients with congenital heart disease: a consensus document. Eur J Cardiovasc Prev Rehabil. 2006;13(3):293–9.
2. Longmuir PE, Brothers JA, de Ferranti SD, Hayman LL, Van Hare GF, Matherne GP, et al. Promotion of physical activity for children and adults with congenital heart disease: a scientific statement from the American Heart Association. Circulation. 2013;127(21):2147–59.
3. Takken T, Giardini A, Reybrouck T, Gewillig M, Hovels-Gurich HH, Longmuir PE, et al. Recommendations for physical activity, recreation sport, and exercise training in paediatric patients with congenital heart disease: a report from the Exercise, Basic & Translational Research Section of the European Association of Cardiovascular Prevention and Rehabilitation, the European Congenital Heart and Lung Exercise Group, and the Association for European Paediatric Cardiology. Eur J Prev Cardiol. 2012;19(5):1034–65.
4. Triedman JK, Newburger JW. Trends in congenital heart disease: the next decade. Circulation. 2016;133(25):2716–33.
5. Tutarel O. Acquired heart conditions in adults with congenital heart disease: a growing problem. Heart. 2014;100(17):1317–21.
6. Tikkanen AU, Oyaga AR, Riano OA, Alvaro EM, Rhodes J. Paediatric cardiac rehabilitation in congenital heart disease: a systematic review. Cardiol Young. 2012;22:1–10.
7. Gomes-Neto M, Saquetto MB, da Silva e Silva CM, Conceicao CS, Carvalho VO. Impact of exercise training in aerobic capacity and pulmonary function in children and adolescents after congenital heart disease surgery: a systematic review with meta-analysis. Pediatr Cardiol. 2016;37(2):217–24.
8. Dulfer K, Helbing WA, Utens E. The influence of exercise training on quality of life and psychosocial functioning in children with congenital heart disease:a review of intervention studies. Sports (Basel). 2017;5(1):E13.
9. Brassard P, Bedard E, Jobin J, Rodes-Cabau J, Poirier P. Exercise capacity and impact of exercise training in patients after a Fontan procedure: a review. Can J Cardiol. 2006;22(6):489–95.
10. Duppen N, Takken T, Hopman MT, Ten Harkel AD, Dulfer K, Utens EM, et al. Systematic review of the effects of physical exercise training programmes in children and young adults with congenital heart disease. Int J Cardiol. 2013;168(3):1779–87.

11. Opotowsky AR, Rhodes J, Landzberg MJ, Bhatt AB, Shafer KM, Yeh DD, et al. A randomized trial comparing cardiac rehabilitation to standard of care for adults with congenital heart disease. World J Pediatr Congenit Heart Surg. 2018;9(2):185–93.
12. Kovacs AH, Kaufman TM, Broberg CS. Cardiac rehabilitation for adults with congenital heart disease: physical and psychosocial considerations. Can J Cardiol. 2018;34(10S2):S270–S7.
13. Dua JS, Cooper AR, Fox KR, Stuart AG. Exercise training in adults with congenital heart disease: feasibility and benefits. Int J Cardiol. 2010;138(2):196–205.
14. Chaix MA, Marcotte F, Dore A, Mongeon FP, Mondesert B, Mercier LA, et al. Risks and benefits of exercise training in adults with congenital heart disease. Can J Cardiol. 2016;32(4):459–66.
15. WHO. Global recommendations on physical activity for health. Geneva: World Health Organization; 2010.
16. Mitchell JH, Haskell W, Snell P, Van Camp SP. Task Force 8: classification of sports. J Am Coll Cardiol. 2005;45(8):1364–7.
17. Kempny A, Dimopoulos K, Uebing A, Moceri P, Swan L, Gatzoulis MA, et al. Reference values for exercise limitations among adults with congenital heart disease. Relation to activities of daily life—single centre experience and review of published data. Eur Heart J. 2012;33(11):1386–96.
18. Sandberg C, Hedstrom M, Wadell K, Dellborg M, Ahnfelt A, Zetterstrom AK, et al. Home-based interval training increases endurance capacity in adults with complex congenital heart disease. Congenit Heart Dis. 2018;13(2):254–62.
19. Opic P, Utens EM, Cuypers JA, Witsenburg M, van den Bosch A, van Domburg R, et al. Sports participation in adults with congenital heart disease. Int J Cardiol. 2015;187:175–82.
20. Dean PN, Gillespie CW, Greene EA, Pearson GD, Robb AS, Berul CI, et al. Sports participation and quality of life in adolescents and young adults with congenital heart disease. Congenit Heart Dis. 2015;10(2):169–79.
21. Dean PN, Battle RW. Congenital heart disease and the athlete: what we know and what we do not know. Cardiol Clin. 2016;34(4):579–89.
22. Diller GP, Dimopoulos K, Okonko D, Li W, Babu-Narayan SV, Broberg CS, et al. Exercise intolerance in adult congenital heart disease: comparative severity, correlates, and prognostic implication. Circulation. 2005;112(6):828–35.
23. Dimopoulos K, Okonko DO, Diller GP, Broberg CS, Salukhe TV, Babu-Narayan SV, et al. Abnormal ventilatory response to exercise in adults with congenital heart disease relates to cyanosis and predicts survival. Circulation. 2006;113(24):2796–802.
24. Swan L, Hillis WS. Exercise prescription in adults with congenital heart disease: a long way to go. Heart. 2000;83(6):685–7.
25. Bille K, Figueiras D, Schamasch P, Kappenberger L, Brenner JI, Meijboom FJ, et al. Sudden cardiac death in athletes: the Lausanne recommendations. Eur J Cardiovasc Prev Rehabil. 2006;13(6):859–75.
26. Budts W, Borjesson M, Chessa M, van Buuren F, Trigo Trindade P, Corrado D, et al. Physical activity in adolescents and adults with congenital heart defects: individualized exercise prescription. Eur Heart J. 2013;34(47):3669–74.
27. Van Hare GF, Ackerman MJ, Evangelista JA, Kovacs RJ, Myerburg RJ, Shafer KM, et al. Eligibility and disqualification recommendations for competitive athletes with cardiovascular abnormalities: task force 4: congenital heart disease: a scientific statement from the American Heart Association and American College of Cardiology. Circulation. 2015;132(22):e281–91.
28. Müller J, Cardiac HA. Exercise physiology in adolescence. In: Schwerzmann M, Thomet C, Moons P, editors. Congenital heart disease and adolescence. Congenital heart disease in adolescents and adults. New York: Springer International Publishing; 2016. p. 43–57.

# Specific Populations: Paediatric and Adolescent Athletes

# 23

Guido E. Pieles, Andrew Maxwell, and Renate Oberhoffer

**Learning Objectives**

1. Understand the specifics of physiological training adaptations in paediatric athletes
2. Learn about diagnostic pathways and tools specific to the paediatric athlete population
3. Differentiate between physiological and pathological cardiac findings in paediatric athletes
4. Learn about the common cardiac problems encountered in paediatric athletes
5. Be aware of the gaps in research and clinical knowledge in paediatric sports cardiology

G. E. Pieles (✉)
Congenital Heart Unit, Bristol Heart Institute, Bristol, UK
e-mail: guido.pieles@bristol.ac.uk

A. Maxwell
Department of Pediatric Cardiology, Heart of the Valley Pediatric Cardiology, Pleasanton, CA, USA
e-mail: amaxwell@heartofthevalley.us

R. Oberhoffer
Department of Preventative Paediatrics, Faculty of Sports and Health Sciences, Technical University of Munich, Munich, Germany
e-mail: renate.oberhoffer@tum.de



A. Pressler, J. Niebauer (eds.), *Textbook of Sports and Exercise Cardiology*,
https://doi.org/10.1007/978-3-030-35374-2_23

## 23.1 Introduction

### 23.1.1 Paediatric Activity Recommendations

Overall, healthy children are more active than adults. Public health guidelines recommend that children should minimise sedentary activity and integrate sports and exercise into their daily lives.

Selected international activity recommendations, adapted from [1]:

- World Health Organisation (WHO 2011, 5–17 years)
  - At least 60 min of moderate to vigorous physical activity daily, >60 min provide additional health benefits. Most physical activity should be aerobic.
  - Vigorous-intensity activities at least 3 days/week.
  - Activities that strengthen muscle and bone at least 3 days/week.
- Canadian Society for Exercise Physiology (CSEP 2012, 5–17 year)
  - 60 min of moderate to vigorous physical activity daily.
  - Vigorous-intensity activities at least 3 days/week,
  - Activities that strengthen muscle and bone at least 3 days/week.
  - Sedentary screen time max. 2 h/day.
- U.S. Department of Health and Human Services (HHS 2008, update 2018, Children and adolescents)
  - At least 60 min of moderate to vigorous physical activity daily
  - Most moderate or vigorous aerobic physical activity,
  - Vigorous-intensity activities at least 3 days/week
  - Activities that strengthen muscle and bone at least 3 days/week.
- UK Department of Health (DoH, 2011, 5–18 years)
  - At least 60 min of moderate to vigorous physical activity daily
  - Activities that strengthen muscle and bone at least 3 days/week.
  - Minimise sedentary time.
- Australian Government Department of Health, 2005, 5–18 years)
  - At least 60 min of moderate to vigorous physical activity daily
  - 2 hours per day maximum time using electronic media for entertainment.

The need for this formal guidance reflects both the overwhelming evidence of health benefit from regular physical exercise and the increasingly sedentary nature of childhood. For example, in the United Kingdom, only 14% of 13–15 year old boys and 9% of girls achieved recommended physical activity levels—a figure which has fallen from 28% in boys and 14% in girls in 2008 [2] (Figs 23.1, 23.2, and 23.3).

At the other end of the activity spectrum, there is a subgroup of paediatric athletes who compete at an increasingly high level. Many elite, competitive paediatric athletes will train for over 20 h per week—a duration of exercise similar to professional adult athletes. Excessive training can have a detrimental effects on the developing musculoskeletal system leading to overuse injuries [3]. Similarly, the syndrome of overtraining and burnout is now well recognised in elite paediatric athletes [4] and this emphasises the need for specialised medical care for the paediatric athlete population.

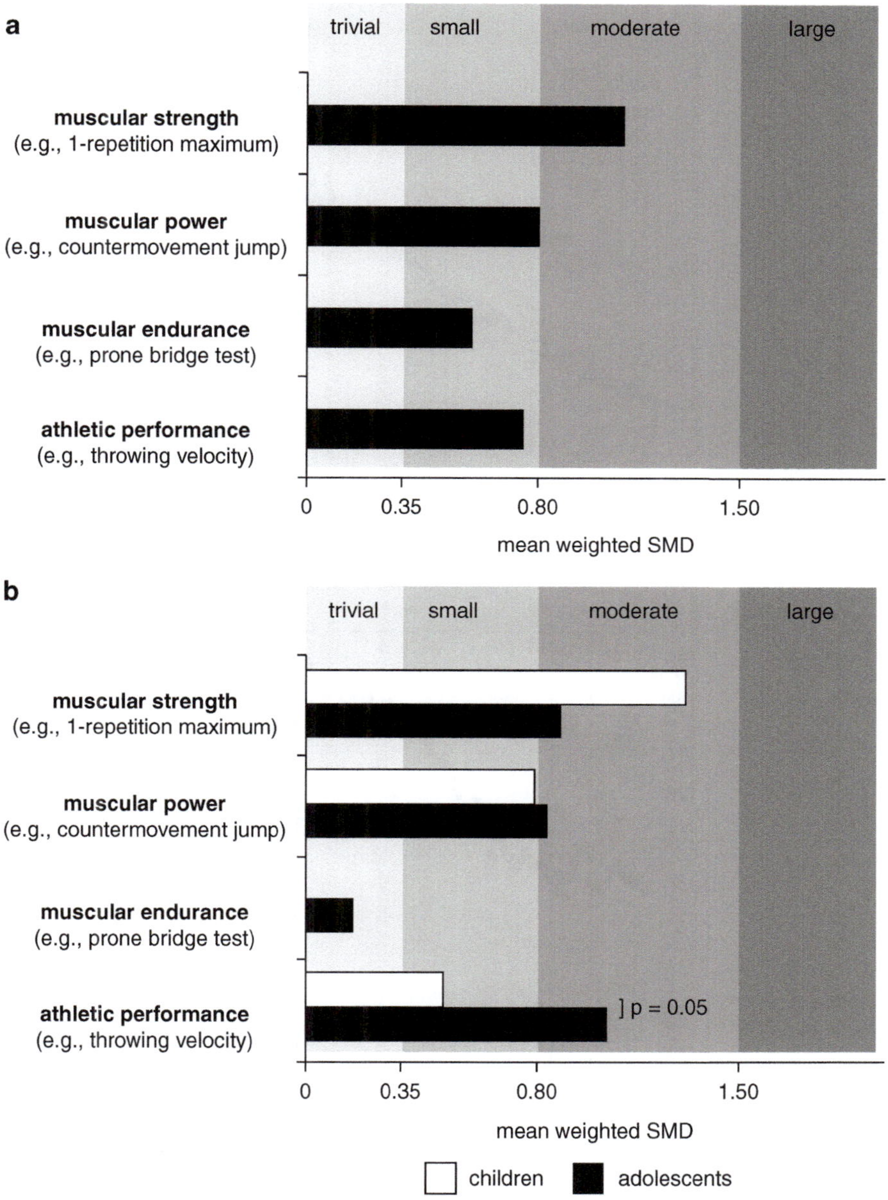


**Fig. 23.1** Effects of resistance training on various measures of muscular strength, derived from a comprehensive analysis of controlled trials. (**a**) shows the overall effects in paediatric athletes aged 6–18 years, whereas (**b**) compares subgroup effects in children vs. adolescents (reprinted with permission from [126]). *SMD* standard mean difference

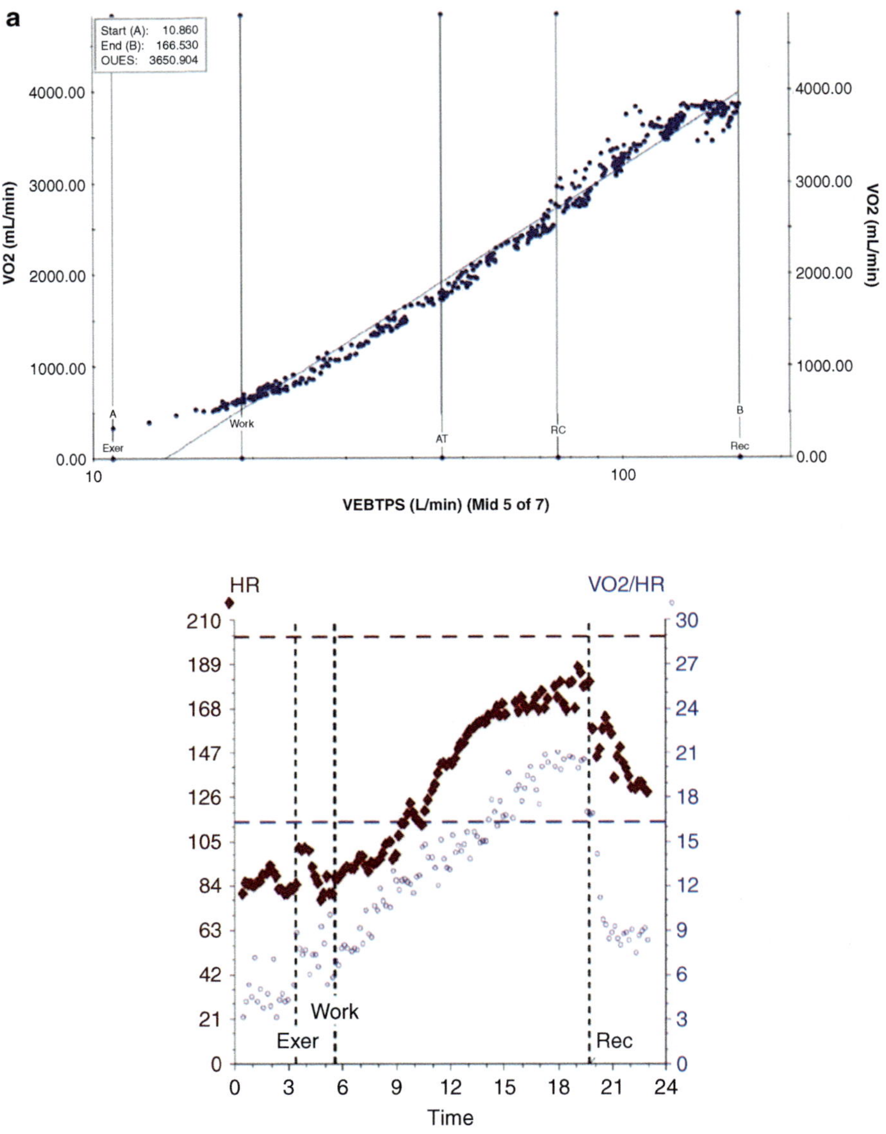


**Fig. 23.2** Oxygen uptake efficiency Slopes, and Heart Rate and Peak Oxygen Pulse Curves of (**a**) an athlete with congenitally absent pericardium and unusually high peak oxygen pulse (surrogate for stroke volume) versus (**b**) a patient with exercise deconditioning with low peak oxygen pulse

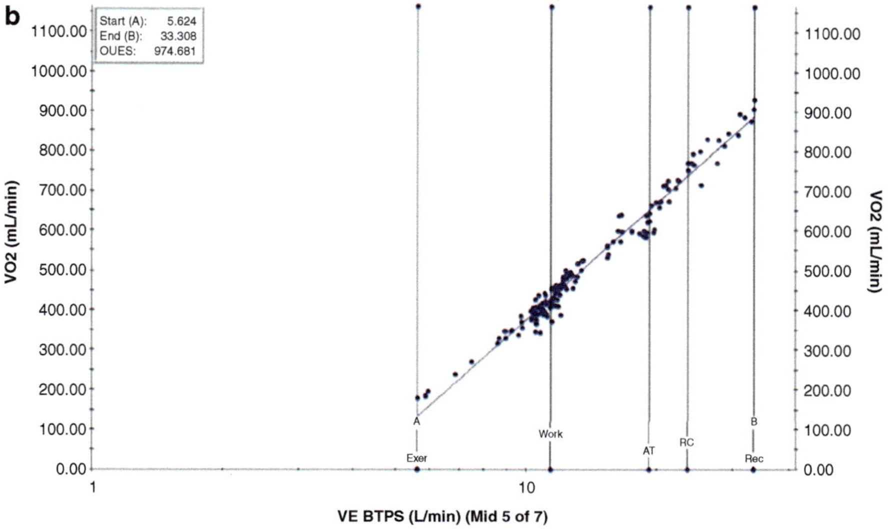


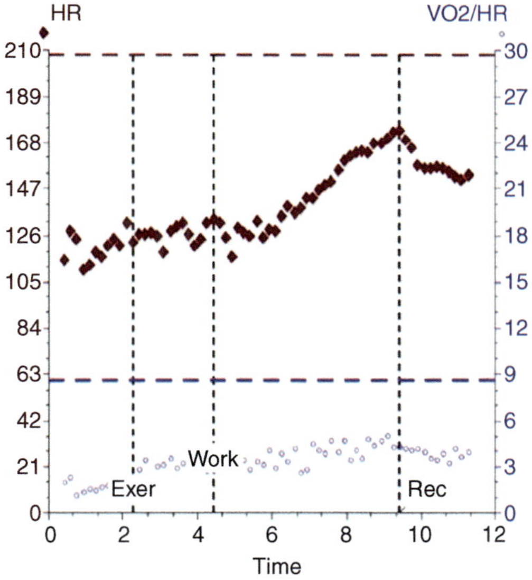


**Fig. 23.2** (continued)

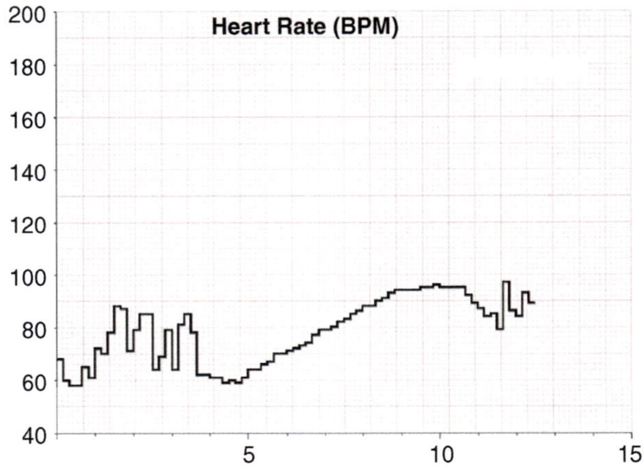


**Fig. 23.3** Heart rate over the course of exercise stress testing in a 10-year-old with a history of SSA-mediated congenital complete heart block that improved by 3 years of age to first-degree and intermittent second-degree heart block at rest. Upon exercise testing, the normal sinus rhythm with first degree block reverts to 2:1 block with intermittent complete heart block

### 23.1.2 Epidemiology of Disease and Sudden Cardiac Death

2000 children die each year from sudden cardiac death (SCD) in the US, the incidence from available studies ranges from 0.6 to 8/100,000 [5, 6]. The prevalence of conditions associated with SCD in young athletes is as high as 0.2–0.7% [7]. The aetiology of SCD in childhood is comparable to those in young adult athletes; however, age of presentation differs for inherited cardiac conditions explaining slightly different aetiological frequencies [8, 9]. The first disease presentation is in 50% sudden cardiac arrest, providing a strong argument of early detection of disease by screening [10, 11]. Despite controversy regarding the most suitable methodology to perform cardiac screening to prevent SCD [12], there is evidence that screening strategies have reduced the number of SCD in childhood, adolescent and young adult athletes [13–15].

Causes of SCD in the paediatric athlete population [16, 17]:

- Structural heart disease (44%):
  - Coronary artery abnormalities (11%)
  - Idiopathic left ventricular hypertrophy/fibrosis (10%)
  - Arrhythmogenic right ventricular cardiomyopathy (6%)
  - Hypertrophic cardiomyopathy (6%)
  - Myocarditis (2%)
  - Other structural diseases (9%)
- Non-structural heart disease (56%; individual incidence uncertain):
  - Long QT syndrome
  - Brugada syndrome
  - Catecholaminergic polymorphic ventricular tachycardia
  - Idiopathic ventricular tachycardia
  - Wolf-Parkinson-White syndrome

## 23.2 Specifics of Cardiac Training Adaptation in the Paediatric Athlete

The management of paediatric athletes is complicated by the fact of somatic growth and psycho-cognitive maturation and peculiar entities of the pediatric age group including legal aspects with integration of the parents. Therefore, an interdisciplinary approach of paediatrics, paediatric cardiology and sports medicine is essential. Commonly, the paediatric patient is defined as an individual of up to 16 years of age, we follow here the following definition.

1. Population and physiological maturation
   (a) Definition of young athlete: 12–17 years old [18]
   (b) Physiological gender related development during this period: puberty growth, hormone dependent bone and muscle mass maturation, changes of motoric entities (endurance, speed, strength, balance), age and weight related heart rate, blood pressure and cardiac output, respiratory capacity, peak oxygen uptake.
   (c) Higher rate of sport related accidents at younger age due to physiological changes of psychological and cognitive system (e.g. self-overestimation at pubertal age).
2. Structural and functional adaptations to exercise
   (a) Adaptation of muscle strength and athletic performance: dependent on age and gender.
   (b) Cardiovascular adaptation: response to regular training (especially endurance) comparable to adult life (decrease of resting heart rate, increase of cardiac output, ventricular cavity size and wall thickness, enlargement of aortic root diameter). Endurance sport at ages <15 years: more pronounced heart rate mediated adaptation and attenuated diastolic function; long term effect unknown [19].
   (c) Development of "athlete's heart" hormone and age dependent, mostly from puberty on and more common in males.
   (d) Corresponding ECG changes also more pronounced >14 years [20].
3. Sport specific adaptations and considerations
   (a) Most pronounced cardiovascular adaptations in classical endurance sports like rowing, triathlon and swimming [21].
   (b) Contact sports: capability of the still flexible thorax to transduce pressure waves conveys a higher risk for commotio cordis (Chap. 27).

## 23.3 Diagnostic Tools and Their Specific Use in the Paediatric Athlete

There has been much of discussion on when, to which extent and if at all the young athlete, especially before puberty, should be screened before participating in competitive sports. However, even if the tragic event of sudden cardiac death is rare, many inherited diseases can be suspected, defined or excluded by experienced paediatric cardiologists. One of the most important and less expensive diagnostic tools are family and the personal medical history and physical examination. The AEPC working group Sports Cardiology, Physical Activity and Prevention stresses this point in its recommendations [22].

### 23.3.1 Medical History

- Number and extent of weekly training and the beginning of the career as an athlete in order to interpret ECG findings, echocardiography and exercise test.
- Recent infections (myocarditis risk) to give advice on training intensity and volume. In general, infections with pyrexia should mandate a break, whereas in simple upper airway infections without severe clinical signs, light endurance training can be continued [23, 24].
- Nutritional aspects: athlete's anorexia is common especially in gymnastics with a female predominance [25]. Moreover, nutritional supplements can show many side effects, like adrenergic overstimulation with the risk of life threatening arrhythmias in energy drinks [26] or the risk of liver adenoma in steroids [27].
- Symptoms of palpitations, exercise dependent respiratory symptoms, dizziness and syncope should be evaluated.
- Medication use needs to be determined, as some medicaments are listed ("Cologne List") equivalent to doping, and some can cause side effects.
- Vaccination status should be documented, and recent vaccinations might influence training recommendations.

### 23.3.2 Family History

- Cardiovascular disease (either congenital or acquired) and risk factors (dyslipidemia, hypertension, diabetes) as well as sudden cardiac death.
- Assessment for syndromes, many are associated with cardiac disease (e.g. signs of connective tissue disease, Marfan syndrome, Williams syndrome, Turner syndrome). This is particularly important when assessing Paralympic athletes.

### 23.3.3 Physical Examination

- Full cardiac examination including pulses in hand and feet (cave: coarctation).
- Assessment for signs of cardiac disease and cardiac compromise.
- Assessment for syndromes.
- Blood pressure measurement. Elevated isolated systolic blood pressure is often found during physical examination of young athletic men and has to be followed up closely after ruling out arterial hypertension by ambulatory blood pressure

monitoring. Central blood pressure should be estimated using an oscillometric or tonometric device: in case it's normal, there is no need for antihypertensive treatment [28]. Exclude aortic pathology (e.g coarctation).

### 23.3.4 12-Lead ECG

The minimum of pre-participation screening besides a proper history and physical examination includes a resting ECG. The interpretation follows routine age- and height-dependent reference values [29] with respect to heart rate, time intervals, heart axis, negative precordial T waves, and signs of hypertrophy. At present, ECG interpretation is based on the international criteria for athlete's ECG [30] (Chap. 8). They have reasonable accuracy in the paediatric athletes [31], but it has to be taken into consideration, that they are valid only from 14 years of age. Thus, in younger age, there is a grey zone regarding young athlete's ECG.

### 23.3.5 Echocardiography

As in the interpretation of the ECG, also echocardiographic examinations should be in the hands of experienced paediatric cardiologists. At least once in the career of a young athlete, at the beginning, congenital heart disease should be ruled out. There is no consensus on frequency of echocardiography in this setting, but there is also no clear evidence, at which time some cardiomyopathies start to develop. There seems to be an influence of testosterone around puberty, so it may be wise to echocardiographically follow up young elite athletes every 2 years. In many cases, it might be difficult to differentiate the cardiac remodelling caused especially by endurance sports from beginning pathological cardiomyopathies. In these cases, more detailed examinations should be undertaken (see below).

Echocardiographic examination should not only rule out congenital heart disease; also signs of myocarditis have to be distinguished. The routine morphometric and functional measurements are age and length dependent [32], should hence be z-scored and should include:

- left and right ventricular dimensions and function (at least shortening fraction, diastolic Doppler and myocardial Doppler parameters like E/A and E/e', left atrial and aortic root diameters, mitral and tricuspid annular plane systolic excursion (MAPSE, TAPSE)).
- assessment of structural and functional adaptation to training. The developmental process (onset, duration) of structural and functional cardiac response to training in the young is still not completely understood, and differentiation is challenging between athlete's heart and early pathological myocardial changings in LV non-compaction (LVNC), hypertrophic cardiomyopathy (HCM), and arrhythmogenic right ventricular cardiomyopathy (ARVC).

- assessment for coronary artery anomalies. This might require cross-sectional imaging in some cases.
- Speckle tracking, tissue Doppler imaging and stress echo as specific methods for further secondary investigations and scientific research.

### 23.3.6 Exercise Assessment

The tools of exercise assessment of athletes are presented in detail in Chap. 11. This section highlights the differences in the paediatric athlete population. Exercise testing in the paediatric athlete differs from that of the adult athlete, as the paediatric athlete demonstrates additional challenges in utilizing various exercise protocols and in attaining similar exercise endpoints compared to adults. They also demonstrate a different cardiovascular response to exercise. Moreover, attaining peak performance may be limited primarily by conditions such as pulmonary disease, arrhythmias, chest wall and spine deformities, and presence of congenital heart disease rather than by signs of myocardial ischaemia.

Exercise testing in the paediatric athlete is usually done to

(a) document physical work capacity.
(b) be a provocative challenge.
(c) provide additional diagnostic information about exercise limitations to guide possible medical management.
(d) allay the concerns for sports participation by parents, coaches, and physical education instructors over cardiac symptoms which have been fuelled by the tragic events of sudden cardiac death [33].

## 23.4 Exercise Stress ECG

The unique cardiopulmonary, vascular, and musculoskeletal variants and pathologies of the paediatric athlete necessitate additional roles of exercise testing. The specific indication will guide the specific procedure selected. In its simplest use, exercise ECG interpretation of electrophysiological changes can assess such pathologies as:

- Impairment in chronotropy due to degrees of heart block and congenital heart disease.
- Ventricular ectopy response with increasing heart rate.
- Functional coronary insufficiency in Kawasaki's disease or congenital coronary anomalies.
- Determination of ventricular repolarization in those with Long QT syndrome, perhaps more accurately than that calculated by sedentary 12-lead [34].
- Changes in antegrade conduction via accessory pathways in WPW [35, 36].

- Elicitation of suspected occult arrhythmias such as catecholaminergic polymorphic ventricular tachycardia (CPVT) [37] or arrythmogenic right ventricular cardiomyopathy (ARVC).

Exercise ECG interpretations can lead to risk stratification allowing clearance for participation, informing on the necessity of interventions before clearance, or the necessity of prohibiting further athletic participation.

## 23.5 Cardio-pulmonary Exercise Testing (CPET)

Adding in pulmonary function assessment and gas exchange, cardio-pulmonary exercise testing (CPET) measures allow more detailed evaluations of various parts of the respiratory chain [38].

- Pulmonary function assessment begins with the airways and lungs identifying the degree of impairment caused by
  - reactive airways disease,
  - pectus excavatum/carinatum [39], or
  - muscular dystrophy.
- Gas exchange measures can identify impairment of
  - stroke volume caused by cardiomyopathy or ventricular dysfunction,
  - pulmonary vascular disease,
  - dysfunction of the autonomic nervous system, or
  - peripheral defects in oxygen transport and oxygen utilization at the working muscle.

## 23.6 Differences in Procedure

- Body size and strength, the developmental age, and individual motivation must be taken into consideration when selecting the best protocol in paediatric athletes:
  - Equipment that is scalable to the size of the athlete (cycle ergometers with height-adjustable seats, reach-adjustable handlebars, and pedal cranks, treadmills with adjustable handrails).
  - Blood pressure cuffs in multiple sizes.
  - Personnel trained at working with young people, paramount to encourage maximal effort [33].
- Testing equipment modalities:
  - Treadmill or cycle ergometer.
  - Crank arm ergometry when handicapped or an injured lower limb [40].
  - Rowing ergometry is also feasible in paediatrics [41].

The choice of modality is based on an athlete's discipline and comfort, familiarity, safety, and the potential for reproducing signs and symptoms that occurred with a similar stress in the ambulatory setting.

## 23.7 Differences in Outcome Variables

The outcome variables assessed by CPET are similar to those used in adults, but there is a different emphasis on some variables (see also Chap. 45).

### 23.7.1 Maximal and Submaximal Exercise Parameters

- **$VO_2$max** is the "gold standard" of physical fitness in adults, but it's difficult to get a paediatric athlete to achieve a *true* $VO_2$max [42].
  - submaximal values are emphasized in paediatrics (e.g. **peak $VO_2$**) which correlate well with predicted $VO_2$max.
  - correlation of predicted peak VO2 is improved by application of correction factors for weight [43].
- **PWC170** measures physical work capacity at a heart rate of 170 bpm achieved by cycle ergometry.
- **Oxygen Uptake Efficiency Slope (OUES)**: Newer concepts have been developed to better assess peak fitness especially in those with congenital heart disease [44–46].
- **Ventilatory Anaerobic Threshold (VAT)**:
  - the measure of $VO_2$ at the point during a progressive exercise test where anaerobic metabolism begins to supplement aerobic efforts [38, 47, 48].
  - better marker for endurance performance than $VO_2$max in paediatrics [49].
  - highly reproducible measure that correlates strongly with peak $VO_2$ and is sensitive enough to detect fitness improvements [50, 51].
  - Specificity of onset of anaerobic metabolism in children and adolescents, e.g. no particular point in young athletes as many mechanisms begin to come into play to convert over to anaerobic metabolism: two distinct ventilatory thresholds, **VAT1** and **VAT2** and the midpoint between the two (**MPVT**; [52, 53]).
- **Peak Oxygen Pulse**:
  - Good indicator of cardiovascular function in the paediatric population.
  - Particularly useful in those with congenital heart disease and with autonomic dysfunction.
  - Because the oxygen pulse is derived by dividing the $VO_2$ by the heart rate at any given time it's a surrogate measure for stroke volume.
- **Maximal Workload**:
  - Metabolic equivalence (METS) in adults and Watts in paediatric athletes.
  - MET is a means of expressing the oxygen requirement of physical activity relative to an assumed resting value (1 MET = 3.5 ml/kg/min).
  - Resting energy expenditure is age- and body mass-dependent.
  - 8–12 year olds have a resting oxygen requirement per kg body weight that is 70% higher than adults [54].
  - Corrections for body weight and fat-free mass have additional utility [55].

- **Ventilatory Efficiency**:
  - Ratio of $V_E/VCO_2$.
  - Improves with age due to a relative increase in alveolar tissue making up tidal volume comparted to increase in dead space (mouth, trachea, bronchi). Thus, $V_D/V_T$ falls with age [56].
  - Ventilatory efficiency slope at submaximal testing correlates with peak $VO_2$ in healthy youths and in paediatric patients with pulmonary vascular disease [57, 58].

### 23.7.2 Pulmonary Function Testing

Assessment of common pathologies (asthma, vocal cord dysfunction syndrome, congenital heart disease surgery-related low lung volume, pectus excavatum, scoliosis).

Common basic parameters:

- Forced vital capacity (FVC), forced expiratory volume in 1 s (FEV1),
- Maximum forced expiratory flow (FEFmax).
- Maximal voluntary ventilation (MVV) measured while stationary.
- Selective analysis of breath to breath tidal volume versus minute ventilation during exertion which further defines the extent of pulmonary limitations in patients with lung disease [59].

## 23.8 Direct Cardiac Assessment During Exercise Stress by Cardiac Imaging

In the paediatric athlete, stress echocardiography can unmask subclinical ventricular dysfunction and valvar stenosis or regurgitation which may not be apparent at rest. Although large scale normative data during exercise stress have not been established, less load dependent parameters, such as myocardial deformation (strain) and Tissue Doppler imaging can provide information on force-frequency relationship and myocardial contractility reserve during exercise stress, and paediatric normative data exist [60, 61]. Exercise stress is superior to dobutamine stress in the assessment of the athlete as it assesses ventricular function in relation to other physiological exercise adaptations and can be combined with cardiopulmonary exercise testing. Dobutamine stress echocardiography can have a role in assessing morphological and functional coronary artery problems.

Indications for exercise stress echocardiography assessing:

- systolic and diastolic function (strain, PW TDI, inflow PW).
- valve function (PW inflow and outflow gradients).
- myocardial exercise reserve (increase in strain, PW TDI, EF).

- wall motion abnormalities in cardiomyopathies and Kawasaki disease (qualitative, strain, TDI).
- interventricular coupling and dyssynchrony assessment (TDI, strain).

Exercise stress cardiac magnetic resonance (CMR) imaging has recently been introduced in the assessment of athletes and is superior to exercise stress echo in assessing cardiac volumes and wall motion abnormalities [62]. While stress CMR using pharmacological agents is standard in adult ischaemic heart disease it does not have a main stream diagnostic role in the paediatric athlete; however, it is becoming a useful secondary investigation in pediatrics [63].

### 23.8.1 Cardiac Magnetic Resonance (CMR) and Computed Tomography (CT)

CMR allows window-independent imaging, accurate delineation of detailed anatomy including 3-D reconstruction, and tissue characterization and is the gold standard in ventricular and regurgitant volume quantification.

Use of CMR in:

- Ventricles: RV and LV volumes, myocardial mass, myocardial scar (which may act as a surrogate for arrhythmia risk).
- Valves and prosthetic material: regurgitation fraction, visualization of prosthetic materials (conduits).
- Myocardial pathologies including fibrosis (HCM, LVNC, ARVC) using contrast.
- Detailed morphological studies (e.g. pulmonary veins, coronary arteries).
- Size and gender specific paediatric centiles are available for both echocardiographic measurements and cardiac MRI [64–66].

Cardiac CT is the imaging modality of choice in the delineation of small anatomical structures such as coronary arteries and collateral arteries and for imaging parenchymal lung pathology. The main disadvantage of CT is lower temporal resolution and radiation, however modern techniques have reduced the exposure to radiation.

### 23.8.2 Mobile Monitoring

While standard functional laboratory tests (exercise stress ECG, CPET, exercise imaging) should always be included in the secondary assessment of the paediatric athlete, mobile monitoring is increasingly becoming a diagnostic tool of choice in certain conditions. Advantages are its use in the athlete specific and chosen training environment, portability and prolonged monitoring during exercise with potentially higher pick up rates of pathology (e.g. arrhythmias). Cableless mobile and app based devices are available for clinical use in children, and early data on feasibility and diagnostic value are encouraging [67].

Indications are:

(a) Cardiac symptoms during exercise,
(b) On-field cableless monitoring during training and competition,
(c) Paroxysmal symptoms of palpitations, dizziness and syncope,
(d) Post-intervention (e.g. arrhythmia ablation) monitoring,
(e) Risk stratification in pathologies (e.g. cardiomyopathies, congenital heart disease),
(f) Continuous monitoring of up to a week.

## 23.9 Common Cardiac Problems, Their Diagnoses and Treatment in the Paediatric Athlete

Congenital heart disease in the paediatric athlete population is discussed in Chap. 22 and will not be discussed here in detail. Activity recommendations for patients with congenital heart disease should be followed [68].

### 23.9.1 Cardiomyopathies

The main differential diagnoses of athlete's heart also in the paediatric athlete are HCM, LVNC and AVC. Echocardiography is the primary imaging tool but does not have optimal sensitivity and specificity in detecting inherited myocardial disease, and young adolescents often have minimal symptoms. CMR is of high value as secondary imaging tool in assessing the presence of cardiomyopathy. CMR is particularly useful in the context of 12-lead ECG T-wave changes that may reflect an ethnically-related variant or mild hypertrophy that seems disproportionate to the level of exercise participation. The presence of late gadolinium enhancement or diastolic dysfunction support the presence of underlying cardiomyopathy, but absence does not exclude it. In the paediatric athlete the developing nature of cardiomyopathies means that a single point assessment does not exclude subsequent manifestation of a genotype positive, phenotype negative inherited cardiomyopathy. Serial annual evaluation is paramount. Index case and family cascade genotyping in paediatric cardiomyopathies should be performed when clinically indicated. However, age of independent—and legal—capacity to consent to genetic testing is debated and a close collaboration with a geneticist and genetic counsellor is recommended. No specific paediatric guidelines for paediatric cardiomyopathy genetic testing exist, but there is emerging evidence, that genotyping can help in risk stratification (reviewed in [69]).

- **Hypertrophic cardiomyopathy**

Diagnosis of HCM in the paediatric athlete population remains a challenge as the majority of cases remain phenotypically dormant during childhood.

- Family history is central.
- First line 12-lead ECG screening should follow the international criteria; their accuracy in paediatric athletes has recently been assessed [31], and subsequent assessment for suspected HCM should follow ESC and AHA guidelines.
- Echocardiography and CMR are the imaging tools of choice.
  LV hypertrophy should be categorised as abnormal if the LV end-diastolic wall thickness z-score is >2. A diagnostic help can be the LV end-diastolic diameter, which is reduced in the majority of phenotypic paediatric HCM [70]; however, mild and developing or subclinical phenotypes in childhood and adolescence are common.
  As in adults, abnormal echocardiographic diastolic tissue Doppler parameters or myocardial systolic strain can be first indicators of an evolving phenotype [70].
- The use of de-training in the paediatric athlete population to ascertain a diagnosis of HCM has not been sufficiently explored and should be used judiciously. Adult sports participation guidelines should be followed [71].

In athletes with suspected HCM, serial annual evaluation is paramount and should include ECG, echocardiogram, exercise testing and CMR.

- **Arrhythmogenic Ventricular Cardiomyopathy** (AVC)

Clinical diagnosis of AVC in the paediatric population is challenging and often delayed until late adolescence and adulthood. The disease can be concealed in childhood, progresses with period bursts rather than continuous progression and signs of disease often mimic changes seen in the healthy young athletic population [72]. Diagnostic criteria have evolved solely based on evidence from the affected adult patient population but are currently also used for paediatric ARVC patients with a lower sensitivity and specificity. Echocardiographic revised task force criteria rarely trigger suspicion in children and adolescents as they rely on adult RV diameters and are less sensitive and specific in paediatric AVC [73] with recent studies suggesting that additional modalities such as 2-D strain are more sensitive in assessing adolescents with AVC [74].

- CMR is the diagnostic imaging modality of choice also in children, but recent studies have shown that predictive parameters differ from those regarded as mainstay in adults [75].

- CPET including exercise ECG can occasionally be helpful in arrhythmia detection, but arrhythmic activity is highly variable in adolescent patients with AVC [76].
- Enlarged cardiac diameters in paediatric athletes can mimic cardiomyopathic changes [77] and tools such as CMR and arrhythmia monitoring need to be performed.
- In AVC, CMR findings such as fatty infiltration and fibrosis are of limited value in children and focus lies on ventricular function, regional wall motion abnormalities and z-scores of RV and LV dimensions [75].
- As with HCM, longitudinal assessment is warranted.

Little data on the onset and incidence of LV involvement in children and adolescents exist. The different phases in the natural history of classic AVC are also found in the paediatric disease:

(a) “concealed”, with subtle RV structural changes, with or without ventricular arrhythmias.
(b) “overt electrical disorder”, with symptomatic life-threatening ventricular arrhythmias associated with obvious RV morpho-functional abnormalities.
(c) “RV failure”, due to progression and extension of RV disease.
(d) “biventricular failure”, caused also by pronounced LV disease [78].

AVC in childhood is less common than in the adult population, it is however important to realise that adult modified task force criteria [79] diagnostic tools are less sensitive and specific in paediatric AVC [74] and this remains true when differentiating athletic adaption (e.g. RV dilatation) from AVC in the paediatric athlete. As for adult athletes with AVC, competition guidelines from ESC and AHA should be followed and paediatric athletes with definite, borderline or even possible diagnosis of AVC are restricted from most competitive sports with the possible exception of low-intensity class IA sports. In athletes monitored for suspicion of AVC, serial annual evaluation is paramount and should include ECG, echocardiogram, exercise testing and CMR.

- **Left-ventricular non-compaction cardiomyopathy (LVNC)**

LVNC in childhood is very heterogeneous and often presents with an undulating phenotype of mild but also severe forms [80]. Left ventricular hypertrabeculation is not uncommon in the healthy adult athlete [81] population. No comparable data exist for the childhood athlete, and a differentiation between physiologically pronounced trabeculation and LVNC disease in this age group is a challenge as accuracy of adult LVNC diagnostic criteria have not been evaluated in children.

- Suspicion of LVNC on echocardiography in the paediatric athlete needs to lead to careful further assessment by CMR and rhythm monitoring.
- Mild hypertrabeculation in the setting of normal function, without CMR features such as wall motion abnormalities or fibrosis, and without evidence of rhythm abnormalities can be regarded as a normal phenomenon, but serial monitoring is advised.
- Advanced echocardiographic imaging tools such as strain can help detect disease [82].

### 23.9.2 Arrhythmia Syndromes

Hereditary primary electrical disorders may account for up to 30% of all SCD between the ages of 5 and 35 years [83]. Details of these syndromes are provided in separate chapters. The following are details specific to the paediatric population. They include the following.

- **Congenital Long QT Syndrome (LQTS)**
  - Although most patients remain asymptomatic throughout life, up to 13% may experience SCD and 36% may experience syncope before the age of 40 years if untreated.
  - The mean age at the time of the first symptom is around 14 years of age.
  - Participation in competitive sports should follow adult guidelines [84].
  - Genetic testing is recommended in all patients with diagnosis of LQTS [85, 86].
- **Short QT Syndrome**
  - Presenting as cardiac arrest resulting in either SCD or aborted SCD, often at a young age, in 34% and a family history of SCD in 15% of those who have it. Up to 60% experience syncope [87–89].
  - A benign variety of the disease has been observed in children with atrial fibrillation and a KCNH2 mutation [90].
  - AHA/ACC and ESC guideline recommendations are discussed in Chap. 20 [84].
- **Early Repolarization Syndrome (ERS)**
  - Distinct from the entity of a short QT syndrome.
  - Heterogeneous group of specific QRS-T junction patterns that are commonly found on the electrocardiograms of young healthy subjects. ERS is defined as >1 mm of J-point elevation in any two contiguous ECG leads, with the exception of the right precordial leads (V1-V3).
  - May be associated with an increased risk of sudden cardiac death and there may be some overlap in pathophysiology with the Brugada syndrome (see below).
  - Diagnosis can be made when the ECG features of ERS are present in an individual with a history of idiopathic VF or polymorphic ventricular tachycardia.
  - Therapy for ERS has been proposed along the lines of that for CPVT [91].

- **Brugada Syndrome (BrS)**
  - May be responsible for 4 to 12% of all SCD [92, 93] and may be has high as 20% of sudden unexplained deaths in infancy and young childhood [94, 95].
  - Strong male predominance with one series being 70% male [96]. A more recent study found a higher frequency of females in the paediatric population [97].
  - In the Asian population, the male to female ratio is nine-fold higher than in Caucasian populations.
  - Although not often identified until the third to fourth decade of life, identification in the paediatric population is common particularly when investigating family cohorts.
  - When found in those under 20 years of age, BrS is drug-induced rather than spontaneous in 2/third of cases.
  - Of those cases occurring spontaneously, most are found on family screening (63%) or as an incidental finding (12%) [98].
  - Often asymptomatic and may remain so, particularly below the age of 20 years.
  - Syncope or sudden cardiac death or aborted death due to a ventricular arrhythmia may happen in up to 42% of those above 20 years of age who are diagnosed [99] while syncope occurs in 14%, aborted sudden death in 6% of those under 20 [98].
  - For the most common type, SCN5A defect, symptoms usually occur when sleeping.
  - About 6% of arrhythmic events occur while febrile with disproportionally higher rates at younger ages, as well as disproportionally higher rates in males and Caucasians [100].
  - Primary prophylaxis is essential with strict antipyresis and even sometimes hospitalization during febrile illnesses, as well as avoidance of contraindicated medications and alcohol.
  - Adult AHA/ACC and ESC sports participation guidelines should be followed [84].
  - Quinidine or hydroquinidine are often used to treat asymptomatic children and these have been found to normalize ECGs, and suppress electric storm and recurrent VF [101, 102]. Mexiletine and beta-blockers are sometimes employed as well.
  - Symptomatic paediatric patients nearly uniformly are recommended for implantable cardioverter defibrillators (ICDs). The rate of inappropriate shock at all ages is high, and children have additional complications of ICDs [103].
- **Catecholaminergic Polymorphic Ventricular Tachycardia (CVPT)**:
  - Presents with the mean age of onset of symptoms and that of diagnosis at about 8 and 10.5 years of age, respectively [104].
  - May cause syncope, convulsions, and sudden death during physical activity or emotional distress, although in about 25% of patients under 20 years life-threatening events occurred during normal wakeful activities [105].

- 18% of patients and 36% of positive first degree relatives had life-threatening symptoms including syncope, aborted SCD or SCD [106].
- Up to 80% will experience arrhythmia and 30% will succumb to SCD [107].
- Regardless of expediency of other therapies, lifestyle modifications should be pursued immediately.
- AHA/ACC and ESC guideline recommendations are discussed in Chap. 20 [84].

### 23.9.3 Supraventricular Arrhythmias

Children with structurally normal hearts have the same mechanisms of arrhythmias than those found in adults but with great differences in prevalence. Accessory pathways, atrial foci, and dual AV nodal physiology represent the vast majority of paediatric supraventricular arrhythmias. Arrhythmias in structural heart disease may be due to the disease or may result from chronic hemodynamic stress or from the surgical intervention [108].

- Prevalence of supraventricular arrhythmias of 2.25 per 1000 persons with an annual incidence of those being diagnosed under 19 years of age of 13 per 100,000.
- Atrioventricular re-entrant tachycardia (AVRT; see below) is by far the most common in the paediatric age group, with 55 to 60% of those with an accessory pathway who undergo EP study manifesting some degree of ventricular pre-excitation consistent with Wolff-Parkinson-White Syndrome (WPW) [109].
- Atrio-fascicular accessory pathways (AFP via Mahaim fibers) and permanent junctional reciprocating tachycardia represent a small proportion of AVRT.
- Atrioventricular nodal re-entrant tachycardia (AVNRT) whereby two distinct pathways exist within the Triangle of Koch (dual AV node pathophysiology) accounts for 17% of children going to EP study.
- Ectopic atrial tachycardia accounts for 4 to 6% in this group.
- Atrial flutter and de novo atrial fibrillation are rare in children.
- Atrial fibrillation as a consequence of a degeneration from an activated accessory pathway is more frequent. However, sudden cardiac death from pre-excitation remains uncommon [110].
- **Atrioventricular Reentrant Tachycardia (AVRT)**
  - Caused by anomalous and accessory AV connections made of muscle bundles breaching the separation of atria from ventricles at any point across the AV junction which can be present in both structurally normal hearts and in those with congenital malformations.
  - The presence of these pathways allows for a circus rhythm to occur usually in an antegrade fashion down the normal AV node and back up through the accessory pathway.
  - Those without pre-excitation may have a normal baseline ECG but a history of paroxysmal tachycardia. The abnormal rhythm can only be detected by capturing an event with event recorder or by EP study.

  - For those with pre-excitation, the accessory pathway is inferred from the baseline ECG with the presence of a short PR interval made short by the onset of delta waves. Identification of the location of the pathway is further inferred from the direction of the deflection of the delta waves across the 12 leads. Such an ECG pattern is found in 0.15 to 0.25% of the population and about one third of these people go on to develop an arrhythmia during a 10-year follow-up [108, 111].
- **Wolff-Parkinson-White Syndrome**
  - The lifetime incidence of SCD from WPW is estimated to be 3–4%. Especially in the paediatric population, VF and SCD can be the first arrhythmic event [112, 113].
  - Regardless of expediency of other therapies, lifestyle modifications should be pursued immediately. Certainly, vagal maneuvers should be taught right away and a medication plan considered. Of those who are symptomatic (in other words, have Wolff-Parkinson-White syndrome), the evaluation and recommendations are more clear-cut and involve catheter ablation.
  - For those that are asymptomatic, the evaluation and treatment remain somewhat controversial.
  - AHA/ACC and ESC guideline recommendations are discussed in Chap. 20 [84].

### 23.9.4 Acquired Arrhythmias

- **Atrial Tachycardias**

  There is some evidence that young athletes are at increased risk of developing atrial fibrillation (AF) and flutter (AFL) and perhaps even atrial ectopic tachycardia (AT) [114–116]. Athletes may be particularly prone because of a particularly high vagal tone, as well as remodelling of the atria including changes in size, pressure, and function. Indeed, atrial function in terms of left and right atrial longitudinal strain may have the strongest relationship with the early onset of AF compared with any other factor involved in atrial remodelling. Increased myocardial inflammation and fibrosis as well as an increased presence of sympathetic tone, alterations in thyroid function, and use of performance-enhancing or stimulatory substances may also contribute [84, 117]. More recent evidence attributes some cause to a disorder in myocardial energy metabolism [118].
  - In elite athletes under age 25 with some sort of arrhythmia, 9% were found to have AF—all being male.
  - AF was the cause of long-lasting palpitations in 40% of these athletes.
  - Nearly half of those with AF have underlying substrate; WPW, arrhythmogenic cardiomyopathy (AC), and post-myocarditis. The other half are considered idiopathic [115].
  - AHA/ACC and ESC guidelines recommendations are discussed in Chap. 18 [84].
  - Athletes identified with atrial ectopic tachycardia are advised to follow the same recommendations as those with re-entrant tachycardia [84].

- **Heart Block**:
  First- and second-degree heart block is diagnosed and managed similar to that in the adult population. There are certain aspects of third-degree heart block that are unique in the paediatric population.
  *Congenital Complete Heart Block (CCHB)*
  - often occurs from exposure to maternal SSA and SSB antibodies in mothers with Sjogren's syndrome or Lupus.
  - Patients with CCHB as part of congenitally corrected transposition (L-TGA) are at high risk for degenerating into a life-threatening arrhythmia and should probably be managed as those with acquired complete heart block [119, 120].
  - AHA/ACC and ESC guideline recommendations are discussed in Chap. 22 [84].

  *Acquired complete heart block (ACHB)*
  - can be a complication of heart surgery or, on occasion, of myocarditis [121] or rarely spontaneously [122].

  Athletes with ACHB and those with CCHB associated with L-transposition of the great vessels should have a permanent pacemaker placed regardless of symptoms, type of structural heart disease, and exercise capacity unless the heart block is attributable to completely reversible causes and resolves completely such as might occur following resolution of myocarditis.
- **Acquired Ventricular Arrhythmias**
  For the most part, the epidemiology, pathophysiology, diagnosis and management of these are similar to that in the adult athlete population. AHA/ACC and ESC guidelines for management of athletes with ventricular arrhythmias are discussed in Chap. 17 [84].
  *Premature Ventricular Complexes (PVCs)*
  - Most commonly benign.
  - Requires evaluation to determine their nature. By various methods, they should be assessed for:
    frequency.
    suppression with increasing heart rate—usually under the effect of exercise testing.
    whether they are monomorphic or polymorphic.
    occur in singlets or having episodes of non-sustained VT.
    occur in isolation or in the presence of more concerning cardiac pathology.

  *Non-sustained Ventricular Tachycardia (NSVT)*
  - Short runs defined as >3 consecutive PVCs up to a maximum duration of 30 s or continued rhythm that does not provoke cardiovascular collapse, may be benign.
  - Their presence should be more concerning for underlying heart disease than single PVCs [123].
  - Evaluation for NSVT should be the same as that for PVCs.

  *Sustained monomorphic Ventricular Tachycardia (SMVT)*
  - may be a benign arrhythmia in the paediatric population, in particular as a benign right ventricular outflow tract tachycardia, but its presence should be more concerning for underlying heart disease as well as e.g. ARVC.
  - workup is similar to that of PVCs and NSVT but must be particularly thorough so as to not miss underlying developing disease.

*Sustained Polymorphic VT, Ventricular Flutter, and Ventricular Fibrillation*

- Are never benign in the paediatric population.
- These patient/athletes require a full evaluation and generally receive an implantable cardioverter-defibrillator except perhaps in the setting of transient inflammatory or electrolyte disorder.

## 23.10 Care of the Paediatric Athlete in the Future

As sports academies undergo increasing professional development, it is imperative to show more diligence to safeguard the development of the paediatric athlete. Whilst the significant progress achieved in adult sports cardiology can guide assessment guidelines and protocols in paediatric sports cardiology, adult normative data and current cardiac pre-participation guidelines cannot be unequivocally applied to the paediatric heart. Future research focusing on the development of gender, growth and age specific normative 12-lead ECG and echocardiographic criteria, will advance paediatric screening and assessment protocols; increasing diagnostic accuracy. At present, too few paediatricians and paediatric cardiologists are sufficiently trained to provide expert opinion [124] and training pathways and a stronger engagement of paediatric and sports governing bodies are needed to improve this. Consequently, an approach requiring synergy between paediatric and sports cardiologists, exercise physiologists, policy makers and sports organisations is required to develop paediatric cardiac monitoring tools and protocols, eventually working towards a child athlete centered specialty (paediatric sports cardiology) that matches the sports professionalism of the current and future paediatric athlete.

**Clinical Pearls**

- No specific paediatric guidelines exist, but current screening guidelines include athletes from 12 to 14 years onwards, they should be followed.
- Normal ECG parameters change during growth and somatic maturation and with ethnicity.
- Athletic cardiac changes can mimick but also mask underlying heart disease also in paediatric athletes.
- Teenage onset of cardiomyopathies (HCM, ARVC, LVNC) is less common, but present.
- Growth and maturation change echocardiographic parameters and need to be accounted for by using z-scores and also pubertal assessment.
- Growth and maturation require serial cardiac assessments, particularly during puberty.
- Dynamic and mobile assessment during exercise is warranted in the diagnostic assessment of suspected pathology.
- Pathological arrhythmias are less often acquired, compared to adults, but more commonly symptoms of an underlying general myocardial disease or arrhythmia syndrome and diagnostic assessment should be meticulous.

- No specific paediatric participation guidelines exist and adult guidelines should be followed, taking into account specifics of age, maturational stage and natural history (time of onset) of myocardial disease and arrhythmia syndromes.
- Close collaboration between paediatricians, sports and paediatric cardiologists, sports physicians and coaching staff is required to provide optimal care.

## Review

### Questions

1. Do paediatric athletes between 12 and 16 years of age show significant training related cardiac adaptations?
2. Can adult cardiac screening and diagnostic criteria and guidelines be applied to paediatric athletes?
3. Do paediatric athletes are at risk of developing the same arrhythmias as adult athletes?

### Answers

1. Recent professionalisation of athletic training in academies has led to training intensity and volumes that can lead to cardiac changes in chamber size and ventricular wall thickness and are also visible in the 12-lead ECG as recently shown in a meta-analysis. As in adults, ethnicity specific changes are detectable, and the sports cardiologist needs to be aware of these [125].
2. No specific cardiac screening guidelines exist, the available recommendations are modelled on adult guidelines [22]. The latest adult athlete ECG screening guidelines (International Criteria) have been evaluated in athletes younger than 16 years of age and found to have moderate accuracy and should be used [31].
3. The incidence and types of arrhythmias in paediatric athletes differ slightly from those found in adult athletes. Accessory pathways such as WPW are most common, congenital heart blocks of varying degrees are more often observed. Importantly, as in adults, cardiac arrest can be the first presentation of a ventricular arrhythmia or a myocardial disease, malignant arrhythmias such as CPVT often present in teenage years, and early diagnosis of ventricular arrhythmias and arrhythmogenic cardiomyopathies remains a particular challenge in paediatric athletes. Atrial fibrillation and flutter are very rare.

## References

1. Pieles GE, Horn R, Williams CA, Stuart AG. Paediatric exercise training in prevention and treatment. Arch Dis Child. 2014;99(4):380–5.
2. Townsend MW, Williams, J.; Bhatnagar, P.; Rayner M, Physical activity statistics 2015. 2015. London: British Heart Foundation.

3. Brenner JS, American Academy of Pediatrics Council on Sports M, Fitness. Overuse injuries, overtraining, and burnout in child and adolescent athletes. Pediatrics. 2007;119(6):1242–5.
4. Gustafsson H, Hill AP, Stenling A, Wagnsson S. Profiles of perfectionism, parental climate, and burnout among competitive junior athletes. Scand J Med Sci Sports. 2016;26(10):1256–64.
5. Atkins DL, Everson-Stewart S, Sears GK, Daya M, Osmond MH, Warden CR, et al. Epidemiology and outcomes from out-of-hospital cardiac arrest in children: the Resuscitation Outcomes Consortium Epistry-Cardiac Arrest. Circulation. 2009;119(11):1484–91.
6. Drezner JA, Rao AL, Heistand J, Bloomingdale MK, Harmon KG. Effectiveness of emergency response planning for sudden cardiac arrest in United States high schools with automated external defibrillators. Circulation. 2009;120(6):518–25.
7. Sharma S. Point/mandatory ECG screening of young competitive athletes. Heart Rhythm. 2012;9(11):1896.
8. Berger S, Kugler JD, Thomas JA, Friedberg DZ. Sudden cardiac death in children and adolescents: introduction and overview. Pediatr Clin N Am. 2004;51(5):1201–9.
9. Maron BJ, Epstein SE, Roberts WC. Causes of sudden death in competitive athletes. J Am Coll Cardiol. 1986;7(1):204–14.
10. Maron BJ, Shirani J, Poliac LC, Mathenge R, Roberts WC, Mueller FO. Sudden death in young competitive athletes. Clinical, demographic, and pathological profiles. JAMA. 1996;276(3):199–204.
11. Corrado D, Basso C, Thiene G, McKenna WJ, Davies MJ, Fontaliran F, et al. Spectrum of clinicopathologic manifestations of arrhythmogenic right ventricular cardiomyopathy/dysplasia: a multicenter study. J Am Coll Cardiol. 1997;30(6):1512–20.
12. Maron BJ, Haas TS, Doerer JJ, Thompson PD, Hodges JS. Comparison of U.S. and Italian experiences with sudden cardiac deaths in young competitive athletes and implications for preparticipation screening strategies. Am J Cardiol. 2009;104(2):276–80.
13. Harmon KG, Zigman M, Drezner JA. The effectiveness of screening history, physical exam, and ECG to detect potentially lethal cardiac disorders in athletes: a systematic review/meta-analysis. J Electrocardiol. 2015;48(3):329–38.
14. Corrado D, Basso C, Pavei A, Michieli P, Schiavon M, Thiene G. Trends in sudden cardiovascular death in young competitive athletes after implementation of a preparticipation screening program. JAMA. 2006;296(13):1593–601.
15. Maron BJ, Doerer JJ, Haas TS, Tierney DM, Mueller FO. Sudden deaths in young competitive athletes: analysis of 1866 deaths in the United States, 1980-2006. Circulation. 2009;119(8):1085–92.
16. Finocchiaro G, et al. Etiology of sudden death in sports: insights from a United Kingdom regional registry. Front Physiol. 2016;67(18):2108–15.
17. Harmon KG, et al. Incidence, cause, and comparative frequency of sudden cardiac death in National Collegiate Athletic Association Athletes: a decade in review. Circulation1. 2015;32(1):10–19.
18. Araujo CG, Scharhag J. Athlete: a working definition for medical and health sciences research. Scand J Med Sci Sports. 2016;26(1):4–7.
19. Hauser M, Petzuch K, Kuhn A, Schon P, Elmenhorst J, Schonfelder M, et al. The Munich Triathlon Heart Study: ventricular function, myocardial velocities, and two-dimensional strain in healthy children before and after endurance stress. Pediatr Cardiol. 2013;34(3):576–82.
20. McClean G, Riding NR, Ardern CL, Farooq A, Pieles GE, Watt V, et al. Electrical and structural adaptations of the paediatric athlete's heart: a systematic review with meta-analysis. Br J Sports Med. 2018;52(4):230.
21. Sharma S, Maron BJ, Whyte G, Firoozi S, Elliott PM, McKenna WJ. Physiologic limits of left ventricular hypertrophy in elite junior athletes: relevance to differential diagnosis of athlete's heart and hypertrophic cardiomyopathy. J Am Coll Cardiol. 2002;40(8):1431–6.
22. Fritsch P, Ehringer-Schetitska D, Dalla Pozza R, Jokinen E, Herceg-Cavrak V, Hidvegi E, et al. Cardiovascular pre-participation screening in young athletes: recommendations of the Association of European Paediatric Cardiology. Cardiol Young. 2017;27(9):1655–60.
23. Dick NA, Diehl JJ. Febrile illness in the athlete. Sports Health. 2014;6(3):225–31.

24. Scharhag J, Meyer T. Return to play after acute infectious disease in football players. J Sports Sci. 2014;32(13):1237–42.
25. Joy E, Kussman A, Nattiv A. 2016 update on eating disorders in athletes: a comprehensive narrative review with a focus on clinical assessment and management. Br J Sports Med. 2016;50(3):154–62.
26. Enriquez A, Frankel DS. Arrhythmogenic effects of energy drinks. J Cardiovasc Electrophysiol. 2017;28(6):711–7.
27. Solimini R, Rotolo MC, Mastrobattista L, Mortali C, Minutillo A, Pichini S, et al. Hepatotoxicity associated with illicit use of anabolic androgenic steroids in doping. Eur Rev Med Pharmacol Sci. 2017;21(1 Suppl):7–16.
28. Saladini F, Palatini P. Isolated systolic hypertension in young individuals: pathophysiological mechanisms, prognostic significance, and clinical implications. High Blood Press Cardiovasc Prev. 2017;24(2):133–9.
29. Park MK, Guntheroth WG. How to read pediatric ECG's. Philadelphia, PA: Mosby; 2006.
30. Drezner JA, Sharma S, Baggish A, Papadakis M, Wilson MG, Prutkin JM, et al. International criteria for electrocardiographic interpretation in athletes: consensus statement. Br J Sports Med. 2017;51(9):704–31.
31. McClean G, Riding NR, Pieles G, Watt V, Adamuz C, Sharma S, et al. Diagnostic accuracy and Bayesian analysis of new international ECG recommendations in paediatric athletes. Heart. 2019;105(2):152–9.
32. Lopez L, Colan S, Stylianou M, Granger S, Trachtenberg F, Frommelt P, et al. Relationship of echocardiographic Z scores adjusted for body surface area to age, sex, race, and ethnicity: the Pediatric Heart Network Normal Echocardiogram Database. Circ Cardiovasc Imaging. 2017;10(11):e006979.
33. Rowland TW, American College of Sports Medicine, North American Society of Pediatric Exercise Medicine. Cardiopulmonary exercise testing in children and adolescents. Champaign, IL: Human Kinetics; 2018. p. xi, 275p.
34. Ahluwalia N, Raju H. Assessment of the QT interval in athletes: red flags and pitfalls. Curr Treat Options Cardiovasc Med. 2018;20(10):82.
35. Ergul Y, Ozturk E, Ozyilmaz I, Unsal S, Carus H, Tola HT, et al. Utility of exercise testing and adenosine response for risk assessment in children with Wolff-Parkinson-White syndrome. Congenit Heart Dis. 2015;10(6):542–51.
36. Wackel P, Irving C, Webber S, Beerman L, Arora G. Risk stratification in Wolff-Parkinson-White syndrome: the correlation between noninvasive and invasive testing in pediatric patients. Pacing Clin Electrophysiol. 2012;35(12):1451–7.
37. Horner JM, Ackerman MJ. Ventricular ectopy during treadmill exercise stress testing in the evaluation of long QT syndrome. Heart Rhythm. 2008;5(12):1690–4.
38. Wasserman K. Principles of exercise testing and interpretation: including pathophysiology and clinical applications. 5th ed. Philadelphia: Wolters Kluwer Health/Lippincott Williams & Wilkins; 2012. p. xiii, 572p.
39. Amăricăi E, Suciu O, Onofrei RR, Miclăuş RS, Caţan L, Cerbu S, et al. Assessment of children with pectus excavatum without surgical correction. Wien Klin Wochenschr. 2019;131(5-6):126–31.
40. Moldover JR, Downey JA. Cardiac response to exercise: comparison of 3 ergometers. Arch Phys Med Rehabil. 1983;64(4):155–9.
41. Gibson PB, Szimonisz SM, Rowland TW. Rowing ergometry for assessment of aerobic fitness in children. Int J Sports Med. 2000;21(8):579–82.
42. Rowland TW. Aerobic exercise testing protocols. In: Rowland TW, editor. Pediatric laboratory exercise testing clinical guidelines. Champaign, IL: Human Kinetics; 1992. p. 195.
43. Heyman E, Briard D, Dekerdanet M, Gratas-Delamarche A, Delamarche P. Accuracy of physical working capacity 170 to estimate aerobic fitness in prepubertal diabetic boys and in 2 insulin dose conditions. J Sports Med Phys Fitness. 2006;46(2):315–21.
44. Baba R, Nagashima M, Goto M, Nagano Y, Yokota M, Tauchi N, et al. Oxygen uptake efficiency slope: a new index of cardiorespiratory functional reserve derived from the relation

between oxygen uptake and minute ventilation during incremental exercise. J Am Coll Cardiol. 1996;28(6):1567–72.
45. Akkerman M, van Brussel M, Hulzebos E, Vanhees L, Helders PJ, Takken T. The oxygen uptake efficiency slope: what do we know? J Cardiopulm Rehabil Prev. 2010;30(6):357–73.
46. Akkerman M, van Brussel M, Bongers BC, Hulzebos EH, Helders PJ, Takken T. Oxygen uptake efficiency slope in healthy children. Pediatr Exerc Sci. 2010;22(3):431–41.
47. Wasserman K, McIlroy MB. Detecting the threshold of anaerobic metabolism in cardiac patients during exercise. Am J Cardiol. 1964;14:844–52.
48. Wasserman K, Whipp BJ, Koyl SN, Beaver WL. Anaerobic threshold and respiratory gas exchange during exercise. J Appl Physiol. 1973;35(2):236–43.
49. Buchheit M, Solano R, Millet GP. Heart-rate deflection point and the second heart-rate variability threshold during running exercise in trained boys. Pediatr Exerc Sci. 2007;19:192–204.
50. Gaskill SE, Ruby BC, Walker AJ, Sanchez OA, Serfass RC, Leon AS. Validity and reliability of combining three methods to determine ventilatory threshold. Med Sci Sports Exerc. 2001;33(11):1841–8.
51. Mucci PB, Baquet G, Nourry C, Deruelle F, Berthoin S, Fabre C. Exercise testing in children: comparison in ventilatory thresholds changes with interval-training. Pediatr Pulmonol. 2012;48(8):809–16.
52. Hebestreit H, Staschen B, Hebestreit A. Ventilatory threshold: a useful method to determine aerobic fitness in children? Med Sci Sports Exerc. 2000;32(11):1964–9.
53. Washington RL, van Gundy JC, Cohen C, Sondheimer HM, Wolfe RR. Normal aerobic and anaerobic exercise data for North American school-age children. J Pediatr. 1988;112(2):223–33.
54. Harrell JS, McMurray RG, Baggett CD, Pennell ML, Pearce PF, Bangdiwala SI. Energy costs of physical activities in children and adolescents. Med Sci Sports Exerc. 2005;37(2):329–36.
55. Gulmans VA, de Meer K, Binkhorst RA, Helders PJ, Saris WH. Reference values for maximum work capacity in relation to body composition in healthy Dutch children. Eur Respir J. 1997;10(1):94–7.
56. Giardini A, Odendaal D, Khambadkone S, Derrick G. Physiologic decrease of ventilatory response to exercise in the second decade of life in healthy children. Am Heart J. 2011;161(6):1214–9.
57. Breithaupt PG, Colley RC, Adamo KB. Using the oxygen uptake efficiency slope as an indicator of cardiorespiratory fitness in the obese pediatric population. Pediatr Exerc Sci. 2012;24(3):357–68.
58. Rausch CM, Taylor AL, Ross H, Sillau S, Ivy DD. Ventilatory efficiency slope correlates with functional capacity, outcomes, and disease severity in pediatric patients with pulmonary hypertension. Int J Cardiol. 2013;169(6):445–8.
59. Santuz P, Baraldi E, Filippone M, Zacchello F. Exercise performance in children with asthma: is it different from that of healthy controls? Eur Respir J. 1997;10(6):1254–60.
60. Pieles GE, Gowing L, Forsey J, Ramanujam P, Miller F, Stuart AG, et al. The relationship between biventricular myocardial performance and metabolic parameters during incremental exercise and recovery in healthy adolescents. Am J Physiol Heart Circ Physiol. 2015;309(12):H2067–76.
61. Cifra B, Mertens L, Mirkhani M, Slorach C, Hui W, Manlhiot C, et al. Systolic and diastolic myocardial response to exercise in a healthy pediatric cohort. J Am Soc Echocardiogr. 2016;29(7):648–54.
62. La Gerche A, Claessen G, Van De Bruaene A, Pattyn N, Van Cleemput J, Gewillig M, et al. Cardiac magnetic resonance imaging: a new gold standard for ventricular volume quantification during high-intensity exercise. Circ Cardiovasc Imaging. 2013;6(2):329–38.
63. Biko DM, Collins RT 2nd, Partington SL, Harris M, Whitehead KK, Keller MS, et al. Magnetic resonance myocardial perfusion imaging: safety and indications in pediatrics and young adults. Pediatr Cardiol. 2018;39(2):275–82.
64. Sarikouch S, Peters B, Gutberlet M, Leismann B, Kelter-Kloepping A, Koerperich H, et al. Sex-specific pediatric percentiles for ventricular size and mass as reference values for

cardiac MRI: assessment by steady-state free-precession and phase-contrast MRI flow. Circ Cardiovasc Imaging. 2010;3(1):65–76.
65. Dallaire F, Slorach C, Hui W, Sarkola T, Friedberg MK, Bradley TJ, et al. Reference values for pulse wave Doppler and tissue Doppler imaging in pediatric echocardiography. Circ Cardiovasc Imaging. 2015;8(2):e002167.
66. Overbeek LI, Kapusta L, Peer PG, de Korte CL, Thijssen JM, Daniels O. New reference values for echocardiographic dimensions of healthy Dutch children. Eur J Echocardiogr. 2006;7(2):113–21.
67. Macinnes M, Martin N, Fulton H, McLeod KA. Comparison of a smartphone-based ECG recording system with a standard cardiac event monitor in the investigation of palpitations in children. Arch Dis Child. 2019;104(1):43–7.
68. Budts W, Borjesson M, Chessa M, van Buuren F, Trigo Trindade P, Corrado D, et al. Physical activity in adolescents and adults with congenital heart defects; individualized exercise prescription. Eur Heart J. 2013;34(47):3669–74.
69. Richard P, Denjoy I, Fressart V, Wilson MG, Carre F, Charron P. Advising a cardiac disease gene positive yet phenotype negative or borderline abnormal athlete: is sporting disqualification really necessary? Br J Sports Med. 2012;46(Suppl 1):i59–68.
70. Lipshultz SE, Orav EJ, Wilkinson JD, Towbin JA, Messere JE, Lowe AM, et al. Risk stratification at diagnosis for children with hypertrophic cardiomyopathy: an analysis of data from the Pediatric Cardiomyopathy Registry. Lancet. 2013;382(9908):1889–97.
71. Pelliccia A, Solberg EE, Papadakis M, Adami PE, Biffi A, Caselli S, et al. Recommendations for participation in competitive and leisure time sport in athletes with cardiomyopathies, myocarditis, and pericarditis: position statement of the Sport Cardiology Section of the European Association of Preventive Cardiology (EAPC). Eur Heart J. 2019;40(1):19–33.
72. Bauce B, Frigo G, Benini G, Michieli P, Basso C, Folino AF, et al. Differences and similarities between arrhythmogenic right ventricular cardiomyopathy and athlete's heart adaptations. Br J Sports Med. 2010;44(2):148–54.
73. Steinmetz M, Krause U, Lauerer P, Konietschke F, Aguayo R, Ritter CO, et al. Diagnosing ARVC in pediatric patients applying the revised task force criteria: importance of imaging, 12-lead ECG, and genetics. Pediatr Cardiol. 2018;39(6):1156–64.
74. Pieles GE, Grosse-Wortmann L, Hader M, Fatah M, Chungsomprasong P, Slorach C, et al. Association of Echocardiographic Parameters of Right Ventricular Remodeling and Myocardial Performance With Modified Task Force Criteria in Adolescents With Arrhythmogenic Right Ventricular Cardiomyopathy. Circ Cardiovasc Imaging. 2019;12(4):e007693.
75. Etoom Y, Govindapillai S, Hamilton R, Manlhiot C, Yoo SJ, Farhan M, et al. Importance of CMR within the Task Force Criteria for the diagnosis of ARVC in children and adolescents. J Am Coll Cardiol. 2015;65(10):987–95.
76. Sequeira IB, Kirsh JA, Hamilton RM, Russell JL, Gross GJ. Utility of exercise testing in children and teenagers with arrhythmogenic right ventricular cardiomyopathy. Am J Cardiol. 2009;104(3):411–3.
77. Popple E, George K, Somauroo J, Sharma S, Utomi V, Lord R, et al. Right ventricular structure and function in senior and academy elite footballers. Scand J Med Sci Sports. 2018;28(12):2617–24.
78. Thiene GNA, Angelini A, Daliento L, Scognamiglio R, Corrado D. Anatomoclinical aspects of arrhythmogenic right ventricular cardiomyopathy. In: Baroldi GCF, Goodwin JF, editors. Advances in cardiomyopathies. Milano: Springer Verlag; 1990. p. 397–408.
79. Marcus FI, McKenna WJ, Sherrill D, Basso C, Bauce B, Bluemke DA, et al. Diagnosis of arrhythmogenic right ventricular cardiomyopathy/dysplasia: proposed modification of the task force criteria. Circulation. 2010;121(13):1533–41.
80. Pignatelli RH, McMahon CJ, Dreyer WJ, Denfield SW, Price J, Belmont JW, et al. Clinical characterization of left ventricular noncompaction in children: a relatively common form of cardiomyopathy. Circulation. 2003;108(21):2672–8.
81. Gati S, Chandra N, Bennett RL, Reed M, Kervio G, Panoulas VF, et al. Increased left ventricular trabeculation in highly trained athletes: do we need more stringent criteria for the diagnosis of left ventricular non-compaction in athletes? Heart. 2013;99(6):401–8.

82. Sabatino J, Di Salvo G, Krupickova S, Fraisse A, Prota C, Bucciarelli V, et al. Left ventricular twist mechanics to identify left ventricular noncompaction in childhood. Circ Cardiovasc Imaging. 2019;12(4):e007805.
83. Puranik R, Chow CK, Duflou JA, Kilborn MJ, McGuire MA. Sudden death in the young. Heart Rhythm. 2005;2(12):1277–82.
84. Zipes DP, Link MS, Ackerman MJ, Kovacs RJ, Myerburg RJ, NAM E 3rd. Eligibility and disqualification recommendations for competitive athletes with cardiovascular abnormalities: Task Force 9: arrhythmias and conduction defects: a scientific statement from the American Heart Association and American College of Cardiology. J Am Coll Cardiol. 2015;66(21):2412–23.
85. Al-Khatib SM, Stevenson WG, Ackerman MJ, Bryant WJ, Callans DJ, Curtis AB, et al. AHA/ACC/HRS guideline for management of patients with ventricular arrhythmias and the prevention of sudden cardiac death: a report of the American College of Cardiology/American Heart Association Task Force on Clinical Practice Guidelines and the Heart Rhythm Society. J Am Coll Cardiol. 2018;72(14):e91–e220.
86. Priori SG, Schwartz PJ, Napolitano C, Bloise R, Ronchetti E, Grillo M, et al. Risk stratification in the long-QT syndrome. N Engl J Med. 2003;348(19):1866–74.
87. Gussak I, Brugada P, Brugada J, Wright RS, Kopecky SL, Chaitman BR, et al. Idiopathic short QT interval: a new clinical syndrome? Cardiology. 2000;94(2):99–102.
88. Giustetto C, Di Monte F, Wolpert C, Borggrefe M, Schimpf R, Sbragia P, et al. Short QT syndrome: clinical findings and diagnostic-therapeutic implications. Eur Heart J. 2006;27(20):2440–7.
89. Mazzanti A, Kanthan A, Monteforte N, Memmi M, Bloise R, Novelli V, et al. Novel insight into the natural history of short QT syndrome. J Am Coll Cardiol. 2014;63(13):1300–8.
90. Bjerregaard P. Diagnosis and management of short QT syndrome. Heart Rhythm. 2018;15(8):1261–7.
91. Priori SG, Wilde AA, Horie M, Cho Y, Behr ER, Berul C, et al. HRS/EHRA/APHRS expert consensus statement on the diagnosis and management of patients with inherited primary arrhythmia syndromes: document endorsed by HRS, EHRA, and APHRS in May 2013 and by ACCF, AHA, PACES, and AEPC in June 2013. Heart Rhythm. 2013;10(12):1932–63.
92. Antzelevitch C, Brugada P, Borggrefe M, Brugada J, Brugada R, Corrado D, et al. Brugada syndrome: report of the second consensus conference. Heart Rhythm. 2005;2(4):429–40.
93. Sarquella-Brugada G, Campuzano O, Iglesias A, Sanchez-Malagon J, Guerra-Balic M, Brugada J, et al. Genetics of sudden cardiac death in children and young athletes. Cardiol Young. 2013;23(2):159–73.
94. Chockalingam P, Wilde A. The multifaceted cardiac sodium channel and its clinical implications. Heart. 2012;98(17):1318–24.
95. Tfelt-Hansen J, Winkel BG, Grunnet M, Jespersen T. Cardiac channelopathies and sudden infant death syndrome. Cardiology. 2011;119(1):21–33.
96. Benito B, Sarkozy A, Mont L, Henkens S, Berruezo A, Tamborero D, et al. Gender differences in clinical manifestations of Brugada syndrome. J Am Coll Cardiol. 2008;52(19):1567–73.
97. Milman A, Gourraud JB, Andorin A, Postema PG, Sacher F, Mabo P, et al. Gender differences in patients with Brugada syndrome and arrhythmic events: data from a survey on arrhythmic events in 678 patients. Heart Rhythm. 2018;15(10):1457–65.
98. Andorin A, Behr ER, Denjoy I, Crotti L, Dagradi F, Jesel L, et al. Impact of clinical and genetic findings on the management of young patients with Brugada syndrome. Heart Rhythm. 2016;13(6):1274–82.
99. Priori SG, Napolitano C, Gasparini M, Pappone C, Della Bella P, Giordano U, et al. Natural history of Brugada syndrome: insights for risk stratification and management. Circulation. 2002;105(11):1342–7.
100. Michowitz Y, Milman A, Sarquella-Brugada G, Andorin A, Champagne J, Postema PG, et al. Fever-related arrhythmic events in the multicenter survey on arrhythmic events in Brugada syndrome. Heart Rhythm. 2018;15(9):1394–401.
101. Mehrotra S, Juneja R, Naik N, Pavri BB. Successful use of quinine in the treatment of electrical storm in a child with Brugada syndrome. J Cardiovasc Electrophysiol. 2011;22(5):594–7.

102. Hermida JS, Denjoy I, Clerc J, Extramiana F, Jarry G, Milliez P, et al. Hydroquinidine therapy in Brugada syndrome. J Am Coll Cardiol. 2004;43(10):1853–60.
103. Viskin S. Brugada syndrome in children: don't ask, don't tell? Circulation. 2007;115(15):1970–2.
104. Celiker A, Erdogan I, Karagoz T, Ozer S. Clinical experiences of patients with catecholaminergic polymorphic ventricular tachycardia. Cardiol Young. 2009;19(1):45–52.
105. Roston TM, Yuchi Z, Kannankeril PJ, Hathaway J, Vinocur JM, Etheridge SP, et al. The clinical and genetic spectrum of catecholaminergic polymorphic ventricular tachycardia: findings from an international multicentre registry. Europace. 2018;20(3):541–7.
106. Broendberg AK, Nielsen JC, Bjerre J, Pedersen LN, Kristensen J, Henriksen FL, et al. Nationwide experience of catecholaminergic polymorphic ventricular tachycardia caused by RyR2 mutations. Heart. 2017;103(12):901–9.
107. Napolitano C, Bloise R, Monteforte N, Priori SG. Sudden cardiac death and genetic ion channelopathies: long QT, Brugada, short QT, catecholaminergic polymorphic ventricular tachycardia, and idiopathic ventricular fibrillation. Circulation. 2012;125(16):2027–34.
108. Brugada J, Blom N, Sarquella-Brugada G, Blomstrom-Lundqvist C, Deanfield J, Janousek J, et al. Pharmacological and non-pharmacological therapy for arrhythmias in the pediatric population: EHRA and AEPC-Arrhythmia Working Group joint consensus statement. Europace. 2013;15(9):1337–82.
109. Van Hare GF, Javitz H, Carmelli D, Saul JP, Tanel RE, Fischbach PS, et al. Prospective assessment after pediatric cardiac ablation: demographics, medical profiles, and initial outcomes. J Cardiovasc Electrophysiol. 2004;15(7):759–70.
110. Santinelli V, Radinovic A, Manguso F, Vicedomini G, Ciconte G, Gulletta S, et al. Asymptomatic ventricular preexcitation: a long-term prospective follow-up study of 293 adult patients. Circ Arrhythm Electrophysiol. 2009;2(2):102–7.
111. Krahn AD, Manfreda J, Tate RB, Mathewson FA, Cuddy TE. The natural history of electrocardiographic preexcitation in men. The Manitoba Follow-up Study. Ann Intern Med. 1992;116(6):456–60.
112. Silva G, de Morais GP, Primo J, Sousa O, Pereira E, Ponte M, et al. Aborted sudden cardiac death as first presentation of Wolff-Parkinson-White syndrome. Rev Port Cardiol. 2013;32(4):325–9.
113. Timmermans C, Smeets JL, Rodriguez LM, Vrouchos G, van den Dool A, Wellens HJ. Aborted sudden death in the Wolff-Parkinson-White syndrome. Am J Cardiol. 1995;76(7):492–4.
114. Sanchis-Gomar F, Perez-Quilis C, Lippi G, Cervellin G, Leischik R, Lollgen H, et al. Atrial fibrillation in highly trained endurance athletes - Description of a syndrome. Int J Cardiol. 2017;226:11–20.
115. Furlanello F, Bertoldi A, Dallago M, Galassi A, Fernando F, Biffi A, et al. Atrial fibrillation in elite athletes. J Cardiovasc Electrophysiol. 1998;9(8 Suppl):S63–8.
116. Dendale P, De Meirleir K, De Wolf D. Ectopic atrial tachycardia in a young athlete. Med Sci Sports Exerc. 1994;26(8):937-40.
117. Hubert A, Galand V, Donal E, Pavin D, Galli E, Martins RP, et al. Atrial function is altered in lone paroxysmal atrial fibrillation in male endurance veteran athletes. Eur Heart J Cardiovasc Imaging. 2018;19(2):145–53.
118. Qiu J, Tu T, Zhou S, Liu Q. Disordered myocardium energy metabolism in the progression of atrial fibrillation in highly trained endurance athletes. Int J Cardiol. 2017;233:95.
119. Simmons MA, Rollinson N, Fishberger S, Qin L, Fahey J, Elder RW. Modern incidence of complete heart block in patients with L-looped ventricles: does univentricular status matter? Congenit Heart Dis. 2015;10(5):E237–42.
120. Yan J, Varma SK, Malhotra A, Menahem S. Congenital complete heart block: single tertiary centre experience. Heart Lung Circ. 2012;21(11):666–70.
121. Wang JN, Tsai YC, Lee WL, Lin CS, Wu JM. Complete atrioventricular block following myocarditis in children. Pediatr Cardiol. 2002;23(5):518–21.

122. Gladman G, Davis AM, Fogelman R, Hamilton RM, Gow RM. Torsade de pointes, acquired complete heart block and inappropriately long QT in childhood. Can J Cardiol. 1996;12(7):683–5.
123. Heidbuchel H, Corrado D, Biffi A, Hoffmann E, Panhuyzen-Goedkoop N, Hoogsteen J, et al. Recommendations for participation in leisure-time physical activity and competitive sports of patients with arrhythmias and potentially arrhythmogenic conditions. Part II: ventricular arrhythmias, channelopathies and implantable defibrillators. Eur J Cardiovasc Prev Rehabil. 2006;13(5):676–86.
124. Drezner JA, Levine BD, Vetter VL. Reframing the debate: screening athletes to prevent sudden cardiac death. Heart Rhythm. 2013;10(3):454–5.
125. McClean G, Riding NR, Ardern CL, Farooq A, Pieles GE, Watt V, et al. Electrical and structural adaptations of the paediatric athlete's heart: a systematic review with meta-analysis. Br J Sports Med. 2018;52(4):230.
126. Granacher U, Lesinski M, Busch D, Muehlbauer T, Prieske O, Puta C, et al. Effects of resistance training in youth athletes on muscular fitness and athletic performance: a conceptual model for long-term athlete development. Front Physiol. 2016;7:164.

# Specific Populations: Female Athletes

# 24

Susanne Berrisch-Rahmel
and Nicole M. Panhuyzen-Goedkoop

**Learning Objectives**

1. Cardiac adaptation in (elite) female athletes.
2. The female hormonal system and exercise.
3. Incidence and causes of sudden cardiac death in female athletes.
4. Pregnancy and exercise (adaptation of the cardiovascular system, safe and unsafe physical activities during pregnancy, exercise and pregnancy in elite athletes)
5. Pre-participation screening in female athletes.

## 24.1 Introduction

Females participating in athletic activities have gained an enormous popularity in recent years. Many women nowadays even participate in typical masculine sports such as boxing, martial arts, soccer and rugby, and the female athletes do not shun to participate in competitive, elite sports or in master athletic activities.

- Women were allowed to participate for the first time during the IXth modern Olympic Games in Amsterdam (1928), but only in track & field.
- Since the XXXth Olympic Games in London (2012) women and males equally participate in all types of sports.

S. Berrisch-Rahmel (✉)
MVZ DaVita CardioCentrum Düsseldorf, Düsseldorf, Germany
e-mail: berrisch-rahmel@t-online.de

N. M. Panhuyzen-Goedkoop
Department of Clinical and Experimental Cardiology, Amsterdam Cardiovascular Sciences, Amsterdam UMC, University of Amsterdam, Heart Center, Meibergdreef, Amsterdam, Germany

Department of Sports Cardiology, Sports Medical Centre Papendal, Arnhem, The Netherlands
e-mail: n.m.panhuyzen@amsterdamumc.nl





A. Pressler, J. Niebauer (eds.), *Textbook of Sports and Exercise Cardiology*,
https://doi.org/10.1007/978-3-030-35374-2_24

- However, even today the financial rewards in commercial sports like soccer, tennis, cycling and golf are lower for female elite athletes compared with male athletes.

Female athletes differ from their male counterparts in several aspects, such as in

1. Anthropometry,
2. The hormonal system,
3. Physiology, and
4. Psychology.

Female athletes tend to have a smaller body size and a lower lean body mass, but a higher body fat-percentage (usually between 20 and 25%). Female athletes have a smaller heart muscle mass, skeletal muscle mass and a lower endurance capacity. Peak oxygen uptake in male athletes is higher, because of a higher cardiac output and higher amounts of hemoglobin transporting oxygen to the muscles. In addition, female athletes have a lower amount of circulation androgens. Furthermore, during the menstrual period loss of blood induces a reduction of hemoglobin transporting oxygen, thereby reducing the physical performance and recovery after exercise. Therefore, the male muscular system can perform better during exercise, and female athletes are less capable in power sports and endurance sports.

In this chapter the sports cardiology issues relevant to female athletes, e.g. physiologic cardiac adaptation, screening for eligibility to participate in exercise, and exercise during pregnancy are discussed. However, despite the increasing popularity of females participating in sports and the clinical relevance of gender differences, a surprisingly low number of sports cardiology studies have been conducted on female athletes so far.

## 24.2 Cardiac Adaptation in (Elite) Female Athletes

Cardiac adaptation to exercise in athletes is regulated by the neurovegetative system (NVS). The NVS regulates the autonomic nervous system (ANS) and the hormonal system. Cardiac adaptation, classified as electrical changes (or electrophysiological remodeling) and structural changes (or morphologic remodeling), induces cardiac functional changes to increase the cardiac output and the maximal oxygen transport ($VO_2$max) required for an optimal physical performance. The determinants of cardiac adaptation in athletes are the type and intensity of sports, gender, age, body size, ethnicity, use of prohibited or illicit drugs, and the existence of inherited or congenital cardiovascular conditions [1]. Female athletes, like male athletes, are capable of exercise-induced electrical and morphologic cardiac changes compared to sedentary controls. However, the cardiac changes differ between female and male athletes.

### 24.2.1 Electrical Cardiac Changes

- The electrical cardiac changes in female athletes differ from their male counterparts. Gender differences are related to the influence of sex hormones on cardiac repolarization and the underlying transmembrane currents. An athlete's ECG reflects vagotonia and the increased dimensions of the cavities and wall sizes of the four cardiac compartments.
- Bjornstad and Storstein et al. found significantly lower heart rates (64 bpm) and voltage criteria for right and left ventricular hypertrophy including taller T-waves among female athletes (n = 542) compared with female sedentary controls [2, 3].
- In a study on computerized ECG measurements in college athletes, Gademan et al. found that the type of sports affected the heart rate, the QRS duration (gymnastics 82 ms, volleyball 95 ms), the QRS axis (basketball vertical axis, golf left axis), and the T-wave amplitude, that was highest in female cross-country skiers (0.80 mV) [4]. Among male athletes this electrical cardiac adaptation was more pronounced, but expressed itself in other ECG findings, which is probably attributed to a higher androgenic hormone level inducing more extensive training-related cardiac remodeling in male athletes.
- In contrast to male athletes, the morphologic cardiac changes among female athletes involve the atria and in few cases the ventricles (see Sect. 24.2.2). Therefore, voltage criteria of ventricular hypertrophy are rarely seen on the ECG.

#### 24.2.1.1 Female Hormones and the ECG

In 1920 Bazett et al. described that the QTc-interval in females was longer compared with males. At birth, the QTc-intervals of both genders are very similar [5]. During the adolescence or young adult period the sex hormones become increasingly active. In males, the testosterone level is high and decreases slowly during adulthood until the age of 50 years. During the adolescent period the QTc-interval in males becomes shorter compared with females (1–20 ms) until it normalizes once the testosterone levels have decreased [6]. The normal QTc values in athletes, described by the International recommendations, are <480 ms for female athletes and <470 ms for male athletes [7].

- **Estrogen** affects the action potential at different levels. Estrogen reaches a high level during the follicular phase. Estrogen prolongs the QTc-interval by reducing the 'repolarization reserve'. The concept of the 'repolarization reserve' hypothesizes that impairment of a transmembrane ion channel induces other repolarizing currents to take over and compensate. Therefore, excessive repolarization changes and, consequently, QTc-prolongation inducing Torsade de Pointes (TdP) arrhythmia do not occur [8]. Therefore, females are more susceptible for drug-induced TdP arrhythmias than males [8].
- **Progesterone** reaches high levels during the luteal phase (after the ovulation). Progesterone reduces the L-type inward calcium current (ICaL) in the plateau phase 2 of the electrical repolarization (Fig. 24.1). The plateau voltage is

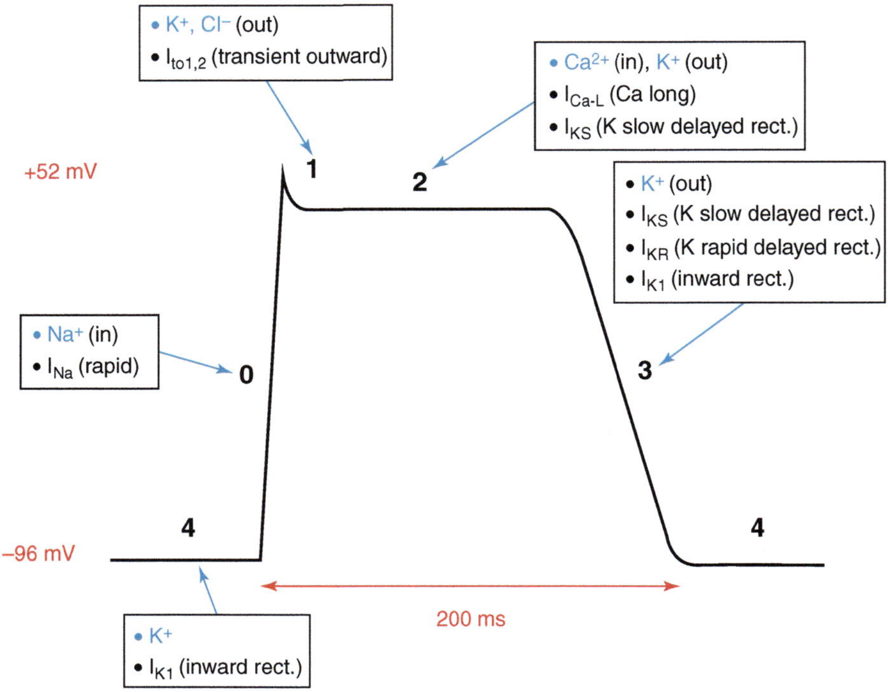


**Fig. 24.1** The influence of the electrical current on the different phases of the action potential (see text for more details)

shifted towards more positive values that may result in enhanced activation of outward potassium currents (IKr and IKs), shortening the repolarization duration [8, 9].

- Estrogen can oppose the effect of progesterone. Estrogen reduces the rapid delayed rectifier potassium current (IKr), thereby increasing after-depolarizations (Fig. 24.1) [8, 9].

In competitive athletes the 'repolarization reserve' can be impaired when an unknown cardiovascular condition (e.g. cardiomyopathy) is present or when illicit substances or drug abuse superimpose on the repolarizing currents inducing lethal cardiac arrhythmias [8].

#### 24.2.1.2 Ethnical Differences

- Rawlins et al. found in a combined British-French study, that African/Afro-Caribbean female athletes show a longer PR interval (162 ± 25), a shorter QRS duration (84 ± 10 ms), a higher prevalence of ST- segment elevation (14%), and a higher prevalence of T-wave inversion (11%) compared with Caucasian female athletes (149 ± 23 ms, 87 ± 1 ms, 2% and 1%, respectively) [10].

**Table 24.1** Electrical cardiac adaptations in female athletes [2, 4, 7, 10]

| | Caucasian | African/Afro-Caribbean |
|---|---|---|
| Heart rate, bpm | <64 | |
| PR interval, ms | 149 ± 23 | 162 ± 25 |
| QRS duration, ms | 87 ± 10 | 84 ± 10 |
| QRS axis | Vertical left | |
| ST-segment elevation, prevalence in % | 2 | 14 |
| T-wave amplitude, mV | <0.80 | |
| T-wave inversions, prevalence in % | 1 | 11 |
| QTc-interval, ms | <480 | <480 |

- There was little difference between both ethnicities regarding the QRS-axis and the QTc-interval duration, and the prevalence of incomplete right bundle branch (iRBBB) [10].
- Voltage criteria for left ventricular hypertrophy (LVH) and for right and left atrial enlargement (RAE/LAE) also differed little among both ethnicities (Afro-Caribbeans 8%, 5%,!3% and Caucasians 12%, 4% and 10%, respectively) [10].

Table 24.1 summarizes electrical cardiac changes in female athletes.

### 24.2.2 Morphologic Cardiac Changes

Structural cardiac changes are less pronounced in female athletes compared with male athletes. Power sports induce an increase in left ventricular wall thickness, as in men, while high dynamic sports commonly induce an increase in LV cavity size. Both types of training induce an increase in LV mass [11]. However, the cardiac dimensions in female athletes mostly are within the normal limits described for the general population. Echocardiography in female athletes:

- The end-diastolic left ventricular cavity size (LVEDD) in elite female athletes (12–49 years of age) rarely exceeded the normal limits of 54 mm (8%), and the wall thickness of the left ventricle (LVWT) seldom exceeded 11 mm [10, 12–14].
- Compared with sedentary controls, the LVEDD and LVWT are larger in female athletes (LVEDD 49 ± 4 mm, LVWT 8.2 ± 0.9 mm; sedentary controls 46 ± 3 mm and 7.2 ± 0.6 mm) [10, 12–14].
- For African/Afro-Caribbean female athletes a LVWT of 12–13 mm was found among 3% [10].
- The systolic deformation parameters of the left ventricle in female power sports and endurance sports participants are within normal limits, with a slightly reduced global longitudinal and circumferential strain in endurance sport [11].
- Similar to the left ventricle, female athletes demonstrate an increased dimension of the right ventricular cavity, measured in the short axis view, exceeding the normal limits in 40% (RVOT diameter >28 mm, 24% of them >51 mm) [15].

**Table 24.2** Morphologic cardiac adaptation in female athletes, transthoracic echocardiographic upper limits of normal (adapted from data presented in [10–18])

| | Caucasian | | African/Afro-Caribbean | |
|---|---|---|---|---|
| | Adolescent (14–18 years) | Adult (>18 years) | Adolescent (14–18 years) | Adult (>18 years) |
| LV enddiastolic diameter, mm | 54 | 56–60 | 56 | 56 |
| LV wall thickness, mm | 11 | 11 | 11 | 12–13 |
| RV enddiastolic diameter, mm | | 49 | | 49 |
| RV outflow tract, mm | | 40 | | 40 |

*LV* left ventricular, *RV* right ventricular

The challenge remains to distinguish pathology from physiologic cardiac adaptation. With cardiac imaging the dimensions of the LVEDD were consistent with those observed in dilated cardiomyopathy (DCM) in 1% of the female athletes (14% in male athletes). However, in no case imaging revealed an abnormal thickening of the LV wall suggesting potential hypertrophic cardiomyopathy (HCM) (2% in Caucasian males, 13% in African/Afro-Caribbean males) [13, 16]. Interestingly, it seems that female endurance athletes develop a more eccentric type of LVH compared with male athletes [17].

- In brief, an LVEDD exceeding 54 mm regardless of ethnicity, and an LVWT exceeding 11 mm in Caucasian female athletes or 13 mm in African/Afro-Caribbean female athletes raises suspicion for a pathological background [18].

Table 24.2 summarizes the upper limits of normal morphologic cardiac changes in female athletes.

## 24.3 Sudden Cardiac Death in Female Athletes

Exercise-related sudden cardiac arrest/death (SCA/SCD) is a tragic but very rare event among athletes (see also Chap. 6).

- The annual incidence rate ranges between 0.6 to 2.85 per 100,000 young athletes (age 12–35 years) [19–28].
- In master athletes (>35 years) the incidence is higher (2–6.7 per 100,000) and is expected to increase with age [26–28].
- Over 90% of all exercise-related SCA/SCD occur among recreational athletes [29, 30].
- Female athletes tend to have a significantly lower risk of SCA/SCD than men. The female-male ratio among young athletes is 1.5:8.5 (<35 years), and among master athletes 0.5:9.5 [20, 22, 24, 30].
- This lower risk among female athletes can be attributed to an increased prevalence and phenotypic expression of high-risk cardiovascular conditions in males, such as inherited cardiomyopathy, electrical disease and coronary artery disease, that are probably induced by high levels of androgen [18, 21, 22, 31].

- Moreover, more male athletes participate in popular sports showing the highest incidence of SCA/SCD, such as soccer and basketball [22].
- Finocchiaro et al. described that the majority (53%) of SCD cases among female athletes had a structurally normal heart, suggesting that an electrical disease is the underlying mechanism [18].

Cardiovascular conditions associated with SCA/SCD differ in young *vs.* master athletes. In young athletes there is a predominance of inherited causes, such as channelopathies and cardiomyopathies, and myocarditis (see also particular chapters). Among master athletes, coronary artery disease and HCM are most common [32]. In addition, among all age groups myocarditis and blunt chest trauma prone for life-threatening ventricular arrhythmia are important causes of SCA/SCD.

- In brief, female athletes die very rarely during exercise. However, when SCA/SCD occurs, an underlying electrical heart disease is the most likely cause.

## 24.4 Pregnancy and Exercise

As more and more women are actively involved in sports, the proportion of pregnant sportswomen and athletes is also rising. For a long time, pregnant women were advised against sports activities. It was feared that physical exertion could lead to a harmful competitive situation of energy resources for both mother and child [33, 34].

- In the 1960s, light physical activity during pregnancy was recommended for the first time. Leisure time physical activity during pregnancy has multiple obstetric benefits apart from the exercise benefits—there were easier birth processes, an improved placental development and a favorable influence on fetal development in sportively active women [35].
- Based on the consistent safety evidence regarding exercise during pregnancy, multiple nations and health care organizations, including the American College of Obstetrics and Gynecology (first in 2002, reaffirmed 2009 and 2015), recommend moderate-intensity exercise for 20–30 min on most if not all days of the week (i.e., 150–180 min per week). Most of these groups additionally recommend muscle- and bone-strengthening activities using major muscle groups twice a week as beneficial.
- Pregnant women who were rather un-athletic before their pregnancy should in any case be motivated to take part in regular sporting activities [36].

### 24.4.1 Benefits of Sports in Pregnancy

1. maintaining fitness at a higher level;
2. improved body control and perception, movement safety despite the growing belly;
3. less back pain;

4. more balanced, less sudden mood swings;
5. less gestational diabetes, especially in overweight women;
6. less development of excessive gestational weight gain;
7. easier recovery of the initial weight;
8. risk reduction of varicose veins and thrombosis;
9. less preeclampsia and reduced cesarean sections.

The Norwegian Mother and Child Cohort Study (MoBa) with 61,098 pregnant women demonstrated lower rates of preterm birth in women exercising 3–5 times per week at 30 weeks [37].

### 24.4.2 Recommendations for Exercise in Pregnancy

- Women who did not exercise before pregnancy should start at low intensity (50% peak oxygen uptake ($VO_2$peak)) with 10-min intervals and 10-min breaks. After 2–4 weeks the duration (slowly up to 30–45 min) and later the intensity of the training program (75% $VO_2$peak) should be increased [38].
- Clapp et al. were able to show that it is possible until delivery to carry out weight-bearing exercise for 20 min, 3–5 times a week at 55–65% intensity of the preconceptional aerobic capacity [39, 40].
- All pregnant women should be advised to perform a light 5-min warm-up before exercise and to cool down after exercise (i.e., gentle walking or cycling).
- Pregnant women who habitually engage in vigorous-intensity aerobic activity or are highly active can continue this activity during pregnancy.
- Healthy trained pregnant women and her fetus can tolerate somewhat higher exercise intensities (85–90% $VO_2$peak). However, prolonged exercise of more than 45 min results in an elevated core maternal and fetal temperature, representing a potential fetal risk.
- Regular medical check-ups are of crucial importance, especially in the case of high-intensity physical exertion and in pregnant women with no sporting experience.

Pregnancy is associated with significant anatomical, hormonal, metabolic, cardiovascular and pulmonary changes/adaptations. In women who have obstetric or medical co-morbidities, exercise regimens should be individualized.

### 24.4.3 Cautions and Concerns for Exercise During Pregnancy

For women at risk of premature birth or fetal growth retardation, exercise beyond the second trimester should be discouraged [41]. According to the current ESC Guidelines for the management of cardiovascular diseases during pregnancy, in the case of known significant cardiovascular diseases as well as in the case of high-risk pregnancies a recommendation for sport should only be given after shared consultation with gynecologists and cardiologists [42]. Table 24.3 summarizes relative and absolute contraindications to exercise during pregnancy [38].

**Table 24.3** Relative and absolute contraindications to exercise during pregnancy (summarized recommendations from [38])

| Relative contraindications | Absolute contraindications |
|---|---|
| Cervical enlargement | Hemodynamically significant cardiac disease |
| Poorly controlled type 1 diabetes | Restrictive lung disease |
| Chronic bronchitis or other respiratory disorders | Incompetent cervix or cerclage |
| Unevaluated maternal cardiac arrhythmia | Multiple gestation at risk of premature labor |
| History of fetal growth restriction, miscarriage, premature birth or labour | Persistent second- or third-trimester bleeding |
| Orthopaedic limitations | Placenta previa after 26 weeks of gestation |
| | Premature labor during the current pregnancy |
| | Ruptured membranes |
| | Pre-eclampsia or pregnancy-induced hypertension |
| | Severe anemia |

### 24.4.4 Changes in the Cardiovascular System During Pregnancy

Pregnancy is associated with significant anatomical, hormonal, metabolic, cardiovascular and pulmonary changes/adaptations. This article focuses on the cardiovascular adaptions [35, 43–46].

- Physiological adaptations of the cardiovascular system begin in the fifth week of pregnancy and can last up to 1 year after birth.
- Cardiac output increases by about 40% due to an increased stroke volume (10–20%) and an increased heart rate (5–10%).
- The blood volume increases by about 40–50% during pregnancy, dependent on iron and folate resources.
- Vascular tone decreases due to increased progesterone concentrations in the plasma.
- The systemic vascular resistance is reduced.

The cardiovascular changes caused by pregnancy are comparable to endurance training. Thus, trained pregnant women at rest have reduced heart rates and increased stroke volumes.

- Athletes who have maintained an adapted workout throughout their pregnancy have significantly improved post-natal fitness parameters and a higher level of performance [34].
- An improved oxygen transport capacity of 15–18% increase in absolute aerobic capacity persists for several months after giving birth [47]. Parameters such as increased stroke volume and reduced resistance can still be found up to one year after birth [39, 40].

The fear of many athletes having to accept a drastic loss of personal performance during pregnancy does not seem to be justified. In contrast, one can even expect an increased level of performance [48].

### 24.4.5 Training Recommendations

Again, according to the American College of Obstetricians and Gynecologists 2015, the following recommendations are applicable:

- Long-term exposure—especially anaerobic exposure—can lead to hyperthermia and dehydration, which can negatively affect the fetus. Thus,
  - before training sufficient food intake and sufficient hydration is recommended to prevent hypoglycemia.
  - a sufficient intake of calories is important to prevent weight loss, which can affect the growth of the fetus.
  - in extremely warm weather conditions with high/humid ambient temperature and humidity, the training duration should be reduced.
  - the training should generally not be perceived as too strenuous (e.g. perceived effort 13–14 on Borg's 6–20 scale; see Chap. 44).

#### 24.4.5.1 Recommended Sports

Sports with regular aerobic activity are recommended:

1. pregnancy gymnastics;
2. rhythmic sports such as gymnastics, yoga, Pilates and dance;
3. sports with regular, aerobic stress such as swimming, walking or cycling (ergometer);
4. Jogging (provided it has been practiced regularly before);
5. Moderate skiing at 2000–2500 m altitude (with appropriate ability);
6. Snorkeling, rowing, recreational tennis and golfing;
7. Swimming and water gymnastics as an effective sport to alleviate pregnancy-induced back pain.

#### 24.4.5.2 Sports That Are Not Recommended

It is not advisable to engage in sports with a risk of overstraining or even injuring the fetus:

1. contact sports such as ice hockey, football or basketball, martial arts, boxing;
2. Sports with increased risk of falling (mountain biking, inline skating, skating, horse riding, surfing, water skiing, trampoline jumping);
3. Extreme sports like bungee jumping, parachuting, paragliding, etc.;
4. Diving below 30 m (danger of decompression sickness for the fetus);
5. Hot Yoga and Hot Pilates;
6. Participation in marathons (cave: increase of the body core temperature).

#### 24.4.5.3 Warning Signs

The following symptoms should prompt immediate termination of exercise, independent of prior well-being:

1. vaginal bleeding;
2. amniotic fluid leakage;
3. decreased fetal movement;
4. contractions more frequent than every 6 min;
5. chest pain;
6. irregular heartbeat;
7. shortness of breath, dizziness, syncope;
8. calf pain, calf swelling.

Only 10–15% of all pregnant women implement training recommendations. Reasons are patient specific and culturally driven and/or obstetric providers who do not recommend regular exercise due to a lack of specific knowledge or motivation [35, 43–45].

The key caveat of the aforementioned recommendations is the phrase "*in the absence of medical or obstetric complications*." However, the majority of U.S. women of reproductive age (20–39 years) are unhealthy prior to conception; for instance, 30% are obese (BMI > 30 kg/m$^2$), 7% have chronic hypertension, 2–3% are diabetic, 15–20% are active smokers, 10–15% are anemic (hemoglobin <10.0 g/L), and 10% have cardiovascular disease [49]. In these circumstances, a good education and care for the pregnant women is of utmost importance.

### 24.4.6 Competition Participation During and After Pregnancy

Competitions in the early pregnancy phase are basically possible [44, 45].

- The pregnancy-induced increase of human chorionic gonadotropin has a positive effect on performance (personal records, all between the 25th and 35th week).
- Given the lack of available research to advice elite athletes who choose to exercise above moderate levels, particular attention should be paid to fetal growth in the second and third trimester.
- 4 weeks after birth, (performance) training can be started again; light physical activities are possible within a few days after delivery in the case of uncomplicated processes.
- Multiple national and international organizations recommend that every neonate should exclusively be breastfed for 6 months and continued to be at least partly breastfed for 12 months or more. It makes sense to breastfeed the child before training to avoid jamming of the milk [46].
- Competitive athletes require frequent and close monitoring as they tend to maintain a strenuous training schedule during pregnancy and resume high-intensity postpartum training earlier than others.

Numerous studies and individual case observations - some of them by prominent female athletes - have shown that adapted training has not only a positive effect on the course of pregnancy, but that significantly improved fitness parameters and a higher level of performance can be observed after birth [50]. Therefore, advice to elite athletes regarding exercise frequency, duration and intensity beyond current guidelines must be individualized with a regular observation of maternal and fetal well-being [51].

**Clinical Pearls**

- Sudden cardiac arrest (SCA) among female athletes is very rare. If SCA occurs, an electrical cardiovascular condition is a common cause.
- Estrogen prolongs the QTc-interval by reducing the 'repolarization reserve'. Female athletes are more susceptible for drug-induced Torsade-de-Pointes arrhythmias.
- The cardiac dimensions of the ventricles among female athletes rarely exceed the normal values, as measured at echocardiography.
- Regular sporting activities during pregnancy have multiple benefits. In women who have obstetric or medical co-morbidities, exercise regimens should be individualized.
- Pregnant women who were sedentary before their pregnancy should be motivated to take part in leisure time physical activity.

## Review

## Questions

1. A 24-year-old elite female volleyball player visits your out-patient sports cardiology clinic. Since two weeks she suffers from near-syncope during training sessions. The family history for SCA and inherited cardiovascular conditions is negative. Her physical examination is normal. The ECG demonstrates a sinus rhythm, no electrical axis deviation, PR-interval 210 ms, QRS duration 90 ms, QTc-interval 490 ms. No voltage criteria of ventricular hypertrophy.
   (a) What is your differential diagnosis?
   (b) Do you require additional cardiac evaluation? If yes, which? If no, why not?
   (c) What is your management, including recommendations for sports continuation?
2. A 28-year-old elite female middle distance runner visits you for a sport examination. She is looking to get pregnant. She is afraid having to stop training and undertaking competitions.
   (a) What is your recommendation?
   (b) Do you have any practical advice? If yes, which?
   (c) What is your management plan for the postpartum training?

3. Four months later the same 28-year-old elite female middle distance runner is pregnant and comes to a visit. She tolerates the training with higher exercise intensities (85–90% $VO_2$peak) well but is exercising no longer than 45 min.
   (a) Which symptoms should prompt immediate termination of exercise, regardless of prior well being?
   (b) Which other sports are not recommended?

## Answers

1. (a) The symptoms may indicate Torsades-de-Pointes in Long QT syndrome. Think of a high estrogen level prolonging the QTc-interval in females. (b) Additional evaluation is required here because of an exercise-related near-syncope: analysis of the QTC interval during with exercise stress testing and rhythm assessment by Holter monitoring; echocardiography to exclude structural causes of near-syncope. (c) In case Long QT syndrome is demonstrated, restrictions apply to this patient as outlined in Chap. 20 on channelopathies.
2. (a) Pregnant women who habitually engage in vigorous intensity aerobic activity or are highly active can continue this activity during pregnancy. It is not advisable to engage in marathons because of the increase of the body core temperature. Regular observation of maternal and fetal well-being is necessary.
   (b) Sufficient food intake and sufficient hydration is recommended before training to prevent hypoglycemia. A sufficient intake of calories is important to prevent weight loss, which can affect the growth of the fetus. In extremely warm weather conditions with high/humid ambient temperature and humidity, the training duration should be reduced.
   (c) Light physical activities are possible within a few days after delivery if there were no complications. Performance training can be started again 4 weeks after birth. Improved fitness parameters and a higher level of performance can be observed after birth.
3. (a) Warning signs to stop exercise are vaginal bleeding, amniotic fluid leakage, decreased fetal movement, contractions more frequent than every 6 min, chest pain, irregular heartbeat, shortness of breath, dizziness, syncope, calf pain, calf swelling.
   (b) It is not advisable to engage in sports with a risk of overstraining or even injuring the fetus:
   - contact sports such as ice hockey, football or basketball, martial arts, boxing;
   - Sports with increased risk of falling (mountain biking, inline skating, skating, horse riding, surfing, water skiing, trampoline jumping);
   - Extreme sports like bungee jumping, parachuting, paragliding, etc.;
   - Diving below 30 m (danger of decompression sickness for the fetus);
   - Hot Yoga and Hot Pilates

## References

1. Wilson MG, Drezner JA, Sharma S. International Olympic Committee—manual of sports cardiology. 1st ed. Hoboken: Wiley-Blackwell; 2016.
2. Bjornstad H, Storstein L, Meen HD, Hals O. Electrocardiographic findings in athletic students and sedentary controls. Cardiology. 1991;79(4):290–305.
3. Storstein L, Bjornstad H, Hals O, Meen HD. Electrocardiographic findings according to sex in athletes and controls. Cardiology. 1991;79(3):227–36.
4. Gademan MG, Uberoi A, Le VV, Mandic S, van Oort ER, Myers J, et al. The effect of sport on computerized electrocardiogram measurements in college athletes. Eur J Prev Cardiol. 2012;19(1):126–38.
5. Stramba-Badiale M, Spagnolo D, Bosi G, Schwartz PJ. Are gender differences in QTc present at birth? MISNES investigators. Multicenter Italian study on neonatal electrocardiography and sudden infant death syndrome. Am J Cardiol. 1995;75(17):1277–8.
6. Rautaharju PM, Zhou SH, Wong S, Calhoun HP, Berenson GS, Prineas R, et al. Sex differences in the evolution of the electrocardiographic QT interval with age. Can J Cardiol. 1992;8(7):690–5.
7. Sharma S, Drezner JA, Baggish A, Papadakis M, Wilson MG, Prutkin JM, et al. International recommendations for electrocardiographic interpretation in athletes. Eur Heart J. 2018;39(16):1466–80.
8. Varro A, Baczko I. Cardiac ventricular repolarization reserve: a principle for understanding drug-related proarrhythmic risk. Br J Pharmacol. 2011;164(1):14–36.
9. Rodriguez I, Kilborn MJ, Liu XK, Pezzullo JC, Woosley RL. Drug-induced QT prolongation in women during the menstrual cycle. JAMA. 2001;285(10):1322–6.
10. Rawlins J, Carre F, Kervio G, Papadakis M, Chandra N, Edwards C, et al. Ethnic differences in physiological cardiac adaptation to intense physical exercise in highly trained female athletes. Circulation. 2010;121(9):1078–85.
11. Doronina A, Edes IF, Ujvari A, Kantor Z, Lakatos BK, Tokodi M, et al. The female athlete's heart: comparison of cardiac changes induced by different types of exercise training using 3D echocardiography. Biomed Res Int. 2018;2018:3561962.
12. Pelliccia A, Culasso F, Di Paolo FM, Maron BJ. Physiologic left ventricular cavity dilatation in elite athletes. Ann Intern Med. 1999;130(1):23–31.
13. Pelliccia A, Maron BJ, Culasso F, Spataro A, Caselli G. Athlete's heart in women. Echocardiographic characterization of highly trained elite female athletes. JAMA. 1996;276(3):211–5.
14. Whyte GP, George K, Sharma S, Firoozi S, Stephens N, Senior R, et al. The upper limit of physiological cardiac hypertrophy in elite male and female athletes: the British experience. Eur J Appl Physiol. 2004;92(4–5):592–7.
15. Zaidi A, Ghani S, Sharma R, Oxborough D, Panoulas VF, Sheikh N, et al. Physiological right ventricular adaptation in elite athletes of African and Afro-Caribbean origin. Circulation. 2013;127(17):1783–92.
16. Papadakis M, Carre F, Kervio G, Rawlins J, Panoulas VF, Chandra N, et al. The prevalence, distribution, and clinical outcomes of electrocardiographic repolarization patterns in male athletes of African/Afro-Caribbean origin. Eur Heart J. 2011;32(18):2304–13.
17. Finocchiaro G, Sharma S. Do endurance sports affect female hearts differently to male hearts? Futur Cardiol. 2016;12(2):105–8.
18. Finocchiaro G, Dhutia H, D'Silva A, Malhotra A, Steriotis A, Millar L, et al. Effect of sex and sporting discipline on LV adaptation to exercise. JACC Cardiovasc Imaging. 2017;10(9):965–72.
19. Bille K, Figueiras D, Schamasch P, Kappenberger L, Brenner JI, Meijboom FJ, et al. Sudden cardiac death in athletes: the Lausanne Recommendations. Eur J Cardiovasc Prev Rehabil. 2006;13(6):859–75.

20. Corrado D, Basso C, Pavei A, Michieli P, Schiavon M, Thiene G. Trends in sudden cardiovascular death in young competitive athletes after implementation of a preparticipation screening program. JAMA. 2006;296(13):1593–601.
21. Corrado D, Basso C, Schiavon M, Thiene G. Screening for hypertrophic cardiomyopathy in young athletes. N Engl J Med. 1998;339(6):364–9.
22. Harmon KG, Asif IM, Klossner D, Drezner JA. Incidence of sudden cardiac death in National Collegiate Athletic Association athletes. Circulation. 2011;123(15):1594–600.
23. Margey R, Roy A, Tobin S, O'Keane CJ, McGorrian C, Morris V, et al. Sudden cardiac death in 14- to 35-year olds in Ireland from 2005 to 2007: a retrospective registry. Europace. 2011;13(10):1411–8.
24. Maron BJ, Doerer JJ, Haas TS, Tierney DM, Mueller FO. Sudden deaths in young competitive athletes: analysis of 1866 deaths in the United States, 1980-2006. Circulation. 2009;119(8):1085–92.
25. Maron BJ, Thompson PD, Ackerman MJ, Balady G, Berger S, Cohen D, et al. Recommendations and considerations related to preparticipation screening for cardiovascular abnormalities in competitive athletes: 2007 update: a scientific statement from the American Heart Association Council on Nutrition, Physical Activity, and Metabolism: endorsed by the American College of Cardiology Foundation. Circulation. 2007;115(12):1643–455.
26. Siscovick DS, Weiss NS, Fletcher RH, Lasky T. The incidence of primary cardiac arrest during vigorous exercise. N Engl J Med. 1984;311(14):874–7.
27. Thompson PD, Funk EJ, Carleton RA, Sturner WQ. Incidence of death during jogging in Rhode Island from 1975 through 1980. JAMA. 1982;247(18):2535–8.
28. Van Camp SP, Bloor CM, Mueller FO, Cantu RC, Olson HG. Nontraumatic sports death in high school and college athletes. Med Sci Sports Exerc. 1995;27(5):641–7.
29. Berdowski J, de Beus MF, Blom M, Bardai A, Bots ML, Doevendans PA, et al. Exercise-related out-of-hospital cardiac arrest in the general population: incidence and prognosis. Eur Heart J. 2013;34(47):3616–23.
30. Marijon E, Tafflet M, Celermajer DS, Dumas F, Perier MC, Mustafic H, et al. Sports-related sudden death in the general population. Circulation. 2011;124(6):672–81.
31. Chandra N, Papadakis M, Sharma S. Preparticipation screening of young competitive athletes for cardiovascular disorders. Phys Sportsmed. 2010;38(1):54–63.
32. Priori SG, Blomstrom-Lundqvist C, Mazzanti A, Blom N, Borggrefe M, Camm J, et al. ESC Guidelines for the management of patients with ventricular arrhythmias and the prevention of sudden cardiac death: The Task Force for the Management of Patients with Ventricular Arrhythmias and the Prevention of Sudden Cardiac Death of the European Society of Cardiology (ESC). Endorsed by: Association for European Paediatric and Congenital Cardiology (AEPC). Eur Heart J. 2015;36(41):2793–867.
33. Kardel KR. Effects of intense training during and after pregnancy in top-level athletes. Scand J Med Sci Sports. 2005;15(2):79–86.
34. Pivarnik JM, Perkins CD, Moyerbrailean T. Athletes and pregnancy. Clin Obstet Gynecol. 2003;46(2):403–14.
35. Bo K, Artal R, Barakat R, Brown W, Dooley M, Evenson KR, et al. Exercise and pregnancy in recreational and elite athletes: 2016 evidence summary from the IOC expert group meeting, Lausanne. Part 2-the effect of exercise on the fetus, labour and birth. Br J Sports Med. 2016;50(21):1297–305.
36. Barakat R, Perales M, Garatachea N, Ruiz JR, Lucia A. Exercise during pregnancy. A narrative review asking: what do we know? Br J Sports Med. 2015;49(21):1377–81.
37. Juhl M, Andersen PK, Olsen J, Madsen M, Jorgensen T, Nohr EA, et al. Physical exercise during pregnancy and the risk of preterm birth: a study within the Danish National Birth Cohort. Am J Epidemiol. 2008;167(7):859–66.
38. Committee opinion no. 650 summary: physical activity and exercise during pregnancy and the postpartum period. Obstet Gynecol. 2015;126(6):1326–7.
39. Clapp JF 3rd. Exercise during pregnancy. A clinical update. Clin Sports Med. 2000;19(2):273–86.

40. Clapp JF 3rd, Kim H, Burciu B, Lopez B. Beginning regular exercise in early pregnancy: effect on fetoplacental growth. Am J Obstet Gynecol. 2000;183(6):1484–8.
41. Davies GA, Wolfe LA, Mottola MF, MacKinnon C. Society of O, gynecologists of Canada SCPOC. Joint SOGC/CSEP clinical practice guideline: exercise in pregnancy and the postpartum period. Can J Appl Physiol. 2003;28(3):330–41.
42. Regitz-Zagrosek V, Roos-Hesselink JW, Bauersachs J, Blomstrom-Lundqvist C, Cifkova R, De Bonis M, et al. 2018 ESC guidelines for the management of cardiovascular diseases during pregnancy. Eur Heart J. 2018;39(34):3165–241.
43. Bo K, Artal R, Barakat R, Brown W, Davies GA, Dooley M, et al. Exercise and pregnancy in recreational and elite athletes: 2016 evidence summary from the IOC expert group meeting, Lausanne. Part 1-exercise in women planning pregnancy and those who are pregnant. Br J Sports Med. 2016;50(10):571–89.
44. Bo K, Artal R, Barakat R, Brown WJ, Davies GAL, Dooley M, et al. Exercise and pregnancy in recreational and elite athletes: 2016/17 evidence summary from the IOC expert group meeting, Lausanne. Part 4-Recommendations for future research. Br J Sports Med. 2017;51(24):1724–6.
45. Bo K, Artal R, Barakat R, Brown WJ, Davies GAL, Dooley M, et al. Exercise and pregnancy in recreational and elite athletes: 2016/17 evidence summary from the IOC Expert Group Meeting, Lausanne. Part 3-exercise in the postpartum period. Br J Sports Med. 2017;51(21):1516–25.
46. Newton ER, May L. Adaptation of maternal-fetal physiology to exercise in pregnancy: the basis of guidelines for physical activity in pregnancy. Clin Med Insights Women's Health. 2017;10:1179562X17693224.
47. Brown W. The benefits of physical activity during pregnancy. J Sci Med Sport. 2002;5(1):37–45.
48. Beilock SL, Feltz DL, Pivarnik JM. Training patterns of athletes during pregnancy and postpartum. Res Q Exerc Sport. 2001;72(1):39–46.
49. Nickens MA, Long RC, Geraci SA. Cardiovascular disease in pregnancy: (women's health series). South Med J. 2013;106(11):624–30.
50. Khan KM. Are 12 systematic reviews on exercise in pregnancy too many? Not for 125 million women who are pregnant every year: Kudos Society of Obstetricians and Gynaecologists of Canada (SOGC) and Canadian Society for Exercise Physiology (CSEP). Br J Sports Med. 2019;53(2):79–80.
51. Martinez-Pascual B, Alvarez-Harris S, Fernandez-de-Las-Penas C, Palacios-Cena D. Pregnancy in Spanish elite sportswomen: a qualitative study. Women Health. 2017;57(6):741–55.

# Specific Populations: Athletes of Afro-Caribbean Origin

# 25

Aneil Malhotra, Michael Papadakis, and Sanjay Sharma

**Learning Objectives**
1. To characterise the electrical differences between the black and white athlete's heart.
2. To outline the cardiac structural differences between the black and white athlete.
3. To understand the effect of age on the ECG and echocardiogram in black and white athletes.
4. To appreciate the regional differences between black athletes from varying parts of the African subcontinent.

## 25.1 Defining Ethnicity

Being of 'black' ethnic origin traditionally refers to individuals of African and Afro-Caribbean descent.

- Athletes from this ethnic background are participating at every level of sport and comprise three-quarters of National Basketball Association (NBA) players in the USA and the majority of the French football World Cup winning team in 2018.

Data from large-scale preparticipation screening programmes have helped further our understanding of variations that exist between black and white (European Caucasian) athletes. Such studies have led to specific electrical variations in the black athlete being classified as a normal variant, such as anterior T wave inversion.

A. Malhotra
Consultant Cardiologist-Inherited Cardiac Conditions and Sports Cardiology, Manchester University Hospitals, University of Manchester, Manchester, London, UK
e-mail: aneil.malhotra@manchester.ac.uk

M. Papadakis (✉) · S. Sharma
Cardiology Clinical Academic Group, St. George's, University of London, London, UK
e-mail: mipapada@sgul.ac.uk; sasharma@sgul.ac.uk



A. Pressler, J. Niebauer (eds.), *Textbook of Sports and Exercise Cardiology*,
https://doi.org/10.1007/978-3-030-35374-2_25

Contemporary screening programmes comprise health questionnaires that more accurately specify which region of Africa or the Caribbean the athlete originates from, and recent evidence has highlighted that repolarization differences, with particular reference to T wave inversion, do exist between black athletes from different regions of Africa.

## 25.2 Sudden Cardiac Death in Black Athletes

Distinction between T-wave inversion ECG patterns associated with ethnically-mediated physiological cardiac adaptation and those representing a potentially fatal disorder is crucial. Identifying subtle forms of cardiomyopathy that can provide the substrate for exercise-induced fatal arrhythmias often poses a conundrum when evaluating black athletes.

- There is a four to six-fold higher incidence of sudden cardiac death (SCD) during exercise among young black athletes (aged 14–35 years) compared with young white athletes [1–3].
- In an American study of National Collegiate Athletic Association (NCAA) student athletes, the risk of SCD was highest among basketball players at an overall rate of 1 in 11,394 person-years.
- Comparative rates among American football was 1 in 38,000.
- Among white basketball players the overall death rate was 1 in 21,824 but much higher in in black males (1 in 5743) [2].
- Increased rates of SCD among male basketball players compared with other athletes were also noted among high-school adolescents [4]. Athletes who play basketball professionally, however, tend to have a certain body habitus in which morphological expression of cardiomyopathy requires a better understanding than is currently known.
- A study of over 11,000 adolescent football players in the UK reported an overall incidence of SCD of 1 in 14,794 person-years but this was much higher among black football players (1 in 3708) than white counterparts (1 in 25,880) [1].

The dynamic component of basketball, similar to football in the UK, may provide adrenergic triggers for an underlying substrate, with a higher participation rate of black athletes in these sports.

## 25.3 Electrical Changes

### 25.3.1 Adult Black Athletes

It is now well-established that both white and black athletes reveal a high prevalence of benign, exercise-related ECG changes, particularly ST segment elevation, voltage criteria for left ventricular hypertrophy (LVH) and early repolarization [5–9]. It is also apparent that black athletes demonstrate a higher prevalence of T wave inversion which would be deemed abnormal in white athletes and often associated with primary cardiomyopathies.

Some recommendations on interpretation of the athlete's ECG had previously deemed T wave inversion beyond V1 as abnormal [10, 11] but in the Seattle criteria, anterior T wave inversion in V1-V2 is considered a normal finding [12, 13]. This is consensus-based with no studies yet done to endorse this.

- In a study of 1959 adult male American football players, T wave inversion was reported by Magalski et al. as 13 times more common in black athletes than white counterparts [7].
- Another study by Papadakis et al. compared the ECGs of 904 black adult male athletes with 1819 white adult male athletes, 119 black sedentary controls and 52 black patients with HCM [5].
  - T wave inversion was more than six times more common in black athletes than white athletes (22.8% vs. 3.7%; $p < 0.0001$).
  - Black controls demonstrated more T wave inversion than white athletes (10.1% vs. 3.7%; $p < 0.001$), suggesting that T wave inversion was an adaptation of exercise rather than ethnicity alone.
  - The T wave inversion in black athletes was mainly found in the anterior leads V1-V4 (12.7%).
  - In nearly two-thirds of these cases, the T wave inversion was preceded by J-point elevation and an ST segment with a convex morphology (Fig. 25.1).

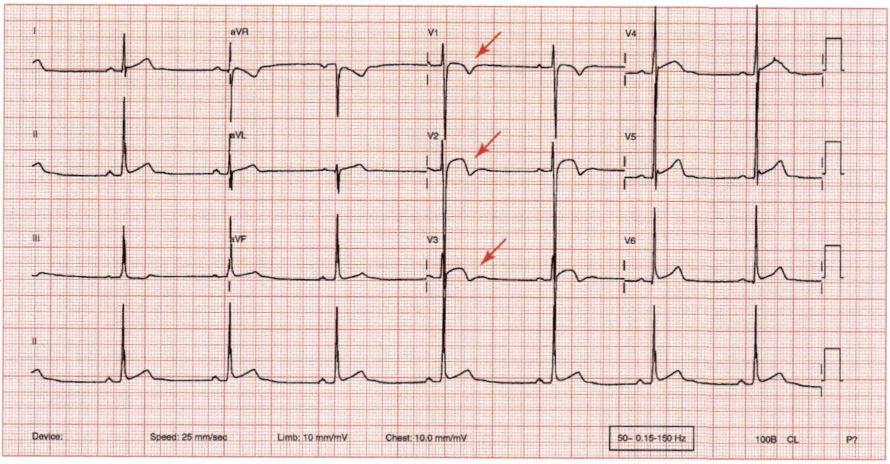


**Fig. 25.1** An example of a black athlete's ECG with T wave inversion V1-V3 preceded by a convex ST segment (red arrows)

- Deep T wave inversion (> −0.02 mv in depth) was more prevalent in black athletes compared with white athletes and black controls (12.1% vs. 1.0% vs. 1.7% respectively; $p < 0.0001$).
- T wave inversion in the inferior leads was 6% and in the lateral leads was 4%.
- The vast majority of black individuals with HCM however, exhibited T wave inversion (87.2%), which was most commonly present the lateral leads (76.9%).
- Isolated anterior T wave inversion was present in only 3.8% of patients and inferior T wave inversion alone was 1.9%.
- The preceding ST segments in black patients with HCM were frequently depressed (50.0%) but ST depression was virtually absent in black athletes (0.4%) and black controls (0%).
- While initial evaluation failed to identify an underlying cardiomyopathy in athletes with T wave inversion, two black athletes and one white athlete were subsequently diagnosed with HCM over a follow-up period of 69.7 ± 29.6 months. All three athletes demonstrated T wave inversion in the inferior and/or lateral leads.

Importantly, none of the black athletes with anterior T wave inversion was diagnosed with a cardiomyopathy, leading to the conclusion that this particular ECG pattern of T wave inversion in V1-V4, when preceded by J point elevation and ST segment elevation with a convex morphology, is now considered a normal ethnic adaptation to exercise [11–13]. T wave inversion in the lateral leads, however, warrants comprehensive evaluation with long-term follow-up (Fig. 25.2). The significance of inferior T wave inversion is as yet undetermined, and hence initial evaluation as a minimum is warranted at least with an echocardiogram.

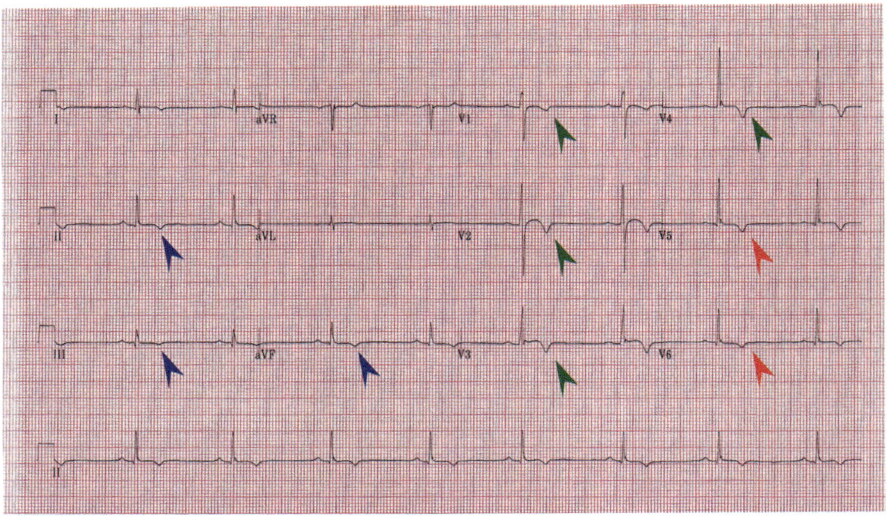


**Fig. 25.2** An ECG showing anterior T wave inversion (green arrows), inferior T wave inversion (blue arrows) and lateral T wave inversion (red arrows). T wave inversion in the inferior and or lateral leads warrants regular surveillance

### 25.3.2 Regional Electrical Variations Within Africa

Further evidence has emerged that the prevalence of T-wave inversion may vary dependent on the geographical origin of an athlete:

- A study of nearly 1698 black male athletes underwent pre-participation ECG and were categorised according as north, east, middle and west African, African American/Caribbean, South American, and west Asian.
  - Repolarization abnormalities were significantly more common among middle (8.5%) and west (6.4%) African athletes than east (1.5%) and north Africans (1.2%).

This highlights that there is variability in the electrical adaptations of 'black' athletes and geographical origin should be taken into consideration.

### 25.3.3 Adolescent Black Athletes

Few studies to date have focused on the black adolescent athlete:

- Di Paulo et al. compared 154 black (African) football players to 62 white football players and reported a higher prevalence of ST segment elevation (91% vs. 56%; $p < 0.001$) and deep T wave inversion (14% vs. 3%; $p < 0.001$) [14].
- In another study on black adolescent athletes, Sheikh et al. studied 329 black adolescent athletes (mean age 16.4 years and 74.5% males), 903 white adolescent athletes (mean age 16.4 years and 81.4% males) and black controls (mean age 15.3 years and 66.5% males) [15].
  - The authors reported a five-fold greater prevalence of T wave inversion in black adolescent athletes compared with white adolescent athletes (22.8% vs. 4.5%; $p < 0.001$).
  - Black sedentary controls demonstrated more T wave inversion than white adolescent athletes (13.4% vs. 45%; $p < 0.001$).
  - As with black adult athletes, T-wave inversion in black adolescents was predominantly confined to the anterior leads V1-V4 (14.3%).
  - Black male adolescent athletes had a higher prevalence of T wave inversion compared with adolescent black female athletes though not deemed statistically significant (24.5% vs. 16.7%; $p = 0.17$).
  - No black female athlete demonstrated deep T wave inversion, compared with 9% of black males in the study suggesting that the presence of deep T wave inversion in a female should warrant further investigation.
  - The prevalence of inferior and lateral T wave inversion was similar to adult counterparts (black adolescent athletes: 6.1% and 2.4% respectively; white adolescent athletes: 1.7% and 0.3% respectively; black controls: 0.7% for both).
  - Further evaluation of T wave inversion failed to reveal any underlying pathology, though given the association of T wave inversion with cardiomyopathy, regular follow-up is warranted.

## 25.4 Structural Changes

### 25.4.1 Adult Black Athletes

Black athletes demonstrate similar quantitative changes in left ventricular (LV) cavity dimensions to white athletes [5, 16]. The main structural difference between white and black athletes, however, is LV wall thickness (LVWT).

- Basavarajaiah et al. reported a greater mean LVWT in 300 black adult male athletes compared with that of 300 white adult male athletes (11.3 ± 1.6 mm vs. 10.0 ± 1.5 mm, $p < 0.001$; Fig. 25.3) [16].
  - Importantly, 18% of black athletes had a LVWT >12 mm which falls within the range of morphologically mild HCM (12–15 mm).
  - Moreover, 3% of black athletes exhibited significant LVH ≥ 15 mm, as opposed to none of the white athletes having an LVWT greater than 14 mm.
  - The pattern of LVH was homogeneous and often associated with LV cavity dilatation between 55 and 66 mm. Further evaluation of all athletes with LVH failed to elucidate underlying HCM.
- These findings were reproduced in a collaborative study between the UK and France of 904 black athletes and 1819 white athletes.
  - 12.4% of black athletes demonstrated a LVWT >12 mm compared with just 1.6% of white athletes [5] (Fig. 25.3).
  - No athlete exhibited a LVWT exceeding 16 mm.
- In a study by Rawlins et al. black female athletes demonstrated greater LVWTs compared with white female athletes (9.2 ± 1.2 mm vs. 8.6 ± 1.2 mm; $p < 0.001$) [16].
  - Only 3% black female athletes revealed a LVWT >11 mm with none >13 mm.
  - None of the white female athletes exceeded 11 mm.

### 25.4.2 Adolescent Black Athletes

Like adult counterparts, adolescent black athletes may also develop LVH to a greater degree than white adolescent athletes.

- Di Paolo et al. reported a greater mean LVWT in black adolescent athletes compared with white adolescent athletes (9.7 ± 1.3 mm vs. 9.2 ± 1.0 mm; $p < 0.001$), with 2.6% black athletes demonstrating LVH > 12 mm compared with 0% white athletes [17].
- In the study by Sheikh et al. evaluating 245 male and 84 female black adolescent athletes, 7% exhibited LVH > 12 mm, compared with 0.6% of 903 white adolescent athletes and none of 134 sedentary black adolescent controls [15].
- While no female adolescent athlete revealed a wall thickness > 13 mm, male adolescent athletes could develop LVH up to 15 mm.
- In those <16 years old, 5.5% black adolescent athletes exhibited LVH compared with none of the white athletes.
- No subject with LVH was subsequently diagnosed with HCM during evaluation or follow-up over a mean period of 99.1 ± 47.6 months.

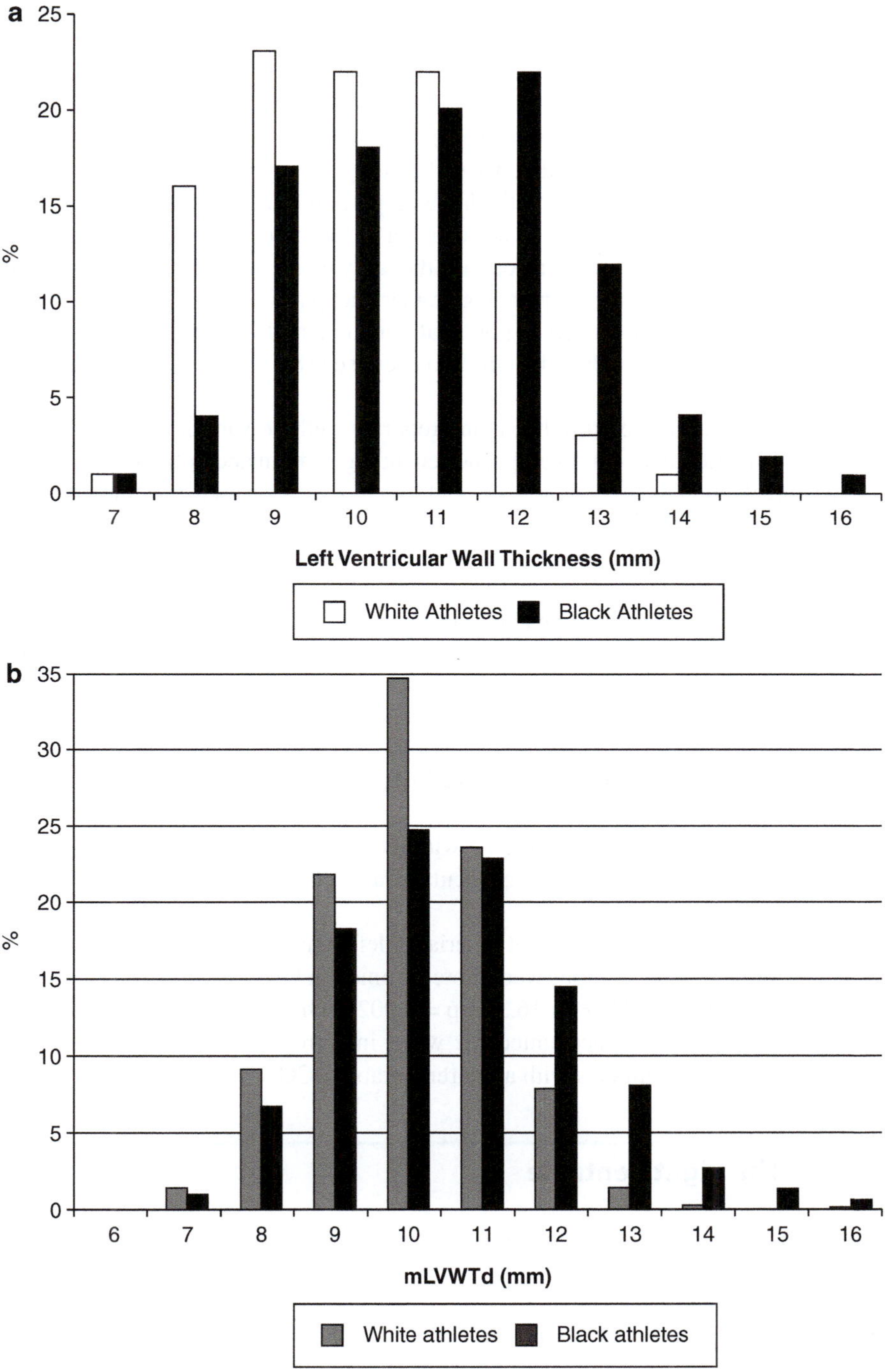


**Fig. 25.3** Bar chart (**a** from [28], and **b** from [5]) illustrating the rightward shift in normal distribution of left ventricular wall thickness in black athletes compared with white athletes

## 25.5 T-Wave Inversion and LV Hypertrophy in Black Athletes

Though T-wave inversion is a hallmark of cardiomyopathy, it is also possible that environmental factors, such as the stresses of cardiac load associated with exercise, could interact with a pathogenic rare variant and expose a concealed disease phenotype which would otherwise have remained concealed or only presented later on in life. When however, consideration is given to the large proportion of black athletes with T-wave inversion, this suggests that in the majority of cases this represents an ethnic variant, or a so-called innocent bystander. In contrast, the rarity of T-wave inversion in white athletes is more likely to represent pathology rather than physiology.

Several studies have eluded to potential genetic targets that may explain ethnic differences in cardiovascular adaptation to exercise [18].

- For example, the literature has many reports of ethnic variation between black and white individuals in several genes encoding sodium and potassium ion channels involved in the pathogenesis of LQTS and Brugada syndrome, including the KCN family and SCN5A, particularly the Y1102 polymorphism and its association with SCD in the black population (see also Chap. 12) [19–22].
- Polymorphisms in some of these targets have been show to influence T-wave parameters including T-wave alternans and repolarisation intervals [21].
- However, as of yet there are no robust reports on potential genetic targets that may specifically influence T-wave inversion.

## 25.6 Increased Trabeculations Among Black Athletes

- In a study of over 1100 athletes without symptoms, 18% demonstrated an increased prevalence of left ventricular trabeculations compared with 7% of controls.
  - Nearly a tenth of athletes met criteria for left ventricular non-compaction [23].
  - Moreover, trabeculations were more common in black athletes compared with white athletes (28.8% vs 16.3%; $p = 0.002$), which again highlights that ethnicity needs to be accounted for when interpreting the echocardiogram of asymptomatic athletes with an unremarkable ECG.

## 25.7 The Right Ventricle

There are few studies reporting the ethnic variation between black and white athletes for the right ventricle.

- One study compared 375 white athletes and 300 black athletes and found that white athletes demonstrated larger right ventricular diameter and outflow tract dimensions [24].
  - While such structural dilatation satisfied criteria for arrhythmogenic right ventricular cardiomyopathy (ARVC), the additional electrical changes of

anterior T-wave inversion were found in 3% of black athletes, reinforcing the clinical suspicion of ARVC.

– While subsequent evaluation did not reveal underlying pathology, the application of these criteria in non-white populations is highlighted.

**Clinical Pearls**

- Ethnicity needs to be accounted for when evaluating the pre-participation ECG and echocardiogram of an athlete.
- Black athletes reveal a greater degree of ECG repolarization changes such as T-wave inversion and left ventricular hypertrophy on echocardiography compared with white athletes.
- The distinction between athlete's heart and underlying mild phenotypic cardiomyopathy is more challenging.

## Review

## Questions

1. An asymptomatic 15-year-old black athlete underwent pre-participation screening. His ECG is displayed below (Fig. 25.4). What is your advice:
   (a) Refer for echocardiogram.
   (b) Reassure and consider repeat evaluation in 1 year.
   (c) Refer for an exercise test.
   (d) Familial evaluation.
   (e) Request a cardiac MRI.

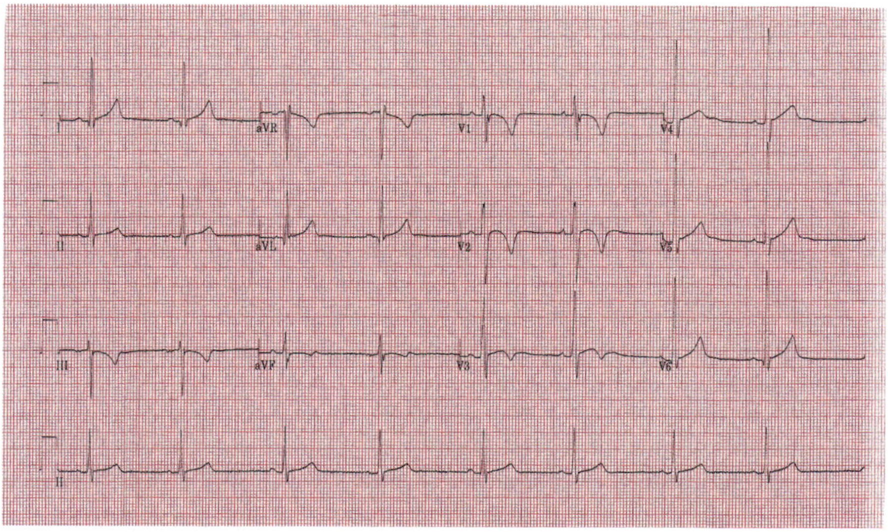


**Fig. 25.4** ECG referring to review question 1

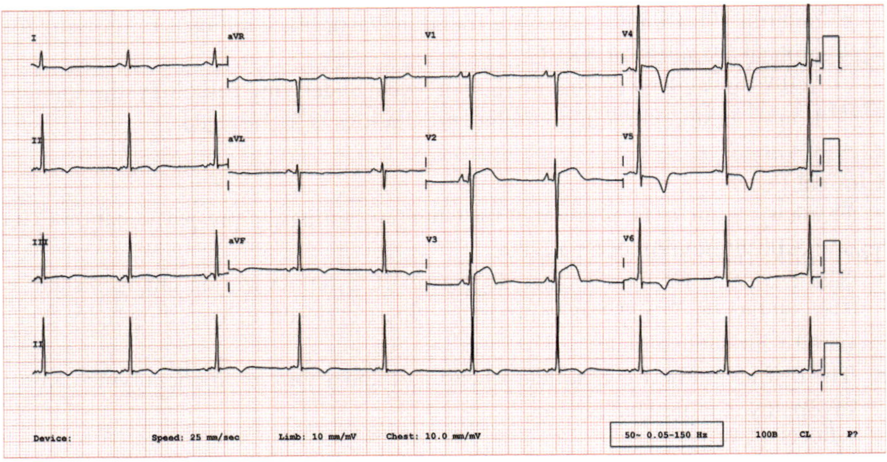


**Fig. 25.5** ECG referring to review question 2

2. A black male athlete of north African origin presented with chest pain and the ECG below (Fig. 25.5). Echocardiography revealed good biventricular systolic function with a left ventricular maximal wall thickness of 14 mm. What would you do next:
   (a) Perform an exercise test and ambulatory ECG.
   (b) Perform a cardiac MRI.
   (c) Perform genetic testing.
   (d) Perform a cardiac MRI, exercise test and ambulatory ECG monitoring.
   (e) Reassure that the LV hypertrophy on echocardiogram is within normal limits.

## Answers

1. Answer is (**b**). Anterior T wave inversion (V1-V3) is present on this ECG which affects up to 13% of **adult** black athletes and is deemed a normal variant when preceded by a convex ST-segment. Among white adult athletes, the prevalence is 0.3%, and given the rarity and extension beyond V2, it warrants further investigation according to the international recommendations [25]. In addition, there are tall amplitude QRS complexes on the ECG that are associated with athletic status and likely lean body habitus.

   In those **under** the age of 16 years, this ECG pattern is considered 'juvenile' and does not warrant further investigation in the absence of symptoms or a significant family history. The prevalence of anterior T-wave inversion in those aged 12 years is up to 15% [26]. A study by Migliore et al. reported a prevalence of T wave inversion of 5.7% among 2765 children aged between 8–18 years who underwent preparticipation screening [27]. The majority of T wave inversion (4.7%) was localized to the right precordial leads and considered a juvenile pattern. This was significantly higher (8.4%) in children aged <14 years old but fell to just 1.7% in those ≥14 years and affects just 0.2% of adults.

2. Answer is (**d**). This patient is symptomatic with chest pain and has an ECG that shows left ventricular hypertrophy meeting Sokolow-Lyon criterion, early repolarization in V3 and V4 with an ascending ST segment morphology, a partial right bundle branch pattern and importantly, lateral T wave inversion in V5-V6 and I and aVL. Additionally, there is an upright T-wave in aVR.

   This distribution of T-wave inversion is found in less than 4% of black athletes and prompts further evaluation given the association with hypertrophic cardiomyopathy. Though the left ventricular maximal wall thickness is 14 mm and reflects the upper limit of normal, further assessment with MRI is indicated. This will enable accurate chamber size and wall thickness quantification as well as highlight any abnormal patterns of fibrosis. Ambulatory ECG monitoring and exercise testing will help establish if any arrhythmias are present as well as the haemodynamic response to exercise. Genetic testing may be useful further down the clinical pathway, particularly if a diagnosis is clinically established, though a negative result does not exclude hypertrophic cardiomyopathy.

## References


1. Malhotra A, Dhutia H, Finocchiaro G, et al. Outcomes of cardiac screening in adolescent soccer players. N Engl J Med. 2018;379(6):524–34.
2. Harmon KG, Asif IM, Klossner D, J a D. Incidence of sudden cardiac death in National Collegiate Athletic Association athletes. Circulation. 2011;123(15):1594–600.
3. Maron BJ, Carney KP, Lever HM, et al. Relationship of race to sudden cardiac death in competitive athletes with hypertrophic cardiomyopathy. J Am Coll Cardiol. 2003;41(6):974–80.
4. Drezner JA, Harmon KG, Marek JC. Incidence of sudden cardiac arrest in innesota high school student athletes: the limitations of catastrophic insurance claims. J Am Coll Cardiol. 2014;63(14):1455–6.
5. Papadakis M, Carre F, Kervio G, et al. The prevalence, distribution, and clinical outcomes of electrocardiographic repolarization patterns in male athletes of African/Afro-Caribbean origin. Eur Heart J. 2011;32(18):2304–13.
6. Choo JK, Abernethy WB, Hutter AM. Electrocardiographic observations in professional football players. Am J Cardiol. 2002;90(2):198–200.
7. Magalski A, Maron BJ, Main ML, et al. Relation of race to electrocardiographic patterns in elite American football players. J Am Coll Cardiol. 2008;51(23):2250–5.
8. Balady GJ, Cadigan JB, Ryan TJ. Electrocardiogram of the athlete: an analysis of 289 professional football players. Am J Cardiol. 1984;53(9):1339–43.
9. Noseworthy P, Weiner R, Kim J, et al. Early repolarization pattern in competitive athletes: clinical correlates and the effects of exercise training. Circ Arrhythm Electrophysiol. 2011;4(4):432–40.
10. Corrado D, Pelliccia A, Heidbuchel H, et al. Recommendations for interpretation of 12-lead electrocardiogram in the athlete. Eur Heart J. 2010;31(2):243–59.
11. Sheikh N, Papadakis M, Ghani S, et al. Comparison of ECG criteria for the detection of cardiac abnormalities in Elite Black and White Athletes. Circulation. 2014;129(16):1637–49.

12. Drezner J, Ackerman MJ, Anderson J, et al. Electrocardiographic interpretation in athletes: the "Seattle criteria". Br J Sports Med. 2013;47(3):122–4.
13. Sharma S, Drezner J, Baggish A, et al. International recommendations for the interpretation of the athlete's ECG. J Am Coll Cardiol. 2017;69(8):1057–75.
14. Di Paolo FM, Schmied C, Zerguini YA, et al. The Athlete's heart in adolescent Africans: an electrocardiographic and echocardiographic study. J Am Coll Cardiol. 2012;59(11):1029–36.
15. Sheikh N, Papadakis M, Carre F, et al. Cardiac adaptation to exercise in adolescent athletes of African ethnicity: an emergent elite athletic population. Br J Sports Med. 2013 Jun;47(9):585–92.
16. Basavarajaiah S, Boraita A, Whyte G, et al. Ethnic differences in left ventricular remodeling in highly-trained athletes relevance to differentiating physiologic left ventricular hypertrophy from hypertrophic cardiomyopathy. J Am Coll Cardiol. 2008;51(23):2256–62.
17. Rawlins J, Carre F, Kervio G, et al. Ethnic differences in physiological cardiac adaptation to intense physical exercise in highly trained female athletes. Circulation. 2010;121(9):1078–85. https://doi.org/10.1161/CIRCULATIONAHA.109.917211.
18. Di Paolo FM, Schmied C, Y a Z, et al. The athlete's heart in adolescent Africans: an electrocardiographic and echocardiographic study. J Am Coll Cardiol. 2012;59(11):1029–36.
19. Montgomery H, Clarkson P, Barnard M, et al. Angiotensin-converting-enzyme gene insertion/deletion polymorphism and response to physical training. Lancet. 1999;353(9152):541–5.
20. Killen S a S, Kunic J, Wang L, et al. SCN5A allelic expression imbalance in African-Americans heterozygous for the common variant p.Ser1103Tyr. BMC Med Genet. 2010;11:74.
21. Van Norstrand DW, Tester DJ, Ackerman MJ. Overrepresentation of the proarrhythmic, sudden death predisposing sodium channel polymorphism S1103Y in a population-based cohort of African-American sudden infant death syndrome. Hear Rhythm. 2008;5(5):712–5.
22. Porthan K, Marjamaa A, Viitasalo M, et al. Relationship of common candidate gene variants to electrocardiographic T-wave peak to T-wave end interval and T-wave morphology parameters. Hear Rhythm. 2010;7(7):898–903.
23. Juang JMJ, Horie M. Genetics of Brugada syndrome. J Arrhythmia. 2016;32(5):418–25.
24. Gati S, Chandra N, Bennett RL, et al. Increased left ventricular trabeculation in highly trained athletes: do we need more stringent criteria for the diagnosis of left ventricular non-compaction in athletes. Heart. 2013;99(6):401–8.
25. Zaidi A, Ghani S, Sharma R, et al. Physiological right ventricular adaptation in elite athletes of African and Afro-Caribbean origin. Circulation. 2013;127(17):1783–92.
26. Malhotra A, Dhutia H, Gati S, et al. Anterior T-wave inversion in young white athletes and nonathletes: prevalence and significance. J Am Coll Cardiol. 2017 Jan 3;69(1):1–9.
27. Ascenzi FD, Anselmi F, Berti B, et al. Prevalence and significance of T-wave inversion in children practicing sport: a prospective, 4-year follow-up study. Int J Cardiol. 2019;279:100–4.
28. Migliore F, Zorzi A, Michieli P, et al. Prevalence of cardiomyopathy in Italian asymptomatic children with electrocardiographic T-wave inversion at preparticipation screening. Circulation. 2012;125(3):529–38.

# Commotio Cordis

# 26

Erik Ekker Solberg and Mark S. Link

**Learning Objectives**

1. Understand the mechanisms behind commotio cordis.
2. What you should do if commotio cordis occurred in the vicinity of you.
3. Learn about mechanisms of sudden cardiac arrest by understanding the vulnerability of the recovery phase of the cardiac cycle.
4. Learn about the usefulness of an experimental model to understand different aspects of the pathophysiology behind commotio cordis.

## 26.1 Introduction

Commotio cordis (CC) is a phenomenon in which sudden cardiac arrest occurs due to a chest wall strike. While thought to be extremely rare a couple decades ago, it is now apparent that CC is a common cause of sudden cardiac death in athletes in the US but is more rare in Europe [1–7]. CC is not a new phenomenon. It was described in workplace accidents in the nineteenth century, and there is evidence of CC occurring in sports in the early twentieth century, even though it was not recognized as such. In a 1900–1910 archival baseball report, there were 19 deaths due to ball strikes over the heart [8].

The original version of this chapter was revised. The correction to this chapter can be found at https://doi.org/10.1007/978-3-030-35374-2_52

E. E. Solberg
Medicals Department, Diakonhjemmet Hospital, Oslo, Norway
e-mail: erik.solberg@diakonsyk.no

M. S. Link (✉)
Department of Medicine, Division of Cardiology, UTSouthwestern Medical Center, Dallas, TX, USA
e-mail: mark.link@utsouthwestern.edu



A. Pressler, J. Niebauer (eds.), *Textbook of Sports and Exercise Cardiology*,
https://doi.org/10.1007/978-3-030-35374-2_26

## 26.2 Commotio Cordis in Sports

### 26.2.1 Epidemiology

- In American youth sports, CC is the second leading cause of death [2].
- According to the National Commotio Cordis Registry created in 1996 and closed in 2010, 224 cases of sudden death from chest impact have accrued during that period [9–12].
- Approximately 75% of these cases occurred in the setting of sport including 50% during competitive - and 25% during recreational sport [13].
- Approximately 25% of cases in the registry occurred during non-sporting activities such as playful fighting between individuals or child discipline [9].

In most cases victims are struck by projectiles normally implemented in the game, such as balls and pucks. The majority of cases occur in sports that involve a small projectile with a dense core that tends to be propelled at a high velocity, such as in baseball, lacrosse, and hockey [9]. All impacts were sustained over the left precordium, directly over the cardiac silhouette [7]. Every year approximately 20 new cases of CC were reported to the registry.

- Solberg et al., by reporting a Norwegian case of CC, suggested that it was underrecognized in Europe [14].
- Cooper et al. confirmed this recently by presenting 17 cases of CC from the UK [15]. 16 of these cases were male, 11 were 18 years old or younger. 11 occurred whilst playing ball sports such as football, cricket and rugby, while 6 involved physical interaction including assault.

Thus, cases of CC in the UK followed a similar circumstantial and age profile as those reported from the US. An incidence number, though, is not possible to establish in a European country due to the lack of proper registration. Information from other parts of the world are lacking.

### 26.2.2 Gender

- Victims are overwhelmingly male.
- A previous explanation for the predominance of males is that they populate the majority of sports in which CC occurs, but it appears quite unlikely that the major predilection for males reflects a 95% incidence of chest wall impact in sports.
- Also, the gender difference in participation in various sports shifts.

We suspect that there may also be some gender related biological susceptibility to chest-wall induced sudden cardiac death. Indeed, other arrhythmic conditions demonstrate gender predilection for arrhythmia, including females with long QT syndrome [16, 17] and males with Brugada syndrome [18]. Genetic differences in ion channels between the sexes or biological modification of these channels by sex hormones may be involved in the male susceptibility to CC [19–21].

### 26.2.3 Age

- CC is most commonly observed in young Americans, with a peak incidence between the ages 11 and 19 years old (median age 14 years old).
- Young individuals may be at higher risk for CC due to an increased compliance of the chest wall as compared to adults [22].
- In addition, maturation of the heart may reduce susceptibility to CC.
- Finally, the predominance of young subjects in the registry likely relates to the high level of participation in youth sports in American culture.

### 26.2.4 Collapse and Arrhythmias

- Half of the subjects in the registry collapsed instantaneously while others experienced brief lightheadedness before losing consciousness [7].
- The initial rhythm seen in the majority of patients with attempted resuscitation was ventricular fibrillation (VF), but in those victims undergoing prolonged resuscitation, asystole has also been reported [9].
- Resuscitation, once thought to be unsuccessful, has now been demonstrated to be successful in up to 60% (Fig. 26.1) [23].

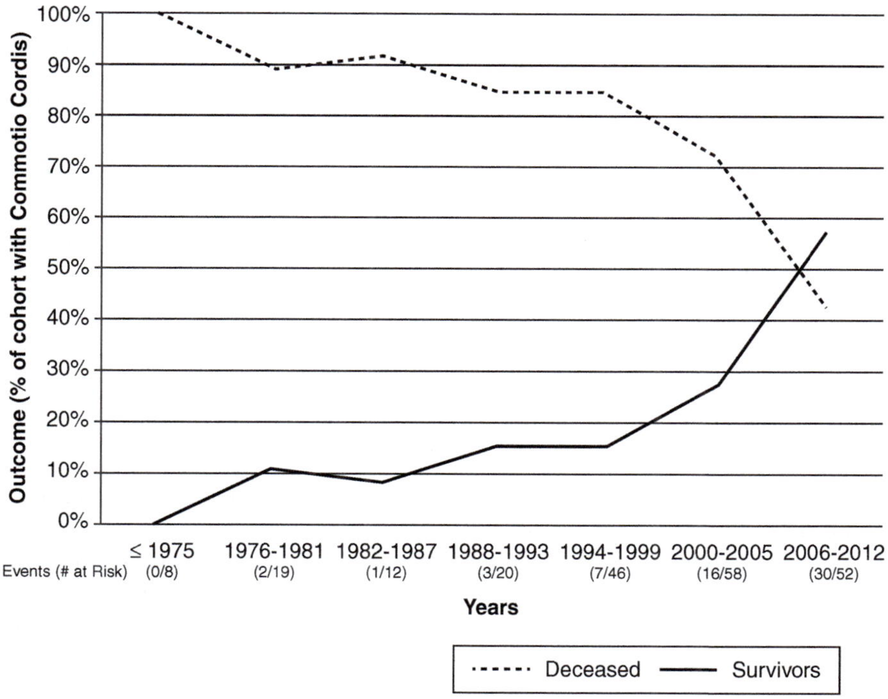


**Fig. 26.1** Mortality compared to survival rates from commotio cordis from before 1975 to 2012 (reprinted with permission from [23])

Whether syncope associated with chest wall impact is an aborted CC event secondary to non-sustained ventricular fibrillation or transient complete heart block is postulated, but not proved.

## 26.3 Pathophysiology

In a model developed by Mark S Link, an anesthetized juvenile swine was placed prone in a sling [24]. Projectiles impacted the chest wall over the cardiac silhouette, speed varied from 32 to 112 km/h. Impacts were gated to the cardiac cycle by a cardiac stimulator which triggered from the surface electrocardiogram of the swine.

- In the initial publication both VF and transient heart block were observed [24].
- Heart block was not related to timing of impact relative to the cardiac cycle and was always transient.
- In subsequent experiments transient heart block was observed rarely.

In the current model, VF is reproducibly induced by chest wall impact if a confluence of factors, including timing relative to the cardiac cycle, is achieved [24, 25].

## 26.4 Variables Important in the Generation of Ventricular Fibrillation

### 26.4.1 Timing

- Only impacts timed to strike during a narrow window of vulnerability during cardiac repolarization (10–30 ms prior to peak T-wave) resulted in VF (Fig. 26.2).
- Impacts at other time periods of the cardiac cycle did not result in VF, but caused other arrhythmic events such as
  - premature ventricular contractions,
  - transient heart block,
  - ST elevation, and
  - bundle-branch block [24].

### 26.4.2 Velocity of Impact

- Higher energy impacts were more likely to cause VF compared to low velocity impacts.
- In animals weighing between 10 and 25 kg, chest impacts induce VF approximately 50% of the time at baseball and lacrosse ball velocities of 64 km/h.
- At impact velocities of 80–112 km/h, an increased incidence of direct thoracic and myocardial damage was observed, suggesting cardiac contusion rather than CC.

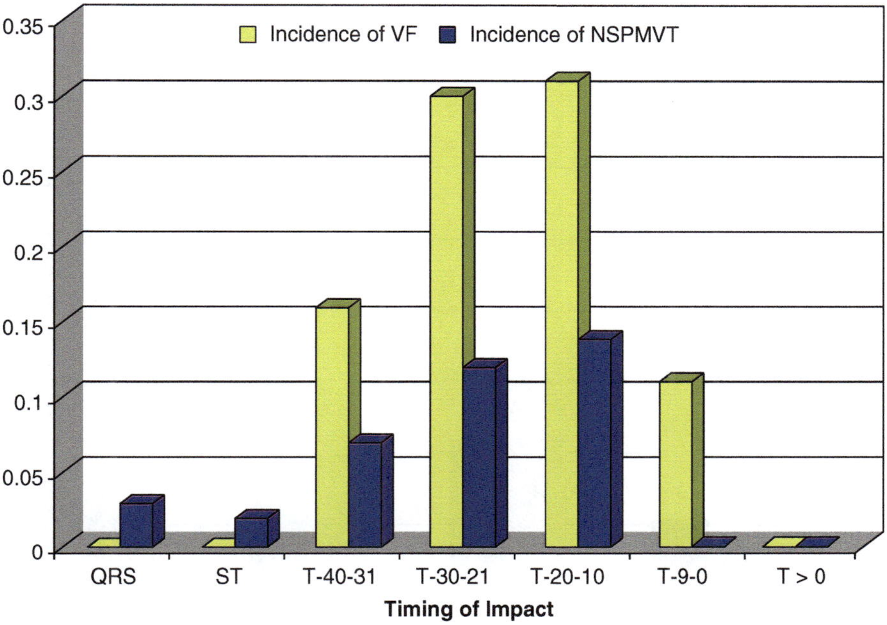


**Fig. 26.2** The timing of impact proved to be one of the most critical variables in the commotio cordis model. Only impacts on a narrow window of the upslope of the T-wave caused ventricular fibrillation (VF). The time window for non-sustained polymorphic ventricular tachycardia (NSPMVT) was slightly wider (reprinted with permission from [3])

### 26.4.3 Impact Location

Consistent with the clinical profile of CC in humans, impact location directly over the cardiac silhouette is necessary for VF induction.

- In fact, 48 km/h impacts at the center of the left ventricle induced VF in 30% while impacts at the base caused VF in 12% and at the apex in 5% [26].
- Impacts that occurred outside the borders of the heart silhouette have *never* resulted in VF induction.

### 26.4.4 Hardness of Impact Object

The harder the object the more likely VF will occur. In the original model a spherical block of wood was utilized [24]. Age-appropriate safety baseballs reduced the risk of VF inverse to their hardness (Fig. 26.3) [24, 27]. Yet the protection is not absolute. Even very soft baseballs, known as T-balls, can produce VF in an animal model and in humans.

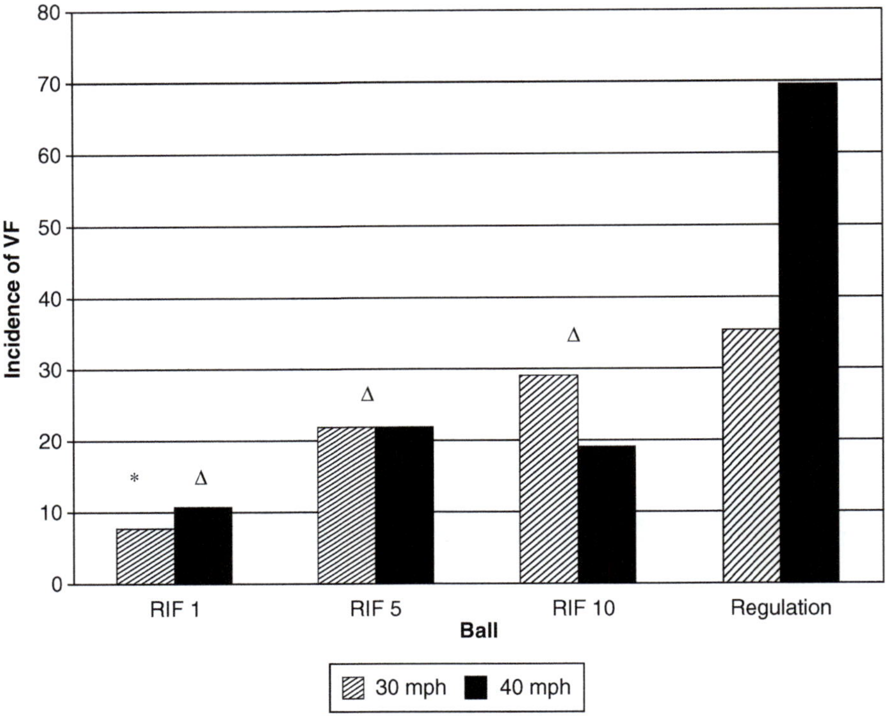


**Fig. 26.3** The risk of ventricular fibrillation (VF) is directly related to the hardness of the baseball. The harder balls have approximately five- to sevenfold the risk for commotio cordis compared to the T-balls, marketed for youth <7 years of age. In addition the intermediate grades of safety baseballs, marked for 8–10 and 11–13 year olds are intermediate in protection from commotio cordis (reprinted with permission from [41]). *RIF* reduced injury factor (balls were composed of a rubber core varying in hardness and covered by a leather exterior varying in stiffness (Newton/cm)

### 26.4.5 Shape

Smaller, more compact objects, such as those shaped like a golf ball, produced VF more frequently than objects with a larger surface that distribute the energy of impact over a wider area [28]. A flat sphere with the diameter of a baseball did not cause VF in the model.

### 26.4.6 Left Ventricular Pressure

Velocity, hardness, shape and impact location are likely related to the creation of a critical threshold pressure in the left ventricle necessary for VF induction.

- Generation of VF with ball impacts was not observed until the LV pressure increased to 250–300 mmHg [26, 29, 30].
- VF was more likely with greater LV pressure increases, and the optimal LV pressure rise was around 500 mmHg to induce VF.

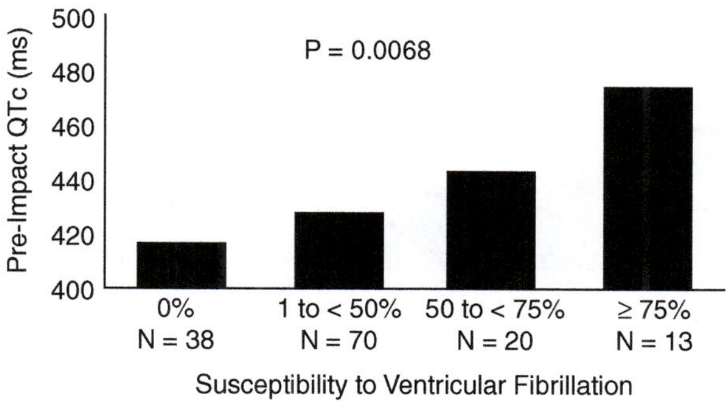


**Fig. 26.4** In our experimental model swine demonstrated a variability in susceptibility to chest blow induced ventricular fibrillation. This variable susceptibility was related to the length of the QTc interval. The longer the QTc the more susceptable the animal to VF with chest blows (reprinted with permission from [20])

### 26.4.7 Individual Susceptibility

- Of 1274 impacts to 139 swine, 360 impacts (28%) resulted in VF.
- The median incidence of VF was 20%; yet there was wide variability in individual animal susceptibility to VF.
- The majority of animals (91; 65%) were relatively resistant to VF (VF < 30% of strikes).
- Only 14% had >50% occurrence of VF with chest wall impacts, and only 7 (5%) had >80% occurrence of chest impacts which induced VF.
- The animals with the longer baseline QTc appeared to be the animals more susceptible to ball induced VF (Fig. 26.4).

## 26.5 Mechanism of Commotio cordis

How physical trauma causes ventricular fibrillation is postulated to be a result of both a chest wall induced increased dispersion of repolarization and a premature ventricular beat (Fig. 26.5). Both of these requirements are caused by the physical blow.

- Physical stimulation of the heart with the production of electrical consequences (such as premature ventricular contractions from cardiac catheters) has been termed *mechano-electric coupling*.

This phenomenon has been attributed to the presence of stretch-sensitive ion channels within cardiac myocytes [31–33]. A candidate stretch-sensitive channel in CC is the $K^{+}_{ATP}$ channel. This channel is responsible for the phenomenon of ST segment elevation and VF in acute myocardial ischemia [29, 33–36]. In the swine model developed by Link et al., $K^{+}_{ATP}$ blockade by the old anti-diabetic drug

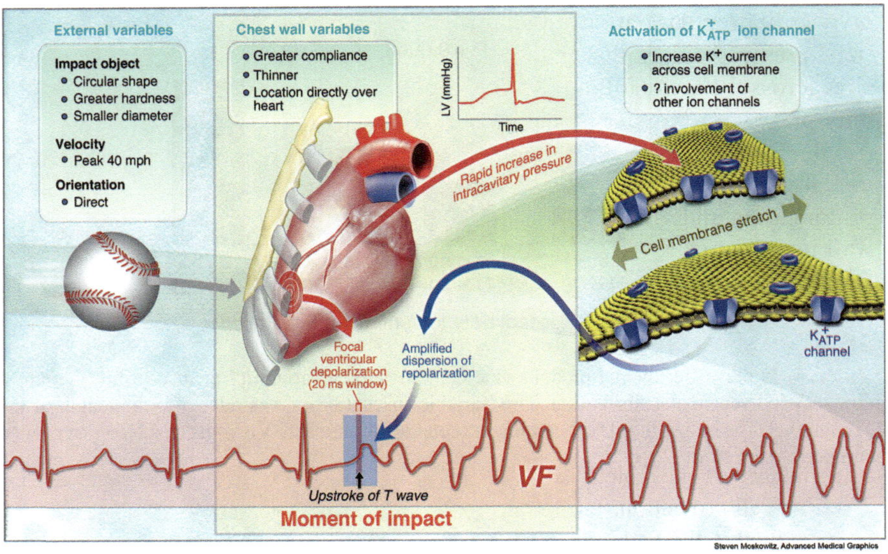


**Fig. 26.5** The confluence of variables and a proposed mechanism necessary for commotio cordis to occur. Important impact object variables are shape, hardness, diameter, and velocity. Human characteristics are the pliability of the chest wall, impact timing, location and orientation of blow, and individual susceptibility, likely carried in ion channels involved in repolarization (reprinted with permission from [4])

Glibenclamide (Daonil) prior to chest wall impact resulted in significantly less VF induction and ST elevation [34]. The potential role of other ion channels remains the targets of ongoing and future research. Of note, double blocking of the autonomic nervous system (by beta blocker and atropine respectively) did not change the frequency of arrhythmias, arguing that abrupt shifts in the autonomic nervous system are not a source of arrhythmia induction [37].

- Despite optimization of the clinical variables for induction of VF, less than 50% of impacts result in VF.
- Of the impacts that do not result in VF, 70% result in premature ventricular contractions, the proposed trigger in CC.

Based on the observation that the trigger is produced, but not VF, it is hypothesized that the necessary alteration in repolarization was not induced by the blow. Studies of VF induction by inflation of a balloon in Langendorff-perfused rabbit hearts revealed that VF could only be induced during a vulnerable time window that corresponded to a period of increased dispersion of myocardial repolarization. In addition, as compared to baseline action potentials, pressure pulses that induced VF further increased repolarization dispersion across the myocardium [34, 38, 39]. Thus, it appears that chest impacts not only provide the trigger for lethal arrhythmia, but also might themselves contribute to the creation of a suitable substrate for VF induction. In the swine model of CC it is likely that repolarization abnormalities manifested by QT prolongation underlie individual animal susceptibility to VF induction by chest wall impacts [20].

## 26.6 Prevention of Commotio Cordis

Prevention is potentially achievable by three means:

1. avoidance of chest blows,
2. chest wall protection, and
3. by softening the ball.

Reducing chest wall impact could be accomplished by coaching and rules changes. In youth baseball some have prohibited the use of the chest to stop the ball. While unpredictable motion of the projectile cannot be prevented, coaching can provide a measure of preparedness and understanding that might allow the participants to avoid unnecessary chest wall impact.

- Of the 125 events that occurred during competitive sport in the National Commotio Cordis Registry, 32% of individuals were wearing some sort of chest protection at the time of impact.
- In some cases, mainly hockey, it appears the chest protector was lifted during play and thus not covering the heart.
- In other cases, such as during baseball and lacrosse, however, impact occurred directly over the heart [7].

Chest protectors are generally not designed to prevent CC, but rather soft tissue injury. In the swine model of CC, seven commercially available lacrosse chest protectors and nine baseball chest protectors did not prevent VF induction (Fig. 26.6) [27, 40].

Age-appropriate softer balls, known as safety baseballs, significantly reduced the incidence of VF induction by chest impacts in the swine model [24, 41]. These data and other clinical data from the United States Consumer Protection Agency have led to calls for the utilization of age-appropriate safety baseballs in sports.

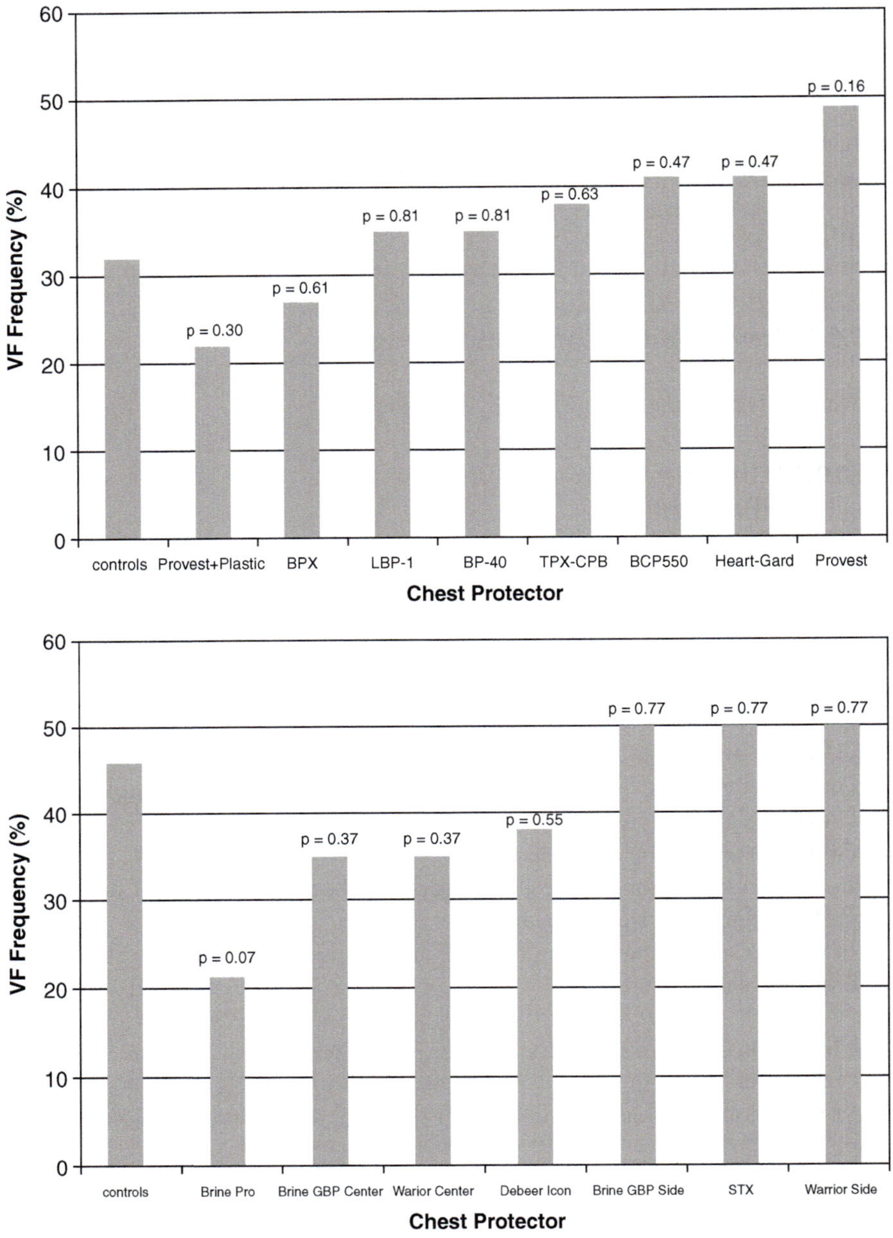


**Fig. 26.6** Effectiveness of various models of chest wall protectors designed for use in either baseball (**upper** panel) or lacrosse (**lower** panel) in preventing ventricular fibrillation triggered by chest blows in an animal model. None of the models tested was able to significantly reduce the incidence of ventricular fibrillation when compared to control conditions (reprinted with permission from [27])

## 26.7 Treatment

CC cases reported early in the literature were nearly universally fatal.

- In the National Registry data reported in 1995 survival was 25% [6, 9, 12, 13].
- More recent data from the registry shows that survival is reaching 60% (Fig. 26.1) [23].

There are several potential reasons for this improved survival. Increased recognition of this phenomenon likely plays the largest role. It is clear that early cardiopulmonary resuscitation and defibrillation of a cardiac arrest victim is the key to survival. The poor survival rates of CC in the past have been in part attributed to delayed recognition and thus therapy [9]. With increased recognition that an individual collapsing after a chest blow is in cardiac arrest, resuscitation can commence earlier [42–46].

- Coaches and trainers as well as the athletes themselves should be able to recognize a cardiac arrest and use an automated external defibrillator (AED), as well as cardiopulmonary resuscitation.

## 26.8 Conclusion

CC is a rare but tragic event that typically occurs in adolescent boys during sports when they are struck in the chest. Because of the American Commotio Cordis Registry and the experimental model, the understanding of CC has evolved considerably over the last 10–15 years. An animal model has been utilized to explore and describe the important variables and mechanism of CC precisely, providing substantial knowledge to the field of arrhythmias. Impact during a narrow window of repolarization causes ventricular fibrillation. Factors such as timing, hardness and shape of the object, object impact velocity, location of impact, and individual susceptibility have been identified. Biological characteristics such as gender, pliability of the chest wall and genetic susceptibility play a role. The induction mechanism of ventricular fibrillation appears to be an increase in heterogeneity of repolarization caused by induced abnormalities of ion channels activated by abrupt increases in left ventricular pressure from the impact. CC is one of the commonest causes of SCA in the US, though it is rare in Europe. This difference is probably due to variation in sports between the continents and that CC may be under-recognized in Europe, one of the reasons why it is additionally important to inform about the condition. Prevention of CC is attainable. Finally, improved recognition and early resuscitation has improved the outcome of CC victims.

**Clinical Pearls**

- Expect the unexpected—would you have recognized that cardiac arrest actually may occur due to a blow to the chest during sports?
- Life is fragile, also an impact to the chest may induce a cascade of bodily processes leading to sudden cardiac arrest.
- Be aware of the vulnerable recovery phase of the cardiac cycle—it is not only adrenergic stress that may lead to sudden cardiac arrest.

## Review

### Questions

1. Which factors protect against commotio cordis?
2. What part of the cardiac cycle is most prone to cardiac arrest as a consequence of a blow to the chest?
3. Does a brisk alteration of the autonomic system play a role in inducing commotio cordis?

### Answers

1. Protection is potentially achievable by three means: avoidance of chest blows, at least on the cardiac silhouette, chest wall protection e.g. by wearing specially designed gear, or using softer balls.
2. 10–30 ms prior to the peak of the T-wave in ECG.
3. No, when double blocking the autonomic system no differences were found in eliciting SCA by a blow.

## References

1. Haq CL. Sudden death due to low-energy chest-wall impact (commotio cordis). N Engl J Med. 1998;339(19):1399.
2. Link MS. Commotio cordis: sudden death due to chest wall impact in sports. Heart. 1999;81(2):109–10.
3. Link MS, Estes NA 3rd. Mechanically induced ventricular fibrillation (commotio cordis). Heart Rhythm. 2007;4(4):529–32.
4. Link MS, Estes NA. Athletes and arrhythmias. J Cardiovasc Electrophysiol. 2010;21(10):1184–9.
5. Maron BJ. Sudden death in young athletes. N Engl J Med. 2003;349(11):1064–75.
6. Maron BJ, Link MS, Wang PJ, Estes NA 3rd. Clinical profile of commotio cordis: an under appreciated cause of sudden death in the young during sports and other activities. J Cardiovasc Electrophysiol. 1999;10(1):114–20.
7. Maron BJ, Poliac LC, Kaplan JA, Mueller FO. Blunt impact to the chest leading to sudden death from cardiac arrest during sports activities. N Engl J Med. 1995;333(6):337–42.
8. Maron BJ, Boren SD, Estes NA 3rd. Early descriptions of sudden cardiac death due to commotio cordis occurring in baseball. Heart Rhythm. 2010;7(7):992–3.

9. Maron BJ, Gohman TE, Kyle SB, Estes NA 3rd, Link MS. Clinical profile and spectrum of commotio cordis. JAMA. 2002;287(9):1142–6.
10. Maron BJ, Shirani J, Poliac LC, Mathenge R, Roberts WC, Mueller FO. Sudden death in young competitive athletes. Clinical, demographic, and pathological profiles. JAMA. 1996;276(3):199–204.
11. Maron BJ, Strasburger JF, Kugler JD, Bell BM, Brodkey FD, Poliac LC. Survival following blunt chest impact-induced cardiac arrest during sports activities in young athletes. Am J Cardiol. 1997;79(6):840–1.
12. Maron BJ, Poliac LC, Kyle SB. Clinical profile of commotio cordis: an under-appreciated cause of sudden cardic death in the young during sporting activities. Circulation. 1997;96:I–755.
13. Maron BJ, Estes NA 3rd. Commotio cordis. N Engl J Med. 2010;362(10):917–27.
14. Solberg EE, Embra BI, Borjesson M, Herlitz J, Corrado D. Commotio cordis—under-recognized in Europe?: a case report and review. Eur J Cardiovasc Prev Rehabil. 2011;18(3):378–83.
15. Cooper S, Woodford NW, Maron BJ, Harris KM, Sheppard MN. A lethal blow to the chest as an underdiagnosed cause of sudden death in United Kingdom sports (football, cricket, rugby). Am J Cardiol. 2019;124(5):808–11.
16. Goldenberg I, Moss AJ, Bradley J, Polonsky S, Peterson DR, McNitt S, et al. Long-QT syndrome after age 40. Circulation. 2008;117(17):2192–201.
17. Zareba W, Moss AJ, Locati EH, Lehmann MH, Peterson DR, Hall WJ, et al. Modulating effects of age and gender on the clinical course of long QT syndrome by genotype. J Am Coll Cardiol. 2003;42(1):103–9.
18. Gehi AK, Duong TD, Metz LD, Gomes JA, Mehta D. Risk stratification of individuals with the Brugada electrocardiogram: a meta-analysis. J Cardiovasc Electrophysiol. 2006;17(6):577–83.
19. Knollmann BC, Roden DM. A genetic framework for improving arrhythmia therapy. Nature. 2008;451(7181):929–36.
20. Alsheikh-Ali AA, Madias C, Supran S, Link MS. Marked variability in susceptibility to ventricular fibrillation in an experimental commotio cordis model. Circulation. 2010;122(24):2499–504.
21. Roden DM. Drug-induced prolongation of the QT interval. N Engl J Med. 2004;350(10):1013–22.
22. Link MS, Maron BJ, Wang PJ, VanderBrink BA, Zhu W, Estes NA 3rd. Upper and lower limits of vulnerability to sudden arrhythmic death with chest-wall impact (commotio cordis). J Am Coll Cardiol. 2003;41(1):99–104.
23. Maron BJ, Haas TS, Ahluwalia A, Garberich RF, Estes NA 3rd, Link MS. Increasing survival rate from commotio cordis. Heart Rhythm. 2013;10(2):219–23.
24. Link MS, Wang PJ, Pandian NG, Bharati S, Udelson JE, Lee MY, et al. An experimental model of sudden death due to low-energy chest-wall impact (commotio cordis). N Engl J Med. 1998;338(25):1805–11.
25. Link MS. Commotio cordis: ventricular fibrillation triggered by chest impact-induced abnormalities in repolarization. Circ Arrhythm Electrophysiol. 2012;5(2):425–32.
26. Link MS, Maron BJ, VanderBrink BA, Takeuchi M, Pandian NG, Wang PJ, et al. Impact directly over the cardiac silhouette is necessary to produce ventricular fibrillation in an experimental model of commotio cordis. J Am Coll Cardiol. 2001;37(2):649–54.
27. Weinstock J, Maron BJ, Song C, Mane PP, Estes NA 3rd, Link MS. Failure of commercially available chest wall protectors to prevent sudden cardiac death induced by chest wall blows in an experimental model of commotio cordis. Pediatrics. 2006;117(4):e656–62.
28. Kalin J, Madias C, Alsheikh-Ali AA, Link MS. Reduced diameter spheres increases the risk of chest blow-induced ventricular fibrillation (commotio cordis). Heart Rhythm. 2011;8(10):1578–81.
29. Link MS. Mechanically induced sudden death in chest wall impact (commotio cordis). Prog Biophys Mol Biol. 2003;82(1-3):175–86.
30. Madias C, Maron BJ, Weinstock J, Estes NA 3rd, Link MS. Commotio cordis—sudden cardiac death with chest wall impact. J Cardiovasc Electrophysiol. 2007;18(1):115–22.

31. Kohl P, Ravens U. Cardiac mechano-electric feedback: past, present, and prospect. Prog Biophys Mol Biol. 2003;82(1-3):3–9.
32. Kohl P, Hunter P, Noble D. Stretch-induced changes in heart rate and rhythm: clinical observations, experiments and mathematical models. Prog Biophys Mol Biol. 1999;71(1):91–138.
33. Kohl P, Nesbitt AD, Cooper PJ, Lei M. Sudden cardiac death by Commotio cordis: role of mechano-electric feedback. Cardiovasc Res. 2001;50(2):280–9.
34. Link MS, Wang PJ, VanderBrink BA, Avelar E, Pandian NG, Maron BJ, et al. Selective activation of the K(+)(ATP) channel is a mechanism by which sudden death is produced by low-energy chest-wall impact (Commotio cordis). Circulation. 1999;100(4):413–8.
35. Madias C, Maron BJ, Supron S, Estes NA 3rd, Link MS. Cell membrane stretch and chest blow-induced ventricular fibrillation: commotio cordis. J Cardiovasc Electrophysiol. 2008;19(12):1304–9.
36. Van Wagoner DR. Mechanosensitive gating of atrial ATP-sensitive potassium channels. Circ Res. 1993;72(5):973–83.
37. Stout CW, Maron BJ, Vanderbrink BA, Estes NA 3rd, Link MS. Importance of the autonomic nervous system in an experimental model of commotio cordis. Med Sci Monit. 2007;13(1):BR11–5.
38. Bode F, Franz MR, Wilke I, Bonnemeier H, Schunkert H, Wiegand UK. Ventricular fibrillation induced by stretch pulse: implications for sudden death due to commotio cordis. J Cardiovasc Electrophysiol. 2006;17(9):1011–7.
39. Fabritz CL, Kirchhof PF, Behrens S, Zabel M, Franz MR. Myocardial vulnerability to T wave shocks: relation to shock strength, shock coupling interval, and dispersion of ventricular repolarization. J Cardiovasc Electrophysiol. 1996;7(3):231–42.
40. Viano DC, Bir CA, Cheney AK, Janda DH. Prevention of commotio cordis in baseball: an evaluation of chest protectors. J Trauma. 2000;49(6):1023–8.
41. Link MS, Maron BJ, Wang PJ, Pandian NG, VanderBrink BA, Estes NA 3rd. Reduced risk of sudden death from chest wall blows (commotio cordis) with safety baseballs. Pediatrics. 2002;109(5):873–7.
42. Drezner JA, Rogers KJ. Sudden cardiac arrest in intercollegiate athletes: detailed analysis and outcomes of resuscitation in nine cases. Heart Rhythm. 2006;3(7):755–9.
43. Friedman FD, Dowler K, Link MS. A public access defibrillation programme in non-inpatient hospital areas. Resuscitation. 2006;69(3):407–11.
44. Link MS, Maron BJ, Stickney RE, Vanderbrink BA, Zhu W, Pandian NG, et al. Automated external defibrillator arrhythmia detection in a model of cardiac arrest due to commotio cordis. J Cardiovasc Electrophysiol. 2003;14(1):83–7.
45. Marenco JP, Wang PJ, Link MS, Homoud MK, Estes NA 3rd. Improving survival from sudden cardiac arrest: the role of the automated external defibrillator. JAMA. 2001;285(9):1193–200.
46. Salib EA, Cyran SE, Cilley RE, Maron BJ, Thomas NJ. Efficacy of bystander cardiopulmonary resuscitation and out-of-hospital automated external defibrillation as life-saving therapy in commotio cordis. J Pediatr. 2005;147(6):863–6.

# Cardiovascular Side Effects of Commonly Prescribed Medications and Performance Enhancing Drugs and Special Considerations for the Athlete

# 27

Maria Joan Brosnan and Paolo Emilio Adami

**Learning Objectives**

1. Understand the cardiovascular side effects of commonly prescribed medications.
2. Understand the cardiovascular effect of performance enhancing drugs.
3. Understand the adverse cardiovascular effects of other non-prescribed, but legal substances such as energy drinks.
4. Understand the implication of legal and illegal substances on exercise performance.

## 27.1 Commonly Prescribed or over the Counter Medications and Supplements

### 27.1.1 Beta Blockers and Antiarrhythmics

All substances discussed in this chapter are also summarized in the Table 27.1. Starting with **beta blockers**, they are banned in skill-based sports such as shooting and archery, due to the performance benefit offered due to a lowering of heart rate and reduction in anxiety and tremor. Conversely, there is a general reluctance amongst athletes and prescribers to use beta blockers in athletes with cardiovascular disease, due to the potentially detrimental effects of lowering of heart rate on

M. J. Brosnan
Department of Cardiology and Sports Cardiology, St Vincent's Hospital and Baker Institute, Melbourne, VIC, Australia
e-mail: maria.brosnan@svha.org.au

P. E. Adami (✉)
Department of Health and Science, World Athletics, Monaco, Monaco
e-mail: paoloemilio.adami@worldathletics.org



A. Pressler, J. Niebauer (eds.), *Textbook of Sports and Exercise Cardiology*,
https://doi.org/10.1007/978-3-030-35374-2_27

**Table 27.1** List of most important substances with cardiovascular side effects. However, substances are not limited to those listed

| Substance category | Pharmacological class |
|---|---|
| Commonly prescribed or over the counter medications and supplements | |
| *Beta blockers and antiarrhythmics* | |
| | Nebivolol, sotalol, atenolol, propranolol |
| | Flecainide |
| *Anti-inflammatory drugs* | |
| | Ibuprofen, naproxen, ketoprofen, diclofenac |
| *Anti-coagulants and antiplatelet* | |
| | Acenocoumarin, warfarin |
| | Dabigratan, Rivaroxaban, Apixaban, Edoxaban |
| | Aspirin, clopidogrel, prasugrel and ticagrelor |
| Performance enhancing substances | |
| *Oxygen-carrying modulators and dissociation curve modulators* | |
| | Blood doping |
| | Recombinant human erythropoietin (rhEPO) |
| | Cobalt chloride |
| | RSR 13 |
| | Sildenafil |
| *Anabolic agents* | |
| | Exogenous and endogenous androgenic anabolic steroids (AAS) like 1-Androstenediol, 1-Testosterone, Danazol, Stanozolol, 5-Androstenedione, Nandrolone, Testosterone |
| | SARMS (synthetic androgen receptor modulators) like andarine, enobosarm |
| | Human Growth Hormone (hGH) |
| *Metabolic modulators* | |
| | L-Carnitine |
| | Meldonium (mildronate) |
| | Beta alanine |
| *Beta 2 agonists* | |
| | Salbutamol, clenbuterol |
| Psychoactive drugs | |
| *Benzodiazepines* | |
| | Triazolam, zolpidem, zopiclone, lorazepam, diazepam |
| *Antidepressants and antipsychotics* | |
| | Amitriptyline, amoxapine, clomipramine, desipramine, doxepin, imipramine, nortriptyline, trimipramine |
| *Selective serotonin reuptake inhibitors (SSRIs)* | |
| | Fluoxetine, sertraline, paroxetine and citalopram |
| *Anticomitials* | |

**Table 27.1** (continued)

| Substance category | Pharmacological class |
|---|---|
| | Sodium valproate, gabapentin, lamotrigine, levetiracetam, oxcarbazepine, tiagabine, topiramate, vigabatrin, zonisamide and carbamazepine |
| *Narcotics* | |
| | Buprenorphine, dextromoramide, diamorphine (heroin), fentanyl and by-products such as: hydromorphone, methadone, morphine, oxycodone, oxymorphone, pentazocine and pethidine |
| *Stimulants* | |
| | Caffeine |
| | Methylphenidate and derivates |
| | Ephedrine-containing compounds |

exercise performance. Interestingly, there appears to be a threshold of 15–20% of heart rate reduction beyond which exercise performance is reduced, but below which aerobic performance may be maintained [1].

- In a small group of healthy, untrained volunteers, nebivolol (a beta 1 selective beta blocker), at a dose of 5 mg daily, was found to result in no significant reduction in peak power output or maximal oxygen consumption as compared to placebo, despite a 14% reduction in peak heart rate [1].
- In the same study, 100 mg of atenolol was shown to result in a 25% reduction in maximum heart rate, and 5% reduction in both peak power output and maximal oxygen consumption, leading the authors to conclude that the lack of impact on performance of nebivolol may have been due to the lesser impact on peak heart rate at the prescribed dose, or perhaps the vasodilatory effects of nebivolol.
- At a dose of 240 mg/day, chronic administration of propranolol (a non-selective beta blocker) in untrained healthy subjects has been shown to reduce peak heart rate by 25%, maximal oxygen consumption by 7.5% and maximum work load by 5% [2].
- Sotalol has been shown to have a dose-dependent reduction on maximum heart rate, with the reduction ranging from a 4% at a dose of 160 mg/24 h to 25% at 640 mg/24 h [3].
- A similar dose dependent relationship with heart rate reduction has been demonstrated for propranolol, with marked individual variability [4].

**Flecainide** is a Class 1c antiarrhythmic used for the suppression of supraventricular and ventricular arrhythmias. It is commonly prescribed preferentially in athletic populations over beta blockers due to the commonly held notion that it does not affect resting heart rate nor exercise performance.

- Whilst flecainide does not lower resting heart rate, it's effect on exercise heart rate was documented in a placebo double blinded trial of 24 non-athletes, in whom exercise heart rate was reduced even at low intensity exercise levels on a dose of 200 mg/day, with a difference of around 15 bpm (9%) at peak exercise, despite no significant reduction in exercise time [5].

Thus, although maximum heart rate is not a surrogate for exercise capacity, there does appear to be a threshold of around 15% heart rate reduction beyond which exercise performance would be expected to be reduced, and individual variability in the dose-heart rate response. Thus, when prescribing beta blockers and antiarrhythmics in athletes, it is prudent to perform maximal exercise tests at baseline and during up-titration of therapy to guide exercise prescription and expectations.

## 27.2 Performance Enhancing Substances

### 27.2.1 Oxygen-Carrying Modulators and Dissociation Curve Modulators

Agents which can increase oxygen availability to the working muscles, either by

1. increasing oxygen content in the blood,
2. improving cardiac output, or
3. improving peripheral oxygen extraction

are theorized to improve endurance performance; however, the evidence for a positive effect on performance for many of these agents is poor.

**Blood doping**, usually consisting of transfusion of autologous blood collected some time earlier to increase red blood cell mass, has been used for decades. There are small, blinded trials which support the notion that oxygen carrying capacity and hence performance are improved with blood doping [6, 7].

- Berglund et al. performed a single blinded study on 6 cross country skiers and observed a mean 6% reduction in 15 km race time both 3 and 14 days after reinfusion of 1350 mL of autologous blood [6].
- Similar results were observed by Brien et al., who performed a double blinded cross-over study on 6 high level amateur 10 km runners, where hematocrit increased by 5% and 10 km race time was reduced by an average of one minute after reinfusion of 400 ml of packed red blood cells, but not post infusion of sham saline [7].

**Recombinant human erythropoietin** (rhEPO) triggers an increase red blood cell mass and hemoglobin concentration similar to that of blood doping, as well as an improvement in maximal oxygen consumption, however good evidence that this translates into a positive effect on performance is lacking [8, 9].

- Birkeland et al. demonstrated an increase in both hematocrit and maximal oxygen consumption ($VO_2$max) following administration of rhEPO over 4 weeks in

a double-blind placebo-controlled study with only a small cohort of trained cyclists (n = 10). This period was needed to demonstrate a large treatment effect (42.7 vs. 50.8% ($p < 0.0001$), and 63.6 vs. 68.1 ml/min/kg ($p < 0.0001$) for hematocrit and $VO_2max$, respectively) [10]. Although this study did not have a direct performance measure, time to exhaustion was increased significantly in the EPO group from 12.8 to 14 min ($p < 0.0001$) as compared to 13.1 to 13.3 min ($p = 0.04$) in the control group who were exposed to the same training effect [10].
- Similar effects on maximal oxygen consumption have been demonstrated in other placebo-controlled, double blind studies of rhEPO administration [9, 11–13]. However, in the study of Heuberger et al., no improvement in a race to Mont Ventoux time was observed despite a 5% improvement in $VO_2max$ [9].

Nevertheless, it is not surprising that different EPO formulations, direct EPO receptor agonists and micro-dosing techniques are used by athletes with the aim of improving performance with minimal risk of being detected.

- The potential negative cardiovascular consequences of such practices are underlined by a prospective cross sectional study of 3000 healthy older adults, which found that each doubling in serum EPO level was independently associated with a 25% increase in risk of incident heart failure over a mean follow up of 10 years [14].

Rather than increasing the blood oxygen content (like rhEPO), theoretically the same effect may be achieved by increasing the amount of $O_2$ that hemoglobin can deliver to the surrounding tissues. A number of agents with these properties have been reportedly used by athletes to aid performance:

- **Cobalt chloride** is a water soluble compound that can stimulate erythropoiesis and angiogenesis, presumably due to activation of hypoxia inducible factor (HIF-1) signaling [15]. Although the direct cardiovascular effects in humans has not been prospectively studied, unintentional ingestion of cobalt has been associated with the development of a dilated cardiomyopathy [16, 17].
- **RSR 13** (right shifting reagent 13, or Efaproxiral) is a synthetic modifier of Hb, with in vivo studies demonstrating a shift in the $Hb/O_2$ dissociation curve to the right, thereby increasing the dissociation of $O_2$ in the peripheral muscles. RSR13 has been shown to increase oxygen consumption in stimulated canine skeletal muscle [18], when inspired $O_2$ was supplemented. However, in humans breathing sea level air, the right-shift of the $O_2$ curve RSR13 causes significant hypoxemia under resting conditions [19] that is likely to be further exacerbated by exercise. The side effects associated with exercising in a hypoxemic state are not known and it is unlikely that the physiology and potential risks are known to the athletes in whom it is being used.

There have also been attempts to improve muscle oxygen delivery by improving cardiac output. Specific pulmonary vasodilators such as **Sildenafil** are rumored to be widely used amongst some endurance athletes. The rationale would seem that by reducing pulmonary vascular resistance it may be possible to reduce cardiac work, particularly of the right ventricle (RV), thereby enabling the heart to maintain a high level of function for longer [20]. This is especially relevant given that exercise seems to place a disproportionate load on the pulmonary circulation and RV [21]. A number of studies have assessed whether pulmonary vasodilators can improve exercise performance in healthy volunteers and athletes.

- Ghofrani et al. documented improvements in exercise capacity in a randomised, double-blind placebo controlled trial in 14 healthy subjects during normobaric hypoxia (10% $O_2$) and at altitude (Mount Everest base camp, 5245 m above sea level) [22].

However, whilst studies using both PDE5 receptor and endothelin antagonists have consistently demonstrated improvements in hemodynamics and exercise performance in *hypoxic* conditions, they have failed to show any benefit in *normoxia* [23–25]. These agents are thus currently not banned by the World Anti-Doping Agency (WADA) who state they are continuing to evaluate the science to assess whether they are performance enhancing.

### 27.2.2 Anabolic Agents

The WADA list of banned **androgenic anabolic steroids** (AAS) is extensive, and identification of these substances are responsible for around 60% of positive doping results. They represent one of the oldest classes of drugs of abuse and, accordingly, its effects have been most extensively investigated.

- When combined with exercise training, AAS increase muscle mass and strength and reduce fat [26, 27].
- Significant increases in strength have been observed in double-blinded randomized trails comparing 12 weeks of AAS vs placebo in small cohorts (n = 10) [28].

A common misconception is that AAS are used exclusively by strength athletes, but they are also used to aid in recovery and strength in endurance pursuits. The concomitant use of anabolic agents with EPO is common both in strength and endurance athletes [29].

Mortality amongst athletes using AAS is estimated to be 6–20 fold that of clean athletes, and around one third of these deaths can be attributed to cardiovascular causes [30]. Well acknowledged cardiovascular side effects of AAS are

1. cardiomyopathy,
2. myocardial infarction,
3. dyslipidaemia,
4. cardiac conduction abnormalities, and
5. coagulation abnormalities [29, 31–33].

A series of post-mortem studies and studies utilising echocardiography and cardiac magnetic resonance imaging (CMR) have confirmed the existence of AAS-induced cardiomyopathy, which shares similar characteristics to hypertrophic cardiomyopathy, with greater cardiac mass, greater left ventricular wall thickness/hypertrophy (LVH), a greater prevalence of cardiac fibrosis and impairment of systolic and diastolic left ventricular function [33–37]. The pathogenesis and prevalence of arrhythmic events in AAS users has not been well detailed, but both myocardial fibrosis and atherogenesis are plausible substrates.

Intriguingly, evidence suggests that AAS may have confounded popular understanding of exercise-induced cardiac remodelling. The Morganroth hypothesis contends that concentric remodelling of the myocardium occurs in response to the heightened afterload of strength training. However, when Luijckx et al. compared power-trained athletes with a history of AAS use with those who had not used AAS, they found that cardiac hypertrophy was only significantly increased in the former group [36].

**SARMS** (synthetic androgen receptor modulators, e.g. thymosin beta 4) are a newer class of drugs, designed to dissociate the androgenic and anabolic effects of AAS, thereby making detection more difficult. Little is known about the cardiovascular side effects of the many peptides designed to modulate androgen receptor activity. It is likely that both the performance enhancement and side effects are less than AAS, but it is very difficult to know for certain.

**Human Growth Hormone** (hGH) is an endogenous neurohormone that is purported to have anabolic effects when used in supra-physiologic doses. Although it is rumoured to be widely used, there is little evidence that recombinant hGH improves performance although it may aid more rapid recovery from soft tissue damage [29]. Little is known about the direct cardiovascular effects of excessive hGH administration in athletes; however, hGH excess in patients with acromegaly results in hypertension, congestive cardiac failure and cardiomyopathy [29].

### 27.2.3 Metabolic Modulators

**L-Carnitine** is an amino acid produced naturally in the body. Supplementation is believed to enhance fatty acid oxidation and stimulate the production of ATP, aiding muscular contraction during prolonged aerobic exercise. However, evidence supporting performance enhancement is not compelling [38].

- There is no evidence of cardiovascular toxicity with L-carnitine.
- Rather, there is some evidence for anti-hypertensive and anti-fibrotic effects in hypertensive mice [39].
- Currently L-carnitine is not on the WADA list of banned substances.

**Meldonium** (mildronate) is licenced for clinical use in some Eastern European countries as an anti-anginal with a mechanism of action that is believed to be modulated, at least in part, by lowering of L-carnitine availability and reducing mitochondrial energy production [40]. Thus, in these two agents that are believed to be widely used by athletes there are opposing mechanisms of action. Neither agent has established efficacy nor safety data for use during strenuous exercise.

- After anecdotal reports of widespread use at the London 2012 Olympics, meldonium was detected in the urine of 9% of athletes at the 2015 European Games [41], and was hence included in the list of banned substances by WADA in January 2016.

**Beta alanine** is a non-essential amino acid that can be synthesised in the liver and obtained through dietary intake of poultry and meat. Several recent studies and meta-analyses have shown that chronic, high-dose oral supplementation with beta-alanine can

1. increase muscle carnosine levels,
2. intramuscular buffering capacity, and
3. improve performance of high intensity and intermittent exercise [42–44].

Studies of adverse cardiovascular effects in humans taking oral beta-alanine supplements are lacking. However, neurotoxicity, myotonia and respiratory distress are clinical features in humans with mitochondrial disorders associated with beta-alanine excess, and in vitro studies in which rat cardiomyocytes and fibroblasts were directly exposed to beta-alanine, oxidative stress and cell apoptosis was observed [45]. Therefore, it seems plausible that excess supplementation may have deleterious cardiovascular effects.

- Currently, beta-alanine supplementation is legal under the WADA code and its use among athletes is widespread, with a self-reported usage of 60% in some sporting codes [46].

### 27.2.4 Beta 2 Agonists

**Beta 2 agonists** such as salbutamol and clenbuterol are prescribed commonly as treatment for asthma, given their bronchodilatory effects on the smooth muscles of the lung.

- In 2011, Pluim et al. performed a meta-analysis of randomised controlled trials comparing inhaled or systemic beta 2 agonists to placebo and concluded that there are no data to support a positive effect on $VO_2max$, peak power output, strength or endurance performance with inhaled beta 2 agonists (salbutamol, albuterol or terburaline) [47].
- There was some weak evidence in support of high dose, oral salbutamol having a positive anaerobic capacity and strength [47], however the doses used would be expected to produce adverse side effects such as tachycardia, ventricular ectopy, tremor and hypokalaemia [48].

Clenbuterol has emerged more recently as a drug of misuse in both elite and recreational athletic circles, due to its effect on beta-3 receptors in adipocytes, resulting in lipolysis and weight loss, a desirable side effect in sports where being lean and/or light weight is desirable [49]. The doses required to achieve these effects are 120–160 μg daily, which is 3–4 times higher than the doses that are generally prescribed for asthmatics [49]. Not surprisingly, side effects such as tachycardia, gastrointestinal disturbances and tremor are common in individuals using clenbuterol in these doses, and even cardiac arrest has been reported [50].

## 27.3 Psychoactive Drugs

### 27.3.1 Benzodiazepines

Often co-administered, **benzodiazepines** differ among one another for kinetics, metabolic destiny, and active metabolites and should not be taken for a period exceeding 3–4 weeks because of the risk of tachyphylaxis and addiction. Chronic use can cause nocturnal hypoventilation, with a decrease in tissue oxygenation and clinical consequences. Particular attention has to be paid to symptoms occurring after withdrawal of the agents (withdrawal syndrome):

- With drugs with a short/medium half-life (t1/2) like triazolam, the withdrawal syndrome is more likely to occur once the treatment is interrupted while it rarely appears after intake cessation of drugs with a long t1/2.
- Withdrawal syndrome is virtually absent with molecules such as zolpidem and zopiclone.
- Symptoms arise proportionally to t1/2 (e.g. 24 h for lorazepam, 3–7 days for diazepam).
- Withdrawal syndrome can cause
  - arrhythmic episodes such as
    sinus tachycardia,
    atrial fibrillation and atrial flutter,
    supraventricular and ventricular cardiac ectopy, and
  - atrial pressure abnormalities such as
    systolic hypertension,
    orthostatic hypotension,
    symptoms of sympathetic hyperactivity with diaphoresis, agitation, anxiety, tremors and delirium.
- A beta-blocker treatment is recommended in case of withdrawal syndrome [51].

### 27.3.2 Antidepressants and Antipsychotics

Classic **tricyclics** (ADT) are, among antidepressant drugs, nonselective inhibitors of serotonin and noradrenaline reuptake. They can cause severe cardiovascular effects.

- The most common effects, usually depending on the dose, are QRS enlargement, AV blocks to different extents, QT lengthening, and negative inotropic effect with a reduction in the ejection fraction.

- They can also cause, especially in older athletes, Raynaud's phenomenon, orthostatic hypotension and sinus tachycardia and bradycardia.
- Some antidepressants and antipsychotics might cause: QT lengthening with the torsadogenic risk of producing LQTS, ventricular arrhythmias, torsade de pointe and sudden death.
- The risk is intended on the base of the single drug or attendant factors such as: age, underlying pathology, hypopotassaemia and drugs coadministration.
- These drugs are ADT such as: amitriptyline, amoxapine, clomipramine, desipramine, doxepin, imipramine, nortriptyline, trimipramine and other antidepressants such as: citalopram, fluoxetine, sertraline (see following section on SSRIs), amoxapine, venlafaxine and doxepin.

Not all antidepressants cause QT lengthening, and the torsadogenic risk increases with higher doses or when drugs are co-administered (e.g. antiarrhythmics, antihistamines, stimulants, antibiotics and antimycotics). It might be also due to familial aggregation, as in 10% of cases [52]. Typical antipsychotics (chlorpromazine, pimozide, thioridazine, perphenazine, trifluoperazine, haloperidol and droperidol) and atypical antipsychotics (clozapine, quetiapine, risperidone, sultopride, ziprasidone and loxapine) are more likely to cause QT lengthening and torsade de pointe. However, the group of atypical antipsychotics is considered to be less hazardous.

- Electrocardiograms show that some tricyclic antidepressants (amitriptyline, desipramine and nortriptyline), other antidepressants (maprotiline and lithium) and some antipsychotic drugs (trifluoperazine and loxapine), might cause even highly arrhythmic Brugada like type 1 and coved type syndrome.
- This is more frequent in familial aggregation cases (Na channel mutation, SCN5A) [52, 53].
- The choice, initiation and continuation of an antidepressants and antipsychotics therapy require a careful ECG evaluation (PR, QRS, QTc, ventricular repolarization specific and nonspecific alterations, bradycardia and supra and ventricular arrhythmias).
- Subjects suffering from underlying incompatible cardiac structure disease, electrolyte disorders (hypo and hyperpotassaemia and hypomagnesemia), liver and hepatic failure [54] and those treated with co-administered synergic drugs are excepted.

### 27.3.3 Selective Serotonin Reuptake Inhibitors (SSRIs)

**SSRIs** include drugs such as fluoxetine, sertraline, paroxetine and citalopram. Their most common CV effects are

1. arterial hypertension,
2. sinus tachycardia,

3. supra and ventricular arrythmias, and
4. heart failure due to myocardial negative inotropic effect [55, 56].

Overdose can lead to secondary brady-tachy syndrome and to systemic arterial hypotension. SSRIs can cause, to different extents (e.g. milder for Escitalopram) CYP3A4 enzymes hepatic inhibition. Treatment with warfarin has to be constantly monitored as the risk of severe haemorrhage is definite and it increases when warfarin is combined with acetylsalicylic acid and other antiplatelet drugs. SSRIs co-administration can lead to lethal hyponatremia.

### 27.3.4 Anticomitials

Young athletes might need prolonged anticomitial treatment. Anticomitials might have pharmacokinetic interactions with other drugs.

- Sodium valproate as hepatic metabolism inhibitor can increase phenobarbital plasma concentrations and favour drowsiness and psychic troubles especially in children.
- Other anticomitials such as phenytoin and carbamazepine can decrease plasma concentration of sodium valproate through the "**enzymatic activity**".
- The list of anticomitials also include gabapentin, lamotrigine, levetiracetam, oxcarbazepine, tiagabine, topiramate, vigabatrin, zonisamide and carbamazepine.
- Therapy with carbamazepine, valproic acid, phenobarbital and phenytoin can be monitored by plasma levels.
- Treatment with anticomitials in athletes always has to be reported and plasma levels measured.
- Serial ECG analysis are necessary to verify tolerance to therapy and, as asymptomatic bradyarrhythmia and nocturnal AV block can occur, Holter monitor might be needed.

### 27.3.5 Narcotics

The WADA list includes buprenorphine, dextromoramide, diamorphine (heroin), fentanyl and by-products such as: hydromorphone, methadone, morphine, oxycodone, oxymorphone, pentazocine and pethidine. **Narcotics** can be used in athletes suffering from post-traumatic pain syndrome. Oxycodone, a strong opioid analgesic, is increasingly used among young students and athletes [57].

- Narcotics can cause psychic troubles, a reduction in the perception of pain and a dangerous false sense of well-being.
- Methadone and levomethadyl can cause QT-lengthening and be torsadogenic [58].

### 27.3.6 Anti-inflammatory Drugs

The intake of "legal" drugs, such as the **non-steroidal anti-inflammatories** (NSAID) is more common in elite athletes than in non-athlete peers [59, 60]. These drugs may cause

1. delayed tissue regeneration,
2. gastrointestinal complications (gastralgia, heartburn, haemorrhage, alvus disorders),
3. disorders of the central nervous system (fatigue, headache, decreased perception of muscle strength),
4. decreased renal blood flow resulting in decreased kidney function (indomethacin, celecoxib), and
5. CV risks (cyclooxygenase inhibitor, Cox-2).

In order to reduce the adverse effects of these anti-inflammatory drugs, topical use (if effective) should be preferred to oral, parenteral or intravenous administration [61].

### 27.3.7 Anti-coagulants and Antiplatelet

One of the most important topics in the management of the athlete in treatment with **anti-coagulants** is the **haemorrhagic risk** during physical activity caused by traumas or collision with opponents, thus mostly in team sports and sports with a high intrinsic risk. Such risk is particularly high for veteran athletes, over 35-year-old and up until 70 years or more, who practice and train with the same intensities as younger athletes.

- It is worth reminding that in subjects treated with Vitamin K antagonists (VKA), like acenocoumarin (Sintrom) and warfarin (Coumadin), an increase in the training intensity or volume can affect the INR values.

VKA achieve their anticoagulant effect by interfering with several coagulative factors like II, V, VII and IX. Their metabolism is significantly affected by substances acting on cytochrome (CYP) P450. AVK require periodic INR control and have a delayed and prolonged effect that lasts even after suspension.

A recently introduced class of anti-coagulants is made of New Oral Anti-Coagulants (NOAC). NOAC are thrombin selective inhibitors (Dabigratan) or of the activated X Factor (Rivaroxaban, Apixaban, Edoxaban).

- It is still unknown if the NOAC's effect is influenced by exercise intensity and volume like VKA.
- NOAC have a short half-life and they are metabolized mostly through renal and hepatic excretion, therefore having a better and safer efficacy profile.

- It is clear that for their pharmacokinetics, bioavailability, efficacy and safety NOAC should be preferably prescribed in physically active and exercising subjects.
- Furthermore, NOAC have very mild interactions with cardiovascular drugs, like atorvastatin, verapamil, diltiazem, quinidine, amiodarone and dronedarone.

Having only recently been introduced, long-term therapy effects still require further investigation, in particular for the possible drug-drug interactions and the inhibiting or promoting effect on CYP3/A/4, that is directly involved in the hepatic clearance, for example, of rivaroxaban and apixaban. Few information is available coming from long-term treatment in a real-world scenario, for instance a significant increase of apixaban and rivaroxaban plasmatic levels have been described in the presence of HIV protease inhibitors.

The most commonly used antiplatelet drugs include aspirin, clopidogrel, prasugrel and ticagrelor. Just like anti-coagulants, antiplatelet medications increase the haemorrhagic risk, particularly in physically active individuals.

When establishing the individual risk, it is important to consider also other age-related CV diseases that might increase the likeliness of CV events such as coronary-artery disease, hypertension and atrial fibrillation. In this group of patients, anticoagulants and antiplatelet drugs reduce the risk of CV events but at the same time increase the risk of exercise-related and spontaneous haemorrhagic events. Thus, when prescribing this drug category to the exercising subject, several factors should be considered:

1. age,
2. sex,
3. coexisting cardiovascular disease (in case of AF the $CHA_2DS_2$-VASc score),
4. type and intensity of the physical activity practiced.

Low intensity and low exercises are preferable in most cases (see Chap. 1).

### 27.3.8 Stimulants

The use of **ergogenic substances** among athletes has been widely documented in anonymous survey studies. These substances, like energy drinks and food supplements, are usually self-prescribed and aim at increasing the physical and cognitive performance.

- Most of energy drinks freely available on the market contain high doses of caffeine and other molecules with a similar stimulating effect.
- Post-mortem and retrospective acceptance and emergency department studies have shown a significant correlation between the abuse of high-caffeine content substances and fatal arrhythmias.

- Although a clear cause-effect relationship between energy drinks and cardiac arrhythmias has not been demonstrated in large population prospective studies, the use of these substances should be limited.

Other stimulants of common use are those prescribed for the treatment of Attention-Deficit/Hyperactivity Disorder (ADHD), a condition of increasingly common diagnosis in North American and Scandinavian countries. The treatment usually relies on methylphenidate or its derivates. The prescription of ADHD treatment is strictly regulated by the World Anti-Doping Agency (WADA), International Sports Federations, and National Anti-Doping Agencies.

- Amphetamine-derived treatment is highly discouraged in subjects with familial or personal history of arrhythmic diseases, in particular those with a genetic background.
- The use of methylphenidate in athletes is allowed upon acceptance of a Therapeutic Use Exemption (TUE) application.

Beside the arrhythmogenic effect of amphetamine-derived substances, these drugs also have shown to increase the risk of *heat-related illnesses*.

- In particular, amphetamines could potentially mask or delay fatigue by slowing down the exercise-induced internal temperature rise.
- This could also impact the thermoregulatory system resulting in a potentially muscle overheating [62].
- The use of dopamine reuptake inhibitors has shown to improve performance but also to cause hyperthermia without any change in the perception of effort or thermal stress potentially increasing the risk of exertional heat injuries [63].
- A similar effect is known for ephedrine-containing compounds, due to the sympathomimetic effect, impairing the body's ability to dissipate heat properly [64].

**Clinical Pearls**

- The use of most commonly prescribed CV medication needs to be tailored to the patients' needs and lifestyle, taking into consideration the type of physical activity performed.
- Commonly prescribed CV medications may have an effect on exercise performance in athletes as well as patients with a very active lifestyle.
- The athletic pursuits of patients should also be considered when prescribing non-cardiac medications such as anti-depressants and stimulants, given the increased risk of heat related illness and arrhythmias.
- Many of the substances taken for performance enhancement such as human growth hormone and stimulants have no clear evidence for performance enhancement, but clear negative impacts on cardiovascular health.
- Over the counter substances such as Energy drinks and other stimulating substances might have an arrhythmogenic effect on predisposed individuals.

## Review

### Questions

1. In which type of sport are beta-blockers not allowed, according to the WADA list of prohibited substances?
2. True or false? The dose-heart rate response to beta blockade has little individual variability.
3. True or false? Pulmonary vasolidators such as sildenafil have been shown to improve exercise performance at sea level.
4. The use of androgenic anabolic agents is associated with cardiovascular side effects which mimic what commonly inherited cardiomyopathy?

### Answers

1. Skill sports.
2. False. There appears to be significant individual variability in the effect of a given dose of beta blocker on the resting and exercise heart rate. Dosing should be slowly uptitrated and exercise testing considered to assess heart rate response and exercise performance in order to tailor prescription to the athletic person's needs.
3. False. There is some evidence for a performance benefit in hypoxic conditions, but this has not been replicated in normoxic (sea level) conditions.
4. Hypertrophic cardiomyopathy.

## References


1. Van Bortel LM, van Baak MA. Exercise tolerance with nebivolol and atenolol. Cardiovasc Drug Ther. 1992;6(239):239–47.
2. Gullestad L, Hallen J, Medbo JI, Gronnerod O, Holme I, Sejersted OM. The effect of acute vs chronic treatment with beta-adrenoceptor blockade on exercise performance, haemodynamic and metabolic parameters in healthy men and women. Br J Clin Pharmacol. 1996;41(1):57–67.
3. Funck-Brentano C, Kibleur Y, Le Coz F, Poirier JM, Mallet A, Jaillon P. Rate dependence of sotalol-induced prolongation of ventricular repolarization during exercise in humans. Circulation. 1991;83(2):536–45.
4. Coltart DJ, Shand DG. Plasma propranolol levels in the quaniitative assessment of beta-adrenergic blockade in man. Br Med J. 1970;3(5725):731–4.
5. Wang JA, Lau CP, Tai YT, Wu BZ. Effects of flecainide on exercise hemodynamics and electrocardiography in patients without structural heart disease. Clin Cardiol. 1995;18(3):140–4.
6. Berglund B, Hemmingson P. Effect of reinfusion of autologous blood on exercise performance in cross-country skiers. Int J Sports Med. 1987;8(3):231–3.
7. Brien AJ, Simon TL. The effects of red blood cell infusion on 10-km race time. JAMA. 1987;257(20):2761–5.
8. Heuberger JA, Cohen Tervaert JM, Schepers FM, Vliegenthart AD, Rotmans JI, Daniels JM, et al. Erythropoietin doping in cycling: lack of evidence for efficacy and a negative risk-benefit. Br J Clin Pharmacol. 2013;75(6):1406–21.

9. Heuberger J, Rotmans JI, Gal P, Stuurman FE, van't Westende J, Post TE, et al. Effects of erythropoietin on cycling performance of well trained cyclists: a double-blind, randomised, placebo-controlled trial. Lancet Haematol. 2017;4(8):e374–e86.
10. Birkeland KI, Stray-Gundersen J, Hemmersbach P, Hallen J, Haug E, Bahr R. Effect of rhEPO administration on serum levels of sTfR and cycling performance. Med Sci Sports Exerc. 2000;32(7):1238–43.
11. Wilkerson DP, Rittweger J, Berger NJ, Naish PF, Jones AM. Influence of recombinant human erythropoietin treatment on pulmonary O2 uptake kinetics during exercise in humans. J Physiol. 2005;568(Pt 2):639–52.
12. Connes P, Perrey S, Varray A, Prefaut C, Caillaud C. Faster oxygen uptake kinetics at the onset of submaximal cycling exercise following 4 weeks recombinant human erythropoietin (r-HuEPO) treatment. Pflugers Arch. 2003;447(2):231–8.
13. Parisotto R, Gore CJ, Emslie KR, Ashenden MJ, Brugnara C, Howe C, et al. A novel method utilising markers of altered erythropoiesis for the detection of recombinant human erythropoietin abuse in athletes. Haematologica. 2000;85(6):564–72.
14. Garimella PS, Katz R, Patel KV, Kritchevsky SB, Parikh CR, Ix JH, et al. Association of serum erythropoietin with cardiovascular events, kidney function decline, and mortality: the health aging and body composition study. Circ Heart Fail. 2016;9(1):e002124.
15. Lippi G, Franchini M, Guidi GC. Cobalt chloride administration in athletes: a new perspective in blood doping? Br J Sports Med. 2005;39(11):872–3.
16. Alexander CS. Cobalt-beer cardiomyopathy. A clinical and pathologic study of twenty-eight cases. Am J Med. 1972;53(4):395–417.
17. Ebert B, Jelkmann W. Intolerability of cobalt salt as erythropoietic agent. Drug Test Anal. 2014;6(3):185–9.
18. Richardson RS, Tagore K, Haseler LJ, Jordan M, Wagner PD. Increased VO2 max with right-shifted Hb-O2 dissociation curve at a constant O2 delivery in dog muscle in situ. J Appl Physiol (1985). 1998;84(3):995–1002.
19. Suh JH, Stea B, Nabid A, Kresl JJ, Fortin A, Mercier JP, et al. Phase III study of efaproxiral as an adjunct to whole-brain radiation therapy for brain metastases. J Clin Oncol. 2006;24(1):106–14.
20. La Gerche A, Claessen G. Is exercise good for the right ventricle? Concepts for health and disease. Canadian. J Cardiol. 2015;31(4):502–8.
21. La Gerche A, Heidbuchel H. Can intensive exercise harm the heart? You can get too much of a good thing. Circulation. 2014;130(12):992–1002.
22. Ghofrani HA, Reichenberger F, Kohstall MG, Mrosek EH, Seeger T, Olschewski H, et al. Sildenafil increased exercise capacity during hypoxia at low altitudes and at Mount Everest base camp: a randomized, double-blind, placebo-controlled crossover trial. Ann Intern Med. 2004;141(3):169–77.
23. Faoro V, Boldingh S, Moreels M, Martinez S, Lamotte M, Unger P, et al. Bosentan decreases pulmonary vascular resistance and improves exercise capacity in acute hypoxia. Chest. 2009;135(5):1215–22.
24. Hsu AR, Barnholt KE, Grundmann NK, Lin JH, McCallum SW, Friedlander AL. Sildenafil improves cardiac output and exercise performance during acute hypoxia, but not normoxia. J Appl Physiol. 2006;100(6):2031–40.
25. Guidetti L, Emerenziani GP, Gallotta MC, Pigozzi F, Di Luigi L, Baldari C. Effect of tadalafil on anaerobic performance indices in healthy athletes. Br J Sports Med. 2008;42(2):130–3.
26. Bhasin S, Storer TW, Berman N, Callegari C, Clevenger B, Phillips J, et al. The effects of supraphysiologic doses of testosterone on muscle size and strength in normal men. N Engl J Med. 1996;335(1):1–7.
27. Forbes GB, Porta CR, Herr BE, Griggs RC. Sequence of changes in body composition induced by testosterone and reversal of changes after drug is stopped. JAMA. 1992;267(3):397–9.
28. Giorgi A, Weatherby RP, Murphy PW. Muscular strength, body composition and health responses to the use of testosterone enanthate: a double blind study. J Sci Med Sport. 1999;2(4):341–55.

29. Pope HG Jr, Wood RI, Rogol A, Nyberg F, Bowers L, Bhasin S. Adverse health consequences of performance-enhancing drugs: an Endocrine Society scientific statement. Endocr Rev. 2014;35(3):341–75.
30. Achar S, Rostamian A, Narayan SM. Cardiac and metabolic effects of anabolic-androgenic steroid abuse on lipids, blood pressure, left ventricular dimensions, and rhythm. Am J Cardiol. 2010;106(6):893–901.
31. Hartgens F, Rietjens G, Keizer HA, Kuipers H, Wolffenbuttel BH. Effects of androgenic-anabolic steroids on apolipoproteins and lipoprotein (a). Br J Sports Med. 2004;38(3):253–9.
32. Thompson PD, Cullinane EM, Sady SP, Chenevert C, Saritelli AL, Sady MA, et al. Contrasting effects of testosterone and stanozolol on serum lipoprotein levels. JAMA. 1989;261(8):1165–8.
33. Darke S, Torok M, Duflou J. Sudden or unnatural deaths involving anabolic-androgenic steroids. J Forensic Sci. 2014;59(4):1025–8.
34. Far HR, Agren G, Thiblin I. Cardiac hypertrophy in deceased users of anabolic androgenic steroids: an investigation of autopsy findings. Cardiovasc Pathol. 2012;21(4):312–6.
35. Baggish AL, Weiner RB, Kanayama G, Hudson JI, Picard MH, Hutter AM Jr, et al. Long-term anabolic-androgenic steroid use is associated with left ventricular dysfunction. Circ Heart Fail. 2010;3(4):472–6.
36. Luijkx T, Velthuis BK, Backx FJ, Buckens CF, Prakken NH, Rienks R, et al. Anabolic androgenic steroid use is associated with ventricular dysfunction on cardiac MRI in strength trained athletes. Int J Cardiol. 2013;167(3):664–8.
37. D'Andrea A, Caso P, Salerno G, Scarafile R, De Corato G, Mita C, et al. Left ventricular early myocardial dysfunction after chronic misuse of anabolic androgenic steroids: a Doppler myocardial and strain imaging analysis. Br J Sports Med. 2007;41(3):149–55.
38. Kim JH, Pan JH, Lee ES, Kim YJ. L-Carnitine enhances exercise endurance capacity by promoting muscle oxidative metabolism in mice. Biochem Biophys Res Commun. 2015;464(2):568–73.
39. Blanca AJ, Ruiz-Armenta MV, Zambrano S, Miguel-Carrasco JL, Arias JL, Arevalo M, et al. Inflammatory and fibrotic processes are involved in the cardiotoxic effect of sunitinib: protective role of L-carnitine. Toxicol Lett. 2016;241:9–18.
40. Dambrova M, Makrecka-Kuka M, Vilskersts R, Makarova E, Kuka J, Liepinsh E. Pharmacological effects of meldonium: Biochemical mechanisms and biomarkers of cardiometabolic activity. Pharmacol Res. 2016;113:771–80.
41. Stuart M, Schneider C, Steinbach K. Meldonium use by athletes at the Baku 2015 European Games. Br J Sports Med. 2016;50(11):694–8.
42. Quesnele JJ, Laframboise MA, Wong JJ, Kim P, Wells GD. The effects of beta-alanine supplementation on performance: a systematic review of the literature. Int J Sport Nutr Exerc Metab. 2014;24(1):14–27.
43. Bellinger PM, Minahan CL. The effect of beta-alanine supplementation on cycling time trials of different length. Eur J Sport Sci. 2016;16:1–8.
44. Bellinger PM, Minahan CL. Performance effects of acute beta-alanine induced paresthesia in competitive cyclists. Eur J Sport Sci. 2016;16(1):88–95.
45. Shetewy A, Shimada-Takaura K, Warner D, Jong CJ, Mehdi AB, Alexeyev M, et al. Mitochondrial defects associated with beta-alanine toxicity: relevance to hyper-beta-alaninemia. Mol Cell Biochem. 2016;416(1–2):11–22.
46. Kelly VG, Leveritt MD, Brennan CT, Slater GJ, Jenkins DG. Prevalence, knowledge and attitudes relating to beta-alanine use among professional footballers. J Sci Med Sport. 2016;20(1):12–6.
47. Pluim BM, de Hon O, Staal JB, Limpens J, Kuipers H, Overbeek SE, et al. beta(2)-Agonists and physical performance: a systematic review and meta-analysis of randomized controlled trials. Sports Med. 2011;41(1):39–57.
48. Sears MR. Adverse effects of beta-agonists. J Allergy Clin Immunol. 2002;110(6 Suppl):S322–8.
49. Milano G, Chiappini S, Mattioli F, Martelli A, Schifano F. beta-2 agonists as misusing drugs? Assessment of both Clenbuterol- and Salbutamol-related European Medicines Agency pharmacovigilance database reports. Basic Clin Pharmacol Toxicol. 2018;123(2):182–7.

50. Brett J, Dawson AH, Brown JA. Clenbuterol toxicity: a NSW poisons information centre experience. Med J Aust. 2014;200(4):219–21.
51. Shader RI, Greenblatt DJ. Use of benzodiazepines in anxiety disorders. N Engl J Med. 1993;328(19):1398–405.
52. Sicouri S, Antzelevitch C. Sudden cardiac death secondary to antidepressant and antipsychotic drugs. Expert Opin Drug Saf. 2008;7(2):181–94.
53. Yap YG, Behr ER, Camm AJ. Drug-induced Brugada syndrome. Europace. 2009;11(8):989–94.
54. Witchel HJ, Hancox JC, Nutt DJ. Psychotropic drugs, cardiac arrhythmia, and sudden death. J Clin Psychopharmacol. 2003;23(1):58–77.
55. Warrington SJ, Padgham C, Lader M. The cardiovascular effects of antidepressants. Psychol Med Monogr Suppl. 1989;16:i–iii, 1–40
56. Shader RI, Greenblatt DJ. Selective serotonin reuptake inhibitor antidepressants: cardiovascular complications—sorting through findings. J Clin Psychopharmacol. 2001;21(5):467–8.
57. Friedman RA. The changing face of teenage drug abuse—the trend toward prescription drugs. N Engl J Med. 2006;354(14):1448–50.
58. Fanoe S, Jensen G, Ege P. Proarrhythmic effect of methadone: an alternative explanation of sudden death in heroine addicts. PACE. 2006;29(Suppl 1):S30.
59. Milberg P, Hilker E, Ramtin S, Cakir Y, Stypmann J, Engelen MA, et al. Proarrhythmia as a class effect of quinolones: increased dispersion of repolarization and triangulation of action potential predict torsades de pointes. J Cardiovasc Electrophysiol. 2007;18(6):647–54.
60. Tscholl P, Feddermann N, Junge A, Dvorak J. The use and abuse of painkillers in international soccer: data from 6 FIFA tournaments for female and youth players. Am J Sports Med. 2009;37(2):260–5.
61. Alaranta A, Alaranta H, Helenius I. Use of prescription drugs in athletes. Sports Med. 2008;38(6):449–63.
62. Roelands B, Hasegawa H, Watson P, Piacentini MF, Buyse L, De Schutter G, et al. The effects of acute dopamine reuptake inhibition on performance. Med Sci Sports Exerc. 2008;40(5):879–85.
63. Keisler BD, Hosey RG. Ergogenic aids: an update on ephedra. Curr Sports Med Rep. 2005;4(4):231–5.
64. Morozova E, Yoo Y, Behrouzvaziri A, Zaretskaia M, Rusyniak D, Zaretsky D, et al. Amphetamine enhances endurance by increasing heat dissipation. Physiol Rep. 2016;4(17):e12955.

# Cardiac Safety in Sports Arenas

# 28

Luis Serratosa, Efraim Kramer, Erik Ekker Solberg, and Mats Börjesson

**Learning Objectives**

1. Learn about the unique characteristics that make emergency medical care at mass gathering sports events different to other emergency medical services.
2. How to organize the emergency medical services in sports stadiums or arenas.
3. Learn that every mass gathering sports event requires a written description of all medical resources needed, the so-called medical action plan, specifically adjusted for each venue and event.
4. How to provide prompt and effective management to any sudden cardiac arrest in any area of the venue.

L. Serratosa (✉)
Rehabilitation, Sports Medicine and Physiotherapy Department, Hospital Universitario Quironsalud Madrid, Madrid, Spain

Ripoll & De Prado Sport Clinic, FIFA Medical Centre of Excellence, Madrid, Spain

E. Kramer
Department of Sports Medicine, University of Pretoria, Pretoria, South Africa
e-mail: efraim.kramer@wits.ac.za

E. E. Solberg
Medical Department, Diakonhjemmet Hospital, Oslo, Norway
e-mail: erik.solberg@diakonsyk.no

M. Börjesson
Neuroscience and Physiology & Center for Health and Performance, University of Gothenburg, Gothenburg, Sweden
e-mail: mats.brjesson@telia.com



A. Pressler, J. Niebauer (eds.), *Textbook of Sports and Exercise Cardiology*,
https://doi.org/10.1007/978-3-030-35374-2_28

## 28.1 Introduction

Illustrating that cardiac care may also be needed in prehospital areas, this chapter describes emergency cardiac care in a geographical area where many people meet for a sports event, the so-called mass gathering sports events.

- Traditionally, mass gathering medical care has been defined as emergency health care services provided to spectators and participants, in events where at least 1000 persons are gathered at a specific location for a defined period of time [1].
- Nevertheless, most published reports have described the medical care coverage for greater than 25,000 attendees [2–4].

As in other mass gathering events, sports stadiums and arenas may gather several thousands of persons during a certain amount of time, creating challenges not only related to the medical care for both athletes and spectators inside the venues, but also affecting the local, non-event related, health care resources (prehospital emergency medical services and hospitals).

Planning medical care for certain mass sports events such as the Olympics, FIFA World Cup or the World Championship Games in Athletics may be particularly challenging as spectators and participants may be spread in multiple sites/arenas, across long distances, and exposed to varied environmental conditions during many days or even weeks [3–6]. Some additional factors may need to be considered when planning medical care for adaptive sports events, especially those related with individual needs of athletes [7]. Ensuring safe participation of athletes and providing adequate medical care for spectators is always one of the main challenges for those organizing sports events in stadiums and arenas.

Among all medical issues, sudden cardiac arrest (SCA) represents the most challenging emergency for which event organizers must be prepared in order to provide a prompt and adequate response to improve chances of survival. Other potentially life-threatening medical conditions, like syncope, spinal cord injuries or concussion must also be handled properly.

- Importantly, the risk of cardiac events may be increased in both athletes [8] and spectators [9–12] with underlying cardiovascular disease, due to the increased physical and/or emotional stress.
- However, the effect of emotional stress on the incidence of cardiac events among spectators is still controversial [13–15].
- The reported incidence of SCA among spectators ranges from 0.17 [16] to 0.38/100,000 spectators [17, 18].
- This means that every medium to large size sports arena is likely to have a number of SCA events per season.
- For example, a total of seven cases of acute coronary syndrome were reported in the Barcelona FC stadium (98,260 spectators) during the 2000–2001 season [19].

A coordinated response with early and effective cardiopulmonary resuscitation (CPR) and defibrillation is key to improve survival from out of hospital SCA [20]. Placing automated external defibrillators (AEDs) in areas where as few as one cardiac arrest per 5 years can be expected, is considered to be cost-effective [20]. By introducing the "chain of survival", enabling rescuers to deliver early and effective CPR and providing access to early defibrillation within 3–5 min of collapse, survival rates from out of hospital SCA can be as high as 70% [20–22].

- In the clinical context of sports arenas, the **German Football League's study** showed impressive resuscitation success rates, with 96% of the 52 patients who suffered a SCA being transported to hospital with spontaneous circulation [17]. These results were related to well organized and adequately trained emergency medical services (EMS) being able to provide short response times and support the need to implement effective strategies for emergency cardiac care in mass gathering sports events.
- Disappointingly, the 2005–2006 season **European Arena study** showed that as many as 28% of the participating First and Second Division clubs did not have an AED available in the arena, 36% did not have a written Medical Action Plan (MAP), and 35% did not have CPR training programme for personnel [16].
- However, a more recent study of the 92 professional football clubs of the top four leagues of the English Football Association showed a better status, with all clubs having an AED on match days and training sessions, and most (83%) having an emergency action plan. Still some improvements in AED training and equipped ambulances availability on match days were identified as necessary in the lower divisions [23].

As a consequence of the Arena study [16], in 2011 the Section of Sports Cardiology of the European Association of Preventive Cardiology (EAPC) published a consensus document regarding cardiovascular safety at sports arenas [24]. Preceding this, the only existing comprehensive document to assist EMS physicians with planning emergency medical care at mass gathering events was published in 2000 by the National Association of Emergency Medical Services Physicians (NAEMSP) of the United States of America (USA) [25]. An update of this position statement [26] and FIFA's recommendations on Mass Gathering Football Emergency Medicine [27] were published in 2015. Based on existing scientific data and expert consensus, all these documents propose minimum standards for delivery of EMS in mass gathering sports events.

The present chapter deals with planning of EMS in sports stadiums and arenas. These are broad based recommendations in order to allow organizers to adapt to the specific needs of the arena according to size, location and architectural characteristics, with the common goal of providing prompt, safe, effective, efficient and coordinated management of any SCA. Mass gathering medical care should also include less acute cardiovascular care and non-cardiac medical care which is not discussed in this chapter.

## 28.2 Medical Action Plan (MAP) and Event Planning

The American Olympic athlete Jackie Joyner-Kersee's axiom, "it is better to look ahead and prepare than to look back and regret", holds true when assuming the responsibility of organizing the healthcare for any mass gathering sports event.

There are several aspects that make mass gathering sports events medical care in arenas different to other EMS, and that should be considered in the planning (Table 28.1) [24].

As in any mass gathering event, organizing the emergency medical care in sports arenas requires a written description of the medical resources needed (the MAP), as well as providing detailed plans for its use.

- This MAP should be specifically tailored for each venue and ideally adjusted for each event.
- It should also be reviewed and updated at least annually.
- Every MAP should address all aspects listed in Table 28.2 and discussed in detail below [24].

Including a detailed map of the venue with locations of all health care resources (advanced life support (ALS) and basic life support (BLS) medical care posts/centres, ambulances and mobile medical teams (MMTs, AEDs, etc.) as well as, if possible, emergency exits and evacuation routes, may be very useful for all the EMS personnel, both as a guide during the event and for pre and post event debriefing meetings (Fig. 28.1).

For practical purposes, the majority of medium or large size stadiums and arenas can be divided into two specific functional areas, namely the *competition* and *non-competition* areas:

**Table 28.1** Unique characteristics of sports mass gathering emergency medical care

| |
|---|
| Medical personnel usually need to navigate large crowds and architectural barriers (i.e. fences, lifts, stairs, etc.) that interfere with adequate emergency medical care and meeting response times |
| Use of motorized transport may be prevented by architectural barriers |
| Evacuation routes may be crowded at certain moments |
| Weather conditions in outdoors events (i.e. rain, snow, extreme temperatures) |
| Patients refusing to receive medical care, and hostility from surrounding spectators or between rival fans, may complicate the working environment |
| Alcohol and drugs consumption |
| Characteristics of athletes, spectators and competition (level, type of sport, adaptive sports, age, language, familiarity with the venue, duration, multiple sites, national, international) |
| VIP medical care |
| Potential for terrorist acts and mass casualty incidents needing greater demand for medical care and initial triage of casualties |
| Communication challenges including prolonged transportation time to hospital |

**Table 28.2** Key aspects that should be addressed in the MAP of every sports arena

| |
|---|
| Responsibilities and contact information of the appointed event medical director |
| Roles and responsibilities of all health care personnel |
| Medical equipment including AEDs |
| ALS and BLS treatment facilities |
| ALS and BLS transportation |
| Communications system |
| Patient contacts documentation system |
| Continuous quality improvement and training (i.e. rehearsals and meetings) |
| Coordination with local health care resources |

*MAP* medical action plan, *AED* automated external defibrillator, *ALS* advanced life support, *BLS* basic life support

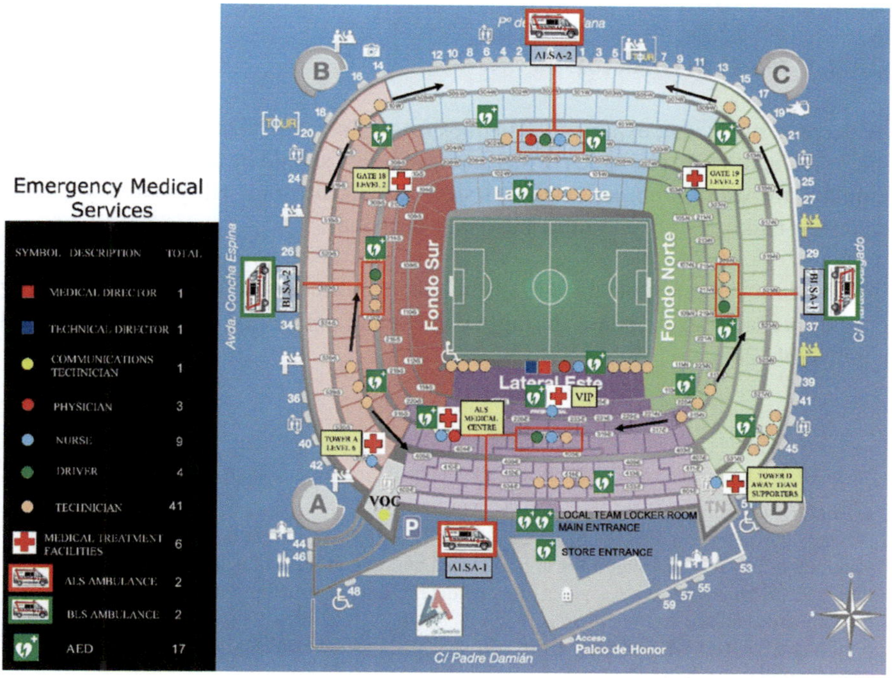


**Fig. 28.1** Map of a large size football stadium (81,000 spectators) with locations of all health care resources

1. The *competition area* comprises those parts of a stadium where the sports activity is actually undertaken, including changing rooms, officials' offices, doping control room, etc. Due to security considerations, accreditation passes are generally required to gain access to these and the VIP areas.
2. The *non-competition area* comprises the spectator seating area, commercial vendor areas, hospitality areas and the parking areas in and around the stadium.

The single most important determining factors for successful SCA management is the time from patient collapse to initiation of CPR and first AED shock, when indicated. Within a sports arena, the overwhelming majority of SCA events will be witnessed, potentially allowing for almost immediate CPR activation and a summoned BLS (CPR + AED) response within the required goal of 3–5 min [28]. In fact, the survival rate of exercise-related SCA has been shown to be considerably higher inside arenas compared to outside [28].

The medical emergency planning must ensure safety of the patient, rescuers and surrounding spectators as well as if needed, the safe and efficient transfer of the patient, away from the site of collapse to the nearest, most appropriate medical facility. The distance and predicted transport times to the nearest hospitals, should be timed and stated in the MAP.

## 28.3 Personnel

### 28.3.1 Medical Director

A licensed physician, experienced in out-of-hospital medical care and familiar with the local health care resources (EMS and hospitals), should be appointed as medical director for every arena of sufficient size, as this measure will positively impact decision-making, transportation and triage decisions.

- The duties and responsibilities of the medical director in the previous planning and preparation, response during the event and post-event analysis are outlined in Table 28.3.

**Table 28.3** Duties and responsibilities of the medical director in a sports mass gathering event

| |
|---|
| Designing, updating and implementing the MAP |
| Actively participate in the organizing committee of every major event taking place at the arena |
| Planning of any remodelling of the arena or even building process of a new stadium, to ensure that medical emergency care aspects (e.g.: medical rooms, evacuation routes, transportation, etc.) are considered |
| Supervising that all EMS personnel are adequately trained and certified in emergency cardiovascular medicine |
| During the event, should be easily identifiable and always available by some form of communication modality to all EMS personnel, and especially to the EMS representative located inside the venue operations centre of large arenas |
| Ensuring that all patient contacts are properly documented |
| Establishing and maintaining communication and collaboration with the local EMS and physicians of interest in nearby hospitals, to improve patient outcomes and allow for follow-up of critically ill patients transported to the hospital |
| Organizing periodic training rehearsals and debriefing meetings (e.g. pre and post-event, post SCA events) with the EMS personnel |
| Acting as a media spokesperson, if required |

*MAP* medical action plan, *EMS* emergency medical services, *SCA* sudden cardiac arrest

### 28.3.2 Medical and Other Healthcare Personnel

The timely response to a collapsed, possible SCA patient with initial cardiac resuscitation and subsequent transfer from the site of collapse, with or without return of spontaneous circulation (ROSC), requires adequate numbers of medical and allied healthcare personnel, sufficiently qualified, skilled and experienced. These must be well adapted to the prehospital medical environment, and specifically to that of a large, multi-level arena, designed to hold a large capacity of participants. The following aspects should be considered when deciding on the number and training level of the emergency medical personnel:

a) arena capacity and predicted attendance of the event (Fig. 28.2),
b) architectural barriers (Fig. 28.3),
c) level of risk of the sport (i.e., contact vs. non-contact sports) and event (i.e., rivalry of opposing teams, familiarity with the arena),
d) weather conditions in conventional outdoors arenas, and
e) transport times to higher levels of medical care.

Presence of at least 1–2 physicians (aside from team physicians)/50,000 spectators, 1 nurse/10000 spectators, ALS certified, and 2 medical technicians

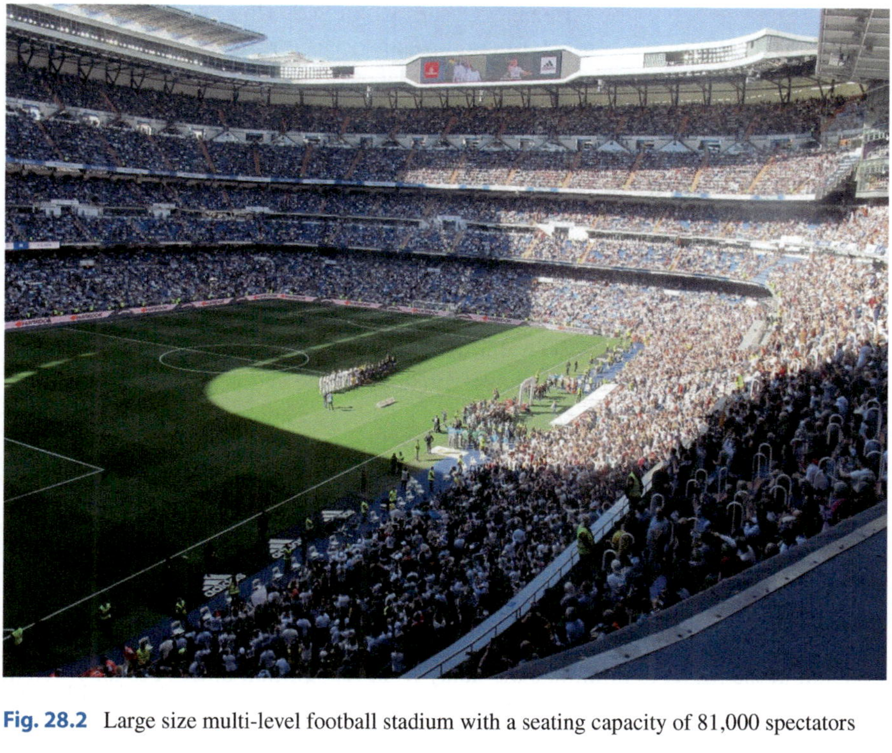

Fig. 28.2 Large size multi-level football stadium with a seating capacity of 81,000 spectators

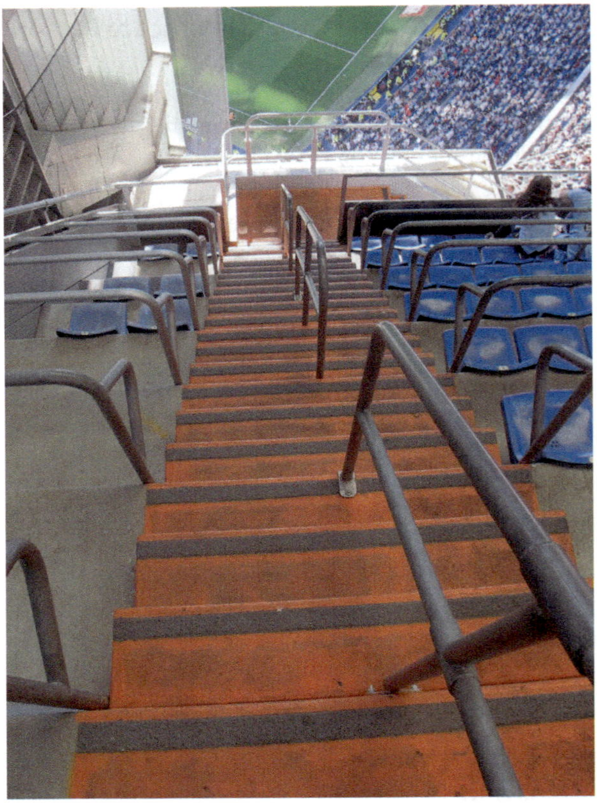

**Fig. 28.3** Stairs and other architectural barriers in the upper deck of a large football stadium

(MTs)/10,000 spectators has been recommended in previous documents [24, 29, 30], but the final number should be adjusted to guarantee prompt CPR and defibrillation, even in those areas of the venue where access is more complicated.

- All the medical and allied healthcare personnel should be at least BLS qualified, encompassing CPR and AED training.
- All EMS personnel need to be dressed in appropriate visible uniforms for immediate identification by the spectators and should be equipped with the necessary BLS or ALS medical and communication equipment, thus promoting expeditious response and treatment (Fig. 28.4).
- Ushers and other non-medical personnel (i.e., security) working at the stadium should be aware of how to alert the on-site EMS and ideally, as many as possible should be trained in CPR and AED use.

The specific roles of each personnel category and hierarchy should be specified in detail in the MAP, to minimize the delay from recognition of SCA to an efficient response with BLS and if needed, ALS.

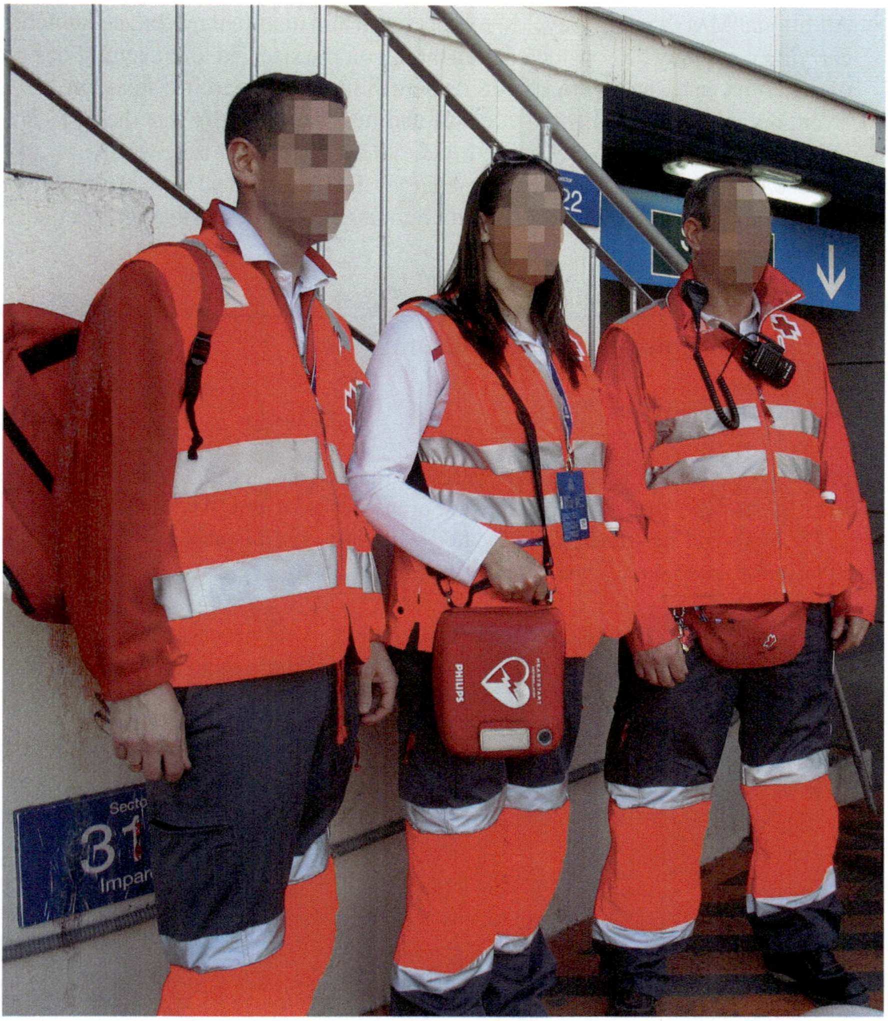


**Fig. 28.4** Mobile medical team with BLS medical and communications equipment

Overall, the first SCA response and resuscitation within a sports stadium will usually be performed by the MMTs, which should be strategically positioned in the venue and depending on their location, could be comprised of two to four members, some including ALS trained personnel. They must be on site and when activated by a patient collapse, these MMTs should be able to speedily and safely respond and gain access to the collapsed patient's side, anywhere within the stadium. Ensuring a safe, satisfactory and successful response, resuscitation and if necessary, transfer of the SCA patient in an often-crowded area of the stadium, while carrying medical bags, a defibrillator and a rigid patient carrying device, requires planning, training and regular rehearsals.

- Additional MMTs using bicycles, motorcycles, and modified motorized stretcher carrying carts may be considered, depending on the size and architectural design of the arena, and any external EMS responsibilities (e.g. parking areas, etc.).
- Event organizers and EMS providers should in advance certify that the EMS and individually all its personnel have sufficient liability insurance coverage.
- In case of being contacted by the media, all EMS personnel should remember that their duty to protect confidentiality remains at all times, also after a patient's death.

## 28.4 Requirements of the Stadium

### 28.4.1 Treatment Facilities

Depending on the size and characteristics of the arena, a number of primary care medical posts and, in medium-large size arenas at least one ALS medical center (Fig. 28.5), should be strategically located with best possible access for spectators, especially for those with physical disabilities.

- If possible, the ALS medical center should have an easy access from the teams' locker rooms and VIP area, and an easy evacuation route to an ALS ambulance.

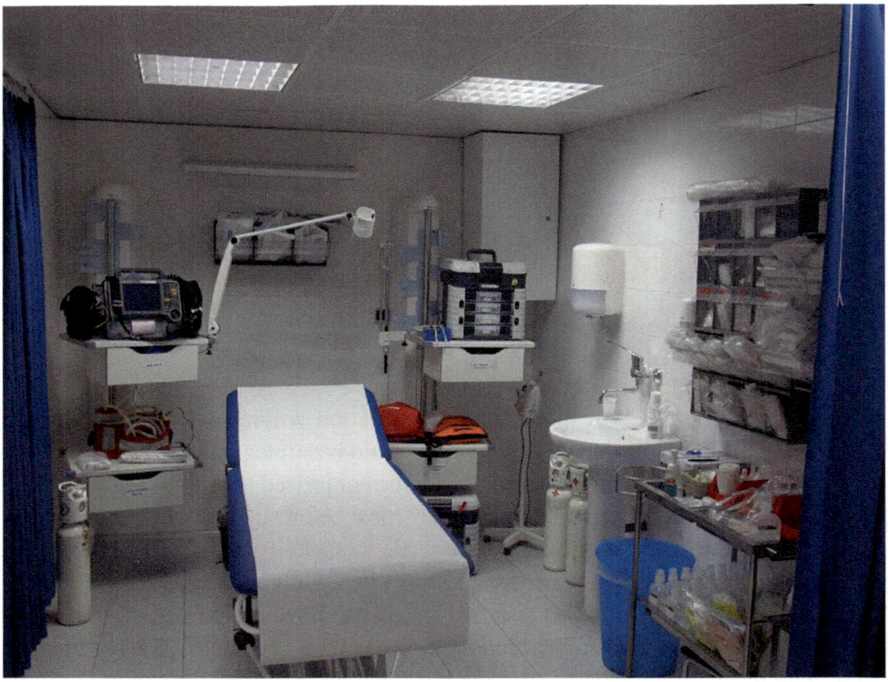

**Fig. 28.5** Medical room with advanced life support medical equipment

- Ideally, there should be at least 1 nurse and 1 MT in every primary care medical post, and at least 1 physician and 1 nurse in the ALS medical center.
- These on-site medical posts may be very useful in large arenas where a high number of patients may occasionally be expected and in locations with prolonged transport times to higher levels of care.

### 28.4.2 Medical Equipment

The appropriate cardiac resuscitation equipment required for management of a SCA within a sports stadium structure encompasses all the equipment carried by the MMTs and the one located within the medical centers of large arenas. This requires, as a minimum, a number of fully functional AEDs and where necessary, such as in the ALS medical center, an ALS type manual multifunctional defibrillator/synchronized cardioverter/transcutaneous pacemaker with accessory diagnostic functions (e.g. pulse oximetry). Older monophasic defibrillators are also acceptable, as is the use of defibrillator paddles and gel, as long as adequate safety precautions are undertaken during defibrillation.

- AEDs should be also widely distributed throughout the arena and the total number can be calculated by using suggested algorithms [31], to make it possible to achieve the goal of first defibrillation in 3–5 min after the patients collapse, in any part of the venue.
- Fixed AEDs should be visible and clearly marked in all maps of the venue.
- Batteries and pads of all AEDs should be checked annually.

The ALS MMTs and medical centers should also have all the emergency care medication needed to adequately treat a SCA. Including stretchers, wheelchairs and stair-chairs should also be considered to assist in patients transport.

A readiness check of all equipment and medication should be performed prior to every event.

In order to ensure safety, there are some aspects that should be considered when using the emergency medical cardiac equipment for the management of SCA within a sports stadium, in specific conditions:

1. CPR + AED use in wet (rain) conditions is considered safe [32].
2. Adequacy of space to position the patient horizontal on a hard surface for effective external chest compressions. This may not be possible if a patient collapses in the seat within the spectators seating area, due to the minimum available space. It may then be necessary to speedily transfer the SCA patient from the seat to the nearest adequate area and lay him/her down horizontally before external chest compressions can be effectively initiated and AED pads applied for rhythm analysis.
3. In case of vomiting or if peripheral venous access is needed, waste and all used items removal should be appropriately handled.

4. Consideration should also be given to the various causes of cardiac arrest which may require various adaptations to the normal clinical protocol practiced, namely lightning strike cardiac arrest, multiple patients cardiac arrest from a stadium stampede, anaphylactic cardiac arrest from stinging insects, etc.

### 28.4.3 Signage and Information Related with Access to Care

- Easily discernible signs should be strategically placed throughout the arena to facilitate quick location of all medical care posts/centers and AEDs (Fig. 28.6).
- Information including a map with location of treatment facilities (BLS and ALS), MMTs, AEDs and ambulances should also be included in the official event programme, team and/or arena websites, as well as in visible posters/wall charts located at teams and referees locker rooms, doping control and delegates rooms, and VIP lounges in the competitions area.
- To maximize visibility, signs, posters/ and program information should be designed with pictograms, bold text and bright colors.
- The MAP should be also available for the sport governing bodies and opposing teams, well in advance of the match or tournament.
- In international events, all signs and information related with access to care should be written in the host country's native language, in English and in any other languages required by the organizing body.

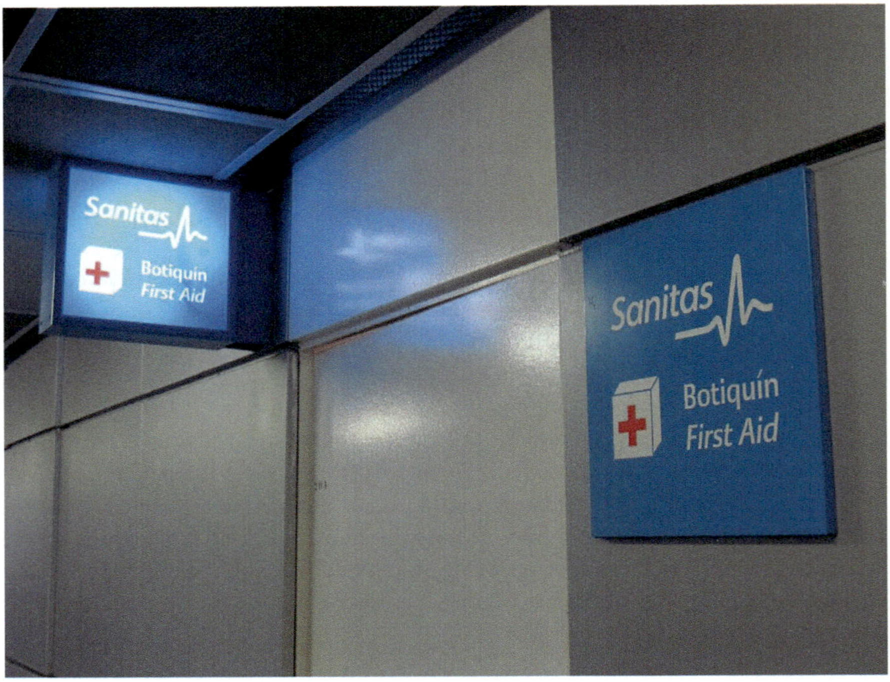


**Fig. 28.6** Signs to facilitate location of medical rooms

### 28.4.4 Patient Transportation

Once cardiac resuscitation has been in progress for a period of time, it may be necessary to plan for evacuation of the patient from the site where resuscitation was initiated. This may require transfer of the patient who has obtained ROSC to the most appropriate medical facility in the stadium (BLS medical post or ALS medical center) or to the nearest hospital, for immediate post resuscitation stabilization and care. However, the patient without ROSC may also be required to be transferred for reasons which may include safety, crowd considerations, need for upgraded clinical management at the ALS medical center or nearest hospital, or termination of resuscitation in privacy.

- In a patient who has gained ROSC, transfer logistics include use of an immobilizing patient carriage device, so that CPR + AED use can be immediately restarted, if ROSC is lost during transfer.
- This entails considering various potential difficulties, namely stairs, ramps, lifts, which if not considered during the planning and practice phase, may cause major logistical problems, to ensure safe, appropriate patient transfer within or out of the stadium to waiting ambulances, which cannot directly access the patient due to structural limitations.
- Carriage of an unconscious patient from the stadium seated area, using a long spinal board type device, maintaining a constant horizontal position, whilst negotiating a steep incline quite frequently of >30° should be planned and practiced beforehand, in order to realize the required manpower necessary.
- Carrying a patient horizontally on a long trauma spinal board may in fact require up to ten persons to undertake the same task in the upper decks of some arenas.

Furthermore, if the SCA patient has not successfully achieved ROSC and transfer is thought most appropriate, this will not only entail carriage of the pulseless patient horizontally on a long, trauma spinal board, but will also require continuous, competent chest compressions, rescue ventilations and AED analysis and shocks.

Safe and relatively unimpeded evacuation routes should be designed, both in the competition and non-competition area, and clearly marked to minimize transport times. Transport times in a full capacity stadium from different parts of the arena to the nearest medical post and ambulance should be measured and stated in the MAP.

Whether an ambulance can enter the field of play, or not, is important to ascertain, so that plans can be appropriately made in advance. Likewise, it is important to establish if the stadium ramps or lifts are accessible for ambulance stretchers, ambulances or modified motorized stretcher carrying carts, all of which need adequate access if they are to be used to convey the patient safely and appropriately away from the site. Although not for SCA patients, wheelchairs and specially stair-chairs may be of help in many arenas.

The ambulance, its crew, medical equipment and medical protocols must have been audited to ensure that safe, effective and efficient CPR can be undertaken in the moving ambulance on-route to the receiving medical facility. Distance and

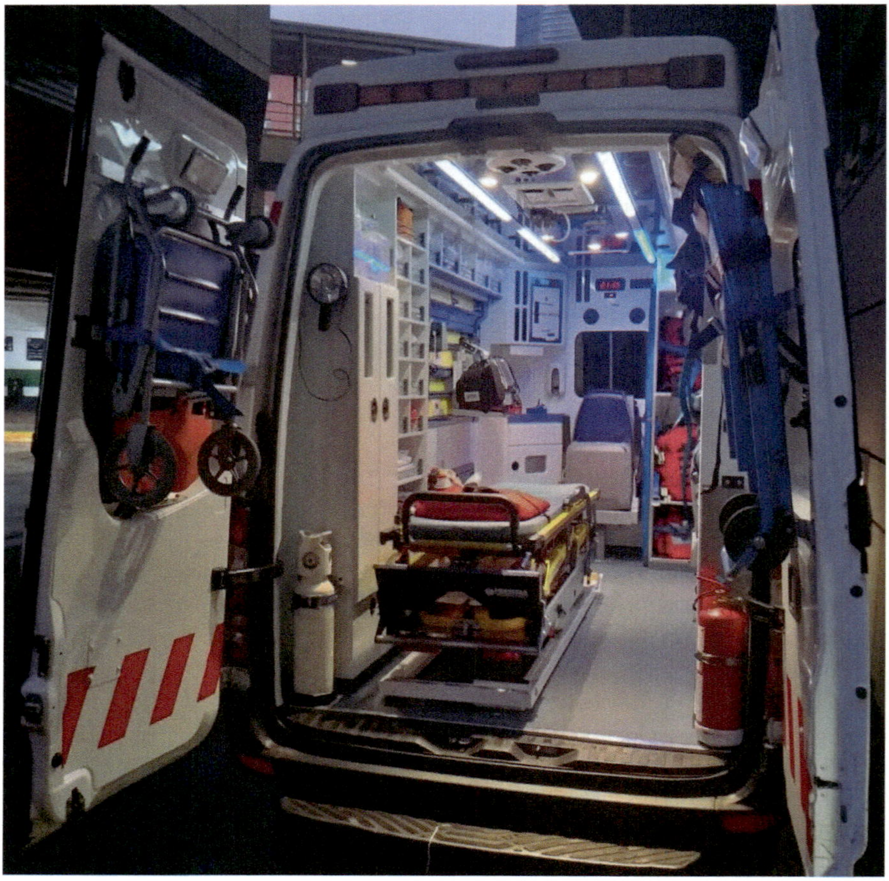

**Fig. 28.7** Large capacity fully equipped Advanced Life Support ambulance

transport times to the nearest hospitals should be measured and stated in the MAP, considering the worst scenarios related with traffic congestion. The fastest evacuation routes should be designed and selected in coordination with the local authorities.

Many medium and large sports arenas will have a designated helicopter landing area, for life threatening medical emergencies. All members of the EMS team who will access the helicopter landing zone must be familiar with the various safety and operational aspects concerned.

The number and type of internal (motorized stretcher carrying carts) and external (BLS and ALS ambulances) transportation resources should be adapted according to the characteristics (size, architecture, location) of the arena/event.

- As a recommendation, a minimum of 1 ALS ambulance (Fig. 28.7) adequately staffed with at least 1 physician, 1 nurse and 1 MT, should be always present during the event if >10,000 spectators are expected [24].

- Replacing, if only one, or making the required changes in the positioning of the ambulances should be also pre-planned in the MAP.
- All vehicles should be clearly described in the medical action plan and marked in the map of the venue (Fig. 28.1).

## 28.5 Communications

No emergency can be effectively managed without adequate communications. In order to ensure a speedy both primary and secondary response, all members involved with a medical emergency in and around the sports stadium should be contactable whenever necessary and have updated information, using either

1. two-way mobile radios,
2. cellphones,
3. land-line phones,
4. pager messages, or
5. similar devices.

In case of a cardiac or other medical emergency, the EMS representative in the venue operations center of large stadiums or the person with these responsibilities in smaller arenas, must be constantly updated with any necessary information, so that medical assistance can be dispatched; transport guided and arranged as required, and other allied emergency services alerted and briefed (e.g. traffic police, referral hospital).

Communication training must be integral to any of the clinical simulated training scenarios to familiarize all medical and healthcare team members with the designated communication devices being used. All communication systems should be tested prior to each event. Ideally, the MAP should list all the relevant cell and land-line phone numbers.

## 28.6 Documentation

All patient contacts should be registered, ideally, in a standardized electronic medical records database, ensuring confidentiality and safety of all the patient's information. If possible, a signed copy of the report should be delivered to the patient or those accompanying him/her. An "against medical advice" section or specific form for patients who refuse treatment will help in reducing the event and/or venue liability.

If the patient is transferred to the hospital, a written report is necessary and should include information on

1. patient's condition,
2. investigations,
3. treatment,

4. location and time of incident,
5. method and timing of transfer, as well as
6. any problems incurred during transport [33].

The medical record may also be used for continuous quality improvement of the EMS, research purposes, and more important, as a legal document, possibly with varying requirements in different national settings.

## 28.7 Planning, Coordination and Continuous Training

The effective and efficient management of any life-threatening cardiac emergency requires planning well in advance, good coordination, cooperation and communication, in order to timeously recognize any patient who has collapsed anywhere within or around the arena's area of responsibility. Coordination and cooperation with the local EMS and nearest Hospitals is also essential to optimize all available resources.

- The MAP should define which local EMS and nearby hospitals, and how, will take care of the patient from the arena medical staff in specific cases such as a cardiac emergency.
- The arena EMS must be ready to provide adequate medical care, with all personnel and ambulances in their assigned positions, before the access gates open, and have to remain available until the last spectator and/or player has left the stadium.
- The sequence of life saving events can only be successfully accomplished if the approved, and regularly audited emergency MAP, is known to all members of the medical and healthcare services and is regularly rehearsed using life-like scenarios with debriefing sessions in order to update and/or correct any weakness in the system.
- Such clinical training scenarios should include practical response to and evaluation of resuscitation and transfer of the victim, in a crowded spectator seating area, or in those other areas of most difficult access inside the venue.
- Debriefing meetings with the EMS team should be also organized before and after every event, and also after every SCA, as they are an excellent opportunity for quality improvement.
- Ideally, the medical director should also attend the periodic meetings with the rest of the key organizational heads of the safety and security committee of the arena.

## 28.8 Local/National Adaptations

There is no current validated, internationally accepted, medical care mass gathering system, although the basic principles are accepted by expert opinion and consensus [24, 26, 27]. Each country may have its own specific regulations that legally mandate the various aspects of medical care mass gathering events, including minimum requirements of medical staff and equipment, mutual emergency services assistance etc.

Local regulations may likewise prescribe the scope and range of prehospital emergency medical practice by specific medical and allied healthcare professionals, influencing who may undertake what particular out-of-hospital emergency medical treatment, in and around the sport stadium. This legislative, and hence logistical, prerequisite may be further influenced by different international sports governing bodies own recommended minimum requirements [27]. All of these regulatory requirements need to be considered, with practical adaptations or modifications, where and when required.

## 28.9 Other "arenas"

Many of the most important aspects previously mentioned for sports arenas MAPs may also be applied in other sporting environments, such as

1. long-distance running races,
2. cross-country ski-races,
3. water sports, etc.

In any mass gathering/participation sport event, prompt delivery of potentially life-saving measures, such as CPR within 1 min and defibrillation within 3–5 min, in case of SCA, should be the main aspect to consider when planning and designing the EMS. In long-distance running competitions, such as marathons, in addition to first aid posts every few killometers, mobile emergency response teams with paramedics who ride bicycles and carry AEDs are also being used to accomplish prompt delivery of CPR and defibrillation [34]. Sports events and competitions in other more remote areas (i.e. desert, mountains, open water, etc.) may create greater challenges to achieve the same level of safety as in more confined sport environments such as arenas (see also Chap. 30).

## 28.10 Conclusions

Emergency medical care at mass gathering sports events has some unique characteristics that makes it different to other EMS. Organizing the EMS in sports arenas requires a detailed MAP that should be specifically tailored for each venue and type of event. The MAP should aim to support safe, coordinated and efficient management of any acute life-threatening event, most importantly SCA. This is ensured by individually tailoring the number of healthcare and related personnel as well as the medical equipment, communications system and emergency transportation logistics, with the goal to achieve CPR in 1 min, and defibrillation in the first 3–5 min of a SCA, in any area of the venue.

**Clinical Pearls**

- The occurrence of Sudden Cardiac Arrest (SCA) in and around the environments of a Sports Stadium or Arena will always exist
- What remains unknown is the timing, the location, the victim and the eventual clinical outcome.
- Of all the previous unknowns mentioned, only the clinical outcome can be positively influenced by ensuring effective and efficient skills training (BLS / ALS / ICU), medical equipping, organizational preplanning and practical simulations of SCA for the designated numbers of personnel that will function, in whatever capacity, in and around the environment of the Sports Stadium or Arena.
- A positive clinical outcome for SCA in Sport Stadiums and Arenas can be enhanced by ensuring that the Medical Action Plan (MAP) initiates CPR on a SCA victim within a 3–5-minute time frame from collapse.
- Likewise, a positive clinical response can also be obtained by a regularly rehearsed MAP, involving simulated SCA scenarios in all areas of the sport structure, including practical training in CPR and AED skill enhancement, communications, manikin stabilisation and ambulance service transfer and post exercise debriefing.

## Chapter Review

### Questions

1. Which of the following factors have a positive effect on the outcome of sudden cardiac arrest within a sports stadium or arena?
   (a) A frequently rehearsed stadium Medical Action Plan
   (b) Adequate quantities of AEDs located within the sport stadium environment
   (c) Training of cardiopulmonary resuscitation to large numbers of personnel working within the sport stadium structure, in whatever capacity
   (d) Highly visible, mobile emergency medical teams on-duty within the sport stadium environment
   (e) All of the above
2. Survival rates from sport stadium (out of hospital) SCA can be as high as 70% if effective CPR and AED use is undertaken within which recommended time period?
   (a) Within 3–5 min of victim collapse
   (b) Within 3–5 min of sport stadium communication centre notification
   (c) Within 3–5 min of mobile medical team activation
   (d) Within 3–5 min of sport stadium ambulance personnel notification
   (e) None of the above
3. Key aspects that should be addressed in the Medical Action Plan of every sports stadium or arena include which of the following?
   (a) Defined roles and responsibilities of all medical and health care personnel

(b) Fully checked, clean, functional medical equipment including AEDs
(c) Functional communication system for all medical and healthcare teams
(d) Coordination and communication with local health care resources
(e) All of the above

4. Which of the following factors may increase the level of risk for the provision of effective and efficient medical services within a sport stadium or arena?
   (a) The architectural design of the stadium
   (b) The level of athlete contacts within the sport type
   (c) The expected weather conditions in conventional outdoor stadiums or arenas
   (d) Rivalry between opposing team fans
   (e) All of the above

## Answers

1. All of the above. All of the above factors have a positive effect of obtaining successful outcomes for any SCA located within a sports stadium or arena environment.
2. Within 3–5 min of victim collapse, as this is the critical time when cardiac output ceases within the victim and restoration of cardiac flow within 3–5 min is the crucial research proven time for achieving successful Return of Spontaneous Circulation
3. All of the above. All of the above factors are key aspects that should be addressed in the Medical Action Plan (MAP) of every sports stadium or arena tournament.
4. All of the above. All of the above-mentioned factors increase the level of risk for the provision of effective and efficient medical services within a sport stadium or arena and need to be compensated for by increasing the levels of medical and healthcare personnel, medical equipment, communication devices etc.

## References

1. De Lorenzo RA. Mass gathering medicine: a review. Prehosp Disaster Med. 1997;12(1):68–72.
2. Milsten AM, Maguire BJ, Bissell RA, Seaman KG. Mass-gathering medical care: a review of the literature. Prehosp Disaster Med. 2002;17(3):151–62.
3. Arliani GG, Lara PHS, Pedrinelli A, Ejnisman B, Leite LMB, Cohen M. Analysis of medical assistance provided to spectators at the 2014 FIFA world cup matches. Acta Ortop Bras. 2018;26(1):33–5.
4. Morimura N, Katsumi A, Koido Y, Sugimoto K, Fuse A, Asai Y, et al. Analysis of patient load data from the 2002 FIFA World Cup Korea/Japan. Prehosp Disaster Med. 2004;19(3):278–84.
5. Hiltunen T, Kuisma M, Maatta T, Tennila A, Hari T, Backman R, et al. Prehospital emergency care and medical preparedness for the 2005 World Championship Games in Athletics in Helsinki. Prehosp Disaster Med. 2007;22(4):304–11.
6. Yancey AH 2nd, Fuhri PD, Pillay Y, Greenwald I. World Cup 2010 planning: an integration of public health and medical systems. Public Health. 2008;122(10):1020–9.

7. Leggit JC, Brundage CD. Adaptive sports event planning. In: De Luigi AJ, editor. Adaptive sports medicine a clinical guide. Cham: Springer International Publishing AG; 2018. p. 359–69.
8. Corrado D, Basso C, Rizzoli G, Schiavon M, Thiene G. Does sports activity enhance the risk of sudden death in adolescents and young adults? J Am Coll Cardiol. 2003;42(11):1959–63.
9. Carroll D, Ebrahim S, Tilling K, Macleod J, Smith GD. Admissions for myocardial infarction and World Cup football: database survey. BMJ. 2002;325(7378):1439–42.
10. Katz E, Metzger JT, Schlaepfer J, Fromer M, Fishman D, Mayer L, et al. Increase of out-of-hospital cardiac arrests in the male population of the French speaking provinces of Switzerland during the 1998 FIFA World Cup. Heart. 2005;91(8):1096–7.
11. Leeka J, Schwartz BG, Kloner RA. Sporting events affect spectators' cardiovascular mortality: it is not just a game. Am J Med. 2010;123(11):972–7.
12. Wilbert-Lampen U, Leistner D, Greven S, Pohl T, Sper S, Volker C, et al. Cardiovascular events during World Cup soccer. N Engl J Med. 2008;358(5):475–83.
13. Barone-Adesi F, Vizzini L, Merletti F, Richiardi L. It is just a game: lack of association between watching football matches and the risk of acute cardiovascular events. Int J Epidemiol. 2010;39(4):1006–13.
14. Niederseer D, Thaler CW, Egger A, Niederseer MC, Ploderl M, Niebauer J. Watching soccer is not associated with an increase in cardiac events. Int J Cardiol. 2013;170(2):189–94.
15. Kloner RA, McDonald S, Leeka J, Poole WK. Comparison of total and cardiovascular death rates in the same city during a losing versus winning super bowl championship. Am J Cardiol. 2009;103(12):1647–50.
16. Borjesson M, Dugmore D, Mellwig KP, van Buuren F, Serratosa L, Solberg EE, et al. Time for action regarding cardiovascular emergency care at sports arenas: a lesson from the Arena study. Eur Heart J. 2010;31(12):1438–41.
17. Luiz T, Preisegger T, Rombach D, Madler C. Cardiac arrest in spectators in German football stadiums. Precautionary measures, frequency and short-term outcome. Anaesthesist. 2014;63(8–9):636–42.
18. Leusveld E, Kleijn S, Umans VA. Usefulness of emergency medical teams in sport stadiums. Am J Cardiol. 2008;101(5):712–4.
19. Serra Grima R, Carreno MJ, Tomas Abadal L, Brossa V, Ligero C, Pons J. Acute coronary events among spectators in a soccer stadium. Rev Esp Cardiol. 2005;58(5):587–91.
20. Perkins GD, Handley AJ, Koster RW, Castren M, Smyth MA, Olasveengen T, et al. European Resuscitation council guidelines for resuscitation 2015: section 2. Adult basic life support and automated external defibrillation. Resuscitation. 2015;95:81–99.
21. Berdowski J, Blom MT, Bardai A, Tan HL, Tijssen JG, Koster RW. Impact of onsite or dispatched automated external defibrillator use on survival after out-of-hospital cardiac arrest. Circulation. 2011;124(20):2225–32.
22. Drezner JA, Toresdahl BG, Rao AL, Huszti E, Harmon KG. Outcomes from sudden cardiac arrest in US high schools: a 2-year prospective study from the National Registry for AED Use in Sports. Br J Sports Med. 2013;47(18):1179–83.
23. Malhotra A, Dhutia H, Gati S, Yeo TJ, Finnochiaro G, Keteepe-Arachi T, et al. Emergency response facilities including primary and secondary prevention strategies across 79 professional football clubs in England. Br J Sports Med. 2019;53(13):813–7.
24. Borjesson M, Serratosa L, Carre F, Corrado D, Drezner J, Dugmore DL, et al. Consensus document regarding cardiovascular safety at sports arenas: position stand from the European Association of Cardiovascular Prevention and Rehabilitation (EACPR), section of Sports Cardiology. Eur Heart J. 2011;32(17):2119–24.
25. Jaslow D, Yancey A 2nd, Milsten A. Mass gathering medical care: the medical director's checklist for the NAEMSP standards and clinical practice committee. National Association of Emergency Medicine Services Physicians: Leneka, KS; 2000.
26. Schwartz B, Nafziger S, Milsten A, Luk J, Yancey A 2nd. Mass gathering medical care: resource document for the National Association of EMS Physicians Position Statement. Prehosp Emerg Care. 2015;19(4):559–68.

27. Dvorak J, Kramer EB, Mandelbaum B, Zideman D, Schmied C, Patricios J, et al. Mass-gathering football medicine. In: Dvorak J, Kramer EB, editors. Football emergency medicine manual. 2nd ed. Zurich: Fédération Internationale de Football Association (FIFA); 2015. p. 72–109.
28. Frisk Torell MSA, Herlitz J, Claesson A, Svensson L, Börjesson M. Outcome of exercise-related out-of-hospital cardiac arrest is dependent on location: sports arenas vs outside of arenas. PLoS One. 2019;14(2):e0211723.
29. Shayne P, Holliman CJ, Wang NE, Parrillo SJ. International emergency medicine reference list. J Emerg Med. 1999;17(1):159–61.
30. Parrillo SJ. EMS and mass gatherings. EMedicine. 2004:1–9.
31. Motyka TM, Winslow JE, Newton K, Brice JH. Method for determining automatic external defibrillator need at mass gatherings. Resuscitation. 2005;65(3):309–14.
32. Lyster T, Jorgenson D, Morgan C. The safe use of automated external defibrillators in a wet environment. Prehosp Emerg Care. 2003;7(3):307–11.
33. Dunn MJ, Gwinnutt CL, Gray AJ. Critical care in the emergency department: patient transfer. Emerg Med J. 2007;24(1):40–4.
34. Kinoshi T, Tanaka S, Sagisaka R, Hara T, Shirakawa T, Sone E, et al. Mobile automated external defibrillator response system during road races. N Engl J Med. 2018;379(5):488–9.

# Part II

# Sports Cardiology in Recreational/Master Athletes

# Medical Supervision of Mass Sporting Events

# 29

Martin Schwellnus and Paolo Emilio Adami

**Learning Objectives**

1. Understand and estimate the risk of medical encounters at mass community-based sports events.
2. Be able to define and classify medical encounters at mass community-based sports events.
3. Understand the exercise benefit-risk paradox.
4. Implement step-wise planning to reduce the risk of medical encounters at mass community-based sports events.
5. Understand the potential role of pre-event medical screening for mass sporting events.
6. Plan and implement medical care on race day for mass community-based sporting events.
7. Develop guidelines to minimize the potential negative effects of environmental stress, including air quality at mass community-based sporting events.
8. Be able to document medical encounters at community-based sporting events.

M. Schwellnus (✉)
Sport, Exercise Medicine and Lifestyle Institute (SEMLI), University of Pretoria, Pretoria, South Africa
e-mail: mschwell@iafrica.com

P. E. Adami
Department of Health and Science, International Association of Athletics Federations – IAAF, Monte Carlo, Monaco
e-mail: paoloemilio.adami@iaaf.org



A. Pressler, J. Niebauer (eds.), *Textbook of Sports and Exercise Cardiology*,
https://doi.org/10.1007/978-3-030-35374-2_29

## 29.1 Introduction

Non-communicable disease (NCDs) of lifestyle are the number one cause of death worldwide and are currently responsible for >70% of all deaths. Physical inactivity is one of the major modifiable risk factors for NCDs. Universal prescription guidelines for physical activity for all individuals include engaging in >150 min of moderate- to high intensity physical exercise weekly.

- Brisk walking, jogging, running, cycling, swimming are common endurance exercise activities that are prescribed to individuals.
- There are an increasing number of sports events around the world where large numbers of individuals engage in organized endurance sports—these can be considered "mass community-based sporting events".
- Mass community-based sporting events include park runs, road races (distances vary from 5 km to ultra-marathons), cycling events, swimming events, and events combining endurance sports e.g. triathlon
- There are data indicating that the profile of participants at these events is changing, with increasing numbers of older individuals and female participants.

There is a known risk of medical complications during moderate- to high intensity exercise, and this risk varies according to the "risk profile" of the individual. These medical complications during exercise can vary from minor to severe life-threatening and also result in death from cardiac arrest and other causes. Medical staff, that are responsible for participant safety at mass community-based sporting events:

1. need to be aware of the risk of medical encounters at events, causes and risk factors associated with medical encounters, and
2. can design and implement strategies to reduce the risk of medical encounters at these events.

### 29.1.1 Risk of Medical Encounters at Mass Sporting Events

- In a recently published international consensus paper, general definitions and more specific definitions of medical encounters (by severity, timing and type) were outlined [1].

#### 29.1.1.1 General Definitions

A mass community-based endurance sports event is defined as

- "*a planned and organised endurance sports event, usually with > 1000 entrants (recreational and/or elite), at a specific location, for a specific purpose, and for a defined period of time (single day/stage or multiple stages/several consecutive days)*" [2, 3].

A "community-based" event is typically planned and organised by a community sports organisation with a committee that includes a race director. We refer to "mass participation" as a mass-gathering with >1000 race entrants [2, 3], but also recognise that events of a smaller size (<1000 race entrants) can be managed and collect data.

An "endurance sports event" is an event that includes one or more of the following sport types:

(a) distance running
(b) cycling
(c) swimming
(d) triathlon
(e) biathlon
(f) duathlon
(g) canoeing/kayaking
(h) cross country skiing
(i) mixed ultra-endurance events
(j) other similar activities that combine any of these disciplines or function with more than one athlete as a team of entrants.

The medical team is defined as

- the "*team responsible for the medical care during the event and is made up by officially designated medical staff (medical physicians, emergency medical and basic first aid providers, registered nurses, physiotherapists, athletic trainers, and others), typically led by a medical director (or equivalent)*".

### 29.1.2 Definitions of Medical Encounters

Athletes participating in endurance events may develop a "medical problem" during the event, and this "medical problem" may or may not be reported by the athlete to the medical team providing medical care at the event. Therefore, not all medical problems are reported by the participants.

- A "non-reported medical problem" is defined as "*a medical problem experienced by an athlete participating in an event, where the athlete decides to either seek no assistance, or seek assistance outside of the event medical team*".

The term "medical encounter" is used as the standardised term to define any reported "medical problem" at an event, including both illnesses and injuries. Medical encounters can be classified by severity into:

(a) minor,
(b) moderate,
(c) serious/life-threatening,

(d) sudden cardiac arrest,
(e) sudden cardiac death, and
(f) sudden death.

The detailed definitions of medical encounters as well as the definitions of medical encounters classified by severity are listed in Table 29.1 and depicted in Fig. 29.1. A medical encounter at a sports event can occur at different times during or following the event, and documenting the timing of the encounter is clinically important. Three time periods for the timing of a medical encounter have been defined:

- *during the event (from the official start to completion of the event).*
- *immediately post-finish (from the time the athlete completes the event to 1 h after the athlete completes the event).*
- *delayed presentation (between 1 and 24 h after the athlete completes the event).*

### 29.1.3 The Exercise Benefit-Risk Paradox

Moderate- to high-intensity regular physical activity, including distance running, is widely recommended for health [4], there is also equally strong evidence that moderate- to high-intensity exercise acutely, and transiently, increases the risk of a range

**Table 29.1** Definitions of medical encounters and medical problems. (Reproduced with permission from [1])

| Terminology | Definition |
|---|---|
| Non-reported medical problem | A medical problem experienced by an athlete participating in an event, where "*the athlete decides athlete decides not to seek assistance from the event medical team, or seeks assistance outside of the event medical team*" |
| Medical encounter | A reported medical problem that is an "*interaction between the medical team and a race participant requiring medical assistance or evaluation* [68, 69], *taking place from the official start of the event, up to 24 h after the official cut-off time of the event*" |
| Minor medical encounter | A medical encounter that:<br>1. *is not significant or severe enough to result in withdrawal of the athlete from the event following assessment by the medical staff,*<br>**<u>or</u>**<br>2. *does not require admission and supervised medical care at race medical facilities (on the race course, or at the end of the event) or transfer to a hospital for supervised medical care* |

**Table 29.1** (continued)

| Terminology | Definition |
|---|---|
| Moderate medical encounter | A medical encounter that:<br>1. *is significant (severe) enough to result in withdrawal of the athlete from the event following assessment by the medical staff,* **or**<br>2. *is non-life threatening but requires medical assessment and admission to the event medical facilities with supervised medical care,* **or**<br>3. *is non-life threatening but requires referral or transfer to a hospital* |
| Serious/life-threatening medical encounter | A medical encounter that is known to be life- threatening and requires immediate emergency medical treatment with<br>1. *either admission to a high-care (intensive care and observation) medical area at the event,* **or**<br>2. *transport (with or without admission) to a hospital* |
| Event related sudden cardiac arrest (SCA) | A medical encounter (cardiac arrest) that requires immediate cardiopulmonary resuscitation (including defibrillation), where the medical problem resulting in cardiac arrest was:<br>1. *deemed to be directly related to the event,* **and**<br>2. *the onset of the medical problem occurred during the event or within 1–24 h of the finish time* [20, 70, 71][a] |
| Event related sudden cardiac death (SCD) | A medical encounter that resulted in sudden cardiac death (SCD) from a SCA, where the medical problem resulting in SCD was:<br>1. *deemed to be directly related to the event,* **and**<br>2. *the onset of the medical problem occurred during the event or within 1–24 h of the finish time* [20, 70, 71][a] |
| Event related sudden death | A medical encounter that resulted in sudden death from non-cardiac causes, where the medical problem resulting in death was:<br>1. *deemed to be directly related to the event,* **and**<br>2. *the onset of the medical problem occurred during the event or within 1–24 h of the finish time* [20, 70, 71][a] |

[a]In order to compare sudden cardiac arrest (SCA), sudden cardiac death (SCD) and event related sudden death data to previously reported data it is critical to record, the timing of the cardiac arrest or death in one of three possible time periods as follows: (a) during the event, (b) immediately after finishing and up to 1 h after the event, and c) between 1 and 24 h after the event

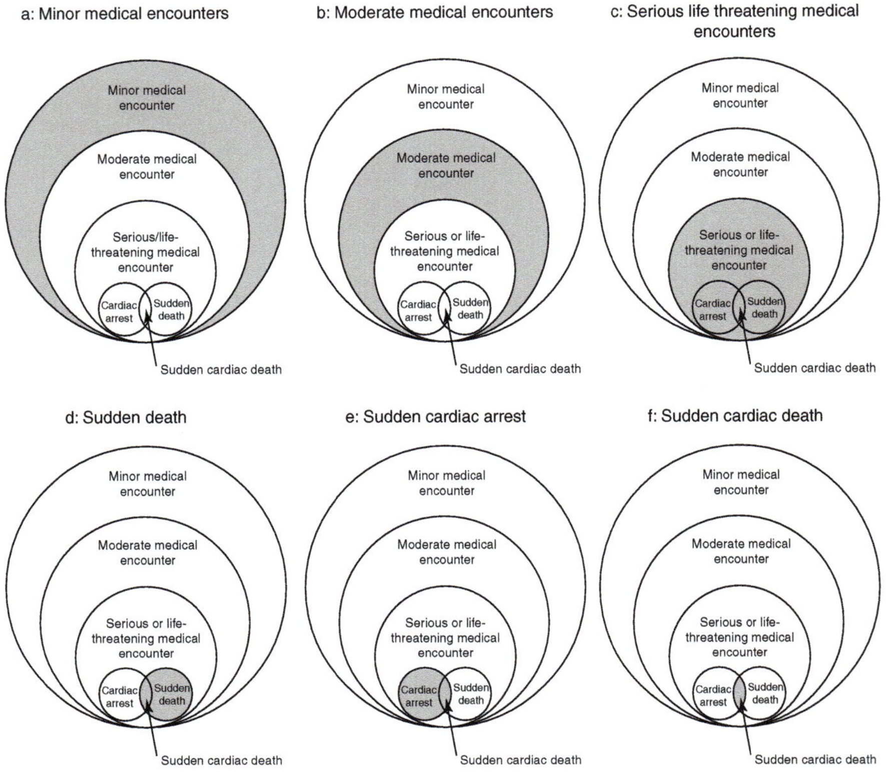


**Fig. 29.1** Classification of medical encounters by severity. (Reproduced with permission from [1])

of acute medical complications [5, 6], including acute myocardial infarction and sudden cardiac death [7–11].

- **Exercise benefit-risk paradox 1**: Regular moderate-to high-intensity physical activity is both associated with substantial long-term health benefits, there are also potential negative health consequences during an acute exercise session [7–11].
- **Exercise benefit-risk paradox 2**: The greatest health benefits of regular exercise are frequently observed in
  - sedentary individuals that transition to becoming physically active, and
  - patients with known chronic disease [12]

but these groups also have a higher risk of potential acute medical complications during an exercise session [7, 9, 13–16].

It is important that the exercise benefit-risk paradoxical observations need to be placed into perspective. Data from >30 meta-analyses unequivocally support the recommendation that, from a population perspective, *the participation in regular physical activity in these two groups of individuals still far outweighs the potential negative health consequences of an acute exercise session* [7–9, 14, 15].

## 29.2 Planning to Reduce the Risk of Medical Encounters at Mass Community-Based Sports Events

Race medical teams/race medical directors have a responsibility to reduce the risk of medical encounters at mass community-based sports events. Three pre-race planning and implementation steps are important to reduce this risk:

1. Quantify the risk of acute medical encounters during exercise.
2. Identify causes, risk factors and the frequency of "at-risk" individuals for medical encounters.
3. Design and implement measures to reduce the risk of acute medical encounters during an exercise session.

### 29.2.1 Step 1: Quantifying the Risk of Acute Medical Encounters During Exercise

Physical exercise can trigger acute cardiovascular in both younger and older athletic populations [7, 11, 13, 17–22]. The relative risk of an acute cardiovascular event during exercise, compared with sedentary activity, varies from 2 times in young athletes [11] to as much as 56 times in older individuals who are at risk for cardiovascular disease or who have existing cardiovascular disease [7, 11, 16]. The absolute risk of an acute cardiovascular event during an exercise session is consistently reported as being very low (1 in 50,000 to 1 in 200,000 annually) [7–9, 11, 14, 15]. The risk of sudden death during mass community-based distance running events such as the half-marathon (21 km) and the marathon (42 km) are well described [11, 17, 23–29], and there is considerable variation in the reported absolute risk of sudden death during marathons and similar races (between 1 in 30,000 to 1 in 250,000 race entrants); generally this risk is 1 in 114,000 race entrants (calculated cumulative risk) [11] and therefore also reported as being very low.

Besides sudden death during marathon running, sudden cardiac arrest (including non-fatal cardiac arrest) and other serious medical complications can also occur. In Table 29.2, the absolute risk of medical complications during distance running by severity (sudden death, sudden cardiac arrest, serious medical complications, and any medical complication) is summarized [30].

- In comparison to sudden death, the risk of sudden cardiac arrest during a marathon race is 2–3 times higher [11].
- In comparison to sudden death, the relative risk of a serious medical complication at a distance running event such as the marathon is 50–100 times higher than sudden death.

**Table 29.2** The absolute risk of medical encounters during distance running by severity (sudden death, sudden cardiac arrest, serious medical encounters, any medical encounter)—rates are expressed per 100,000 race entrants and number of entrants per single incident. (Reproduced with permission from [30])

| Severity of medical encounter | Event/s | Absolute risk (per 100,000 race entrants) | Absolute risk (number of race entrants per 1 incident) |
|---|---|---|---|
| Sudden cardiac death (SCD) | US Marathons (1976–1994) [72] | 1.8 | 55,556 |
| | US Marathons (1995–2004) [73] | 0.5 | 200,000 |
| | US marathons (1976–2009) [24] | 0.58 | 171,005 |
| | UK marathons (1981–2006) [74] | 1.5 | 66,667 |
| | RACER registry—US marathons and half-marathons (2000–2010) [26] | 0.4 | 250,000 |
| | Two Oceans races (SA)(2008–2011) [29] | 3.4 | 29,412 |
| | French marathons and half marathons (RACE)(2006–2012) [75] | 0.4 | 250,000 |
| | Tel Aviv races (2007–2013) [76] | 1.4 | 69,000 |
| Sudden cardiac arrest (SCA) | US Marathons (1976–1994) [72] | 2.3 | 43,478 |
| | US Marathons (1995–2004) [73] | 1.8 | 55,556 |
| | US marathons (1976–2009) [24] | 1.75 | 57,002 |
| | Two popular US marathons (1982–2009) [23] | 2.6 | 38,461 |
| | UK marathons (1981–2006) [74] | 2.5 | 40,000 |
| | RACER registry—US marathons and half-marathons (2000–2010) [26] | 0.5 | 200,000 |
| | Two Oceans races (SA)(2008–2011) [29] | 4.6 | 21,739 |
| | French marathons and half marathons (RACE)(2006–2012) [75] | 1.8 | 55,556 |
| Serious medical encounter[a] | Vancouver International Marathon (2006–2011) [31] | 53 | 1887 |
| | Baltimore Marathon (2002–2005) [31] | 47 | 2128 |
| | Baltimore Marathon (2001) [31] | 155 | 645 |
| | Twin Cities Marathon (1983–1994) [31] | 35 | 2857 |
| | Two Oceans races (SA)(2008–2011) [29] | 56 | 1786 |
| | Tel Aviv races (2007–2013) [76] | 16.7 | 5988 |
| Any medical encounter[b] | Vancouver International Marathon (2006–2011) [31] | 4449 | 22 |
| | Baltimore Marathon (2002–2005) [31] | 3395 | 29 |
| | Baltimore Marathon (2001) [31] | 2282 | 44 |
| | Twin Cities Marathon (1983–1994) [31] | 1908 | 52 |
| | Two Oceans races (SA)(2008–2011) [29] | 827 | 121 |

[a]Variable definitions: generally the number of patients transferred by any means by the medical team for further investigation and/or management (Medical Transfer Rate—MTR) [31]

[b]Variable definition: generally the number of athletes that are attended to on site by the medical team (Patient Presentation Rate—PPR) [31]

- The absolute risk of any medical complication during a marathon race also varies between 1 in 22 to 1 in 121 entrants, but generally is about 1 in 50 runners.
- The clinical relevance of these data is that in a marathon with a large field of 50,000 runners, the medical staff will, on average, encounter a:
  - sudden death every 2–3 years,
  - sudden cardiac arrest every year,
  - 25 runners that present with a serious medical complication requiring specialized management or hospitalization, and
  - 1000 runners that require medical attention (Fig. 29.2) [30].

This risk continuum is an important consideration in planning medical coverage at large mass community-based sports events. Providing this coverage is a considerable undertaking and requires careful planning long in advance of the event, recruitment of a large team of specialized medical staff [31], the establishment of considerable infrastructure, and securing sophisticated equipment at race medical facilities to ensure race safety.

Many factors determine the risk of a medical encounter during mass community-based sports events including:

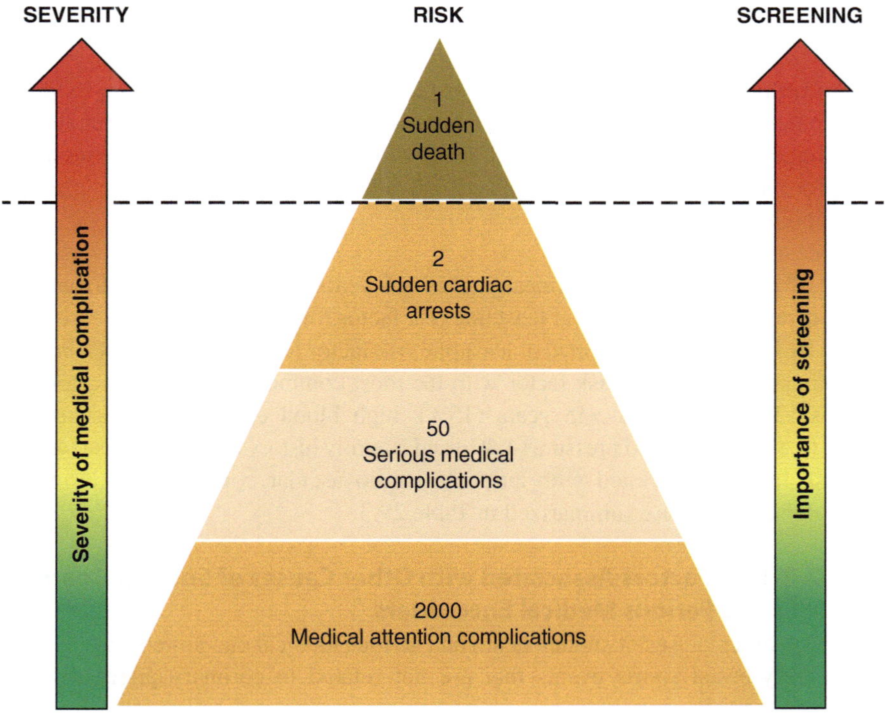


**Fig. 29.2** Risk of medical complications, severity and screening continuum—estimated absolute risk (per 100,000 race entrants) of medical complications in distance running events. (Reproduced with permission from [30])

- environmental conditions on race day,
- the course and race distance, and
- the "risk" demographics of the running population (runner experience, runner education, and runners with risk factors for acute medical complications during exercise),

all of which may influence the incidence of these complications at a specific race [31].

### 29.2.2 Step 2: Identify Causes, Risk Factors and the Frequency of "at-risk" Individuals for Medical Encounters

The demographics of participants in mass community-based sports events is changing. In the distance running population, demographics changed over the past two to three decades, with almost 50% of current marathon entrants being older than 40 years.

#### 29.2.2.1 Risk Factors Associated with Acute Cardiovascular Encounters

The most common cause of sudden death or cardiac arrest in older marathon runners is coronary artery disease.

- According to the European guidelines [32, 33], older runners (males >45 years; females >55 years) with one or more risk factors for CVD, and runners of younger age with two or more risk factors for CVD, require medical assessment before engaging in moderate- to high-intensity exercise such as distance running.
- Recently, it was shown that:
  - 10% of Master athletes (mean age 50 ± 9 years) have existing cardiovascular disease, and 64% have at least one risk factor for cardiovascular disease [34].
  - 16.1% of runners reported at least one risk factor for CVD, with 13.4% reporting more than one risk factor with the most common specific risk factors for CVD being males >45 years (15%), high blood cholesterol concentration (5.8%), high blood pressure (4.4%) and a family history of heart disease (4.4%).
- Risk factors associated with an acute cardiovascular complication during an exercise session are summarized in Table 29.3.

#### 29.2.2.2 Risk Factors Associated with Other Causes of Sudden Death and Serious Medical Encounters

There are other causes of sudden death and serious medical encounters during mass community-based sports events that are not related to coronary artery disease, including the following:

(a) severe fluid and electrolyte abnormalities (mainly hyponatremia)
(b) acute renal failure

**Table 29.3** Risk factors associated with an increased relative risk of acute cardiovascular complications during moderate- to high-intensity exercise. (Reproduced with permission from [30])

| Risk factor | Sub-category with increased relative risk |
|---|---|
| Sex [9, 13, 14] | • Males |
| Age [9, 13] | • Older age (> 35 years) |
| Habitual exercise status [9, 13–15, 31] | • Sedentary (no exercise sessions per week) (novice runner) |
| Exercise duration [31] | • Unaccustomed prolonged exercise |
| Exercise intensity [15] | • Unaccustomed high-intensity exercise (> 80% maximum capacity) |
| Underlying chronic disease (known or unknown) [9, 13, 15] | • Cardiovascular disease, metabolic disease including diabetes mellitus, renal disease, other chronic disease |
| Presence of risk factors for chronic disease [13] | • Family history of premature CVD, dyslipidemia, increased BMI, smoking status, hypertension |
| Symptoms of cardiovascular disease [9, 15, 32] | • Chest pain including discomfort in the chest, neck, jaw, arms or other areas, shortness of breath at rest or with mild exertion, dizziness or syncope, orthopnea or paroxysmal nocturnal dyspnea, ankle edema, palpitations or tachycardia, intermittent claudication, know heart murmur, unusual fatigue or shortness of breath with usual activities |
| Acute illness and inflammation [18, 77] | • Inflammation and increased risk of plaque rupture<br>• Infective illness associated with myo-pericarditis<br>• Infective illness associated with exertional heatstroke<br>• Infective illness associated with exertional rhabdomyolysis |
| Drugs and medication use [78–80] | • Arrhythmogenic drugs (including performance enhancing drugs, social drugs, prescribed medication)<br>• Drugs associated with rhabdomyolysis<br>• Drugs increasing the risk of severe electrolyte abnormalities resulting in arrhythmias (e.g. hyponatremia, hypokalemia) |
| Education [31] | • Poor runner education |

(c) exertional heat stroke
(d) other serious encounters

Risk factors for these other non-cardiac encounters should also be considered in an intervention strategy to reduce the risk of acute medical encounters during exercise (Table 29.4). Race participants may have several intrinsic risk factors that can predispose them to serious acute cardiovascular (Table 29.3) or other serious non-cardiac medical complications (Table 29.4) on race day. The risk of a medical complication on race day in the "at risk" runner is also influenced by other extrinsic factors such as

- exposure to adverse environmental conditions (heat and humidity, altitude, pollution),
- the race distance, and
- course characteristics.

**Table 29.4** Risk factors associated with an increased relative risk of other serious medical complications during moderate- to high-intensity exercise. (Reproduced with permission from [30])

| Medical complication | Risk factors |
|---|---|
| Hyponatremia [81–83] | • Overdrinking (water, sports drinks and other hypotonic beverages)<br>• Exercise duration >4 h<br>• Event inexperience or inadequate training<br>• Slow running or performance pace<br>• High or low body mass index<br>• Readily available fluids<br>• Drugs and medication<br>• Skeletal muscle damage (rhabdomyolysis) |
| Acute kidney injury and renal failure [84–87] | • Underlying chronic renal disease<br>• Renal hypouricemia,<br>• Sickle cell disease<br>• Latent myopathy<br>• Rhabomyolysis<br>• Acute illness (viral, bacterial)<br>• Drugs and medication (NSAIDs, analgesics)<br>• Dehydration |
| Exertional heatstroke [88–92] | • History of heatstroke<br>• Fever<br>• Acute infective illness (upper respiratory, gastrointestinal)<br>• Diarrhea, vomiting<br>• Sweat gland dysfunction<br>• Sunburn<br>• Dehydration<br>• Medications (diuretics, anti-depressants)<br>• Sleep loss<br>• Advanced age<br>• Excessive alcohol use<br>• Lack of heat acclimatization<br>• Sedentary lifestyle (low physical fitness)<br>• Overweight/obesity<br>• Cardiovascular dysfunction<br>• Hypokalemia |

#### 29.2.2.3 How Common Are Risk Factors Associated with Medical Encounters in Race Participants?

Over the past two decades, the demographics of the marathon participant shifted to older runners and female runners [13]. There is an increase of >12-fold in overall participation in marathon runners since 1976, with a notable increase in participation in the older age groups (>40 years); in 2015, 49% of all runners completing marathons in the USA were masters (>40 years old).

- The prevalence of risk factors in 21 km and 56 km runners was recently documented through an online pre-participation screening tool, and showed the following:
  - 2.3% of all runners reported known existing cardiovascular disease (CVD)

  - the most common CVD's were coronary artery disease (0.5%), followed by arrhythmia (0.4%)
  - 1.8% runners reported symptoms that may be suggestive of CVD.
- Four risk categories for medical encounters during participation (very high risk, high risk, intermediate risk and low risk) in participants that underwent screening with criteria, recommended interventions and frequency in runners have been published [35, 36] (Table 29.5).

#### 29.2.2.4 Prescription Medication as a Risk Factor for Medical Encounters During Exercise

The use of prescription medication is extremely common among mass races participants (47.2% of runners) and is among the most common criteria identified by the current European guidelines [32, 33], for recommending consulting a physician before exercise. The potential risk of a medical complication during exercise, as a result of prescription medication, can vary greatly and is related to the underlying medical condition for which the medication is prescribed, and the side effect profile of the medication.

Pharmacological agents may be associated with an increased risk of developing medical complications during exercise as follows:

(a) cardiac arrhythmias [37–40]
(b) renal complications including acute renal failure [41], rhabdomyolysis [42, 43]
(c) gastrointestinal bleeding [44–46]
(d) risk of tendon injuries including acute tendon rupture [47, 48].

- **Analgesic and anti-inflammatory medications** (AAIM) use is particularly frequent among athletes due to the high injury rate (SAFER VI). A considerable number of runners (15.6%) reported ingestion of pharmacological agents, mainly anti-inflammatory medication (7.8%) and more specifically NSAIDs (4.9%), in the 7 days before or during races is of concern.
- **Stimulants** such as methylphenidate and dextroamphetamine-AMP, commonly prescribed for the treatment of attention deficit hyperactivity disorder can have severe consequences when exercising for a prolonged period of time in a hot environment. These substances increase the availability of dopamine, masking the signs and symptoms of fatigue, and allowing for a longer duration of exercise. This might lead to elevated temperature in excess of 40 °C and increased heart rate, thus predisposing to exertional heat illness [49].
- **Anti-depressants**, in particular selective serotonin reuptake inhibitors (SSRIs), have a significant impact on body temperature regulation. Thermoregulation is controlled by dopamine and serotonin. When the neurotransmitters' balance is impaired, the hypothalamic set temperature could be impacted, increasing the risk of exertional heat illness [50]. Furthermore, SSRIs have been found to reduce the serum sodium concentrations, thus, thirst. This could lead to an increased dehydration during exercise in the heat [51].

**Table 29.5** Risk categories, clinical categories, and criteria for risk stratification in distance runner entrants. (Reproduced with permission from [1])

| Risk category | Clinical category | Criteria for risk stratification |
|---|---|---|
| Very high risk | Existing CVD or symptoms of CVD | 1. Any runner who answered "yes" to *one (or more)* of the following questions (below):<br>(a) Have you ever suffered from any heart or blood vessel conditions including heart attack, undiagnosed chest pain, coronary artery bypass operation, angioplasty (balloon), heart failure, heart transplant, cardiac arrhythmia (abnormal heart beat), rheumatic fever, heart murmur, cardiomyopathy, myocarditis, use of a pacemaker, or inherited heart defect?<br>(b) Do you use any prescribed medication on a daily weekly or monthly basis to treat heart rhythm, heart failure, or other heart disease?<br>(c) Do you currently suffer from any symptoms of heart or blood vessel disease, including any of the following: shortness of breath when sitting or lying down, shortness of breath with mild exercise, waking up with shortness of breath at night, palpitations that make you dizzy, chest pain when sitting or performing exercise or when you are emotionally stressed, pain (or discomfort) in the neck jaw arms at rest or during exercise, dizziness during exercise or fainting spells)? |
| High risk | Risk factors for CVD | 1. Any male runner ≥45 years or female runner ≥55 years, who answered "yes" to any **one** of the following questions (below):<br>2. Any runner (other than male runners ≥45 years or female runners ≥55 years) who answered "yes" to **two or more** of the following questions (below):<br>(a) Are you aware or have you ever been diagnosed with any risk factors for heart or blood vessel disease including high blood cholesterol a family member with heart disease cigarette smoking lack of physical activity high blood pressure being overweight or having diabetes mellitus (sugar sickness)?<br>(b) Do you use any prescribed medication on a daily weekly or monthly basis to treat high blood cholesterol, blood pressure, treat diabetes (tables or insulin)? |

| | | |
|---|---|---|
| Intermediate risk | One risk factor for CVD **or** existing other chronic disease **or** use of prescription medication **or** use of medication before and during races **or** history of collapse during training/racing **or** known current injury **or** history of EAMC | 1. Any male runner ≥45 years OR female runner ≥55 years<br>2. Any runner who answered “yes” to **one** of the components in the following question (below):<br>(a) Are you aware or have you ever been diagnosed with any risk factors for heart or blood vessel disease including high blood cholesterol a family member with heart disease cigarette smoking lack of physical activity high blood pressure being overweight or having diabetes mellitus (sugar sickness)?<br>3. Any runner who answered “yes” to **one (or more)** of the following questions (below):<br>(a) Do you currently suffer from any metabolic or hormonal disease including diabetes mellitus thyroid gland disorders hypoglycemia (low blood sugar) hyperglycemia (high blood sugar) or heat intolerance?<br>(b) Do you suffer from any respiratory (lung) disease including asthma emphysema (COPD) wheezing cough postnasal drip hay fever or repeated flu like illness?<br>(c) Do you suffer from any gastrointestinal disease including heartburn nausea vomiting abdominal pain weight loss or gain (>5 kg) a change in bowel habits chronic diarrhea blood in the stools or past history of liver or gallbladder disease?<br>(d) Do you suffer from any diseases of the nervous system including past history of stroke or transient ischemic attack (TIA) frequent headaches epilepsy depression anxiety attacks muscle weakness nerve tingling loss of sensation or chronic fatigue?<br>(e) Do you suffer from any disease of the kidney or bladder including past history of kidney or bladder disease blood in the urine loin pain kidney stones frequent urination or burning during urination?<br>(f) Do you suffer from any disease of the blood or immune system including anemia recurrent infections HIV/AIDS leukemia or are you using any immunosuppressive medication?<br>(g) Do you suffer from any growths or cancer including a past history of cancer?<br>(h) Do you suffer from any allergies including a past history of allergies to medication plant material or animal material?<br>(i) At the moment do you use any prescribed medication on a daily weekly or monthly basis to treat chronic (long-term) medical conditions or injuries?<br>(j) Have you ever in your running career used medicines to treat injuries in the week before a race—including anti-inflammatory drugs cortisone (pills or injection) or painkillers?<br>(k) Have you ever in your running career used medicines to treat injuries during a race—including anti-inflammatory drugs cortisone (pills or injection) or pain killer?<br>(l) Do you, or did you suffer from any symptoms of a running injury (muscles tendons bones ligaments or joints) in the last 12 months?<br>(m) Have you ever collapsed (fell down not because of an accident needing medical attention) during at the finish or after a race or training session?<br>(n) Have you ever in your running career suffered from muscle cramping (painful spontaneous sustained spasm of a muscle) during or immediately (within 6 h) after running (in training or competition)? |
| Low risk | No reported medical history | 1. Any runner who answered “**no**” to **all** the medical screening questions |

*CVD* cardiovascular disease, *EAMC* exercise associated muscle cramp

- **Statins** are the most effective and frequently prescribed medications for the management of high concentrations of low-density lipoprotein cholesterol (LDL-C). Inhibition of HMG-CoA-reductase prevents the production of mevalonic acid. Mevalonate is also produced in response to heat stress and an increased production of mevalonate is associated to a greater tolerance to heat at cellular level. Therefore, preventing the production of mevalonate could potentially place an individual at risk of exertional heat stress.

The cardiovascular effects of commonly prescribed substances are extensively presented in another chapter in this book; therefore, readers are invited to refer to that specific chapter (Chap. 28). Nevertheless, some substances are particularly relevant for endurance events participants, for the severe side effects they can have.

#### 29.2.2.5 Step 3: Design and Implement Measures to Reduce the Risk of Medical Encounters During Exercise

##### Introduction to Pre-exercise Screening

International guidelines to reduce the risk of acute cardiovascular risk during exercise have been developed and implemented by many sports federations [10, 52], and international bodies including the International Olympic Committee (IOC) [53] and the International Paralympic Committee (IPC) either mandate or recommend pre-participation screening [10]. However, currently these screening programs focus mostly on screening younger elite athletes [21, 54, 55], and concentrate almost exclusively on pre-participation *cardiac* screening (including a resting ECG) to reduce the risk of acute cardiovascular complications.

- In Canada, the Physical Activity Readiness Questionnaire (PAR-Q+) and the Physical Activity Readiness Medical Examination (ePARMed-X+) were developed as primary front-line pre-participation tools for physical activity [56], and are based on a systematic review of evidence (see Chap. 7) [57, 58].
- Similarly, the American Heart Association (AHA) [59] and the American College of Sports Medicine (ACSM) [15] have recommendations for pre-participation screening.
- The European Society of Cardiology together with the European Association of Cardiovascular Prevention and Rehabilitation [32] specifically developed recommendations, by consensus, for the pre-participation screening of masters and leisure athletes.
- The first step in the recommended screening process is a "self-assessment of risk", and this is based on the American Heart Association (AHA)/American College of Sports Medicine (ACSM) pre-participation screening questionnaire for individuals at Health/Fitness facilities [60] and the PAR-Q [32].
- The European guidelines recommend that this initial "self-assessment of risk" can be conducted by the individual and consists of health information related to:
  - any history of known cardiovascular disease, cardiovascular symptoms, medication use, and other health issues (Sect. 29.1), and

- known risk factors for cardiovascular disease including male gender, older age, hypertension, smoking, hypercholesterolemia, diabetes or hyperglycemia, and obesity (Sect. 29.2).

Based on the responses to questions in Sect. 29.1 (any one positive response to a question) and Sect. 29.2 (presence of ≥2 risk factors), it is then recommended that individuals undergo a thorough medical assessment by a qualified physician before participating in moderate- to high-intensity exercise, such as distance running [32].

- In one study, the ESC/EACPR screening guidelines have been applied to adult participants >40 years of age, who participated in the National Health and Nutrition Examination Survey (2001–2004) [61]. Based on "self-assessment of risk", approximately 95% of women and 93.5% were advised to consult a physician before embarking on exercise [20].
- In two other studies, full pre-participation screening incorporating medical histories, physical examination and special investigations (electrocardiography, echocardiography and blood tests) effectively identified middle-aged athletes with risk factors of cardiovascular disease (CVD) [62, 63].

However, neither study identified the links between the "risk self-assessment" and the outcome of the full screening. Although ideal, full screening of every leisure athlete older than 45 years who participate in large community events would not be cost-effective or logistically feasible.

#### 29.2.2.6 What Is the Role of Pre-event Medical Screening for Mass Sporting Events?

A potential strategy to reduce the number of medical encounters is the development of an online pre-participation "self-assessment of risk", as currently recommended by European guidelines, during pre-race registration in community-based mass sports participation (distance running) event. International pre-exercise screening recommendations in leisure athletes [15, 32, 33] are currently not applied at community-based mass participation events and there are few data that these guidelines are indeed appropriate for pre-event medical screening of leisure athletes.

- In one study involving >15,000 recreational distance runners, the pre-race screening tool (Table 29.6) identified that over 30% of entrants for this event would, according to current European guidelines, require referral for a full medical assessment prior to participation in the distance races (moderate-to-high intensity exercise).

#### 29.2.2.7 Does Pre-event Screening Reduce Medical Encounters?

International medical associations have produced consensus-based recommendations/guidelines to screen individuals prior to engaging in moderate- to high-intensity exercise [15, 32, 33, 56, 59]. Pre-screening must be accompanied by an individualized educational intervention program.

**Table 29.6** Summary: main elements of the pre-race medical screening tool. (Reproduced with permission from [1])

| Medical screening tool: self-assessment of risk[a] |
|---|
| 1. Have you ever suffered from any heart or blood vessel conditions including heart attack, undiagnosed chest pain, coronary artery bypass operation, angioplasty (balloon), heart failure, heart transplant, cardiac arrhythmia (abnormal heart beat), rheumatic fever, heart murmur, cardiomyopathy, myocarditis, use of a pacemaker, or inherited heart defect? |
| 2. Do you currently suffer from any symptoms of heart or blood vessel disease, including any of the following: shortness of breath when sitting or lying down, shortness of breath with mild exercise, waking up with shortness of breath at night, palpitations that make you dizzy, chest pain when sitting or performing exercise or when you are emotionally stressed, pain (or discomfort) in the neck jaw arms at rest or during exercise, dizziness during exercise or fainting spells)? |
| 3. Are you aware or have you ever been diagnosed with any risk factors for heart or blood vessel disease including high blood cholesterol, a family member with heart disease, cigarette smoking, lack of physical activity, high blood pressure, being overweight, or having diabetes mellitus (sugar sickness)? |
| 4. Do you currently suffer from any metabolic or hormonal disease including diabetes mellitus thyroid gland disorders hypoglycemia (low blood sugar) hyperglycemia (high blood sugar), or heat intolerance? |
| 5. Do you suffer from any respiratory (lung) disease including asthma, emphysema (COPD), wheezing, cough, postnasal drip, hay fever, or repeated flu like illness? |
| 6. Do you suffer from any gastrointestinal disease including heartburn, nausea, vomiting, abdominal pain, weight loss or gain (> 5 kg), a change in bowel habits, chronic diarrhea, blood in the stools, or past history of liver or gallbladder disease? |
| 7. Do you suffer from any diseases of the nervous system including past history of stroke or transient ischemic attack (TIA), frequent headaches, epilepsy, depression, anxiety attacks, muscle weakness, nerve tingling, loss of sensation, or chronic fatigue? |
| 8. Do you suffer from any disease of the kidney or bladder including past history of kidney or bladder disease, blood in the urine, loin pain, kidney stones, frequent urination, or burning during urination? |
| 9. Do you suffer from any disease of the blood or immune system including anemia, recurrent infections, HIV/AIDS, leukemia, or are you using any immunosuppressive medication? |
| 10. Do you suffer from any growths or cancer, including a past history of cancer? |
| 11. Do you suffer from any allergies including a past history of allergies, to medication, plant material, or animal material? |
| 12. At the moment do you use any prescribed medication on a daily weekly or monthly basis to treat chronic (long-term) medical conditions or injuries? |
| 13. Have you ever collapsed (fell down not because of an accident needing medical attention) during at the finish or after a race or training session? |
| 14. Do you, or did you suffer from any symptoms of a running injury (muscles tendons bones ligaments or joints) in the last 12 months? |
| 15. Have you ever in your running career suffered from muscle cramping (painful spontaneous sustained spasm of a muscle) during or immediately (within 6 h) after running (in training or competition)? |

[a]Once a participant answered "yes" to any of the main screening questions, further details were obtained using "dropdown" boxes with additional questions

- In one recently published study, such a pre-race screening and educational intervention was shown to be associated with the following [36]:
  - A reduction in overall medical encounters of 29% (21.1 km race—reduction by 19%; 56 km race—reduction by 39%).

- A reduction in serious life-threatening medical encounters by 64%.
- Registration numbers increased in the intervention period, and overall % race starters (81.5%) were similar in the control (81.0%) and intervention period (81.8%).
- The wet bulb globe temperature (WBGT) was similar in the control and intervention period.

### 29.2.3 Planning Medical Care on Race Day for Mass Community-Based Sporting Events

#### 29.2.3.1 Pre-race Planning

- Race organizers should appoint a Medical Director as head of the Medical Team.
- The Medical Director is ultimately responsible for all health care services provided at all official sites, venues and accommodation areas.
- The Medical Director is in charge of the overall coordination of medical organization and represents the Medical Team of the Organising Committee.
- The Medical Director's responsibilities include:
  - Ensure recruitment and supervision of the various medical personnel.
  - Design a comprehensive health care system, making sure that adequate facilities, supplies and equipment are available for medical care at all official sites.
  - Co-ordination of community medical resources, including emergency transport services, emergency room(s) and hospital admissions.

#### 29.2.3.2 Planning Health Care Services on Race Day

The scope of health care services on race day includes:

(a) critical care,
(b) first-aid,
(c) treatment for environmental illnesses, and
(d) general medical problems associated with endurance events.

The extent of services depends on the location, duration and type of competition, as well as the type and number of participants expected, and the nature of the injuries or illnesses which are predictable.

Health Care Services include, but are not limited to the following:

- Adequate facilities available for medical services to cover all people and all competition sites;
- Provision of primary and emergency care to all above mentioned people at the various venues and areas of the event, at no charge to all eligible persons;
- Provision of other medical support services needed to ensure the safety and health of the aforementioned, and of the spectators;
- Coordinating service with the hospital network and emergency services;
- Supervision of environmental, meteorological health and safety at all sites.

## 29.3 Guidelines to Minimize the Potential Negative Effects of Environmental Stress, Including Air Quality

### 29.3.1 Heat Stress

The risk of heat illness increases above 21 °C (70 °F) and 50% relative humidity. The WBGT, which measures the combined thermal stress from the wet bulb (WBT), dry bulb (DBT), and black globe (BGT) thermometers has been widely used to assess environmental heat stress. Several thermal stress indexes have been developed through the years and provide with further information, like the Physiologically Equivalent Temperature (PET), the modified PET (mPET) and Universal Thermal Climate (UTCI) indexes.

The thermal index and colour coded flags to indicate the risks of thermal stress are:

| | |
|---|---|
| BLACK FLAG: | Extreme Risk—WBGT >28 °C (82 °F), PET >35 °C |
| RED FLAG: | High Risk—WBGT is 23–28 °C (73–82 °F), PET is 29–35 °C |
| YELLOW FLAG: | Moderate Risk—WBGT is 18–23 °C (65–73 °F), PET is 23–29 °C |
| GREEN FLAG: | Low Risk—WBGT is below 18 °C (65 °F), PET is 18–23 °C |
| WHITE FLAG: | No Risk for heat stress but increasing risk for hypothermia when—WBGT is below 10 °C (50 °F), PET 18 °C. |

A recent publication [64] has clarified and established the relationship between environmental parameters on race day and the risk of not completing the race due to excessive heat stress. This relationship has been described through the following formula (*t*, temperature):

$$\%\text{Do Not Finish} = -0.59 \times t^{\circ}\text{C} + 0.02 \times t^{\circ}\text{C}^2 + 5.75$$

In general, particularly considering endurance events, better performance and less adverse results are obtained when the environmental conditions are going to improve, rather than worsen, during the event. As an example, in hot environmental conditions, start times would be better set for late afternoon rather than early morning (increased thermal stress in sunny morning), for road racing.

#### 29.3.1.1 Air Quality

- The health impact of living and exercising in highly polluted environments have been widely demonstrated in the scientific literature [65–67].
- Therefore, the monitoring programmes of local pollution and pollen ratings before and during an endurance event should be implemented.
- Daily average of main pollutants ($NO_2$, $O_3$, particulate matter (PM2.5, PM10), CO) should be provided, before and for the entire duration of the event.

### 29.3.2 Medical Facilities on Race Day

Medical services must be available on the race course, and available to all participants. The medical areas should include:

(a) a pre-starting line treatment area;
(b) medical first-aid teams along the course, ideally every 5 km or located in strategic positions;
(c) a triage/emergency area at the finish line;
(d) the main treatment area at the finish line (with ambulances stationed near-by).

Advanced life support emergency ambulance with AED coverage should be available along the whole course, up to the finish line. The first-aid teams should evacuate all injured or sick athletes from the course at the earliest time, and transfer all of them to the main treatment area at the finish line. The evaluation and treatment of environmental and exercise related medical problems like dehydration, hyperthermia, hypothermia, exercise associated collapse, and problems associated with road racing, including allergic responses such as anaphylactic shock, hives, asthma exacerbation, and diabetic insulin reactions is of notable importance.

## 29.4 Aid Stations

- Aid stations should be located every 5 km or at pre-defined medical points along the course.
- AED and first-aid kits shall be available.
- Equipment and supplies for obtaining vital signs, performing BLSD and ACLS should be available at major on-course medical stations.

## 29.5 Roving Medical Vehicles and Critical Care Teams

- Roving medical vehicles and mobile medical aid, though they are impeded by runners, offer the best solution for rapid response to a collapsed athlete on a road course.
- The use of fully-equipped ambulances on the course is advantageous and increases the medical response capabilities.
- Equipment and supplies for obtaining vital signs, performing Basic Life Support—Defibrillation (BLSD) and Advanced Cardiac Life Support (ACLS) should be available in the roving medical vehicles.

## 29.6 First Response Teams

- AED-equipped motorcycles or bicycles have rapid access to collapsed athletes with potential cardiac arrest.
- Operators must be trained in the use of AED, and the team must be integrated with the local emergency medical system.
- Several teams must be assigned along the course to follow the main pack and separated by 2–4 km giving rapid access to most runners.
- First response teams should be prepared to evaluate and treat cardiac arrest, exertional heat stroke, hyponatremia, diabetic insulin shock, status asthma, and exercise-or allergic anaphylaxis.

## 29.7 Finish Line Area

It has been widely demonstrated that the number of medical encounters in the final quarter of the race is significantly higher in respect to other segments. Therefore, in the last 2 km of the course, medical staff and supplies should be increased. Usually at this stage of the race runners are tired but still try to increase their pace as they approach the finish line, thus the number of collapses increase.

- The last 500 m should have several medical staff deployed along the course to act as spotters for runners in distress.
- This is particularly important for mass road races. Equipment and supplies for obtaining vital signs, performing BLSD and ACLS should be available at the finish line.
- The finish line is usually where most medical encounters occur.
- This is the location where the majority of medical staff and volunteers should be.
- The finish line team should include:
  - A Triage Officer and team to direct the flow of casualties to the proper area for care; and
  - Sweep team/field medical personnel divided into medical care teams that can spot runners as soon as they show signs of distress, transporting them to the closest medical point or manage medical illnesses or injuries on site.

Dedicated medical areas may be organised for participants based on injury or illness. The triage team should direct runners to the proper care centre.

## 29.8 Documenting Medical Encounters at Community-Based Sporting Events

General race data and medical encounter data at mass community-based endurance sport events should be collected in a standardised format and this has been covered extensively in a recently published international consensus statement [1]. Research methods related to event data collection, athlete demographics, sport code, sport participation history, medical incident data collection procedures and reporting of the data are critical for quality of any scientific studies in this field. The following categories of general race data should be collected (Table 29.7):

- race day data,
- athlete demographics,
- athlete race performance, and
- geographical data of the course.

**Table 29.7** Data collection (essential and additional data) on race day, athlete demographics, athlete race performance, course geography, and environmental conditions on race day. (Reproduced with permission from [1])

| Category | Minimum/essential data | Additional data |
|---|---|---|
| Race day data | • Location (nearest city)<br>• Date of the race (dd:mm:yyyy)<br>• Official starting time (hh:mm:ss)<br>• Official cut-off (finish) time (hh:mm:ss)<br>• Number of registrants (entrants): The number of athletes who register to participate in the event.<br>• Number of starters: The number of registered athletes who start the event.<br>• Number of finishers: The number of registered starting athletes who finish the event | |
| Athlete demographics (individual athlete data) | • Age (on registration day)<br>• Sex | • Height (cm)<br>• Body weight (kg) |
| Athlete race performance (individual athlete data) | • Race discipline (if applicable – different sporting codes)<br>• Race registered for (if applicable – different race distances)<br>• Race starting time (hh:mm:ss)<br>• Race finishing time (hh:mm:ss)<br>• Calculated total race time (hh:mm:ss) | • Previous participation in this event type (number of previous races in this event type)<br>• No. of times previously participated in this race (number)<br>• Personal best time for this race (hh:mm)<br>• Qualifying time for this race (if applicable: event and time—hh:mm:ss)<br>• No. of races participated in, in previous year (number)<br>• Date of last race participated in (dd:mm:yyyy)<br>• Personal best time for this event in the last 12 months year (hh:mm:ss)<br>• Average regular training in the last 12 months (h/w)? Split times [distance (km) from the start line should be recorded in conjunction with the split time (hh:mm:ss)] |

(continued)

**Table 29.7** (continued)

| Category | Minimum/essential data | Additional data |
|---|---|---|
| Geographical data of the course | • Total course distance (m)<br>• Individual course sections (if applicable e.g. triathlons) (m)<br>• Altitude (m) (mean, range)<br>• Total elevation of the event course (m)<br>• Change in elevation (m) | • Type of surface of the event course (if applicable) (tar, asphalt, off-road, grass/, gravel, sand etc.)<br>• Nature of the event course surface (wet, dry) |
| Environmental conditions on race day | • Ambient temperature (°C)<br>• Relative humidity (%)<br>• Wind speed (km/hr)<br>• Wind direction (degrees)<br>• Precipitation (mm)<br>• Wet Bulb Globe Temperature (WBGT) Index (°C) (at the start and finish of the race) | • Wet Bulb Globe Temperature (WBGT) Index (°C) (continuously throughout the race)<br>• Pollution (air quality index) (numeric air quality index (AQI) or ppbv/ppmv or $mg.m^{-3}/\mu g.m^{-3}$ for $PM_{10}$, $PM_{2.5}$, $PM_{0.1}$) (e.g. $NO_2$, $O_3$)<br>• Pollen count (grains/$m^3$)<br>• Ultraviolet (UV) radiation Index<br>• PET (Physiological Equivalent Temperature) index. The PET utilizes i.e. air temperature, air humidity (relative humidity, specific humidity or any other measure of air humidity), wind speed, global radiation and geographical information (latitude, longitude and elevation, sky view factor (SVF) and ground surface characteristics). |
| Medical team data | • Size of the medical team (total number of staff)<br>• Qualified medical doctors(number)<br>• Number of allied health professionals (number)<br>• Number of nursing staff (number)<br>• Number of first aiders (number)<br>• Number of fixed medical stations on route (number)<br>• Number of mobile medical stations on route (number)<br>• Medical station at finish (yes/no)<br>• Number of AED's on route<br>• High care/intensive care facility at finish (yes/no) | • Medical race director/deputies (number)<br>• Medical doctor (Sport and Exercise Medicine specialist) (number)<br>• Medical doctor (Emergency Medicine/Intensive Care specialist) (number)<br>• Medical doctor (Cardiologist) (number)<br>• Medical doctor (Other specialist) (number)<br>• Medical doctor (General Practitioner/ Family Physician) (number)<br>• Physiotherapist (number)<br>• Athletic trainer(number)<br>• First Aider (Advance Life Support) (number)<br>• First Aider (Basic Life Support) (number) |

Medical encounters at mass community-based endurance sports events can be broadly classified into two main diagnostic categories:

1. *illness-related* and
2. *injury-related* medical encounters.

*Illness-related* medical encounters are usually classified by major organ system affected, while *injury-related* encounters are usually classified by major anatomical regions affected.

### 29.8.1 Illness-Related Medical Encounters

- The use of a diagnostic classification system of illness-related medical encounters by main organ system is recommended (Table 29.8).
- The severity of illness-related medical encounters can further be classified as minor, moderate, serious/life-threatening, and sudden cardiac arrest/death using the definitions described above.
- Additional information can also be collected including the following:
  - the location of the illness on the course (e.g. related to hills, course conditions),

**Table 29.8** Diagnostic categories of illness-related medical encounters by main organ system and more common specific types/diagnosis of medical encounters. (Reproduced with permission from [1])

| Main organ system | Illness type/diagnosis |
|---|---|
| Multiple organ systems | |
| | Heat Illness |
| | Hypothermia |
| | Hyperthermia/exertional heat stroke |
| | Sunburn |
| | Rhabdomyolysis |
| | Fluid and electrolyte disorders |
| | Dehydration (mild: <5% body weight loss) |
| | (moderate: >5% to <7% body weight loss) |
| | (severe: >7% body weight loss) |
| | Hyponatraemia |
| | Acid-base disorders |
| | Other electrolyte disorders |
| | Infection |
| | Systemic Infection (excluding pathogens localised to one area) |
| Cardiovascular system | |
| | Exercise Associated Postural Hypotension (EAPH) |
| | Syncope (non-specific) |
| | Chest pain (non-specific) |
| | Ischaemic heart disease |
| | Acute coronary syndrome (myocardial infarction, angina) |
| | Stable angina |
| | Cardiac arrest |
| | Sudden cardiac death |
| | Cardiac arrest (successfully resuscitated) |
| | Conduction abnormality including arrhythmias |
| | Supraventricular tachycardia |
| | Ventricular tachycardia |
| | Frequent ventricular extra-systoles |
| | Other significant arrhythmia |
| | Other abnormality on ECG (including non-specific) |

(continued)

**Table 29.8** (continued)

| Main organ system | Illness type/diagnosis |
|---|---|
| | Congestive heart failure |
| | Hypertrophic cardiomyopathy and other cardiomyopathies |
| | Other congenital/inherited cardiovascular disease |
| | Murmurs/Valvular disease |
| | Acute myocarditis (viral) |
| | Acute pericarditis |
| | Venous disease |
| | Deep venous thrombosis |
| | Other venous disease including calf/ankle oedema, cause unknown |
| | Peripheral vascular disease |
| | Other cardiovascular disease |
| Respiratory disease and ENT (ear, nose/throat) systems | |
| | Respiratory tract infection (bacterial or viral) |
| | Other upper respiratory tract infection |
| | Other lower respiratory tract infection |
| | Asthma and/or allergy |
| | Allergy—rhinitis/sinusitis/hay fever (for urticaria see MDUX) |
| | Asthma—allergic |
| | Asthma—exercise induced only |
| | Pneumothorax |
| | Acute pulmonary embolus |
| | Vocal cord dysfunction |
| | Other respiratory illness not otherwise specified |
| Central nervous system (CNS) | |
| | Exercise Associated Muscle Cramps (EAMC) |
| | Mild EAMC (localised, no altered mental status, no systemic symptoms) |
| | Severe EAMC (generalized, altered mental status or with systemic symptoms |
| | Dizziness/nausea (non-specific) |
| | Coma (cause unknown) |
| | Confusion (non-specific) |
| | Stroke/Cerebrovascular Accident (CVA) |
| | Epilepsy |
| | Headaches |
| | Exercise related headache |
| | Migraine |
| | Cluster headaches |
| | Headache not otherwise specified |
| | Other neurological problem |
| | Generalised tight muscles/spasticity |
| Rheumatological system | |
| | Joint pain (non-specific) |
| | Joint infection—septic arthritis (excluding complications of surgery or perforating lacerations) |
| | Infection of bone—osteomyelitis |
| | Osteoarthritis (OA)—generalised (not isolated to one joint) |

**Table 29.8** (continued)

| Main organ system | Illness type/diagnosis |
|---|---|
| | Gout |
| | Pseudogout |
| | Seronegative arthritis |
| | Rheumatoid arthritis |
| | Fibromyalgia/multiple sore muscle areas |
| | Rheumatological disease other/undiagnosed |
| Gastrointestinal system | |
| | Nausea/vomiting (non-specific) |
| | Abdominal pain (non-specific) |
| | Gastrointestinal infection |
| | Gastroenteritis (including food poisoning) |
| | Other gastrointestinal infection |
| | Gastritis |
| | Exercise associated gastritis/reflux |
| | Non-steroidal anti-inflammatory drug (NSAID) associated gastritis/peptic ulceration |
| | Gastritis/peptic ulceration—non exercise/NSAID related |
| | Diarrhoea |
| | Runner's diarrhoea |
| | Gastrointestinal bleeding (upper gastrointestinal tract) including hematemesis |
| | Gastrointestinal bleeding (lower gastrointestinal tract) including melena |
| | Surgical bowel problem (acute bowel) |
| | Other gastrointestinal illness |
| Genitourinary system (excluding infections) | |
| | Genitourinary infection |
| | Cystitis |
| | Other genitourinary infection |
| | Acute kidney injury |
| | Acute renal failure |
| | Other urinary Illness |
| | Haematuria |
| | Pregnancy |
| Haematological system and nutritional deficiencies | |
| | Anaemia |
| | Sickle-cell trait |
| Endocrine/metabolic system | |
| | Thyroid disorder |
| | Hypothyroid |
| | Hyperthyroid |
| | Hypoglycaemia (non-specific) |
| | Diabetes mellitus |
| | Type I (insulin dependent) |
| | Type II (non-insulin dependent) |
| | Other endocrine disorder |
| Dermatological system (excluding infections, skin lesions/tumours and sunburn MVHX) | |
| | Sunburn |
| | Skin Infection/Cellulitis/Abscess/Infected Bursa |
| | Skin chafing/blister |

(continued)

**Table 29.8** (continued)

| Main organ system | Illness type/diagnosis |
|---|---|
| | Abrasion |
| | Laceration |
| | Urticaria |
| | Dermatitis |
| | Other rash not otherwise mentioned or undiagnosed |
| Ophthalmological system (excluding trauma) | |
| Dental illness | |
| Psychological/psychiatric illness | |
| | Anxiety/panic disorder, including hyperventilation |
| | Other psychological/psychiatric disorder not otherwise specified |
| Tumours/malignancies | |
| Drug use/overdose/poisoning | |
| Medical illness (OTHER or undiagnosed) | |
| | Tired athlete (non-specific) |
| | Other medical illness |

  - pre-race medical history (e.g. pre-race acute illness, use of medications prior or during the event), and
  - other factors possibly contributing to the illness (e.g. weather conditions, equipment failure, athlete inexperience)

### 29.8.2 Injury-Related Medical Encounters

- The use of an injury-related medical encounter classification by the main anatomical region affected by the injury, is recommended (Table 29.9).
- The severity of injury-related medical encounters can further be classified as minor, moderate, serious/life-threatening, or death using the definitions described above.
- For injury-related medical encounters, additional information related to
  - the location of the injury on the course (e.g. related to hills, course conditions),
  - onset of the injury (acute injury, chronic injury, acute exacerbation of a chronic injury),
  - mechanism of the injury (e.g. traumatic, non-traumatic, contact or non-contact, nature of the contact), and
  - other factors contributing to the injury (e.g. violation of rules, weather conditions, equipment failure, athlete inexperience)

could also be collected.

The adoption of a uniform data collection procedure at the event medical facilities to record all medical encounters is recommended. Recently, a standardised

**Table 29.9** Diagnostic categories of injury-related medical encounters by main anatomical region and more common injury types/diagnosis. (Reproduced with permission from [1])

| Main anatomical region | Injury type/diagnosis |
|---|---|
| Head injuries | |
| | Head/Facial Bruising/Haematoma |
| | Head laceration/abrasion |
| | Facial Muscle and/or Tendon strain/spasm/trigger points |
| | Facial Joint sprain/injury |
| | Facial Dislocation |
| | Head/Facial fracture |
| | Concussion/Brain Injury |
| | Concussion |
| | Intracranial bleed |
| | Head Organ Damage (including eye, ear, mouth injury; excluding haematoma, laceration) |
| | Eye injury/trauma |
| | Ear trauma |
| | Dental Injury |
| | Head Pain/Injury (Other/not specified) |
| Neck Injuries | |
| | Neck Soft Tissue Bruising/Haematoma |
| | Neck Laceration/Abrasion |
| | Whiplash |
| | Neck muscle and/or tendon strain/spasm/trigger points |
| | Cervical Spine Facet Joint injuries |
| | Cervical Disc Injury |
| | Neck Fracture |
| | Cervical Fracture/s |
| | Laryngeal fracture |
| | Neck Organ Damage |
| | Neurological Neck Injury |
| | Cervical nerve root compression/stretch (proximal burner/stinger) |
| | Cervical spinal cord injury |
| | Cervical spinal column degenerative disc disease/arthritis |
| | Cervical Vascular Injury |
| | Neck Pain/Injury (Other/not specified) |
| Shoulder Injuries | |
| | Shoulder Soft Tissue Bruising/Haematoma |
| | AC Joint contusion |
| | Shoulder Soft Tissue Laceration/Abrasion |
| | Shoulder muscle strain/spasm/trigger points |
| | Shoulder Tendon Overuse Injury/Strain |
| | Acute Shoulder Sprains/Subluxation |
| | Glenohumeral joint sprains |
| | Acromioclavicular joint sprain |
| | Shoulder Osteochondral Lesion |
| | Acute Shoulder Dislocation |
| | Anteroinferior shoulder dislocation |
| | Inferior shoulder dislocation |
| | Posterior shoulder dislocation |
| | Chronic Shoulder instability |
| | Shoulder impingement/Synovitis |
| | Shoulder Fractures |

(continued)

**Table 29.9** (continued)

| Main anatomical region | Injury type/diagnosis |
|---|---|
| | Clavicular fracture |
| | Scapula fracture |
| | Humerus Fracture |
| | Shoulder Neurological/vascular injury (excl. Non mechanical nerve problems—see MNXX) |
| | Shoulder Osteoarthritis |
| | Shoulder Pain/Injury (Other/not specified) |
| Upper Arm Injuries (between the shoulder and the elbow) | |
| | Upper Arm Soft Tissue Bruising/Haematoma |
| | Upper Arm Laceration/Abrasion |
| | Upper Arm Muscle Strain/Spasm/Trigger points |
| | Upper Arm Tendon Injury |
| | Upper Arm Fracture |
| | Upper Arm Bony Stress/Overuse Injury |
| | Other Upper Arm Overuse Injury |
| | Upper Arm neurological injury |
| | Upper Arm Vascular Injury |
| | Upper Arm Pain/Injury not otherwise specified |
| Elbow Injuries | |
| | Elbow Soft Tissue Bruising/Haematoma |
| | Elbow Laceration/Abrasion |
| | Elbow Muscle Strain/Spasm/Trigger Points |
| | Elbow Tendon Injury |
| | Lateral epicondylopathy |
| | Medial epicondylopathy |
| | Elbow Joint Ligament Sprain |
| | Elbow Osteochondral Injury |
| | Elbow Dislocation |
| | Anterior elbow dislocation |
| | Posterior elbow dislocation |
| | Dislocated radial head |
| | Elbow Instability |
| | Elbow Impingement/Synovitis |
| | Elbow Stress/Overuse Injuries including stress fractures |
| | Elbow Neurological Injury/Entrapment |
| | Elbow Osteoarthritis |
| | Elbow Pain/Injury (Other/not specified) |
| Forearm Injuries (between Elbow and Wrist) | |
| | Forearm Soft Tissue Bruising/Haematoma |
| | Forearm Laceration/Abrasion |
| | Forearm Muscle Injury |
| | Forearm Tendon Injury |
| | Forearm fracture(s) |
| | Fracture radius and ulna midshaft |
| | Fracture radius midshaft |
| | Fractured ulna midshaft |
| | Other Stress/Overuse injuries to Forearm |
| | Forearm Neurological Injury |
| | Forearm Vascular Injury |
| | Forearm Pain/Injury (Other/not specified) |

**Table 29.9** (continued)

| Main anatomical region | Injury type/diagnosis |
|---|---|
| Wrist Injuries | |
| | Wrist and Hand Soft Tissue Bruising/Haematoma |
| | Wrist and Hand Laceration/Abrasion |
| | Wrist and Hand Muscle Injury |
| | Wrist and Hand Tendon Injury |
| | Wrist and Hand Joint Injury (including minor avulsion fracture) |
| | Wrist and Hand Osteochondral/Chondral Injury |
| | Wrist and Hand Dislocations (including minor avulsion fractures) |
| | Chronic Wrist or Hand Instability |
| | Wrist and Hand Impingement/Synovitis |
| | Wrist and Hand Fractures |
| | Fracture of distal radius +/− ulna |
| | Fracture of distal ulna |
| | Scaphoid fracture |
| | Fractured hamate |
| | Fractured trapezium |
| | Fracture other carpal bone |
| | Fractured thumb |
| | Fracture metacarpals 2–5 |
| | Fracture finger(s) (excluding avulsion fractures |
| | Wrist and Hand Stress/Overuse Injuries (including stress fractures) |
| | Wrist and Hand Neurological Injury |
| | Wrist and Hand Vascular Injury |
| | Wrist and Hand Osteoarthritis |
| | Other Wrist and Hand Pain/Injury (Other/not specified) |
| Chest Injury | |
| | Chest Wall Soft Tissue Bruising/Haematoma |
| | Chest Wall laceration/Abrasion |
| | Chest Muscle or Tendon strain/spasm/trigger points |
| | Chest Joint Sprains |
| | Sternoclavicular Sprain |
| | Chest Dislocations |
| | Sternoclavicular Dislocation |
| | Chest Joint Instability |
| | Synovitis of Chest Joint |
| | Chest Fracture(s) |
| | Rib Fracture(s) |
| | Sternal fracture |
| | Fracture of costochondral margin |
| | Chest Cavity Injury |
| | Pneumothorax |
| | Haemothorax |
| | Cardiac Contusion Injury |
| | Chest injury (Other/not specified) |
| Trunk and Abdominal Injury | |
| | Abdominopelvic Soft Tissue Bruising/Haematoma (excluding bruised organs) |
| | Truncal Laceration/Abrasion |
| | Truncal Muscle Strain/Spasm/Trigger points |
| | Abdominal Tendon Injury |

(continued)

**Table 29.9** (continued)

| Main anatomical region | Injury type/diagnosis |
|---|---|
| | Abdominal Biomechanical Injury |
| | Abdominal Organ Injury |
| | Spleen trauma |
| | Intestinal trauma |
| | Liver trauma |
| | Pancreatic trauma |
| | Kidney trauma |
| | Multiple organ trauma |
| | Other organ trauma not otherwise specified |
| | Pelvic Organ Injury |
| | Genital Injury |
| | Bladder trauma |
| | Abdominal pain (Other/not specified) |
| Thoracic Spine Injury (including Thoracolumbar Junction) | |
| | Thoracic Soft Tissue Bruising/Haematoma |
| | Thoracic Laceration/Abrasion |
| | Thoracic Muscle and Tendon Strain/Spasm/Trigger Points |
| | Thoracic spine Joint Injury |
| | Thoracic Disc Injury |
| | Thoracic Spine Fracture |
| | Thoracic Postural Syndrome |
| | Thoracic spine Osteoarthritis |
| | Thoracic Pain/Injury (Other/not specified) |
| Lumbar Spine Injury | |
| | Lumbar Soft Tissue Bruising/Haematoma |
| | Lumbar Laceration/Abrasion |
| | Lumbar Spine muscle and Tendon Strain/Spasm/Trigger Points |
| | Lumbar Spine Joint Injury |
| | Lumbar facet joint sprain |
| | Lumbar ligament Sprain |
| | Lumbar Disc Injury (excluding degenerative disc disease) |
| | Lumbar Instability |
| | Spondylolisthesis any Level |
| | Lumbar Spine Facet Joint Pain/Stiffness |
| | Lumbar Spine Fracture |
| | Lumbar spine vertebral body fracture |
| | Lumbar spine transverse process fracture |
| | Lumbar spinous process fracture |
| | Lumbar pars interarticularis acute fracture |
| | Lumbar pedicle fracture |
| | Multiple lumbar spine fractures |
| | Other lumbar spine fracture |
| | Complication of lumbar fracture (including non-union, excluding spinal injury) |
| | Lumbar Stress Fracture |
| | Lumbar Spine Neurological Injury |
| | Lumbar spinal fracture with associated neurological injury |
| | Lumbar disc injury with associated neurological injury |
| | Lumbosacral Nerve root impingement due to foraminal stenosis bony and disc |

**Table 29.9** (continued)

| Main anatomical region | Injury type/diagnosis |
|---|---|
| | Lumbar Spinal canal stenosis |
| | Lumbosacral nerve stretch/traction injury |
| | Other lumbosacral nerve injury |
| | Osteoarthritis Lumbosacral spine |
| | Lumbar Pain/Injury (Other/not specified) |
| Pelvis/Buttock Injuries (excluding groin) | |
| | Pelvis/Buttock Soft Tissue Bruising/Haematoma |
| | Pelvic/Buttock Laceration/Abrasion |
| | Pelvic/Buttock Muscle Strain/Spasm/Trigger Points |
| | Buttock/Pelvis Tendon Injury |
| | Sacroiliac Joint Injury (excluding L5/S1 injury) |
| | Sacroiliac Joint Instability |
| | Buttock and Pelvis Synovitis/Bursitis |
| | Pelvic fracture(s) (excluding growth plate fractures) |
| | Fractured Ilium |
| | Fractured sacrum |
| | Fractured coccyx |
| | Fractured ischium |
| | Multiple fractures pelvis and sacrum |
| | Pelvic Stress Fracture(s) |
| | Buttock/Pelvic Nerve Injury |
| | Pelvic/Buttock Pain (Other/not specified) |
| Hip and Groin Injuries | |
| | Hip and Groin Soft Tissue Bruising/Haematoma |
| | Hip and Groin Laceration/Abrasion |
| | Hip and Groin Muscle Strain/Tear |
| | Hip and Groin Tendon Injuries (including hernia, excluding avulsion injuries in the paediatric population) |
| | Trochanteric syndrome |
| | Hip Joint Sprain |
| | Hip Joint Chondral/Osteochondral Injury |
| | Hip Joint Dislocation |
| | Hip Joint Inflammation/Synovitis/Other Biomechanical Lesion |
| | Hip/Groin Fractures |
| | Femoral fracture |
| | Acetabular fracture |
| | Fracture pubic ramus |
| | Hip/Groin Stress Fracture |
| | Other Stress/Overuse Injury Hip and Groin |
| | Femoroacetabular impingement |
| | Groin Neurovascular Injuries |
| | Groin Organ Damage |
| | Hip/Groin Arthritis |
| | Hip/Groin Pain (Other/not specified) |
| Thigh Injuries | |
| | Thigh Soft Tissue Bruising/Haematoma |
| | Thigh Laceration/Abrasion |
| | Thigh Muscle strain/Spasm/Trigger Points |
| | Proximal hamstring tendinopathy |
| | Hamstring muscle strain |

(continued)

**Table 29.9** (continued)

| Main anatomical region | Injury type/diagnosis |
|---|---|
| | Quadriceps muscle Strain |
| | Adductor tendinopathy |
| | Adductor muscle strain |
| | Thigh muscle cramping during exercise |
| | Hamstring cramping during exercise |
| | Quadricep cramping during exercise |
| | Adductor muscle cramping during exercise |
| | Thigh muscle trigger points |
| | Thigh muscle wasting |
| | Femoral Fracture |
| | Femoral Stress Fracture |
| | Other stress/Overuse Injuries to Thigh |
| | Thigh Neurological Injury |
| | Thigh Vascular Injury |
| | Thigh pain/Injury (Other/not specified) |
| Knee Injuries | |
| | Knee Soft Tissue Bruising/Haematoma |
| | Knee Laceration/Abrasion |
| | Knee Muscle Strain/Spasm/Trigger Points |
| | Knee Tendon Injury |
| | Patellar tendinopathy |
| | Quadriceps tendinopathy |
| | Iliotibial band syndrome (ITBS) |
| | Popliteus tendinopathy |
| | Pes anserinus tendinopathy |
| | Proximal gastrocnemious tendinopathy |
| | Biceps femoris tendinopathy |
| | Patellofemoral pain (Anterior knee pain) syndrome |
| | Knee Sprains/Ligament Injuries |
| | Acute ACL injury |
| | Acute PCL injury |
| | MCL injury knee |
| | Patellar subluxation |
| | Combined ligament injuries knee |
| | Knee Dislocation |
| | Patellar dislocation |
| | Tibio-femoral dislocation |
| | Knee Instability (chronic or recurrent subluxations) |
| | Knee Impingement/Synovitis/Biomechanical Lesion not associated with other conditions |
| | Knee Fractures |
| | Patellar fracture |
| | Distal femoral fracture |
| | Proximal tibial fracture |
| | Knee Stress Fracture |
| | Knee Osteoarthritis |
| | Knee Pain/Injury (Other/not specified) |
| Lower Leg Injuries | |
| | Leg Soft Tissue Bruising/Haematoma |
| | Lower Leg Laceration/Abrasion |

**Table 29.9** (continued)

| Main anatomical region | Injury type/diagnosis |
|---|---|
| | Lower leg muscle Injury |
| | Anterior compartment muscle injury |
| | Lateral compartment muscle injury |
| | Gastrocnemius muscle injury/strain |
| | Soleus Injury/strain |
| | Calf cramping during exercise |
| | Lower Leg Tendon Injuries (see knee or ankle depending on tendon location) |
| | Lower Leg Fractures |
| | Fractured Midshaft Tibia |
| | Fractured fibula |
| | Medial Tibial Stress Syndrome |
| | Lower Leg Stress Fractures |
| | Tibial Stress Fracture |
| | Fibular Stress Fracture |
| | Other Leg Overuse Injury |
| | Neurological Injury of Lower Leg |
| | Lower Leg Vascular Injury |
| | Popliteal Artery Entrapment Syndrome |
| | Other Lower Leg Pain/Injury (Other/not specified) |
| Ankle Injuries | |
| | Ankle Soft Tissue Bruising/Haematoma |
| | Ankle Laceration/Abrasion |
| | Ankle Tendon Injury |
| | Achilles tendinopathy (insertional) |
| | Achilles tendinopathy (mid-substance) |
| | Achilles tendon rupture |
| | Extensor tendon injuries at ankle |
| | Tibialis anterior injuries |
| | Tibialis posterior injuries |
| | Flexor hallucis tendon injury |
| | Peroneal tendon injury |
| | Ankle Sprains |
| | Ankle syndesmosis sprain |
| | Ankle lateral ligament sprain |
| | Ankle deltoid ligament sprain |
| | Ankle multiple ligaments sprain |
| | Ankle Osteochondral Injuries |
| | Ankle Dislocation |
| | Chronic Ankle Instability |
| | Chronic medial instability |
| | Chronic lateral instability |
| | Ankle Synovitis/Impingement/Bursitis not otherwise specified |
| | Ankle Fracture |
| | Fracture tibia and fibula at ankle joint |
| | Fractured talus |
| | Fractured calcaneus |
| | Ankle Stress Injuries/Stress Fractures |
| | Nerve Injury at Ankle |
| | Ankle Vascular Injury |

(continued)

**Table 29.9** (continued)

| Main anatomical region | Injury type/diagnosis |
|---|---|
| | Osteoarthritis of Ankle/Subtalar Joint |
| | Ankle Pain/Injury (Other/not specified) |
| Foot Injuries | |
| | Foot Soft Tissue Bruising/Haematoma |
| | Foot Laceration/Abrasion |
| | Foot Muscle Strain/Spasm/trigger Points |
| | Foot Tendon Injuries |
| | Foot Joint Sprain |
| | Foot Chondral/Osteochondral Lesion |
| | Foot Dislocation |
| | Synovitis/Impingement/Biomechanical Lesion of Foot |
| | Plantar Fasciopathy (Fasciitis) |
| | Foot Fractures |
| | Fracture tarsal bone |
| | Fracture Metatarsal(s) |
| | Fracture great toe |
| | Fracture lesser toes (2—5) |
| | Complication of fractured foot including non-union |
| | Stress Reactions/Fractures in Foot |
| | Foot Osteoarthritis |
| | Sesamoid injuries |
| | Foot Neurological Injury |
| | Foot Vascular Injury |
| | Foot Pain/Injury (Other/not specified) |
| Injuries Location Unspecified or Crossing Anatomical Boundaries | |
| | Soft Tissue Bruising/Haematoma Location Unspecified or Crossing Anatomical Boundaries |
| | Laceration/Abrasion Location Unspecified or Crossing Anatomical Boundaries |
| | Laceration/abrasion upper limb |
| | Laceration/abrasion lower limb |
| | Muscle Strain/Spasm/Trigger Points Location Unspecified or Crossing Anatomical Boundaries |
| | Muscle strain upper limb |
| | Muscle strain lower limb |
| | Muscle strain spine |
| | Tendon Injury Location Unspecified or Crossing Anatomical Boundaries |
| | Sprain Location Unspecified |
| | Chondral/Osteochondral injury Location Unspecified |
| | Dislocation Location Unspecified |
| | Upper limb joint dislocation |
| | Lower limb joint dislocation |
| | Instability of Joint Location Unspecified |
| | Upper limb joint instability |
| | Lower limb joint instability |
| | Fracture Location Unspecified or Crossing Anatomical Boundaries |
| | Fracture upper limb |
| | Fracture lower limb |

**Table 29.9** (continued)

| Main anatomical region | Injury type/diagnosis |
|---|---|
| | Stress Fracture Location Unspecified or Crossing Anatomical Boundaries |
| | Postural Syndrome |
| | Upper limb synovitis/impingement lesion |
| | Lower limb synovitis/impingement lesion |
| | Neurological lesion Location Unspecified or Crossing Anatomical Boundaries |
| | Spinal injury location unspecified or crossing anatomical boundaries |
| | Upper limb neurological injury |
| | Lower limb neurological injury |
| | Vascular Injury Location Unspecified or Crossing Anatomical Boundaries |
| | Upper limb vascular injury |
| | Lower limb vascular injury |
| | Osteoarthritis Location Unspecified or Crossing Anatomical Boundaries (excluding generalised OA) |
| | Upper limb osteoarthritis |
| | Lower limb osteoarthritis |

**R**ace **M**edical **E**ncounter **D**ata (R-MED) form for illness-related medical encounters (Table 29.10) and injury-related medical encounters (Table 29.11) was suggested [1].

**Clinical Pearls**

- The health benefits of regular moderate- to high-intensity physical activity are undisputed, but during such activity there is an increased risk of medical encounters.
- Mass community-based sports events are increasing in popularity, with greater participation among older athletes—this may increase the risk of medical encounters at these events.
- Medical encounters at mass community-based sports events can vary in severity, from sudden cardiac arrest or death, to minor medical encounters.
- Planning to reduce the risk of medical encounters is the responsibility of the race medical director and requires a step-wise approach.
- Pre-race medical screening and educational intervention may reduce the risk of medical encounters.
- The potential negative effects of environmental stress, including air quality, on athlete health can be reduced by careful pre-race planning.

**Table 29.10** Illness-related Race Medical Encounter Data (R-MED) form—endurance sport events. (Reproduced with permission from [1])

**<EVENT NAME>**

**Illness-Related Race Medical Encounter Data (R-MED) Form**

| | | | |
|---|---|---|---|
| **1. RACE DETAILS: <Pre-populate before the event>** | | | |
| <Race name> | Date: dd/mm/yyyy | Official start time: | Official finish time: |

| |
|---|
| **2. LOCATION OF THE MEDICAL FACILITY:** |
| ☐ Course Q1 ☐ Course Q2 ☐ Course Q3 ☐ Course Q4 ☐ At finish ☐ Sweeper bus ☐ Hospital ☐ Other |

| | | | |
|---|---|---|---|
| **3. ATHLETE DEMOGRAPHIC DETAILS:** | | | |
| Race Number: | Male ☐ Female ☐ | Race finisher: YES ☐ NO ☐ | |
| Arrival time at medical facility (hh/mm): | | | |

| | | | | | |
|---|---|---|---|---|---|
| **4. ATHLETE ILLNESS-RELATED MEDICAL HISTORY:** | | | | | |
| **4a. Pre-race history:** | | | | | |
| Did the athlete suffer from any pre-race acute illness/symptoms (gastro/acute illness or infective illness? | | | | YES ☐ NO ☐ | |
| Details of pre-race illness or injury (Type) | | | | | |
| ☐ URT symptoms with no systemic symptoms | | ☐ URT symptoms with systemic symptoms | | ☐ LRT symptoms | |
| ☐ Nausea/vomiting and diarrhoea | | ☐ Nausea only | | ☐ Nausea and vomiting | |
| ☐ Diarrhoea | | ☐ Other infective illness | | ☐ Other pre-raceillness | |
| Onset of pre-race illness | ☐ Race day | ☐ 1 day before | ☐ 2-7 days before | ☐ 8-14 days before | ☐ > 15days before |
| Analgesics/NSAIDs use **<u>0-24 hours before</u>** the race?YES ☐ NO ☐ | | | Analgesics/NSAIDs use **<u>during</u>** the race? YES ☐ NO ☐ | | |
| Prescription medication use (list please): YES ☐ NO ☐ | | | Reason for medication use: | | |

| | | | |
|---|---|---|---|
| **4b. Presenting complaint:** | | | |
| ☐ Collapse (pre-finish) | ☐ Collapse (post-finish) | ☐ Confused | ☐ Muscle cramps (localized) |
| ☐ Chest pain | ☐ Palpitations | ☐ Fatigue/exhaustion | ☐ Muscle cramps (systemic) |
| ☐ Abdominal cramps/pain | ☐ Diarrhoea | ☐ Nausea/vomiting | ☐ Seizure |
| ☐ Headache | ☐ Hot (suspected hyperthermia) | ☐ Cold (suspected hypothermia) | ☐ Difficulty breathing |
| ☐ Wheeze | ☐ Coughing | ☐ Skin (chafing/ blisters) | ☐ Skin (cut / laceration) |
| ☐ Skin (other) | ☐ Musculoskeletal (head/neck) | ☐ Musculoskeletal (chest/trunk) | ☐ Musculoskeletal (upper limb) |
| ☐ Musculoskeletal (spine/back) | ☐ Musculoskeletal (hip/pelvis) | ☐ Musculoskeletal (lower limb) | ☐ Deep Chest/Abdominal trauma |
| ☐ Other: | | | |
| Additional clinical notes: | | | |

| | | |
|---|---|---|
| **4c. Location of the medical encounter on the course:** | | |
| ☐ Not known or not applicable | Distance from the start (km) | Nearest distance marker (km) |

| | | | | |
|---|---|---|---|---|
| **5. CLINICAL EXAMINATION:** | | | | |
| 5.1. Mental status (APVU): | ☐ Alert | ☐ Responds to voice | ☐ Responds to pain | ☐ Unresponsive |
| 5.2. Glasgow Coma Scale: /15 | Eye: /4 | Verbal: /5 | Motor: /6 | |
| 5.3. Hydration: | ☐ Normal (clinically) | ☐ Dry mouth (mucosa) | ☐ Oedema (swollen periphery) | ☐ Poor skin turgor |
| Fluid intake during race (ml): | Pre-race weight (kg): | Postrace weight (kg): | % Weight change: % | |
| 5.4.Vital signs | | | | |

| Time of measurement | Pulse | BP Systolic/diastolic) | Core Temp | % Sats | Glucose | Other |
|---|---|---|---|---|---|---|
| Admission | | | | | | |
| | | | | | | |
| | | | | | | |
| | | | | | | |
| | | | | | | |
| | | | | | | |

**Table 29.10** (continued)

| 5.5. Other clinical findings: |
|---|
| |
| |
| |

| 6. ORDERS/ INVESTIGATIONS: | | | | |
|---|---|---|---|---|
| ☐ Admit to ICU/resuscitation (medical tent or hospital) | ☐ Admit medical tent for treatment | ☐ Elevate legs | ☐ Fluids (Oral) | ☐ Fluids (IV) |
| ☐ Cooling | ☐ Warming | ☐ Wound care | ☐ Other: | |
| ☐ Lab tests (glucose) | ☐ Lab tests (sodium) | ☐ Lab tests (potassium) | ☐ Lab tests (urea/creat) | ☐ Lab tests (blood gas) |
| ☐ Lab tests (Hct/Hb) | ☐ Lab tests (ECG) | ☐ Lab tests (Ultrasound) | ☐ Lab tests (Other) | |

| 7. LABORATORY / INVESTIGATION RESULTS (ATTACH): | | | | |
|---|---|---|---|---|
| ☐ Lab tests (glucose) | ☐ Lab tests (sodium) | ☐ Lab tests (potassium) | ☐ Lab tests (urea/creat) | ☐ Lab tests (blood gas) |
| ☐ Lab tests (Hct/Hb) | ☐ Lab tests (ECG) | ☐ Lab tests (Ultrasound) | ☐ Lab tests (Other) | |

| 8. TREATMENT: | | | |
|---|---|---|---|
| 8.1. Fluids | | | |
| Oral Fluid (volume ml): | Type: Water:☐ Sports drink:☐ Hypertonic saline:☐ Other: | | |
| IV Fluid (volume ml): | Type: | Rate: ml over min | Start time: End time: |
| 8.2. Medication | | | |
| Type: | Dosage: | Route (po/IM/IV): | Time (given): |
| Type: | Dosage: | Route (po/IM/IV): | Time (given): |
| 8.3. Other treatment: | | | |

| 9. PRE-DISCHARGE ASSESSMENT: | | | |
|---|---|---|---|
| Conscious/orientated YES☐; No ☐; N/A ☐ | Ambulatory YES☐; No ☐; N/A ☐ | Asymptomatic YES☐; No ☐; N/A ☐ | Passed urine: YES☐; No ☐; N/A ☐ |

| 10. FINAL DIAGNOSIS OF ILLNESS-RELATED MEDICAL ENCOUNTER: | | | |
|---|---|---|---|
| **Main organ system** | | | |
| Multiple organs☐ | Cardiovascular system ☐ | Respiratory / ENT system ☐ | Central nervous system ☐ |
| Rheumatological system ☐ | Gastrointestinal system ☐ | Genitourinary system ☐ | Haematology / Nutrition ☐ |
| Endocrine / Metabolic ☐ | Dermatological system ☐ | Ophthalmological system ☐ | Dental illness ☐ |
| Psychological / Psychiatric ☐ | Tumour / malignancy ☐ | Drug use / Overdose ☐ | Other medical illness ☐ |
| **Final diagnosis / illnesstype:** | **<Enter code from Table>** | | |

| 11. ILLNESS-RELATED MEDICAL ENCOUNTER SEVERITY: | | |
|---|---|---|
| Minor encounter ☐ | Moderate encounter ☐ | Serious / life threatening encounter ☐ |
| Sudden cardiac arrest (SCA) during race ☐ | Sudden cardiac arrest (SCA) < 1hr post race☐ | Sudden cardiac arrest (SCA) 1-24hrs post race ☐ |
| Sudden cardiac death (SCD)during race ☐ | Sudden cardiac death (SCD) < 1hr post race☐ | Sudden cardiac death (SCD) 1-24hrs post race ☐ |
| Non-cardiac sudden death during race ☐ | Non-cardiac sudden death< 1hr post race ☐ | Non-cardiac sudden death1-24hrs post race ☐ |

| 12. DISCHARGE INFORMATION: | | | |
|---|---|---|---|
| ☐ Discharged | ☐ Hospital transfer | ☐ Follow-up care needed | ☐ Refusal of care |
| ☐ Follow up call by race medical team needed YES ☐ NO ☐ | | ☐ Other special instruction: | |

| 13. TRANSPORT INFORMATION: | Authorized by: Dr |
|---|---|
| Hospital name: | Transported by: |
| Receiving doctor: | Receiving doctor's contact details: |
| Family / Next of Kin notified: YES ☐ NO ☐ | Who was notified? |

| 14. ADDITIONAL CLINICAL NOTES: |
|---|
| |
| |

| 15: DOCTOR / CLINICIAN DETAILS: | | |
|---|---|---|
| **Doctor/ Clinician name:** | **Signature:** | **Date: Time:** |

**Table 29.11** Injury-related Race Medical Encounter Data (R-MED) form—endurance sport events. (Reproduced with permission from [1])

| | | | |
|---|---|---|---|
| **<EVENT NAME>**<br>**Injury-Related Race Medical Encounter Data (R-MED) Form** | | | |
| | | | |
| **1. RACE DETAILS <Pre-populate before the event>** | | | |
| <Race name> | Date: dd/mm/yyyy | Official start time: | Official finish time: |
| | | | |
| **2. LOCATION OF THE MEDICAL FACILITY** | | | |
| ☐ Course Q1 ☐ Course Q2 ☐ Course Q3 ☐ Course Q4 ☐ At finish ☐ Sweeper bus ☐ Hospital ☐ Other | | | |
| | | | |
| **3. ATHLETE DEMOGRAPHIC DETAILS** | | | |
| Race Number: | Male ☐ Female☐ | Race finisher: YES ☐ NO ☐ | |
| Arrival time at medical facility (hh/mm): | | | |
| | | | |
| **4. ATHLETE MEDICAL HISTORY** | | | |
| **4a. Injury history:** | | | |
| **Onset of Injury:** | | | |
| ☐ Acute | ☐ Chronic (pre-existing) | ☐ Acute exacerbation of chronic injury | |
| **Mechanism of Injury:** | | | |
| ☐Traumatic-contact with another athlete | ☐ Traumatic – contact with moving object | ☐ Traumatic – contact with immobile object | |
| ☐ Traumatic non-contact | ☐ Overuse injury | ☐ Other | |
| **Location of the injury on the course:** | | | |
| ☐ Not known or not applicable | Distance from the start (km) | Nearest distance marker (km) | |
| **Factors Contributing to the mechanism of injury:** | | | |
| ☐ Violation of rules | ☐ Weather conditions | ☐ Equipment failure | |
| ☐ Course/field of play conditions | ☐ Fatigue | ☐ Psychological | |
| ☐ Other: | | | |
| **4b. Presenting complaint:** | | | |
| ☐ Pain | ☐ Loss of function | ☐ Swelling | ☐ Confusion |
| ☐ Unresponsive (coma) | ☐ Head/neck injury | ☐ Chest injury | ☐ Trunk injury |
| ☐ Upper limb injury | ☐ Spine/back injury | ☐ Hip/pelvis injury | ☐ Lower limb injury |
| ☐ Abdominal injury | ☐ Injury multiple anatomical areas: | ☐ Other injury: | |
| Additional clinical notes: | | | |
| | | | |
| **5. CLINICAL EXAMINATION** | | | |
| 5.1. Mental status (APVU): ☐ Alert | ☐ Responds to voice | ☐ Responds to pain | ☐ Unresponsive |
| 5.2. Glasgow Coma Scale: /15 | Eye: /4 | Verbal: /5 | Motor: /6 |
| 5.3. Hydration: ☐ Normal (clinically) | ☐ Dry mouth (mucosa) | ☐ Oedema (swollen periphery) | ☐ Poor skin turgor |
| Fluid intake during race (ml): | Pre-race weight (kg): | Post-race weight (kg): | % Weight change: % |
| 5.4. Vital signs | | | |

| Time of measurement | Pulse | BP Systolic/diastolic) | Respiratory rate | % Sats | Other |
|---|---|---|---|---|---|
| Admission | | | | | |
| | | | | | |
| | | | | | |
| | | | | | |
| | | | | | |
| | | | | | |
| | | | | | |

| | | | |
|---|---|---|---|
| 5.5. Other clinical findings: | | | |
| | | | |
| | | | |
| | | | |
| | | | |
| **6. ORDERS/ RECOMMENDED INVESTIGATIONS** | | | |
| ☐ Admit to ICU/resuscitation (medical tent or hospital) | | ☐ Admit to medical tent | |
| ☐ Splint / brace | ☐ Warming | ☐ Wound care | ☐ Other: |

**Table 29.11** (continued)

| | | | |
|---|---|---|---|
| ☐ Lab tests (Ultrasound) | ☐ Lab tests (Radiology – X Rays) | ☐ Lab tests (MRI scan) | ☐ Lab tests (CT scan) |
| | | | |
| **7. LABORATORY RESULTS** | | | |
| Clinical notes: | | | |
| **8. TREATMENT** | | | |
| 8.1. Wound care | ☐ Wound dressing | ☐ Suture laceration | Other: |
| 8.2. Fluids | | | |
| Oral Fluid (volume ml): | Type: Water: ☐ Sports drink: ☐ Hypertonic saline: ☐ Other: | | |
| IV Fluid (volume ml): | Type: | Rate: ml over min | Start time: End time: |
| 8.3. Medication | | | |
| Type: | Dosage: | Route (po/IM/IV): | Time (given): |
| Type: | Dosage: | Route (po/IM/IV): | Time (given): |
| 8.4. Other treatment: | | | |
| | | | |
| **9. PRE-DISCHARGE ASSESSMENT:** | | | |
| Conscious/orientated YES ☐; No ☐; N/A ☐ | Ambulatory YES ☐; No ☐; N/A ☐ | Asymptomatic YES ☐; No ☐; N/A ☐ | Passed urine: YES ☐; No ☐; N/A ☐ |
| | | | |
| **10. FINAL DIAGNOSIS OF INJURY-RELATED MEDICAL ENCOUNTER** | | | |
| **Main anatomical area** | | | |
| Head injury ☐ | Neck injury ☐ | Shoulder injury ☐ | Upper arm injury ☐ |
| Elbow injury ☐ | Forearm injury ☐ | Chest injury ☐ | Trunk / abdominal injury ☐ |
| Lumbar spine injury ☐ | Pelvis / buttock injury ☐ | Hip / groin injury ☐ | Thigh injury ☐ |
| Knee injury ☐ | Lower leg injury ☐ | Ankle injury ☐ | Foot injury ☐ |
| Injury location unspecified or crossing anatomical boundaries: | | | |
| **Final diagnosis / injury type:** | **<Enter code from Table>** | | |
| | | | |
| **12. INJURY-RELATED MEDICAL ENCOUNTER SEVERITY:** | | | |
| Minor encounter ☐ | Moderate encounter ☐ | Serious / life threatening ☐ | |
| Non-cardiac sudden death during race ☐ | Non-cardiac sudden death< 1hr post race ☐ | Non-cardiac sudden death 1-24hrs post race ☐ | |
| | | | |
| **12. DISCHARGE INFORMATION:** | | | |
| ☐ Discharged | ☐ Hospital transfer | ☐ Follow-up care needed | ☐ Refusal of care |
| ☐ Follow up call by race medical team needed YES ☐ NO ☐ | | ☐ Other special instruction: | |
| | | | |
| **13. TRANSPORT INFORMATION** | | **Authorized by: Dr** | |
| Hospital name: | | Transported by: | |
| Receiving doctor: | | Receiving doctor's contact details: | |
| Family / Next of Kin notified: YES ☐ NO ☐ | | Who was notified? | |
| | | | |
| **14. ADDITIONAL CLINICAL NOTES:** | | | |
| | | | |
| | | | |
| | | | |
| **15: DOCTOR / CLINICIAN DETAILS:** | | | |
| **Doctor's / Clinician Name:** | **Signature:** | **Date:** | **Time:** |

## Review

### Questions

1. You are appointed as the chief race medical director for a large half-marathon (21.1 km) running event, where the expected number of race starters are about 45,000. The race will be held in a European city in May, and the city is at sea level. Based on current scientific data, which of the following statements are true for the type and severity of medical encounters that you may expect at this race?
   (a) I can expect that there will be 1–2 runners with sudden cardiac arrest during the race
   (b) About 5–10 runners will develop serious life-threatening medical encounters
   (c) I need to plan that there about 2000 runners will require medical attention
   (d) If the race is held at 2 pm in the afternoon rather than early in morning, it is likely that there will be fewer medical encounters
2. In your preparations for the race above (in question 1), where you are the chief medical director responsible for the medical care, which of the following are important considerations at the finish line area?
   (a) I need to deploy more medical resources and more staff at the finish line than along the course
   (b) At the finish line area, there should be a dedicated Triage Officer and team to direct the flow of casualties to the proper area for care
   (c) Equipment and supplies for obtaining vital signs, performing BLSD and ACLS should be available at the finish line.
   (d) There should be a high-care medical facility at the finish line
3. A 56-year-old female runner enters for a marathon for the first time. In preparation for the race she trained for about 10 weeks, with a weekly training distance that averages at 25 km per week. She is a type 2 diabetic, takes anti-depressant medication and has a chronic left rotator cuff impingement in the shoulder for which she uses occasional NSAIDs. What risk factors does this runner have of developing a medical complication during the race? What advice would you give her?

### Answers

1. Question
   (a) Yes: The incidence of sudden death is about 1 in 100,000 entrants, but sudden cardiac arrest is 2–3 higher i.e. 1 in 30,000 to 1 in 50,000
   (b) No. The incidence of serious life-threatening medical encounters varies but is about 1 in 2000 race starters. Therefore, for a race with about 50,000 starters, you can expect about 25 serious life-threatening medical encounters
   (c) Yes. The incidence of moderate medical encounters (requiring medical attention) is about 1 in 50. You can expect about 1000 runners that will require medical attention

   (d) No. If the race is held at 2 pm in the afternoon, it is likely that the environmental conditions will be less favourable in May (spring to early summer in Europe). It is likely that the WBGT will be higher, and if it is above 18°, the risk of medical encounters increases (moderate risk). Higher WBGT will increase the risk even more.

2. Question
   (a) Yes. The number of medical encounters in the final quarter of the race is significantly higher in respect to other segments. Therefore, in the last 2 km of the course, medical staff and supplies should be increased.
   (b) Yes. A Triage Officer at the finish line area is very important to direct runners with medical complications to the appropriate treatment area—this should be a senior medical doctor with previous race medical care experience.
   (c) Yes. Equipment and supplies for obtaining vital signs, performing BLSD and ACLS should be available at the finish line.
   (d) Yes. There should be a high-care medical facility at the finish line.
3. Question

   This runner has a number of factors that increase her risk of an acute medical complication during the marathon. She is over 55 years, and is a diabetic and therefore, according to international guidelines, has ≥2 risk factors. The advice would be that she requires a full medical assessment before participating in moderate- to high intensity exercise. It is also important to determine if she has concomitant cardiovascular disease and other complications associated with diabetes. She also uses medications that may increase her risk of a medical complications during exercise, including anti-depressants and NSAIDs. Finally, her training and preparation for a marathon is not optimal because she only started 10 weeks before the marathon, and her weekly training of 25 km is less that what is advised to prepare for a marathon.

## References


1. Schwellnus M, Kipps C, Roberts WO, Drezner JA, D'Hemecourt P, Troyanos C, et al. Medical encounters (including injury and illness) at mass community-based endurance sports events: an international consensus statement on definitions and methods of data recording and reporting. Br J Sports Med. 2019;53(17):1048–55.
2. Ranse J, Hutton A, Turris SA, Lund A. Enhancing the minimum data set for mass-gathering research and evaluation: an integrative literature review. Prehosp Disaster Med. 2014;29(3):280–9.
3. Lund A, Turris SA, Bowles R, Steenkamp M, Hutton A, Ranse J, et al. Mass-gathering health research foundational theory: part 1—population models for mass gatherings. Prehosp Disaster Med. 2014;29(6):648–54.
4. Warburton DE, Bredin SS. Reflections on physical activity and health: what should we recommend? Can J Cardiol. 2016;32(4):495–504.
5. Sanchez LD, Corwell B, Berkoff D. Medical problems of marathon runners. Am J Emerg Med. 2006;24(5):608–15.
6. Schwabe K, Schwellnus MP, Derman W, Swanevelder S, Jordaan E. Older females are at higher risk for medical complications during 21 km road race running: a prospective study in 39 511 race starters—SAFER study III. Br J Sports Med. 2014;48(11):891–7.

7. Thompson PD, Franklin BA, Balady GJ, Blair SN, Corrado D, Estes NA 3rd, et al. Exercise and acute cardiovascular events placing the risks into perspective: a scientific statement from the American Heart Association Council on Nutrition, Physical Activity, and Metabolism and the Council on Clinical Cardiology. Circulation. 2007;115(17):2358–68.
8. Eijsvogels TM, Molossi S, Lee DC, Emery MS, Thompson PD. Exercise at the extremes: the amount of exercise to reduce cardiovascular events. J Am Coll Cardiol. 2016;67(3):316–29.
9. Goodman JM, Burr JF, Banks L, Thomas SG. The acute risks of exercise in apparently healthy adults and relevance for prevention of cardiovascular events. Can J Cardiol. 2016;32(4):523–32.
10. Mont L, Pelliccia A, Sharma S, Biffi A, Borjesson M, Brugada Terradellas J, et al. Pre-participation cardiovascular evaluation for athletic participants to prevent sudden death: position paper from the EHRA and the EACPR, branches of the ESC. Endorsed by APHRS, HRS, and SOLAECE. Eur J Prev Cardiol. 2017;24(1):41–69.
11. Day SM, Thompson PD. Cardiac risks associated with marathon running. Sports Health. 2010;2(4):301–6.
12. Hoffmann TC, Maher CG, Briffa T, Sherrington C, Bennell K, Alison J, et al. Prescribing exercise interventions for patients with chronic conditions. Can Med Assoc J. 2016;188(7):510–8.
13. Chugh SS, Weiss JB. Sudden cardiac death in the older athlete. J Am Coll Cardiol. 2015;65(5):493–502.
14. Sanchis-Gomar F, Santos-Lozano A, Garatachea N, Pareja-Galeano H, Fiuza-Luces C, Joyner MJ, et al. My patient wants to perform strenuous endurance exercise. What's the right advice? Int J Cardiol. 2015;197:248–53.
15. Riebe D, Franklin BA, Thompson PD, Garber CE, Whitfield GP, Magal M, et al. Updating ACSM's recommendations for exercise preparticipation health screening. Med Sci Sports Exerc. 2015;47(11):2473–9.
16. Siscovick DS, Weiss NS, Fletcher RH, Schoenbach VJ, Wagner EH. Habitual vigorous exercise and primary cardiac arrest: effect of other risk factors on the relationship. J Chronic Dis. 1984;37(8):625–31.
17. Siegel AJ. Pheidippides redux: reducing risk for acute cardiac events during marathon running. Am J Med. 2012;125(7):630–5.
18. Harmon KG, Asif IM, Maleszewski JJ, Owens DS, Prutkin JM, Salerno JC, et al. Incidence and etiology of sudden cardiac arrest and death in high school athletes in the United States. Mayo Clin Proc. 2016;91(11):1493–502.
19. Harmon KG, Asif IM, Maleszewski JJ, Owens DS, Prutkin JM, Salerno JC, et al. Incidence, cause, and comparative frequency of sudden cardiac death in national collegiate athletic association athletes: a decade in review. Circulation. 2015;132(1):10–9.
20. Harmon KG, Drezner JA, Wilson MG, Sharma S. Incidence of sudden cardiac death in athletes: a state-of-the-art review. Br J Sports Med. 2014;48(15):1185–92.
21. Drezner JA, O'Connor FG, Harmon KG, Fields KB, Asplund CA, Asif IM, et al. AMSSM position statement on cardiovascular preparticipation screening in athletes: current evidence, knowledge gaps, recommendations and future directions. Br J Sports Med. 2017;51(3):153–67.
22. Lawless CE, Asplund C, Asif IM, Courson R, Emery MS, Fuisz A, et al. Protecting the heart of the American athlete: proceedings of the American College of Cardiology Sports and Exercise Cardiology Think Tank October 18, 2012, Washington, DC. J Am Coll Cardiol. 2014;64(20):2146–71.
23. Roberts WO, Roberts DM, Lunos S. Marathon related cardiac arrest risk differences in men and women. Br J Sports Med. 2013;47(3):168–71.
24. Webner D, DuPrey KM, Drezner JA, Cronholm P, Roberts WO. Sudden cardiac arrest and death in United States marathons. Med Sci Sports Exerc. 2012;44(10):1843–5.
25. Mathews SC, Narotsky DL, Bernholt DL, Vogt M, Hsieh YH, Pronovost PJ, et al. Mortality among marathon runners in the United States, 2000-2009. Am J Sports Med. 2012;40(7):1495–500.
26. Kim JH, Malhotra R, Chiampas G, d'Hemecourt P, Troyanos C, Cianca J, et al. Cardiac arrest during long-distance running races. N Engl J Med. 2012;366(2):130–40.

27. Cohen SI, Ellis ER. Death and near death from cardiac arrest during the Boston Marathon. Pacing Clin Electrophysiol. 2012;35(2):241–4.
28. Finn SE, Coviello J. Myocardial infarction & sudden death in recreational master marathon runners. Nurse Pract. 2011;36(2):48–53.
29. Schwabe K, Schwellnus M, Derman W, Swanevelder S, Jordaan E. Medical complications and deaths in 21 and 56 km road race runners: a 4-year prospective study in 65 865 runners—SAFER study I. Br J Sports Med. 2014;48(11):912–8.
30. Schwellnus MP. Premarathon evaluations: is there a role for runner prerace medical screening and education to reduce the risk of medical complications? Curr Sports Med Rep. 2017;16(3):129–36.
31. Turris SA, Lund A, Mui J, Wang P, Lewis K, Gutman SJ. An organized medical response for the Vancouver International Marathon (2006-2011): when the rubber hits the road. Curr Sports Med Rep. 2014;13(3):147–54.
32. Borjesson M, Urhausen A, Kouidi E, Dugmore D, Sharma S, Halle M, et al. Cardiovascular evaluation of middle-aged/senior individuals engaged in leisure-time sport activities: position stand from the sections of exercise physiology and sports cardiology of the European Association of Cardiovascular Prevention and Rehabilitation. Eur J Cardiovasc Prev Rehabil. 2011;18(3):446–58.
33. Corrado D, Schmied C, Basso C, Borjesson M, Schiavon M, Pelliccia A, et al. Risk of sports: do we need a pre-participation screening for competitive and leisure athletes? Eur Heart J. 2011;32(8):934–44.
34. Shapero K, Deluca J, Contursi M, Wasfy M, Weiner RB, Lewis GD, et al. Cardiovascular risk and disease among masters endurance athletes: insights from the Boston MASTER (Masters Athletes Survey To Evaluate Risk) initiative. Sports Med Open. 2016;2(1):29.
35. Schwabe K, Schwellnus M, Swanevelder S, Jordaan E, Derman W, Bosch A. Leisure athletes at risk of medical complications: outcomes of pre-participation screening among 15,778 endurance runners—SAFER VII. Phys Sportsmed. 2018;46(4):405–13.
36. Schwellnus M, Swanevelder S, Derman W, Borjesson M, Schwabe K, Jordaan E. Prerace medical screening and education reduce medical encounters in distance road races: SAFER VIII study in 153 208 race starters. Br J Sports Med. 2019;53(10):634–9.
37. Behr ER, Roden D. Drug-induced arrhythmia: pharmacogenomic prescribing? Eur Heart J. 2013;34(2):89–95.
38. Tamargo J, Caballero R, Delpon E. Drug-induced atrial fibrillation. Expert Opin Drug Saf. 2012;11(4):615–34.
39. Granier M, Massin F, Pasquie JL. Pro- and anti-arrhythmic effects of anti-inflammatory drugs. Antiinflamm Antiallergy Agents Med Chem. 2013;12(1):83–93.
40. Evans B, Cox A, Nicol E, Patil Mead M, Behr E. Drug-associated arrhythmia in the military patient. J R Army Med Corps. 2015;161(3):253–8.
41. Lange ML, Skansing TB. Acute renal failure after participation in high endurance sport. Ugeskr Laeger. 2016;178(3):V08150682.
42. Szczepanik ME, Heled Y, Capacchione J, Campbell W, Deuster P, O'Connor FG. Exertional rhabdomyolysis: identification and evaluation of the athlete at risk for recurrence. Curr Sports Med Rep. 2014;13(2):113–9.
43. Sandhu RS, Como JJ, Scalea TS, Betts JM. Renal failure and exercise-induced rhabdomyolysis in patients taking performance-enhancing compounds. J Trauma. 2002;53(4):761–3; discussion 3-4
44. Alaranta A, Alaranta H, Helenius I. Use of prescription drugs in athletes. Sports Med. 2008;38(6):449–63.
45. Waterman JJ, Kapur R. Upper gastrointestinal issues in athletes. Curr Sports Med Rep. 2012;11(2):99–104.
46. Shoor S. Athletes, nonsteroidal anti-inflammatory drugs, coxibs, and the gastrointestinal tract. Curr Sports Med Rep. 2002;1(2):107–15.
47. Melhus A. Fluoroquinolones and tendon disorders. Expert Opin Drug Saf. 2005;4(2):299–309.

48. van der Linden PD, Nab HW, Simonian S, Stricker BH, Leufkens HG, Herings RM. Fluoroquinolone use and the change in incidence of tendon ruptures in the Netherlands. Pharm World Sci. 2001;23(3):89–92.
49. Lakhan SE, Kirchgessner A. Prescription stimulants in individuals with and without attention deficit hyperactivity disorder: misuse, cognitive impact, and adverse effects. Brain Behav. 2012;2(5):661–77.
50. Epstein Y, Albukrek D, Kalmovitc B, Moran DS, Shapiro Y. Heat intolerance induced by antidepressants. Ann N Y Acad Sci. 1997;813:553–8.
51. Stollberger C, Lutz W, Finsterer J. Heat-related side-effects of neurological and non-neurological medication may increase heatwave fatalities. Eur J Neurol. 2009;16(7):879–82.
52. Thunenkotter T, Schmied C, Dvorak J, Kindermann W. Benefits and limitations of cardiovascular pre-competition screening in international football. Clin Res Cardiol. 2010;99(1):29–35.
53. Ljungqvist A, Jenoure P, Engebretsen L, Alonso JM, Bahr R, Clough A, et al. The International Olympic Committee (IOC) Consensus Statement on periodic health evaluation of elite athletes March 2009. Br J Sports Med. 2009;43(9):631–43.
54. Drezner JA, Harmon KG, Asif IM, Marek JC. Why cardiovascular screening in young athletes can save lives: a critical review. Br J Sports Med. 2016;50(22):1376–8.
55. Chatard JC, Mujika I, Goiriena JJ, Carre F. Screening young athletes for prevention of sudden cardiac death: practical recommendations for sports physicians. Scand J Med Sci Sports. 2016;26(4):362–74.
56. Bredin SS, Gledhill N, Jamnik VK, Warburton DE. PAR-Q+ and ePARmed-X+: new risk stratification and physical activity clearance strategy for physicians and patients alike. Can Fam Physician. 2013;59(3):273–7.
57. Warburton DE, Jamnik VK, Bredin SS, McKenzie DC, Stone J, Shephard RJ, et al. Evidence-based risk assessment and recommendations for physical activity clearance: an introduction. Appl Physiol Nutr Metab. 2011;36(Suppl 1):S1–2.
58. Warburton DE, Gledhill N, Jamnik VK, Bredin SS, McKenzie DC, Stone J, et al. Evidence-based risk assessment and recommendations for physical activity clearance: consensus document 2011. Appl Physiol Nutr Metab. 2011;36 Suppl 1:S266–98.
59. Maron BJ, Araujo CG, Thompson PD, Fletcher GF, de Luna AB, Fleg JL, et al. Recommendations for preparticipation screening and the assessment of cardiovascular disease in masters athletes: an advisory for healthcare professionals from the working groups of the World Heart Federation, the International Federation of Sports Medicine, and the American Heart Association Committee on Exercise, Cardiac Rehabilitation, and Prevention. Circulation. 2001;103(2):327–34.
60. Balady GJ, Chaitman B, Driscoll D, Foster C, Froelicher E, Gordon N, et al. Recommendations for cardiovascular screening, staffing, and emergency policies at health/fitness facilities. Circulation. 1998;97(22):2283–93.
61. Whitfield GP, Pettee Gabriel KK, Rahbar MH, Kohl HW 3rd. Application of the American Heart Association/American College of Sports Medicine adult preparticipation screening checklist to a nationally representative sample of US adults aged >=40 years from the National Health and Nutrition Examination Survey 2001 to 2004. Circulation. 2014;129(10):1113–20.
62. Aagaard P, Sahlen A, Bergfeldt L, Braunschweig F. Preparticipation evaluation of novice, middle-age, long-distance runners. Med Sci Sports Exerc. 2013;45(1):130–7.
63. Menafoglio A, Di Valentino M, Porretta AP, Foglia P, Segatto JM, Siragusa P, et al. Cardiovascular evaluation of middle-aged individuals engaged in high-intensity sport activities: implications for workload, yield and economic costs. Br J Sports Med. 2015;49(11):757–61.
64. El Helou N, Tafflet M, Berthelot G, Tolaini J, Marc A, Guillaume M, et al. Impact of environmental parameters on marathon running performance. PLoS One. 2012;7(5):e37407.
65. Giorgini P, Rubenfire M, Bard RL, Jackson EA, Ferri C, Brook RD. Air pollution and exercise: a review of the cardiovascular implications for health care professionals. J Cardiopulm Rehabil Prev. 2016;36(2):84–95.
66. Sharman JE, Cockcroft JR, Coombes JS. Cardiovascular implications of exposure to traffic air pollution during exercise. QJM. 2004;97(10):637–43.

67. Carlisle AJ, Sharp NC. Exercise and outdoor ambient air pollution. Br J Sports Med. 2001;35(4):214–22.
68. Roberts WO. A 12-yr profile of medical injury and illness for the twin cities marathon. Med Sci Sports Exerc. 2000;32(9):1549–55.
69. Roberts WO, Nicholson WG. Youth marathon runners and race day medical risk over 26 years. Clin J Sport Med. 2010;20(4):318–21.
70. Solberg EE, Borjesson M, Sharma S, Papadakis M, Wilhelm M, Drezner JA, et al. Sudden cardiac arrest in sports—need for uniform registration: a position paper from the sport cardiology section of the European Association for Cardiovascular Prevention and Rehabilitation. Eur J Prev Cardiol. 2016;23(6):657–67.
71. Landry CH, Allan KS, Connelly KA, Cunningham K, Morrison LJ, Dorian P, et al. Sudden cardiac arrest during participation in competitive sports. N Engl J Med. 2017;377(20):1943–53.
72. Maron BJ, Poliac LC, Roberts WO. Risk for sudden cardiac death associated with marathon running. J Am Coll Cardiol. 1996;28(2):428–31.
73. Roberts WO, Maron BJ. Evidence for decreasing occurrence of sudden cardiac death associated with the marathon. J Am Coll Cardiol. 2005;46(7):1373–4.
74. Tunstall Pedoe DS. Marathon cardiac deaths: the London experience. Sports Med. 2007;37(4–5):448–50.
75. Gerardin B, Collet JP, Mustafic H, Bellemain-Appaix A, Benamer H, Monsegu J, et al. Registry on acute cardiovascular events during endurance running races: the prospective RACE Paris registry. Eur Heart J. 2016;37(32):2531–41.
76. Yankelson L, Sadeh B, Gershovitz L, Werthein J, Heller K, Halpern P, et al. Life-threatening events during endurance sports: is heat stroke more prevalent than arrhythmic death? J Am Coll Cardiol. 2014;64(5):463–9.
77. Dick NA, Diehl JJ. Febrile illness in the athlete. Sports Health. 2014;6(3):225–31.
78. Deligiannis A, Bjornstad H, Carre F, Heidbuchel H, Kouidi E, Panhuyzen-Goedkoop NM, et al. ESC study group of sports cardiology position paper on adverse cardiovascular effects of doping in athletes. Eur J Cardiovasc Prev Rehabil. 2006;13(5):687–94.
79. Hoogsteen J, Bennekers JH, van der Wall EE, van Hemel NM, Wilde AA, Crijns HJ, et al. Recommendations and cardiological evaluation of athletes with arrhythmias: part 1. Neth Heart J. 2004;12(4):157–64.
80. Fragakis N, Vicedomini G, Pappone C. Endurance sport activity and risk of atrial fibrillation—epidemiology, proposed mechanisms and management. Arrhythm Electrophysiol Rev. 2014;3(1):15–9.
81. Hew-Butler T, Rosner MH, Fowkes-Godek S, Dugas JP, Hoffman MD, Lewis DP, et al. Statement of the 3rd International Exercise-Associated Hyponatremia Consensus Development Conference, Carlsbad, California, 2015. Br J Sports Med. 2015;49(22):1432–46.
82. Chlibkova D, Knechtle B, Rosemann T, Tomaskova I, Novotny J, Zakovska A, et al. Rhabdomyolysis and exercise-associated hyponatremia in ultra-bikers and ultra-runners. J Int Soc Sports Nutr. 2015;12:29.
83. Urso C, Brucculeri S, Caimi G. Physiopathological, epidemiological, clinical and therapeutic aspects of exercise-associated hyponatremia. J Clin Med. 2014;3(4):1258–75.
84. Patel DR, Gyamfi R, Torres A. Exertional rhabdomyolysis and acute kidney injury. Phys Sportsmed. 2009;37(1):71–9.
85. Clarkson PM. Exertional rhabdomyolysis and acute renal failure in marathon runners. Sports Med. 2007;37(4–5):361–3.
86. Patel DR, Torres AD, Greydanus DE. Kidneys and sports. Adolesc Med Clin. 2005;16(1):111–9, xi
87. Sural S, Chakraborty S. Acute kidney injury in hereditary renal hypouricaemia—a case report and review of literature. J Indian Med Assoc. 2013;111(8):556–7.
88. Casa DJ, Armstrong LE, Kenny GP, O'Connor FG, Huggins RA. Exertional heat stroke: new concepts regarding cause and care. Curr Sports Med Rep. 2012;11(3):115–23.
89. Oh RC, Henning JS. Exertional heatstroke in an infantry soldier taking ephedra-containing dietary supplements. Mil Med. 2003;168(6):429–30.

90. Coris EE, Ramirez AM, Van Durme DJ. Heat illness in athletes: the dangerous combination of heat, humidity and exercise. Sports Med. 2004;34(1):9–16.
91. American College of Sports M, Armstrong LE, Casa DJ, Millard-Stafford M, Moran DS, Pyne SW, et al. American College of Sports Medicine position stand. Exertional heat illness during training and competition. Med Sci Sports Exerc. 2007;39(3):556–72.
92. Sithinamsuwan P, Piyavechviratana K, Kitthaweesin T, Chusri W, Orrawanhanothai P, Wongsa A, et al. Exertional heatstroke: early recognition and outcome with aggressive combined cooling—a 12-year experience. Mil Med. 2009;174(5):496–502.

# Incidence and Causes of Sudden Cardiac Death in Recreational Athletes

# 30

Xavier Jouven, Kumar Narayanan, and Eloi Marijon

**Learning Objectives**

1. To understand the current burden of recreational sports related SCD using incidence data from observational studies and registries.
2. Summarize the current information available on causes of sports related SCD, from autopsy data and from survivors via population-based studies.
3. Describe the specific characteristics of sports related SCD.
4. Outline strategies to reduce SCD burden related to sports.

## 30.1 Introduction

Participating athletes in competitive sport events as well as sports participants in general are usually healthy and perceived to be fit. It is also accepted that regular sports activity is beneficial in reducing long-term overall as well as cardiovascular mortality, including sudden cardiac death (SCD) [1–7]. However, the occasional instance of SCD during a sporting event in full public glare serves as a grim reminder of the small but definite arrhythmic risk of extreme exercise. This paradox of

X. Jouven · E. Marijon (✉)
Paris-Sudden Death Expertise Center (Paris-SDEC), Paris, France

Paris Descartes University, Paris, France

Cardiology Department, European Georges Pompidou Hospital, Paris, France

Paris-Cardiovascular Research Center (Inserm U970), Paris, France
e-mail: xavier.jouven@inserm.fr

K. Narayanan
Paris-Sudden Death Expertise Center (Paris-SDEC), Paris, France

Cardiology Department, Medicover Hospitals, Hyderabad, India
e-mail: kumar.narayanan@inserm.fr



A. Pressler, J. Niebauer (eds.), *Textbook of Sports and Exercise Cardiology*,
https://doi.org/10.1007/978-3-030-35374-2_30

exercise has been described for more than 20 years [1, 4, 6], wherein, although regular physical activity has proven benefits for cardiovascular health, vigorous exercise could increase the short-term risk of dying suddenly (during or shortly after exercise).

- Therefore, fairly extensive attention has focused on physical exertion as a potential trigger for SCD.
- To add to the complexity, the risk of sports-related SCD decreases with regular exercise training [7, 8].

Notwithstanding these facts, the occurrence of such unexpected and tragic events among athletes, who epitomize health and well-being, invariably begs the question as to whether they cannot be prevented or better managed. The ability to screen athletes to prevent such events has been the subject of considerable scientific attention and controversy [9–11]. The devastating and traumatic consequences of sports-related SCD, therefore, mandate a thorough understanding of this phenomenon across the general population [12, 13].

In this review, we summarize the current knowledge in this field, to provide an overview of the connection between sports and SCD, and to place into perspective the current thoughts on screening and other measures to improve outcomes.

## 30.2 Sports Activity: Conclusively Beneficial for Long-Term Sudden Cardiac Death Risk

The cardiovascular advantages of physical activity are well-established, and the excessive attention often focused on sports-related SCD should not overshadow the broad issue that regular exercise has irrefutable benefits [14]. Several studies have demonstrated a strong and consistent reduction of risk through regular physical activity with regard to

(a) Cardiovascular mortality [3].
(b) Atrial fibrillation [15].
(c) Coronary artery disease [16].

with the last mentioned being described more than 35 years ago [17]. Considering that coronary artery disease is one of the major underlying causes of SCD [especially during sports activity in subjects over 30 years of age [18, 19]], regular physical activity could, through reduction of coronary artery disease, lead to a decreased SCD risk. Concordant with this, studies have clearly established that regular physical activity is associated with a lower long-term risk of SCD [7, 20–24]. Therefore, there is scientific consensus that a certain amount of physical activity is strongly recommended to reduce overall mortality [25], including SCD.

In contrast, for sports-related SCD, an analogy of "drug overdosage" [26] has been used, considering that sports (exercise) is in fact an effective "drug" for SCD risk reduction. This analogy suggests that the association between sports and mortality may follow a U-curve [27]: moderate sports would confer a lower overall mortality, whereas strenuous sports activity would be associated with a similar mortality as a non-exercising population owing to a counter-balancing effect of short-term SCD risk. However, this concept remains controversial: for instance, recent data from healthy elite athletes (French participants in the Tour de France) reported a significantly lower mortality when compared with the general population [28]. Such results need careful interpretation, considering the potential selection bias in a population of elite athletes [29].

## 30.3 Sudden Death in the Young Competitive Athlete: The Apparent Part of the Iceberg

A young competitive athlete is traditionally defined as any person 10–35 years old who participates in an organized sports program (team or individual sport) that requires regular competition and training [9, 18, 30–32]. SCD occurring among young competitive athletes has always attracted major media attention, with emblematic examples in footballers [33] or, more recently, cyclists [34]. To date, the large majority of data on sports-related SCD have focused on the burden among young competitive athletes and the extent to which intensive physical activity may be actually harmful. The focus on healthy young athletes is highly understandable given the substantial social and emotional impact of sudden and unexpected deaths in this population.

However, there are some noteworthy facts in this regard:

- Sudden death in competitive athletes is a very low-frequency event [35, 36].
- Furthermore, several studies published on this subject included not only sudden deaths owing to cardiovascular causes, but also trauma [10] or even suicide [37].
- Other studies included SCD occurring in circumstances unassociated with sport [10].

Overall, although an accurate estimation of the incidence of sports-related SCD among young competitive athletes is challenging, it is estimated to be fewer than 10 per million per year in a recent meta-analysis [35]. In contrast, considering the burden of sports participation in the general population, focusing on competitive athletes alone could lead to a rather biased perspective on sports-related SCD.

## 30.4 Sudden Cardiac Death Among Recreational Sports Participants: The Majority of Sports-Related Sudden Cardiac Death

Sports-related SCD accounts for a small but significant proportion of all SCD, with recent studies consistently reporting around 5% of overall SCD occurring during sporting activity [38, 39]. Because the incidence of SCD is around 300,000 cases per year in Europe [40, 41] and North America [42, 43], it may be estimated that

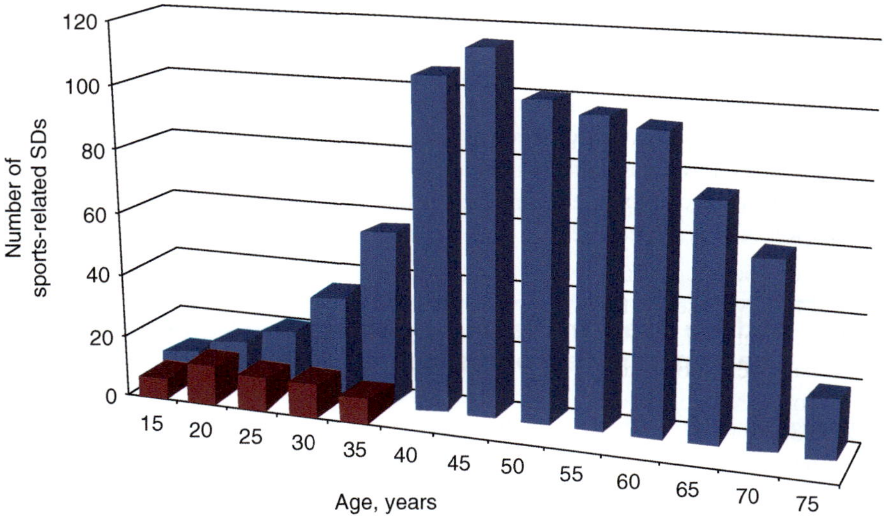


**Fig. 30.1** Distribution by age of sports-related sudden cardiac death in young competitive athlete (red) and general population (blue) (reprinted with permission from [31]). *SD* sudden death

sports-related SCD likely accounts for 15,000 cases annually in North America and in Europe. This estimation underlines the important magnitude of this entity. Literature on sports-related SCD, during recreational sports activities in the community, remains relatively sparse. The emphasis on young competitive athletes as opposed to recreational sports participants is discordant with the relative magnitudes of the respective problems, which was recently highlighted by a population-based registry [31].

- Overall, among all sports-related SCD, only 6% occurred in young competitive athletes, opposed to 94% among recreational sports participants (Fig. 30.1) [31].

This is intuitive, given the large pool of recreational sports participants as compared with competitive athletes. Thus, there is a crucial need to focus attention on this large at-risk population of subjects.

## 30.5 Sports-Related Sudden Cardiac Death Presents with Highly Homogenous Characteristics

Results from three large population-based registries recently published have elucidated the fairly uniform characteristics of sports-related SCD [31, 38, 39]. This form of SCD usually affects middle-aged patients, with a striking male predominance (>90% of cases), even after consideration of differences in participation rate according to sex. This predominance is notably higher than observed in non-sports-related SCD [44–46]. Several hypotheses can be advanced as an explanation for this [47, 48]:

- First, this difference can be related to sex differences in the extent and type of sports participation (e.g., beyond the lower participation rate of women in sports, a lower duration or intensity of physical activity).
- Second, an intrinsic physiologic difference related to sex is possible, considering the sex-specific prevalence of coronary heart disease.
  - Moreover, sex differences can also involve differences in arrhythmogenic substrate, trigger, or autonomic modulators. As an example, vagal activation has been shown to be more common in women than in men during abrupt coronary occlusion [49] and may have beneficial antiarrhythmic effects.
  - Sex-based differences with regard to nutritional factors and adherence to healthy life-styles may be implicated as well.
- Finally, the contribution of other medical conditions (comorbidities) and treatments received may also have played a role in this observed difference.

In terms of medical history, a significant fraction of patients have previous heart disease [31, 39] and, interestingly, several patients present with symptoms (chest pain, dyspnea) during the week before the event [39] (similar to non-sports-related SCD [50]. In fact, up to one-third of sports-related SCD patients report warning symptoms in the days before the event [39], which are usually neglected. Attention to this could potentially create room for subacute prevention, with better identification of high-risk patients and education for self-assessment of risk.

Regarding circumstances, most sports-related SCD occur in public places [51], and a large majority of cases (around 90%) are witnessed by bystanders, with often multiple witnesses. This almost-universal presence of a bystander permits precise phenotyping of sports-related SCD (often difficult with other cases of SCD), with precise information on presentation and delays (including from collapse to cardiopulmonary resuscitation [CPR]). Rates of bystander CPR are also substantially higher than that described in the non-sports setting, ranging from 30% to 80%, and an initial shockable rhythm is found in 50% to 80% of cases [as compared with three- to fourfold lower in a non-sports setting [45, 52]]. However, rates of automated external defibrillator (AED) use are disappointingly low, especially in France (<1% of cases [31] vs. 36% in the Netherlands [38, 53, 54]. This consistent phenotype has provided a reliable model to study determinants of survival in this population, and to identify areas for improvement.

Owing to these characteristics, survival is notably higher in sports-related SCD, ranging from 16% to 45% in multiple international reports [31, 38] compared with less than 10% for overall SCD [41, 45]. In fact, several studies have reported even higher survival rates, for example, up to 85% in US high school subjects [55]. The opportunities to intervene early in this form of SCD suggest that these figures can be improved on.

## 30.6 How to Tackle Sports-Related Sudden Cardiac Death?

Strategies to reduce the burden of sports-related SCD can be considered under two approaches, namely, primary prevention (through pre-participation screening and population education) and improved management of the SCD event (to increase survival rate). These approaches should ideally complement each other to achieve best results.

Primary prevention of sports-related SCD relies on the prior screening of sports participants, as well as education of participants and other stakeholders in sporting events. However, the concept of universal screening remains controversial; while early identification of asymptomatic structural or electrical cardiac abnormalities has postulated benefits, cost effectiveness remains uncertain [9] [56]. A seemingly attractive and logical way for prevention would be to screen patients for asymptomatic cardiac lesions before sports participation. Toward this end, an understanding of the usual underlying causes of sports-related SCD is crucial.

- In a retrospective analysis of 1500 forensic autopsies, Tabib and colleagues [19] reported different etiologic patterns according to the age of occurrence of the sports-related SCD event.
  - Under 30 years of age, the main causes were heritable diseases, such as hypertrophic cardiomyopathy and arrhythmogenic right ventricular cardiomyopathy.
  - Over 30 years of age, atherosclerotic coronary disease strongly predominated.

Guidelines regarding cardiovascular evaluation before sports activity [57] suggest that in order to assess sport-related SCD risk among older sports participants, the main issues to consider are

(a) Medical history
(b) Level of physical activity
(c) Previous exercise training

To further enhance screening, especially among young competitive athletes, strategies based on systematic performance of 12-lead electrocardiogram have been proposed [9, 58–60]. Although this measure has had some promising results, there is significant ongoing controversy about such an approach with regard to cost effectiveness, false-positive rates, and the potential psychological impact on a young target population (see Chap. 8) [56, 61]. Notwithstanding these issues, considering the potential benefits, current guidelines advocate preparticipation electrocardiographic screening [62].

Although even governmental legislation has been considered, for instance, with regard to sports participation, this debate has been often emotionally fraught and a difficult dilemma for clinicians. A universal and undifferentiated strategy of screening is probably not an effective approach. However, identification of select subgroups that might benefit from such screening remains problematic. One would need to start with certain broad areas of focus, such as among middle-aged men, where, considering the greater risk, effective ways to enhance pre-participation screening need to be actively sought. Considering the recent data that previous warning symptoms were present in several instances of sports-related SCD [39], systematic assessment of such symptoms, and education of participants to identify them and take appropriate action, seems to be necessary [63]. This could indeed be an easy and cost-effective intervention to identify patients at increased risk.

SCD occurring during sports activity offers a particularly suitable setting to achieve a favorable outcome that needs to be capitalized upon. Compared with other SCD, survival is relatively high after sports-related SCD, which can reach even up to 80% with immediate use of AEDs. However, one needs to bear in mind that this overall picture often masks major regional disparities in survival across regions, varying, for instance, from less than 10% to almost 50% (Fig. 30.2) in France [64].

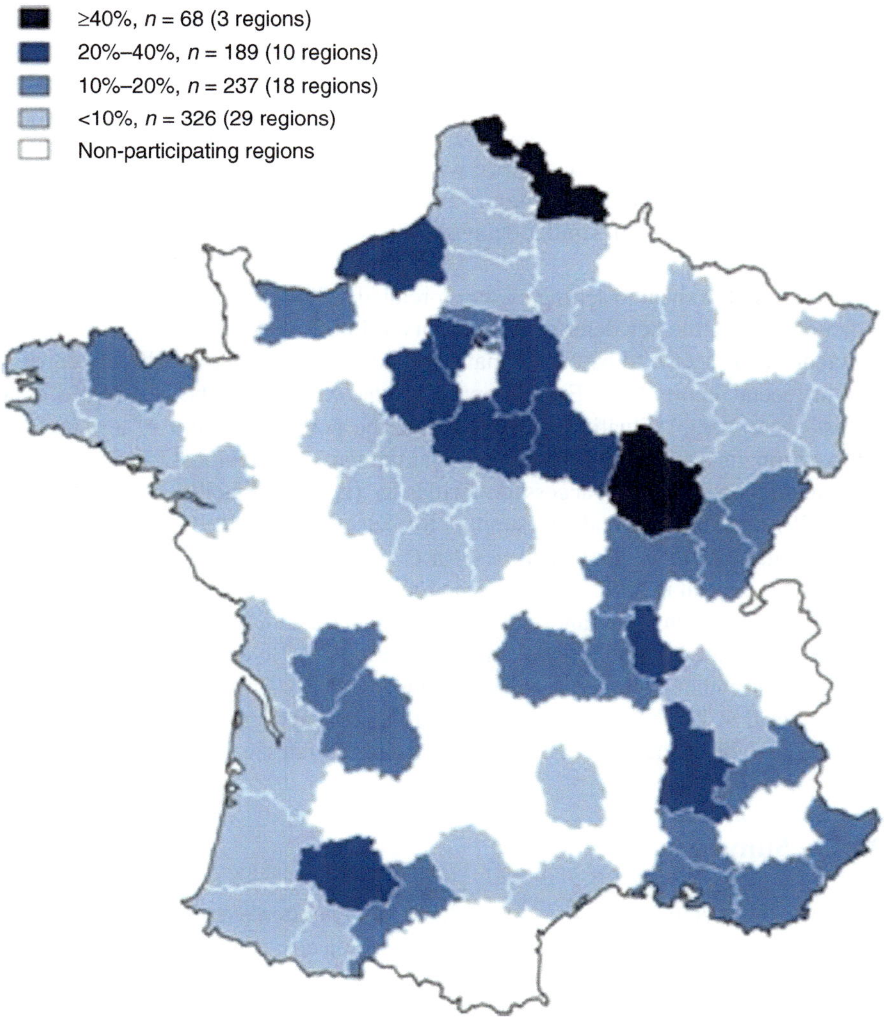


**Fig. 30.2** Survival rates after sport-related sudden cardiac death across districts in France (reprinted with permission from [64])

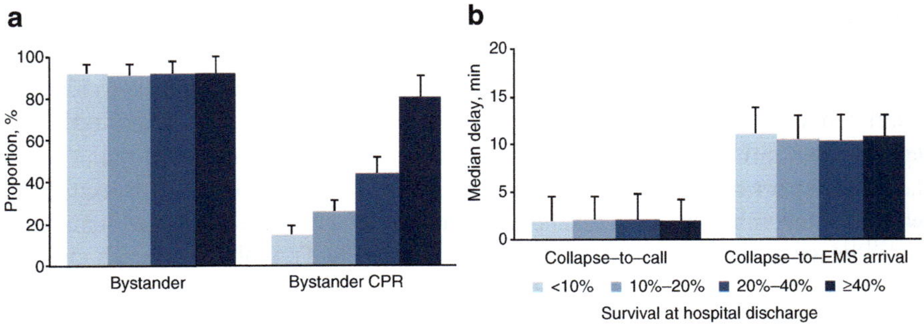


**Fig. 30.3** Factors associated with rates of survival at hospital discharge after sport-related sudden cardiac death. (**a**) Progressive increase in rates of survival at hospital discharge with increasing bystander CPR but not by bystander presence alone. (**b**) No significant difference in the Collapse-to-Call and Collapse-to-EMS Arrival times across survival strata (reprinted with permission from [64]). *CPR* cardiopulmonary resuscitation, *EMS* emergency medical services

This heterogeneity in survival rates is similar to results from studies performed in overall SCD [65]. However, in contrast with all SCD occurring in the general population, sports-related SCD consistently presents with homogenous characteristics (almost always witnessed, similar delays to intervention, similar rates of shockable rhythm) [64].

Therefore, the specific setting of sports-related SCD offers a unique opportunity to better analyze the key determinants of survival in SCD (Fig. 30.3). Interestingly, bystander CPR seems to be one of main prognostic factors, a result highly consistent in recent reports [41]. Finally, sports-related SCD could be considered as a "quasi-experimental"situation to demonstrate the potential benefit of a particular intervention in a relatively controlled environment, as previously described for implementation of public access defibrillation (in sports facilities [66–68]; see Chap. 29) or extracorporeal life support for selected cases [69]. The widespread deployment of AEDs in sport facilities, for example, may be a major tool available to enhance survival in sports-related SCD [66, 67].

To this end, recent guidelines advocated that AEDs should be widely distributed throughout the arena or on mobile emergency responders to achieve the goal of first defibrillation within 5 min of a witnessed collapse [67]. Thus, although survival in sports-related SCD is better than for all SCD, room for improvement clearly remains in the form of public education, improved bystander CPR rates, and greater AED access.

## 30.7 Summary

Although the specific entity of sports-related SCD is often a devastating and emotionally charged event in a young individual, exercise in general is clearly beneficial and has a role in the prevention and therapy of cardiac disease, and even in long-term prevention of sports-related SCD. Therefore, the goal for health care providers should certainly not be to discourage sports participation. However, there should be concerted efforts to enhance prevention and management of sports-related SCD, which seems to be a particularly suitable model for specific therapies. Targeted prevention through tailored and individualized pre-participation screening and an enhanced focus on middle-aged men during recreational sports could be of particular benefit.

**Clinical Pearls**

- While regular physical activity has long term cardiovascular benefits, including SCD risk reduction, there is a small but definite SCD risk during extreme exercise, which constitutes the paradox of exercise.
- SCD occurring in competitive athletes accounts for a minority of all sports-related SCD, while SCD during recreational sports constitutes the majority of these cases.
- Sports-associated SCD presents with relatively homogeneous characteristics, occurring mostly in middle-aged males, mostly witnessed and with better survival compared to overall SCD.
- Coronary artery disease is the most common pathology underlying sports SCD and a good proportion of subjects have prior warning symptoms, making sub-acute prevention feasible.
- Strategies to reduce sports SCD burden include prevention through targeted screening and improving survival rates through public education, enhanced bystander CPR and greater public AED access.

## Review

### Questions

1. A 45-year-old male with diagnosed coronary artery disease recently underwent coronary angiography and stenting. He is presently asymptomatic. He seeks your advice regarding playing recreational tennis in the evenings, as he is worried after reading about instances of people dying suddenly while playing. Would you advise him to play sports?
2. The owner of a fitness center chain contacts you for advice as there was a recent case of a person having a sudden cardiac arrest while exercising in one of his facilities. He asks you to suggest some measures which would be useful to prevent such events in the future. What are some practically useful measures which you can suggest?

### Answers

1. Yes. While there is a transient small risk of SCD associated with vigorous physical activity, this should not overshadow the fact that regular exercise/sports have irrefutable cardiovascular benefits. Therefore, a blanket prohibition of sports in this case is not warranted. However, a thorough discussion and patient education

is mandatory, with advice to gradually build up the activity level and to pay attention to any warning symptoms during exercise which can often precede an SCD event.

2. Strategies to prevent sports related SCD include targeted screening of individuals, public education and better AED access. Some practical measures which the fitness chain owner can implement could include arranging educational talks by experts for participants in the centers, focusing on cardiovascular prevention, early evaluation of any potential symptoms and also stressing the importance of early response in case of a witnessed cardiac arrest. Training in CPR can be arranged for interested volunteers and lastly AEDs can be made available in all centers. These strategies should help reduce instances of SCD during exercise and improve rates of bystander CPR and early AED use, two key determinants of survival after SCD.

## References

1. Albert CM, Mittleman MA, Chae CU, Lee IM, Hennekens CH, Manson JE. Triggering of sudden death from cardiac causes by vigorous exertion. N Engl J Med. 2000;343(19):1355–61.
2. Conraads VM, Beckers P, Vaes J, Martin M, Van Hoof V, De Maeyer C, et al. Combined endurance/resistance training reduces NT-proBNP levels in patients with chronic heart failure. Eur Heart J. 2004;25(20):1797–805.
3. Lee DC, Pate RR, Lavie CJ, Sui X, Church TS, Blair SN. Leisure-time running reduces all-cause and cardiovascular mortality risk. J Am Coll Cardiol. 2014;64(5):472–81.
4. Maron BJ. The paradox of exercise. N Engl J Med. 2000;343(19):1409–11.
5. Sharma S, Merghani A, Mont L. Exercise and the heart: the good, the bad, and the ugly. Eur Heart J. 2015;36(23):1445–53.
6. Siscovick DS, Weiss NS, Fletcher RH, Lasky T. The incidence of primary cardiac arrest during vigorous exercise. N Engl J Med. 1984;311(14):874–7.
7. Whang W, Manson JE, Hu FB, Chae CU, Rexrode KM, Willett WC, et al. Physical exertion, exercise, and sudden cardiac death in women. JAMA. 2006;295(12):1399–403.
8. Dahabreh IJ, Paulus JK. Association of episodic physical and sexual activity with triggering of acute cardiac events: systematic review and meta-analysis. JAMA. 2011;305(12):1225–33.
9. Corrado D, Basso C, Pavei A, Michieli P, Schiavon M, Thiene G. Trends in sudden cardiovascular death in young competitive athletes after implementation of a preparticipation screening program. JAMA. 2006;296(13):1593–601.
10. Maron BJ, Doerer JJ, Haas TS, Tierney DM, Mueller FO. Sudden deaths in young competitive athletes: analysis of 1866 deaths in the United States, 1980–2006. Circulation. 2009;119(8):1085–92.
11. Maron BJ, Shirani J, Poliac LC, Mathenge R, Roberts WC, Mueller FO. Sudden death in young competitive athletes. Clinical, demographic, and pathological profiles. JAMA. 1996;276(3):199–204.
12. Jouven X, Bougouin W, Karam N, Marijon E. Epidemiology of sudden cardiac death: data from the Paris sudden death expertise center registry. Rev Prat. 2015;65(7):916–8.
13. Waldmann V, Bougouin W, Karam N, Albuisson J, Cariou A, Jouven X, et al. Sudden cardiac death: a better understanting for a better prevention. Ann Cardiol Angeiol (Paris). 2017;66(4):230–8.
14. Arena R, Guazzi M, Lianov L, Whitsel L, Berra K, Lavie CJ, et al. Healthy lifestyle interventions to combat noncommunicable disease-a novel nonhierarchical connectivity model for

key stakeholders: a policy statement from the American Heart Association, European Society of Cardiology, European Association for Cardiovascular Prevention and Rehabilitation, and American College of Preventive Medicine. Eur Heart J. 2015;36(31):2097–109.
15. Morseth B, Graff-Iversen S, Jacobsen BK, Jorgensen L, Nyrnes A, Thelle DS, et al. Physical activity, resting heart rate, and atrial fibrillation: the Tromso study. Eur Heart J. 2016;37(29):2307–13.
16. Tanasescu M, Leitzmann MF, Rimm EB, Willett WC, Stampfer MJ, Hu FB. Exercise type and intensity in relation to coronary heart disease in men. JAMA. 2002;288(16):1994–2000.
17. Morris JN, Everitt MG, Pollard R, Chave SP, Semmence AM. Vigorous exercise in leisure-time: protection against coronary heart disease. Lancet. 1980;2(8206):1207–10.
18. Marijon E, Bougouin W, Jouven X. Sports-related sudden death: lessons from the French registry. Rev Prat. 2015;65(7):919–23.
19. Tabib A, Miras A, Taniere P, Loire R. Undetected cardiac lesions cause unexpected sudden cardiac death during occasional sport activity. A report of 80 cases. Eur Heart J. 1999;20(12):900–3.
20. Chiuve SE, Fung TT, Rexrode KM, Spiegelman D, Manson JE, Stampfer MJ, et al. Adherence to a low-risk, healthy lifestyle and risk of sudden cardiac death among women. JAMA. 2011;306(1):62–9.
21. Deo R, Albert CM. Epidemiology and genetics of sudden cardiac death. Circulation. 2012;125(4):620–37.
22. Deo R, Vittinghoff E, Lin F, Tseng ZH, Hulley SB, Shlipak MG. Risk factor and prediction modeling for sudden cardiac death in women with coronary artery disease. Arch Intern Med. 2011;171(19):1703–9.
23. Lemaitre RN, Siscovick DS, Raghunathan TE, Weinmann S, Arbogast P, Lin DY. Leisure-time physical activity and the risk of primary cardiac arrest. Arch Intern Med. 1999;159(7):686–90.
24. Wannamethee G, Shaper AG, Macfarlane PW, Walker M. Risk factors for sudden cardiac death in middle-aged British men. Circulation. 1995;91(6):1749–56.
25. Wen CP, Wai JP, Tsai MK, Yang YC, Cheng TY, Lee MC, et al. Minimum amount of physical activity for reduced mortality and extended life expectancy: a prospective cohort study. Lancet. 2011;378(9798):1244–53.
26. O'Keefe JH, Lavie CJ. Run for your life ... at a comfortable speed and not too far. Heart. 2013;99(8):516–9.
27. Schnohr P, O'Keefe JH, Marott JL, Lange P, Jensen GB. Dose of jogging and long-term mortality: the Copenhagen City Heart Study. J Am Coll Cardiol. 2015;65(5):411–9.
28. Marijon E, Tafflet M, Antero-Jacquemin J, El Helou N, Berthelot G, Celermajer DS, et al. Mortality of French participants in the tour de France (1947–2012). Eur Heart J. 2013;34(40):3145–50.
29. Zaidi A, Sharma S. Reduced mortality in former tour de France participants: the benefits from intensive exercise or a select genetic tour de force? Eur Heart J. 2013;34(40):3106–8.
30. Corrado D, Basso C, Rizzoli G, Schiavon M, Thiene G. Does sports activity enhance the risk of sudden death in adolescents and young adults? J Am Coll Cardiol. 2003;42(11):1959–63.
31. Marijon E, Tafflet M, Celermajer DS, Dumas F, Perier MC, Mustafic H, et al. Sports-related sudden death in the general population. Circulation. 2011;124(6):672–81.
32. Pelliccia A, Di Paolo FM, Corrado D, Buccolieri C, Quattrini FM, Pisicchio C, et al. Evidence for efficacy of the Italian national pre-participation screening programme for identification of hypertrophic cardiomyopathy in competitive athletes. Eur Heart J. 2006;27(18):2196–200.
33. Dvorak J. A lion never dies: pro memoria of Marc-Vivien foe. Br J Sports Med. 2009;43(9):628.
34. Myngheer D. Cycling mourns second Belgian death. 2016. http://www.bbc.com/sport/cycling/35914893.
35. Gerardin B, Collet JP, Mustafic H, Bellemain-Appaix A, Benamer H, Monsegu J, et al. Registry on acute cardiovascular events during endurance running races: the prospective RACE Paris registry. Eur Heart J. 2016;37(32):2531–41.
36. Kim JH, Malhotra R, Chiampas G, d'Hemecourt P, Troyanos C, Cianca J, et al. Cardiac arrest during long-distance running races. N Engl J Med. 2012;366(2):130–40.

37. Harmon KG, Asif IM, Klossner D, Drezner JA. Incidence of sudden cardiac death in National Collegiate Athletic Association athletes. Circulation. 2011;123(15):1594–600.
38. Berdowski J, de Beus MF, Blom M, Bardai A, Bots ML, Doevendans PA, et al. Exercise-related out-of-hospital cardiac arrest in the general population: incidence and prognosis. Eur Heart J. 2013;34(47):3616–23.
39. Marijon E, Uy-Evanado A, Reinier K, Teodorescu C, Narayanan K, Jouven X, et al. Sudden cardiac arrest during sports activity in middle age. Circulation. 2015;131(16):1384–91.
40. Berdowski J, Berg RA, Tijssen JG, Koster RW. Global incidences of out-of-hospital cardiac arrest and survival rates: systematic review of 67 prospective studies. Resuscitation. 2010;81(11):1479–87.
41. Hasselqvist-Ax I, Riva G, Herlitz J, Rosenqvist M, Hollenberg J, Nordberg P, et al. Early cardiopulmonary resuscitation in out-of-hospital cardiac arrest. N Engl J Med. 2015;372(24):2307–15.
42. Kudenchuk PJ, Brown SP, Daya M, Rea T, Nichol G, Morrison LJ, et al. Amiodarone, Lidocaine, or placebo in out-of-hospital cardiac arrest. N Engl J Med. 2016;374(18):1711–22.
43. Mozaffarian D, Benjamin EJ, Go AS, Arnett DK, Blaha MJ, Cushman M, et al. Heart disease and stroke statistics—2015 update: a report from the American Heart Association. Circulation. 2015;131(4):e29–322.
44. Adrie C, Cariou A, Mourvillier B, Laurent I, Dabbane H, Hantala F, et al. Predicting survival with good neurological recovery at hospital admission after successful resuscitation of out-of-hospital cardiac arrest: the OHCA score. Eur Heart J. 2006;27(23):2840–5.
45. Bougouin W, Lamhaut L, Marijon E, Jost D, Dumas F, Deye N, et al. Characteristics and prognosis of sudden cardiac death in greater Paris: population-based approach from the Paris sudden death expertise center (Paris-SDEC). Intensive Care Med. 2014;40(6):846–54.
46. Grasner JT, Meybohm P, Lefering R, Wnent J, Bahr J, Messelken M, et al. ROSC after cardiac arrest—the RACA score to predict outcome after out-of-hospital cardiac arrest. Eur Heart J. 2011;32(13):1649–56.
47. Marijon E, Bougouin W, Celermajer DS, Perier MC, Dumas F, Benameur N, et al. Characteristics and outcomes of sudden cardiac arrest during sports in women. Circ Arrhythm Electrophysiol. 2013;6(6):1185–91.
48. Marijon E, Bougouin W, Perier MC, Celermajer DS, Jouven X. Incidence of sports-related sudden death in France by specific sports and sex. JAMA. 2013;310(6):642–3.
49. Airaksinen KE, Ikaheimo MJ, Linnaluoto M, Tahvanainen KU, Huikuri HV. Gender difference in autonomic and hemodynamic reactions to abrupt coronary occlusion. J Am Coll Cardiol. 1998;31(2):301–6.
50. Marijon E, Uy-Evanado A, Dumas F, Karam N, Reinier K, Teodorescu C, et al. Warning symptoms are associated with survival from sudden cardiac arrest. Ann Intern Med. 2016;164(1):23–9.
51. Marijon E, Bougouin W, Karam N, Beganton F, Lamhaut L, Perier MC, et al. Survival from sports-related sudden cardiac arrest: In sports facilities versus outside of sports facilities. Am Heart J. 2015;170(2):339–45 e1.
52. Rea TD, Eisenberg MS, Becker LJ, Murray JA, Hearne T. Temporal trends in sudden cardiac arrest: a 25-year emergency medical services perspective. Circulation. 2003;107(22):2780–5.
53. Karam N, Narayanan K, Bougouin W, Benameur N, Beganton F, Jost D, et al. Major regional differences in automated external defibrillator placement and basic life support training in France: further needs for coordinated implementation. Resuscitation. 2017;118:49–54.
54. Karam N, Pechmajou L, Marijon E, Jouven X. How often does athlete sudden cardiac death occur outside the context of exertion? J Am Coll Cardiol. 2016;68(19):2125–6.
55. Drezner JA, Toresdahl BG, Rao AL, Huszti E, Harmon KG. Outcomes from sudden cardiac arrest in US high schools: a 2-year prospective study from the National Registry for AED use in sports. Br J Sports Med. 2013;47(18):1179–83.
56. Halkin A, Steinvil A, Rosso R, Adler A, Rozovski U, Viskin S. Preventing sudden death of athletes with electrocardiographic screening: what is the absolute benefit and how much will it cost? J Am Coll Cardiol. 2012;60(22):2271–6.

57. Borjesson M, Urhausen A, Kouidi E, Dugmore D, Sharma S, Halle M, et al. Cardiovascular evaluation of middle-aged/senior individuals engaged in leisure-time sport activities: position stand from the sections of exercise physiology and sports cardiology of the European Association of Cardiovascular Prevention and Rehabilitation. Eur J Cardiovasc Prev Rehabil. 2011;18(3):446–58.
58. Corrado D, Pelliccia A, Bjornstad HH, Vanhees L, Biffi A, Borjesson M, et al. Cardiovascular pre-participation screening of young competitive athletes for prevention of sudden death: proposal for a common European protocol. Consensus statement of the study Group of Sport Cardiology of the working Group of Cardiac Rehabilitation and Exercise Physiology and the working Group of Myocardial and Pericardial Diseases of the European Society of Cardiology. Eur Heart J. 2005;26(5):516–24.
59. Mont L, Pelliccia A, Sharma S, Biffi A, Borjesson M, Brugada Terradellas J, et al. Pre-participation cardiovascular evaluation for athletic participants to prevent sudden death: position paper from the EHRA and the EACPR, branches of the ESC. Endorsed by APHRS, HRS, and SOLAECE. Eur J Prev Cardiol. 2017;24(1):41–69.
60. Sharma S, Drezner JA, Baggish A, Papadakis M, Wilson MG, Prutkin JM, et al. International recommendations for electrocardiographic interpretation in athletes. J Am Coll Cardiol. 2017;69(8):1057–75.
61. Wheeler MT, Heidenreich PA, Froelicher VF, Hlatky MA, Ashley EA. Cost-effectiveness of preparticipation screening for prevention of sudden cardiac death in young athletes. Ann Intern Med. 2010;152(5):276–86.
62. Corrado D, Schmied C, Basso C, Borjesson M, Schiavon M, Pelliccia A, et al. Risk of sports: do we need a pre-participation screening for competitive and leisure athletes? Eur Heart J. 2011;32(8):934–44.
63. Karam N, Marijon E, Jouven X. Opening a new front in the fight against sudden cardiac death: is it time for near-term prevention? Int J Cardiol. 2017;237:10–2.
64. Marijon E, Bougouin W, Celermajer DS, Perier MC, Benameur N, Lamhaut L, et al. Major regional disparities in outcomes after sudden cardiac arrest during sports. Eur Heart J. 2013;34(47):3632–40.
65. Girotra S, van Diepen S, Nallamothu BK, Carrel M, Vellano K, Anderson ML, et al. Regional variation in out-of-hospital cardiac arrest survival in the United States. Circulation. 2016;133(22):2159–68.
66. Borjesson M, Dugmore D, Mellwig KP, van Buuren F, Serratosa L, Solberg EE, et al. Time for action regarding cardiovascular emergency care at sports arenas: a lesson from the Arena study. Eur Heart J. 2010;31(12):1438–41.
67. Borjesson M, Serratosa L, Carre F, Corrado D, Drezner J, Dugmore DL, et al. Consensus document regarding cardiovascular safety at sports arenas: position stand from the European Association of Cardiovascular Prevention and Rehabilitation (EACPR), section of sports cardiology. Eur Heart J. 2011;32(17):2119–24.
68. Page RL, Husain S, White LY, Rea TD, Fahrenbruch C, Yin L, et al. Cardiac arrest at exercise facilities: implications for placement of automated external defibrillators. J Am Coll Cardiol. 2013;62(22):2102–9.
69. Lebreton G, Pozzi M, Luyt CE, Chastre J, Carli P, Pavie A, et al. Out-of-hospital extracorporeal life support implantation during refractory cardiac arrest in a half-marathon runner. Resuscitation. 2011;82(9):1239–42.

# Potential Cardiac Damage Induced by Strenuous Exercise

# 31

Stefan Möhlenkamp and Axel Pressler

**Learning Objectives**

1. Learn that intensive endurance exercise may induce or accelerate "structural cardiac damage" that is different from physiological adaptations in the athletes' heart.
2. Become familiar with the presence and clinical significance of increased coronary artery calcification as a consequence of long-term intensive endurance exercise.
3. Acknowledge, that it is currently not clear if coronary artery calcification in athletes generally represents "healthy hardening" and stable plaque or if it indicates an elevated CAD/CVD risk.
4. Be informed that long-term repetitive strenuous exercise may induce and/or accelerate myocardial fibrosis as evidenced by late gadolinium enhancement using magnetic resonance imaging.
5. Learn about the different etiologies, potential clinical backgrounds and clinical consequences of different patterns of LGE in athletes.

## 31.1 Introduction

This chapter refers to cardiac damage that is potentially induced by strenuous exercise itself, as opposed to damage that is induced by diseases and abnormalities that lead to cardiac damage in physically active and inactive persons alike, such as

S. Möhlenkamp (✉)
Clinic of Cardiology and Intensive Care Medicine, Bethanien Hospital Moers, Moers, Germany
e-mail: stefan.moehlenkamp@bethanienmoers.de

A. Pressler
Private Center of Sports & Exercise Cardiology, Munich, Germany
e-mail: axel.pressler@kardiologie-mit-herz.de



A. Pressler, J. Niebauer (eds.), *Textbook of Sports and Exercise Cardiology*,
https://doi.org/10.1007/978-3-030-35374-2_31

coronary artery disease (CAD), myocarditis, myocardial bridging, etc. The sequelae of these and other diseases for physically active persons are addressed elsewhere in this book (see particular chapters referring to these entities).

- There is ample evidence beyond doubt that regular extensive exercise at moderate intensity is cardio-protective [1].
- It prevents cardiovascular disease (CVD) such as myocardial infarction or stroke and reduces morbidity and mortality from CVD and other diseases such as cancer.

Further, it is well-established that regular physical exercise leads to cardiac adaptations that are summarized as "athlete's heart" (see Chap. 3). Such alterations may be discernable in persons performing ≥5 h of sports per week but are frequently seen particularly in endurance athletes performing 15–30 h of weekly training. The term "athletes' heart" is used to indicate a physiological response to exercise that usually recedes after training cessation. The term "cardiac damage" is used here to denote pathophysiological alterations that may not be "healthy" and may potentially be linked to adverse clinical events. We present evidence that long-term high-intensity strenuous exercise can induce or accelerate structural damage that may in part counteract the benefits conveyed by regular moderate-intensity exercise. It is acknowledged, though, that structural damage and CVD events are most likely a consequence of a complex interplay of various contributing factors (Fig. 31.1) [2]. It also has to be noted that this chapter mainly refers to increased coronary artery calcium (CAC) and the prevalence of myocardial fibrosis. Other potential consequences of long-term intensive endurance exercise such as atrial fibrillation are outlined in other parts of this book.

It should finally be noted and always kept in mind that many of the studies on these issues have evaluated marathon runners as a primary target group, a term which should be regarded with caution when referring to intensive athletic activity and long-term endurance exercise training. Although some may have finished many marathon or ultramarathon races, the majority of runners have primarily to be classified as recreational. This is due to the fact that a substantial part of them has started marathon training and participation only later in life, with a much greater likelihood of having been exposed to unhealthier lifestyles beforehand, as compared to the more traditional understanding of the term "athlete" (see Chaps. 1 and 33).

## 31.2 Coronary Atherosclerosis

### 31.2.1 Prevalence of Coronary Artery Calcium

It was first recognized in 2008 that recreational master marathon runners can have an increased burden of subclinical coronary artery calcification [3, 4]:

- Compared to age-matched controls from the general population, these endurance athletes were more often free from coronary atherosclerosis (Table 31.1).

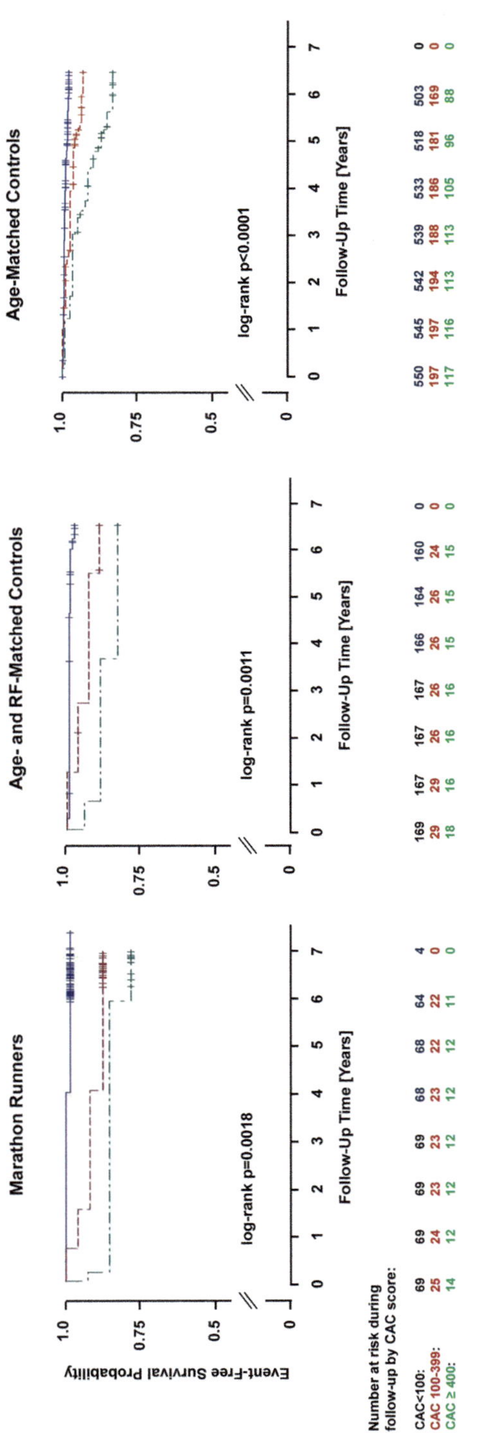


**Fig. 31.1** A complex interaction of multiple factors is likely necessary for an athlete to develop structural cardiac disease and CVD events (Modified from [2])

**Table 31.1** Distribution of coronary artery calcification (CAC) measures in marathon runners and non-active controls (adapted from [4])

| | | Participants of the Heinz Nixdorf Recall Study | | | |
|---|---|---|---|---|---|
| | Marathon runners (group I) | Age-matched controls (8:1) (group II) | Controls matched for age and risk factors (2:1) (group III) | p-Value group I vs. II | p-Value group I vs. III |
| $Log_2$(CAC + 1) [mean ± SD] | 4.1 ± 3.6 | 4.9 ± 3.3 | 3.8 ± 3.4 | =0.28 | =0.02 |
| CAC [Q1, median, Q3] | 0/36/217 | 3/38/187 | 0/12/78 | =0.36 | =0.02 |
| Zero CAC [%] | 28.7 | 18.4 | 31.5 | =0.01 | =0.50 |
| CAC > 75th percentile [%] | 25.0 | 24.2 | 14.8 | =0.85 | =0.01 |
| CAC 0 to <10 | 40.74 | 34.61 | 48.61 | =0.52 | =0.02 |
| CAC 10 to <100 | 23.15 | 29.05 | 29.63 | | |
| CAC 100 to <400 | 23.15 | 22.80 | 13.43 | | |
| CAC ≥ 400 | 12.96 | 13.54 | 8.33 | | |

Comparisons in continuous or binary measures adjusted for matching factors (age for group I/II, age, BMI, Framingham risk, smoking status for group I/III)

- If CAC was present, their burden was much higher than expected, given their half Framingham risk score [3, 4].
- Compared to controls matched for age and risk factors, i.e. compared to men who presumably had a beneficial risk factor profile throughout their lives, marathon runners even had higher CAC scores (Table 31.1).
- A CAC-score > 100, a threshold that has been proposed to raise risk awareness [5], was observed in 36% of runners.
- A CAC score < 15, a threshold considered safe for high-intensity physical activity [5], was present in only 43% of runners.

These findings are in line with observations from the Twin-Cities-Marathon in Minneapolis/St. Paul [6]:

- Fifty men aged 59 ± 7 years who had completed at least one marathon each year for 25 consecutive years underwent CVD risk assessment including coronary CT imaging.
- Compared with 23 sedentary controls, runners had increased calcified plaque volumes (84 vs. 44 mm$^3$, $p < 0.0001$) [6].

These findings were supported by a large primary prevention study, where CAC scores increased significantly with increasing categories of physical activity [7]:

- Men with at least 3000 MET-min per week were more likely to have prevalent CAC of at least 100 Agatston Units (AU; relative risk = 1.11 (95%CI, 1.03–1.20)) compared with less physically activity men.

### 31.2.2 Coronary Atherosclerosis and Prognosis in Athletes

An increasing burden of subclinical atherosclerosis predicts future CAD/CVD events in various general populations [8, 9]. It is unclear, if this also holds true for individuals undergoing endurance exercise. Importantly for this context, Criqui et al. [10] showed that

1. CAC *volume* was positively and independently predictive of future events.
2. At any given level of CAC volume, CAC *density* was inversely and significantly associated with CAD/CVD events.

Data on this issue are currently lacking for athletes. Hence, the question remains, whether increases in CAC burden due to regular strenuous exercise represent "healthy hardening" and stabilized plaque of coronary arteries or if it should be considered as an indicator of elevated risk comparable to that in other cohorts. Data from the aforementioned marathon study support the latter: while overall CVD and all-cause mortality risk was low as expected, it was observed that the 6.5-year coronary event rate in marathon runners was similar to that in the general population for every given category in CAC burden (Fig. 31.2) [11]. These findings have been attributed to a previously unfavorable risk factor profile, including smoking [12]. However, if previous exposure to traditional risk factors would be a prerequisite for CAC to develop in athletes, then lifestyle conversion may reduce, but not eliminate the risk arising from this risk factor exposure, and risk factor assessment during active training can be misleading.

**Fig. 31.2** Kaplan–Meier event-free survival curves in marathon runners, age-matched controls, and age- and risk factor-matched controls (Reproduced with permission from [11])

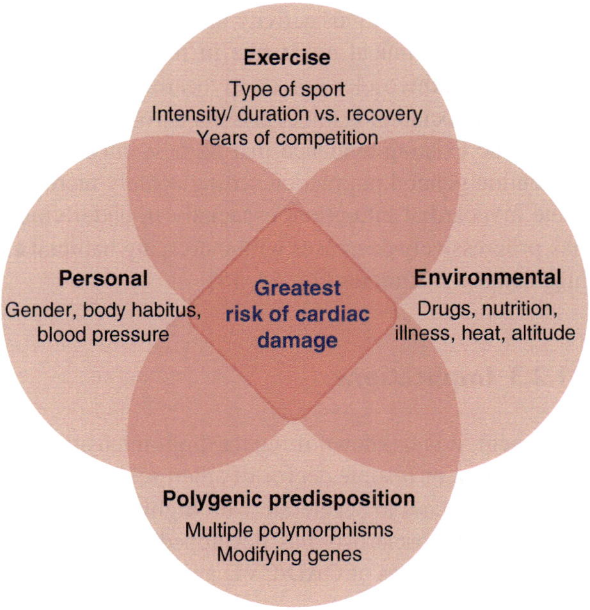

Data from the Cooper Clinic Longitudinal Study do not support an elevated all-cause and CVD mortality risk associated with strenuous exercise in individuals with increased CAC burden:

- As expected, in each category of physical activity, men with CAC > 100 AU had much higher CVD and all-cause mortality risk than those with CAC < 100.
- Physically highly active men (>3000 MET-min/week) with comparatively low CAC scores (<100 AU) were half as likely to die than men with low levels of physical activity (<1500 MET-min/week) (HR (95%CI): 0.52 (0.29–0.91)) [7].
- In men with CAC scores >100 AU, the reduced risk of all-cause and CVD mortality with increasing physical activity did not reach statistical significance. It was still lower but somewhat attenuated in the highest category of physical activity.
- At other CAC-thresholds, i.e. CAC > 0 AU and CAC > 400 AU, findings were similar.

Unfortunately, DeFina et al. [7] did not match physically highly active men with controls showing similarly low traditional risk factor profiles but lower physical activity levels.

Others have suggested an inverse J-shaped curve for the association of long-term high-intensity strenuous exercise and event risk (see Chap. 42):

- In the Copenhagen City Heart Study, light and moderate joggers had a lower mortality risk than non-joggers, whereas strenuous joggers had a mortality rate not statistically different from that of the sedentary group [13].

That study was much debated, partly because of the very few events in the highest category of strenuous activity that may lead to a misinterpretation and overestimation of the clinical event rate in highly active joggers; moreover, the rate of sub-clinical atherosclerosis or myocardial fibrosis was unknown. Also, such a J-shaped association is not consistent across studies [13]. Nonetheless, the findings add to the existing evidence that highest-intensity physical exercise in a primary prevention general population setting acutely increases the risk of sudden death or acute myocardial infarction, especially in underlying subclinical disease. Yet, this risk progressively decreases with increasing habitual exercise, apparently also at its high-intensity extremes [12, 14, 15].

### 31.2.3 Implications

At present, it is unknown if regular high-intensity exercise *induces* coronary artery calcification, or if some degree of atherosclerosis at baseline is required for the calcification process to accelerate with highly strenuous exercise. Irrespective of how coronary atherosclerosis has developed, an advanced CAC burden is associated with increased rates of CAD/CVD events at least in some master athletes, just as in other populations. CAD/CVD event rates are low, but they clearly do occur in physically highly active persons, especially at an advanced age, even though we still have difficulties in predicting these events.

It is prudent that CAC imaging is considered as part of an advanced risk assessment especially in persons >50 years with present or past risk factors intending to commence or continue intensive exercise training. If CAC is present, risk factor optimization including statins and blood pressure control should be considered depending on its distribution and the non-calcified plaque morphology.

## 31.3 Myocardial Fibrosis

### 31.3.1 Etiology and Prevalence

Several diseases such as CAD, myocarditis, cardiomyopathy, hypertension, or valvular heart disease may lead to disintegrated myocardium, alterations in the interstitial myocardial space, and/or increased micro-vascular permeability. This may eventually result in increased fibrosis, i.e. an increase in myocardial collagen volume, via inflammation, myocardial strain, or ischemia. Such alterations, irrespective of being acute or chronic, cause gadolinium to reside within the myocardial interstitial space, which can be visualized as late gadolinium enhancement (LGE) using magnetic resonance imaging (MRI).

- Myocardial fibrosis has previously been reported at autopsy or biopsy in athlete case series [16], but its MRI-prevalence in vivo was first reported in 2008, being 12% in athletes aged >50 years [4].
- Wilson et al. reported a prevalence of 50% in a smaller cohort [17].
- In comparison, LGE-prevalence in the general population ranges between 4% and 10% but has been described to be as high as 20% in older adults [18–21].

Interestingly, marathon participation was associated with presence of LGE: doubling the number of marathon competitions led to a 65% increase in LGE-prevalence [4]. This was supported by a study in 12 life-long veteran athletes [17]. In that study, LGE presence was significantly associated with

(a) The number of years spent in training ($p < 0.001$)
(b) The number of previously finished competitive marathons ($p < 0.001$)
(c) The number of ultra-endurance (>50 miles) marathons ($p < 0.007$) completed

In competitive triathletes, exercise-induced hypertension and again competition history were independently predictive of LGE [22].

LGE in endurance athletes was not consistently confirmed across other studies for various reasons, mostly due to younger age [23–25]. Bohm et al. recently studied LGE in 33 athletes aged 47 years with a training history of 30 years. These authors found no LGE except for one athlete with presumed subclinical pericarditis

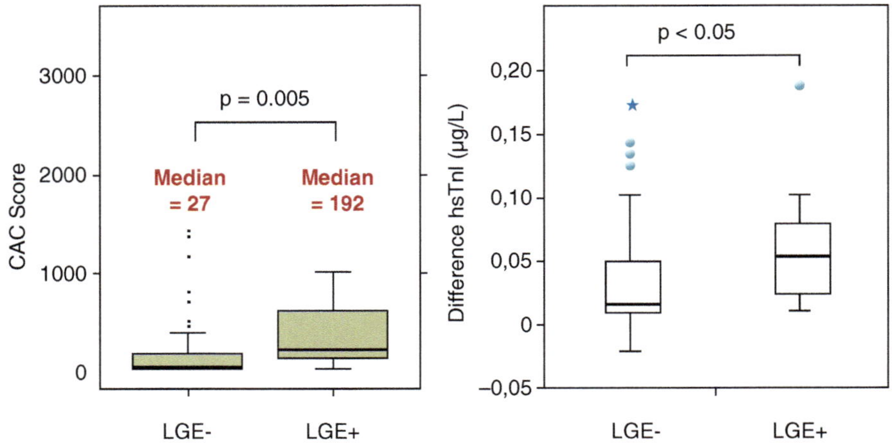


**Fig. 31.3** CAC Scores (left) and increase in cardiac troponin-values during a marathon race (right) by presence or absence of Late Gadolinium Enhancement (LGE) indicating myocardial fibrosis on Magnetic Resonance Imaging (MRI) in Marathon runners (right panel) (Reproduced with permission from [40])

[26]. These athletes were 10 years younger than the ones in the above-mentioned studies and it remains a matter of debate if long-term repetitive strenuous endurance exercise itself may *induce* myocardial fibrosis. It is likely, though, that myocardial fibrosis formation is *accelerated* by concomitant diseases such as hypertension, diabetes, coronary artery disease, or myocarditis, which do occur subclinically. This is supported by the observation that master marathon runners with LGE also had significantly more CAC than those without LGE (Fig. 31.3a), indicating a pathophysiological link between epicardial coronary disease, the intramyocardial microvasculature, and myocardial fibrosis.

### 31.3.2 Cardiac Biomarkers and Cardiac Function After Endurance Competitions

This paragraph addresses physiologic responses to endurance exercise, to better relate these findings to potentially pathologic observations (see below). Across various studies, about 50% of participants of endurance exercise competitions show cardiac troponin (cTn) elevation [27]. The possible mechanisms include exercise-induced increased myocardial cell permeability and stress-related myocardial cell necrosis. An association of cTn elevations with post-exercise cardiac dysfunction is not consistent across studies [27]. In 60 non-elite middle-aged marathon participants, Neilan et al. demonstrated significant increases in cTn and also NT-proBNP after the race, which correlated with post-race left ventricular diastolic and right ventricular dysfunction [28]. Interestingly, participants with lower training mileage had higher increases in cardiac biomarkers. These transient increases in biomarkers [29] and cardiac injury likely reflect cardiac fatigue, but it may be speculated that these responses to endurance exercise could have a role in fibrosis formation, if repeated often and intensely enough.

### 31.3.3 Myocardial Fibrosis and Cardiac Troponin

Marathon runners with LGE had higher cardiac troponin increases after a marathon competition (Fig. 31.3b). It is unclear though, if troponin was released from previously fibrotic myocardial arrays, or if troponin release in these runners indicated myocardial stress and strain that may eventually lead to cell death and increased collagen formation if only repeated often and intensely enough. Minor release of troponin is almost invariably seen after bouts of endurance exercise, possibly due to increased cell permeability in healthy athletes [14, 30]. Elevated troponin values usually normalize within 72 h [31]. In patients with CVD, such increases in troponin are much higher, and troponin kinetics are different. Future studies on the association of strenuous exercise, troponin release and myocardial fibrosis should therefore include repeat troponin measurements beyond 72 h.

### 31.3.4 Distribution of Myocardial Fibrosis

Another important aspect of myocardial fibrosis in athletes is its distribution. An **ischemic** subendocardial localization is usually distinguished from a **non-ischemic** mid-ventricular patchy pattern of LGE distribution, which is typically seen in myocarditis, cardiomyopathy, sarcoidosis etc. Overall, the LGE-patterns are as heterogeneous as their etiology.

Fibrosis unrelated to CVD may typically be located at the right ventricular septal insertion points. These sites seem particularly susceptible to functional strain during intense endurance exercise [32]:

- In 40 athletes aged 37 years (90% males), an acute reduction in RV function increased with race duration and correlated with increases in biomarkers of myocardial injury.
- LGE was again more prevalent in those athletes with a longer history of competitive sport [32].

### 31.3.5 Myocardial Fibrosis and Prognosis

LGE on MRI in athletes may have prognostic implications, especially in concurrence with evidence of subclinical CAD.

- In the Marathon study, runners with coronary events had a higher prevalence of LGE than those without events (57 versus 8%, $p = 0.003$), consistent with a Kaplan-Meier analysis (log-rank, $p < 0.0001$) [11].

- Others suggest that "myocardial fibrosis detected by LGE in cardiac studies of asymptomatic athletes performed for other non-clinical reasons should be treated as an incidental finding and not pursued" [16].

Indeed, data derived from a research setting should not result in clinical decisions. Given the generally excellent prognosis of asymptomatic athletes, and outcome data being limited to one study with few events [11], there is currently no clinical action required.

However, apart from athletic activity, in various other cohorts the presence of myocardial fibrosis as detected by MRI was indeed associated with substantially higher event rates. This was shown for

(a) Suspected myocarditis [33]
(b) Biopsy-proven myocarditis [34]
(c) Dilated cardiomyopathy [35]
(d) Hypertrophic cardiomyopathy [36]
(e) Sudden cardiac death survivors [37]
(f) Coronary artery disease [38]

It would thus be surprising if athletes without CAD were among the few groups in whom the presence of myocardial fibrosis was not linked to adverse events. Until better evidence is available, especially in older athletes, it seems prudent that advanced risk stratification in older athletes with ECG- or echo-abnormalities, especially when cardiac symptoms are present, or who simply are at an elevated CVD risk for other reasons, should include consideration of MRI with LGE. The implications of LGE in athletes at risk include

- Avoiding extreme bouts of exercise
- Wearing an ECG-watch during exercise, or
- Undergoing implantation of an event recorder.

## 31.4 Summary

Evidence accumulates that strenuous endurance exercise is associated with higher CAC burden. From all we know about the protective mechanisms of regular exercise [1], it seems unlikely that any intensity of exercise has a role in *inducing* the atherosclerotic process, but longitudinal studies are lacking. Strenuous endurance exercise may accelerate calcification in the presence of early or advanced atherosclerosis resulting from the exposure to current or past traditional CVD risk factors. Different from atherosclerosis, initial evidence suggests that repeat strenuous exercise may indeed induce and—once present—aggravate myocardial fibrosis, without presence of pre-clinical cardiac disease as a prerequisite. It has been acknowledged "that high-volume and -intensity training in the setting of pre-existing CAD or even remote and undiagnosed myocarditis can lead to adverse outcomes" [12]. With modern imaging techniques such as cardiac CT and cardiac MRI it is possible to visualize these pre-clinical disease states.

The question then is how to define "healthy"? How healthy does an athlete have to be for intensive exercise to cause no harm? Is intensive endurance exercise only healthy in the very healthy? Indeed, rates of myocardial infarction or revascularization are low in athletes, and mortality rates are even lower [7, 11]. Therefore, large longitudinal studies are needed to determine a dose-response- and cause-effect-relationship between repeated bouts of strenuous exercise, structural cardiac damage, and CVD events [39].

**Clinical Pearls**

- Long-term strenuous endurance exercise may induce or accelerate "structural cardiac damage" that is different from physiological adaptations in athletes' heart.
- Coronary artery calcification (CAC) may accelerate as a consequence of long-term endurance exercise. It is currently not clear if CAC in athletes generally represents "healthy hardening" and stable plaque or if it indicates an elevated CAD/CVD risk.
- Long-term repetitive strenuous exercise may induce and accelerate myocardial fibrosis. Myocardial fibrosis—as evidenced by late gadolinium enhancement using magnetic resonance imaging—has been linked with CAC and cardiac troponin after endurance exercise, and also with impaired outcome.

## Review

## Questions

1. An asymptomatic 65-year-old marathon runner presents for general cardiovascular check-up. He has already undergone coronary artery calcium (CAC) scoring because of a positive family history and a high-normal resting blood pressure. His Agatston Score is 529 (=high). What are the clinical implications?
   (a) A CAC score of 529 in an asymptomatic marathon runner has no clinical relevance. As he is asymptomatic, he can continue running without restriction.
   (b) The risk of a significant coronary artery stenosis is high. He should therefore directly undergo invasive coronary angiography and probably coronary artery stenting.
   (c) The Agatston score indicates calcified atherosclerosis. He may have an elevated risk of future coronary events. Additional testing for (subclinical) ischemia and risk factor modification should be considered.
   (d) The marathon runner is at elevated risk of a coronary event. He must be advised to stop running and rather pursue physical activity that is less strenuous at heart rates below 80% of maximum heart rate for age and sex.
   (e) The higher the Agatston score, the less likely it is for plaque to rupture. Therefore, he has "healthy hardening" and can be advised to continue running.

2. (I) Late gadolinium enhancement (LGE) in an endurance athlete is likely of no prognostic relevance
   Because
   (II) LGE in athletes often occurs at the hinge points where the right ventricular wall inserts into the interventricular septum.
   Which of the following combinations is true?
   (a) Statement (I) is correct, statement (II) is correct, the link is correct.
   (b) Statement (I) is incorrect, statement (II) is correct.
   (c) Statement (I) is correct, statement (II) is correct, the link is incorrect.
   (d) Statement (I) is correct, statement (II) is incorrect.
   (e) Both Statements are incorrect.

## Answers

1. Correct Answer: "C"
   Explanation:
   (a) This statement is false because a very high Agatston score, i.e. >400, is associated with a higher risk of coronary events. Therefore, a thorough risk factor assessment is warranted, and risk factors should be modified according to guidelines.
   (b) Even though the risk of luminal narrowing >50% somewhere in the coronary tree is high, there is no need for invasive angiography or stenting unless there is a relevant ischemic area at risk, i.e. >10% of myocardium.
   (c) This statement is correct. There is calcified plaque (most likely accompanied by non-calcified plaque) in the coronary arteries and a considerable risk of stenosis relevant for ischemia during strenuous exercise. Additional ischemia testing should hence be considered, and risk factors should be modified according to guidelines.
   (d) This statement is not true. There is currently no evidence that ceasing endurance exercise improves prognosis in asymptomatic cohorts even in the presence of advanced subclinical atherosclerosis. Quite the opposite: regular exercise at moderate intensity and duration prevents events also in persons with CAD.
   (e) This statement is false. A high plaque density has been suggested to be somewhat protective of plaque rupture, but this cannot be concluded from the Agatston score, which is an index derived from calcified plaque area and density.
2. Correct Answer: "B"
   Explanation:
   Even though evidence is still limited, the presence of LGE has been shown to increase cardiac event risk in many clinical entities, including CAD, cardiomyopathy, myocarditis, sarcoidosis, etc. Initial evidence suggests that this also holds in master athletes without a history of CAD. It is likely that this elevated risk associated with LGE is generally true. Evidence accumulates that LGE in

athletes often occurs at the insertion points of the RV wall into the interventricular septum, but this depends on the age and history of the cohort studied. Other patterns and locations have been published.

## References


1. Schuler G, Adams V, Goto Y. Role of exercise in the prevention of cardiovascular disease: results, mechanisms, and new perspectives. Eur Heart J. 2013;34(24):1790–9.
2. La Gerche A, Heidbuchel H. Can intensive exercise harm the heart? You can get too much of a good thing. Circulation. 2014;130(12):992–1002.
3. Mohlenkamp S, Schmermund A, Kroger K, Kerkhoff G, Brocker-Preuss M, Adams V, et al. Coronary atherosclerosis and cardiovascular risk in masters male marathon runners. Rationale and design of the "marathon study". Herz. 2006;31(6):575–85.
4. Mohlenkamp S, Lehmann N, Breuckmann F, Brocker-Preuss M, Nassenstein K, Halle M, et al. Running: the risk of coronary events : prevalence and prognostic relevance of coronary atherosclerosis in marathon runners. Eur Heart J. 2008;29(15):1903–10.
5. Thompson PD, Balady GJ, Chaitman BR, Clark LT, Levine BD, Myerburg RJ. Task force 6: coronary artery disease. J Am Coll Cardiol. 2005;45(8):1348–53.
6. Schwartz RS, Kraus SM, Schwartz JG, Wickstrom KK, Peichel G, Garberich RF, et al. Increased coronary artery plaque volume among male Marathon runners. Mo Med. 2014;111(2):89–94.
7. DeFina LF, Radford NB, Barlow CE, Willis BL, Leonard D, Haskell WL, et al. Association of all-cause and cardiovascular mortality with high levels of physical activity and concurrent coronary artery calcification. JAMA Cardiol. 2019;4:174–81.
8. Erbel R, Mohlenkamp S, Moebus S, Schmermund A, Lehmann N, Stang A, et al. Coronary risk stratification, discrimination, and reclassification improvement based on quantification of subclinical coronary atherosclerosis: the Heinz Nixdorf Recall Study. J Am Coll Cardiol. 2010;56(17):1397–406.
9. Yeboah J, McClelland RL, Polonsky TS, Burke GL, Sibley CT, O'Leary D, et al. Comparison of novel risk markers for improvement in cardiovascular risk assessment in intermediate-risk individuals. JAMA. 2012;308(8):788–95.
10. Criqui MH, Denenberg JO, Ix JH, McClelland RL, Wassel CL, Rifkin DE, et al. Calcium density of coronary artery plaque and risk of incident cardiovascular events. JAMA. 2014;311(3):271–8.
11. Mohlenkamp S, Leineweber K, Lehmann N, Braun S, Roggenbuck U, Perrey M, et al. Coronary atherosclerosis burden, but not transient troponin elevation, predicts long-term outcome in recreational marathon runners. Basic Res Cardiol. 2014;109(1):391.
12. Levine BD. Can intensive exercise harm the heart? The benefits of competitive endurance training for cardiovascular structure and function. Circulation. 2014;130(12):987–91.
13. Schnohr P, O'Keefe JH, Marott JL, Lange P, Jensen GB. Dose of jogging and long-term mortality: the Copenhagen City Heart Study. J Am Coll Cardiol. 2015;65(5):411–9.
14. Eijsvogels TM, Molossi S, Lee DC, Emery MS, Thompson PD. Exercise at the extremes: the amount of exercise to reduce cardiovascular events. J Am Coll Cardiol. 2016;67(3):316–29.
15. Maron BJ. The paradox of exercise. N Engl J Med. 2000;343(19):1409–11.
16. van de Schoor FR, Aengevaeren VL, Hopman MT, Oxborough DL, George KP, Thompson PD, et al. Myocardial fibrosis in athletes. Mayo Clin Proc. 2016;91(11):1617–31.
17. Wilson M, O'Hanlon R, Prasad S, Deighan A, Macmillan P, Oxborough D, et al. Diverse patterns of myocardial fibrosis in lifelong, veteran endurance athletes. J Appl Physiol (1985). 2011;110(6):1622–6.
18. Barbier CE, Bjerner T, Johansson L, Lind L, Ahlstrom H. Myocardial scars more frequent than expected: magnetic resonance imaging detects potential risk group. J Am Coll Cardiol. 2006;48(4):765–71.

19. Breuckmann F, Mohlenkamp S, Nassenstein K, Lehmann N, Ladd S, Schmermund A, et al. Myocardial late gadolinium enhancement: prevalence, pattern, and prognostic relevance in marathon runners. Radiology. 2009;251(1):50–7.
20. Schelbert EB, Cao JJ, Sigurdsson S, Aspelund T, Kellman P, Aletras AH, et al. Prevalence and prognosis of unrecognized myocardial infarction determined by cardiac magnetic resonance in older adults. JAMA. 2012;308(9):890–6.
21. Turkbey EB, Nacif MS, Guo M, McClelland RL, Teixeira PB, Bild DE, et al. Prevalence and correlates of myocardial scar in a US cohort. JAMA. 2015;314(18):1945–54.
22. Tahir E, Starekova J, Muellerleile K, von Stritzky A, Munch J, Avanesov M, et al. Myocardial fibrosis in competitive triathletes detected by contrast-enhanced CMR correlates with exercise-induced hypertension and competition history. JACC Cardiovasc Imaging. 2018;11(9):1260–70.
23. Hanssen H, Keithahn A, Hertel G, Drexel V, Stern H, Schuster T, et al. Magnetic resonance imaging of myocardial injury and ventricular torsion after marathon running. Clin Sci (Lond). 2011;120(4):143–52.
24. Mousavi N, Czarnecki A, Kumar K, Fallah-Rad N, Lytwyn M, Han SY, et al. Relation of biomarkers and cardiac magnetic resonance imaging after marathon running. Am J Cardiol. 2009;103(10):1467–72.
25. Trivax JE, Franklin BA, Goldstein JA, Chinnaiyan KM, Gallagher MJ, deJong AT, et al. Acute cardiac effects of marathon running. J Appl Physiol (1985). 2010;108(5):1148–53.
26. Bohm P, Schneider G, Linneweber L, Rentzsch A, Kramer N, Abdul-Khaliq H, et al. Right and left ventricular function and mass in male elite master athletes: a controlled contrast-enhanced cardiovascular magnetic resonance study. Circulation. 2016;133(20):1927–35.
27. Shave R, Baggish A, George K, Wood M, Scharhag J, Whyte G, et al. Exercise-induced cardiac troponin elevation: evidence, mechanisms, and implications. J Am Coll Cardiol. 2010;56(3):169–76.
28. Neilan TG, Januzzi JL, Lee-Lewandrowski E, Ton-Nu TT, Yoerger DM, Jassal DS, et al. Myocardial injury and ventricular dysfunction related to training levels among nonelite participants in the Boston marathon. Circulation. 2006;114(22):2325–33.
29. Scharhag J, Herrmann M, Urhausen A, Haschke M, Herrmann W, Kindermann W. Independent elevations of N-terminal pro-brain natriuretic peptide and cardiac troponins in endurance athletes after prolonged strenuous exercise. Am Heart J. 2005;150(6):1128–34.
30. Scharhag J, Urhausen A, Schneider G, Herrmann M, Schumacher K, Haschke M, et al. Reproducibility and clinical significance of exercise-induced increases in cardiac troponins and N-terminal pro brain natriuretic peptide in endurance athletes. Eur J Cardiovasc Prev Rehabil. 2006;13(3):388–97.
31. Scherr J, Braun S, Schuster T, Hartmann C, Moehlenkamp S, Wolfarth B, et al. 72-h kinetics of high-sensitive troponin T and inflammatory markers after marathon. Med Sci Sports Exerc. 2011;43(10):1819–27.
32. La Gerche A, Burns AT, Mooney DJ, Inder WJ, Taylor AJ, Bogaert J, et al. Exercise-induced right ventricular dysfunction and structural remodelling in endurance athletes. Eur Heart J. 2012;33(8):998–1006.
33. Grani C, Eichhorn C, Biere L, Murthy VL, Agarwal V, Kaneko K, et al. Prognostic value of cardiac magnetic resonance tissue characterization in risk stratifying patients with suspected myocarditis. J Am Coll Cardiol. 2017;70(16):1964–76.
34. Grun S, Schumm J, Greulich S, Wagner A, Schneider S, Bruder O, et al. Long-term follow-up of biopsy-proven viral myocarditis: predictors of mortality and incomplete recovery. J Am Coll Cardiol. 2012;59(18):1604–15.
35. Halliday BP, Gulati A, Ali A, Guha K, Newsome S, Arzanauskaite M, et al. Association between Midwall late gadolinium enhancement and sudden cardiac death in patients with dilated cardiomyopathy and mild and moderate left ventricular systolic dysfunction. Circulation. 2017;135(22):2106–15.

36. Chan RH, Maron BJ, Olivotto I, Pencina MJ, Assenza GE, Haas T, et al. Prognostic value of quantitative contrast-enhanced cardiovascular magnetic resonance for the evaluation of sudden death risk in patients with hypertrophic cardiomyopathy. Circulation. 2014;130(6):484–95.
37. Neilan TG, Farhad H, Mayrhofer T, Shah RV, Dodson JA, Abbasi SA, et al. Late gadolinium enhancement among survivors of sudden cardiac arrest. JACC Cardiovasc Imaging. 2015;8(4):414–23.
38. Kwong RY, Chan AK, Brown KA, Chan CW, Reynolds HG, Tsang S, et al. Impact of unrecognized myocardial scar detected by cardiac magnetic resonance imaging on event-free survival in patients presenting with signs or symptoms of coronary artery disease. Circulation. 2006;113(23):2733–43.
39. Mohlenkamp S, Heusch G, Erbel R. Letter by Mohlenkamp et al regarding articles, "can intensive exercise harm the heart? The benefits of competitive endurance training for cardiovascular structure and function" and "can intensive exercise harm the heart? You can get too much of a good thing". Circulation. 2015;131(23):e524.
40. Mohlenkamp S, Heusch G, Erbel R. Cardiovascular risks of strenuous physical exercise. Aktuell Kardiol. 2014;3(6):355–60.

# The Role of Imaging

# 32

Axel Pressler and Stefan Möhlenkamp

**Learning Objectives**

1. Indications for the stepwise integration of advanced imaging techniques in the diagnostic work-up of recreational/master athletes.
2. Cardiovascular risks during sports participation particularly pertaining to recreational/master athletes and how to optimally implement advanced imaging as part of risk stratification.
3. Differentiating athlete's heart from conditions that are of particular relevance in recreational/master athletes, such as hypertension.
4. Significance of findings during advanced imaging with respect to continued sports participation, e.g. increased coronary calcium burden or myocardial fibrosis.

## 32.1 Introduction

At least in symptomatic athletes or in those with equivocal findings during basic screening examinations, the appropriate application of further imaging techniques is crucial to detect, graduate and potentially treat cardiac conditions that may pose an increased risk for continued sports participation [1]. This primarily refers to the prevention of acute cardiac events such as sudden cardiac death (SCD) during sports, but also involves both negative and positive effects on the development and the clinical course of chronic cardiac disorders. This is of particular relevance in

A. Pressler
Private Center of Sports & Exercise Cardiology, Munich, Germany
e-mail: axel.pressler@kardiologie-mit-herz.de

S. Möhlenkamp (✉)
Clinic of Cardiology and Intensive Care Medicine, Bethanien Hospital Moers, Moers, Germany
e-mail: stefan.moehlenkamp@bethanienmoers.de



A. Pressler, J. Niebauer (eds.), *Textbook of Sports and Exercise Cardiology*,
https://doi.org/10.1007/978-3-030-35374-2_32

recreational/master athletes, since these individuals very often perform strenuous and high-intensity activities such as marathon or triathlon in a non-organized and non-supervised fashion, and the number of individuals participating in these events has increased massively over the past decades [2]. In addition, recreational/master athletes are usually at least middle-aged and have very often been exposed to elevated cardiovascular risk factor profiles over a longer period of time as compared to young competitive athletes. Therefore, advanced imaging rather focuses on improved risk stratification and the detection of coronary artery disease (CAD) as the main cause of SCD in this cohort than on detecting inherited or acquired cardiomyopathies [2].

Thus, this chapter particularly focuses on the role of advanced imaging techniques as part of the clinical and diagnostic work-up of recreational/master athletes and the differences to young competitive athletes; regarding the latter, the reader is referred to Part 1 of this book.

## 32.2 Echocardiography

In recreational/master athletes, similar to young competitive athletes (see Chap. 9), echocardiography mainly aims at detecting any structural or functional disorder that may be associated with an increased risk of sports participation. While in young athletes this usually pertains to cardiomyopathies at risk of SCD, middle-aged athletes are likely to show a much higher prevalence of chronic alterations as a consequence of longstanding exposure to cardiovascular risk factors, such as degenerative valvular heart disease and, in particular, hypertension [2]. Thus, a rather common clinical scenario in this subgroup of athletes is to determine the pathophysiologic background of mild left ventricular hypertrophy, which can either be induced by

(a) Intensive endurance exercise
(b) Early hypertensive heart disease, or
(c) Even moderate aortic valve stenosis

In addition, increased left atrial size or enlarged diameters of the ascending aorta may also represent a diagnostic conundrum, which could result in serious long-term consequences if not diagnosed and treated adequately [1, 3].

However, in contrast to the wealth of literature on the differentiation of athlete's heart from underlying pathologies in young competitive athletes, there is still a surprising paucity of studies focusing solely on recreational/master athletes. In light of this, usually the same reference values for cardiac dimensions as well as accepted upper limits of normal are applied (see Chap. 9).

Nonetheless, both parameters of diastolic and systolic left ventricular function appear to be useful in differentiating sports-induced hypertrophy from hypertensive heart disease according to at least small studies:

- *Limongelli* et al. compared 30 master athletes (age 43.9 ± 5.9 years) to 20 age-matched hypertensive non-athletes, 20 patients with hypertrophic cardiomyopathy (HCM), and 30 healthy individuals with respect to allometrically scaled left ventricular mass (LVM/height$^{2.7}$). Athletes had higher LVM than controls, but lower values compared to patients; systolic function assessed by fractional shortening and ejection fraction was normal in athletes, but lower in hypertensive and higher in HCM patients. Regarding diastolic function, an abnormal relaxation pattern was observed in almost all patients but in no athlete or control subject [4].
- Galanti et al. compared 80 master athletes with 80 sedentary hypertensive control subjects matched for wall thickness, all of which showing normal traditional diastolic relaxation patterns. However, application of tissue-Doppler derived parameters of diastolic function clearly discriminated between groups: values were normal in master athletes (E′ 9.4 ± 3.1 cm/s; E/E′ 7.8 ± 2.1) but significantly lower/higher in hypertensive subjects (E′ 7.2 ± 2.4 cm/s; E/E′ 10.6 ± 3.2; $p < 0.001$) indicating impaired diastolic function in the latter group [5].
- Using speckle-tracking echocardiography, Galderisi et al. compared 22 elite rowers to 18 newly diagnosed, untreated age-matched hypertensive patients and 19 sedentary controls. Both rowers and hypertensive patients showed higher LVM indices, but annular systolic (s′) and early diastolic (e′) velocities were significantly higher, and E/e′ was lower in patients ($p < 0.0001$). In addition, global longitudinal strain (GLS) was significantly lower in hypertensive subjects (−17.5 ± 2.8%) as compared to athletes (−22.2 ± 2.7%) and controls (−21.2 ± 2.0%; $p < 0.0001$). Both GLS and E/e′-ratio were statistically accurate in discriminating patients with hypertension from athletes and controls [6].

These studies confirm that left ventricular hypertrophy in recreational/master athletes as a consequence of long-term intensive sports participation does usually not result in impaired systolic and diastolic function, as assessed by both traditional and novel echocardiographic parameters.

### 32.2.1 Indications for Echocardiography in Recreational/Master Athletes

Echocardiography is not regarded as an essential part of pre-participation screening in the majority of countries. Nonetheless it may be of more value in recreational/master athletes who are very likely to having accumulated a higher cardiovascular risk during their lifetime when compared to young competitive athletes. According to the latest recommendations of the European Association of Preventive Cardiology (EAPC) and the European Association of Cardiovascular Imaging (EACVI) [1], the indications to perform echocardiography (and other examinations) are summarized in the Table 32.1.

**Table 32.1** Indications for advanced cardiac imaging in athletes as recommended by the European Association of Preventive Cardiology (EAPC) and the European Association of Cardiovascular Imaging (EACVI) (modified from data presented in [1])

| | Echocardiography | CCT | CMR | Nuclear imaging |
|---|---|---|---|---|
| *Clinical history* | | | | |
| SCD or known cardiomyopathy in the family | + | | + | |
| Palpitations | + | | | |
| Syncope | | | + | |
| Chest pain | + | + | + | + |
| *Physical examination* | | | | |
| Cardiac murmurs or abnormal cardiac sound | + | | | |
| Marfanoid habitus | + | + | + | |
| *12-leads ECG* | | | | |
| T wave inversion | + | | + | |
| ST segment depression | + | | + | |
| Pathologic Q waves | + | | + | |
| Complete LBBB | + | + | + | + |
| Bifascicular block (RBBB and LAH) | + | | | |
| Non-specific intraventricular conduction delay | + | | | |
| Minor non-voltage criteria for LV or RV hypertrophy (atrial enlargement and QRS axis deviation) | + | | | |
| Abnormal exercise testing (repolarization abnormalities/symptoms/arrhythmias) | + | + | + | + |

*CCT* coronary computed tomography, *CMR* cardiac magnetic resonance imaging, *SCD* sudden cardiac death, *ECG* electrocardiogram, *LBBB* left bundle branch block, *RBBB* right bundle branch block, *LAH* left anterior hemiblock, *LV* left ventricle, *RV* right ventricle

## 32.3 Exercise Echocardiography

In the diagnostic work-up of recreational/master athletes, exercise stress echocardiography is primarily applied as a reliable non-invasive methodology to provide information on cardiac function, contractile reserve, exercise capabilities, and arrhythmias, which can be combined with clinical and ECG data and contribute to detect cardiac abnormalities. It is usually recommended to perform exercise stress echocardiography rather than applying pharmacologic agents such as dobutamine, since the latter may not adequately reproduce physical exertion [3].

### 32.3.1 Indications for Exercise Echocardiography in Recreational/ Master Athletes

- Evaluation of global and regional cardiac function during exercise in cases of suspected CAD or coronary anomalies, in individuals with chest pain symptoms, abnormal ECG or doubtful ECG stress testing [3].
- Assessment of ventricular function during exercise, particularly in cases of mildly reduced ventricular systolic function and/or equivocally dilated chambers.

In these cases, exercise echocardiography enables the assessment of contractile reserve of the dilated ventricles, with a significant improvement in contractility during physical exertion, suggesting a physiological response [3, 7].

- Assessment of hemodynamic responses during exercise in valvular heart disease, such as changing pressure gradients or increasing pulmonary artery pressure. This may be helpful in evaluating whether exertional dyspnea may be attributed to a particular valve defect and in guiding advice on continued sports participation [3, 7, 8].

## 32.4 Coronary Computed Tomography

Coronary computed tomography (CCT) allows high-resolution imaging of coronary atherosclerosis and other coronary pathology, such as abnormal origin of coronary arteries or myocardial bridging [9–12]. Moreover, CCT allows additional visualization and quantification of vessel wall morphology including plaque imaging. Since CAD is the main cause of SCD in the mostly middle-aged group of recreational/master athletes (see Chap. 6), CCT plays a major role in the expanded diagnostic work-up of this particular group; many of these athletes may show an elevated risk profile due to an unhealthy lifestyle prior to regular sports participation. In contrast, in young competitive athletes CCT finally confirms or excludes coronary artery anomalies, if this is suspected either due to symptoms or due to equivocal echocardiographic findings in asymptomatic athletes (see Chaps. 9 and 22) [13–15].

### 32.4.1 Indications for CCT in Recreational/Master Athletes

Basically, the indications for CCT as part of clinical work-up do not differ from non-athletes (see also the Table 32.1); they are based on

(a) Additional work-up of symptoms suggestive of relevant CAD such as chest pain or discomfort.
(b) Additional work-up of asymptomatic athletes in case of pathologic findings in previous examinations indicative of relevant CAD [12, 16–18].
(c) Additional work-up of asymptomatic athletes as part of improved risk stratification.

According to the *2010 ACCF/AHA Guideline for Assessment of Cardiovascular Risk in Asymptomatic Adults*, particularly in asymptomatic adults at intermediate risk (10–20% 10-year risk) (Class IIa B), and—with less certainty—in individuals at low to intermediate risk (6–10% 10-year risk) (Class IIb B) CCT may contribute to risk stratification by virtue of quantifying coronary artery calcium [10].

However, it is still a matter of debate whether data from general populations are also valid for an athletic population and which athletes may benefit from CCT with regard to diagnostic and therapeutic implications [13, 19, 20].

**Coronary artery calcium scoring (CAC)** is a non-invasive measure of the presence, localization and extent of coronary atherosclerosis; in contrast, it is not a marker of rupture-prone plaque or the degree of potential coronary artery stenosis at the site of CAC.

- Several studies have demonstrated that the presence and extent of calcified plaque burden is closely linked with future CVD events [21–23].
- Surprisingly, several studies in recent years have shown that in recreational/master athletes there may be a higher degree of CAC burden when compared to non-athletes (Fig. 32.1) [24]; this is also referred to in more detail the previous Chap. 32.
- Usually, various studies have proposed a CAC-score > 100 as a threshold raising increased risk awareness [25] and initiate statin treatment.
- According to recent AHA guidelines on the management of dyslipidaemias, CAC is suggested in patients with elevated 10-year-risk of CVD to help guiding the decision on statin treatment [26].
- Long-term follow-up data further suggest that increased coronary plaque burden, as measured by coronary CT, is associated with worse outcome also in athletes [27].
  - Marathon runners had a similar coronary event rate for every given category of CAC as controls matched for age or age- and risk-factors [27].

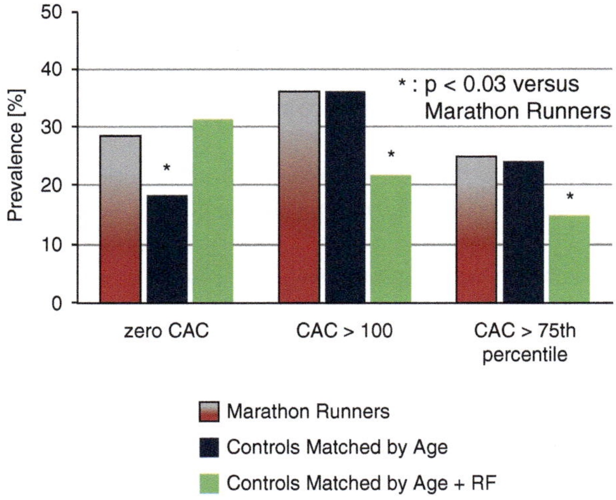


**Fig. 32.1** Calcified coronary plaque burden (coronary artery calcium, CAC) as measured by coronary CT in athletes. Marathon runners (red) had more often no CAC compared to age-matched controls (black) but similar prevalence of advanced CAC, as determined by clinically established thresholds of CAC > 100 and CAC > 75th percentile. However, controls that were matched by age and risk factors, i.e. those who presumably have had a beneficial risk factor profile throughout their lives, had less CAC compared to athletes [24]

**Coronary Computed Tomography Angiography (CCTA)** has been evaluated in only a few studies in athletes (see also Chap. 32):

- *Schwartz* et al. assessed 50 runners having participated in at least one annual marathon race over the past 25 years [28]. Compared to sedentary controls (n = 23), athletes had increased total plaque volumes (200 vs. 126 mm$^3$, $p < 0.01$), calcified plaque volumes (84 vs. 44 mm$^3$, $p < 0.0001$), and non-calcified plaque volumes (116 vs. 82 mm$^3$, $p = 0.04$).
- *Tsiflikas* et al. invited 50 male runners aged >45 years (mean 53 ± 6 years) to undergo CCTA, standard risk assessment and pre-participation screening [29]. The runners had completed a mean of 13.8 marathons (range: 1–72). Despite low PROCAM risk scores (1.9% in 10 years; range 0.39–8.5%), 48% of runners had some degree of atherosclerosis, and 10% had a CAC score > 100. Athletes with CAD on CCTA were 3.5 years older and had slightly higher blood pressures, PROCAM-scores, and individual best finishing times.
- Karlstedt et al. recruited 25 elite marathon runners (55 ± 4 years, 84% males) having finished ≥3 marathons during the preceding 2 years [30]. Participants had to be free of hypertension, dyslipidaemia, and diabetes and had to be never-smokers, but still two runners (8%) showed >70% stenosis on CCTA.
- *Ermolao* et al. evaluated 940 consecutive asymptomatic athletes (aged 45 ± 7 years, 84% males) and performed treadmill- or bicycle-stress-testing prior to high-intensity, mostly competitive sports activities [31]. Only those athletes with pathologic or equivocal ST-segment or repolarization changes (n = 46 (4.9%)) underwent CCTA. Of those, 52% did not have evidence of CAD, but 32% had CAD. The latter were 10 years older (not significant), had more hypertension and a higher risk score. Coronary anomalies were detected in n = 5 athletes (11.4%). Six athletes (14%) had significant (>50%) proximal stenosis.

Recently, high-risk plaque features on high-resolution CCTA were characterized. These include

(a) Low attenuation plaques (0–30 HU) suggestive of lipid-rich plaque
(b) Positive remodelling >110% reflecting the Glagov-phenomenon
(c) Spotty calcification/napkin ring sign, which has been associated with thin-cap fibroatheroma (TCFA) and increased coronary event rates [32, 33]

In addition, measuring fractional flow reserve (FFR) using cardiac CT imaging ($FFR_{CT}$) has been proposed as a non-invasive tool to assess functional consequences of epicardial stenoses on CT images [34]. Whether these additional morphologic and functional CT-derived parameters contribute to a more accurate diagnosis, to guide therapy and to improve outcomes in athletes remains to be shown.

### 32.4.2 Additional Considerations

The goal of advanced imaging is to avoid CVD events at appropriately low side-effects and costs. Regarding CCT, the following issues have to be considered:

- **Radiation**: CCT imaging exposes the athlete to radiation (<1 mSv for CAC scoring, and <1 up to ~10 mSv for CCTA, with low values for lean athletes with low heart rates) [35, 36].
- **Contrast agent**: CCTA requires administration of ~100 cc of contrast agent and necessitates normal thyroid and (near-)normal kidney function.
- **Costs and availability**: Both issues, as well as expertise in the use of CCT imaging in athletes, can vary considerably and must be weighed against the expected improvement in prognosis due to imaging.
  - To date, no studies have analysed cost-effectiveness of CCT imaging in athletes.
  - Initial data from clinical cohorts suggest that CCT imaging may be cost-effective under limited conditions [37–39].
  - Thus, it is not recommended as a broad screening tool in low-risk cohorts but should be considered as a second-line technology in athletes.

## 32.5 Nuclear Imaging

Myocardial perfusion imaging by means of scintigraphy (SPECT) is an established non-invasive method for detecting CAD [40, 41].

1. It is a powerful prognostic indicator in patients with known or suspected CAD [42].
2. It improves risk stratification in individuals without known CAD [43] and in those with high exercise tolerance, i.e. above 12 METs on the Bruce treadmill protocol [44].
3. A normal nuclear stress test is associated with an excellent prognosis for CAD or CVD events.

Likewise, SPECT is not a first line diagnostic test because of costs and radiation (~3–10 mSv) [36]. Few small-sized studies have addressed the role of SPECT imaging specifically in athletes [3]:

- In 18 young male elite athletes, myocardial perfusion defects were associated with left ventricular hypertrophy, resulting in low specificity in athletes with chest pain [45], which is in line with another study [46].
- Because of several unexpected cardiac deaths in Swedish orienteers in the 1980s, Andersson et al. used Thallium-201 perfusion imaging at rest to search for evidence of myocardial fibrosis. Perfusion defects were associated with left ventricular mass and body weight in orienteers and athlete controls but were unrelated to wall-motion abnormalities on echocardiography [47].

- Others have used nuclear imaging techniques such as [$^{18}$F]-FDG positron emission tomography (PET) or $^{123}$I-MIBG scintigraphy in athletes especially in research settings, but the clinical role of these imaging modalities is uncertain, especially in asymptomatic athletes [3].
- Siegel et al. used myocardial scintigraphy to exclude relevant myocardial cell necrosis in marathon runners with elevated post-race CK-MB or cardiac troponin levels [48, 49].

Yet, nuclear imaging has not been shown in larger studies to allow identification of coronary or myocardial disease in symptomatic or asymptomatic athletes. Similar to stress echocardiography, it should be noted that positive findings in athletes undergoing nuclear imaging might be missed if pharmacologic agents are used or if they are not encouraged to attain maximal exhaustion.

Single case studies suggest a mismatch between advanced coronary atherosclerosis burden and comparatively small myocardial perfusion defects in athletes:

- A 64-year-old asymptomatic marathon runner underwent CCTA due to unexpected signs of ischemia on exercise testing, which revealed relevant atherosclerosis with >50% stenosis (Fig. 32.2a). An additional SPECT demonstrated no evidence of ischemia (Fig. 32.2b). He received aggressive risk factor control [20], but RCA-stenting was performed 2 years later at a different clinic.
- A 57-year-old asymptomatic runner underwent CAC as a study participant (score = 210 (77th percentile)). He had elevated blood pressure and Lp(a) levels, but LDL-cholesterol was only 107 mg/dl; blood pressure lowering medication was initiated. Four years later, he suffered from atypical chest pain radiating to his left shoulder during running (but not during high-intensity cycling). His CAC score had increased to 416 (79th percentile). On 99mTc-MIBI scintigraphy he had very mild reversible ischemia (6–10%) (Fig. 32.3a). Nonetheless, CCTA revealed severe LAD-stenosis and myocardial bridging, confirmed by subsequent invasive coronary angiography (Fig. 32.3b) [27].

These cases indicate a discrepancy of no or minimal findings on SPECT imaging despite the presence of advanced coronary artery disease. Interestingly, others have observed the opposite, i.e. relevant ischemia in the absence of coronary atherosclerosis or other pathology (“Athlete’s Syndrome X”) [50]:

- A well-trained 55-year-old male athlete complained of reduced exercise capacity.
  - History of infectious mononucleosis at 23, positive family history for CAD.
  - SPECT revealed frequency-dependent left bundle branch block and ischemia in antero-septal and inferior regions in four of the 18 segments, but coronary angiography showed no atherosclerosis.
  - Statin and calcium antagonist treatment was initiated.

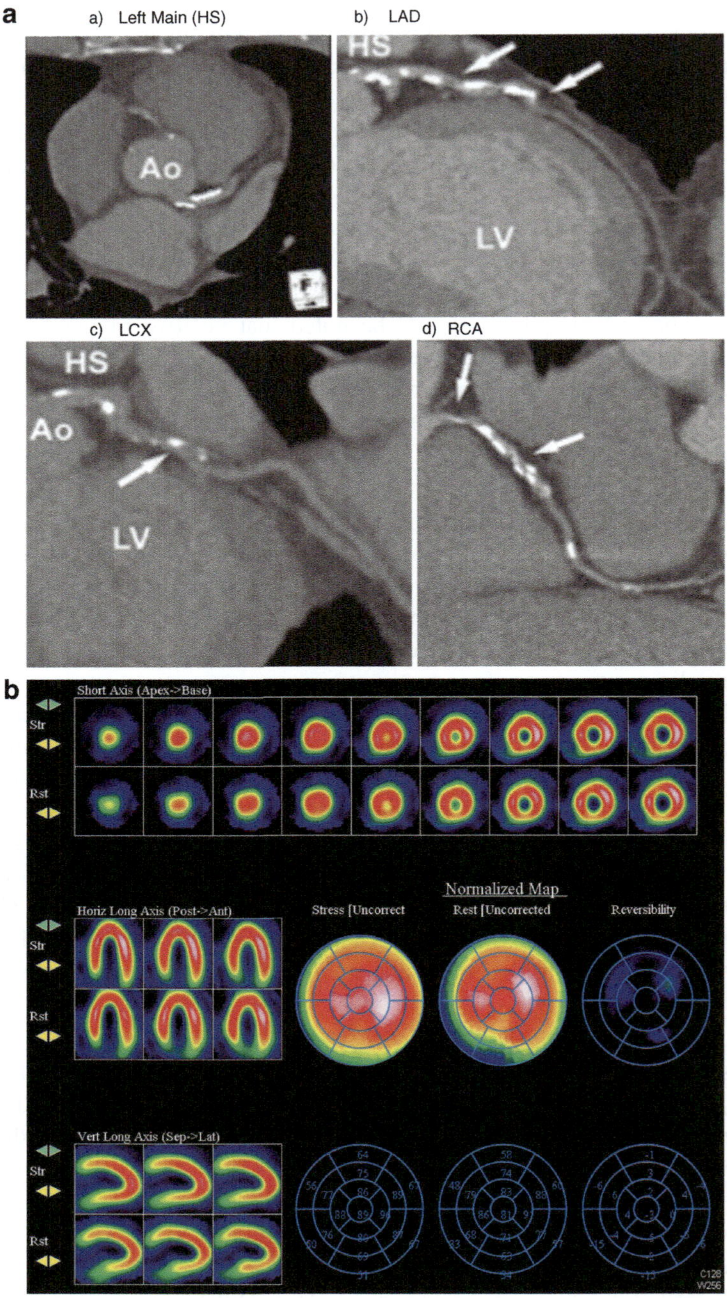


**Fig. 32.2** (**a**) Multi-slice CT-angiography with multiplanar reconstruction of all coronary arteries showing severe calcification especially in the proximal segments including the left main. A detailed analysis showed no left main obstruction, but high suspicion of significant stenoses in several segments (white arrows). (**b**) Myocardial scintigraphy during bicycle stress testing up to 225 W showing no evidence of stress-induced reversible perfusion deficit (Reproduced with permission from [20]). *Ao* aortic root, *HS* left main, *LV* left ventricle

- Seven years later, this athlete was admitted with exercise-induced aborted sudden death. CMR was completely normal, and there was no evidence for a channelopathy.
- He received an automated external defibrillator, but the pathophysiological background remained unclear.

Overall, normal findings on SPECT may not necessarily rule out even severe coronary artery disease in athletes. However, pathologic findings may indicate severe cardiac disease despite the absence of atherosclerosis or cardiomyopathy; evidence if ischemia during SPECT thus requires careful and regular clinical follow-up of athletes.

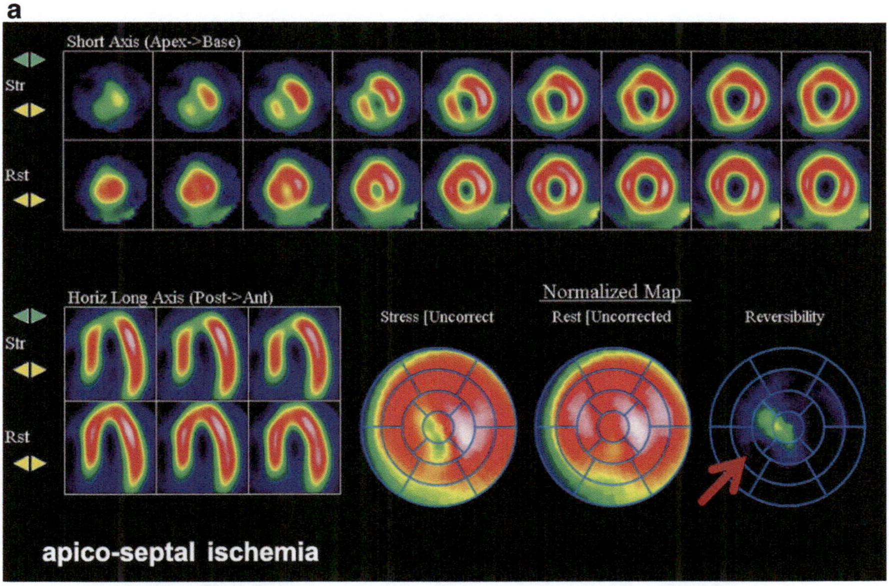


**Fig. 32.3** (**a**) Myocardial perfusion scintigraphy in a runner with exertional fatigue, mild late gadolinium enhancement on MRI, and high coronary artery calcium (CAC) scores. A small ischemic array at the apex and the apico-septal segment, suggesting that life-style and risk factor modification may be sufficient in this runner (see text for details). (**b**) This same runner underwent invasive angiography showing several severe stenoses (>75%, red arrows top) and a long myocardial bridge of the LAD (red arrows, bottom). This runner did not receive PTCA/stents or coronary artery bypass grafts (CABG) (Reproduced with permission from [27])

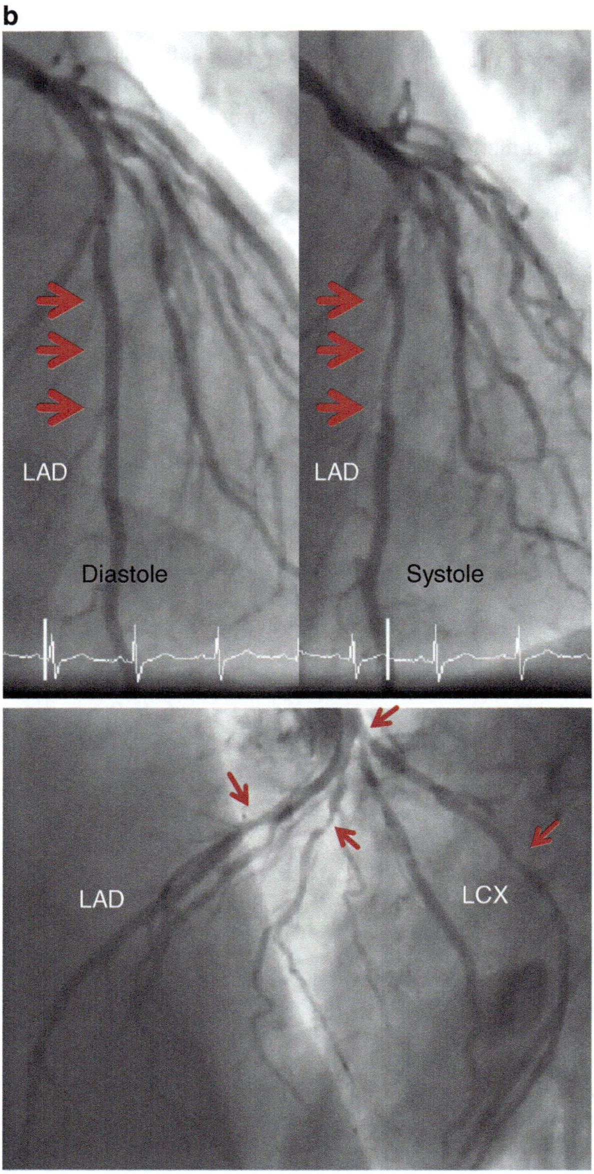


Fig. 32.3 (continued)

## 32.6 Cardiac Magnetic Resonance Imaging (CMR)

CMR imaging is a second-line diagnostic tool, but its application has steadily increased in recent years since

1. It is considered the gold standard to confirm or to largely exclude inherited or acquired cardiomyopathies.
2. Its diagnostic value goes beyond echocardiography, e.g. in the work-up of pathological ECG alterations, the morphologic correlates of which may be missed by traditional ultrasound techniques (Table 32.1).
3. It is increasingly applied to more accurately define chamber sizes and ventricular function or to characterize the amount and degree of hypertrabeculation, with the primary intention to establish baseline findings for comparative follow-up examinations.

Of note, CMR usually shows larger cardiac dimensions and volumes, lower ejection fractions and smaller wall thickness and mass, compared with echocardiography [51]. Reference values derived from echocardiography should thus not uncritically be applied to CMR results in athletes.

In recreational/master athletes the indication and interpretation of CMR results in cases of suspected cardiomyopathy do basically not differ from young competitive athletes, and the reader is referred to the Table 32.1, to Chap. 10 and to the chapters on specific diseases. However, these athletes usually show a higher prevalence of myocardial fibrosis (see Chap. 32), making CMR imaging particularly important in this population.

The traditional method to detect myocardial replacement fibrosis as a possible sign of previous cardiac damage has been **late gadolinium enhancement (LGE)** [52–54]. Using this technique, different patterns of LGE distribution have been reported, enabling at least a basic differentiation between various aetiologies of fibrosis development (Fig. 32.4) [55, 56]:

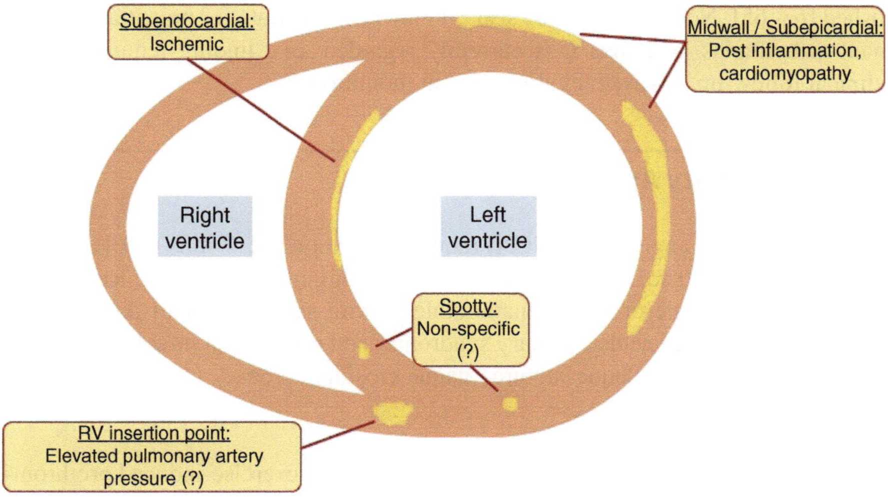


**Fig. 32.4** Schematic depiction of diverse patterns of myocardial fibrosis that have been observed in athletes in recent years, and potential pathophysiologic backgrounds. *RV* right ventricle

- Ischemic pattern: located in the subendocardial regions, usually indicative of underlying CAD (though not always confirmed by invasive coronary angiography).
- Non-ischemic pattern: commonly involving the mid-wall and the subepicardium, usually attributable to inflammatory disease (myocarditis, sarcoidosis, and collagen vascular diseases) or cardiomyopathy-related necrosis or scars (commonly observed concomitant to altered ventricular dimensions).
- LGE at the right ventricular septal insertion point: has been discussed to represent a potential sign of increased right ventricular strain induced by elevated pulmonary artery pressure as a consequence of repeated intensive bouts of exercise over years [56, 57].
- Spotty patterns: have occasionally been reported in endurance athletes not showing any other obvious disease [58].
- Mixed, atypical patterns (diffuse subendocardial, subepicardial basal, and intramyocardial LGE): have been observed in rare forms of cardiomyopathies such as amyloidosis, Anderson-Fabry disease, and mitochondrial myopathy, which should always be taken into consideration as differential diagnoses [59, 60].

**T1 mapping** has recently evolved as a new CMR method for the assessment of the extracellular volume and diffuse rather than localized fibrosis. This technique can potentially be important in myocardial diseases where LGE is less sensitive [61]. This has for example recently been observed in competitive middle-aged triathletes and has been linked to cumulated competition distances and exaggerated blood pressure response to exercise [62] (see Chap. 32).

Overall, the clinical relevance of focal or diffuse myocardial fibrosis, particularly when observed accidentally in otherwise healthy hearts, has not fully been established [63–65]. Nonetheless, as a "scar" it may be a substrate for potentially malignant arrhythmias, and thus it is currently regarded as a finding requiring close clinical follow-up, always including rhythm monitoring.

## 32.7 Coronary Angiography

Invasive coronary angiography (ICA) requires radiation (~2–7 mSv) [36] and contrast agent (~50–70 cc) and is not a first-line imaging modality for clinical evaluation of asymptomatic or symptomatic athletes with suspected heart disease. It is used in sports-related acute coronary syndromes and myocardial infarction [66–72] mostly demonstrating plaque rupture, plaque erosion, coronary vasospasm, thrombosis, or a combination of these.

- In athletes, this may specifically be explained by an exercise-induced prothrombotic/fibrinolytic dysbalance [73, 74] and a burst of inflammation [74, 75] in the presence of CAD.
- Traumatic coronary artery dissection on coronary angiography is possible but rare [76, 77].

Causes of hypercoagulation that have been linked with coronary thrombus formation in athletes and that were visualized by coronary angiography include

(a) High altitude [71]
(b) Epinephrine abuse [78]
(c) Antithrombin III deficiency [79], or
(d) Coronary left main aneurysm [80]

Occasionally, Tako-Tsubo cardiomyopathy (chest pain, apical ballooning, troponin elevation but normal, non-obstructed coronary arteries) has been observed in association with exercise testing [81–85], in swimmers, divers and in relation to anabolic steroid abuse [86–89]. However, although being commonly induced by physical or emotional stress, the overall pathophysiology of this entity remains incompletely understood, and athletes cannot be regarded as a specific population at risk.

### 32.7.1 Myocardial Bridging

A number of case reports and case series describe coronary events associated with coronary anomalies or myocardial bridging in athletes, the majority of which have used ICA to confirm the diagnosis (see Chap. 22) [17, 90–93].

- Myocardial bridging is characterized by systolic compression of the tunnelled segment. Mild cases are reported in <5% of ICA, but the prevalence increases up to 40% in individuals with chest pain in the absence of CAD [94].
  - Due to intracoronary pressure changes and consecutive alterations in the vessel wall, severe systolic coronary compression may represent an anatomic risk factor of myocardial infarction [95, 96], but the majority of affected patients and athletes have a benign prognosis [94, 97].
  - Individuals with asymptomatic myocardial bridging and no evidence of myocardial ischemia need not generally be restricted from vigorous activity [97].
  - It appears prudent that athletes with a myocardial bridge as the only explanation for chest pain, who intend to engage in vigorous sports activities, require careful counselling, medication and may even need surgery for definite treatment [94].

### 32.7.2 Intracoronary Imaging

Additional intracoronary artery imaging helps to better understand the coronary microvascular adaptations to exercise [98–100]. It allows detailed assessment of high-risk plaque features and functional evaluation of epicardial stenosis and its myocardial sequelae.

- In an asymptomatic runner in whom significant CAD was detected in a research setting (Fig. 32.5a) [101], intravascular ultrasound-based virtual histology (IVUS-VH) revealed high-risk plaque features, i.e. TCFA-lesions (Fig. 32.5b), which are associated with higher adverse CAD event rates [102].

- The reason for this runner being asymptomatic was most likely due to above-normal microvascular function, as seen in the unobstructed RCA, and still a near-normal coronary flow reserve (CFR) of 2.8 in the LAD (Fig. 32.5c) [100, 103].
- Many mechanisms, including epicardial flow-mediated vasodilation, arteriogenesis, angiogenesis and reduced arterial stiffness contribute to these findings (see Chap. 41) [98, 99].

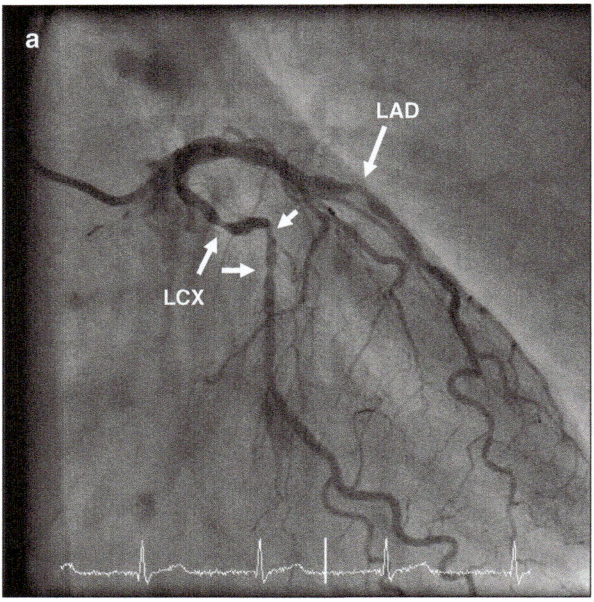


**Fig. 32.5** (**a**) Coronary angiography demonstrating relevant lumen reduction in the mid-LAD and mid-LCX. The RCA showed no stenosis (not shown). (**b**) Intravascular ultrasound (IVUS) image of the LAD using a 2.9 F, 20 MHz catheter (Eagle-Eye©, Volcano, US). Automated pullback was performed at 0.5 mm/s beginning in the distal LAD. Radiofrequency data analysis of the IVUS signal was used for virtual histology (IVUS-VH) assessment. The IVUS-VH study in this runner demonstrates a high amount of necrotic core plaque component (14%, red). Fibrous tissue is marked in dark green (61%), fibro-fatty tissue (21%) in light green and calcified plaque in white (4%). The plaque area at this non-culprit lesion site is 62%. (**c**) Intracoronary Doppler ultrasound (ICD) in the distal LAD and during pull-back. Doppler flow velocity spectra are measured at the tip of the Doppler wire. The FloMap or FloMod system (Endosonics) was used to automatically detect maximum coronary blood flow (CBF) and calculate absolute coronary flow reserve (CFR) as the ratio of average peak velocity (APV) during maximum adenosine-induced hyperemia divided by baseline APV. Coronary blood flow (CBF) increased from 14 to 39 cm/s, i.e. a near-normal CFR of 2.8 (a, top left). During pull-back, CBF increased 5.75-fold at the lesion site (b, top right). After stenting, maximum average peak velocity (APV) during adenosine doubled to 81 cm/s (c, bottom left). In comparison, CFR in the right coronary artery was 5.1, i.e. an increase in APV from 16 to 82 cm/s (d, bottom right). A CFR > 5 and a flow >80 cm/s has been observed in <1% of subjects in a series of patients with normal coronary arteries [103], indicating improved microvascular function in this marathon runner, consistent with observations from others [100] (reproduced with permission from [101])

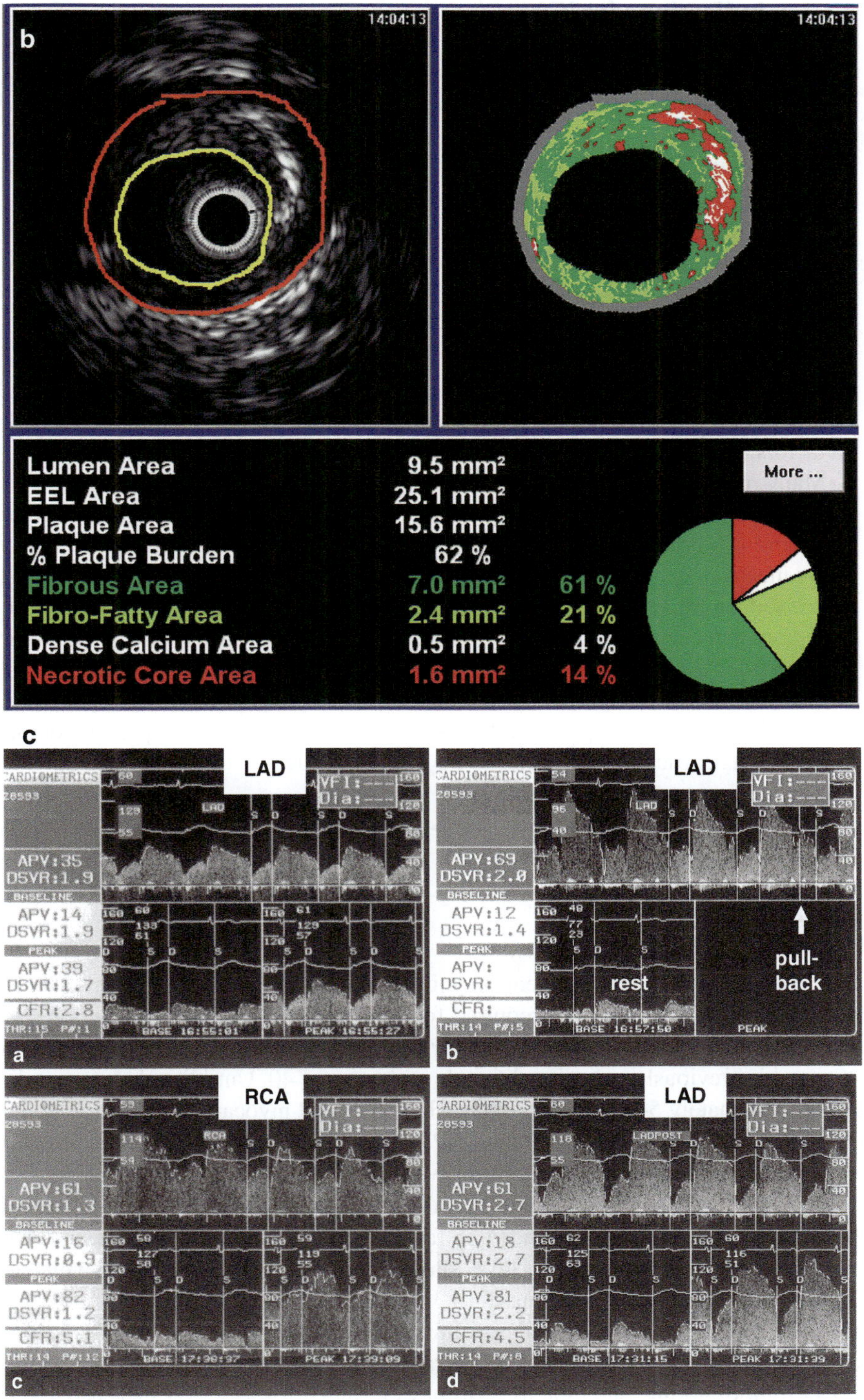


**Fig. 32.5** (continued)

### 32.7.3 Indications for ICA

Overall, ICA is usually only applied in symptomatic athletes with clinical suspicion of CAD that presumably requires interventional therapy, i.e. mainly in acute coronary syndrome and myocardial infarction. It is also used as a stepwise approach following pathological findings during non-invasive work-up indicating a high probability of relevant CAD. If the cause of chest pain cannot readily be identified on ICA, advanced intracoronary artery imaging including intravascular ultrasound (IVUS) and intracoronary Doppler ultrasound (ICD) can help to identify epicardial and intramyocardial microvascular causes of symptoms.

**Clinical Pearls**

- Recreational/master athletes differ from young competitive athletes with respect to a higher prevalence and longer exposure to traditional cardiovascular risk factors.
- Many recreational/master athletes may suffer from clinically inapparent atherosclerosis, thus advanced imaging focuses on risk stratification and the detection of coronary artery disease rather than on inherited or acquired cardiomyopathies.
- By means of echocardiography, assessing tissue-Doppler- and speckle-tracking-derived parameters of systolic and diastolic function may facilitate the differentiation between exercise- or hypertension-induced mild left ventricular hypertrophy.
- Using advanced imaging, an increased coronary plaque burden or myocardial fibrosis may become apparent, the significance of which with respect to continued sports participation remains to be fully elucidated.

## Review

## Questions

A 55-year-old male runner presents in your department for a health exam in order to get written medical clearance required for participation in his next marathon. He had finished 2–3 marathons per year over the past 14 years, after having decided to change his previously unhealthy lifestyle at the age of 40. Until then he was smoking approximately 5–10 cigarettes/day. His father had myocardial infarction at the age of 58. Occasional blood pressure (BP) measurements at his general practitioner had partly revealed borderline systolic values between 130 and 145 mmHg, but when using his wife's device at home values had always been "normal". Thus, no medication had been recommended so far. Physical examination was normal, BP was 147/86 mmHg, and resting ECG showed an isolated increased QRS voltage. His LDL-cholesterol was 167 mg/dl (4.3 mmol/l). You decide to perform exercise testing, showing a maximal blood pressure of 230/90 mmHg and a normal ECG. You also decide to perform an echocardiogram, revealing left ventricular size at the upper limit of normal and mild hypertrophy (12 mm).

1. How do you interpret these findings?
2. How could you add additional information regarding the etiology of left ventricular hypertrophy?
3. How would you estimate this runner's overall cardiovascular risk?
4. Does this patient need additional examinations based on advanced imaging techniques?

In case you have decided to perform CAC, imagine this runner would have a score of 123.

5. Would you treat this patient with statins?
6. Would you advise against continued marathon running?
7. Would you perform additional imaging testing, and if yes, which technique would you use?
8. Would you act different if calcium score was 567?

## Answers

1. The runner was a former smoker but had quit 15 years ago. On the other hand, he has a positive family history of coronary artery disease, and the previous BP measurements were at least borderline, which is regarded high-normal in Europe but already stage I hypertension in the US. The ECG does not further add to these considerations, since isolated increased QRS voltage does at least in young athletes not require additional testing; nonetheless, it could be a sign of BP-induced hypertrophy. Both exercise testing and echocardiography support the suspicion of clinically relevant hypertension.
2. This athlete has a history of longstanding endurance exercise, which may be a sufficient explanation for mild hypertrophy. The assessment of left ventricular diastolic function using tissue Doppler, as well as measuring global longitudinal strain could add to the differentiation between athlete's heart and hypertensive heart disease (although the latter is still not fully excluded in case of normal values).
3. Given the elevated LDL level, the calculated 10-year-risk using the ASCVD score is 8.2%, and thus relevantly elevated.
4. Apart from ambulatory BP monitoring, which is clearly recommended in this case, additional imaging modalities beyond echocardiography are not absolutely indicated. Nonetheless, according to the latest AHA guidelines on the management of blood cholesterol [26], assessment of CAC maybe considered in this situation and should be discussed with the patient.
5. Studies have suggested a CAC cut-off value of >100 to at least raise increased risk awareness, and a benefit of statin treatment has basically been shown for these patients. Given the positive family history of myocardial infarction, a statin should be recommended to the patient.
6. No, there is generally no contraindication to continued running with respect to these findings, providing the BP situation has been clarified and eventually treated.

7. You could think about performing exercise echocardiography due to its higher sensitivity and specificity in confirming or ruling out ischemia as compared to common exercise testing.
8. The athlete is asymptomatic, and thus there is still no clear indication to further expand the diagnostic work-up, since CAC does not allow any conclusion on the presence of severe coronary stenosis. Nonetheless, this score indicates a high likelihood of a cardiovascular event within the following 2–5 years, and it would be prudent to perform exercise echocardiography, nuclear imaging or perhaps even CCTA if local expertise is available.

## References


1. Pelliccia A, Caselli S, Sharma S, Basso C, Bax JJ, Corrado D, et al. European Association of Preventive Cardiology (EAPC) and European Association of Cardiovascular Imaging (EACVI) joint position statement: recommendations for the indication and interpretation of cardiovascular imaging in the evaluation of the athlete's heart. Eur Heart J. 2018;39(21):1949–69.
2. Chugh SS, Weiss JB. Sudden cardiac death in the older athlete. J Am Coll Cardiol. 2015;65(5):493–502.
3. Galderisi M, Cardim N, D'Andrea A, Bruder O, Cosyns B, Davin L, et al. The multi-modality cardiac imaging approach to the Athlete's heart: an expert consensus of the European Association of Cardiovascular Imaging. Eur Heart J Cardiovasc Imaging. 2015;16(4):353–353r.
4. Limongelli G, Verrengia M, Pacileo G, Da Ponte A, Brancaccio P, Canonico R, et al. Left ventricular hypertrophy in Caucasian master athletes: differences with hypertension and hypertrophic cardiomyopathy. Int J Cardiol. 2006;111(1):113–9.
5. Galanti G, Toncelli L, Del Furia F, Stefani L, Cappelli B, De Luca A, et al. Tissue Doppler imaging can be useful to distinguish pathological from physiological left ventricular hypertrophy: a study in master athletes and mild hypertensive subjects. Cardiovasc Ultrasound. 2009;7:48.
6. Galderisi M, Lomoriello VS, Santoro A, Esposito R, Olibet M, Raia R, et al. Differences of myocardial systolic deformation and correlates of diastolic function in competitive rowers and young hypertensives: a speckle-tracking echocardiography study. J Am Soc Echocardiogr. 2010;23(11):1190–8.
7. Lancellotti P, Pellikka PA, Budts W, Chaudhry FA, Donal E, Dulgheru R, et al. The clinical use of stress echocardiography in non-Ischaemic heart disease: recommendations from the European Association of Cardiovascular Imaging and the American Society of Echocardiography. J Am Soc Echocardiogr. 2017;30(2):101–38.
8. Claessen G, La Gerche A, Voigt JU, Dymarkowski S, Schnell F, Petit T, et al. Accuracy of echocardiography to evaluate pulmonary vascular and RV function during exercise. JACC Cardiovasc Imaging. 2016;9(5):532–43.
9. Cho I, Chang HJ, Shin S, Sung JM, Lin FY, et al. Incremental prognostic utility of coronary CT angiography for asymptomatic patients based upon extent and severity of coronary artery calcium: results from the COronary CT angiography EvaluatioN for clinical outcomes InteRnational multicenter (CONFIRM) study. Eur Heart J. 2015;36(8):501–8.
10. Greenland P, Alpert JS, Beller GA, Benjamin EJ, Budoff MJ, Fayad ZA, et al. 2010 ACCF/AHA guideline for assessment of cardiovascular risk in asymptomatic adults: a report of the American College of Cardiology Foundation/American Heart Association Task Force on Practice Guidelines. J Am Coll Cardiol. 2010;56(25):e50–103.
11. Mohlenkamp S, Lehmann N, Moebus S, Schmermund A, Dragano N, Stang A, et al. Quantification of coronary atherosclerosis and inflammation to predict coronary events and all-cause mortality. J Am Coll Cardiol. 2011;57(13):1455–64.

12. Task Force M, Montalescot G, Sechtem U, Achenbach S, Andreotti F, Arden C, et al. ESC guidelines on the management of stable coronary artery disease: the Task Force on the management of stable coronary artery disease of the European Society of Cardiology. Eur Heart J. 2013;34(38):2949–3003.
13. La Gerche A, Baggish AL, Knuuti J, Prior DL, Sharma S, Heidbuchel H, et al. Cardiac imaging and stress testing asymptomatic athletes to identify those at risk of sudden cardiac death. JACC Cardiovasc Imaging. 2013;6(9):993–1007.
14. Maron BJ, Zipes DP, Kovacs RJ, American Heart Association E, Arrhythmias Committee of Council on Clinical Cardiology CoCDiYCoC, Stroke Nursing CoFG, et al. Eligibility and disqualification recommendations for competitive athletes with cardiovascular abnormalities: preamble, principles, and general considerations: a scientific statement from the American Heart Association and American College of Cardiology. Circulation. 2015;132(22): e256–61.
15. Mohlenkamp S. Coronary computed tomography. In: Pelliccia A, Heidbuchel H, Corrado D, Börjesson M, Sharma S, editors. The ESC textbook of sports cardiology. Oxford: Oxford University Press; 2019. p. 153–9.
16. Achenbach S, Barkhausen J, Beer M, Beerbaum P, Dill T, Eichhorn J, et al. Consensus recommendations of the German radiology society (DRG), the German cardiac society (DGK) and the German Society for Pediatric Cardiology (DGPK) on the use of cardiac imaging with computed tomography and magnetic resonance imaging. Rofo. 2012;184(4):345–68.
17. Attili A, Hensley AK, Jones FD, Grabham J, DiSessa TG. Echocardiography and coronary CT angiography imaging of variations in coronary anatomy and coronary abnormalities in athletic children: detection of coronary abnormalities that create a risk for sudden death. Echocardiography. 2013;30(2):225–33.
18. Van Hare GF, Ackerman MJ, Evangelista JK, Kovacs RJ, Myerburg RJ, Shafer KM, et al. Eligibility and disqualification recommendations for competitive athletes with cardiovascular abnormalities: Task Force 4: congenital heart disease: a scientific statement from the American Heart Association and American College of Cardiology. J Am Coll Cardiol. 2015;66(21):2372–84.
19. Lauer MS. Elements of danger—the case of medical imaging. N Engl J Med. 2009;361(9): 841–3.
20. Plicht B, Erbel R, Mohlenkamp S. Is there a preventive value in non-invasive cardiac imaging? Debate on the case of a marathon runner. Dtsch Med Wochenschr. 2009;134(40):e1–5.
21. Detrano R, Guerci AD, Carr JJ, Bild DE, Burke G, Folsom AR, et al. Coronary calcium as a predictor of coronary events in four racial or ethnic groups. N Engl J Med. 2008;358(13): 1336–45.
22. Erbel R, Mohlenkamp S, Moebus S, Schmermund A, Lehmann N, Stang A, et al. Coronary risk stratification, discrimination, and reclassification improvement based on quantification of subclinical coronary atherosclerosis: the Heinz Nixdorf Recall study. J Am Coll Cardiol. 2010;56(17):1397–406.
23. Yeboah J, McClelland RL, Polonsky TS, Burke GL, Sibley CT, O'Leary D, et al. Comparison of novel risk markers for improvement in cardiovascular risk assessment in intermediate-risk individuals. JAMA. 2012;308(8):788–95.
24. Mohlenkamp S, Lehmann N, Breuckmann F, Brocker-Preuss M, Nassenstein K, Halle M, et al. Running: the risk of coronary events : prevalence and prognostic relevance of coronary atherosclerosis in marathon runners. Eur Heart J. 2008;29(15):1903–10.
25. Thompson PD, Balady GJ, Chaitman BR, Clark LT, Levine BD, Myerburg RJ. Task Force 6: coronary artery disease. J Am Coll Cardiol. 2005;45(8):1348–53.
26. Grundy SM, Stone NJ, Bailey AL, Beam C, Birtcher KK, Blumenthal RS, et al. AHA/ACC/AACVPR/AAPA/ABC/ACPM/ADA/AGS/APhA/ASPC/NLA/PCNA guideline on the management of blood cholesterol: executive summary: a report of the American College of Cardiology/American Heart Association Task Force on Clinical Practice Guidelines. J Am Coll Cardiol. 2019;73(24):3168–209.

27. Mohlenkamp S, Leineweber K, Lehmann N, Braun S, Roggenbuck U, Perrey M, et al. Coronary atherosclerosis burden, but not transient troponin elevation, predicts long-term outcome in recreational marathon runners. Basic Res Cardiol. 2014;109(1):391.
28. Schwartz RS, Kraus SM, Schwartz JG, Wickstrom KK, Peichel G, Garberich RF, et al. Increased coronary artery plaque volume among male Marathon runners. Mo Med. 2014;111(2):89–94.
29. Tsiflikas I, Thomas C, Fallmann C, Schabel C, Mangold S, Ketelsen D, et al. Prevalence of subclinical coronary artery disease in middle-aged, male Marathon runners detected by cardiac CT. Rofo. 2015;187(7):561–8.
30. Karlstedt E, Chelvanathan A, Da Silva M, Cleverley K, Kumar K, Bhullar N, et al. The impact of repeated marathon running on cardiovascular function in the aging population. J Cardiovasc Magn Reson. 2012;14:58.
31. Ermolao A, Roman F, Gasperetti A, Varnier M, Bergamin M, Zaccaria M. Coronary CT angiography in asymptomatic middle-aged athletes with ST segment anomalies during maximal exercise test. Scand J Med Sci Sports. 2016;26(1):57–63.
32. Hecht HS, Achenbach S, Kondo T, Narula J. High-risk plaque features on coronary CT angiography. JACC Cardiovasc Imaging. 2015;8(11):1336–9.
33. Otsuka K, Fukuda S, Tanaka A, Nakanishi K, Taguchi H, Yoshikawa J, et al. Napkin-ring sign on coronary CT angiography for the prediction of acute coronary syndrome. JACC Cardiovasc Imaging. 2013;6(4):448–57.
34. Douglas PS, Pontone G, Hlatky MA, Patel MR, Norgaard BL, Byrne RA, et al. Clinical outcomes of fractional flow reserve by computed tomographic angiography-guided diagnostic strategies vs. usual care in patients with suspected coronary artery disease: the prospective longitudinal trial of FFR(CT): outcome and resource impacts study. Eur Heart J. 2015;36(47):3359–67.
35. Mahabadi AA, Achenbach S, Burgstahler C, Dill T, Fischbach R, Knez A, et al. Safety, efficacy, and indications of beta-adrenergic receptor blockade to reduce heart rate prior to coronary CT angiography. Radiology. 2010;257(3):614–23.
36. Meinel FG, Nance JW Jr, Harris BS, De Cecco CN, Costello P, Schoepf UJ. Radiation risks from cardiovascular imaging tests. Circulation. 2014;130(5):442–5.
37. Galper BZ, Wang YC, Einstein AJ. Strategies for primary prevention of coronary heart disease based on risk stratification by the ACC/AHA lipid guidelines, ATP III guidelines, coronary calcium scoring, and C-reactive protein, and a global treat-all strategy: a comparative—effectiveness modeling study. PLoS One. 2015;10(9):e0138092.
38. Pletcher MJ, Pignone M, Earnshaw S, McDade C, Phillips KA, Auer R, et al. Using the coronary artery calcium score to guide statin therapy: a cost-effectiveness analysis. Circ Cardiovasc Qual Outcomes. 2014;7(2):276–84.
39. Roberts ET, Horne A, Martin SS, Blaha MJ, Blankstein R, Budoff MJ, et al. Cost-effectiveness of coronary artery calcium testing for coronary heart and cardiovascular disease risk prediction to guide statin allocation: the multi-ethnic study of atherosclerosis (MESA). PLoS One. 2015;10(3):e0116377.
40. Maddahi J, Kiat H, Van Train KF, Prigent F, Friedman J, Garcia EV, et al. Myocardial perfusion imaging with technetium-99m sestamibi SPECT in the evaluation of coronary artery disease. Am J Cardiol. 1990;66(13):55E–62E.
41. Mohlenkamp S. Nuclear imaging. In: Pelliccia A, Heidbuchel H, Corrado D, Börjesson M, Sharma S, editors. The ESC textbook of sports cardiology. Oxford: Oxford University Press; 2019. p. 159–62.
42. Berman DS, Hachamovitch R, Kiat H, Cohen I, Cabico JA, Wang FP, et al. Incremental value of prognostic testing in patients with known or suspected ischemic heart disease: a basis for optimal utilization of exercise technetium-99m sestamibi myocardial perfusion single-photon emission computed tomography. J Am Coll Cardiol. 1995;26(3):639–47.
43. Hachamovitch R, Berman DS, Kiat H, Cohen I, Cabico JA, Friedman J, et al. Exercise myocardial perfusion SPECT in patients without known coronary artery disease: incremental prognostic value and use in risk stratification. Circulation. 1996;93(5):905–14.

44. Chatziioannou SN, Moore WH, Ford PV, Fisher RE, Lee VV, Alfaro-Franco C, et al. Prognostic value of myocardial perfusion imaging in patients with high exercise tolerance. Circulation. 1999;99(7):867–72.
45. Bartram P, Toft J, Hanel B, Ali S, Gustafsson F, Mortensen J, et al. False-positive defects in technetium-99m sestamibi myocardial single-photon emission tomography in healthy athletes with left ventricular hypertrophy. Eur J Nucl Med. 1998;25(9):1308–12.
46. Bouvier F, Nejat M, Berglund B, Brodin LA, Jorfeldt L, Juhlin-Dannfelt A, et al. High incidence of scintigraphic myocardial uptake defects at rest and during exercise in male elite runners. Heart. 1997;77(3):252–5.
47. Andersson LG, Henriksen E, Damm S, Jonason T, Niklasson U, Wesslen L, et al. Thallium-201 myocardial imaging at rest in male orienteers and other endurance athletes. Ups J Med Sci. 2001;106(1):59–66.
48. Siegel AJ, Lewandrowski KB, Strauss HW, Fischman AJ, Yasuda T. Normal post-race antimyosin myocardial scintigraphy in asymptomatic marathon runners with elevated serum creatine kinase MB isoenzyme and troponin T levels. Evidence against silent myocardial cell necrosis. Cardiology. 1995;86(6):451–6.
49. Siegel AJ, Silverman LM, Holman BL. Normal results of post-race thallium-201 myocardial perfusion imaging in marathon runners with elevated serum MB creatine kinase levels. Am J Med. 1985;79(4):431–4.
50. van de Sande DA, Hoogsteen J, Liem IH, Kemps HM. Athlete's syndrome X. Int J Cardiol. 2014;177(2):e49–50.
51. Prakken NH, Teske AJ, Cramer MJ, Mosterd A, Bosker AC, Mali WP, et al. Head-to-head comparison between echocardiography and cardiac MRI in the evaluation of the athlete's heart. Br J Sports Med. 2012;46(5):348–54.
52. Fieno DS, Kim RJ, Chen EL, Lomasney JW, Klocke FJ, Judd RM. Contrast-enhanced magnetic resonance imaging of myocardium at risk: distinction between reversible and irreversible injury throughout infarct healing. J Am Coll Cardiol. 2000;36(6):1985–91.
53. Kim RJ, Fieno DS, Parrish TB, Harris K, Chen EL, Simonetti O, et al. Relationship of MRI delayed contrast enhancement to irreversible injury, infarct age, and contractile function. Circulation. 1999;100(19):1992–2002.
54. Moon JC, Reed E, Sheppard MN, Elkington AG, Ho SY, Burke M, et al. The histologic basis of late gadolinium enhancement cardiovascular magnetic resonance in hypertrophic cardiomyopathy. J Am Coll Cardiol. 2004;43(12):2260–4.
55. Aquaro GD, Perfetti M, Camastra G, Monti L, Dellegrottaglie S, Moro C, et al. Cardiac MR with late gadolinium enhancement in acute myocarditis with preserved systolic function: ITAMY Study. J Am Coll Cardiol. 2017;70(16):1977–87.
56. van de Schoor FR, Aengevaeren VL, Hopman MT, Oxborough DL, George KP, Thompson PD, et al. Myocardial fibrosis in athletes. Mayo Clin Proc. 2016;91(11):1617–31.
57. La Gerche A, Burns AT, Mooney DJ, Inder WJ, Taylor AJ, Bogaert J, et al. Exercise-induced right ventricular dysfunction and structural remodelling in endurance athletes. Eur Heart J. 2012;33(8):998–1006.
58. Breuckmann F, Mohlenkamp S, Nassenstein K, Lehmann N, Ladd S, Schmermund A, et al. Myocardial late gadolinium enhancement: prevalence, pattern, and prognostic relevance in marathon runners. Radiology. 2009;251(1):50–7.
59. Maron MS. Clinical utility of cardiovascular magnetic resonance in hypertrophic cardiomyopathy. J Cardiovasc Magn Reson. 2012;14:13.
60. Yilmaz A, Sechtem U. Diagnostic approach and differential diagnosis in patients with hypertrophied left ventricles. Heart. 2014;100(8):662–71.
61. Moon JC, Messroghli DR, Kellman P, Piechnik SK, Robson MD, Ugander M, et al. Myocardial T1 mapping and extracellular volume quantification: a Society for Cardiovascular Magnetic Resonance (SCMR) and CMR working Group of the European Society of cardiology consensus statement. J Cardiovasc Magn Reson. 2013;15:92.
62. Tahir E, Starekova J, Muellerleile K, von Stritzky A, Munch J, Avanesov M, et al. Myocardial fibrosis in competitive triathletes detected by contrast-enhanced CMR correlates

with exercise-induced hypertension and competition history. JACC Cardiovasc Imaging. 2018;11(9):1260–70.
63. Hendel RC, Patel MR, Kramer CM, Poon M, Hendel RC, Carr JC, et al. ACCF/ACR/SCCT/SCMR/ASNC/NASCI/SCAI/SIR 2006 appropriateness criteria for cardiac computed tomography and cardiac magnetic resonance imaging: a report of the American College of Cardiology Foundation quality strategic directions committee appropriateness criteria working group, American College of Radiology, Society of Cardiovascular Computed Tomography, Society for Cardiovascular Magnetic Resonance, American Society of Nuclear Cardiology, north American Society for Cardiac Imaging, Society for Cardiovascular Angiography and Interventions, and Society of Interventional Radiology. J Am Coll Cardiol. 2006;48(7):1475–97.
64. Pennell DJ, Sechtem UP, Higgins CB, Manning WJ, Pohost GM, Rademakers FE, et al. Clinical indications for cardiovascular magnetic resonance (CMR): consensus panel report. Eur Heart J. 2004;25(21):1940–65.
65. Yoon YE, Hong YJ, Kim HK, Kim JA, Na JO, Yang DH, et al. 2014 Korean guidelines for appropriate utilization of cardiovascular magnetic resonance imaging: a joint report of the Korean Society of Cardiology and the Korean Society of Radiology. Korean J Radiol. 2014;15(6):659–88.
66. Albano AJ, Thompson PD, Kapur NK. Acute coronary thrombosis in Boston marathon runners. N Engl J Med. 2012;366(2):184–5.
67. Ciampricotti R, el Gamal MI, Bonnier JJ, Relik TH. Myocardial infarction and sudden death after sport: acute coronary angiographic findings. Catheter Cardiovasc Diagn. 1989;17(4):193–7.
68. Ciampricotti R, El-Gamal M, Relik T, Taverne R, Panis J, de Swart J, et al. Clinical characteristics and coronary angiographic findings of patients with unstable angina, acute myocardial infarction, and survivors of sudden ischemic death occurring during and after sport. Am Heart J. 1990;120(6 Pt 1):1267–78.
69. Cuneo A, Oeckinghaus R, Tebbe U. Leisure sport activity as a trigger for acute coronary events in men without known coronary artery disease : a single-center case study. Herz. 2011;36(7):637–42.
70. Halna du Fretay X, Akoudad H, Nejjari M, Benamer H. Myocardial infarction related to sport. Acute clinical and coronary angiographic characteristics in 16 cases. Ann Cardiol Angeiol (Paris). 2013;62(6):398–403.
71. Indermuehle A, Cook S, Marty H. A young mountaineer surviving sudden cardiac arrest at high altitude. BMJ Case Rep. 2010;2010:pii: bcr0720092130.
72. Mohlenkamp S. Coronary angiography. In: Pelliccia A, Heidbuchel H, Corrado D, Börjesson M, Sharma S, editors. The ESC textbook of sports cardiology. Oxford: Oxford University Press; 2019. p. 162–5.
73. Bartsch P. Platelet activation with exercise and risk of cardiac events. Lancet. 1999;354(9192):1747–8.
74. Siegel AJ, Stec JJ, Lipinska I, Van Cott EM, Lewandrowski KB, Ridker PM, et al. Effect of marathon running on inflammatory and hemostatic markers. Am J Cardiol. 2001;88(8):918–20.
75. Suzuki K, Nakaji S, Yamada M, Liu Q, Kurakake S, Okamura N, et al. Impact of a competitive marathon race on systemic cytokine and neutrophil responses. Med Sci Sports Exerc. 2003;35(2):348–55.
76. Kalaga RV, Malik A, Thompson PD. Exercise-related spontaneous coronary artery dissection: case report and literature review. Med Sci Sports Exerc. 2007;39(8):1218–20.
77. Van Mieghem NM, van Weenen S, Nollen G, Ligthart J, Regar E, van Geuns RJ. Traumatic coronary artery dissection: potential cause of sudden death in soccer. Circulation. 2013;127(3):e280–2.
78. Kranjec I, Cerne A, Noc M. Ephedrine-induced acute myocardial infarction in a young athlete: a case of thrombus management. Angiology. 2009;60(2):254–8.

79. Peovska I, Maksimovic J, Kalpak O, Pejkov H, Bosevski M. Recurrent myocardial infarction in a young football player with antithrombin III deficiency. Cardiol J. 2008;15(5): 463–6.
80. Park SH, Kim SE, Ryu SK. Left main coronary artery aneurysm with chronic total occlusion of both left coronary arteries in a young athlete. Heart. 2001;85(1):1e, 11.
81. Dhoble A, Abdelmoneim SS, Bernier M, Oh JK, Mulvagh SL. Transient left ventricular apical ballooning and exercise induced hypertension during treadmill exercise testing: is there a common hypersympathetic mechanism? Cardiovasc Ultrasound. 2008; 6:37.
82. Digne F, Paillole C, Pilliere R, Elayi SC, Gerardin B, Dib JC, et al. Tako-Tsubo syndrome after an exercise echocardiography. Int J Cardiol. 2008;127(3):420–2.
83. Dorfman T, Aqel R, Allred J, Woodham R, Iskandrian AE. Takotsubo cardiomyopathy induced by treadmill exercise testing: an insight into the pathophysiology of transient left ventricular apical (or midventricular) ballooning in the absence of obstructive coronary artery disease. J Am Coll Cardiol. 2007;49(11):1223–5.
84. Vasconcelos Filho FJ, Gomes CA, Queiroz OA, Barreto JE. Dobutamine stress echocardiography-induced broken heart syndrome (Takotsubo syndrome). Arq Bras Cardiol. 2009;93(1):e5–7.
85. Vertesaljai M, Szoke S, Szonyi T, Piroth Z, Fontos G, Szuts K, et al. Transient left ventricular apical akinesis with systolic dysfunction after physical exercise: a form of tako-tsubo syndrome. Orv Hetil. 2008;149(15):687–90.
86. Chenaitia H, Coullange M, Benhamou L, Gerbeaux P. Takotsubo cardiomyopathy associated with diving. Eur J Emerg Med. 2010;17(2):103–6.
87. De Gennaro L, Brunetti ND, Ruggiero M, Rutigliano D, Campanella C, Santoro F, et al. Adrift: Takotsubo cardiomyopathy in an old woman in distress while taking a swim off coast. Int J Cardiol. 2014;177(3):e161–2.
88. Madias JE. Adrift while swimming and Takotsubo syndrome: the vagotonia connection. Int J Cardiol. 2014;177(1):123.
89. Placci A, Sella G, Bellanti G, Margheri M. Anabolic androgenic steroid-induced Takotsubo cardiomyopathy. BMJ Case Rep. 2015;2015:pii: bcr2014209089.
90. Basso C, Maron BJ, Corrado D, Thiene G. Clinical profile of congenital coronary artery anomalies with origin from the wrong aortic sinus leading to sudden death in young competitive athletes. J Am Coll Cardiol. 2000;35(6):1493–501.
91. Joggerst S, Monge J, Uribe C, Sherron S, Angelini P. Sudden cardiac arrest at the finish line: in coronary ectopia, the cause of ischemia is from intramural course, not ostial location. Tex Heart Inst J. 2014;41(2):212–6.
92. Maron BJ. Sudden death in young athletes. N Engl J Med. 2003;349(11):1064–75.
93. Vogt S, Koenig D, Prettin S, Pottgiesser T, Allgeier J, Dickhuth HH, et al. Unusual cause of exercise-induced ventricular fibrillation in a well-trained adult endurance athlete: a case report. J Med Case Rep. 2008;2:120.
94. Mohlenkamp S, Hort W, Ge J, Erbel R. Update on myocardial bridging. Circulation. 2002;106(20):2616–22.
95. Erbel R, Ge J, Mohlenkamp S. Myocardial bridging: a congenital variant as an anatomic risk factor for myocardial infarction? Circulation. 2009;120(5):357–9.
96. Kurt IH. A case of muscular bridge resulting in myocardial infraction following heavy effort: a case report. Cases J. 2009;2(1):135.
97. Gowd BM, Thompson PD. Isolated myocardial bridging and exercise-related cardiac events. Int J Sports Med. 2014;35(14):1145–50.
98. Kojda G, Hambrecht R. Molecular mechanisms of vascular adaptations to exercise. Physical activity as an effective antioxidant therapy? Cardiovasc Res. 2005;67(2): 187–97.
99. Schuler G, Adams V, Goto Y. Role of exercise in the prevention of cardiovascular disease: results, mechanisms, and new perspectives. Eur Heart J. 2013;34(24):1790–9.

100. Windecker S, Allemann Y, Billinger M, Pohl T, Hutter D, Orsucci T, et al. Effect of endurance training on coronary artery size and function in healthy men: an invasive followup study. Am J Physiol Heart Circ Physiol. 2002;282(6):H2216–23.
101. Mohlenkamp S, Bose D, Mahabadi AA, Heusch G, Erbel R. On the paradox of exercise: coronary atherosclerosis in an apparently healthy marathon runner. Nat Clin Pract Cardiovasc Med. 2007;4(7):396–401.
102. Stone GW, Maehara A, Lansky AJ, de Bruyne B, Cristea E, Mintz GS, et al. A prospective natural-history study of coronary atherosclerosis. N Engl J Med. 2011;364(3):226–35.
103. Wieneke H, Haude M, Ge J, Altmann C, Kaiser S, Baumgart D, et al. Corrected coronary flow velocity reserve: a new concept for assessing coronary perfusion. J Am Coll Cardiol. 2000;35(7):1713–20.

# Endurance Exercise and Atrial Fibrillation

# 33

Mahdi Sareban, Eduard Guasch, and Lluis Mont

**Learning Objectives**

1. Understand the epidemiological data linking endurance exercise and risk of atrial fibrillation.
2. Understand pathophysiological mechanisms linking endurance exercise to increased risk of atrial fibrillation.
3. Become familiar with diagnostic modalities in detecting atrial fibrillation in endurance athletes.
4. Be able to individualize treatment options for endurance athletes with atrial fibrillation.

## 33.1 Introduction

Atrial fibrillation (AF) is the most frequent sustained arrhythmia and a major cause of morbidity and mortality [1]. Increasing physical activity has convincingly shown to reduce the risk of AF [2–4]. However, repetitive bouts of prolonged and vigorous endurance exercise has recently emerged as a risk factor for AF in middle-aged male athletes [5].

- Thus, a growing body of literature supports a U-shaped relation between lifetime-accumulated high-intensity endurance training and AF in men [6].

M. Sareban
University Institute of Sports Medicine, Prevention and Rehabilitation, Paracelsus Medical University, Salzburg, Austria
e-mail: m.sareban@salk.at

E. Guasch · L. Mont (✉)
Arrhythmia Unit, Cardiology Department, Hospital Clínic/IDIBAPS, Barcelona, Spain
e-mail: eguasch@clinic.cat; lmont@clinic.cat



A. Pressler, J. Niebauer (eds.), *Textbook of Sports and Exercise Cardiology*,
https://doi.org/10.1007/978-3-030-35374-2_33

The pathophysiology underlying this relation poses a puzzling question with multiple hypothesized mechanisms, which probably in combination create the necessary substrate and trigger for AF onset. Presumably adaptive atrial changes secondary to long-standing endurance training as part of the "athlete's heart" add special considerations as they build up a grey zone of diagnostic uncertainty with atrial changes seen in individuals with AF. Evolving functional diagnostic modalities may re-shape this diagnostic grey zone and facilitate diagnostic workup. Initiating management of AF requires documentation of an AF episode, which can be challenging in athletes as it usually occurs intermittent. New wearable devices hold promise to facilitate early documentation and follow-up, but their reliability still has to be established, especially during exercise. When counseling competitive athletes and highly active people regarding treatment options of AF, special considerations should be taken into account to reduce risk associated with AF but also sustain the numerous health benefits of regular exercise and the lifestyle of being a competitive endurance athlete.

## 33.2 Epidemiology of Atrial Fibrillation in Endurance Athletes

### 33.2.1 Prevalence

At the present time, in the general population the prevalence of AF

- Is about 2% and double than reported in the last decade [7]
- Varies with age and is present in 0.12–0.16% of those younger than 49 years, in 3.7–4.2% of those aged 60–70 years, and in 10–17% of those aged 80 years or older [7].
- Until 2060 these numbers are projected to double, and thus AF will become one of the most important public health problems [8].

Controlled studies with former professional cyclists aged 60–70 years indicate that the prevalence of AF is 6–10% and considerably higher than the control population [9]. Thus, the prevalence of AF seems to be higher within a cohort of individuals practicing long-term and vigorous endurance activities. Taking into account the rising number of master athletes, commonly known as individuals older than 35 years of age participating in ultra-endurance events [10], the number of athletes at risk for AF will rise. Notably, endurance exercise has a gender-specific association with AF risk, as women performing intense exercise were found to have 28% lower risk of AF compared to individuals with a sedentary lifestyle [11].

### 33.2.2 Relationship Between Exercise Dose and Atrial Fibrillation

Early case reports documented tachyarrhythmias in healthy individuals with above-normal exercise capacity without signs of cardiovascular disease [12]. Subsequently,

- Case–control studies reported a higher incidence of AF in endurance athletes [13–15].
- A meta-analysis published in 2009 including six case–control studies reported that the overall risk of AF was significantly higher in athletes than in controls, with an odds ratio of 5.3 [5].
- The next scientific evidence derived from a selected cohort comprising 52,755 finishers of the Vasaloppet, a 90 km cross-country skiing event, indicating that the risk for AF increases with number of completed races and faster finishing time [16].
- And recently, in a prospective study with 115 patients with lone AF, that is AF in the absence of other cardiovascular diseases, and age-matched healthy controls, a history of high volume of vigorous lifetime endurance training was associated with increased risk for lone AF [6].

Considering that the abovementioned studies recruited predominantly males and taking into account a meta-analysis investigating gender differences [11], the increase in AF risk with increasing number of vigorous endurance bouts does not seem to apply for women. It remains unclear why intense physical activity does not increase the AF risk women. Hypotheses that might explain this gender difference include [17]:

1. Fewer comorbidities
2. Shorter duration of exposure to vigorous exercise
3. Impact of sex hormones released in response to exercise
4. Less pronounced atrial structural remodeling
5. Lower sympathetic tone
6. Lower blood pressure

With regard to the well-established protective effect of low to moderate exercise volume and intensity in reducing the risk for AF in both sexes, a U-shaped relation between lifetime-accumulated high-intensity endurance training and AF risk can be drawn as illustrated in Fig. 33.1 for male endurance athletes. Different cutoffs for

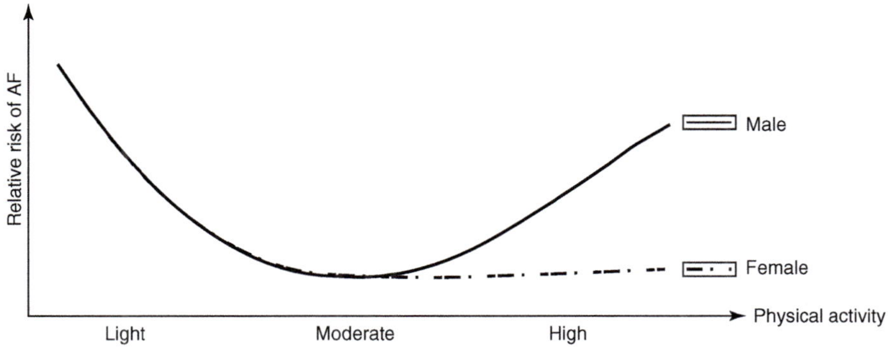


**Fig. 33.1** U-shaped relationship between exercise dose and the relative risk of developing AF. While light-to-moderate exercise decreases AF risk [2, 3, 6], this benefit may be lost or even reverted with higher loads [6, 11, 109]

the ascending flank of the U-curve have been proposed in male athletes, starting from 5 h/week of vigorous intensity exercise at 30 years of age [18] and an accumulated sport practice of above 1500 h [15].

Based on the abovementioned evidence, current guidelines for the management of AF advocate that athletes should be counselled that long-lasting intense sports participation can promote AF [1]. Still, although lifetime-accumulated hours of vigorous activity seem to be a predictor for exercise-induced AF, several further factors should be taken into account:

- The overall risk of exercise-related AF is small
- Competitive endurance exercise at the highest level has numerous health benefits and reduces overall mortality [19]
- Training/AF-risk dose-response curve shows a high inter-individual variability and thus establishing an upper limit of 'safe' endurance training is elusive [6]

Having said this, to improve risk stratification and individualizing counselling, it is necessary to understand the pathophysiologic mechanisms that underlie the increased risk of AF secondary to long-lasting and vigorous endurance exercise.

## 33.3 Pathophysiology of Atrial Fibrillation in Endurance Athletes

The potentially most important determinants of AF in athletes are depicted in Fig. 33.2.

### 33.3.1 Atrial Enlargement

In the general population, there is a well-established relationship between increased LA size and the incidence of AF [20, 21], with arterial hypertension being the most important risk factor for atrial dilatation and AF. Endurance activities demand the generation and maintenance of high cardiac output, imposing a volume challenge that triggers an adaptive response, i.e. enlargement of all cardiac chambers [22]. Consequently, endurance athletes have larger LA dimensions compared with sedentary controls when evaluated by either LA diameter or LA volume indexed for body surface area [23, 24]. Mechanistic hypotheses that describe the relation between LA size with increased risk of AF are the following:

- Atrial enlargement is directly related to mechanical wall stress, according to Laplace's law. This holds especially true for the atria, as they have thinner myocardial wall compared to the ventricles.
- Hidden hypertension or hypertension during exercise bouts may further exacerbate this increase in atrial wall stress [25].

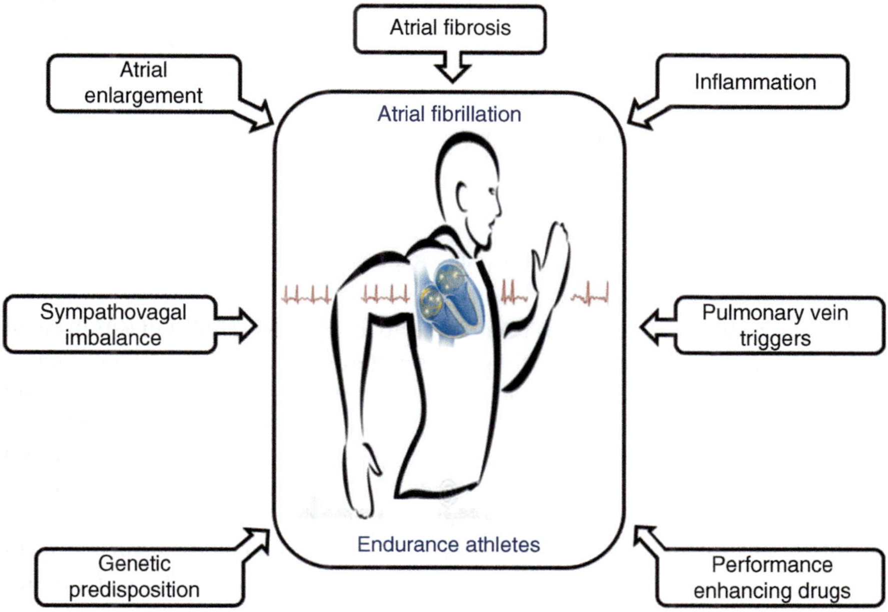


**Fig. 33.2** Schematic representation of the potential mechanisms underlying exercise-induced atrial fibrillation represented

- An increase in atrial mass, which may facilitate re-entrant electrical activity and thus AF [26].
- Conduction heterogeneities in the dilated atria [27].

However, if the athlete's atria undergo the same pathophysiologic changes is currently unknown. In addition, it is currently unknown whether atrial dilatation geometry, which impacts local wall stress, differs between athletes and patients with underlying cardiovascular disease. Of note, some studies documented an association of height and the risk of AF [28]. In understanding the male predominance observed in AF, sex may indeed be secondary to that association. Although it is tempting to assume that LA dilatation imposes the same prognostic implications among endurance athletes and non-athletes, no confirmatory studies support this hypothesis. By now, it is only safe to say that athletes have larger LAs than their sedentary counterparts.

### 33.3.2 Atrial Inflammation and Fibrosis

Although regular physical activity has been demonstrated to establish an anti-inflammatory status, *acute bouts* of vigorous and prolonged exercise transiently

- Increase neutrophil count
- Induce the release of pro-inflammatory cytokines
- Provoke transient increase of cardiac necrosis markers [29, 30]

In humans, a transient p-wave prolongation after ultra-distance races was observed independently of atrial size, leading the authors to postulate that transient inflammatory infiltration or edema could cause such conduction disturbances [31].

Tissue fibrosis results from an accumulation of fibrillar collagen deposits, occurring most commonly as a reparative process. Atrial fibrosis in athletes are hypothesized to be the consequence of

- Increased atrial stretch
- Inflammation that incompletely recover between bouts [32]

Increased atrial wall stress has been shown to trigger TNF-mediated activation of local inflammation, eventually leading to atrial fibrosis in an animal exercise model [33]. Of note, blocking TNF-α did prevent exercise-induced atrial fibrosis and inducibility [33]. In a rat model, 16-weeks of intense training increased atrial interstitial fibrosis and AF inducibility in an electrophysiological test [34]. TGF-β1 and Angiotensin II seem to be centrally involved in the stimulators of collagen synthesis by cardiac fibroblasts [35]. From a mechanistic standpoint, atrial fibrosis disrupts normal electrical conduction in the atrium, and conduction heterogeneity seems to play a decisive role [27] by facilitating the establishment of re-entries and, eventually, AF [35]. Furthermore, there is biochemical evidence of favoring fibrosis in veteran athletes [36]. Still, confirmatory evidence for exercise-induced fibrosis in athletes and that increased wall stretch contribute to myocardial fibrosis pathology is lacking.

### 33.3.3 Atrial Function

Until recently, atrial function was not getting much scientific attention as the atria were thought to be passive transport chambers only. But current literature indicates that the atria actively modulate ventricular filling and thus contribute to global cardiac performance via three repetitive functional phases [37], that is

- LA reservoir phase, in which the LA stores pulmonary venous return during left ventricular contraction and isovolumetric relaxation.
- LA conduit phase, in which the LA passively transfers blood into the LV.
- LA contraction phase, in which the LA actively contracts and thereby contributes to LV filling during the final phase of diastole.

Recent advances in echocardiographic imaging such as speckle tracking echocardiography [38] enabled a more independent insight into atrial function by visualizing and calculating each of the three phases separately [39]. Exercise studies with endurance athletes using an imaging approach underline the contribution of increased atrial function for generating the necessary cardiac output to perform endurance tasks [40, 41]. But there is no evidence for compromised atrial function, which might contribute to the increased risk of AF in healthy and well-hydrated endurance athletes, following a prolonged exercise protocol [42]. Still, master endurance athletes with documented paroxysmal AF, i.e. the very beginning step of AF, have decreased LA reservoir- as well as contractile function compared to endurance athletes without documented AF [43]. Notably, in that study, LA strain assessment was more robust than the assessment of LA volumes and ECG parameters for differentiating between master endurance with AF and healthy controls. Thus, functional assessment of the LA holds promises to identify endurance athletes at risk of developing AF, especially in the diagnostic work-up of athletes with structural LA changes.

### 33.3.4 Autonomic Characteristics

Autonomic tone imbalance is an increasingly recognized factor governing AF initiation and maintenance. Remarkably, the balance between the sympathetic and parasympathetic tone fluctuates during daily life in most individuals, even more in athletes:

- Regular physical activity promotes chronic cardiac parasympathetic enhancement at rest in athletes, thereby inducing sinus bradycardia [32] and yielding ventricular antiarrhythmic properties [44].
- Moderate to intense exercise bouts promote a transient activation of the sympathetic tone and retrieval of the parasympathetic tone in order to rapidly increase cardiac output and peripheral oxygen supply. After physical activity is stopped, parasympathetic tone rapidly increases, followed by a delayed and slow retrieval of the sympathetic tone [45].
- In addition to changes in the autonomic tone balance, experimental [46] and clinical [32, 47] data in recent years suggest that intrinsic electrophysiological remodeling of the sinus node could contribute to sinus bradycardia in athletes.

Both sympathetic and parasympathetic tone shorten the atrial refractory period through ion channel regulation and activation, thereby decreasing wavelength and facilitating the establishment of reentries [48]. Notably, the parasympathetic tone yields deeper arrhythmogenic consequences due to a more heterogeneous and patchy effect throughout the atria [49]. The sympathetic tone increases systolic calcium influx in the cardiomyocytes, facilitating calcium-dependent triggered activity [50]. Simultaneous activation of the parasympathetic and sympathetic tone synergistically shortens atrial refractory period and promotes calcium overload [51]. This combination, which might occur during recovery after physical activity, evolves as particularly arrhythmogenic in the pulmonary veins [51, 52]. Of note, sinus bradycardia itself, independent of the autonomic tone balance, may also contribute to AF incidence [53], likely because of increased spatial refractoriness heterogeneity.

- In conclusion, both augmented sympathetic and parasympathetic tone associate with a higher risk of AF in athletes:

– Athletes with AF usually present arrhythmic relapses in predominantly vagal situations (e.g., post-prandial, at night or immediately after each exercise bout [20, 54, 55]). Animal models [34] and works in athletes [56] suggest that chronically elevated parasympathetic tone plays an important role in exercise-induced AF.
– Some athletes may present with AF during physical activity [57], commonly associating to a decrease in exercise performance.

### 33.3.5 Pulmonary Veins

Pulmonary veins are considered central in AF pathology since the initial work of the Haissaguerre group showing that pulmonary vein isolation decreases AF burden [58]. The pulmonary veins electrophysiological and structural properties make them particularly vulnerable to develop ectopic activity and anchoring re-entries:

- Ectopic activity from the pulmonary veins is justified by their distinct cellular electrophysiological properties [59] and sensitivity to autonomic tone changes [52]. Ectopic activity may present as frequent atrial premature beats that could trigger AF in the presence of an atrial arrhythmogenic substrate, or as rapid firing sustaining AF [60].
- The short action potential duration [59] and abrupt changes in fiber orientation [61] in the pulmonary veins favor reentry formation and anchoring, thereby sustaining AF [62].

Even if the contribution of the pulmonary veins to AF is well accepted, it is currently unknown whether, and if so how, they participate in AF pathology in athletes. Pulmonary vein isolation has been shown to effectively reduce AF burden in athletes [63, 64]. In a small work including 11 athletes undergoing AF ablation, most did show focal activity in the pulmonary veins [57], but these data has not been reproduced. It is currently unknown whether athletes show an increased atrial premature beat burden in comparison to non-athletes [34, 56].

### 33.3.6 Genetic Susceptibility and Performance Enhancing Drugs

There is evolving evidence for a genetic component of AF in the general population, as the individual's risk of developing lone AF at a young age,

- Increases drastically with both increasing number of relatives with lone AF
- Decreasing age at onset of the disease in these relatives [65]

*KCNQ1* was the first disease gene identified for familial AF and encodes a subunit of the potassium channel, which contributes to repolarization of the cardiac action potential. The N-terminal domain of KCNQ1 is also involved in cellular responses to mechanical stretch. Thus, it is hypothesized that such a mutation in combination with exercise-induced atrial stretch may cause AF, especially when other factors as exercise-induced arterial hypertension further promote atrial stretch and finally unmask the inherited ion channel defect [66]. Unfortunately, to date, there are insufficient genetic data that reliably identify those athletes who are at risk of exercise-induced AF.

Performance enhancing drugs are used to push physiology beyond normal limits. Thus, it is biologically evident that their effect may also exaggerate adaptive changes or even initiate potential maladaptive changes that promote AF as chamber dilatation/fibrosis and parasympathetic tone (see also Chap. 28).

## 33.4 Diagnosis of Atrial Fibrillation in Endurance Athletes

### 33.4.1 Resting-, Stress- and Holter-ECG

An electrocardiographic recording displaying the typical characteristics of AF is required to diagnose AF (Fig. 33.3):

(a) Absence of p waves
(b) Irregular atrial activity
(c) Irregular QRS rhythm if atrio-ventricular conduction is preserved (i.e., in the absence of complete AV block).

The most appropriate method to record AF depends on the type, duration and specificity of symptoms [67]:

- *Twelve-lead ECG* may be useful in athletes complaining of long-lasting symptoms that allow them to seek for medical attention. Moreover, AF may be found in asymptomatic athletes undergoing 12-lead ECG-based pre-participation screening [68].
- Longer recording periods may be needed in athletes reporting short duration symptoms during daily life that preclude them from obtaining a conventional 12-lead ECG recording. Several recording methods are available, from *continuous* (e.g., Holter) to *external loop recorders*, typically lasting from 24 h to 1 month. These may also be used to screen for AF in athletes with unspecific symptoms who are deemed to be at high risk of AF (e.g., high burden of atrial premature beats). Of note, a large percentage of false positive findings has been demonstrated for some external loop recorders [69]. *Implantable loop recorders* are very rarely indicated to screen for AF in athletes.
- Some athletes will complain of relatively specific (e.g., palpitations) or unspecific (e.g., decreased performance) symptoms exclusively occurring during physical activity. In these cases, recording cardiac rhythm during the physical activity that triggers symptoms is desirable. Continuous or loop recorders, or specifically dedicated devices [70] may serve for this purpose. It should be noted, though,

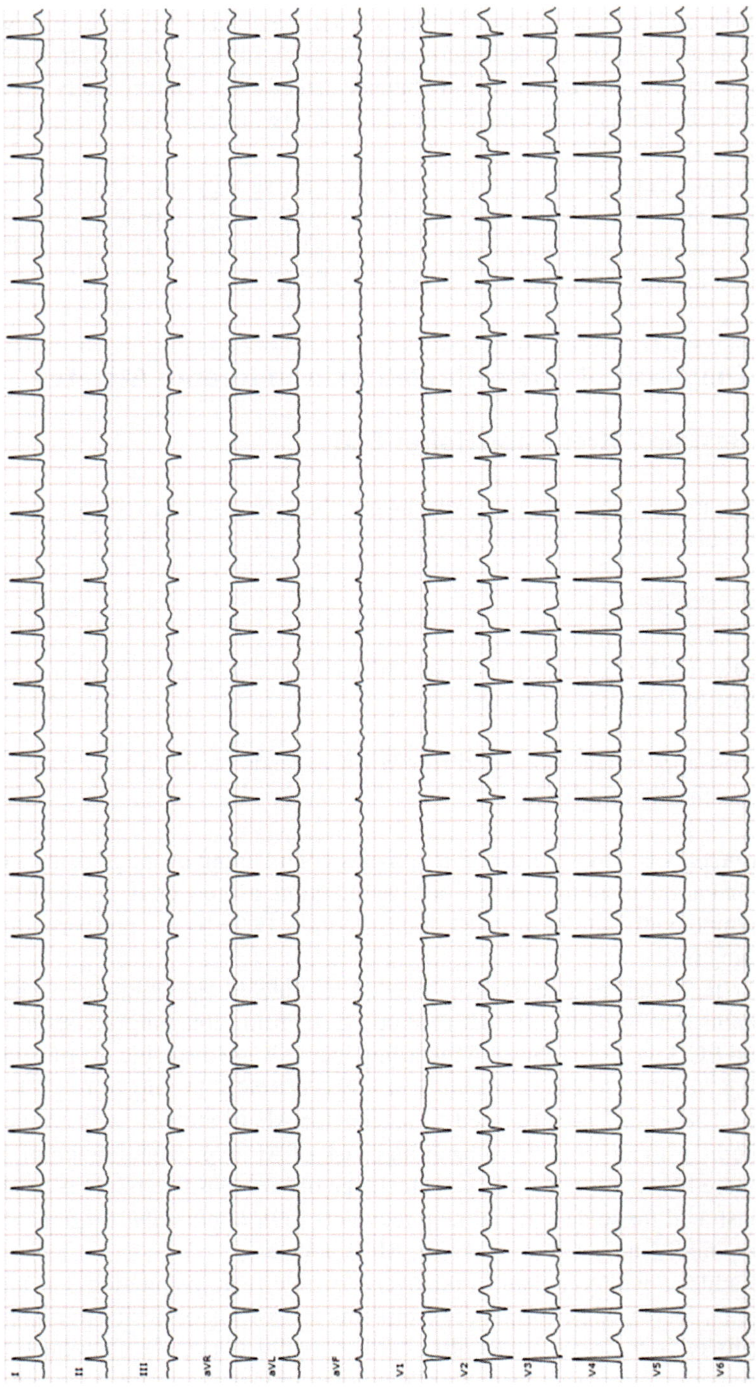


**Fig. 33.3** ECG displaying the typical characteristics of AF

that unstable or noisy recordings during field exercise may lead to inaccurate interpretation and AF overdiagnosis [69]. Alternatively, a stress test mimicking the type, intensity and duration of the physical effort might trigger and diagnose AF. Also, in those athletes with permanent AF who are willing to remain competitive after antiarrhythmic drugs have been initiated, stress test may provide additional information on exercise capacity, hemodynamic behavior and peak heart rate (HR).

### 33.4.2 Novel Wearable Devices

For the last decades, endurance athletes have been recording their HR at rest and during sports to monitor their recovery and exercise intensity using chest strap-based HR watches. Recently, technological advances vastly extended the amount of physiologic data that miniaturized sensors may provide, not only to control training but also to monitor cardiac health. These days,

- Commercially available chest straps provide additional information on RR intervals [71] and even record single channel ECGs from which information about arrhythmias as AF can be derived
- Chest strap-based HR monitors are increasingly replaced by optical sensors, built in smartwatches (e.g. AliveCor, KardiaBand; Fig. 33.4a) which detect pulsatile signals using photoplethysmography
- ECG sensors built in textiles (e.g. CardioSense wearable ECG sensor, Fig. 33.4b) promise use of a wearable ECG recorder over longer periods

These approaches have already shown their utility in not only documenting but also automatically differentiating between AF from sinus rhythm with high accuracy using machine learning-based algorithms [72–74]. Nevertheless, although currently photoplethysmography and other techniques based on RR irregularity may be valuable screening tools, an ECG is always required to reach a definitive AF diagnosis [1, 67]. In addition,

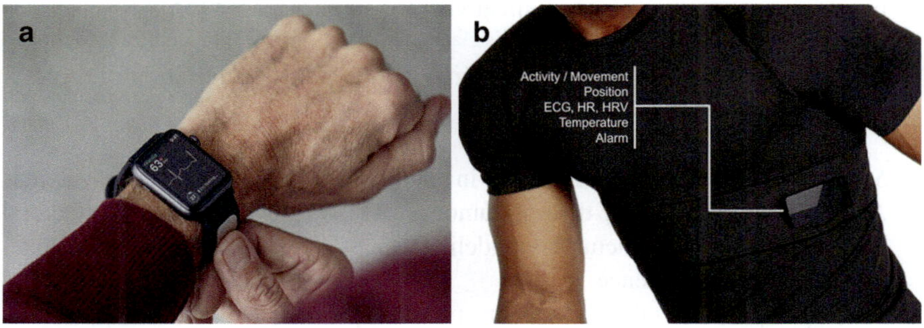


**Fig. 33.4** Novel wearable technology. Panel **a**: AliveCor, KardiaBand (Courtesy of AliveCor), Panel **b**: CardioSense (Courtesy of 2M Engineering)

- The integration of small electronic devices into iOS and Android compatible clothing is rapidly emerging and single-lead ECG derived from a biomedical shirt has already achieved high diagnostic accuracy [75, 76].

All the above-mentioned approaches enable wireless and real-time transmission of the data to a dedicated platform for further analysis. Still, noisy electrode readings due to motion artefacts are still an issue, especially in optical-based devices. However, it is expected that accuracy will continue to improve and also overcome additional challenges as security of individual data. Overall, increased usage of medical wearables among endurance athletes seems to be a natural progression and thus, these devices will help to detect endurance athletes at increased risk or even diagnose unrecognized AF.

## 33.5 Symptoms and Complications of Atrial Fibrillation in Endurance Athletes

Inhomogeneous atrial electrical activation in AF patients results in the loss of atrial contraction and pulse irregularity, which substantiates most of AF symptoms and complications. Overall, athletes with AF report a lower quality of life than non-affected athletes [77].

- *Palpitations* is the most specific symptom of AF; on the other hand, AF is amongst the most frequent causes of sustained, long-lasting palpitations in athletes [78].
- *Decreased physical performance* due to the loss of the atrial contribution to ventricular filling and cardiac output, is a common complaint of athletes with AF [55, 57]. Atrial contraction contributes to cardiac output by 15% at rest [79], and this value increases during exercise [80, 81]. Atrial fibrillation is associated with a decrease in physical performance in the majority of affected athletes [57].
- Some athletes may present with *unspecific symptoms* such as chest tightness, sleeping difficulties, and psychosocial distress [1].
- In very few athletes, AF is completely *asymptomatic* and is only diagnosed during a screening program or a medical visit for another reason [55].

Rarely, one of the AF complications may be the first manifestation of a previously undiagnosed AF:

- *Stroke* risk is increased fivefold in individuals affected by non-valvular AF. However, risk largely diverges amongst AF patients. Some clinical factors, biomarkers [82] and structural remodeling [83, 84] have been associated with an increased stroke incidence.
  - No prospective studies have been specifically conducted in athletes, but current data from retrospective studies support that stroke risk is more than twice as high in athletes with AF than those without AF [77, 85].

- A small, cross-sectional study from Norway reported a similar prevalence of stroke in athletes and non-athletes with confirmed AF (10% vs. 12%, respectively), although the latter had a higher burden of cardiovascular risk factors [77]. In this study, athletes without AF showed a remarkably lower stroke prevalence (4%) [77].
- In another study, Swedish individuals with previous high cross-country skiing activity were compared to the general population with respect to stroke rate and history of AF [85]. Overall, first-time stroke incidence was lower in skiers, but an AF history was more common in skiers than non-skiers, highlighting the larger relative contribution of AF to stroke burden in a low risk population [85]. Although skiers had a lower recurrent stroke risk than the general population, likely accounting for a lower burden of cardiovascular risk factors, AF was still associated with a worse prognosis during follow-up in skiers [85].

- *Heart failure*: A positive interaction is known to occur between heart failure and AF. Roughly one fourth of patients with AF show left ventricular dysfunction, and half of heart failure patients will develop AF [86, 87]. Such a strong association may be explained by a variety of factors:
  - Both AF and heart failure share some etiological risk factors, including hypertension, ischemic heart disease and several cardiomyopathies.
  - Sustained rapid rates in asymptomatic AF may eventually evolve into LV dysfunction and heart failure (so called '*tachycardiomyopathy*'), particularly in those individuals presenting an underlying predisposition [88].
  - Heart failure induces a pro-inflammatory environment and a hemodynamic overload that increase atrial stretch and promote structural and electrophysiological abnormalities. These changes may eventually maintain AF [89].

In the clinical setting, reasonable therapeutic issues may arise in those patients initially presenting with AF and left ventricular dysfunction not attributable to other causes: did heart failure precede AF or vice versa? In this regard, it is worth noting that AF ablation is effective in heart failure patients, either with [90] or without [91] an underlying structural heart disease. In general, AF ablation may be a good choice for patients with heart failure and AF [92].

## 33.6 Treatment and Prognosis of Atrial Fibrillation in Endurance Athletes

Current therapeutic strategies in athletes with AF require a detailed evaluation of the affected athlete and an individualized approach heavily relying into shared-decision. Initial decision should be targeted at:

1. Evaluation of the need for anticoagulation to prevent thromboembolic complications. As for the general population [1], the indication for anticoagulation in

athletes with AF should be based on the $CHA_2DS_2$-VASc score. The $CHA_2DS_2$-VASc score adds one or two points for each of the following:
- **C**ongestive heart failure: 1 point
- **H**ypertension: 1 point
- **A**ge >75 years: 2 points
- **D**iabetes: 1 point
- History of **S**troke: 2 points
- **V**asculopathy: 1 point
- **A**ge >65 years: 1 point
- **S**ex **c**ategory: 1 point for female sex

  In the absence of absolute contraindications, men with ≥1 point and women with ≥2 points might be considered for anticoagulation, preferably with non-vitamin K oral anticoagulants; men adding ≥2 points and women adding ≥3 points should receive anticoagulants [1]. Athletes with AF are usually middle-aged men not accruing other cardiovascular risk factors, and thus long-term anticoagulation is usually not required. Nevertheless, short-term peri-procedural anticoagulation may be occasionally required (i.e., anticoagulation will be required in those athletes undergoing cardioversion or AF ablation).
- Bleeding risk should be assessed in athletes requiring either long- or short-term anticoagulation, and high-contact sports should then be discouraged or prohibited [1, 93].
- Although intermittent anticoagulation has been suggested for athletes with venous thromboembolism, no data is available for athletes with AF [94].
- Non-pharmacological antithrombotic therapies such as LA appendage occluders appear as an attractive choice for athletes engaged in contact sports requiring anticoagulation. Nevertheless, current evidence is insufficient to support their use as a first-line alternative to anticoagulant drugs [1].

2. Decision on whether the antiarrhythmic approach to AF should target sinus rhythm conversion and maintenance (i.e., *rhythm control*), or an adequate rate when accepting AF as the baseline rhythm (i.e., *rate control*). Currently, we do not have robust data to support either rhythm or rate control approach in all patients. This should rather be based on a series of factors including, among others:
   - Frequency and intensity of symptoms.
   - Athlete preferences, including his/her willingness to remain competitive.
   - Experience of the treating physician/medical center on ablation procedures.
   - Specific issues of antiarrhythmic drugs when prescribed to athletes, such as potential hemodynamic disturbances or limitations imposed by antidoping rules released by the World Anti-Doping Agency (WADA).
   - Prevalence of comorbidities.
   - Expected success rate of a rhythm control strategy on the basis of factors such as atrial size [95] or fibrosis burden [96].

Atrial fibrillation commonly impairs physical activity performance [57] and should be specifically inquired in competitive athletes. In general, a rhythm control approach will thus be adequate for most athletes who choose to remain competitive.

The selected antiarrhythmic agent will drive the choice of pharmacological and non-pharmacological therapies. Of note, such decision may change during follow-up:

- An athlete initially selected for a rhythm control strategy might switch to rate control in the presence of serious side effects, intolerance or low efficacy of antiarrhythmic drugs.
- An athlete initially undergoing a rate control strategy might switch to rhythm control if a proper rate control cannot be achieved with a conventional approach.

In a **rhythm control approach** the main therapeutic objective is to achieve and maintain sinus rhythm. Electrical or pharmacological cardioversion may occasionally be needed to restore sinus rhythm. Our available armamentarium includes:

- *Pharmacological approach*: Antiarrhythmic drugs are generally considered as the first line approach to patients with AF. General guidelines should be followed [1], but some considerations should be taken into account in athletes:
  - *Class Ia antiarrhythmics*: disopyramide yields anticholinergic properties that may be particularly convenient in athletes who present cholinergically-mediated AF [1, 97, 98]. Of note, use of low doses and close ECG monitoring is advised because of the potential of ventricular arrhythmogenicity and increased risk of death [99].
  - *Class Ic antiarrhythmics* (e.g., flecainide, procainamide): A combination with AV node blocking agents is encouraged to prevent conversion to a 1:1 flutter that could degenerate into ventricular fibrillation. In those athletes with infrequent relapses, a pill-in-the-pocket strategy [1, 100] may be a safe and convenient strategy. In these patients, current guidelines [1] recommend refraining from sports until AF has reverted and at least until two half-lifes of the antiarrhythmic drug have elapsed (i.e., on average 2 x 20 h for flecainide [101], 2 × 2–10 h for propafenone).
  - *Amiodarone:* although amiodarone effectively prevents relapses of AF, its QT-prolongation and pulmonary, liver, thyroid, cutaneous and visual systemic side effects discourage its use, particularly in young individuals in whom other choices are available.
  - *Dronedarone*, an amiodarone analogue, does not show thyroid side effects and may be useful to maintain sinus rhythm in patients without heart failure, but retains pulmonary and liver side effects.
- *Non-pharmacological approach:* ablation procedures targeting pulmonary veins are a cornerstone of the modern therapeutic arsenal for AF patients. In athletes, AF ablation:
  - is effective and safe [63, 64],
  - allows return to training [57, 102], and
  - may be considered as a first-line approach [1].
- *Reducing physical activity load*: data supporting a potential therapeutic effect is scarce and relies on a very low level of evidence based on a retrospective study [103] and animal models [34]. Economic dependence on sport may further jeopardize its applicability in professional athletes [67].

A **rate control strategy** accepts AF as the baseline rhythm, and the therapeutic objective is to maintain absence of symptoms. The target in these patients should be [1, 104]:

- A resting HR of 80 beats per minute and a heart rate during moderate exercise <110 beats per minute.
- A resting HR of up to 110 beats per minute may be acceptable in the absence of symptoms.

These targets are commonly achieved by means of antiarrhythmic drugs:

- *Pharmacological approach*: is based on the use of AV node blocking drugs, including:
  - Beta-blockers and non-dihydropyridine calcium channel blockers are first line drugs. Robust evidence supporting the use of one pharmacological group over the other is lacking. Nevertheless, some small studies suggest that calcium channel blockers improve HR control [105] and exercise capacity [106] in comparison to beta-blockers, but conflicting data on this issue has also been published [107].
  - Digoxin has relatively low efficacy in controlling HR during exercise [108].
  - Amiodarone yields mild AV node blocking properties, but its systemic side effects greatly limit their use, and thus this agent should be considered as a very last option in young individuals.
- *Non-pharmacological approach*: in these patients this refers to a strategy of "pace and ablate", that is, implanting a pacemaker followed by radiofrequency AV node ablation. Fortunately, this is very rarely required, particularly in athletes.

Independent of the strategy selected, it is advisable to perform an exercise test after therapy has been established, particularly if symptoms during physical effort were the referring symptom, to test the appearance of AF, hemodynamic behavior and peak heart rate.

## 33.7 Outlook

Taking into account the rising number of athletes participating in ultra-endurance events, endurance sport-associated AF is likely to become increasingly prevalent in near future. Current data are still insufficient to adopt specific preventative, diagnostic or prognostic strategies. Thus, longitudinal-designed research in this area will be critical to further elucidate the mechanisms by which it develops and to improve treatment. Novel technological advances may assist the growing sports cardiology community in improving counseling of endurance athletes at risk for AF. At present, in light of our current knowledge, the potential risk of AF should not be used to limit the amount of physical activity.

**Clinical Pearls**

- A growing body of literature supports a U-shaped relation between lifetime-accumulated high-intensity endurance training and AF in men.
- The pathophysiology underlying this relation is hypothesized to be a combination of different mechanisms. Atrial enlargement, atrial inflammation/fibrosis and changes in autonomic tone are some of these mechanisms.
- When counseling highly active people regarding treatment options of AF, special considerations should be taken into account to reduce risk associated with AF but also sustain the numerous health benefits of regular exercise.

## Review

## Questions

1. Regarding the prevalence and relative risk of AF in endurance athletes, which of the following statements is true?
   (a) The prevalence of AF is decreasing in the general population and is projected to further decrease in the next decades.
   (b) The prevalence of AF is higher within a middle-aged cohort of male individuals practicing long-term and vigorous endurance activities compared to the general population.
   (c) Even endurance activities with moderate intensity increase the risk for AF.
   (d) Increased AF risk with increasing number of vigorous endurance activities applies similarly in women and men.
   (e) There is a well-established cutoff where the risk for AF in endurance athletes increases.
2. Regarding the mechanisms of AF in endurance athletes, which of the following statements is true?
   (a) Functional assessment of the LA holds promise to identify endurance athletes at risk of developing AF.
   (b) There is no link between atrial inflammation and atrial fibrosis.
   (c) Regular endurance activities do not promote resting cardiac autonomic activity changes.
   (d) There is no evidence for a genetic component of AF.
   (e) LA dilatation has the same prognostic implications among endurance athletes and non-athletes.
3. Regarding the therapeutic approach to patients with AF, which of the following statements is not true?
   (a) Athletes willing to remain competitive may opt for a rhythm control approach to preserve their physical performance.
   (b) In athletes less than 65 years old who have no other comorbidities, planned cardioversion can be safely performed without anticoagulation.
   (c) The pill-in-the-pocket approach should be considered in those athletes with infrequent AF recurrences.

(d) Although plausible, clinical evidence for a deconditioning benefit on AF burden is scarce.
(e) Amiodarone should be considered a second-line option because of its systemic side effects.

## Answers

1. Answer *b* is correct: There is mounting evidence that middle-aged male endurance athletes are at increased risk for AF compared to sedentary individuals.
2. Answer *a* is correct: New imaging technologies as speckle tracking echocardiography give detailed insights in phasic atrial function and hold promise to identify endurance athletes at risk of developing AF.
3. Answer *b* is not correct: Although athletes with AF usually are at a low thromboembolic risk (i.e., low $CHA_2DS_2VASc$ score), peri-procedural anticoagulation should be administered when undergoing cardioversion or AF ablation.

## References


1. Kirchhof P, Benussi S, Kotecha D, Ahlsson A, Atar D, Casadei B, et al. 2016 ESC guidelines for the management of atrial fibrillation developed in collaboration with EACTS. Eur Heart J. 2016;37:2893–962.
2. Mozaffarian D, Furberg CD, Psaty BM, Siscovick D. Physical activity and incidence of atrial fibrillation in older adults: the cardiovascular health study. Circulation. 2008;118:800–7.
3. Qureshi WT, Alirhayim Z, Blaha MJ, Juraschek SP, Keteyian SJ, Brawner CA, et al. Cardiorespiratory fitness and risk of incident atrial fibrillation: results from the Henry Ford Exercise Testing (FIT) Project. Circulation. 2015;131:1827–34.
4. Morseth B, Graff-Iversen S, Jacobsen BK, Jørgensen L, Nyrnes A, Thelle DS, et al. Physical activity, resting heart rate, and atrial fibrillation: the Tromsø Study. Eur Heart J. 2016;37:2307–13.
5. Abdulla J, Nielsen JR. Is the risk of atrial fibrillation higher in athletes than in the general population? A systematic review and meta-analysis. Europace. 2009;11:1156–9.
6. Calvo N, Ramos P, Montserrat S, Guasch E, Coll-Vinent B, Domenech M, et al. Emerging risk factors and the dose-response relationship between physical activity and lone atrial fibrillation: a prospective case-control study. Europace. 2016;18:57–63.
7. Zoni-Berisso M, Lercari F, Carazza T, Domenicucci S. Epidemiology of atrial fibrillation: European perspective. Clin Epidemiol. 2014;6:213–20.
8. Krijthe BP, Kunst A, Benjamin EJ, Lip GYH, Franco OH, Hofman A, et al. Projections on the number of individuals with atrial fibrillation in the European Union, from 2000 to 2060. Eur Heart J. 2013;34:2746–51.
9. Baldesberger S, Bauersfeld U, Candinas R, Seifert B, Zuber M, Ritter M, et al. Sinus node disease and arrhythmias in the long-term follow-up of former professional cyclists. Eur Heart J. 2008;29:71–8.
10. da Fonseca-Engelhardt K, Knechtle B, Rüst CA, Knechtle P, Lepers R, Rosemann T. Participation and performance trends in ultra-endurance running races under extreme conditions - "Spartathlon" versus "Badwater". Extrem Physiol Med. 2013;2:15.
11. Mohanty S, Mohanty P, Tamaki M, Natale V, Gianni C, Trivedi C, et al. Differential association of exercise intensity with risk of atrial fibrillation in men and women: evidence from a meta-analysis. J Cardiovasc Electrophysiol. 2016;27:1021–9.

12. Fleischmann P, Kellermann JJ. Persistent irregular tachycardia in a successful athlete without impairment of performance. Isr J Med Sci. 1969;5:950–2.
13. Karjalainen J, Kujala UM, Kaprio J, Sarna S, Viitasalo M. Lone atrial fibrillation in vigorously exercising middle aged men: case-control study. BMJ. 1998;316:1784–5.
14. Molina L, Mont L, Marrugat J, Berruezo A, Brugada J, Bruguera J, et al. Long-term endurance sport practice increases the incidence of lone atrial fibrillation in men: a follow-up study. Europace. 2008;10:618–23.
15. Elosua R, Arquer A, Mont L, Sambola A, Molina L, García-Morán E, et al. Sport practice and the risk of lone atrial fibrillation: a case-control study. Int J Cardiol. 2006;108:332–7.
16. Andersen K, Farahmand B, Ahlbom A, Held C, Ljunghall S, Michaëlsson K, et al. Risk of arrhythmias in 52 755 long-distance cross-country skiers: a cohort study. Eur Heart J. 2013;34:3624–31.
17. Myrstad M, Aarønæs M, Graff-Iversen S, Nystad W, Ranhoff AH. Does endurance exercise cause atrial fibrillation in women? Int J Cardiol. 2015;184:431–2.
18. Drca N, Wolk A, Jensen-Urstad M, Larsson SC. Atrial fibrillation is associated with different levels of physical activity levels at different ages in men. Heart. 2014;100:1037–42.
19. Marijon E, Tafflet M, Antero-Jacquemin J, El Helou N, Berthelot G, Celermajer DS, et al. Mortality of French participants in the Tour de France (1947–2012). Eur Heart J. 2013;662833848:1–6.
20. Mont L, Tamborero D, Elosua R, Molina I, Coll-Vinent B, Sitges M, et al. Physical activity, height, and left atrial size are independent risk factors for lone atrial fibrillation in middle-aged healthy individuals. Europace. 2008;10:15–20.
21. Arriagada G, Berruezo A, Mont L, Tamborero D, Molina I, Coll-Vinent B, et al. Predictors of arrhythmia recurrence in patients with lone atrial fibrillation. Europace. 2008;10:9–14.
22. Baggish AL, Wood MJ. Athlete's heart and cardiovascular care of the athlete: scientific and clinical update. Circulation. 2011;123:2723–35.
23. Iskandar A, Mujtaba MT, Thompson PD. Left atrium size in elite athletes. JACC Cardiovasc Imaging. 2015;8:753–62.
24. Sareban M, Winkert K, Sperlich B, Berger MM, Niebauer J, Steinacker JM, et al. Speckle tracking-derived bi-atrial strain before and after eleven weeks of training in elite rowers. Sci Rep. 2018;8:14300.
25. Leischik R, Spelsberg N, Niggemann H, Dworrak B, Tiroch K. Exercise-induced arterial hypertension – an independent factor for hypertrophy and a ticking clock for cardiac fatigue or atrial fibrillation in athletes? F1000Research. 2014;3:105.
26. Zou R, Kneller J, Leon LJ, Nattel S. Substrate size as a determinant of fibrillatory activity maintenance in a mathematical model of canine atrium. Am J Physiol Heart Circ Physiol. 2005;289:H1002–12.
27. Neuberger H-R, Schotten U, Blaauw Y, Vollmann D, Eijsbouts S, van Hunnik A, et al. Chronic atrial dilation, electrical remodeling, and atrial fibrillation in the goat. J Am Coll Cardiol. 2006;47:644–53.
28. Rosenberg MA, Patton KK, Sotoodehnia N, Karas MG, Kizer JR, Zimetbaum PJ, et al. The impact of height on the risk of atrial fibrillation: the cardiovascular health study. Eur Heart J. 2012;33:2709–17.
29. Neubauer O, König D, Wagner K-H. Recovery after an Ironman triathlon: sustained inflammatory responses and muscular stress. Eur J Appl Physiol. 2008;104:417–26.
30. Scharhag J, George K, Shave R, Urhausen A, Kindermann W. Exercise-associated increases in cardiac biomarkers. Med Sci Sports Exerc. 2008;40:1408–15.
31. Wilhelm M, Zueger T, De Marchi S, Rimoldi SF, Brugger N, Steiner R, et al. Inflammation and atrial remodeling after a mountain marathon. Scand J Med Sci Sports. 2014;24:519–25.
32. Guasch E, Mont L. Diagnosis, pathophysiology, and management of exercise-induced arrhythmias. Nat Rev Cardiol. 2017;14:88–101.
33. Aschar-Sobbi R, Izaddoustdar F, Korogyi AS, Wang Q, Farman GP, Yang F, et al. Increased atrial arrhythmia susceptibility induced by intense endurance exercise in mice requires TNFα. Nat Commun. 2015;6:6018.

34. Guasch E, Benito B, Qi X, Cifelli C, Naud P, Shi Y, et al. Atrial fibrillation promotion by endurance exercise: demonstration and mechanistic exploration in an animal model. J Am Coll Cardiol. 2013;62:68–77.
35. Burstein B, Nattel S. Atrial fibrosis: mechanisms and clinical relevance in atrial fibrillation. J Am Coll Cardiol. 2008;51:802–9.
36. Lindsay MM, Dunn FG. Biochemical evidence of myocardial fibrosis in veteran endurance athletes. Br J Sports Med. 2007;41:447–52.
37. Blume GG, Mcleod CJ, Barnes ME, Seward JB, Pellikka PA, Bastiansen PM, et al. Left atrial function: physiology, assessment, and clinical implications. Eur J Echocardiogr. 2011;12:421–30.
38. Mondillo S, Galderisi M, Mele D, Cameli M, Lomoriello VS, Zacà V, et al. Speckle-tracking echocardiography: a new technique for assessing myocardial function. J Ultrasound Med. 2011;30:71–83.
39. Saraiva RM, Demirkol S, Buakhamsri A, Greenberg N, Popović ZB, Thomas JD, et al. Left atrial strain measured by two-dimensional speckle tracking represents a new tool to evaluate left atrial function. J Am Soc Echocardiogr. 2010;23:172–80.
40. Wright S, Sasson Z, Gray T, Chelvanathan A, Esfandiari S, Dimitry J, et al. Left atrial phasic function interacts to support left ventricular filling during exercise in healthy athletes. J Appl Physiol. 2015;119:328–33.
41. Gabrielli L, Bijnens BH, Brambila C, Duchateau N, Marin J, Sitges-Serra I, et al. Differential atrial performance at rest and exercise in athletes: potential trigger for developing atrial dysfunction? Scand J Med Sci Sports. 2016;26:1444–54.
42. Sareban M, Zügel D, Hartveg P, Zügel M, Gary T, Niebauer J, et al. Preserved left atrial mechanics following a 5-h laboratory triathlon in euhydrated athletes. Int J Sports Med. 2019;40:88–94.
43. Hubert A, Galand V, Donal E, Pavin D, Galli E, Martins RP, et al. Atrial function is altered in lone paroxysmal atrial fibrillation in male endurance veteran athletes. Eur Heart J Cardiovasc Imaging. 2018;19:145–53.
44. Vaseghi M, Salavatian S, Rajendran PS, Yagishita D, Woodward WR, Hamon D, et al. Parasympathetic dysfunction and antiarrhythmic effect of vagal nerve stimulation following myocardial infarction. JCI Insight. 2017;2:pii: 86715.
45. Michael S, Graham KS, Oam GMD. Cardiac autonomic responses during exercise and post-exercise recovery using heart rate variability and systolic time intervals-a review. Front Physiol. 2017;8:1–19.
46. D'Souza A, Bucchi A, Johnsen AB, Logantha SJRJ, Monfredi O, Yanni J, et al. Exercise training reduces resting heart rate via downregulation of the funny channel HCN4. Nat Commun. 2014;5:3775.
47. Stein R, Medeiros CM, Rosito GA, Zimerman LI, Ribeiro JP. Intrinsic sinus and atrioventricular node electrophysiologic adaptations in endurance athletes. J Am Coll Cardiol. 2002;39:1033–8.
48. Nattel S. New ideas about atrial fibrillation 50 years on. Nature. 2002;415:219–26.
49. Liu L, Nattel S. Differing sympathetic and vagal effects on atrial fibrillation in dogs: role of refractoriness heterogeneity. Am J Physiol. 1997;273:H805–16.
50. Chen P-S, Chen LS, Fishbein MC, Lin S-F, Nattel S. Role of the autonomic nervous system in atrial fibrillation: pathophysiology and therapy. Circ Res. 2014;114:1500–15.
51. Burashnikov A, Antzelevitch C. Reinduction of atrial fibrillation immediately after termination of the arrhythmia is mediated by late phase 3 early afterdepolarization-induced triggered activity. Circulation. 2003;107:2355–60.
52. Patterson E, Po SS, Scherlag BJ, Lazzara R. Triggered firing in pulmonary veins initiated by in vitro autonomic nerve stimulation. Heart Rhythm. 2005;2:624–31.
53. Grundvold I, Skretteberg PT, Liestl K, Erikssen G, Engeseth K, Gjesdal K, et al. Low heart rates predict incident atrial fibrillation in healthy middle-aged men. Circ Arrhythm Electrophysiol. 2013;6:726–31.

54. Mont L, Sambola A, Brugada J, Vacca M, Marrugat J, Elosua R, et al. Long-lasting sport practice and lone atrial fibrillation. Eur Heart J. 2002;23:477–82.
55. Hoogsteen J, Schep G, Van Hemel NM, Van Der Wall EE. Paroxysmal atrial fibrillation in male endurance athletes. A 9-year follow up. Europace. 2004;6:222–8.
56. Wilhelm M, Roten L, Tanner H, Wilhelm I, Schmid J-P, Saner H. Atrial remodeling, autonomic tone, and lifetime training hours in nonelite athletes. Am J Cardiol. 2011;108: 580–5.
57. Yamaguchi T, Tsuchiya T, Nagamoto Y, Miyamoto K, Takahashi N. Characterization of atrial fibrillation and the effect of pulmonary vein antrum isolation in endurance athletes. J Arrhythmia. 2012;28:175–81.
58. Haïssaguerre M, Shah DC, Jaïs P, Hocini M, Yamane T, Deisenhofer I, et al. Electrophysiological breakthroughs from the left atrium to the pulmonary veins. Circulation. 2000;102:2463–5.
59. Ehrlich JR, Cha T, Zhang L, Chartier D, Melnyk P, Hohnloser SH, et al. Cellular electrophysiology of canine pulmonary vein cardiomyocytes: action potential and ionic current properties. J Physiol. 2003;551:801–13.
60. Chen YJ, Chen SA, Chen YC, Yeh H-II, Chan P, Chang M-SS, et al. Effects of rapid atrial pacing on the arrhythmogenic activity of single cardiomyocytes from pulmonary veins: implication in initiation of atrial fibrillation. Circulation. 2001;104:2849–54.
61. Hocini M, Ho SY, Kawara T, Linnenbank AC, Potse M, Shah D, et al. Electrical conduction in canine pulmonary veins: electrophysiological and anatomic correlation. Circulation. 2002;105:2442–8.
62. Arora R, Verheule S, Scott L, Navarrete A, Katari V, Wilson E, et al. Arrhythmogenic substrate of the pulmonary veins assessed by high-resolution optical mapping. Circulation. 2003;107:1816–21.
63. Calvo N, Mont L, Tamborero D, Berruezo A, Viola G, Guasch E, et al. Efficacy of circumferential pulmonary vein ablation of atrial fibrillation in endurance athletes. Europace. 2010;12:30–6.
64. Koopman P, Nuyens D, Garweg C, La Gerche A, De Buck S, Van Casteren L, et al. Efficacy of radiofrequency catheter ablation in athletes with atrial fibrillation. Europace. 2011;13:1386–93.
65. Oyen N, Ranthe MF, Carstensen L, Boyd HA, Olesen MS, Olesen S-P, et al. Familial aggregation of lone atrial fibrillation in young persons. J Am Coll Cardiol. 2012;60:917–21.
66. Otway R, Vandenberg JI, Guo G, Varghese A, Castro ML, Liu J, et al. Stretch-sensitive KCNQ1 mutation. A link between genetic and environmental factors in the pathogenesis of atrial fibrillation? J Am Coll Cardiol. 2007;49:578–86.
67. San Antonio R, Guasch E, Tolosana JM, Mont L. Determining the best approach to reduce the impact of exercise-induced atrial fibrillation: prevention, screening, or symptom-based treatment? Expert Rev Cardiovasc Ther. 2018;17:14779072.2019.1550720.
68. Mont L, Pelliccia A, Sharma S, Biffi A, Borjesson M, Terradellas JB, et al. Pre-participation cardiovascular evaluation for athletic participants to prevent sudden death: Position paper from the EHRA and the EACPR, branches of the ESC. Endorsed by APHRS, HRS, and SOLAECE. Europace. 2017;19:139–63.
69. Sejr MH, Nielsen JC, Damgaard D, Sandal BF, May O. Atrial fibrillation detected by external loop recording for seven days or two-day simultaneous Holter recording: a comparison in patients with ischemic stroke or transient ischemic attack. J Electrocardiol. 2017;50:287–93.
70. Fabregat-Andres O, Munoz-Macho A, Adell-Beltran G, Ibanez-Catala X, Macia A, Facila L. Evaluation of a new shirt-based electrocardiogram device for cardiac screening in soccer players: comparative study with treadmill ergospirometry. Cardiol Res. 2014;5:101–7.
71. Müssigbrodt A, Richter S, Wetzel U, Van Belle Y, Bollmann A, Hindricks G. Diagnosis of arrhythmias in athletes using leadless, ambulatory HR monitors. Med Sci Sports Exerc. 2013;45:1431–5.
72. Bumgarner JM, Lambert CT, Hussein AA, Cantillon DJ, Baranowski B, Wolski K, et al. Smartwatch algorithm for automated detection of atrial fibrillation. J Am Coll Cardiol. 2018;71:2381–8.

73. Chan P-H, Wong C-K, Poh YC, Pun L, Leung WW-C, Wong Y-F, et al. Diagnostic performance of a smartphone-based photoplethysmographic application for atrial fibrillation screening in a primary care setting. J Am Heart Assoc. 2016;5:pii: e003428.
74. Rozen G, Vaid J, Hosseini SM, Kaadan MI, Rafael A, Roka A, et al. Diagnostic accuracy of a novel mobile phone application for the detection and monitoring of atrial fibrillation. Am J Cardiol. 2018;121:1187–91.
75. Perez de Isla L, Lennie V, Quezada M, Guinea J, Arce C, Abad P, et al. New generation dynamic, wireless and remote cardiac monitorization platform: a feasibility study. Int J Cardiol. 2011;153:83–5.
76. Despang HG, Netz S, Heinig A, Holland HJ, Fischer WJ. Wireless long-term ECG integrated into clothing. Biomed Technol (Berl). 2008;53:270–8.
77. Myrstad M, Aarønæs M, Graff-Iversen S, Ariansen I, Nystad W, Ranhoff AH. Physical activity, symptoms, medication and subjective health among veteran endurance athletes with atrial fibrillation. Clin Res Cardiol. 2016;105:154–61.
78. Furlanello F, Bertoldi A, Dallago M, Galassi A, Fernando F, Biffi A, et al. Atrial fibrillation in elite athletes. J Cardiovasc Electrophysiol. 1998;9:S63–8.
79. Stefanadis C, Dernellis J, Toutouzas P. A clinical appraisal of left atrial function. Eur Heart J. 2001;22:22–36.
80. Channer KS, Jones JV. The contribution of atrial systole to mitral diastolic blood flow increases during exercise in humans. J Physiol. 1989;411:53–61.
81. Nishikawa Y, Roberts JP, Tan P, Klopfenstein CE, Klopfenstein HS. Effect of dynamic exercise on left atrial function in conscious dogs. J Physiol. 1994;481(Pt 2):457–68.
82. Hijazi Z, Lindbäck J, Alexander JH, Hanna M, Held C, Hylek EM, et al. The ABC (age, biomarkers, clinical history) stroke risk score: a biomarker-based risk score for predicting stroke in atrial fibrillation. Eur Heart J. 2016;37:1582–90.
83. Bisbal F, Gomez-Pulido F, Cabanas-GrandÍo P, Akoum N, Calvo M, Andreu D, et al. Left atrial geometry improves risk prediction of thromboembolic events in patients with atrial fibrillation. J Cardiovasc Electrophysiol. 2016;27:804–10.
84. King JB, Azadani PN, Suksaranjit P, Bress AP, Witt DM, Han FT, et al. Left atrial fibrosis and risk of cerebrovascular and cardiovascular events in patients with atrial fibrillation. J Am Coll Cardiol. 2017;70:1311–21.
85. Hållmarker U, Åsberg S, Michaëlsson K, Ärnlöv J, Hellberg D, Lindbäck J, et al. Risk of recurrent stroke and death after first stroke in long-distance ski race participants. J Am Heart Assoc. 2015;4:e002469.
86. Stewart S, Hart CL, Hole DJ, McMurray JJV. A population-based study of the long-term risks associated with atrial fibrillation: 20-year follow-up of the renfrew/Paisley study. Am J Med. 2002;113:359–64.
87. Santhanakrishnan R, Wang N, Larson MG, Magnani JW, McManus DD, Lubitz SA, et al. Atrial fibrillation begets heart failure and vice versa: temporal associations and differences in preserved versus reduced ejection fraction. Circulation. 2016;133:484–92.
88. Wijesurendra RS, Liu A, Eichhorn C, Ariga R, Levelt E, Clarke WT, et al. Lone atrial fibrillation is associated with impaired left ventricular energetics that persists despite successful catheter ablation. Circulation. 2016;134:1068–81.
89. Li D, Fareh S, Leung TK, Nattel S. Promotion of atrial fibrillation by heart failure in dogs: atrial remodeling of a different sort. Circulation. 1999;100:87–95.
90. De Potter T, Berruezo A, Mont L, Matiello M, Tamborero D, Santibanez C, et al. Left ventricular systolic dysfunction by itself does not influence outcome of atrial fibrillation ablation. Europace. 2010;12:24–9.
91. Calvo N, Bisbal F, Guiu E, Ramos P, Nadal M, Maria Tolosana J, et al. Impact of atrial fibrillation-induced tachycardiomyopathy in patients undergoing pulmonary vein isolation. Int J Cardiol. 2013;168:4093–7.
92. Marrouche NF, Brachmann J, Andresen D, Siebels J, Boersma L, Jordaens L, et al. Catheter ablation for atrial fibrillation with heart failure. N Engl J Med. 2018;378:417–27.

93. Zipes DP, Link MS, Ackerman MJ, Kovacs RJ, Myerburg RJ, Estes NAM. Eligibility and disqualification recommendations for competitive athletes with cardiovascular abnormalities: task force 9: arrhythmias and conduction defects: a scientific statement from the American Heart Association and American College of Cardiology. J Am Coll Cardiol. 2015;66:2412–23.
94. Berkowitz JN, Moll S. Athletes and blood clots: individualized, intermittent anticoagulation management. J Thromb Haemost. 2017;15:1051–4.
95. Berruezo A, Tamborero D, Mont L, Benito B, Tolosana JM, Sitges M, et al. Pre-procedural predictors of atrial fibrillation recurrence after circumferential pulmonary vein ablation. Eur Heart J. 2007;28:836–41.
96. Marrouche NF, Wilber D, Hindricks G, Jais P, Akoum N, Marchlinski F, et al. Association of atrial tissue fibrosis identified by delayed enhancement MRI and atrial fibrillation catheter ablation: the DECAAF study. JAMA. 2014;311:498–506.
97. de Vos CB, Nieuwlaat R, Crijns HJGM, Camm AJ, LeHeuzey J-Y, Kirchhof CJ, et al. Autonomic trigger patterns and anti-arrhythmic treatment of paroxysmal atrial fibrillation: data from the Euro Heart Survey. Eur Heart J. 2008;29:632–9.
98. Moore SC, Lee I-M, Weiderpass E, Campbell PT, Sampson JN, Kitahara CM, et al. Association of leisure-time physical activity with risk of 26 types of cancer in 1.44 million adults. JAMA Intern Med. 2016;176:816–25.
99. Lafuente-Lafuente C, Mouly S. L-TMAB. Antiarrhythmics for maintaining sinus rhythm after cardioversion of atral fibrillation. Cochrane Database Syst Rev. 2015;3:CD005049.
100. Alboni P, Botto GL, Baldi N, Luzi M, Russo V, Gianfranchi L, et al. Outpatient treatment of recent-onset atrial fibrillation with the "pill-in-the-pocket" approach. N Engl J Med. 2004;351:2384–91.
101. Holmes B, Heel RC. Flecainide. A preliminary review of its pharmacodynamic properties and therapeutic efficacy. Drugs. 1985;29:1–33.
102. Furlanello F, Lupo P, Pittalis M, Foresti S, Vitali-Serdoz L, Francia P, et al. Radiofrequency catheter ablation of atrial fibrillation in athletes referred for disabling symptoms preventing usual training schedule and sport competition. J Cardiovasc Electrophysiol. 2008;19:457–62.
103. Heidbüchel H, Anné W, Willems R, Adriaenssens B, Van de Werf F, Ector H. Endurance sports is a risk factor for atrial fibrillation after ablation for atrial flutter. Int J Cardiol. 2006;107:67–72.
104. Van Gelder IC, Groenveld HF, Crijns HJGM, Tuininga YS, Tijssen JGP, Alings AM, et al. Lenient versus strict rate control in patients with atrial fibrillation. N Engl J Med. 2010;362:1363–73.
105. Ulimoen SR, Enger S, Carlson J, Platonov PG, Pripp AH, Abdelnoor M, et al. Comparison of four single-drug regimens on ventricular rate and arrhythmia-related symptoms in patients with permanent atrial fibrillation. Am J Cardiol. 2013;111:225–30.
106. Ulimoen SR, Enger S, Pripp AH, Abdelnoor M, Arnesen H, Gjesdal K, et al. Calcium channel blockers improve exercise capacity and reduce N-terminal Pro-B-type natriuretic peptide levels compared with beta-blockers in patients with permanent atrial fibrillation. Eur Heart J. 2014;35:517–24.
107. Farshi R, Kistner D, Sarma JSM, Longmate JA, Singh BN. Ventricular rate control in chronic atrial fibrillation during daily activity and programmed exercise: a crossover open-label study of five drug regimens. J Am Coll Cardiol. 1999;33:304–10.
108. Matsuda M, Matsuda Y, Yamagishi T, Takahashi T, Haraguchi M, Tada T, et al. Effects of digoxin, propranolol, and verapamil on exercise in patients with chronic isolated atrial fibrillation. Cardiovasc Res. 1991;25:453–7.
109. Aizer A, Gaziano JM, Cook NR, Manson JE, Buring JE, Albert CM. Relation of vigorous exercise to risk of atrial fibrillation. Am J Cardiol. 2009;103:1572–7.

# Sport in Extreme Environments: Cardiovascular Issues

# 34

Martin Burtscher and Kay Tetzlaff

**Learning Objectives**

1. General physiological responses to extreme temperatures, i.e. cold or heat.
2. General physiological responses to hypobaria (hypobaric hypoxia, high altitude) or hyperbaria (underwater diving).
3. Cardiovascular risks when exercising in cold or hot environments.
4. Cardiovascular risks while exercising at high-altitude or underwater diving.
5. Most important measures to prevent cardiovascular events when exercising in extreme environments.

## 34.1 Introduction

Humans have been attracted by extreme environments since long times. It were and still are the remotest places on earth like the poles, the highest mountain peaks, the hottest desert, or the deepest sea being particularly fascinating. Although the most extreme environments remain rather reserved to a few extraordinary people, improved access and infrastructure nowadays permit millions of visitors to perform recreational outdoor activities and even competitions at high altitude, in extremely cold or hot regions and to dive into deep waters [1, 2]. Hypobaric hypoxia and cold at high altitudes, heat of the desert, and hyperbaria when diving represent considerable challenges to the human body. It is recalled that humans are homeothermic and extremely dependent on an adequate oxygen supply. Consequently, the human body has to be continuously supplied with sufficient oxygen, and its core temperature has

M. Burtscher (✉)
Department of Sports Sciences, University of Innsbruck, Innsbruck, Austria
e-mail: martin.burtscher@uibk.ac.at

K. Tetzlaff
Department of Sports Medicine, University of Tübingen, Tübingen, Germany
e-mail: kay.tetzlaff@klinikum-tuebingen.de



A. Pressler, J. Niebauer (eds.), *Textbook of Sports and Exercise Cardiology*,
https://doi.org/10.1007/978-3-030-35374-2_34

to be regulated within a relatively narrow range to ensure optimal physiological function and survival. However, human beings are also endowed with the capability to coping with specific environmental stressors by various adaptive biological processes and specific behavioural responses [1]. Initially, the activation of the hypothalamic-pituitary-adrenocortical axis and of the sympathetic nervous system is characteristic for of all these environmental stressors [3]. Usually, adaptation occurs with repeated exposures to those stressors. However, the risk of cardiovascular adverse events may steeply increase in individuals with pre-existing diseases. The adaptive capacity differs considerably between individuals, cardiovascular fitness being an important explanatory variable for those differences [4]. This fact becomes particularly relevant in the light of an increasing sport participation of elderly subjects suffering from cardiovascular diseases. Therefore, aims of this chapter include

- The delineation of general responses to extreme environmental conditions.
- Cardiovascular responses to exercise and associated risks in healthy individuals and in those with cardiovascular diseases.
- Recommendations for prevention.

## 34.2 Demographic Aspects

Worldwide, recreational outdoor sports activities and sport competitions in extreme environments are becoming more and more popular. Such activities include sports like hiking, running, cycling, climbing, skiing and diving performed

(a) Under extreme temperatures (cold, hot)
(b) At terrestrial altitude (hypobaric hypoxia) or
(c) In hyperbaric surroundings

Some examples:

- Worldwide, more than 100 million tourists visit altitudes above 2000 m each year [5].
- Moreover, there are 2000 downhill ski areas spread across 67 countries with an estimated 400 million skier days annually [6].
- Also, competitions at moderate or high altitudes have become extremely popular during previous years, e.g. events like
  - The soccer championships in La Paz (3600 m)
  - The road cycling championships in Bogotá (2640 m)
  - The Pasco Marathon (4380 m)—officially the highest in the world
  - The Ladakh Marathon (3500 m) where participants increased from 1500 Participants in the 1st edition to almost 5500 in the 6th edition in 2017 or
  - The Khardung La Challenge—an ultramarathon (72 km) event, which starts near 4000 m, reaches 5370 m and ends at 3504 m

Events at high altitudes are typically associated with hypoxic but often also with cold conditions. Whereas the North Pole Marathon as well as some open water swim events are characterized by extremely cold conditions, a very hot environment is challenging the participants in desert events such as the Petra Marathon, the Oman Marathon or the multi-day Marathon des Sables through the Moroccan Sahara.

## 34.3 Exercising in the Cold

### 34.3.1 General Physiological Responses to Cold Exposure

Humans are homeotherms, indicating that their core temperature has to be held constant within a relatively narrow range (35.0–37.5 °C). Exposure to cold air or cold water is associated with the risk of becoming hypothermic (core temperature below 35 °C), which is much more pronounced in water since the convective heat loss in water is about 20 times greater compared to air. However, this difference becomes narrower when wearing wet clothes and/or in windy conditions. Sudden exposure to cold, typically immersion into cold water, triggers the cold shock response, characterized by a reflex inspiratory gasp and subsequent uncontrollable hyperventilation and tachycardia. It is noteworthy that the cold shock response is considerably reduced after repeated short-term cold exposures [7].

Heat loss in the cold can be prevented by behavioural responses like the use of protecting clothes and/or voluntary thermogenesis by physical activity and/or by powerful homeostatic responses including

1. Cutaneous vasoconstriction.
2. Involuntary thermogenesis by shivering [1, 8].

The extent of these effector responses (Fig. 34.1) differs depending on the type (air or water), duration and severity of the cold exposure and previous cold adaptation but also on individual characteristics like

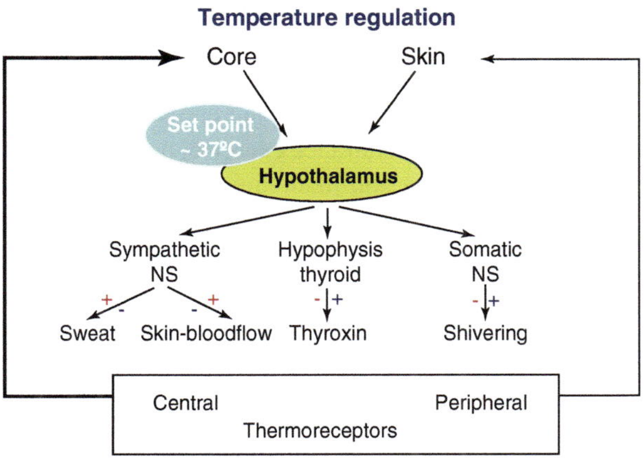


**Fig. 34.1** Schematic presentation of regulatory mechanisms involved in temperature homeostasis. *NS* nervous system

(a) Cardiovascular fitness
(b) Age
(c) Gender
(d) Body composition [9]

1. **Peripheral vasoconstriction** promotes insulation and reduces heat loss from the body when the skin temperature decreases below 35 °C. However, this also promotes rapid cooling especially of the unprotected face, the fingers and toes associated with impaired manual dexterity, tactile sensitivity and gross motor function, and with enhanced risk of cold injury (frostbite) [10]. Remarkably, vasoconstriction of these body parts is interrupted by periodical vasodilatation (hunting response) likely representing some protection from cold injury [10].
2. **Shivering** (rhythmic skeletal muscle contractions) may increase the whole-body metabolic rate up to or even exceeding 350 W [8]. Importantly, the maximal heat production corresponds to almost 50% of the individual's aerobic capacity (maximal oxygen uptake, $VO_2max$) [11]. Subjects with larger fat mass show a delayed shivering response to cold exposure. The decrease of deep body temperature is inversely related to subcutaneous fat thickness [8]. Cold tolerance of older individuals may be reduced due to their lower cardiovascular fitness but also because of a diminished vasoconstrictor response. Sex differences of cold tolerance are primarily explained by anthropometric characteristics. Women have more subcutaneous fat but lower muscle mass and probably also a somewhat lower thermoregulatory response. Thus, the larger surface area to mass ratio and reduced shivering capacity make women more susceptible to prolonged cold stress [12].

### 34.3.2 Cardiovascular Responses and Associated Risk When Exercising in the Cold

Exercising in the cold is associated with considerable heat production preventing a dangerous drop of body temperature, provided exercise intensity is high enough. Heat production during exercise in the cold, corresponding to an intensity exceeding about 60% $VO_2max$, prevents the risk of hypothermia, however, inactivity due to injury or fatigue dramatically increases this risk. Related to the large heat production during intense endurance exercise, moderate cold ambient temperatures facilitate heat dissipation and maintaining optimal body temperature and performance. Ambient temperatures around 10 °C seem to be optimal for fast marathon finishing times [13]. More extreme cold temperatures or lower exercise intensities in the cold may profoundly affect cardiovascular functioning during exercise.

Physiological responses differing in the cold from those in normothermic environment include cardiovascular parameters such as

(a) Heart rate
(b) Stroke volume

(c) Total peripheral resistance
(d) Mean arterial pressure
(e) Requirements of myocardial oxygen consumption.

- Heart rates are reduced during submaximal and maximal exercise. Maximal heart rate and related $VO_2max$ decrease when core temperature is reduced by 0.5–2.0 °C [14].
- In contrast, stroke volume is increased due to peripheral vasoconstriction and the accompanied elevation of the central venous pressure.
- Peripheral vasoconstriction and elevated systemic vascular resistance cause an increase of systemic arterial blood pressure and myocardial oxygen consumption, determined by the so-called double product (systolic blood pressure times heart rate). These responses do not appear to have a relevant impact on performance in healthy subjects [8] but may provoke cold-induced angina attacks in patients suffering from coronary artery disease (CAD), in particular in those with an abnormal baroreceptor function [15].
- Elevated cardiac workload and reduced myocardial perfusion also impair exercise performance in CAD and heart failure patients when exercising in the cold [16].
- Elevated blood pressure at baseline and a pronounced response to cold combined with autonomic dysfunction compromise exercise capacity [17] and put hypertensive patients at greater risk.
- Moreover, exposure to extreme cold was shown to increase the risk of both ischemic and hemorrhagic stroke [18].
- Antianginal and antihypertensive medication lower systemic blood pressure (without affecting the cardiovascular response to cold) and may improve exercise performance in the cold in subjects suffering from hypertension, CAD or heart failure [16].

In general, superficial cooling increases sympathetic activity and may alter cardiac function and consequently increase the risk of arrythmias and cardiac events [19]. Moreover, a lesser reduction of vagal tone during ultra-marathon running in extreme cold was related to superior performance [20].

### 34.3.3 Preventive Aspects

- An appropriate level of physical fitness related to the challenges of the specific physical activity in the cold environment represents an important prerequisite for safe and joyful participation in such activities.
- Exercise testing and sports medical advice (including suitable medication) will support effective preparatory measures.
- Preceding cold exposures (habituation) can effectively reduce cardiovascular responses and probably also associated adverse event. Habituation occurs already after a few exposures associated with more comfortable feeling and diminished and/or delayed cardiovascular and metabolic changes at rest and when exercising in the cold [1].

- Moreover, the use of appropriate clothing contributes importantly to the prevention of adverse events during exercise in the cold.

## 34.4 Exercising in the Heat

### 34.4.1 General Physiological Responses to Heat Exposure

Heat exposure may provoke the risk of hyperthermia (core temperature above 37.5 °C), which is especially pronounced during exercise. As in the cold, preventive strategies include behavioural measures and physiological responses. Behavioural measures comprise the use of appropriate clothing, seeking shadow, rest, cooling by water and/or wind. Physiological responses are characterized by mechanisms including elevation of skin blood flow and sweating to facilitate heat dissipation but also the initiation of circulatory adaptation supporting the maintenance of central blood pressure by an increase in plasma volume and cardiac output [21] (Fig. 34.1).

These mechanisms are extremely powerful as

- Skin blood flow can increase from about 0.5 l/min to over 7 l/min.
- Sweat rates may be above 1.5 l/h resulting in an evaporative heat loss exceeding 1 kW in a 70 kg human [22].

Consequently, systemic vascular resistance, systemic blood pressure and (more pronounced) central venous pressure decrease and cardiac output increases, due to a rise of heart rate. With inadequate rehydration, the body becomes dehydrated. Clinical dehydration occurs with a loss of body water exceeding 3% of body mass, presenting with early symptoms of heat-related disorders such as light-headedness [22]. Thermoregulation is compromised by dehydration (hypohydration) with the consequences of reduced sweating rates and skin blood flow and enhanced heat storage [23]. The rising core temperature evokes

(a) Hyperventilation
(b) Cerebral dysfunction (e.g. confusion), and finally
(c) Cardiovascular collapse [22].

Heat tolerance varies greatly between individuals, e.g. cardiovascular fitness, age, health status, medication, hydration, acclimatization to heat, previous heat disorders, etc. may all modify individual tolerance.

### 34.4.2 Cardiovascular Responses and Associated Risk When Exercising in the Heat

The primary cardiovascular challenge during exercise in hot ambient temperature is to provide appropriate blood volume to the working skeletal muscle and to simultaneously increase the skin blood flow to support heat dissipation [23]. Thus, during exercise in the heat there is a competition between thermoregulatory (skin blood flow) and metabolic (skeletal muscle blood flow) demands finally resulting in a performance decline [24]. In athletes, but also in patients suffering from cardiovascular diseases this competition surpasses the pumping capacity (maximal cardiac output) of the heart.

This situation becomes exacerbated with progressive dehydration, particularly fostered in hot conditions, and is accompanied by profound decreases of the

- End-diastolic volume
- Stroke volume
- Cardiac output
- Blood flow to exercising muscles
- Associated $VO_2max$ [25]

Heart rate is higher for any given cardiac output during exercise in the heat. Cardiac output cannot be increased above a certain level, thus vasodilatation in and blood flow to exercising muscles are limited to prevent severe hypotension. In general, this seems to be achieved by the activity of baroreflex and metaboreflexes (originating in the working muscle); however, in hot conditions, thermoregulatory reflexes may additionally be involved [26]. Assuming that neural responses are primarily controlled by activity of the sympathetic nervous system, this has been termed a "hyperadrenergic state" [27], which may contribute to cardiovascular adverse events. Fatigue experience in hot environments is not resulting from diminished muscle blood flow but rather from the elevated brain temperature.

Heat-related disorders are more common

1. In elderly subjects with reduced thermoregulatory ability
2. In patients suffering from cardiovascular diseases
3. In individuals taking drugs interacting with central nervous function, or
4. In those who experienced previous heat illness [22]

Heat tolerance is reduced in patients with cardiovascular diseases, especially in those with impaired ventricular function, due to an impaired vasodilation response to heat exposure, while the sweating response seems to be preserved [28]. Both exercise training and heat exposure may provide cardioprotection by upregulation of myocardial heat shock protein 70 (HSP 70) [29]. There is one study claiming that fatal heat stroke would even be more prevalent than arrhythmic death during endurance events in hot conditions [30]. Fluid-electrolyte disturbances, like hypernatremia and hyponatremia, at least partly as a consequence of inappropriate fluid (and electrolyte) intake (too much or too little), cause similar symptoms like confusion and disorientation and, if untreated, will progress to coma and death. Exertional dysnatremia was diagnosed in about 30% of collapsed marathon runners [31].

### 34.4.3 Preventive Aspects

- Again, appropriate physical fitness (assessed by exercise testing) may considerably help to reduce the risk of heat-related emergencies.
- Education on appropriate fluid (and salt) intake during long endurance events in the heat or suitable therapy in the case of an emergency are of utmost importance.
- Importantly, several days of heat exposure induce effective acclimatization process, contributing to the prevention of adverse events during subsequent exercise in the heat.
- Already 3–6 exposure days result in the elevation of the plasma volume and the reduction of submaximal heart rates [32].
- After 10–14 days heat acclimatization will be completed associated with increased skin blood flow and sweating capability contributing to cardiovascular stability and improved exercise performance [32].

## 34.5 Exercising at Terrestrial Altitude (in Hypobaric Hypoxia)

### 34.5.1 General Physiological Responses to Altitude (Hypoxia) Exposure

Acute exposure to high altitude provokes the development of high-altitude illnesses, which can largely be prevented by appropriate acclimatization. Barometric pressure and in parallel also partial pressure of oxygen decrease with increasing altitude (hypobaric hypoxia). For instance, at an altitude of 5000 m these pressures constitute only about half of the pressure at sea level (Fig. 34.2).

The reduced oxygen in the inspired air ($PiO_2$) results in a drop of

- The alveolar pressure of oxygen ($PAO_2$) in the lungs and consequently also of
- The arterial pressure of oxygen ($PaO_2$) in the blood and of
- The arterial oxygen saturation ($SaO_2$)

Reduced oxygen in the blood is termed "hypoxemia", and within tissues "hypoxia". Increases in ventilation (hyperventilation) and cardiac output are acute responses to (at least partly) counteract the diminished oxygen supply. A pronounced hyperventilatory response to hypoxia (hypoxic ventilatory response, HVR) can powerfully increase $PAO_2$, $PaO_2$ and $SaO_2$ at a given altitude, however, at the expense of the alveolar and arterial pressure of carbon dioxide ($PACO_2$ and $PaCO_2$) [33]. The HVR is mediated by the activity of peripheral chemoreceptor afferents of the carotid bodies augmenting ventilation and sympathetic activity (contributing to heart rate elevation) [34]. Hyperventilation increases over days at altitude due to the rising sensitivity of the peripheral chemoreceptors (ventilatory acclimatization) [33]. In addition, also systemic blood pressure may at least temporarily be elevated [35]. Increased diuresis at altitude causes loss of bicarbonate (renal compensation of the respiratory alkalosis), but also haemoconcentration due to a reduction in plasma volume accompanied by lowering of the stroke volume. Related to these changes with acclimatization, cardiac

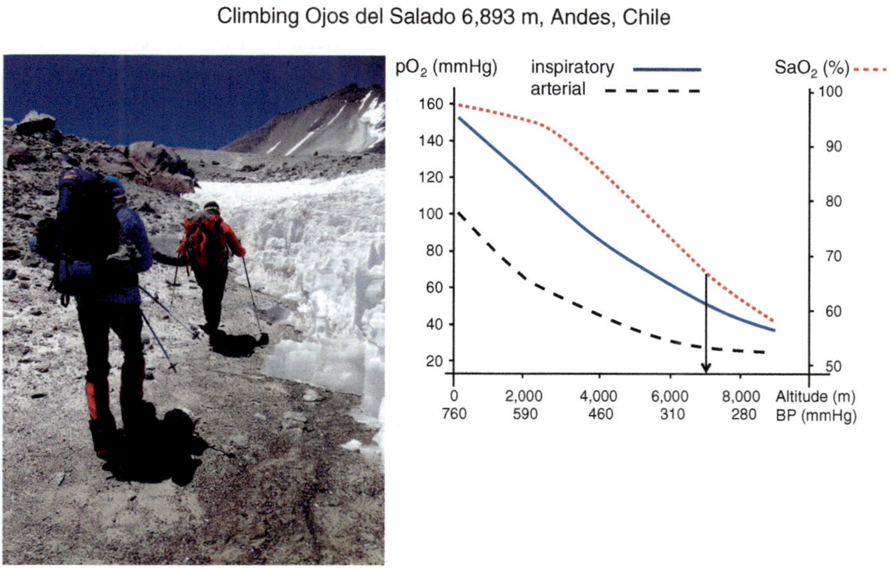


**Fig. 34.2** Altitude-related decrease of inspiratory and arterial oxygen pressure ($pO_2$) and arterial oxygen saturation ($SaO_2$). *BP* barometric pressure

output returns to baseline but heart rate remains elevated because of the lower stroke volume [35]. Pulmonary artery pressure increases at high altitude and remains increased due to hypoxic vasoconstriction in the lung (hypoxic pulmonary vasoconstriction, HPV), which seems to be particularly profound in elderly individuals [36]. All these responses may considerably vary between individuals and do not completely compensate for the reduce $PiO_2$, especially at higher altitudes. The resulting hypoxia negatively not only affects exercise performance but also represents the main cause for the development of high-altitude illnesses like

(a) Acute mountain sickness (AMS)
(b) High altitude cerebral edema (HACE) or
(c) High altitude pulmonary edema (HAPE) [37]

### 34.5.2 Cardiovascular Responses and Associated Risk When Exercising at Altitude (in Hypoxia)

Aerobic capacity, defined as maximal pulmonary oxygen uptake ($VO_2max$) during incremental exercise testing, declines with increasing altitude.

- The decline of $VO_2max$ amounts to about 1.5–3.5% every 300 m of gain in altitude above 1500 m [38].This decline varies individually depending on various factors and is more pronounced in fitter subjects [39].

- According to the Fick principle ($VO_2 = CO \times 1.34[Hb] \times (SaO_2 - SvO_2)$; see Chap. 3), $VO_2$max is closely related to $SaO_2$, meaning that preventing a large drop of $SaO_2$ by hyperventilation will also prevent a large decline in $VO_2$max. Lower levels of ventilation and reduced CO due to HPV and associated insufficiency to fully oxygenate the blood when passing through the pulmonary capillaries can partly explain the more pronounced lowering of $VO_2$max in highly-trained individuals. However, $VO_2$max may also be profoundly affected in patients suffering from lung disease, e.g. COPD or pulmonary hypertension, or from heart disease, e.g. heart failure.
- Related to the increasing ventilation and haemoconcentration with acclimatization, $SaO_2$ and haematocrit contribute to improved arterial oxygen content ($CaO_2$) and oxygen delivery to working muscles, increased arterio-venous oxygen difference, and in particular submaximal exercise performance [40].
- Maximal heart rate drops with acute high-altitude exposure without essential changes during acclimatization.
- In contrast, stroke volume and cardiac output decline further with acclimatization, and improved $CaO_2$ cannot fully compensate for this decline and thus cannot restore sea level $VO_2$max.

Maher and colleagues studied changes in exercise performance during a 12-day high-altitude (4300 m) sojourn in well-trained young men. No improvements were seen for $VO_2$max but submaximal performance rose by 45% during acclimatization (time to exhaustion) [41].

Leisure time activities at altitude like mountain hiking and downhill skiing seem to be associated with relatively high risk of cardiac events, i.e. sudden cardiac death [5]. Males older than 34 years and pre-existing risk factors constitute the main risk group. Prior myocardial infarction has been established to be the most important risk factor. However, the impact of altitude per se on the risk for cardiac events remains unclear. It is probably the unaccustomed physical activity combined with extreme environmental conditions (hypoxia, cold, etc.) that may trigger sudden cardiac death [42]. Beside sudden cardiac death, hypoxia may cause or exacerbate symptoms in CAD patients, but also other conditions associated with high altitude and exercise like

- Cold
- Dehydration
- Sleep disturbances
- Change in diet
- Emotional stress, etc.

may provoke acute coronary events [43]. For instance, the Tenth Mountain Division Study demonstrated reduced exercise performance in elderly subjects exposed to acute moderate altitude, which was associated with acute myocardial ischemia triggered by hypoxemia, sympathetic activation, and pulmonary hypertension [44]. However, after 5 days of acclimatization to simulated moderate altitude, those subjects showed similar exercise performance, sympathetic activation and endothelial function as observed at sea level.

It has to be noted, that high-altitude activities are often performed in remote areas meaning difficult-to-access places and delayed emergency medical assistance.

### 34.5.3 Preventive Aspects

- Both exercise training to achieve an appropriate cardiovascular fitness and acclimatization to altitude by supervised exposure to simulated altitude, e.g. hypoxia room, and/or to real altitude are important preventive measures not only for patients.
- Exercise testing before going to high altitude enables the assessment of the individual cardiovascular fitness and clinical decision making.
- Slow rates of ascent and rest or only low intensity exercise on the first days at altitude help to prevent high altitude illness.
- In certain cases, e.g. known susceptibility or more rapid ascent, preventive medication may be used.
- Ascents to altitude are often related to cold exposure, thus additional habituation to cold is recommended.
- Moreover, adequate behaviour at altitude (individually tailored exercise intensity, resting days, periodic pauses, food and fluid intake) will contribute to the prevention of cardiovascular adverse events.

## 34.6 Exercising at Depth (Diving)

### 34.6.1 General Aspects of Diving Physics and Physiology

The hostile underwater environment is prohibiting humans from prolonged exposures, as essential oxygen supply needs to be maintained by artificial means, e.g., self-contained underwater breathing apparatus (scuba). Without breathing gas supply, exposures are limited to individual breath-hold time.

This environment is mainly characterized by submersion in water and elevated ambient pressure, which elicits multiple effects on human physiology. Hydrostatic pressure adds to ambient pressure at sea level, doubling at a depth of 10 m, and increasing by approximately 100 kPa (1 bar) every additional 10 m of seawater column. When breathing air underwater, nitrogen will dissolve in body tissues upon pressure increase (or descent). Conversely, gas bubbles will form upon pressure decrease or ascent from depth. These gas microbubbles will reach the alveolar bed by venous return to the heart and eventually be dissolved through diffusion. Gas density will increase with ambient pressure. Gas partial pressures (e.g., $pO_2$, $pN_2$) will increase according to ambient pressure. When using air as breathing gas, the scuba-diver is exposed to hyperbaric hyperoxia at depth.

- Acute toxic effects of elevated $pO_2$ may occur at depths beyond 70 m. For instance, a scuba-diver breathing air at 40 m is exposed to inspiratory $pO_2$ roughly equivalent to breathing 100% oxygen at sea level.
- Narcotic effects of high $pN_2$ may emerge at depths beyond 30 m.

Diving gear and posture will add resistive loading to ventilation at depth, in addition to impaired gas flow due to increased density. Thus, hypercapnia may result from altered ventilatory pattern at depth.

Exercising under these environmental conditions will be limited by the respiratory system's ability to cope with the consequences of increased inspiratory resistance and airflow limitation. Exercise while diving may compromise safety for various reasons:

- Increased ventilation during exercise will lead to higher nitrogen take-up, thus, enhanced tissue inert gas load and risk of gas phase liberation during decompression.
- Increased filling of thoracic blood vessels may increase the risk of immersion pulmonary edema due to increased transmural pressures when exercising,

### 34.6.2 Cardiovascular Responses and Associated Risk to Diving

Several factors unique to the underwater environment will significantly affect the cardiovascular system, such as

(a) The diving response (bradycardia)
(b) Immersion/submersion (thoracic blood pooling)
(c) Temperature (heat loss)
(d) Diving gear, e.g. scuba, garment (increased breathing resistance)
(e) Hyperoxia
(f) Hyperbaria (gas density)

The human diving response, considered to have an oxygen conserving role, elicits cardiovascular changes. It involves bradycardia, vasoconstriction of selected vascular beds, reduced blood flow to peripheral capillary beds, and increased sympathetic outflow to the periphery [45].

Head-out immersion causes a blood shift of approximately 700 ml into the thorax [46], leading to increased end-diastolic filling of the right heart and lung vessels, with an increase in pulmonary artery and capillary pressure. This end-diastolic volume increase will increase stroke volume and decrease heart rate. Cardiac output increases according to the water level of immersion in the erect posture; the reported 32–62% cardiac output increase is due to an enlarged stroke volume, dominating over a decrease in heart rate [47]; mean arterial pressure is unchanged. The increased venous return and atrial stretch lead to attenuated secretion of anti-natriuretic hormones and vasopressin which result in a diuresis and natriuresis.

Temperature is another modulator of physiological responses to the aquatic environment. Enhanced conduction and convection will accelerate heat loss in water, resulting in increased vascular resistance of subcutaneous tissues, as well as muscle (vasoconstriction). On the contrary, a limited ability to eliminate heat by evaporation in warm or hot water may raise body temperature to dangerous levels, particularly during exercise.

Hyperoxia induces a reduction in blood flow though vasoconstriction; this has been observed in various vascular beds, including the heart, skeletal muscle, and brain [48]. Reductions in coronary blood velocity have been reported by echocardiography compared with normoxia.

Hyperbaria per se is not known to affect the cardiovascular system. It may, however, in combination with immersion add to further blood shift with increasing water depth.

### 34.6.3 Preventive Aspects

Given the aforementioned physiological challenges, safety precautions have been recommended for recreational scuba-diving, such as training certifications and diving medicals. Assessment of the cardiovascular system is of particular importance for diving safety. While the young and healthy heart may tolerate significant increases in cardiac pre- and afterload, the physiologic challenges on the body imposed by the unique underwater environment may lead to cardiac decompensation in the state of disease. Indeed, diving accident statistics reveal that cardiac conditions are a prominent root cause of diving fatalities, besides technical and equipment issues [49].

The general approach to prevention in diving is that medical conditions which increase the risk of injury should preclude diving. For some conditions, the risk may be acceptable under certain precautions. For example, the risk of right-to-left-shunting of venous gas microbubbles in an individual with a patent foramen ovale can be minimized by avoidance of diving profiles that increase the risk of bubble generation. Selected cardiac conditions are displayed below:

- **Arterial hypertension**: Any symptomatic or unstable hypertension precludes diving. Divers who have demonstrated adequate control of blood pressure and have no secondary organ damage may be allowed to dive. Possible side effects of antihypertensives (e.g. bradycardia for beta-blockers) must be considered when clearing divers.
- **Coronary artery disease**: Symptomatic coronary artery disease is a contraindication to safe diving. Subjects with asymptomatic disease, including those with a known history of myocardial infarction or therapeutic catheterization, may be cleared for low-stress sport diving after 6–12 months of healing and stabilization. Fitness to dive should be based on the patient's exercise tolerance.
- **Congestive heart failure**: Congestive heart failure precludes diving.
- **Rhythm disorders**: Ventricular tachycardia and many types of atrial rhythm disturbances are incompatible with diving, given the risk of unconsciousness and

drowning. Most dysrhythmias that require medication are medically disqualifying. Patients with pre-excitation disorders, such as Wolf-Parkinson-White, may be permitted to dive if they have never experienced symptoms or cardiac arrhythmias.
- **Patent foramen ovale (PFO)**: Subjects with PFO may be allowed to dive. Certain precautions, e.g. avoiding dives that require decompression stops, limiting bottom time, or appropriate use of oxygen-enriched breathing gas mixture, may mitigate risk.
- **Valvular heart disease**: Valvular heart disease is a relative contraindication; individuals with normal hemodynamics and asymptomatic exercise tolerance may be fit to dive.
- **Reduced ejection fraction** is a relative contraindication to diving. Due to the hemodynamic changes from submersion, patients should be aware that diving can precipitate acute pulmonary edema.

Careful consideration must be given to the individual's ability to manage exercise demands when heart disease might compromise exercise capacity.

## 34.7 Conclusion

Unquestionable, regular exercise contributes to health and well-being but may also be associated with cardiovascular risks especially with insufficient cardiovascular fitness and/or pre-existing diseases. Due to the greater health risk when exercising under extreme conditions, pre-exposure medical assessment of exercise performance and cardiorespiratory functioning are of utmost importance. Both exercise training to achieve an appropriate cardiovascular fitness and habituation/acclimatization to the specific environmental conditions are important preventive measures for athletes and patients as well.

**Clinical Pearls**
- Individuals not sufficiently adapted to extreme environmental conditions, i.e. heat, cold, hypobaric hypoxia (altitude), or hyperbaria (depth) are at risk to suffer from cardiovascular adverse events, in particular elderly people and those with pre-existing diseases.
- Assessment of the cardiovascular system including exercise testing and appropriate medical advice are among the most important preventive measures.

## Review

### Questions

1. Which are the most effective homeostatic responses of the human organism when exposed to cold and how are they related to the individual aerobic capacity ($VO_2max$)?

2. How many days are needed for heat acclimatization and physiological changes associated with heat acclimatization?
3. How does acclimatization to high altitude affect maximal and submaximal aerobic exercise performance?
4. Which are the main factors limiting exercise capacity at depth?

## Answers

1. Most effective homeostatic responses to cold exposure are cutaneous vasoconstriction and involuntary thermogenesis by shivering; the maximal heat production corresponds to the individual's aerobic capacity ($VO_2max$).
2. After 10–14 days heat acclimatization will be completed associated with increased skin blood flow and sweating capability contributing to cardiovascular stability and improved exercise performance.
3. Whereas maximal aerobic capacity ($VO_2max$) is hardly affected by acclimatization to high altitude, submaximal exercise performance improves considerably.
4. Increased gas density and increased breathing resistance will restrict ventilation at depth.

## References


1. Burtscher M, Gatterer H, Burtscher J, Mairbäurl H. Extreme terrestrial environments: life in thermal stress and hypoxia. A narrative review. Front Physiol. 2018;9:572.
2. Tetzlaff K, Thorsen E. Breathing at depth: physiologic and clinical aspects of diving while breathing compressed gas. Clin Chest Med. 2005;26(3):355–80.
3. Münzel T, Daiber A. Environmental stressors and their impact on health and disease with focus on oxidative stress. Antioxid Redox Signal. 2018;28(9):735–40.
4. Burtscher M. Exercise limitations by the oxygen delivery and utilization systems in aging and disease: coordinated adaptation and deadaptation of the lung-heart muscle axis – a mini-review. Gerontology. 2013;59(4):289–96.
5. Burtscher M, Ponchia A. The risk of cardiovascular events during leisure time activities at altitude. Prog Cardiovasc Dis. 2010;52(6):507–11.
6. Vanat L. International report on snow & mountain tourism. 2018. http://vanat.ch/RM-world-report-2018.pdf.
7. Eglin CM, Tipton MJ. Repeated cold showers as a method of habituating humans to the initial responses to cold water immersion. Eur J Appl Physiol. 2005;93(5-6):624–9.
8. Castellani JW, Tipton MJ. Cold stress effects on exposure tolerance and exercise performance. Compr Physiol. 2015;6(1):443–69.
9. Stocks JM, Taylor NA, Tipton MJ, Greenleaf JE. Human physiological responses to cold exposure. Aviat Space Environ Med. 2004;75(5):444–57.
10. Cheung SS. Responses of the hands and feet to cold exposure. Temperature (Austin). 2015;2(1):105–20.
11. Golden FS, Hampton IF, Hervey GR, Knibbs AV. Shivering intensity in humans during immersion in cold water [proceedings]. J Physiol. 1979;290(2):48P.
12. McArdle WD, Magel JR, Gergley TJ, Spina RJ, Toner MM. Thermal adjustment to cold-water exposure in resting men and women. J Appl Physiol Respir Environ Exerc Physiol. 1984;56(6):1565–71.

13. El Helou N, Tafflet M, Berthelot G, Tolaini J, Marc A, Guillaume M, et al. Impact of environmental parameters on marathon running performance. PLoS One. 2012;7(5):e37407.
14. Pendergast DR. The effect of body cooling on oxygen transport during exercise. Med Sci Sports Exerc. 1988;20(5 Suppl):S171–6.
15. Marchant B, Donaldson G, Mridha K, Scarborough M, Timmis AD. Mechanisms of cold intolerance in patients with angina. J Am Coll Cardiol. 1994;23(3):630–6. https://doi.org/10.1016/0735-1097(94)90747-1.
16. Ikäheimo TM. Cardiovascular diseases, cold exposure and exercise. Temperature (Austin). 2018;5(2):123–46.
17. Mazic S, Suzic Lazic J, Dekleva M, Antic M, Soldatovic I, Djelic M, et al. The impact of elevated blood pressure on exercise capacity in elite athletes. Int J Cardiol. 2015;180:171–7.
18. Luo Y, Li H, Huang F, Van Halm-Lutterodt N, Qin X, Wang A, et al. The cold effect of ambient temperature on ischemic and hemorrhagic stroke hospital admissions: a large database study in Beijing, China between years 2013 and 2014-utilizing a distributed lag non-linear analysis. Environ Pollut. 2018;232:90–6.
19. Vaseghi M, Shivkumar K. The role of the autonomic nervous system in sudden cardiac death. Prog Cardiovasc Dis. 2008;50(6):404–19.
20. Rundfeldt LC, Maggioni MA, Coker RH, Gunga HC, Riveros-Rivera A, Schalt A, et al. Cardiac Autonomic modulations and psychological correlates in the Yukon Arctic Ultra: the longest and the coldest ultramarathon. Front Physiol. 2018;9:35.
21. Taylor NA. Human heat adaptation. Compr Physiol. 2014;4(1):325–65.
22. Donaldson GC, Keatinge WR, Saunders RD. Cardiovascular responses to heat stress and their adverse consequences in healthy and vulnerable human populations. Int J Hyperthermia. 2003;19(3):225–35.
23. Sawka MN, Leon LR, Montain SJ, Sonna LA. Integrated physiological mechanisms of exercise performance, adaptation, and maladaptation to heat stress. Compr Physiol. 2011;1(4):1883–928.
24. Rowell LB. Human cardiovascular adjustments to exercise and thermal stress. Physiol Rev. 1974;54(1):75–159.
25. Stöhr EJ, González-Alonso J, Pearson J, Low DA, Ali L, Barker H, et al. Dehydration reduces left ventricular filling at rest and during exercise independent of twist mechanics. J Appl Physiol (1985). 2011;111(3):891–7.
26. González-Alonso J, Crandall CG, Johnson JM. The cardiovascular challenge of exercising in the heat. J Physiol. 2008;586(1):45–53.
27. Rowell LB. Hyperthermia: a hyperadrenergic state. Hypertension. 1990;15(5):505–7.
28. Cui J, Arbab-Zadeh A, Prasad A, Durand S, Levine BD, Crandall CG. Effects of heat stress on thermoregulatory responses in congestive heart failure patients. Circulation. 2005;112(15):2286–92.
29. Harris MB, Starnes JW. Effects of body temperature during exercise training on myocardial adaptations. Am J Physiol Heart Circ Physiol. 2001;280(5):H2271–80.
30. Yankelson L, Sadeh B, Gershovitz L, Werthein J, Heller K, Halpern P, et al. Life-threatening events during endurance sports: is heat stroke more prevalent than arrhythmic death? J Am Coll Cardiol. 2014;64(5):463–9.
31. Siegel AJ, d'Hemecourt P, Adner MM, Shirey T, Brown JL, Lewandrowski KB. Exertional dysnatremia in collapsed marathon runners: a critical role for point-of-care testing to guide appropriate therapy. Am J Clin Pathol. 2009;132(3):336–40.
32. Périard JD, Travers GJS, Racinais S, Sawka MN. Cardiovascular adaptations supporting human exercise-heat acclimation. Auton Neurosci. 2016;196:52–62.
33. Lenfant C, Sullivan K. Adaptation to high altitude. N Engl J Med. 1971;284(23):1298–309.
34. Bärtsch P, Gibbs JS. Effect of altitude on the heart and the lungs. Circulation. 2007;116(19):2191–202.
35. Naeije R. Physiological adaptation of the cardiovascular system to high altitude. Prog Cardiovasc Dis. 2010;52(6):456–66.

36. Balanos GM, Pugh K, Frise MC, Dorrington KL. Exaggerated pulmonary vascular response to acute hypoxia in older men. Exp Physiol. 2015;100(10):1187–98.
37. Netzer N, Strohl K, Faulhaber M, Gatterer H, Burtscher M. Hypoxia-related altitude illnesses. J Travel Med. 2013;20(4):247–55.
38. Buskirk ER, Kollias J, Akers RF, Prokop EK, Reategui EP. Maximal performance at altitude and on return from altitude in conditioned runners. J Appl Physiol. 1967;23(2):259–66.
39. Ferretti G, Moia C, Thomet JM, Kayser B. The decrease of maximal oxygen consumption during hypoxia in man: a mirror image of the oxygen equilibrium curve. J Physiol. 1997;498(Pt 1):231–7.
40. Horstman D, Weiskopf R, Jackson RE. Work capacity during 3-wk sojourn at 4,300 m: effects of relative polycythemia. J Appl Physiol Respir Environ Exerc Physiol. 1980;49(2):311–8.
41. Maher JT, Jones LG, Hartley LH. Effects of high-altitude exposure on submaximal endurance capacity of men. J Appl Physiol. 1974;37(6):895–8.
42. Burtscher M. Risk and protective factors for sudden cardiac death during leisure activities in the mountains: an update. Heart Lung Circ. 2017;26(8):757–62.
43. Levine BD. Going high with heart disease: the effect of high altitude exposure in older individuals and patients with coronary artery disease. High Alt Med Biol. 2015;16(2):89–96.
44. Levine BD, Zuckerman JH, deFilippi CR. Effect of high-altitude exposure in the elderly: the tenth mountain division study. Circulation. 1997;96(4):1224–32.
45. Foster GE, Sheel AW. The human diving response, its function, and its control. Scand J Med Sci Sports. 2005;15(1):3–12.
46. Arborelius M, Ballidin UI, Lilja B, Lundgren CE. Hemodynamic changes in man during immersion with the head above water. Aerosp Med. 1972;43(6):592–8.
47. Pendergast DR, Lundgren CE. The underwater environment: cardiopulmonary, thermal, and energetic demands. J Appl Physiol (1985). 2009;106(1):276–83.
48. Brugniaux JV, Coombs GB, Barak OF, Dujic Z, Sekhon MS, Ainslie PN. Highs and lows of hyperoxia: physiological, performance, and clinical aspects. Am J Physiol Regul Integr Comp Physiol. 2018;315(1):R1–R27.
49. Bove AA. The cardiovascular system and diving risk. Undersea Hyperb Med. 2011;38(4):261–9.

# Part III

# Exercise in Primary Prevention of Cardiovascular Disease

# Epidemiology: Physical Activity, Exercise and Mortality

# 35

Martin Bahls and Marcus Dörr

**Learning Objectives**

1. Understand the difference between physical activity and cardiorespiratory fitness.
2. Evidence for mortality risk reduction in CVD subpopulations with higher cardiorespiratory fitness.
3. Understand the distinct associations of physical activity and cardiorespiratory fitness on mortality.
4. Appreciate the different domains of physical activity and their relation to mortality.
5. Evidence that physical activity is protective of disease, while sedentarism is causal for disease development.

## 35.1 Introduction

Cardiovascular diseases (CVD) and cardiometabolic diseases like Type 2 Diabetes Mellitus (T2DM) are the main driver of morbidity and mortality worldwide [1, 2]. In order to reduce the risk of these diseases in the future effective prevention strategies are essential. We generally differentiate between *primary* and *secondary* disease prevention.

- *Primary disease prevention* typically applies to individuals at high risk of developing a first cardiovascular event.
- *Secondary prevention* targets at people with already established CVD.

M. Bahls · M. Dörr (✉)
Department of Internal Medicine B, University Medicine Greifswald, Greifswald, Germany
e-mail: martin.bahls@uni-greifswald.de; marcus.doerr@uni-greifswald.de





A. Pressler, J. Niebauer (eds.), *Textbook of Sports and Exercise Cardiology*,
https://doi.org/10.1007/978-3-030-35374-2_35

Lifestyle modifications, e.g. a healthy diet accompanied by sufficient levels of physical activity (PA) and exercise, are important for both prevention approaches, while pharmacological treatments are mainly but not exclusively used during secondary prevention. This chapter focuses on the importance and beneficial effects of PA and exercise for cardiovascular and cardiometabolic health and prognosis.

An important risk factor for cardiometabolic diseases is physical inactivity (sedentarism). Bed rest studies have identified a causal link between sedentary behaviors and rapidly appearing adverse cardiovascular and metabolic sequelae. For example, 60 days of bed rest decrease plasma volume and left ventricular volume resulting in cardiac left ventricular muscle atrophy [3]. PA, on the other hand, may delay most of or partly reverse these adaptations. For instance, 1 year of intense exercise results in an initially concentric left ventricular remodeling with subsequent dilation to restore baseline mass to volume ratio [4] (see also Chap. 3).

Importantly, exercise is recommended by current guidelines for patients with coronary artery disease, heart failure with reduced as well as with preserved ejection fraction and dilated cardiomyopathy. However, exercise is not recommended during or immediately after acute cardiovascular events. Further, even though there are some reports that too much exercise may result in adverse cardiac adaptations by increasing the risk for atrial fibrillation (see Chap. 34), this is unlikely to be a concern for the general population and patients with cardiometabolic diseases. In addition, one needs to recognize and appreciate the clinical value of cardiorespiratory exercise testing [5]. This chapter focuses on the epidemiological evidence which supports causal links between sedentarism and the protective role of regular PA and exercise as well as higher cardiorespiratory fitness (CRF) on mortality.

## 35.2 Sedentarism, Physical Activity and Cardiorespiratory Fitness

Sedentary behavior has not just been associated with adverse left ventricular cardiac remodeling, but also with the incidence of heart failure.

- In 1,985 black and white adults aged 45 years and older, individuals in the highest quartile for sedentary behavior had a more than twofold greater risk for all-cause mortality compared to individuals with the lowest sedentary time. Further, the sedentary bout duration was also inversely associated with all-cause mortality [6]. This suggests that not only total sedentary but also prolonged and uninterrupted bouts of physical inactivity induce severely adverse outcomes.
- During a 10-year follow-up of the California Men's Health Study (n = 82,695) the risk to develop heart failure was 52% and 17% higher in the group with the lowest and medium level of PA compared to the highest level of PA, respectively [7].
- In the Framingham Heart Study low levels of PA were associated with an increased risk to develop heart failure with reduced as well as preserved ejection fraction in the elderly [8]

Even though the terms PA and cardiorespiratory fitness (CRF) are sometimes used interchangeably, both parameters are not the same.

- Already in the 1970s Paffenbarger et al. reported that weekly caloric energy expenditure was inversely related to all-cause mortality in Harvard alumni [9, 10].
- The first large analysis which demonstrated that low CRF is a better predictor for mortality compared to most other clinical patient characteristics was published in the New England Journal of Medicine by Jonathan Myers in 2002 [11]. In 6,213 men each one metabolic equivalent task (MET; see Chap. 1) increase in CRF was associated with a 12% lower mortality risk. Importantly, this relationship was found for healthy subjects as well as patients with previous cardiopulmonary- and metabolic manifestations (i.e. hypertension, chronic obstructive pulmonary disease, diabetes) or subjects with cardiovascular risk factors (i.e., smokers, obesity or low-density lipoprotein concentration > 220mg/dl).
- In 498,135 UK-Biobank participants a one standard deviation decrease in PA was associated with a 5% greater risk for all-cause mortality. Similarly, a CRF below one standard deviation was associated with a 22% greater risk for all-cause mortality [12]. However, there was no significant correlation between PA and CRF. Hence, the beneficial effects of PA and CRF may be separate from each other. Further, in the same cohort every MET increase was related with a 4% lower risk for vascular disease [13].
- In a 46-year follow-up of the Copenhagen Male Study each 1 ml/kg/min higher peak oxygen uptake ($VO_2$peak) as a measure of CRF was associated with a 45 day longer life [14].
- Of 6,213 men referred for exercise testing between 1987 and 2000, 842 underwent an assessment of adulthood activity patterns. While CRF and PA were both associated with lower all-cause mortality, CRF was a stronger predictor for mortality compared to PA. An increase in 1,000 kcal energy expenditure per week due to physical activity was equivalent to a one MET higher CRF and a mortality benefit by 20% [15].
- The relative risk for coronary heart or cardiovascular disease was compared in seven cohorts which assessed CRF and in 16 cohorts that measured PA with a total of 1,325,004 persons years follow-up. The risk for coronary heart disease or overall cardiovascular disease decreased linearly with increasing levels of PA, in contrast to CRF, where a significant drop occurred before the 25th percentile. Further, the reductions associated with more PA and higher CRF were significantly different (Fig. 35.1) [16].
- The Veteran Affairs (VA) medical centers provide a superb resource for epidemiological research on the associations of CRF with the development of subsequent cardiovascular diseases as well as mortality. In 6,749 black and 8,911 white men with an average age of 60 years, each MET increase in CRF was associated with a 13% lower risk for mortality [17]. In addition, during a median follow-up of 11 years in 20,590 men, each one MET increase was related with a 16% lower risk for major adverse cardiovascular events (MACE) defined as the first occurrence of

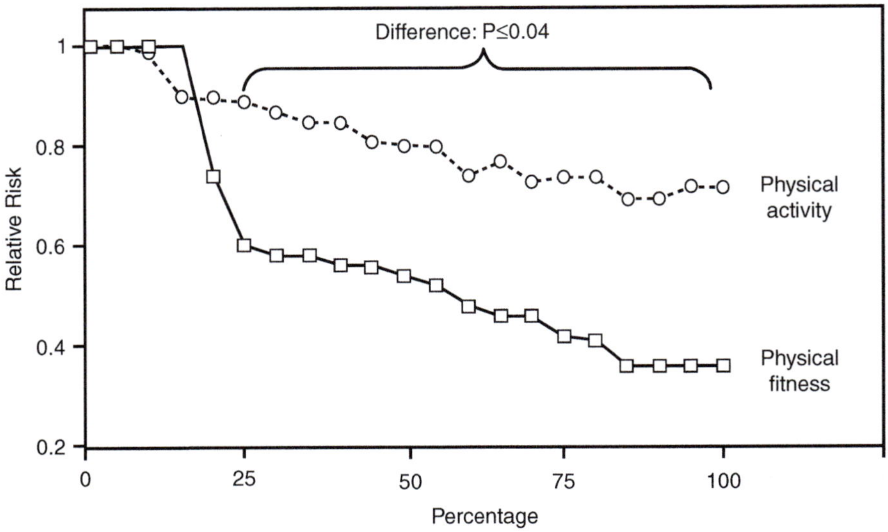


**Fig. 35.1** Estimated dose-response curve for the relative risk of either coronary heart disease or CVD by sample percentage of fitness and PA. Studies weighted by person-years of experience (Reprinted with permission from [16])

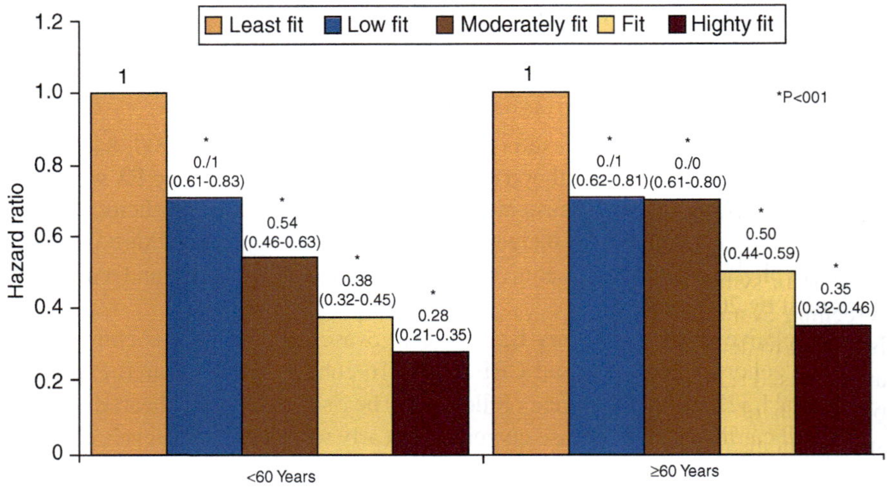


**Fig. 35.2** Adjusted risk for having a major cardiovascular event according to age and fitness categories (Reprinted with permission from [17])

myocardial infarction (fatal and nonfatal), chronic heart failure, coronary artery bypass grafts, or cerebrovascular accidents (fatal and nonfatal) [18]. Importantly, the benefits of a high CRF were observed independent of age (Fig. 35.2).

Even though PA and CRF act through different biological mechanisms, there is a large amount of evidence, that, independent of an individual's health status (e.g.

blood lipid levels, blood pressure and smoking as well as dietary habits), higher levels of PA and CRF improve the overall CVD risk profile [19]. Although the protective effect of a higher CRF is undisputed, important questions regarding its modifiability by PA remain open.

- In the 1990s Bouchard et al. conducted the HERITAGE study which provided significant inside into the complex genetic determinants of resting CRF and changes in CRF due to exercise training [20]. During the initial study 429 sedentary individuals (170 parents and 259 of their offsprings) were recruited and participated in a cardiopulmonary exercise test. The results indicated that more than 50% of the resting CRF was genetically determined. In a second part of the HERITAGE trial the siblings participated in a structured exercise protocol to assess potential changes in CRF due to exercise (i.e., trainability). Interestingly, 47% of this training response was genetically determined and independent of resting CRF [21].
- In 122,007 patients of a tertiary academic medical center, all-cause mortality was lowest in individuals in the highest CRF quartile. When subjects in the highest CRF quartile were compared to the lowest quartile, a fivefold increase in risk for all-cause mortality was observed after a median-follow-up of 8.4 years (Fig. 35.3) [22]. These beneficial effects were also observed in elderly patients and in those with hypertension.
- In a large meta-analysis including 102,980 patients from 33 studies, each one MET higher level of CRF was associated with a 13% and 15% lower risk for all-cause and CVD mortality, respectively. However, the authors also report a high degree of heterogeneity between studies [23].
- In 4,527 adults with no previous history of cardiovascular or lung disease, cancer and hypertension or use of anti-hypertensive medication, a one MET higher $VO_2$peak was associated with a 15% lower risk for incident coronary heart disease [24].
- In 3,926 patients of the Finnish Cardiovascular Study (FINCAVAS) and 2,683 men from the Kuopio Ischaemic Heart Disease study (KIHD) the Duke Treadmill score was inversely associated with mortality [25]. In these studies, METs, which are used to calculate this score, were again linked with prognosis. Specifically, a one MET increase was associated with a 20% and 18% lower risk for cardiovascular mortality in both FINCAVAS and KIHD, respectively.
- In more than 40,000 men who participated in cardiorespiratory exercise testing at the Cooper Clinic in Texas, high CRF attenuated the effect of a triglyceride/high density lipoprotein ratio [26]. A similar observation has been made for body mass index (BMI), where overweight and obese men with moderate CRF had mortality risks similar to normal weight subjects with a very high CRF [27]. Therefore, a high CRF may compensate for other CVD risk factors.
- In 55,456 subjects from the Aerobic Center Longitudinal Study (prospective observational investigation from January 2nd 1974 to December 31st 2002) a one MET higher CRF was associated with a 14% lower risk for sudden cardiac death [28].
- In 2,153 hypertensive elderly males (mean age 75 years), for one MET higher CRF all-cause mortality decreased by 11% [29].

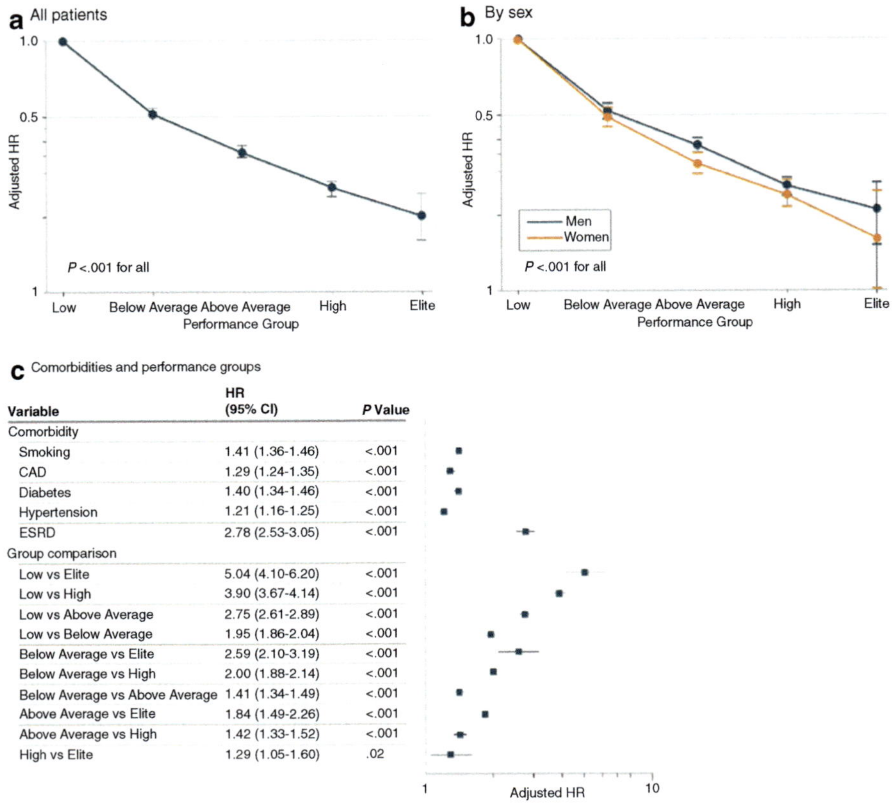


**Fig. 35.3** Risk-adjusted all-cause mortality according to CRF groups. Adjusted hazard ratios (HRs) for all-cause mortality compared with low performers in all patients (**a**) and by sex (**b**) (P values are for comparisons with low performers). (**c**) Adjusted HRs for comorbidities and between performance groups. Error bars indicate 95% CIs. *CAD* coronary artery disease, *ESRD* end-stage renal disease

### 35.2.1 Summary

1. *Sedentary behavior (physical inactivity) or, in other words, the lack of regular exercise causes many cardiometabolic diseases and increases the risk for all-cause and cause-specific mortality.*
2. *Higher levels of PA and CRF may be used as a treatment to prevent many of these cardiometabolic diseases and thereby lower all-cause and cause-specific mortality independent of patient population.*

## 35.3 Do Abnormally High Levels of PA Potentially Result in Adverse Outcomes?

In recent years, studies on the association of very high levels of PA or exercise (such as repeated marathon running over years) with adverse cardiovascular alterations have suggested a potential upper limit beyond which PA may no longer transfer into beneficial outcomes (Fig. 35.4; see also Chaps. 34 and 42) [30]. From an epidemiological perspective, the following observations have been made in a general population:

- In 37,855 subjects of the Henry Ford Exercise Testing Project (The FIT Project) free of known CVD and with an CRF of at least ten METs, the group of patients with 12–13 METs and the group with 14 or more METs showed a 32% and 61% lower risk for all-cause mortality compared to subjects in the 10–11 METs group [31]. Thus, in these study population there was no upper limit for the benefits of a high CRF.

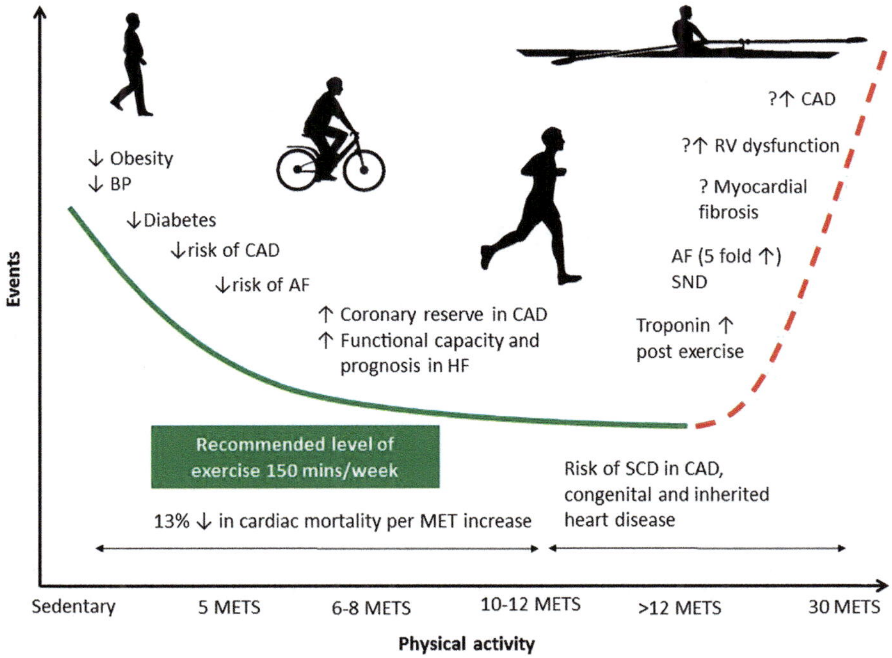


**Fig. 35.4** The U-shaped curve: moderate exercise is superior to no exercise, but extreme exercise is at least discussed to be harmful (Reprinted with permission from [30]). *CAD* coronary heart disease, *BP* blood pressure, *AF* atrial fibrillation, *SND* sinus node disease, *RV* right ventricular

- In the UK Biobank, high levels of CRF were associated with lower mortality but increased risk for atrial fibrillation [13].

The above-mentioned, potentially adverse outcomes do thus not appear to be applicable to the normal population, as more than 50 MET-h per week or more than seven workout sessions per week over a prolonged period would be required for an increased CVD risk [32]. Further, some epidemiological analyses [22] incorrectly classify individuals with a high CRF, on a population level, as "elite", although professional endurance athletes would even reach much higher levels of CRF.

- Participants of the Nord-Trøndelag Health Study (HUNT3) with a very low 10-year CVD risk showed a 15% lower risk for coronary heart disease with each 1 MET higher CRF. This was observed across the whole fitness continuum [24].

### 35.3.1 Summary

1. *Abnormal high levels of PA may have adverse consequences and do increase the risk for atrial fibrillation. In the general population only very few individuals will reach these levels. However, at least for cardiologists working with elite athletes, an increased CVD risk may be of concern.*

## 35.4 Domains of Physical Activity

Even though the benefits of regular PA are generally accepted as being of relevance to lower all-cause, CVD and cancer mortality, PA may occur in different domains. For example, activities may take place

(a) During leisure time (LTPA)
(b) In a sport setting (SPA) or
(c) Be work related (WPA)

This section will thus focus on the associations of LTPA, SPA and WPA with all-cause and CVD mortality. Physical activity in the different domains is generally assessed using either questionnaires or actimetry measurements. With regards to questionnaires, a large meta-analysis which included data from more than 1.3 million individuals concluded that higher levels of PA independent of a particular domain is associated with lower all-cause mortality [33]. However, while the results are very stringent, they also include a significant amount of heterogeneity.

1. Objectively assessed physical activity (accelerometry)
   - In 2,295 adults aged 20–85 years from the National Health and Nutrition Examination (NHANES), above-median levels of moderate to vigorous

physical activity (MVPA) levels were related with a 65% lower risk for all-cause mortality [34].
- In a 10-year follow-up of 962 participants of the Study of the Coronary Artery Risk Development in Young Adults Study (CARDIA study) with a mean age of 45 years, objectively measured PA decreased significantly independent of race or sex [35]
- Data from the NHANES trial suggests that despite the proven benefits of regular PA, patients with cardiometabolic disease are significantly less active compared to a reference group [36].
- Data from the same cohort also demonstrated that high levels of sedentary time and low levels of MVPA are strong and independent predictors for all-cause and cause-specific mortality [37].

2. Physical activity during leisure time
   - In 2,262 Taiwanese CVD patients LTPA was inversely related to all-cause mortality [38]. In elderly Taiwanese subjects a similar trend was observed [39].
   - A recent meta-analysis comprising data of more than 1.5 million participants showed a 23% and 24% lower risk of CVD mortality for moderate and high LTPA, compared to low LTPA, respectively [40]. This association was true for subjects with and without CVD as well as irrespective of age and sex.
   - In 31,818 men and 10,555 women of the Aerobic Center Longitudinal Study, LTPA was only inversely associated with mortality when the model was not adjusted for CRF [41]. This finding suggests that a high CRF is related to a lower risk for all-cause mortality independent of PA.
   - The Study of Health in Pomerania (SHIP) and The Cardiovascular Disease, Living and Ageing in Halle (CARLA) study demonstrated that higher levels of LTPA and SPA were associated with a lower risk for all-cause, CVD and cancer mortality [42].
   - In a large population-based sample from the U.K. (EPIC-Norfolk) a combination of LTPA and WPA was inversely associated risk for all-cause and CVD mortality [43, 44].
   - In the population-based "Cooperative Health Research in the Region of Augsburg" (KORA) study, LTPA was inversely associated with all-cause, CVD and cancer mortality [45]
   - In Switzerland, self-reported physical activity was inversely associated with all-cause and CVD mortality in a dose-response relationship [46].
3. Physical activity in a sports setting
   - When the mortality risk for 1,098 ambitious joggers was compared to 3,950 sedentary non-joggers in the Copenhagen City Heart Study, only 1–2.4 h of jogging per week was related to a 71% lower risk for all-cause mortality [47].
4. Physical activity at work

   Interestingly, WPA was used in the classical studies to demonstrate a positive relationship between PA in general and subsequent risk for CVD incidence. Specifically, in the 1950s Morris and colleagues reported that walking bus conductors and mail carriers had lower incidences of coronary heart disease compared to sedentary bus drivers and civil servants [48, 49]. In another classical study from the 1970s, Pfaffenbarger et al. reported that there was no difference in all-cause mortality risk between longshoremen and sedentary controls [50]. The discussion regarding the association of WPA with mortality is still ongoing today. Hence, this section provides an overview of the current literature.

- In 12,093 Danish nurses with an age between 45 and 64 years, a U-shaped relationship was found for the association between WPA and incident ischemic heart disease during a 15 year follow-up [51].
- In the above-mentioned study on 2,262 Taiwanese CVD patients, domestic and WPA was inversely related to all-cause mortality [38].
- In the Belgian Physical Fitness Study including 1,456 workers aged 40–55 years, workers with low levels of LTPA and WPA as well as workers with low LTPA but high WPA had twofold higher risks for all-cause mortality [52].
- Findings from the Copenhagen City Heart Study on 2,190 males and 2,534 females corroborate these observations. Specifically, individuals with high WPA had a 45% higher risk for all-cause mortality compared to low WPA (Fig. 35.5) [53].
- In 2,133 elderly Taiwanese adults WPA was not at all related to all-cause mortality [39]. Similar results were reported for the EPIC-Norfolk study as well as the previously mentioned study from Switzerland [44, 46].
- Further, in SHIP and CARLA also no significant relation between WPA and mortality was found [42].
- Results from the Cardiovascular Occupational Risk Factor Determination in Israel Study show an increased risk for future CVD events in subjects with high WPA [54].
- In KORA, high WPA was associated with a lower risk for all-cause, CVD and cancer mortality [45].

### 35.4.1 Summary

1. *There is sufficient evidence that LTPA and SPA are inversely associated with all-cause and cause-specific mortality.*
2. *The relationship between WPA and mortality is currently unclear. The heterogeneous findings may be explained by different assessment methods for WPA.*

**Clinical Pearls**

- Physicians should encourage a lifelong physically active lifestyle independent of age.
- In the general population and in patient settings there is no upper limit for the benefits of physical activity and higher levels of cardiorespiratory fitness.
- Cardiologists working with elite athletes should be aware of the increased risk for atrial fibrillation in this population.

| Variables | No. of Participants | Adjusted for age and sex: Events, No. (%) | Adjusted for age and sex: Hazard ratio (95% CI) | Adjusted for age, sex, smoking, body mass index, diabetes, household income, alcohol, and leisure time physical activity: Events, No. (%) | Adjusted for age, sex, smoking, body mass index, diabetes, household income, alcohol, and leisure time physical activity: Hazard ratio (95% CI) |
|---|---|---|---|---|---|
| **Cardiorespiratory fitness** | **4724** | **257 (6.8%)** | | **250 (6.9%)** | |
| High (reference) | 1246 | 49 (5.1%) | 1.00 (reference) | 49 (5.2%) | 1.00 (reference) |
| Moderate | 2837 | 161 (7.0%) | 1.78 (1.29-2.45)*** | 154 (7.0%) | 1.37 (0.98-1.91). |
| Low | 641 | 47 (9.3%) | 3.27 (2.18-4.90)*** | 47 (9.6%) | 2.17 (1.40-3.38)*** |
| **Occupational physical activity** | **4724** | **257 (6.8%)** | | **250 (6.9%)** | |
| Low (reference) | 1623 | 66 (5.4%) | 1.00 (reference) | 63 (5.3%) | 1.00 (reference) |
| Moderate | 1539 | 83 (7.2%) | 1.11 (0.80-1.54) | 81 (7.3%) | 1.16 (0.83-1.63) |
| High | 1562 | 108 (7.9%) | 1.61 (1.19-2.19)** | 106 (8.0%) | 1.45 (1.05-2.00)* |
| **Cardiorespiratory fitness** | **4724** | **257 (6.8%)** | | **250 (6.9%)** | |
| High (reference) | 1246 | 49 (5.1%) | 1.00 (reference) | 49 (5.2%) | 1.00 (reference) |
| Moderate | 2837 | 161 (7.0%) | 1.81 (1.31-2.49)*** | 154 (7.0%) | 1.39 (0.99-1.95). |
| Low | 641 | 47 (9.3%) | 3.53 (2.35-5.30)*** | 47 (9.6%) | 2.34 (1.51-3.63)*** |
| **Occupational physical activity** | **4724** | **257 (6.8%)** | | **250 (6.9%)** | |
| Low (reference) | 1623 | 66 (5.4%) | 1.00 (reference) | 63 (5.3%) | 1.00 (reference) |
| Moderate | 1539 | 83 (7.2%) | 1.15 (0.83-1.59) | 81 (7.3%) | 1.18 (0.84-1.65) |
| High | 1562 | 108 (7.9%) | 1.75 (1.29-2.39)*** | 106 (8.0%) | 1.56 (1.12-2.16)** |
| **High cardiorespiratory fitness** | | | | | |
| **Occupational physical activity** | **1246** | **49 (5.1%)** | | **49 (5.2%)** | |
| Low (reference) | 408 | 8 (2.7%) | 1.00 (reference) | 8 (2.8%) | 1.00 (reference) |
| Moderate | 405 | 18 (5.8%) | 1.77 (0.76-4.10) | 18 (6.1%) | 1.54 (0.65-3.66) |
| High | 433 | 23 (6.6%) | 2.37 (1.06-5.31)* | 23 (6.7%) | 1.66 (0.71-3.86) |
| **Moderate cardiorespiratory fitness** | | | | | |
| **Occupational physical activity** | **2837** | **161 (7.0%)** | | **154 (7.0%)** | |
| Low (reference) | 956 | 45 (5.9%) | 1.00 (reference) | 42 (5.8%) | 1.00 (reference) |
| Moderate | 919 | 50 (7.2%) | 0.98 (0.66-1.47) | 48 (7.3%) | 1.10 (0.72-1.68) |
| High | 962 | 66 (7.9%) | 1.46 (1.00-2.13). | 64 (7.9%) | 1.30 (0.87-1.95) |
| **Low cardiorespiratory fitness** | | | | | |
| **Occupational physical activity** | **641** | **47 (9.3%)** | | **47 (9.6%)** | |
| Low (reference) | 259 | 13 (7.6%) | 1.00 (reference) | 13 (7.7%) | 1.00 (reference) |
| Moderate | 215 | 15 (9.2%) | 1.38 (0.65-2.91) | 15 (9.5%) | 1.01 (0.45-2.24) |
| High | 167 | 19 (11.7%) | 2.90 (1.42-5.94)** | 19 (12.2%) | 2.83 (1.24-6.46)* |
| **Cardiorespiratory fitness / Occupational physical activity** | **4724** | **257 (6.8%)** | | **250 (6.9%)** | |
| High / Low (reference) | 408 | 8 (2.7%) | 1.00 (reference) | 8 (2.8%) | 1.00 (reference) |
| High / Moderate | 405 | 18 (5.8%) | 1.80 (0.78-4.14) | 18 (6.1%) | 1.57 (0.68-3.63) |
| High / High | 433 | 23 (6.6%) | 2.36 (1.05-5.27)* | 23 (6.7%) | 1.68 (0.75-3.79) |
| Moderate / Low | 956 | 45 (5.9%) | 2.75 (1.30-5.83)** | 42 (5.8%) | 1.78 (0.82-3.83) |
| Moderate / Moderate | 919 | 50 (7.2%) | 2.69 (1.27-5.68)** | 48 (7.3%) | 1.87 (0.88-4.00) |
| Moderate / High | 962 | 66 (7.9%) | 4.01 (1.92-8.35)*** | 64 (7.9%) | 2.27 (1.07-4.80)* |
| Low / Low | 259 | 13 (7.6%) | 3.91 (1.62-9.45)** | 13 (7.7%) | 2.03 (0.82-5.02) |
| Low / Moderate | 215 | 15 (9.2%) | 5.07 (2.15-11.98)*** | 15 (9.5%) | 2.61 (1.07-6.34)* |
| Low / High | 167 | 19 (11.7%) | 10.31 (4.50-23.60)*** | 19 (12.2%) | 6.22 (2.67-14.49)*** |

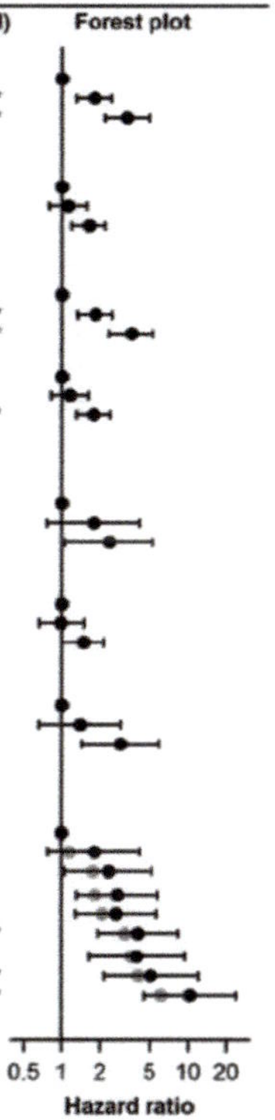


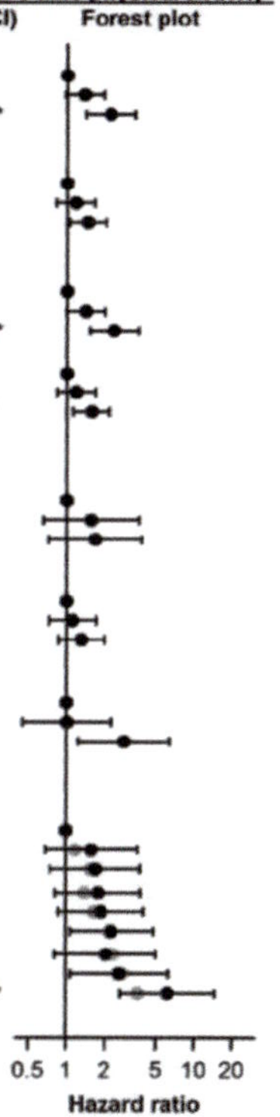


**Fig. 35.5** Shows univariable and multivariable Cox proportional hazards regression and Forest plots of the independent, mutually adjusted, stratified and combined categories of self-reported cardiorespiratory fitness and occupational physical activity from 1991 to 1994 as predictors of all-cause mortality with a median follow-up of 18.5 and 19.8 years among 2,190 males and 2,534 females without a history of cardiovascular disorders in the Copenhagen City Heart Study. (Percentages are 100% minus the Kaplan-Meier estimate of being event-free. The grey dots represent the estimated hazard ratios based on the model with the two main effects and no interaction term. P < 0.10; ∗P < 0.05; ∗∗P < 0.01; ∗∗∗P < 0.001)

## Review

### Questions

1. Explain the difference between sedentarism, PA and CRF with regards to all-cause and CVD mortality.
2. Are there adverse consequences of high levels of PA and CRF?
3. Can you describe the relation between PA in different domains, and why is this differentiation important?

### Answers

1. Sedentary behavior is casually linked with adverse remodeling of the CV system and is a driver of higher all-cause and CVD mortality. PA and CRF are inversely related to all-cause and CVD mortality. A plethora of studies with different ethnicities, age groups and patients with CVD consistently demonstrated that with each MET increase all-cause mortality decreases by approximately 10%.
2. Very high levels of PA are associated with an increased risk of atrial fibrillation and potentially with all-cause and CVD mortality. However, the current data suggesting these associations are mainly of concern for cardiologists who work with elite endurance athletes as high levels of 50 MET-h per week or more are unlikely to be observed in the general population.
3. PA may take place in different domains. Specifically, people may be physically active during leisure time (LTPA), in a sports setting (SPA) or at work (WPA). A large number of studies have explored the relation between domain specific PA and mortality. The data for LTPA and SPA is very strong in demonstrating a dose-depended inverse relationship with all-cause mortality. The currently available literature does not provide a clear direction for WPA.

## References

1. Roth GA, Johnson C, Abajobir A, Abd-Allah F, Abera SF, Abyu G, et al. Global, regional, and national burden of cardiovascular diseases for 10 causes, 1990 to 2015. J Am Coll Cardiol. 2017;70(1):1–25.
2. Wang H, Naghavi M, Allen C, Barber RM, Bhutta ZA, Carter A, et al. Global, regional, and national life expectancy, all-cause mortality, and cause-specific mortality for 249 causes of death, 1980–2015: a systematic analysis for the Global Burden of Disease Study 2015. Lancet. 2016;388(10053):1459–544.
3. Westby CM, Martin DS, Lee SMC, Stenger MB, Platts SH. Left ventricular remodeling during and after 60 days of sedentary head-down bed rest. J Appl Physiol. 2016;120(8):956–64.
4. Arbab-Zadeh A, Perhonen M, Howden E, Peshock RM, Zhang R, Adams-Huet B, et al. Cardiac remodeling in response to 1 year of intensive endurance training. Circulation. 2014;130(24):2152–61. CIRCULATIONAHA. 114.010775.
5. Ross R, Blair SN, Arena R, Church TS, Despres JP, Franklin BA, et al. Importance of assessing cardiorespiratory fitness in clinical practice: a case for fitness as a clinical vital sign: a scientific statement from the American Heart Association. Circulation. 2016;134(24):e653–e99.

6. Diaz KM, Howard VJ, Hutto B, Colabianchi N, Vena JE, Safford MM, et al. Patterns of sedentary behavior and mortality in U.S. middle-aged and older adults: a national cohort study. Ann Intern Med. 2017;167(7):465–75.
7. Young DR, Reynolds K, Sidell M, Brar S, Ghai NR, Sternfeld B, et al. Effects of physical activity and sedentary time on the risk of heart failure. Circ Heart Fail. 2014;7(1):21–7.
8. Kraigher-Krainer E, Lyass A, Massaro JM, Lee DS, Ho JE, Levy D, et al. Association of physical activity and heart failure with preserved vs. reduced ejection fraction in the elderly: the Framingham Heart Study. Eur J Heart Fail. 2013;15(7):742–6.
9. Paffenbarger RS Jr, Wing AL, Hyde RT. Physical activity as an index of heart attack risk in college alumni. Am J Epidemiol. 1978;108(3):161–75.
10. Paffenbarger RS Jr, Hyde RT, Wing AL, Hsieh CC. Physical activity, all-cause mortality, and longevity of college alumni. N Engl J Med. 1986;314(10):605–13.
11. Myers J, Prakash M, Froelicher V, Do D, Partington S, Atwood JE. Exercise capacity and mortality among men referred for exercise testing. N Engl J Med. 2002;346(11):793–801.
12. Celis-Morales CA, Lyall DM, Anderson J, Iliodromiti S, Fan Y, Ntuk UE, et al. The association between physical activity and risk of mortality is modulated by grip strength and cardiorespiratory fitness: evidence from 498 135 UK-Biobank participants. Eur Heart J. 2017;38(2):116–22.
13. Steell L, Ho FK, Sillars A, Petermann-Rocha F, Li H, Lyall DM, et al. Dose-response associations of cardiorespiratory fitness with all-cause mortality and incidence and mortality of cancer and cardiovascular and respiratory diseases: the UK Biobank cohort study. Br J Sports Med. 2019;53(21):1371–8.
14. Clausen JSR, Marott JL, Holtermann A, Gyntelberg F, Jensen MT. Midlife cardiorespiratory fitness and the long-term risk of mortality: 46 years of follow-up. J Am Coll Cardiol. 2018;72(9):987–95.
15. Myers J, Kaykha A, George S, Abella J, Zaheer N, Lear S, et al. Fitness versus physical activity patterns in predicting mortality in men. Am J Med. 2004;117(12):912–8.
16. Williams PT. Physical fitness and activity as separate heart disease risk factors: a meta-analysis. Med Sci Sports Exerc. 2001;33(5):754–61.
17. Kokkinos P, Myers J, Kokkinos JP, Pittaras A, Narayan P, Manolis A, et al. Exercise capacity and mortality in black and white men. Circulation. 2008;117(5):614–22.
18. Kokkinos PF, Faselis C, Myers J, Narayan P, Sui X, Zhang J, et al. Cardiorespiratory fitness and incidence of major adverse cardiovascular events in US veterans: a cohort study. Mayo Clin Proc. 2017, 92(1):39–48.
19. Myers J, McAuley P, Lavie CJ, Despres JP, Arena R, Kokkinos P. Physical activity and cardiorespiratory fitness as major markers of cardiovascular risk: their independent and interwoven importance to health status. Prog Cardiovasc Dis. 2015;57(4):306–14.
20. Bouchard C, Daw EW, Rice T, Perusse L, Gagnon J, Province MA, et al. Familial resemblance for VO2max in the sedentary state: the HERITAGE family study. Med Sci Sports Exerc. 1998;30(2):252–8.
21. Bouchard C, An P, Rice T, Skinner JS, Wilmore JH, Gagnon J, et al. Familial aggregation ofV˙o 2 max response to exercise training: results from the HERITAGE Family Study. J Appl Physiol (1985). 1999;87(3):1003–8.
22. Mandsager K, Harb S, Cremer P, Phelan D, Nissen SE, Jaber W. Association of cardiorespiratory fitness with long-term mortality among adults undergoing exercise treadmill testing. JAMA Netw Open. 2018;1(6):e183605.
23. Kodama S, Saito K, Tanaka S, et al. Cardiorespiratory fitness as a quantitative predictor of all-cause mortality and cardiovascular events in healthy men and women: a meta-analysis. JAMA. 2009;301(19):2024–35.
24. Letnes JM, Dalen H, Vesterbekkmo EK, Wisloff U, Nes BM. Peak oxygen uptake and incident coronary heart disease in a healthy population: the HUNT Fitness Study. Eur Heart J. 2019;40(20):1633–9.
25. Salokari E, Laukkanen JA, Lehtimaki T, Kurl S, Kunutsor S, Zaccardi F, et al. The Duke treadmill score with bicycle ergometer: exercise capacity is the most important predictor of cardiovascular mortality. Eur J Prev Cardiol. 2018;2018:2047487318804618.

26. Farrell SW, Finley CE, Barlow CE, Willis BL, DeFina LF, Haskell WL, et al. Moderate to high levels of cardiorespiratory fitness attenuate the effects of triglyceride to high-density lipoprotein cholesterol ratio on coronary heart disease mortality in men. Mayo Clin Proc. 2017;92(12):1763–71.
27. McAuley PA, Kokkinos PF, Oliveira RB, Emerson BT, Myers JN. Obesity paradox and cardiorespiratory fitness in 12,417 male veterans aged 40 to 70 years. Mayo Clin Proc. 2010;85(2):115–21.
28. Jimenez-Pavon D, Artero EG, Lee DC, Espana-Romero V, Sui X, Pate RR, et al. Cardiorespiratory fitness and risk of sudden cardiac death in men and women in the United States: a prospective evaluation from the aerobics center longitudinal study. Mayo Clin Proc. 2016;91(7):849–57.
29. Faselis C, Doumas M, Pittaras A, Narayan P, Myers J, Tsimploulis A, et al. Exercise capacity and all-cause mortality in male veterans with hypertension aged >/=70 years. Hypertension. 2014;64(1):30–5.
30. Merghani A, Malhotra A, Sharma S. The U-shaped relationship between exercise and cardiac morbidity. Trends Cardiovasc Med. 2016;26(3):232–40.
31. Feldman DI, Al-Mallah MH, Keteyian SJ, Brawner CA, Feldman T, Blumenthal RS, et al. No evidence of an upper threshold for mortality benefit at high levels of cardiorespiratory fitness. J Am Coll Cardiol. 2015;65(6):629–30.
32. Eijsvogels TMH, Molossi S, Lee D-C, Emery MS, Thompson PD. Exercise at the extremes. The amount of exercise to reduce cardiovascular events. J Am Coll Cardiol. 2016;67(3):316–29.
33. Samitz G, Egger M, Zwahlen M. Domains of physical activity and all-cause mortality: systematic review and dose-response meta-analysis of cohort studies. Int J Epidemiol. 2011;40(5):1382–400.
34. Edwards MK, Loprinzi PD. All-cause mortality risk as a function of sedentary behavior, moderate-to-vigorous physical activity and cardiorespiratory fitness. Phys Sportsmed. 2016;44(3):223–30.
35. Pettee Gabriel K, Sidney S, Jacobs DR Jr, Whitaker KM, Carnethon MR, Lewis CE, et al. Ten-year changes in accelerometer-based physical activity and sedentary time during midlife: the CARDIA study. Am J Epidemiol. 2018;187(10):2145–50.
36. Evenson KR, Butler EN, Rosamond WD. Prevalence of physical activity and sedentary behavior among adults with cardiovascular disease in the United States. J Cardiopulm Rehabil Prev. 2014;34(6):406–19.
37. Schmid D, Ricci C, Leitzmann MF. Associations of objectively assessed physical activity and sedentary time with all-cause mortality in US adults: the NHANES study. PLoS One. 2015;10(3):e0119591.
38. Ku PW, Chen LJ, Fox KR, Chen YH, Liao Y, Lin CH. Leisure-time, domestic, and work-related physical activity and their prospective associations with all-cause mortality in patients with cardiovascular disease. Am J Cardiol. 2018;121(2):177–81.
39. Chen L-J, Fox KR, Ku P-W, Sun W-J, Chou P. Prospective associations between household-, work-, and leisure-based physical activity and all-cause mortality among older taiwanese adults. Asia Pac J Public Health. 2012;24(5):795–805.
40. Cheng W, Zhang Z, Cheng W, Yang C, Diao L, Liu W. Associations of leisure-time physical activity with cardiovascular mortality: a systematic review and meta-analysis of 44 prospective cohort studies. Eur J Prev Cardiol. 2018;2018:2047487318795194.
41. Lee DC, Sui X, Ortega FB, Kim YS, Church TS, Winett RA, et al. Comparisons of leisure-time physical activity and cardiorespiratory fitness as predictors of all-cause mortality in men and women. Br J Sports Med. 2011;45(6):504–10.
42. Bahls M, Groß S, Baumeister SE, Völzke H, Gläser S, Ewert R, et al. Association of domain-specific physical activity and cardiorespiratory fitness with all-cause and cause-specific mortality in two population-based cohort studies. Sci Rep. 2018;8(1):16066.
43. Khaw K-T, Jakes R, Bingham S, Welch A, Luben R, Day N, et al. Work and leisure time physical activity assessed using a simple, pragmatic, validated questionnaire and incident cardiovascular

disease and all-cause mortality in men and women: the European Prospective Investigation into Cancer in Norfolk prospective population study. Int J Epidemiol. 2006;35(4):1034–43.
44. Besson H, Ekelund U, Brage S, Luben R, Bingham S, Khaw K-T, et al. Relationship between subdomains of total physical activity and mortality. Med Sci Sports Exerc. 2008;40(11):1909–15.
45. Autenrieth CS, Baumert J, Baumeister SE, Fischer B, Peters A, Döring A, et al. Association between domains of physical activity and all-cause, cardiovascular and cancer mortality. Eur J Epidemiol. 2011;26(2):91–9.
46. Wanner M, Tarnutzer S, Martin BW, Braun J, Rohrmann S, Bopp M, et al. Impact of different domains of physical activity on cause-specific mortality: a longitudinal study. Prev Med. 2014;62:89–95.
47. Schnohr P, O'Keefe JH, Marott JL, Lange P, Jensen GB. Dose of jogging and long-term mortality: the Copenhagen City Heart Study. J Am Coll Cardiol. 2015;65(5):411–9.
48. Morris JN, Heady JA, Raffle PA, Roberts CG, Parks JW. Coronary heart-disease and physical activity of work. Lancet. 1953;265(6796):1111–20.
49. Morris JN, Heady JA, Raffle PA, Roberts CG, Parks JW. Coronary heart-disease and physical activity of work. Lancet. 1953;265(6795):1053–7.
50. Paffenbarger RS Jr, Laughlin ME, Gima AS, Black RA. Work activity of longshoremen as related to death from coronary heart disease and stroke. N Engl J Med. 1970;282(20):1109–14.
51. Allesoe K, Holtermann A, Aadahl M, Thomsen JF, Hundrup YA, Sogaard K. High occupational physical activity and risk of ischaemic heart disease in women: the interplay with physical activity during leisure time. Eur J Prev Cardiol. 2015;22(12):1601–8.
52. Clays E, Lidegaard M, De Bacquer D, Van Herck K, De Backer G, Kittel F, et al. The combined relationship of occupational and leisure-time physical activity with all-cause mortality among men, accounting for physical fitness. Am J Epidemiol. 2014;179(5):559–66.
53. Holtermann A, Marott JL, Gyntelberg F, Sogaard K, Mortensen OS, Prescott E, et al. Self-reported occupational physical activity and cardiorespiratory fitness: importance for cardiovascular disease and all-cause mortality. Scand J Work Environ Health. 2016;42(4):291–8.
54. Harari G, Green MS, Zelber-Sagi S. Combined association of occupational and leisure-time physical activity with all-cause and coronary heart disease mortality among a cohort of men followed-up for 22 years. Occup Environ Med. 2015;72(9):617–24.

# Impact of Exercise on Cardiovascular Risk Factors: Arterial Hypertension

36

Paolo Palatini and Véronique Cornelissen

**Learning Objectives**

1. Be aware that the blood pressure response during exercise varies according to the characteristics of the exercise bout.
2. Know the variables that impact acute and chronic changes in left ventricular dimensions and function in response to exercise.
3. Become familiar with the safety measures for prescribing exercise therapy to hypertensive patients.
4. Have knowledge on the chronic response of blood pressure to different exercise modalities, and on how exercise program characteristics can affect the blood pressure response.
5. Be acquainted with the eligibility criteria for competitive sports activities in hypertensive athletes.

## 36.1 Blood Pressure Response During Exercise

Up to now, the haemodynamic changes caused by exercise in humans have mostly been studied in laboratory tests using bicycle ergometry or treadmill testing to reproduce dynamic exercise and hand-grip with a dynamometer to simulate isometric activities. During dynamic exercise, the need for increasing oxygen delivery to the working muscles is fulfilled by a local vasodilatation [1–3]. A simultaneous vasoconstriction occurs in the non-working muscles and splanchnic bed. The venous return rapidly increases with a consequent rapid rise in cardiac filling. The

P. Palatini (✉)
Department of Medicine, University of Padua, Padua, Italy
e-mail: palatini@unipd.it

V. Cornelissen
Department of Rehabilitation Sciences, KU Leuven, Leuven, Belgium
e-mail: Veronique.cornelissen@kuleuven.be



A. Pressler, J. Niebauer (eds.), *Textbook of Sports and Exercise Cardiology*,
https://doi.org/10.1007/978-3-030-35374-2_36

simultaneous increase in stroke volume (SV) and heart rate causes a marked rise in cardiac output (CO). The net integration of cardiac haemodynamics with the progressive decline in total peripheral resistance (TPR) produce considerable changes in BP which differ according to the type and length of exercise. Static (or isometric) exercise, defined as a sustained muscle contraction without change in muscle length, causes a parallel increase of systolic and diastolic BP [1–3]. A reflex increase in sympathetic activity, possibly related to early recruitment of type II fibres, seems to be the main determinant of the cardiovascular response to isometric effort [4]. It has to be pointed out that the shape and magnitude of the sphygmic waves vary according to the site of measurement [3, 5]. As the BP measurement site moves distally, systolic BP increases due to wave reflection. The progressive peripheral augmentation of systolic BP and pulse pressure is magnified by exercise [6]. In contrast, mean BP does not vary from central to peripheral sites throughout rest and exercise.

## 36.2 Blood Pressure Response to Dynamic Exercise

### 36.2.1 BP Changes During Ergometry with Incremental Workload

Dynamic exercise performed with multistage standard ergometry with incremental workload causes a progressive rise in systolic BP and little changes in diastolic BP.

- During bicycle ergometry there is a progressive increase in systolic BP ranging from 50 to 70 mmHg at peak exercise [6–8].
- Diastolic BP tends to increase during a bicycle test although some authors have found little or no change.

During treadmill exercise, usually systolic BP does not exceed 190 mmHg in normotensive subjects [9, 10]. However, a wide subject-to-subject variability may be observed. Diastolic BP remains substantially unchanged or slightly decreases with a 4–8 mmHg decline reported by most investigators.

In hypertensive subjects, systolic BP during ergometry performed with either bicycle or treadmill testing reaches much higher values than in normotensive subjects [7–10]. However, the absolute increase in BP is similar in hypertensive and normotensive subjects. In both groups, BP at peak exercise is proportional to BP level at baseline.

### 36.2.2 BP Changes During Prolonged Steady-State Exercise

BP changes during prolonged exercise at steady-state workload differ from those during exercise at incremental workload. Palatini et al. compared intra-arterial BP changes during a 1-h long exercise on a semi-recumbent position conducted at the anaerobic threshold with those during traditional bicycle ergometry in a group of normotensive and a group of hypertensive joggers [11]. In both groups the traditional ergometric test to exhaustion caused parallel changes in systolic and diastolic BP with a gradual increase up to peak exercise. A different BP pattern was observed during prolonged exercise. In all individuals, a sharp and parallel rise in systolic BP reaching maximum values during the first minutes after the start was recorded, followed by a progressive decline throughout the rest of the effort. The BP changes during the first 20 min of exercise were similar in the two groups, but thereafter the between-group BP difference tended to decline and at the end of the exercise it was no longer significant. A poor relationship was observed between the BP values at peak exercise and baseline levels. These results showed that the BP increase with strenuous steady-state effort is reduced in hypertensive individuals at peak exercise, probably because of latent impairment of cardiac performance (see below). At the end of exercise there was a sudden drop in BP which slowly returned to pre-exercise levels.

### 36.2.3 BP Response During Sports Activities

The present knowledge on BP changes during sports activities is almost exclusively based on data obtained with laboratory stress testing. However, traditional ergometry can only give a rough estimate of the BP changes which actually occur during sports performed on the field. Ergometric protocols usually imply progressive increments of the workload, a situation which does not reflect any real sports activity. Measuring BP during outdoor activities is not possible with current non-invasive ambulatory techniques, because the cuffing method requires a stationary position of the subject during the measurement. Only an intra-arterial method coupled to a Holter technique or a telemetering system can provide BP measurements in unrestricted subjects. The first invasive recordings in people performing various types of physical activity (jogging, swimming, diving and skiing) were obtained over 50 years ago by Bachmann et al. [12] However, a systematic investigation on the pressor effect of various sports was performed only in the eighties by means of a portable technique consisting in a miniaturized transducer-peristaltic-pump unit connected to the radial artery and a minirecorder worn around the waist [2, 3, 13–15].

#### 36.2.3.1 BP Changes During Running

A peculiar BP pattern has been observed during long-distance running [14, 15].

- Rhythmic oscillations of pulse pressure unrelated to respiration were often observed whose frequency varied from 6 to 27 $min^{-1}$, according to heart rate and pace frequency.
- The source of these pressure oscillations were the periodic shakes received by the heart and the great vessels during the run whose frequency was similar to that of heart rate, thereby generating a 'beat phenomenon'.
- Maximum BP values during running were attained during the first minutes of warm-up, in spite of the lower running velocity [11, 14].

- Subsequently, due to the vasodilatation, a progressive decrease in BP could be observed, so that after 20–30 min of running, BP declined to below pre-exercise values.

A completely different BP pattern could be observed in sprinters in whom a short-lasting noticeable increase in BP was observed [13], similar to that caused by heavy-resistance exercise (see below).

By comparing the BP behaviour in two groups of normotensive and hypertensive athletes, similar results to those achieved in the laboratory during prolonged semi-supine bicycle ergometry were obtained [16]. The between-group BP difference present at rest gradually flattened, so that at the end of the effort the two pressure curves were almost superimposed. This is attributable to a depressed left ventricular diastolic filling in the hypertensive subjects during strenuous effort [16].

#### 36.2.3.2 BP Changes During Cycling

Cycling requires a greater muscular force than running and thus entails a greater isometric component. This is reflected by the greater left ventricular (LV) mass and the more concentric oriented remodelling of the left ventricle of cyclists compared to runners [17]. Due to the larger compression of vessels by muscle activity during cycling, peripheral resistance cannot fall to the same degree as in running.

- Indeed, a higher increase in diastolic BP has been recorded with the intra-arterial method during road cycling than during track running [13].
- The highest BP levels during bicycling were recorded when the subjects pedalled uphill or at high speed on the flat.
- The BP levels achieved by the athletes during road cycling proved to be much higher than those recorded in the same subjects during standard bicycle ergometry, indicating that the laboratory test is not a good predictor of the BP changes which actually occur in outdoor activities.

## 36.3 Blood Pressure Response to Isometric Exercise

### 36.3.1 Laboratory Testing

The most popular test used to study BP changes during an isometric effort is the hand grip which is performed grasping a dynamometer. Several protocols have been proposed generally using 30–50% of the maximal voluntary contraction.

- Isometric exercise causes an increase of both systolic and diastolic BP in either normotensive or hypertensive subjects [18–20].
- The BP rise is due to increases in heart rate and CO with little or no changes in SV and TPR [21].

The magnitude of the increase in BP during isometric exercise depends on several factors. The size of muscle mass employed during the effort is considered a main determinant of the BP response [22, 23]. However, some authors did not find any relationship between the size of active muscle mass and the increase in BP during isometric exercise [24]. The duration of exercise is another factor which affects the magnitude of the BP rise [22, 23] which is proportional to the exercise length. The strength applied to the dynamometer also contributes to increasing BP during the hand grip [22]. In everyday life many isometric activities are performed with concomitant isotonic activities such as carrying heavy weights. In these activities, the typical isometric BP pattern changes because the increase in diastolic BP is completely offset [25].

### 36.3.2 Heavy-Resistance Sports

Heavy resistance sports imply an important isometric component that causes marked short-lasting increases in both systolic and diastolic BP. The pressor effects of heavy-resistance sports have been studied especially in subjects performing weight-lifting with the use of intra-arterial recording:

- In a Canadian study average values of 320/250 mmHg have been recorded with peak values as high as 480/390 mmHg during exercises involving the legs [26].
- Lower peak values were recorded by other investigators ranging from 197/156 to 345/245 mmHg [27].

BP levels reached during weight lifting are proportional to the muscle mass employed in the exercises and are higher when the effort is carried out in the upright position than in the supine [26, 27]. One main determinant for the remarkable BP rises during this type of sport is thought to be the potent Valsalva manoeuvre, which accompanies heavy weight lifts and the consequent increase in intrathoracic and intra-abdominal pressures [20, 26, 27]. This mechanism was actually shown to be operative in a study in which intra-arterial BP and intrathoracic and abdominal pressures were simultaneously measured by two balloon catheter systems (positioned one in the midoesophagus and one in the stomach) [27]. In both body compartments remarkable pressure elevations, parallel to those of BP and proportional to the load, were recorded (Fig. 36.1). Values as high as 170 mmHg were recorded for intra-abdominal pressure which reached greater values than intrathoracic pressure (maximum value 75 mmHg). Much lower BP levels and little or no increase in intracavitary pressures were recorded after abolition of the Valsalva manoeuvre providing direct evidence that the increase in intracavitary pressures is the main determinant of the BP elevations which occur during weight-lifting. On the other hand, the remarkable increases in abdominal pressure caused by the lifts exert a protective effect on the cerebral vessels. Intra-abdominal pressure is transmitted to the cerebrospinal fluid through the intervertebral foramina, thereby reducing the actual transmural pressure across cerebral vessels [28]. The potent pressor reflex originating from tendons stretching and the mechanical compression of the arteries by the contracting muscles are other factors that contribute to elevating BP during heavy-resistance exercise [26, 29].

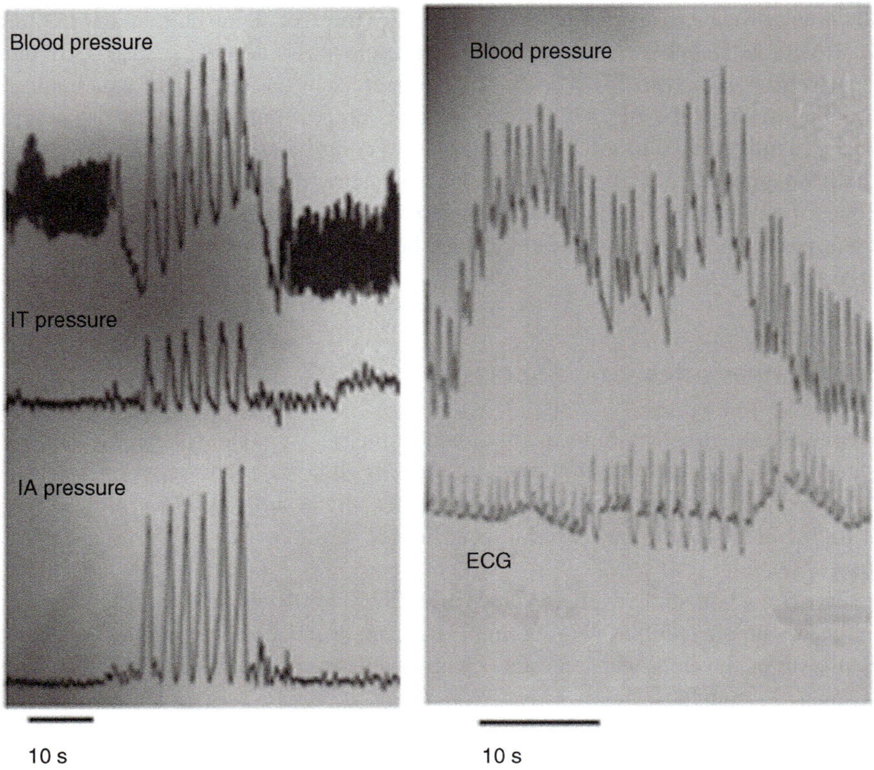


**Fig. 36.1** Intraarterial blood pressure measurement during weight lifting. Left panel: simultaneous recording of intraarterial, intrathoracic (IT), and intraabdominal (IA) pressures during squatting (5 repetitions) in a 25-year-old man. Right panel: intraarterial blood pressure and electrocardiographic (ECG) recording during squatting (one repetition) in a 28-year-old woman. Soon after exercise cessation, an episode of ventricular bigeminy becomes apparent

## 36.4 Left Ventricular Dimensions and Performance During Exercise

There is general agreement that the exercise induced increase in LV ejection fraction is mainly determined by a decrease in end-systolic volume. Instead, there has been much controversy in the literature about the role of the Frank-Starling mechanism during exercise. Part of the controversy is due to the fact that the exercise-induced changes in LV end-diastolic volume are dependent on several clinical variables that can affect LV dimensions:

- *Position of the body***.** Experimental evidence suggests that the increase in CO that occurs during supine exercise results predominantly from an increase in heart rate, with little changes in SV and end-diastolic volume [30, 31], even though some authors observed a small but significant increase in end-diastolic volume [32]. In contrast to the supine position, in the upright posture the end-diastolic volume and SV are decreased in resting conditions, mainly due to peripheral pooling, but they rapidly increase at the onset of exercise [30].

- *Between-sex differences.* It is known that maximal exercise CO is greater in men than in women at any given age [33]. Several studies demonstrated a smaller increase in LV ejection fraction from rest to peak exercise in women than in men over a wide age range [34]. This was due to a more modest decrease in end-systolic volume with exercise in female subjects. Some authors found a different behaviour of the end-diastolic volume between the two sexes during supine exercise, as diastolic volume showed a decline in men and constant dimensions in women [34].
- *Effect of age.* A large number of studies have shown that ageing is associated with a decline in CO during exercise [35, 36]. In older individuals CO during exercise appears to be maintained by a combination of increased heart rate and the Frank-Starling mechanism and in younger ones chiefly by increased heart rate [36, 37]. The well-known age-related decrease in LV compliance seems to account for the use of the Frank-Starling mechanism in older individuals [37, 38].
- *Effect of physical training.* End-systolic LV diameter appears to decrease to the same extent in trained and untrained individuals during exercise [39]. Instead, controversy still exists as regards exertional end-diastolic diameter. According to some authors [39] the Frank-Starling mechanism is operative to the same extent during exercise in trained and untrained subjects. However, according to other investigators [32] end-diastolic volume increases more in sedentary than in trained individuals, according to others [40] only rises in the sedentary subject, and according to yet others [41] only increases in the athlete.
- *Short versus prolonged exercise***.** There is general agreement that CO increases more during a short maximal effort than during prolonged exhausting exercise [42, 43]. According to some authors [44], the lower CO at the end of prolonged exercise is due to a lower utilization of the Frank-Starling mechanism, while LV systolic performance does not differ during short- and long-lasting exercise. However, other authors [42, 43] found a decreased LV performance during the recovery from prolonged exercise indicating that prolonged strenuous exercise results in impaired LV function. A limitation of all the studies which found a depressed LV performance with prolonged exercise is that LV dimensions were measured during the recovery period. Studies which investigated LV performance throughout the exercise session [16] found that after an initial increase LV function remained stable up to the end of a 1 h-long vigorous exercise, without a tendency to decline. Instead, a sharp fall in performance was observed soon after stopping exercise. These findings indicate that data obtained during the recovery cannot be extrapolated to exercise LV performance and that most of the available information on cardiac function during prolonged exercise should be reconsidered.

### 36.4.1 Left Ventricular Performance in Hypertensive Subjects

Although a dysfunction of LV chamber may occur in hypertension, it is not clear at what stage of the disease depressed performance may develop. LV function at rest has been found to be normal or even supernormal in the early stage of hypertension [45]. However, subtle abnormalities of LV performance can be detected during strenuous exercise [42, 43]. As mentioned above the BP increase with long-lasting strenuous effort is reduced in hypertensive compared to normotensive individuals, probably because of latent impairment of cardiac performance.

This hypothesis was tested by Palatini et al. [16] by means of M-mode echocardiography during prolonged in-door exercise to exhaustion. Greater LV ejection fraction ($p = 0.018$), systolic BP/end-systolic volume ($p < 0.0001$) and stress/end-systolic volume ($p = 0.027$) were found in a group of young hypertensive than a group of normotensive individuals throughout the test documenting the existence of an increased ejective performance in the former.

However, LV contractility may be overestimated by the measurement of fractional shortening at the endocardium [46–48].

- Using midwall fractional shortening to evaluate LV performance, some investigators demonstrated that in hypertensive subjects LV contractility was actually depressed at rest [49, 50].
- Using the same exercise protocol, in a later experiment the same group of investigators [51] found that the hypertensives were able to increase their SV and CO adequately during bycicle ergometry through an increase in LV ejective performance.
- However, LV contractility measured at midwall was actually depressed throughout rest ($p = 0.04$) and exercise ($p = 0.004$).
- LV concentric remodelling was the key factor accounting for the reduced LV contractility.

These findings indicate that increased LV ejective performance on a background of depressed LV contractility can temporarily preserve CO but leads to an unfavorable structural LV pattern with deleterious consequences for the left ventricle in the long run.

## 36.5 Physical Activity, Physical Fitness and Future Hypertension: Data from Observational Studies

The last decade, large prospective cohort studies, which allowed for age and anthropometric characteristics, have yielded consistent findings showing an inverse relation between the incidence of hypertension and habitual levels of physical activity, assessed by means of questionnaire or an interview [52].

This finding was confirmed in a recent meta-analysis by Liu et al. [53], pooling data from 21 prospective studies comparing high versus low levels of leisure time physical activity:

- They reported a pooled relative risk (RR) for hypertension of 0.84 [95% confidence interval (CI) 0.78–0.90] in the most active individuals.
- Furthermore, there seems to be no evidence of a nonlinear dose-response association of physical activity and hypertension.
- Namely the risk of hypertension was reduced by 6% (RR 0.94; CI 0.92–0.96) with each ten Metabolic Equivalent of task (MET)-hours/week increment of leisure time physical activity [53], which corresponds to meeting the recommended minimum physical activity level of 150 min/week.
- With twice this amount of activity, the risk was further reduced by 12% [RR 0.88 (0.83–0.92)] [53].
- As, overweight and obesity have been shown to be important and independent risk factors for the development of hypertension [54], it has been hypothesized that increasing physical activity might reduce BP through decreased body weight or improved body composition. However, Liu et al. found that risk estimates were only about 3–4% weaker from studies with than without adjustment for body mass index (BMI) [53].
- Furthermore, high levels of physical activity were associated with lower risk of hypertension in both BMI subgroups, i.e. $<25$ and $\geq 25$ kg/m$^2$ [53].
- Hence, the effect of physical activity on hypertension cannot be explained solely by a change in BMI.

Fewer studies have investigated the effect of physical fitness and incident hypertension:

- Blair et al. were the first to show that low fit individuals had an increased risk (RR 1.52) for the development of hypertension compared to high fit individuals [55].
- Alike, in the recent Coronary Artery Risk Development in Young adults (CARDIA) study [56] baseline physical fitness, estimated based on the duration of a symptom-limited graded exercise test, was shown to be inversely associated with incident hypertension over a 20 year period (hazard ratio 0.63 per 2.9 min longer) and this was present in all race and sex groups [56].
  - More importantly, when both physical activity and physical fitness were included in the same model, results revealed that fitness remained significantly and independently associated with lower likelihood of developing hypertension, while activity attenuated to non-significance [56].
  - Further, activity was only significantly inversely associated with the development of hypertension in the highest category of fitness.

These results suggest that physical activity levels that increase fitness may lead to the greatest benefit [56].

Finally, also improvements in physical activity [57] and physical fitness [58] have been shown to be associated with smaller increments in BP over time.

- E.g. Williams et al. reported that reduction of vigorous physical activity over a 7.4-year period of follow-up increased the odds of developing hypertension.

- Moreover, it was shown that the odds of developing hypertension depended on the follow-up running distance without relation to baseline activity, which implies that success in motivating the population to become more active will not yield its expected anti-hypertensive effect if the activity is not maintained lifelong.

## 36.6 Exercise in the Prevention, Treatment and Management of Hypertension: Data from Randomised Controlled Trials

A difficulty in the interpretation of the epidemiological data is distinguishing cause and effect: that is to ascribe differences in BP or in the incidence of hypertension to differences in levels of physical activity or fitness because of confounding factors that cannot be accounted for [59]. Furthermore, questions on the role of each of the FITT (frequency, intensity, type and time) characteristics of physical activity in the prevention and treatment of hypertension are difficult to answer based on epidemiological data, yet are of utmost importance for optimal exercise prescription. Therefore, randomized controlled trials are needed, since they can evaluate the effectiveness of exercise while controlling for each of the confounders. However, it should be acknowledged that randomized controlled studies assessing the impact of exercise interventions on BP are often limited by their small sample sizes. Meta-analyses, which pool the results of these individual studies, increase the statistical power and can provide greater precision of point estimates with regard to the anti-hypertensive potency of exercise.

For the purpose of this chapter, we will rely on meta-analyses that have investigated the effect of aerobic endurance training [60–62], dynamic resistance training [63, 64], isometric resistance training [65, 66] and alternative types [67–71] of exercise training on BP during the last decade. Common inclusion criteria of these meta-analyses are:

1. Inclusion of a randomized sedentary control group or phase
2. Exercise training as the sole intervention
3. Exercise intervention for a minimum of 4 weeks
4. Inclusion of participants who were sedentary normotensive and/or hypertensive adults with no other concomitant disease
5. Published in a peer-reviewed journal

### 36.6.1 Dynamic Aerobic Endurance Training and Blood Pressure

Dynamic aerobic endurance exercise involves large muscle groups in dynamic repetitive activities (e.g. walking, cycling, running, stair climbing) that result in substantial increases in heart rate and energy expenditure aiming to increase cardiorespiratory fitness. In almost all national and international treatment guidelines for the primary and secondary treatment of hypertension, aerobic endurance exercise has received a Class 1 recommendation with a level A of evidence [72]. This recommendation is supported by bountiful evidence consistently showing the BP lowering effect of aerobic endurance training.

- In the largest meta-analysis to date [61], including 105 endurance training interventions, a reduction of [−3.5 mmHg (95% CI −4.6 to −2.3), $p < 0.0001$]/[−2.5 mmHg (−3.2 to −1.7), $p < 0.0001$] in office BP was found after a median intervention duration of 10 weeks (range 4-52), involving aerobic exercise three times per week (range: 1–7) at an intensity between 35 and 95% of peak oxygen uptake (Fig. 36.2).
- The fact that Cornelissen et al. [73] found a similar reduction in daytime ambulatory BP [−3.2 mmHg, (−5.0 to −1.3)]/[−2.7 mmHg (−3.9 to −1.5)] by pooling data of 16 aerobic endurance training studies adds further support to the BP lowering potential of aerobic endurance training.
- It is noteworthy that endurance training does not seem to affect night-time BP [60, 61].
- In addition, Cornelissen et al. [60] identified 8 randomized controlled trials measuring BP during cycle ergometer exercise at a median work load of 100 W

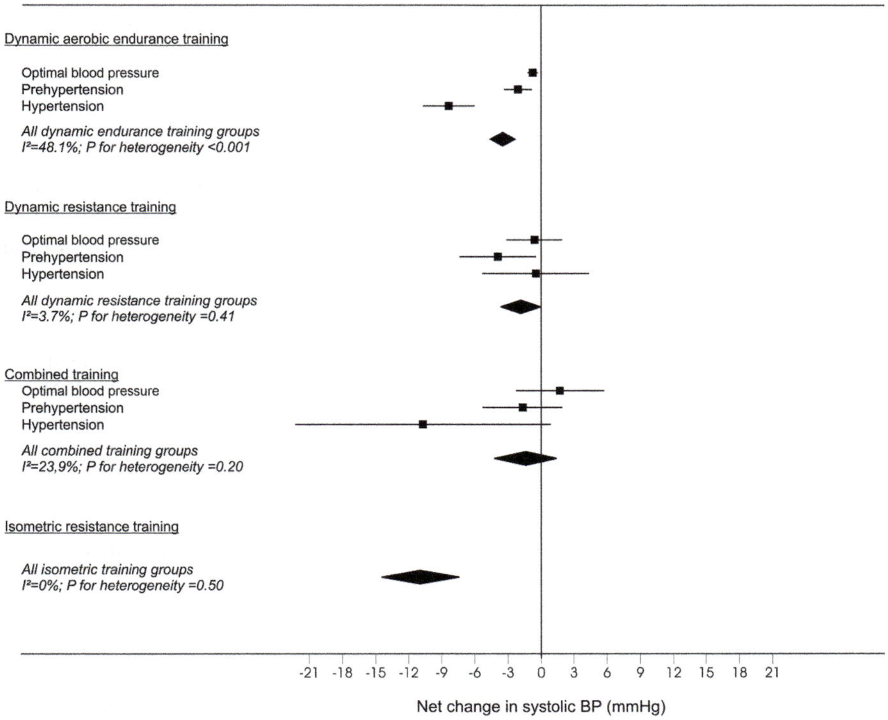


**Fig. 36.2** Net changes in systolic (upper panel) and diastolic (lower panel) blood pressure after different exercise modalities using random-effects analyses. Data are reported as net mean changes, adjusted for control data (95% confidence limits) (Reprinted from [61])

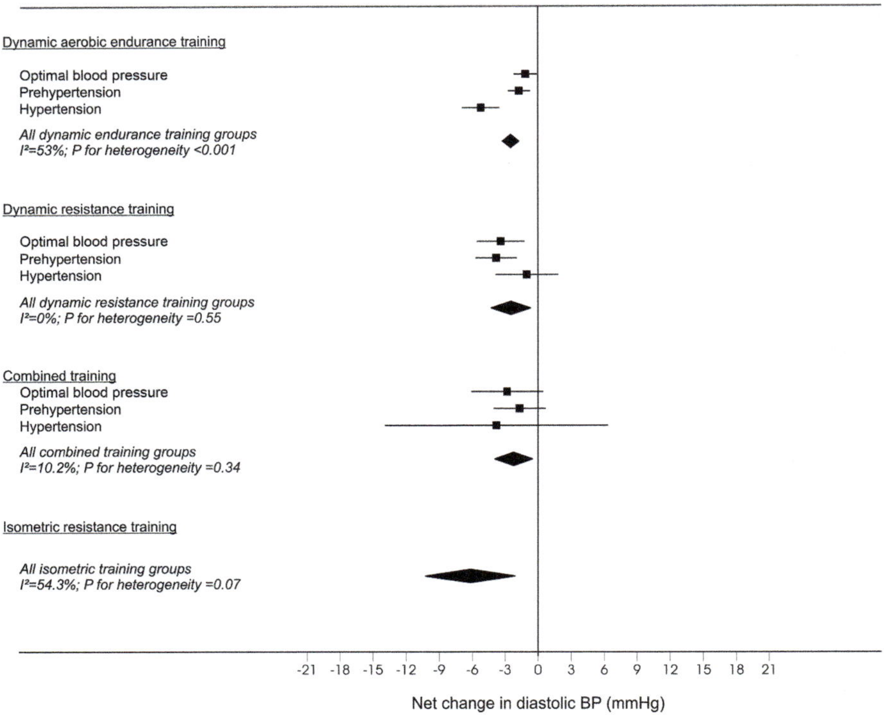


**Fig. 36.2** (continued)

(range 60–140 W) or during treadmill exercise at approximately four METS and reported a reduction of 7 mmHg from a baseline BP of 180 mmHg.

- When the effects of endurance training on office BP were analysed according to the Seventh Report of the Joint National Committee on Prevention, Detection, Evaluation, and Treatment of High Blood Pressure [74], Cornelissen et al. [61] found BP decreases to be most pronounced in 26 study groups with hypertensive participants [−8.3 mmHg (−10.7 to −6.0)]/[−5.2 mmHg (−6.8 to −3.4)] as compared to the 50 groups of prehypertensive subjects [−2.1 (−3.3 to −0.83)]/[−1.7 (−2.7 to −0.68)] and the 29 groups of subjects with normal BP levels [−0.75 (−2.2 to +0.69)]/[−1.1 (−2.2 to −0.068)]. Although this could not be confirmed by subgroup analysis on ambulatory BP data, this is most likely due to the fact that only 6 studies have investigated the effect of endurance exercise among hypertensive patients significantly reducing the statistical power.

*Do gender or ethnicity affect the BP response to aerobic endurance training?* With regard to **ethnicity**,

- A meta-analysis of Whelton et al. [75] found that black participants had significantly greater reduction in systolic BP, and Asian participants had significantly greater reduction in diastolic BP compared with white participants.

- At variance, only recently, did Igarashi et al. [76] find pooled net changes in systolic BP and diastolic BP of −4.7 and −3.2 mmHg, respectively from a baseline BP of 138.2/80.5 mmHg in 1456 East Asian individuals.
- Further, only four studies have investigated the BP lowering potency of exercise in black patients [75], all involving hypertensive patients.

With regard to **gender**,

- Cornelissen and Smart [61] found that BP decreases were most pronounced in male participants, which was in contrast to
- Kelley et al. [77] and Igarashi et al. [76] who reported BP reductions of similar magnitude in men and women

However, given the lack of adjustment for important confounders in these subgroup analyses and the absence of direct comparison studies between men and women or patients of different ethnic origin, clearly further research is needed to study how and why ethnic and/or gender differences in the BP response to endurance training exist, if they exist at all.

Even more important with regard to optimal exercise prescription is the knowledge on how each of the individual exercise characteristics affects the BP response.

- In univariate weighted regression analysis [60] and subgroup analyses [61], weekly training *frequency* did not contribute significantly to explain the inter-study variance of the BP response to aerobic exercise training, i.e. training frequencies between 3 and 7 days per week lowered BP [60].
- However, comparative studies found that the fall in BP was significantly greater in 3 versus 5 days walking group [78] or 1 versus 7 days per week schedules [79].

Yet, current guidelines [80] recommend exercise on most, if not all, days of the week. This is because it has been shown that a single bout of aerobic exercise (10–50 min at 40–100% peak oxygen uptake) results in an immediate reduction in BP of 5–7 mmHg compared to resting BP than can be sustained for up to 24 h after completion of the exercise [81]. This physiological response is termed postexercise hypotension [82]. This acute effect may add significant benefits to the BP treatment of the hypertensive patients by lowering their BP into normotensive ranges for some periods of the day. Furthermore, it might contribute to the BP reductions resulting from exercise training [80]. This underlines the importance of recommending daily aerobic exercise, especially in the hypertensive patients.

Further, with regard to *intensity*, moderate intensity aerobic exercise (40–60% HRR) is recommended to prevent and manage high BP [80]. However, many hypertensive patients are overweight or older who are limited in the level of physical activity they can undertake. In this context, it is of note that Cornelissen et al. [83] found equal reductions in office BP, BP during submaximal exercise and during recovery from exercise in older sedentary individuals following 10 weeks of aerobic exercise at 33% Heart rate reserve (HRR) versus 66% HRR. Similarly, post exercise hypotension already occurs after a single bout of aerobic exercise at 40% of peak oxygen uptake [84, 85]. Therefore, the antihypertensive effect of aerobic exercise seems a low threshold phenomenon with BP reductions already occurring at lower intensity.

However, larger BP reductions are obtained when exercise, acute [84, 85] or chronic [83], is performed at a higher intensity. This was also confirmed by subgroup analyses [61] documenting smaller BP reductions after low-intensity endurance training (<40% HRR) compared with moderate- or high intensity training. In this context, the BP lowering potential of high intensity interval training has increasingly been studied in recent years. Surprisingly, when pooling data from studies comparing isocaloric high intensity interval and moderate intensity continuous training, comparable reductions in resting BP in adults with pre- to established hypertension were observed, despite high intensity interval being associated with greater improvements in peak oxygen uptake [62]. This could suggest that the total volume, and not intensity of exercise, determines the BP response to aerobic exercise.

### 36.6.2 Dynamic Resistance Training and Blood Pressure

Dynamic resistance training involves concentric and/or eccentric contractions of muscles while both the length and the tension of muscle change. To date, the level of evidence upon which the dynamic resistance recommendations are made is weaker [80], which is mainly due to the scarcity of primary level studies investigating the effect of dynamic resistance exercise as antihypertensive treatment, particularly in hypertensive patients.

- To look at the effect of dynamic resistance exercise on BP, Cornelissen et al. [63] pooled data from 30 dynamic resistance trials:
- The majority (90%) of studies used weight or resistance training machines to train the muscles of upper and/or lower body with only two reporting the use of dynabands.
- Study duration varied from 6 to 52 weeks (median 16).
- Training frequency was three sessions per week, with a range from two to three sessions weekly.
- Average training intensity was between 30% and 100% of one repetition maximum (median 76).
- Overall, resistance-training programs targeted the whole body with on average eight exercises/session.
- The training programmes resulted in a significant reduction of [−2.8 mmHg (−4.3 to −1.3)]/[−2.7 mmHg (−3.8 to −1.7)].
- It is noteworthy that aerobic power increased by 11% (+2.6 to +18.6) confirming the dynamic aspect of this mode of training.
- More recently, MacDonald et al. [64] showed that dynamic resistance training elicited BP reductions that were comparable to those previously reported with aerobic training, advising as such the potential of dynamic resistance training as a stand-alone antihypertensive therapy.

The above findings confirmed earlier controlled trials [86, 87] directly comparing the effectiveness of aerobic exercise training versus dynamic resistance training showing BP reductions of similar magnitude.

- In line with aerobic endurance training, the greatest BP reductions occur among samples with higher resting BP (i.e., −6/−5 mmHg for hypertension, and 0/−1 mmHg for normal BP (p = 0.01)).
- Likewise, a single dynamic resistance training session at 40–80% of one RM resulted in similar post exercise hypotension [88] with the reduction in office BP being more pronounced in hypertensive patients and when using larger muscle groups.

Nonetheless, dynamic resistance training studies in hypertensive patients remain scant and data on the effectiveness on ambulatory BP are lacking. Therefore, more RCT are needed to more definitively determine whether dynamic resistance training can act as an equal alternative to aerobic endurance training in the hypertensive patients.

### 36.6.3 Isometric Resistance Training and Blood Pressure

In 2013, the American Heart Association reported that there was emerging evidence supporting the use of isometric resistance training (IRT) for blood pressure management (Class IIB, Level of Evidence C) [89]. Isometric training involving exercises with the arm or leg, in which a muscle develops tension with no visible joint movement, has been increasingly studied the last decade after small proof of concept studies demonstrating large reductions in office BP in normotensive and medicated hypertensive participants. These trials encouraged interest as IRT can be performed easily at any place and any time and requires a smaller investment of time from participants (approximately 12–40 min per week).

- The overall benefit of IRT has been confirmed in a recent meta-analysis pooling data of 16 IRT trials [65]. Compared with control groups, IRT groups showed statistically significant positive effects on systolic (−5.23 mmHg) and diastolic BP (−1.64 mmHg) after 3–12 weeks of isometric handgrip (n = 9) or leg exercise (n = 7) at an average intensity of 5–35% of one repetition maximum for 3–5 times/week.
- Notably, the magnitude of the observed changes in BP was lower than those found in the earliest meta-analysis [61], but in line with more recent meta-analysis [66, 90].
- Further, although the reductions in diastolic BP are no longer clinically relevant, the positive effect of IRT on systolic BP are comparable with changes observed from the aerobic training and dynamic resistance training.
- Further, whereas Inder et al. [66] found unilateral isometric resistance exercise to be superior to bilateral exercise in reducing systolic BP and longer programs inducing higher reductions, this could no longer be confirmed by López-Valenciano [65].

Of note, the number of studies performed in female and patients with hypertension is extremely small, making it difficult to quantify any sex-related and clinical status related differences regarding the anti-hypertensive effect of IRT and to generalize the results to the overall population. As such, clearly, further research is warranted to explore the promising merits of low intensity isometric training as a viable BP lowering therapy.

### 36.6.4 Other Modes of Exercise Training and Blood Pressure

Whereas aerobic training supplemented with dynamic (isometric) resistance training are the prevailing recommendations for hypertensive individuals, there is a growing interest in alternative modes of exercise therapy that can be of added value to an antihypertensive lifestyle in those that lack interest, motivation or the ability to what is called more traditional forms of exercise training. Especially in Asia, Yoga, Tai Chi, Baduanjin and other qigong therapies are favoured by middle aged and eldery hypertensive patients. These alternative modes of exercise are also increasingly being practiced in Western Societies.

- ***Tai chi*** is a mind-body exercise origination in China. It incorporates slow dance-like movements and integrates musculoskeletal, breathing and meditation training [69]. A total of five trials have examined the antihypertensive effect of Tai Chi/Qigong on BP documenting significant and clinically relevant benefits of Tai Chi over no intervention with mean group BP changes of −15.5/−10.6 mmHg.
- Deriving from ancient Indian philosophy, ***yoga*** is a complementary medicine of physical activity and lifestyle modification. This exercise modality is based on isometric, stretching and breathing exercise, deep relaxation techniques and meditation, all of which can be beneficial to hypertensive patients. A systematic review by Cramer [69] pooling data from seven randomized controlled trials concluded that there is emerging but low-quality evidence that yoga, especially yoga breathing, can be a useful adjunct intervention in the management of hypertension. Systolic and diastolic BP were reduced by an average of −9.6/−7.2 mmHg. Effects were larger when only hypertensive patients were included, and yoga breathing exercises were more effective than those that included physical postures [70].
- Further, the antihypertensive effect of ***Baduanjin***, a famous ancient Chinese mind-body exercise characterized by simple, slow relaxing movements, has been recently summarized by Xiong et al. [68]. When used alone, 3–12 months of Baduanjin demonstrated a clinically meaningful improvement on BP (−13/−6.1 mmHg) compared to a no intervention group.
- The results of four trials investigating the potency of ***dance therapy*** to lower BP in hypertensive patients have been summarized by Conceiçao et al. [71]. Dance therapy was defined as twice weekly Ola Hou for 60 minutes (n = 1), 45 min of dance aerobics thrice weekly (n = 2) or 50 min of dance movement therapy two times per week for 4 weeks (n = 1). After a median intervention duration of 12 weeks (range 4–12 weeks) the BP of dancers was −12/−3.4 mmHg lower

compared to control subjects. The small number of trials, the lack of a clear description of the FITT characteristics and the high heterogeneity warrant further research.

- Finally, also ***swimming and aquatic exercises*** have grown in popularity in the last decade, especially among elderly and women. Pooled net changes [67] of aerobic endurance training (n = 7 trials) in water showed significant greater reductions in systolic BP (−8.9 mmHg) and diastolic BP (−3.4 mmHg) compared to previous meta-analyses involving mainly land-based exercise [61]. This is in contrast with direct comparative trials by Colado et al. [91] and Arca et al. [92] who reported that BP decreased to the same extent after aquatic and land-based exercise. Of note, swimming training alone (n = 3 trials) did not lower BP [67]. Clearly, further research is needed to elucidate whether aquatic endurance exercise would be more beneficial as antihypertensive exercise therapy compared to land-based exercise, and why it is different from swimming therapy.

## 36.7 Effect of Regular Exercise Training on Cardiac Structure in Hypertension

Left ventricular hypertrophy (LVH) has been shown to be an important predictor of cardiovascular events in hypertension, independent of BP level [93]. Physical training in normotensive individuals promotes an increase in LV mass. Thus, in hypertensive individuals, regular physical activity could facilitate the development of LVH, offsetting the beneficial effects on BP. However, a number of studies have shown a reduction of LV mass in hypertensive patients after a period of aerobic training [94–96].

- Baglivo et al. observed a decrease of LV mass in a small group of middle-aged hypertensive subjects after 16 months of endurance exercise training [94].
- This finding was confirmed by Kokkinos et al. in a group of African-American men with severe hypertension performing a shorter period of training (16 weeks of aerobic exercise) [95].
- Other authors observed a reduction in both LV mass and wall thickness in patients with mild hypertension [96].

The above findings were confirmed by long-lasting observational studies [97, 98].

- In a cohort of young-to-middle-age subjects, the physically active subjects were less likely to develop LVH than their sedentary counterparts during a median follow-up of 8.3 years with an adjusted OR of 0.24 (CI, 0.07–0.85) [97]. In particular, no athlete involved in competitions developed LVH during the 8 years of observation.
- Similar results were obtained in older hypertensive patients with LVH from the LIFE study [98]. Compared to sedentary individuals, physically active subjects had lower LV mass index and thinner ventricular septum and left posterior wall.

- At variance with the above data, negative results were reported by Hinderliter et al. in overweight individuals with mildly elevated BP after regular endurance exercise [99] and by Reid et al. after 12 weeks of exercise, weight loss, or both in 23 obese individuals [100].

Thus, the majority of the published studies have shown a paradoxical effect of exercise on the left ventricle in hypertensive subjects with favourable changes in LV structure and mass.

Several mechanisms may account for the beneficial effects of physical activity on the heart. Reduction in BP, TPR, large artery stiffness, blood volume and CO are known to occur after a program of physical activity [60]. Also, improvement of several humoral factors such as enhanced endothelial vasodilator function, suppression of the activity of the renin-angiotensin-aldosterone system, reduction of insulin resistance and reduction in sympathetic nervous system activity may be implicated in determining the cardiac effects of exercise [60]. Physical activity in hypertension would induce a direct stimulus to LVH but would also determine an activation of those mechanisms which may attenuate the LV growth. One main mechanism seems to be the reduction of the sympathetic tone that causes beneficial effects on heart rate, BP and other components of the metabolic syndrome [101, 102]. In addition, a reduction of BP reactivity to stressors has been described in physically active individuals [103, 104]. A study of untreated hypertensive patients demonstrated that even a short period of moderate intensity aerobic exercise training significantly reduced muscle sympathetic discharge in subjects with increased central sympathetic activation [105].

## 36.8 Eligibility for Competitive Athletics

The above findings underscore the beneficial effects of physical activity for the prevention and treatment of hypertension. However, it is also known that sports activities are a potential source of significant health hazards. High heart rate and elevated BP during exercise produce a noticeable increase in myocardial oxygen consumption, which may enhance the risk of coronary events which are more common in patients with hypertension [106]. Another potential risk to the hypertensive subject may come from the high BP levels that are reached during heavy resistance physical activities [27, 106]. A sudden increase in BP during exercise may trigger coronary plaque rupture or cerebral events [107, 108]. Thus, exercise prescription and eligibility to competitive athletics should be based on careful clinical assessment of all cardiovascular risk factors and target organ involvement in order to establish the global level of cardiovascular risk (see Chap. 13) [108]. An update of previous European recommendations representing the consensus of an international panel of experts appointed by the European Association of Preventive Cardiology, an association of the European Society of Cardiology, has been recently released [109]. The aim of the panel was to formulate recommendations which represent the best possible balance between risks and benefits inherent with competitive sports participation and to provide a practical document for advising competitive sports activity in people with hypertension.

- According to the panel, caution should be used in subjects with stage 2 to stage 3 hypertension (BP ≥ 160/100 mmHg) for whom temporary activity restriction should be applied until normal BP is achieved with pharmacological treatment.
- Every hypertensive athlete should be thoroughly investigated to exclude target organ damage and coronary artery disease. To this end, the same examination procedure should be applied as in the general population.
- In addition, echocardiography and exercise stress testing (including ECG and BP monitoring) should be performed in all subjects to rule out LV hypertrophy, cardiomyopathies, cardiac ischemia, or valvular disease.

The management of subjects exhibiting isolated high BP response to exercise is still under scrutiny because of lack of data about the prognostic significance of this clinical feature [110]. In the absence of prognostic data, these subjects should receive periodical accurate follow-ups, with special attention to CV risk factors, but should not be restricted from competitive sports. Ambulatory BP monitoring is a useful tool for the assessment of the hypertensive athlete. In case of elevated in-office BP level, this technique is recommended, particularly when "white-coat" hypertension is suspected or if a hypertensive response during exercise testing is present.

Recommendations for participation in competitive sports in athletes with hypertension are based on risk stratification and should be given when the clinical condition is stable with the understanding that general recommendations for the management of hypertension are observed. It is opinion of the expert panel that there is no contraindication for competitive sport participation in athletes if no associated clinical conditions or target organ damage is present and their BP and other cardiovascular risk factors are well controlled with non-pharmacological measures and/or pharmacological treatment [109]. Also, in patients with high-risk in whom control of BP has been achieved, participation in all competitive sports is possible with the exception of power-oriented sports. If BP values are not well controlled by treatment, temporary restriction from competitive sport is recommended. Ambulatory BP monitoring should be performed to verify the actual BP control with treatment.

## 36.9 Safety Precautions During Exercise Therapy in Patients with Arterial Hypertension

Safety measures when prescribing exercise have been recently outlined in the Exercise Prescription in Patients with Different Combinations of Cardiovascular Disease Risk Factors—EXPERT tool [111]. Exercise prescription recommendations for people with hypertension broadly follow guidelines that are known to promote and maintain health in the general adult population [112].

- Only high risk individuals with hypertension (i.e., symptomatic or with known disease) planning to engage in moderate or vigorous intensity exercise are recommended to have a medically supervised exercise stress test prior to beginning an exercise program [112].
- Further, as patients with hypertension have an increased risk for ischemic heart disease, they should be informed about the nature of cardiac prodromal symptoms and exercise-related warning symptoms including chest pain or discomfort, abnormal dyspnea, dizziness or malaise and should seek prompt medical care if such symptoms develop.
- Moreover, the initial total risk evaluation performed after diagnosis should be regularly updated.
- During execution of exercises, it is very important to avoid sudden increases in BP. Therefore, avoiding elevated workloads or excessive short intervals that creates elevated fatigue is strongly recommended.

One of the most common errors in the exercise executions is the *Valsalva manoeuvre*. Avoidance of the Valsalva manoeuvre, which consists in the abrupt inspiration and its interruption causing significant rises in the thoracic pressure, is particularly warranted.

With regard to medication, diuretics are common secondary treatment for hypertension and may lead to dehydration in exercising individuals, especially in warm temperatures and may lead to hypokalaemia [113]. There is also a greater likelihood for sudden excessive hypotension in the immediate post exercise period among patients taking alpha blockers, calcium channel blockers or vasodilatory drugs. The implementation of an extended cool down period of light activity and avoidance of suddenly stopping exercise might decrease the potential for hypotensive-related adverse events [113].

## 36.10 Summary of Exercise Recommendations

Overall, these findings suggest a clear role for exercise in the prevention and daily management of high BP. The magnitude of the BP reductions observed across the different exercise modalities are comparable to the changes obtained with first-line antihypertensive medication [114]. In addition, these BP reductions have been associated with an improvement of cardiovascular risk.

- It has been estimated that a 2 mmHg-reduction of systolic BP results in a 6% reduction in stroke mortality and a 4% reduction in mortality attributable to coronary heart disease.
- The percentage reductions amount to 14% and 9%, respectively, for a 5 mmHg-decrease of BP [74].
- Furthermore a recent network meta-analysis of major exercise and drug trials showed not statistically detectable difference between exercise and drug intervention in mortality outcomes for coronary heart disease [115].

As the majority of well-conducted and conclusive evidence is derived from aerobic endurance training studies, endurance training at low to moderate intensity on most days of the week remains the first choice of exercise therapy. Despite the growing number of studies with dynamic and isometric resistance training, there remains a lack of data in hypertensive patients and therefore both types of resistance training should only be recommended as an adjunct therapy to aerobic endurance training. Finally, other modalities of exercise are emerging and should be welcomed as new antihypertensive lifestyle interventions. However, further research remains needed to allow optimal and personalized exercise prescription.

**Clinical Pearls**

- Blood pressure response during exercise largely depends on modality and intensity of exercise.
- Numerous epidemiological studies have observed inverse relationships between dose of physical activity and blood pressure.
- Randomized controlled trials evidence that regular exercise training decreases systolic and diastolic blood pressure in all populations.

## Review

### Questions

1. A female patient aged 56 years presents at your consultation with an office blood pressure of 139/92 mmHg but otherwise healthy with no other co-morbidities or risk factors. Based on the current available evidence, what type, intensity and frequency of exercise would you preferentially prescribe for her?
2. A 48-year-old competitive football player presents at your consultation for a preparticipation cardiovascular screening. His office BP is 148/90 mmHg and in line with a recent measurement by his GP. Otherwise he has a normal resting ECG, no family history of CV disease and no other risk factors. Can he compete?

### Answers

1. This patient should be recommended to perform aerobic endurance exercise, at least 5 days per week at a moderate intensity for a total of 150 min per week. Dynamic resistance training at moderate intensity could be added as an adjunct, two times per week.
2. According to current guidelines, this player cannot compete as he has a grade I hypertension. Therefore, lifestyle changes and/or medical therapy are advised. From the moment his BP is controlled (<1 40/85 mmHg) and in the absence of any target organ damage or associated clinical conditions, he can return to competition.

## References


1. Zabetakis PM. Profiling the hypertensive patient in sports. Clin Sports Med. 1984;3(1):137–52.
2. Palatini P. Blood pressure behaviour during physical activity. Sports Med. 1988;5(6):353–74.
3. Palatini P. Exercise haemodynamics in the normotensive and the hypertensive subject. Clin Sci (Lond). 1994;87(3):275–87.
4. Mitchell JH, Reardon WC, McCloskey DI. Reflex effects on circulation and respiration from contracting skeletal muscle. Am J Phys. 1977;233(3):H374–8.
5. Rowell LB, Brengelmann GL, Blackmon JR, Bruce RA, Murray JA. Disparities between aortic and peripheral pulse pressures induced by upright exercise and vasomotor changes in man. Circulation. 1968;37(6):954–64.
6. Radice M, Alli C, Avanzini F, Di Tullio M, Mariotti G, Taioli E, et al. Role of blood pressure response to provocative tests in the prediction of hypertension in adolescents. Eur Heart J. 1985;6(6):490–6.
7. Palatini P, Pessina AC, Ardigò A, Veronese P, Dal Palù C. Response to some pressor tests in patients with labile and stable hypertension, before and after administration of atenolol. Boll Soc Ital Cardiol. 1977;22(8):1477–84.
8. Rowell LB. Blood pressure regulation during exercise. Ann Med. 1991;23(3):329–33.
9. Irving JB, Bruce RA, DeRouen TA. Variations in and significance of systolic pressure during maximal exercise (treadmill) testing. Am J Cardiol. 1977;39(6):841–8.
10. Levy AM, Tabakin BS, Hanson JS. Hemodynamic responses to graded treadmill exercise in young untreated labile hypertensive patients. Circulation. 1967;35(6):1063–72.
11. Palatini P, Mos L, Mormino P, Munari L, Del Torre M, Valle F, et al. Intra-arterial blood pressure monitoring in the evaluation of the hypertensive athlete. Eur Heart J. 1990;11(4): 348–54.
12. Bachmann KZR, Riess PJ, Zoloch KA. Blutddrucktelemetrie: kontinuerliche, directe blutdruckmessungen im altag und beim sport. Dts Med Wochenschr. 1970;14:741–7.
13. Palatini P, Mormino P, Mos L, Di Marco A, Munari L, Del Torre M, et al. Blood pressure changes during physical exercise (the beat phenomenon). J Hypertens Suppl. 1988;6(4):S88–90.
14. Palatini P, Mos L, Mormino P, Di Marco A, Munari L, Fazio G, et al. Blood pressure changes during running in humans: the "beat" phenomenon. J Appl Physiol (1985). 1989;67(1):52–9.
15. Palatini P, Mos L, Munari L, Mormino P, Del Torre M, Valle F, et al. Beats modulate blood pressure during running. Am J Hypertens. 1989;2(11 Pt 1):872–4.
16. Palatini P, Bongiovì S, Mario L, Schiraldi C, Mos L, Pessina AC. Above-normal left ventricular systolic performance during exercise in young subjects with mild hypertension. Eur Heart J. 1995;16(2):232–42.
17. Fagard R, Aubert A, Staessen J, Eynde EV, Vanhees L, Amery A. Cardiac structure and function in cyclists and runners. Comparative echocardiographic study. Br Heart J. 1984;52(2):124–9.
18. Chaney RH, Arndt S. Predictability of blood pressure response to isometric stress. Am J Cardiol. 1983;51(5):787–90.
19. Jones RI, Lahiri A, Cashman PM, Dore C, Raftery EB. Left ventricular function during isometric hand grip and cold stress in normal subjects. Br Heart J. 1986;55(3):246–52.
20. Sullivan J, Hanson P, Rahko PS, Folts JD. Continuous measurement of left ventricular performance during and after maximal isometric deadlift exercise. Circulation. 1992;85(4):1406–13.
21. Bezucha GR, Lenser MC, Hanson PG, Nagle FJ. Comparison of hemodynamic responses to static and dynamic exercise. J Appl Physiol Respir Environ Exerc Physiol. 1982;53(6):1589–93.
22. Seals DR, Washburn RA, Hanson PG, Painter PL, Nagle FJ. Increased cardiovascular response to static contraction of larger muscle groups. J Appl Physiol Respir Environ Exerc Physiol. 1983;54(2):434–7.
23. Seals DR, Hanson PG, Washburn RA, Painter PL, Ward A, Nagle FJ. Cardiovascular response to static contraction in borderline hypertension. Clin Cardiol. 1985;8(6):348–52.
24. McCloskey DI, Streatfeild KA. Muscular reflex stimuli to the cardiovascular system during isometric contractions of muscle groups of different mass. J Physiol. 1975;250(2):431–41.

25. Silke B, Watt SJ, Taylor SH. The circulatory response to lifting and carrying and its modification by beta-adrenoceptor blockade. Int J Cardiol. 1984;6(4):527–36.
26. MacDougall JD, Tuxen D, Sale DG, Moroz JR, Sutton JR. Arterial blood pressure response to heavy resistance exercise. J Appl Physiol (1985). 1985;58(3):785–90.
27. Palatini P, Mos L, Munari L, Valle F, Del Torre M, Rossi A, et al. Blood pressure changes during heavy-resistance exercise. J Hypertens Suppl. 1989;7(6):S72–3.
28. Hamilton WFWR, jr HHT. Arterial cerebrospinal and venous pressures in man during cough and strain. Am J Phys. 1944;141:42–50.
29. Fleck SJ, Dean LS. Resistance-training experience and the pressor response during resistance exercise. J Appl Physiol (1985). 1987;63(1):116–20.
30. Poliner LR, Dehmer GJ, Lewis SE, Parkey RW, Blomqvist CG, Willerson JT. Left ventricular performance in normal subjects: a comparison of the responses to exercise in the upright and supine positions. Circulation. 1980;62(3):528–34.
31. Steingart RM, Wexler J, Slagle S, Scheuer J. Radionuclide ventriculographic responses to graded supine and upright exercise: critical role of the Frank-Starling mechanism at submaximal exercise. Am J Cardiol. 1984;53(11):1671–7.
32. Fisman EZ, Frank AG, Ben-Ari E, Kessler G, Pines A, Drory Y, et al. Altered left ventricular volume and ejection fraction responses to supine dynamic exercise in athletes. J Am Coll Cardiol. 1990;15(3):582–8.
33. ASTRAND I. Aerobic work capacity in men and women with special reference to age. Acta Physiol Scand Suppl. 1960;49(169):1–92.
34. Adams KF, Vincent LM, McAllister SM, el-Ashmawy H, Sheps DS. The influence of age and gender on left ventricular response to supine exercise in asymptomatic normal subjects. Am Heart J. 1987;113(3):732–42.
35. Julius S, Amery A, Whitlock LS, Conway J. Influence of age on the hemodynamic response to exercise. Circulation. 1967;36(2):222–30.
36. Younis LT, Melin JA, Robert AR, Detry JM. Influence of age and sex on left ventricular volumes and ejection fraction during upright exercise in normal subjects. Eur Heart J. 1990;11(10):916–24.
37. Mann DL, Denenberg BS, Gash AK, Makler PT, Bove AA. Effects of age on ventricular performance during graded supine exercise. Am Heart J. 1986;111(1):108–15.
38. Bongiovì S, Palatini P, Macor F, Visentin P, Pessina AC. Age and blood-pressure-related changes in left ventricular diastolic filling. J Hypertens Suppl. 1992;10(2):S25–30.
39. Ginzton LE, Conant R, Brizendine M, Laks MM. Effect of long-term high intensity aerobic training on left ventricular volume during maximal upright exercise. J Am Coll Cardiol. 1989;14(2):364–71.
40. Tomai F, Ciavolella M, Gaspardone A, De Fazio A, Basso EG, Giannitti C, et al. Peak exercise left ventricular performance in normal subjects and in athletes assessed by first-pass radionuclide angiography. Am J Cardiol. 1992;70(4):531–5.
41. Fagard R, Van den Broeke C, Amery A. Left ventricular dynamics during exercise in elite marathon runners. J Am Coll Cardiol. 1989;14(1):112–8.
42. Vanoverschelde JL, Younis LT, Melin JA, Vanbutsele R, Leclercq B, Robert AR, et al. Prolonged exercise induces left ventricular dysfunction in healthy subjects. J Appl Physiol (1985). 1991;70(3):1356–63.
43. Seals DR, Rogers MA, Hagberg JM, Yamamoto C, Cryer PE, Ehsani AA. Left ventricular dysfunction after prolonged strenuous exercise in healthy subjects. Am J Cardiol. 1988;61(11):875–9.
44. Upton MT, Rerych SK, Roeback JR, Newman GE, Douglas JM, Wallace AG, et al. Effect of brief and prolonged exercise on left ventricular function. Am J Cardiol. 1980;45(6):1154–60.
45. Hartford M, Wikstrand JC, Wallentin I, Ljungman SM, Berglund GL. Left ventricular wall stress and systolic function in untreated primary hypertension. Hypertension. 1985;7(1):97–104.
46. Aurigemma GP, Silver KH, Priest MA, Gaasch WH. Geometric changes allow normal ejection fraction despite depressed myocardial shortening in hypertensive left ventricular hypertrophy. J Am Coll Cardiol. 1995;26(1):195–202.

47. Palatini P, Visentin P, Nicolosi G, Mione V, Stritoni P, Michieletto M, et al. Endocardial versus midwall measurement of left ventricular function in mild hypertension: an insight from the Harvest Study. J Hypertens. 1996;14(8):1011–7.
48. Palatini P, Visentin P, Mormino P, Pietra M, Piccolo D, Cozzutti E, et al. Left ventricular performance in the early stages of systemic hypertension. HARVEST Study Group Hypertension and Ambulatory Recording Venetia Study. Am J Cardiol. 1998;81(4):418–23.
49. Shimizu G, Hirota Y, Kita Y, Kawamura K, Saito T, Gaasch WH. Left ventricular midwall mechanics in systemic arterial hypertension. Myocardial function is depressed in pressure-overload hypertrophy. Circulation. 1991;83(5):1676–84.
50. de Simone G, Devereux RB, Roman MJ, Ganau A, Saba PS, Alderman MH, et al. Assessment of left ventricular function by the midwall fractional shortening/end-systolic stress relation in human hypertension. J Am Coll Cardiol. 1994;23(6):1444–51.
51. Palatini P, Frigo G, Visentin P, Mario L, Mormino P, Pessina AC. Left ventricular contractile performance in the early stage of hypertension in humans. Eur J Appl Physiol. 2001;85(1-2):118–24.
52. Huai P, Xun H, Reilly KH, Wang Y, Ma W, Xi B. Physical activity and risk of hypertension: a meta-analysis of prospective cohort studies. Hypertension. 2013;62(6):1021–6.
53. Liu X, Zhang D, Liu Y, Sun X, Han C, Wang B, et al. Dose-response association between physical activity and incident hypertension: a systematic review and meta-analysis of cohort studies. Hypertension. 2017;69(5):813–20.
54. Haslam DW, James WP. Obesity. Lancet. 2005;366(9492):1197–209.
55. Blair SN, Goodyear NN, Gibbons LW, Cooper KH. Physical fitness and incidence of hypertension in healthy normotensive men and women. JAMA. 1984;252(4):487–90.
56. Carnethon MR, Evans NS, Church TS, Lewis CE, Schreiner PJ, Jacobs DR, et al. Joint associations of physical activity and aerobic fitness on the development of incident hypertension: coronary artery risk development in young adults. Hypertension. 2010;56(1):49–55.
57. Williams PT. A cohort study of incident hypertension in relation to changes in vigorous physical activity in men and women. J Hypertens. 2008;26(6):1085–93.
58. Sawada S, Tanaka H, Funakoshi M, Shindo M, Kono S, Ishiko T. Five year prospective study on blood pressure and maximal oxygen uptake. Clin Exp Pharmacol Physiol. 1993;20(7-8):483–7.
59. Fagard RH, Cornelissen VA. Effect of exercise on blood pressure control in hypertensive patients. Eur J Cardiovasc Prev Rehabil. 2007;14(1):12–7.
60. Cornelissen VA, Fagard RH. Effects of endurance training on blood pressure, blood pressure-regulating mechanisms, and cardiovascular risk factors. Hypertension. 2005;46(4):667–75.
61. Cornelissen VA, Smart NA. Exercise training for blood pressure: a systematic review and meta-analysis. J Am Heart Assoc. 2013;2(1):e004473.
62. Costa EC, Hay JL, Kehler DS, Boreskie KF, Arora RC, Umpierre D, et al. Effects of high-intensity interval training versus moderate-intensity continuous training on blood pressure in adults with pre- to established hypertension: a systematic review and meta-analysis of randomized trials. Sports Med. 2018;48(9):2127–42.
63. Cornelissen VA, Fagard RH, Coeckelberghs E, Vanhees L. Impact of resistance training on blood pressure and other cardiovascular risk factors: a meta-analysis of randomized, controlled trials. Hypertension. 2011;58(5):950–8.
64. MacDonald HV, Johnson BT, Huedo-Medina TB, Livingston J, Forsyth KC, Kraemer WJ, et al. Dynamic resistance training as stand-alone antihypertensive lifestyle therapy: a meta-analysis. J Am Heart Assoc. 2016;5(10)
65. López-Valenciano A, Ruiz-Pérez I, Ayala F, Sánchez-Meca J, Vera-Garcia FJ. Updated systematic review and meta-analysis on the role of isometric resistance training for resting blood pressure management in adults. J Hypertens. 2019;
66. Inder JD, Carlson DJ, Dieberg G, McFarlane JR, Hess NC, Smart NA. Isometric exercise training for blood pressure management: a systematic review and meta-analysis to optimize benefit. Hypertens Res. 2016;39(2):88–94.
67. Igarashi Y, Nogami Y. The effect of regular aquatic exercise on blood pressure: a meta-analysis of randomized controlled trials. Eur J Prev Cardiol. 2018;25(2):190–9.

68. Xiong X, Wang P, Li S, Zhang Y, Li X. Effect of Baduanjin exercise for hypertension: a systematic review and meta-analysis of randomized controlled trials. Maturitas. 2015;80(4):370–8.
69. Lauche R, Peng W, Ferguson C, Cramer H, Frawley J, Adams J, et al. Efficacy of Tai Chi and qigong for the prevention of stroke and stroke risk factors: a systematic review with meta-analysis. Medicine (Baltimore). 2017;96(45):e8517.
70. Cramer H, Haller H, Lauche R, Steckhan N, Michalsen A, Dobos G. A systematic review and meta-analysis of yoga for hypertension. Am J Hypertens. 2014;27(9):1146–51.
71. Conceição LS, Neto MG, do Amaral MA, Martins-Filho PR, Oliveira Carvalho V. Effect of dance therapy on blood pressure and exercise capacity of individuals with hypertension: a systematic review and meta-analysis. Int J Cardiol. 2016;220:553–7.
72. Pescatello LS, MacDonald HV, Ash GI, Lamberti LM, Farquhar WB, Arena R, et al. Assessing the existing professional exercise recommendations for hypertension: a review and recommendations for future research priorities. Mayo Clin Proc. 2015;90(6):801–12.
73. Cornelissen VA, Buys R, Smart NA. Endurance exercise beneficially affects ambulatory blood pressure: a systematic review and meta-analysis. J Hypertens. 2013;31(4):639–48.
74. Chobanian AV, Bakris GL, Black HR, Cushman WC, Green LA, Izzo JL, et al. Seventh report of the Joint National Committee on Prevention, Detection, Evaluation, and Treatment of High Blood Pressure. Hypertension. 2003;42(6):1206–52.
75. Whelton SP, Chin A, Xin X, He J. Effect of aerobic exercise on blood pressure: a meta-analysis of randomized, controlled trials. Ann Intern Med. 2002;136(7):493–503.
76. Igarashi Y, Akazawa N, Maeda S. Regular aerobic exercise and blood pressure in East Asians: a meta-analysis of randomized controlled trials. Clin Exp Hypertens. 2018;40(4):378–89.
77. Kelley GA, Kelley KS. Aerobic exercise and resting blood pressure in women: a meta-analytic review of controlled clinical trials. J Womens Health Gend Based Med. 1999;8(6):787–803.
78. Tully MA, Cupples ME, Hart ND, McEneny J, McGlade KJ, Chan WS, et al. Randomised controlled trial of home-based walking programmes at and below current recommended levels of exercise in sedentary adults. J Epidemiol Community Health. 2007;61(9):778–83.
79. Jennings G, Nelson L, Nestel P, Esler M, Korner P, Burton D, et al. The effects of changes in physical activity on major cardiovascular risk factors, hemodynamics, sympathetic function, and glucose utilization in man: a controlled study of four levels of activity. Circulation. 1986;73(1):30–40.
80. Pescatello LS, MacDonald HV, Lamberti L, Johnson BT. Exercise for hypertension: a prescription update integrating existing recommendations with emerging research. Curr Hypertens Rep. 2015;17(11):87.
81. Cornelissen VA, Fagard RH. Exercise intensity and postexercise hypotension. J Hypertens. 2004;22(10):1859–61.
82. Kenney MJ, Seals DR. Postexercise hypotension. Key features, mechanisms, and clinical significance. Hypertension. 1993;22(5):653–64.
83. Cornelissen VA, Arnout J, Holvoet P, Fagard RH. Influence of exercise at lower and higher intensity on blood pressure and cardiovascular risk factors at older age. J Hypertens. 2009;27(4):753–62.
84. Eicher JD, Maresh CM, Tsongalis GJ, Thompson PD, Pescatello LS. The additive blood pressure lowering effects of exercise intensity on post-exercise hypotension. Am Heart J. 2010;160(3):513–20.
85. Pescatello LS, Guidry MA, Blanchard BE, Kerr A, Taylor AL, Johnson AN, et al. Exercise intensity alters postexercise hypotension. J Hypertens. 2004;22(10):1881–8.
86. Cononie CC, Graves JE, Pollock ML, Phillips MI, Sumners C, Hagberg JM. Effect of exercise training on blood pressure in 70- to 79-yr-old men and women. Med Sci Sports Exerc. 1991;23(4):505-11.
87. Collier SR, Kanaley JA, Carhart R, Frechette V, Tobin MM, Hall AK, et al. Effect of 4 weeks of aerobic or resistance exercise training on arterial stiffness, blood flow and blood pressure in pre- and stage-1 hypertensives. J Hum Hypertens. 2008;22(10):678–86.

88. Casonatto J, Goessler KF, Cornelissen VA, Cardoso JR, Polito MD. The blood pressure-lowering effect of a single bout of resistance exercise: a systematic review and meta-analysis of randomised controlled trials. Eur J Prev Cardiol. 2016;23(16):1700–14.
89. Brook RD, Appel LJ, Rubenfire M, Ogedegbe G, Bisognano JD, Elliott WJ, et al. Beyond medications and diet: alternative approaches to lowering blood pressure: a scientific statement from the american heart association. Hypertension. 2013;61(6):1360–83.
90. Carlson DJ, Inder J, Palanisamy SK, McFarlane JR, Dieberg G, Smart NA. The efficacy of isometric resistance training utilizing handgrip exercise for blood pressure management: a randomized trial. Medicine (Baltimore). 2016;95(52):e5791.
91. Colado JC, Triplett NT, Tella V, Saucedo P, Abellán J. Effects of aquatic resistance training on health and fitness in postmenopausal women. Eur J Appl Physiol. 2009;106(1):113–22.
92. Arca EA, Martinelli B, Martin LC, Waisberg CB, Franco RJ. Aquatic exercise is as effective as dry land training to blood pressure reduction in postmenopausal hypertensive women. Physiother Res Int. 2014;19(2):93–8.
93. Casale PN, Devereux RB, Milner M, Zullo G, Harshfield GA, Pickering TG, et al. Value of echocardiographic measurement of left ventricular mass in predicting cardiovascular morbid events in hypertensive men. Ann Intern Med. 1986;105(2):173–8.
94. Baglivo HP, Fabregues G, Burrieza H, Esper RC, Talarico M, Esper RJ. Effect of moderate physical training on left ventricular mass in mild hypertensive persons. Hypertension. 1990;15(2 Suppl):I153–6.
95. Kokkinos PF, Narayan P, Colleran JA, Pittaras A, Notargiacomo A, Reda D, et al. Effects of regular exercise on blood pressure and left ventricular hypertrophy in African-American men with severe hypertension. N Engl J Med. 1995;333(22):1462–7.
96. Zanettini R, Bettega D, Agostoni O, Ballestra B, del Rosso G, di Michele R, et al. Exercise training in mild hypertension: effects on blood pressure, left ventricular mass and coagulation factor VII and fibrinogen. Cardiology. 1997;88(5):468–73.
97. Palatini P, Visentin P, Dorigatti F, Guarnieri C, Santonastaso M, Cozzio S, et al. Regular physical activity prevents development of left ventricular hypertrophy in hypertension. Eur Heart J. 2009;30(2):225–32.
98. Boman K, Gerdts E, Wachtell K, Dahlöf B, Nieminen MS, Olofsson M, et al. Exercise and cardiovascular outcomes in hypertensive patients in relation to structure and function of left ventricular hypertrophy: the LIFE study. Eur J Cardiovasc Prev Rehabil. 2009;16(2):242–8.
99. Hinderliter A, Sherwood A, Gullette EC, Babyak M, Waugh R, Georgiades A, et al. Reduction of left ventricular hypertrophy after exercise and weight loss in overweight patients with mild hypertension. Arch Intern Med. 2002;162(12):1333–9.
100. Reid CM, Dart AM, Dewar EM, Jennings GL. Interactions between the effects of exercise and weight loss on risk factors, cardiovascular haemodynamics and left ventricular structure in overweight subjects. J Hypertens. 1994;12(3):291–301.
101. Palatini P. Cardiovascular effects of exercise in young hypertensives. Int J Sports Med. 2012;33(9):683–90.
102. Thompson PD, Buchner D, Pina IL, Balady GJ, Williams MA, Marcus BH, et al. Exercise and physical activity in the prevention and treatment of atherosclerotic cardiovascular disease: a statement from the Council on Clinical Cardiology (Subcommittee on Exercise, Rehabilitation, and Prevention) and the Council on Nutrition, Physical Activity, and Metabolism (Subcommittee on Physical Activity). Circulation. 2003;107(24):3109–16.
103. Pescatello LS, Bairos L, Vanheest JL, Maresh CM, Rodriguez NR, Moyna NM, et al. Postexercise hypotension differs between white and black women. Am Heart J. 2003;145(2):364–70.
104. Palatini P, Bratti P, Palomba D, Saladini F, Zanatta N, Maraglino G. Regular physical activity attenuates the blood pressure response to public speaking and delays the development of hypertension. J Hypertens. 2010;28(6):1186–93.
105. Laterza MC, de Matos LD, Trombetta IC, Braga AM, Roveda F, Alves MJ, et al. Exercise training restores baroreflex sensitivity in never-treated hypertensive patients. Hypertension. 2007;49(6):1298–306.

106. Fagard RH. Athletes with systemic hypertension. Cardiol Clin. 2007;25(3):441–8vii.
107. Laukkanen JA, Khan H, Kurl S, Willeit P, Karppi J, Ronkainen K, et al. Left ventricular mass and the risk of sudden cardiac death: a population-based study. J Am Heart Assoc. 2014;3(6):e001285.
108. Black HR, Sica D, Ferdinand K, White WB. American Heart Association Electrocardiography and Arrhythmias Committee of Council on Clinical Cardiology CoCDiY, Council on Cardiovascular and Stroke Nursing, Council on Functional Genomics and Translational Biology, and American College of Cardiology. Eligibility and disqualification recommendations for competitive athletes with cardiovascular abnormalities: task force 6: hypertension: a scientific statement from the American Heart Association and the American College of Cardiology. Circulation. 2015;132(22):e298–302.
109. Niebauer J, Börjesson M, Carre F, Caselli S, Palatini P, Quattrini F, et al. Recommendations for participation in competitive sports of athletes with arterial hypertension: a position statement from the sports cardiology section of the European Association of Preventive Cardiology (EAPC). Eur Heart J. 2018;39(40):3664–71.
110. Palatini P. Exaggerated blood pressure response to exercise: pathophysiologic mechanisms and clinical relevance. J Sports Med Phys Fitness. 1998;38(1):1–9.
111. Hansen D, Niebauer J, Cornelissen V, Barna O, Neunhäuserer D, Stettler C, et al. Exercise prescription in patients with different combinations of cardiovascular disease risk factors: a consensus statement from the EXPERT working group. Sports Med. 2018;48(8):1781–97.
112. Borjesson M, Urhausen A, Kouidi E, Dugmore D, Sharma S, Halle M, et al. Cardiovascular evaluation of middle-aged/senior individuals engaged in leisure-time sport activities: position stand from the sections of exercise physiology and sports cardiology of the European Association of Cardiovascular Prevention and Rehabilitation. Eur J Cardiovasc Prev Rehabil. 2011;18(3):446–58.
113. Sharman JE, La Gerche A, Coombes JS. Exercise and cardiovascular risk in patients with hypertension. Am J Hypertens. 2015;28(2):147–58.
114. AOaCftACRGTAaL-LTtPHA T. Major outcomes in moderately hypercholesterolemic, hypertensive patients randomized to pravastatin vs usual care: the Antihypertensive and Lipid-Lowering Treatment to Prevent Heart Attack Trial (ALLHAT-LLT). JAMA. 2002;288(23):2998–3007.
115. Naci H, Ioannidis JP. Comparative effectiveness of exercise and drug interventions on mortality outcomes: metaepidemiological study. BMJ. 2013;347:f5577.

# Impact of Exercise on Cardiovascular Risk Factors: Dyslipidemia

# 37

Axel Pressler and Mats Börjesson

**Learning Objectives**

1. Be informed about adequate risk stratification in patients and athletes based on lipid levels.
2. Get to know the effects of physical activity or exercise training on the different traditional lipid parameters such as HDL, LDL or triglycerides.
3. Be informed about the most important studies having evaluated these effects on either an epidemiological or a randomized basis.
4. Understand the nature of various interventions (exercise training alone or as part of dietary or multimodal lifestyle interventions) and their different impact on lipid profiles.
5. Learn on the effects of statins in combination with athletic activity and rehabilitative exercise.

## 37.1 Physiological Background and Risk Stratification

### 37.1.1 Lipid Metabolism and Targets of Exercise

Atherosclerosis is a chronic, progressive disease, starting early in life, and is the most common etiology for cardiovascular disease (CVD). Starting with the diffusion of LDL-cholesterol from the blood into the vessel wall, and its oxygenation and formation of an inflammatory process, atherosclerosis leads to the formation of

A. Pressler (✉)
Private Center of Sports & Exercise Cardiology, Munich, Germany
e-mail: axel.pressler@kardiologie-mit-herz.de

M. Börjesson
Neuroscience and Physiology & Center for Health and Performance, University of Gothenburg and Sahlgrenska University Hospital/Ostra, Gothenburg, Sweden
e-mail: mats.brjesson@telia.com



A. Pressler, J. Niebauer (eds.), *Textbook of Sports and Exercise Cardiology*,
https://doi.org/10.1007/978-3-030-35374-2_37

foam-cells from macrophages [1]. This in turn leads to the formation of plaques in the vessel wall, consisting of a core of lipids (mainly cholesterol) and a cap, which could rupture, leading to aggravated atherosclerosis or acute thrombus formation, resulting in acute events such as stroke, myocardial infarction or even sudden cardiac death (SCD).

The main non-modifiable risk factors for atherosclerosis are age and gender, while the most important modifiable risk factor may be dyslipidemia [2]. Dyslipidemia refers to abnormal levels of various lipids and lipid fractions, usually defined as values above a certain normal level for each lipid, for instance high total cholesterol >5.2 mmol/L (200 mg/dl) or hypertriglyceridemia >1.7 mmol/l (150 mg/dl) [3]. Dyslipidemia is usually subclinical and asymptomatic and is thus sometimes not detected before clinical manifestations of CVD are present.

On the contrary, fat is a necessary part of our diet, as it contains the fat-soluble vitamins A, D, E and K, and it is also an important substrate for energy production:

- Triglycerides (TG) consist of three fatty acids and one glycerol molecule and constitute the main energy stores of the body. TGs are also an integral part of the cell membrane.
- Cholesterol is produced in the liver or is absorbed from our food in the intestine. Cholesterol is part of the cell membrane and is also a precursor to sex hormones (testosterone and progesterone).

In order to be transported in the blood, fat molecules must bind to proteins and form water-soluble complexes, the so-called *lipoproteins*. These lipoproteins are defined according to size and density into different classes:

(a) Chylomicrons
(b) Very low-density lipoprotein (VLDL)
(c) Low-density lipoprotein (LDL)
(d) High density lipoprotein (HDL)

or even more divided into intermediate-density lipoprotein (IDL) and lipoprotein (a) (Lp(a)). The latter is a variant of LDL with the addition of a glycoproteins (ApoA1 or ApoB). The sum of LDL-, VLDL-, IDL- and HDL-cholesterol is what is measured as total cholesterol. LDL contains the absolute majority of the serum-cholesterol.

- Dyslipidemia may be the result of genetic susceptibility and/or lifestyle related risk factors, such as physical inactivity, smoking, overweight/obesity and diabetes mellitus.
- The most important dietary factor may be the intake of saturated fat, which mainly increases the LDL-cholesterol levels.
  - Healthy food, including fruit, vegetables, reduced saturated fat and moderate alcohol intake [4], is associated with better lipid levels.

- Genetic factors do play a major role for some patients, such as familiar hypercholesterolemia [5], which can be associated with extremely high LDL-cholesterol levels (>5 mmol/L).
  - Depending on the severity of dyslipidemia, these patients could have a very high risk of early manifestations of CVD, including stroke and myocardial infarction in young age.
- In turn, HDL-cholesterol is typically lower in patients with diabetes mellitus, in those with overweight/obesity, those being physically inactive and among smokers [6], and is higher in women compared to men.
- The TG levels are usually the result of unfavorable lifestyle factors, with excessive alcohol intake and physical inactivity being very important.
  - However, hypertriglyceridemia is also seen in diabetes mellitus type 2 and hypothyroidism.

In summary, physical activity has the potential to reverse dyslipidemia, with the most obvious targets being HDL-cholesterol (increase), ApoB/ApoA1 (lower ratio) [7] and TG (decrease) (Table 37.1).

### 37.1.2 Lipids and Cardiovascular Risk

Abnormal lipid levels (dyslipidemia) are highly associated with increased CVD-risk [8]:

1. Most commonly, increased levels of these lipoprotein complexes are associated with CVD-risk: Total-cholesterol, LDL-cholesterol, VLDL-cholesterol, IDL-cholesterol and Lp(a).
2. Conversely, increased levels of HDL-cholesterol are associated with lower CVD-risk, at least on an epidemiological basis [9]. For instance, HDL transports cholesterol to the liver and decreases LDL-oxidation (protective effect).
3. High levels of TG are not considered to be an independent risk factor for CVD, but it may be, if associated with low HDL-cholesterol and/or extremely high levels (>10 mmol/L), as part of a familiar hypertriglyceridemia.
4. The levels of ApoA1 and ApoB approximately equal the levels of HDL-cholesterol and LDL-cholesterol, respectively. The ApoB/ApoA1 ratio is a stronger predictor than LDL/HDL [2]. In two patients with the same levels of LDL, the one with higher ApoB (as a measure of total atherogenic particles) has the higher risk.

**Table 37.1** Brief overview of the effects of physical activity / exercise to be expected on different lipid parameters

| Lipid parameter | Effect of physical activity/exercise |
|---|---|
| Total-cholesterol | 0/– |
| LDL | 0/– |
| HDL | + |
| TG | – |
| ApoB/apoA1 | – |

*0* no effect, + mild increase, – mild decrease

### 37.1.3 Risk Stratification in Athletes with Dyslipidemia

As dyslipidemia is one of the most important risk factors for atherosclerosis in general, this is also true for coronary artery disease (CAD). As discussed in more detail in Chap. 46, older and less fit individuals may take part in high-intensity endurance training and competition [10]. This means that athletes and patients wishing to take part in sports, especially at older age, will very likely have an underlying dyslipidemia or even (subclinical) CAD.

- Therefore, it is important to assess to total risk profile for underlying CAD, in each individual with dyslipidemia, e.g. using the established ESC SCORE models [3].
- In cases of individuals with increased overall risk, further evaluation should be applied (see Chap. 46), usually including a maximal exercise test.
- In cases with established CAD, it is important to achieve a comprehensive risk factor control, as well as regular follow-ups of the clinical picture and risk factor levels.

The prognosis of any individual with dyslipidemia will be dependent on the lipid levels, as discussed above. The first line of treatment includes smoking cessation and dietary advice, including "healthy food" (see above). In addition, physical activity may have multiple positive effects, potentially accentuated by healthy food/diet. Frequently, also pharmaceutical treatment has to be applied, based on the total risk profile and thus the total risk for CVD-events, according to SCORE.

## 37.2 Scientific Evidence

### 37.2.1 Epidemiological Studies

When interpreting the evidence derived from epidemiological studies, it is important to once again differ between physical activity (PA) and exercise training (ET). Although somewhat arbitrarily defined and often not clearly separated, these terms usually refer to different intensities of physical efforts:

- PA refers to light to moderate activities performed every day without aiming at specifically increasing cardiorespiratory fitness. This includes activities such as active commuting (e.g. by foot or bicycle), walking, household or garden activities or cycling to stores.
- ET usually refers to a goal-oriented physical training regimen with the clear aim to improve exercise capacity and physical performance in general or in specific types of sport, as such resulting in a more pronounced energy expenditure compared with PA.

Evidence for the associations of PA and increased fitness levels induced by ET with lipid profiles has been derived from epidemiological observations in large patient populations. Although this has expanded our knowledge, the limitations of this approach must be kept in mind, since PA habits or ET regimens are mostly measured only indirectly and inaccurately (usually by questionnaires). Results may thus statistically be confounded, questioning the casual relationships of the reported results.

With respect to increased PA, favorable effects have been reported on reduced mortality [11], presented in detail in Chap. 36 of this book. However, only few studies have focused on the independent effect of PA on lipid levels:

- *Women's Health Study:* included 27,158 asymptomatic females (age 55 ± 7 years), PA was assessed by questionnaire, and activity categories were derived [12].
  - A significantly lower proportion of women classified as "active" had HDL values <50 mg/dl as compared to inactive women, independent of body mass index (BMI) category.
  - Normal-weight, active women were significantly less likely to show LDL levels >130 mg compared to their sedentary counterparts; however, this was not confirmed in higher BMI categories (Fig. 37.1).

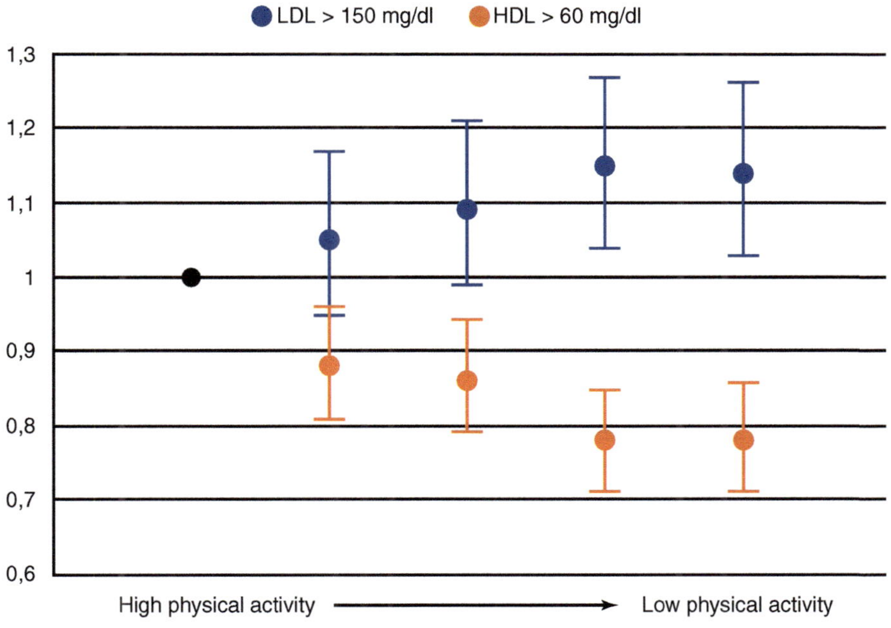


**Fig. 37.1** Adjusted odds ratios and their 95% confidence intervals of showing favorable lipid profiles according to the level of physical activity in the Women's Health Study, with high physical activity being the reference. The risk of showing an elevated LDL-cholesterol level increased alongside decreasing physical activity levels, whereas the likelihood of showing a beneficial HDL-level decreased in less active women (Created from data presented in [12])

  - Beneficial lipid profiles contributed approximately 20% to the cardiovascular risk reduction associated with increased PA [13].
- *CARDIA Study:* included 12,364 middle-aged adults (45 years) 20 years after initial evaluation. Active commuting (walking or cycling to work; assessed by questionnaire) was linked to improved TG levels in men but had no effects on other lipids, and no effects in women [14].
- *National runners' and walkers' health cohorts:* compared 33,060 runners with 15,945 walkers (51 ± 11 years). The amount of risk reduction for incident hypercholesterolemia was similar among groups when similar energy expenditures had been achieved [15]. This indicates that frequent walking may equal the effects of at least short bouts of running.
- In 8800 Australian adults (53 ± 14 years), a television viewing time of <2 h/day was associated with more favorable lipid profiles compared to ≥2 h, although absolute differences were small [16].

Overall, findings from epidemiological studies on different patterns of PA are inconsistent with respect to single lipid parameters, but results suggest that at least 'something is better than nothing'.

Regarding effects of ET or cardiorespiratory fitness, the commonest approach has been to link the maximum workload attained during a single exercise test (usually termed "fitness") to long-term mortality outcomes.

- In 6213 men (59 ± 11 years), a significantly reduced mortality risk was observed in the subgroup with the highest fitness as compared to the lowest fitness group, independent of a total cholesterol (TC) level > 220 mg [17].
- In 5721 women (52 ± 8 years), a higher fitness was associated with reduced mortality after adjustment for the Framingham Risk Score, which includes TC and HDL levels [18].

Findings from these two studies indicate that a high "fitness" as assessed by exercise testing appears to mitigate the unfavorable effects of elevated cholesterol levels in both middle-aged men and women.

- In 11,418 healthy males (44 ± 9 years), the impact of fitness on the age-related longitudinal changes of lipid levels over the life course was investigated [19]. A higher fitness level was associated with a delayed development of abnormal lipid profiles as compared to participants with low fitness.
- In 3148 men (42 ± 8 years) undergoing preventive examinations at two different time points, both a loss in fitness and a gain in fatness (BMI) were associated with the development of hypercholesterolemia [20]. In contrast, improving fitness was independently associated with a 30% lower risk for hypercholesterolemia.

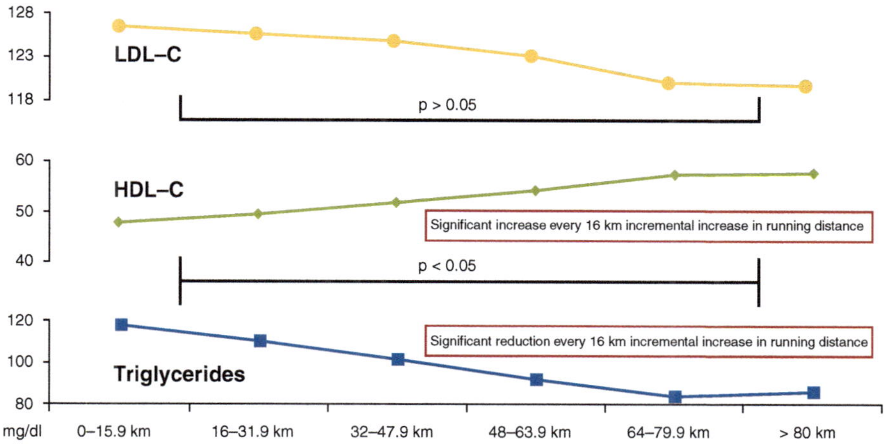


**Fig. 37.2** Schematic depiction of data from the *National Runners' Health Study* showing the course of lipid parameters according to different weekly running distances. Regarding HDL a significant increase and regarding triglyceride levels, a significant reduction was achieved with every 16 km incremental increase in running distance, whereas observed decreases in LDL levels did not reach statistical significance (Created from data presented in [21])

Further epidemiological studies conducted already during the 1990s provided evidence on the volume of endurance exercise required to improve lipid profiles:

- In 8283 male recreational runners (45 ± 10 years), weekly running distances (obtained by questionnaire) were linked to individual lipid profiles [21].
  - Runners with a weekly distance of >80 km showed significantly higher HDL and lower TG levels compared to those running <16 km.
  - Again, differences in LDL levels were less pronounced (Fig. 37.2).
- Similar findings were obtained, at least with respect to increases in HDL, in a cohort 1837 female runners [22].

These observations are of some interest, but few patients will be convinced of the benefits of running >80 km/week. In addition, recent data did not show additional mortality benefits with increasing running distances per week [23], indicating that epidemiological associations based on evaluations at single time points do not always transfer into improved clinical outcomes.

Less evidence is available on the associations of fitness levels with Lp(a) or familial hypercholesterolemia (FAH):

- Regarding Lp(a), in an observational study on diabetic men (55 ± 8 years), higher fitness as assessed by exercise testing was associated with significantly lower levels of Lp(a), but no clinical outcomes were reported [24].
- Regarding FAH, in an observational study on 639 affected-patients free of cardiovascular disease at baseline, decreased exercise capacity assessed by exercise testing at baseline significantly predicted incident coronary events during follow-up [25].

Summary of findings from epidemiological studies:

Studies indicate beneficial effects of high physical activity or fitness levels on lipid profiles, mostly pertaining to mildly improved HDL and TG levels; less effects are observed on LDL levels. However, although mortality risk is reduced in subjects with higher baseline fitness, it cannot definitely be derived from this data whether these effects are at least partly mediated by exercise-induced lipid profile improvements.

### 37.2.2 Randomized or Observational Trials

Few randomized controlled trials (RCT) of sufficient quality have focused on lipid levels as primary outcome of PA or ET interventions; they are by far more often assessed as secondary variables, lacking adequate statistical power. Other studies have focused on the effect of specific types of exercise on lipid levels, presented further below. Three relevant RCT applying ET or PA interventions are listed here:

- Eighty-one men (30–55 years) were randomized 1:1 to a regular moderate running program (70–85% peak oxygen uptake ($VO_2$peak)) over 1 year or to a non-exercising control group [26].
  - Lipid profiles in runners improved in absolute terms, but group differences were not significant.
  - Only runners with weekly distances >13 km showed significant increases in HDL.
  - However, running longer distances per week was significantly associated with further improvements in HDL and LDL levels.
- *HERITAGE family study*: In this non-controlled observational study, 675 participants from black and white families (17–65 years) underwent 20 weeks of moderate aerobic exercise training on cycle ergometers at 75% $VO_2$peak [27].
  - A modest, but significant increase in HDL in males and females and a significant reduction of TG in males was observed; other lipid levels remained unchanged.
  - Interestingly, the lipid response to exercise correlated significantly within family members [28], indicating a contribution of genetic factors to the extent of exercise-induced effects.
- Following a PA counseling intervention in 179 type 2 diabetic subjects (62 ± 1 years), lipid profiles improved alongside weekly increases in energy expenditure; statistical significance was reached when values corresponding to 2.5 h of walking were exceeded [29].

Thus, PA or ET interventions may result in improved lipid levels, with mild increases in HDL and reductions of TG levels as the leading effect. However, long bouts of moderate aerobic exercise are required to induce these changes, and LDL levels remain largely unaffected.

### 37.2.3 Different Types of Exercise

With respect to different types of exercise, resistance training (RT) or high-intensity interval training (HIIT) may represent alternative approaches beyond moderate aerobic exercise in selected patients (Chap. 44). Studies were mostly small in size, thus particularly effects of RT can better be derived from meta-analyses (see below). Regarding exercise at higher intensities or a classic HIIT protocol, the following two studies have evaluated its particular effect on lipid levels:

- In a landmark study evaluating the effect of amount vs. intensity of exercise on a variety of lipid parameters [30], a total of 84 sedentary, overweight-to-obese, dyslipidemic men and women (51 ± 8 years) were randomized to three subgroups differing by pre-defined amounts and intensities of exercise, or to a non-exercising control group.
  - After 8 months of training, a significant increase in HDL was observed only in the group performing high amount and high intensity exercise.
  - No effects on TC and LDL were observed.
  - Summarizing the absolute group-effects on all investigated lipoprotein parameters, there was a clear association with the amount, but not with the intensity of exercise.
- In 32 patients with the Metabolic Syndrome (52 ± 4 years), moderate exercise was compared with a 4 × 4 min HIIT protocol. Improvements were only observed for HDL levels, and interestingly this was restricted to the moderate exercise group [31].

Results from these trials are inconsistent, but both interventions indicate that moderate aerobic exercise appears to play a more pivotal role in improving lipid levels than increased intensities.

### 37.2.4 Effects of Exercise on Particle Size and Structure

Due to the classic epidemiological association of high HDL and low LDL levels with reduced mortality, exercise intervention studies have traditionally focused on improving the absolute quantity of these parameters. However, changes in their "quality", namely particle size and structure, have also been linked to an increased risk for developing atherosclerotic disease. Regarding LDL subfractions, this particularly pertains to the proportion of particles of small density, whereas risk appears reduced with increasing LDL particle size (Fig. 37.3). Regarding HDL, research has in the meantime also focused on functional components rather than simply measuring absolute levels:

- In the randomized controlled study on amount and intensity of exercise presented above [30], no changes in total LDL levels, but significant reductions of small dense particles and increases in particle size were observed, indicating beneficial exercise effects on a molecular level.

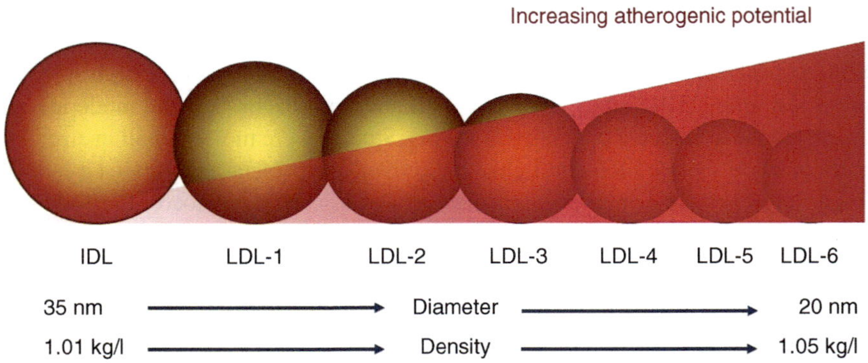


**Fig. 37.3** Size and density of LDL subfractions. With decreasing particle size and increasing density the atherogenic potential increases, with the smallest particles showing the highest risk. Studies have shown a shift towards larger (and thus more beneficial) particles induced by a higher fitness level or an active exercise training intervention (see text for more details)

- In another observational study, a significantly lower proportion of LDL small dense subfractions were observed in fit vs. in unfit hypercholesterolemic men (as assessed by exercise testing) [32].
- In the population-based *Dallas Heart Study*, HDL efflux capacity (defined as the ability of HDL to accept cholesterol from macrophages), but not baseline HDL level was inversely associated with incident cardiovascular events after adjustment for baseline risk factors [33].
- In heart failure patients, the ability of HDL to promote endothelial function by stimulating the production of nitric oxide in vascular endothelial cells [34] was shown to be impaired compared with healthy controls.
  - However, after 12 weeks of aerobic exercise training, this functional property of HDL was restored, which was, in turn, clinically linked to improved flow-mediated dilatation.

Apart from these observations, a key clinical problem remains unresolved: drug-induced massive HDL increases have not consistently resulted in a reduction of cardiovascular events as compared to placebo. Thus, at this point of time, it is equivocal whether the comparably small increases in HDL levels induced by exercise will transfer into any clinical significance at all. On the other hand, it can also not be excluded that exercise may confer a more beneficial effect on HDL structure than drugs do. More research will be required to elucidate the role of lipid subfractions or functional properties within cardiovascular risk reduction.

Summary of findings from randomized and observational studies:

Moderate aerobic exercise appears superior to high-intensity interval or resistance training regimens with respect to improvements of HDL and TC levels. When selectively intending to improve lipid levels, performing long bouts of moderate, dynamic exercise should be preferred over short, intensive bouts, including resistance training. No consistent effect is reported on LDL levels.

### 37.2.5 Systematic Reviews and Meta-Analyses

Several systematic reviews and meta-analyses have summarized the specific effects of PA or ET interventions on lipid levels, either assessed as primary or as secondary outcomes in the studies included. The results are presented in Table 37.2.

Summary of findings from systematic reviews and meta-analyses:

**Table 37.2** Summary of findings from systematic reviews and meta-analyses evaluating the effect of physical activity and exercise training interventions on lipid levels

| No. of studies included | No. of patients included | Age (years) | Type of intervention | Duration of intervention (weeks) | Main results | References |
|---|---|---|---|---|---|---|
| 25 | 1176 | 49 ± 14 | Walking | >8 | Significant reduction of LDL (−5.5 ± 2.2 mg/dl); no effect on other lipids | [46] |
| 25 | 1404 | 23–75 | Moderate aerobic exercise | >8 | Significant HDL-increase (+2.53 mg/dl) only when exceeding >120 min exercise per week; other lipids not tested | [47] |
| 13 | 613 (overweight and obese) | 31–63 | Moderate aerobic exercise | ≥8 | Significant 16% reduction of TG; no effect on other lipids | [48] |
| 10 | 1260 (coronary artery disease) | 50–67 | Moderate aerobic exercise | ≥4 | Modest but significant HDL increase (+3.7 ± 1.3 mg/dl) and TG reduction (−19.3 ± 5.4 mg/dl); no changes in TC and LDL | [49] |
| 29 | 1329 | 20–75 | Resistance training | ≥4 | Modest but significant improvements in TC (−2.7%), LDL (−4.6%) and TG (−6.4%); no effect on HDL | [50] |
| 34 | N/A | N/A | Moderate aerobic exercise, resistance training or both | >8 | No effect of resistance training alone; together with aerobic exercise significant TG reduction (−26.5 mg/dl); no effect on other lipids | [51] |

(continued)

**Table 37.2** (continued)

| No. of studies included | No. of patients included | Age (years) | Type of intervention | Duration of intervention (weeks) | Main results | References |
|---|---|---|---|---|---|---|
| 14 | 661 | N/A | High-intensity interval training | ≥2 | Significant HDL increase in only three of 14 studies; no effect on other lipids | [52] |
| 6 | 445 | 51–69 (mean ages) | Tai chi | >12 | Significant TG reduction (−16.8 mg/dl); no effect on other lipids | [53] |

*TC* total cholesterol, *HDL* high-density lipoprotein cholesterol, *LDL* low-density lipoprotein cholesterol, *TG* triglycerides, *N/A* no information on this variable provided

Similar to results from single studies, HDL and TG levels have been identified as primary targets of physical activity or exercise training interventions in both primary and secondary prevention settings. Likewise, moderate aerobic exercise has been shown to be superior to high-intensity interval or resistance training.

### 37.2.6 Exercise Alone vs. Exercise and Diet

Several studies have compared the effects of PA or ET alone with either diet alone or with a combined diet and ET intervention:

- In the epidemiologic *WHITEHALL-II-study*, the independent effects of either lipid-lowering medication, diet or PA on LDL levels were investigated in 4469 patients (39–62 years) over a follow-up period of 11.3 years [35].
  - As expected, the greatest LDL reduction was induced by initiating medical treatment.
  - Both improving diet (e.g. increased intake of unsaturated fatty acids) and increasing PA induced a less pronounced (vs. medication), but similar amount of reduction.
- In an RCT, 264 overweight subjects (25–49 years) were randomized to either hypocaloric diet or hypocaloric diet and ET groups or to a control group over a period of 12 months [36].
  - Participants in both intervention groups successfully reached dietary goals, but significant improvements in HDL and TG (in women also LDL) levels compared to controls were only observed in the diet and ET group.
- Similar observations were obtained in a subsequent RCT by the same group, randomizing 377 participants (30–64 years) to either diet or ET alone, diet and ET combined or to a control group (difference to the former study was an ET alone group) [37].

- After 12 months, a significant reduction of LDL levels was only observed in the combined group, whereas an observed increase of HDL after ET alone did not reach statistical significance.

Findings from these studies at least partly confirm the potential of ET alone to primarily induce an increase in HDL levels. Regarding LDL, significant reductions may be induced by both diet and ET alone, but they only reach statistical significance when both modalities are combined.

### 37.2.7 Multimodal Lifestyle Interventions

Apart from the aforementioned studies comparing ET with dietary interventions, other approaches offer multimodal lifestyle interventions and evaluate their effect against standard medical care. These programs consist of structured, supervised interventions of different frequencies, intensities and duration, usually including PA, dietary and psychological advice. Typically, these interventions have been applied to (pre-)diabetic patients, aiming at delaying either the incidence or the clinical progress of type 2 diabetes. Since these programs are referred to in more detail in Chap. 39, only one example focusing on changes in lipid profiles is presented here:

- In the multicenter RCT Look AHEAD, 5145 overweight or obese patients with type 2 diabetes were assigned to either participate in an intensive lifestyle intervention that promoted weight loss through decreased caloric intake and increased PA (intervention group) or to receive diabetes support and education (control group).
  - The primary endpoint, a reduction of cardiovascular mortality, was missed and the study was terminated early after 9.6 years follow-up [38].
  - However, in the first years of the study significant improvements in HDL and TG levels were observed but diminished over time alongside a decrease in the number of supervised educational sessions [39].
  - In contrast, LDL cholesterol was not different between groups.

Importantly, the mean level of fitness measured in the Look AHEAD participants was increased in the first year, but went back to baseline after that, strongly indicating that participants decreased being active [39]. This once again underlines the difficulty of a long-term adherence to a lifestyle-related behavior change, which would otherwise perhaps have resulted in maintained improvements in lipid levels and perhaps even in a reduction in mortality.

## 37.3 Statin Treatment and Exercise

Depending on the risk profiles, many patients will be candidates for both ET interventions and statin treatment. Statins and PA or ET may be a particularly good combination as their main effects on lipid levels complement each other, with

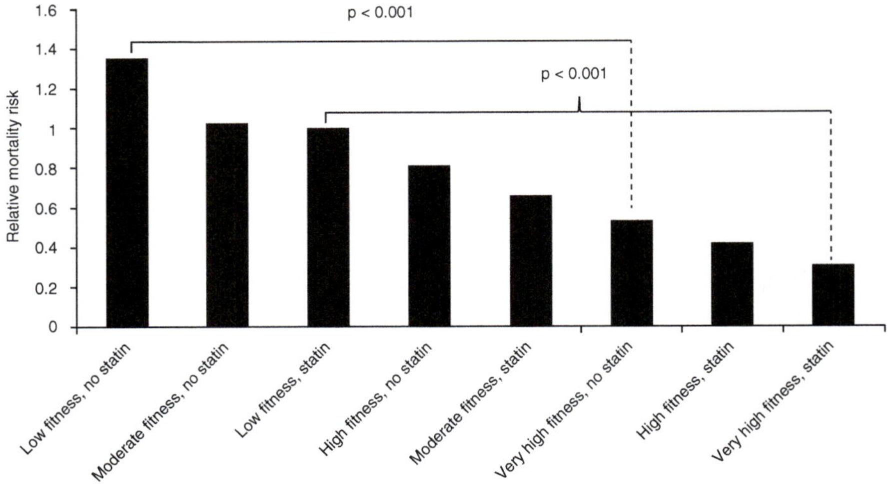


**Fig. 37.4** Distribution of relative mortality risk reduction in patients with different fitness levels as assessed by exercise testing and the presence or absence of statin treatment (Created from data presented in [40]. Printed with authorization from: Pressler A. A run a day keeps lipids at bay? Regular exercise as a treatment of dyslipidaemias. Dtsch Z Sportmed. 2017; 68: 253–260)

exercise having a more pronounced effect on those fractions (TG, HDL) that statins show lower effects on, and vice versa (LDL). Since statins may induce negative effects on muscle integrity, several studies have evaluated combined effects of medical treatment and ET:

- In 10,043 men (59 ± 11 years) with and without cardiovascular disease [40], the combined effect of fitness (assessed by exercise test) and statin therapy were evaluated.
  - A total of 2318 deaths were noted during a follow-up of 10 years, and both high fitness and statin therapy were independently associated with reduced mortality.
  - If both modalities were present, risk reduction was more than doubled, indicating an exponential beneficial effect of combining exercise and statins at least from an epidemiological perspective (Fig. 37.4).
- In a cardiac rehabilitation setting, no differences in changes in $VO_2$peak after 3 months of ET were observed between patients with (n = 968) or without (n = 233) statin treatment [41].
- In contrast, in patients with the Metabolic Syndrome, 37 participants (43 ± 11 years) were randomized to 12 weeks of aerobic ET alone or to ET and simvastatin 40 mg [42]. $VO_2$peak increased significantly in the exercise-only group, but was blunted in the combined group, indicating an unfavorable interaction between statins and exercise in this small population.

Thus, statin therapy may attenuate the effects induced by regular exercise in single cases, but the overall evidence suggests neutral or even beneficial effects of combining both treatments. It is therefore not justified to withhold statin treatment (if indicated according to current guidelines) in patients exercising regularly, or vice versa.

Statins are usually the first-line treatment in all types of dyslipidemia, having their strongest effect in reducing LDL-cholesterol levels. As the effects of statins on HDL-improvement and TG-reduction is much weaker, the combination of PA or ET and statins may be extremely useful in patients with dyslipidemia. In modern society, a lipid profile with low HDL and hypertriglyceridemia is more common than extremely high LDL-levels, making the combination of PA and statins particularly useful. In patients with extremely elevated levels of LDL, i.e. familiar hypercholesterolemia, statins may have to be combined with other (modern) lipid lowering drugs.

In athletes being treated with statins, it is important to acknowledge the association of statins and muscular side-effects:

- Muscle pain (benign) is overall not uncommon
- Myopathy, pain, weakness and major increments in muscle creatinkinase (CK) as a marker of severe muscle damage [43]

If any muscle symptoms are experienced during statin treatment in an exercising individual, the physical activity should be stopped and a clinical control, including CK, should be initiated. In case of benign muscle symptoms, an alternative statin or an alternative lipid-lowering drug can be tried. Training may be resumed when the patient is symptom-free and CK has returned to baseline (www.fyss.se).

## 37.4 Practical Recommendations

### 37.4.1 What Do Current Guidelines Advice?

According to the significance of appropriate lipid management, guidelines are updated in close intervals, with the latest recommendations of the European Society of Cardiology in association with either the European Atherosclerosis Society [8] (EAS; focusing on dyslipidemia) and the European Association of Cardiovascular Prevention and Rehabilitation [3] (focusing on prevention) having been published in 2019 and in 2016. Both guidelines almost exclusively focus on LDL as the primary treatment target, in line with the latest guidelines from the American Heart Association [44]. Although the favorable epidemiological effect of elevated HDL levels on mortality is still acknowledged, recent efforts to reduce mortality risk by actively elevating HDL levels using various agents have mostly failed, despite substantial increases induced by these drugs [45].

In these guidelines, ET is mentioned within the sections on non-pharmacological treatment options but is largely embedded into the evidence for combined effects of multi-modal lifestyle interventions. Nonetheless, single evidence grades for exercise are provided in the EAS guidelines, with the highest evidence for increasing HDL (+++A), followed by reducing triglycerides (TG; ++A); instead, lowering LDL by exercise is less well established (LDL; +B) [8].

It is generally recommended that individuals with dyslipidemia engage in a minimum of 150 min per week of moderate PA, or at least 75 min of vigorous activities, the latter being comparable to active ET. It is, however, emphasized that, in order to achieve greater benefits, a gradual increase up to 300 min per week of moderate and 150 min per week of vigorous PA should be targeted. Combinations of moderate and vigorous activities are of course possible, with a minimum duration of exercise of 10 min (shorter sessions may be preferred in deconditioned individuals). Importantly, a regular assessment of individual fitness is highly recommended. With special regards to patients with dyslipidemia, again longer bouts of exercise of up to 60–90 min per day are recommended, according to the evidence presented in this chapter. Independent of lipid levels, resistance training is recommended in moderate intensities at least on 2 days per week (see Chaps. 44 and 45 for more details on calculating suitable intensities from measured parameters and on the modalities of prescription).

## 37.5 Conclusion

Summarizing the current evidence, effects of regular exercise on lipid levels are at best modest, and many studies have yielded rather disappointing results. Long bouts of moderate aerobic exercise are preferred over resistance or high-intensity interval exercise. Small improvements in HDL and TG are most frequently observed, the clinical significance of which remains to be established. LDL is rarely affected in absolute terms, but exercise-induced reductions of atherogenic small dense subfractions indicate that future research should additionally focus on changes in lipid quality rather than quantity. Elevated LDL levels should be treated according to current guidelines, which in many cases will include early-onset statin therapy. Apart from individual side effects pertaining to symptoms of myalgia, the overall evidence supports a favorable effect of combining exercise and statin therapy. Finally, as stated in the introduction, the present article focuses on the effects of exercise on lipid levels as a single intervention. Since in many patients abnormal lipid profiles are part of a combination of various risk factors, exercise training as a key component of multi-modal lifestyle interventions remains a cornerstone of non-pharmacological therapies and should be implemented into treatment strategies wherever possible.

**Clinical Pearls**

- Patients with dyslipidemia should be motivated to increase their physical activity habits but should be informed that effects will be more pronounced with more vigorous activities.
- High fitness levels are associated with improved lipid profiles or mitigate unfavorable effects of increased lipids, independent of changes in body weight.
- Studies and meta-analyses mostly indicate beneficial effects of increased physical activity habits, exercise training or high fitness levels on lipid profiles, usually pertaining to mildly improved HDL and TG levels; less effects are observed on LDL levels.

- Long bouts of moderate continuous exercise are preferred over high-intensity interval or resistance training interventions.
- Multimodal lifestyle interventions improve lipid profiles, but long-term adherence is required to maintain these effects.
- Statin therapy may attenuate the effects induced by regular exercise in single cases, but the overall evidence suggests neutral or even beneficial effects of combining both treatments

## Review

### Questions

1. A 49-year-old female overweight patient presents in your outpatient clinic, wishing to begin a regular exercise program in order to decrease her lipid levels and reduce weight. Her LDL is 197 mg/dl (5.12 mmol/l), her HDL 67 mg/dl (1.74 mmol/l) and her triglycerides are 234 mg/dl (2.67 mmol/l). She would prefer shorter bouts of high intensity exercise or resistance training in a gym due to a lack of time. Her father suffered from coronary artery disease diagnosed at the age of 55 years; blood pressure and glucose level are normal, and she has never smoked. What would be your first step? What do you tell her about the expected effect of her preferred type of exercise? Would you prescribe a statin in addition to lifestyle advice?
2. Which of the following combinations best describes the effects of exercise on lipid levels?
   (a) Moderate continuous exercise—LDL decrease
   (b) High intensity interval exercise—LDL increase
   (c) Resistance exercise—HDL increase
   (d) Moderate continuous exercise—Triglyceride decrease
   (e) Moderate continuous exercise—HDL decrease
3. A 55-year-old male patient is planning to start regular resistance training. Due to increased LDL levels and significant carotid plaques he is prescribed atorvastatin 20 mg. After several weeks of training he presents with muscle pain in both legs several hours after exercise, lasting for several hours. His creatinkinase is elevated (800 U/l). What are your next steps?

### Answers

1. This patient clearly shows a relevantly increased risk of premature cardiovascular disease due to the high LDL level and the positive family history of coronary artery disease, both indicating a possible genetic background (familial hypercholesterolemia). This is independent of the lack of other risk factors, although it should be noted that these may mitigate the overall risk. Thus, the first step should be a risk stratification and an extensive diagnostic work-up focusing on

the presence of at least subclinical cardiovascular disease, including exercise testing and also possibly coronary calcium scoring. If a significant atherosclerotic disease is ruled out, exercise should be recommended as asked for by the patient. However, this patient should be informed that a relevant effect on LDL levels cannot be expected on average, but that HDL and Triglyceride levels may benefit; she should also be informed that these benefits will be more pronounced through performing moderate continuous exercise rather than high intensity or resistance exercise. To achieve lower LDL levels, exercise should be combined with a dietary intervention. According to the AHA/ACC guidelines, a statin should be prescribed if LDL levels exceed 190 mg/dl (5 mmol/l); this could only be debated if extensive work-up does not yield any sign of atherosclerotic disease. Close, annual follow-ups are reasonable.

2. The correct answer is (**d**). Findings from the majority of randomized studies, confirmed by meta-analyses, have shown a rather good response of triglyceride levels to moderate aerobic, continuous exercise, whereas effects on LDL levels of either type of exercise is inconsistent. Moderate continuous exercise usually also results in a mild increase, not decrease, of HDL levels.
3. This is a rather typical, but not an easy case. Both the newly initiated resistance training and the statin may be responsible for muscle pain, either alone or in combination, and this also holds true for the increased CK level. However, such high values are usually more typically induced by resistance training. A possible additional statin side effect could be an elevation of liver enzymes, but this may also be observed after resistance exercise. A reasonable approach would be to at least reduce or totally interrupt one of the interventions (preferably starting with the resistance training, since it is likely that chosen weights might have been too heavy). After 2–3 weeks, a clinical and laboratory follow-up should be performed, and depending on the change in symptoms and CK levels, exercise could be started again at lower intensities. Otherwise, the same procedure is required for the statin treatment. If with atorvastatin the symptoms and increased CK levels will recur, a change to an alternative statin would be a first option; however, achieving a risk-adapted LDL level remains an important target.

## References


1. Palmefors H, DuttaRoy S, Rundqvist B, Borjesson M. The effect of physical activity or exercise on key biomarkers in atherosclerosis – a systematic review. Atherosclerosis. 2014;235(1):150–61.
2. Yusuf S, Hawken S, Ounpuu S, Dans T, Avezum A, Lanas F, et al. Effect of potentially modifiable risk factors associated with myocardial infarction in 52 countries (the INTERHEART study): case-control study. Lancet. 2004;364(9438):937–52.
3. Piepoli MF, Hoes AW, Agewall S, Albus C, Brotons C, Catapano AL, et al. European guidelines on cardiovascular disease prevention in clinical practice: The Sixth Joint Task Force of the European Society of Cardiology and Other Societies on Cardiovascular Disease Prevention in Clinical Practice (constituted by representatives of 10 societies and by invited experts)

Developed with the special contribution of the European Association for Cardiovascular Prevention & Rehabilitation (EACPR). Eur Heart J. 2016;37(29):2315–81.
4. Estruch R, Ros E, Salas-Salvado J, Covas MI, Corella D, Aros F, et al. Primary prevention of cardiovascular disease with a Mediterranean diet. N Engl J Med. 2013;368(14):1279–90.
5. Marks D, Thorogood M, Neil HA, Humphries SE. A review on the diagnosis, natural history, and treatment of familial hypercholesterolaemia. Atherosclerosis. 2003;168(1):1–14.
6. Forde OH, Thelle DS, Arnesen E, Mjos OD. Distribution of high density lipoprotein cholesterol according to relative body weight, cigarette smoking and leisure time physical activity. The cardiovascular disease study in Finnmark 1977. Acta Med Scand. 1986;219(2):167–71.
7. Behre C, Bergstrom G, Schmidt C. Moderate physical activity is associated with lower ApoB/ApoA-I ratios independently of other risk factors in healthy, middle-aged men. Angiology. 2010;61(8):775–9.
8. Mach F, Baigent C, Catapano AL, Koskinas KC, Casula M et al. ESC/EAS guidelines for the management of dyslipidaemias: lipid modification to reduce cardiovascular risk. Eur Heart J. 2019;00:1–78. https://doi.org/10.1093/eurheartj/ehz455. [Epub ahead of print].
9. Gordon T, Castelli WP, Hjortland MC, Kannel WB, Dawber TR. High density lipoprotein as a protective factor against coronary heart disease. The Framingham Study. Am J Med. 1977;62(5):707–14.
10. Aagaard P, Sahlen A, Braunschweig F. Performance trends and cardiac biomarkers in a 30-km cross-country race, 1993–2007. Med Sci Sports Exerc. 2012;44(5):894–9.
11. Lear SA, Hu W, Rangarajan S, Gasevic D, Leong D, Iqbal R, et al. The effect of physical activity on mortality and cardiovascular disease in 130 000 people from 17 high-income, middle-income, and low-income countries: the PURE study. Lancet. 2017;390:2643–54.
12. Mora S, Lee IM, Buring JE, Ridker PM. Association of physical activity and body mass index with novel and traditional cardiovascular biomarkers in women. JAMA. 2006;295(12):1412–9.
13. Mora S, Cook N, Buring JE, Ridker PM, Lee IM. Physical activity and reduced risk of cardiovascular events: potential mediating mechanisms. Circulation. 2007;116(19):2110–8.
14. Gordon-Larsen P, Boone-Heinonen J, Sidney S, Sternfeld B, Jacobs DR Jr, Lewis CE. Active commuting and cardiovascular disease risk: the CARDIA study. Arch Intern Med. 2009;169(13):1216–23.
15. Williams PT, Thompson PD. Walking versus running for hypertension, cholesterol, and diabetes mellitus risk reduction. Arterioscler Thromb Vasc Biol. 2013;33(5):1085–91.
16. Dunstan DW, Barr EL, Healy GN, Salmon J, Shaw JE, Balkau B, et al. Television viewing time and mortality: the Australian diabetes, obesity and lifestyle study (AusDiab). Circulation. 2010;121(3):384–91.
17. Myers J, Prakash M, Froelicher V, Do D, Partington S, Atwood JE. Exercise capacity and mortality among men referred for exercise testing. N Engl J Med. 2002;346(11):793–801.
18. Gulati M, Pandey DK, Arnsdorf MF, Lauderdale DS, Thisted RA, Wicklund RH, et al. Exercise capacity and the risk of death in women: the St James women take heart project. Circulation. 2003;108(13):1554–9.
19. Park YM, Sui X, Liu J, Zhou H, Kokkinos PF, Lavie CJ, et al. The effect of cardiorespiratory fitness on age-related lipids and lipoproteins. J Am Coll Cardiol. 2015;65(19):2091–100.
20. Lee DC, Sui X, Church TS, Lavie CJ, Jackson AS, Blair SN. Changes in fitness and fatness on the development of cardiovascular disease risk factors hypertension, metabolic syndrome, and hypercholesterolemia. J Am Coll Cardiol. 2012;59(7):665–72.
21. Williams PT. Relationship of distance run per week to coronary heart disease risk factors in 8283 male runners. The National Runners' health study. Arch Intern Med. 1997;157(2):191–8.
22. Williams PT. High-density lipoprotein cholesterol and other risk factors for coronary heart disease in female runners. N Engl J Med. 1996;334(20):1298–303.
23. Lee DC, Pate RR, Lavie CJ, Sui X, Church TS, Blair SN. Leisure-time running reduces all-cause and cardiovascular mortality risk. J Am Coll Cardiol. 2014;64(5):472–81.

24. Jae SY, Heffernan KS, Lee MK, Fernhall B, Park WH. Relation of cardiorespiratory fitness to inflammatory markers, fibrinolytic factors, and lipoprotein(a) in patients with type 2 diabetes mellitus. Am J Cardiol. 2008;102(6):700–3.
25. Pitsavos CH, Chrysohoou C, Panagiotakos DB, Kokkinos P, Skoumas J, Papaioannou I, et al. Exercise capacity and heart rate recovery as predictors of coronary heart disease events, in patients with heterozygous familial hypercholesterolemia. Atherosclerosis. 2004;173(2):347–52.
26. Wood PD, Haskell WL, Blair SN, Williams PT, Krauss RM, Lindgren FT, et al. Increased exercise level and plasma lipoprotein concentrations: a one-year, randomized, controlled study in sedentary, middle-aged men. Metabolism. 1983;32(1):31–9.
27. Leon AS, Rice T, Mandel S, Despres JP, Bergeron J, Gagnon J, et al. Blood lipid response to 20 weeks of supervised exercise in a large biracial population: the HERITAGE family study. Metabolism. 2000;49(4):513–20.
28. Rice T, Despres JP, Perusse L, Hong Y, Province MA, Bergeron J, et al. Familial aggregation of blood lipid response to exercise training in the health, risk factors, exercise training, and genetics (HERITAGE) family study. Circulation. 2002;105(16):1904–8.
29. Di Loreto C, Fanelli C, Lucidi P, Murdolo G, De Cicco A, Parlanti N, et al. Make your diabetic patients walk: long-term impact of different amounts of physical activity on type 2 diabetes. Diabetes Care. 2005;28(6):1295–302.
30. Kraus WE, Houmard JA, Duscha BD, Knetzger KJ, Wharton MB, McCartney JS, et al. Effects of the amount and intensity of exercise on plasma lipoproteins. N Engl J Med. 2002;347(19):1483–92.
31. Tjonna AE, Lee SJ, Rognmo O, Stolen TO, Bye A, Haram PM, et al. Aerobic interval training versus continuous moderate exercise as a treatment for the metabolic syndrome: a pilot study. Circulation. 2008;118(4):346–54.
32. Halle M, Berg A, König D, Keul J, Baumstark MW. Differences in the concentration and composition of low-density lipoprotein subfraction particles between sedentary and trained hypercholesterolemic men. Metabolism. 1997;46(2):186–91.
33. Rohatgi A, Khera A, Berry JD, Givens EG, Ayers CR, Wedin KE, et al. HDL cholesterol efflux capacity and incident cardiovascular events. N Engl J Med. 2014;371(25):2383–93.
34. Adams V, Besler C, Fischer T, Riwanto M, Noack F, Höllriegel R, et al. Exercise training in patients with chronic heart failure promotes restoration of high-density lipoprotein functional properties. Circ Res. 2013;113(12):1345–55.
35. Bouillon K, Singh-Manoux A, Jokela M, Shipley MJ, Batty GD, Brunner EJ, et al. Decline in low-density lipoprotein cholesterol concentration: lipid-lowering drugs, diet, or physical activity? Evidence from the Whitehall II study. Heart. 2011;97(11):923–30.
36. Wood PD, Stefanick ML, Williams PT, Haskell WL. The effects on plasma lipoproteins of a prudent weight-reducing diet, with or without exercise, in overweight men and women. N Engl J Med. 1991;325(7):461–6.
37. Stefanick ML, Mackey S, Sheehan M, Ellsworth N, Haskell WL, Wood PD. Effects of diet and exercise in men and postmenopausal women with low levels of HDL cholesterol and high levels of LDL cholesterol. N Engl J Med. 1998;339(1):12–20.
38. Look ARG, Wing RR, Bolin P, Brancati FL, Bray GA, Clark JM, et al. Cardiovascular effects of intensive lifestyle intervention in type 2 diabetes. N Engl J Med. 2013;369(2):145–54.
39. Look ARG, Wing RR. Long-term effects of a lifestyle intervention on weight and cardiovascular risk factors in individuals with type 2 diabetes mellitus: four-year results of the Look AHEAD trial. Arch Intern Med. 2010;170(17):1566–75.
40. Kokkinos PF, Faselis C, Myers J, Panagiotakos D, Doumas M. Interactive effects of fitness and statin treatment on mortality risk in veterans with dyslipidaemia: a cohort study. Lancet. 2013;381(9864):394–9.
41. Rengo JL, Savage PD, Toth MJ, Ades PA. Statin therapy does not attenuate exercise training response in cardiac rehabilitation. J Am Coll Cardiol. 2014;63(19):2050–1.
42. Mikus CR, Boyle LJ, Borengasser SJ, Oberlin DJ, Naples SP, Fletcher J, et al. Simvastatin impairs exercise training adaptations. J Am Coll Cardiol. 2013;62(8):709–14.

43. Laufs U, Scharnagl H, Halle M, Windler E, Endres M, Marz W. Treatment options for statin-associated muscle symptoms. Dtsch Arztebl Int. 2015;112(44):748–55.
44. Stone NJ, Robinson JG, Lichtenstein AH, Bairey Merz CN, Blum CB, Eckel RH, et al. 2013 ACC/AHA guideline on the treatment of blood cholesterol to reduce atherosclerotic cardiovascular risk in adults: a report of the American College of Cardiology/American Heart Association Task Force on Practice Guidelines. J Am Coll Cardiol. 2014;63(25 Pt B):2889–934.
45. Keene D, Price C, Shun-Shin MJ, Francis DP. Effect on cardiovascular risk of high density lipoprotein targeted drug treatments niacin, fibrates, and CETP inhibitors: meta-analysis of randomised controlled trials including 117,411 patients. BMJ. 2014;349:g4379.
46. Kelley GA, Kelley KS, Tran ZV. Walking, lipids, and lipoproteins: a meta-analysis of randomized controlled trials. Prev Med. 2004;38(5):651–61.
47. Kodama S, Tanaka S, Saito K, Shu M, Sone Y, Onitake F, et al. Effect of aerobic exercise training on serum levels of high-density lipoprotein cholesterol: a meta-analysis. Arch Intern Med. 2007;167(10):999–1008.
48. Kelley GA, Kelley KS, Vu Tran Z. Aerobic exercise, lipids and lipoproteins in overweight and obese adults: a meta-analysis of randomized controlled trials. Int J Obes. 2005;29(8):881–93.
49. Kelley GA, Kelley KS, Franklin B. Aerobic exercise and lipids and lipoproteins in patients with cardiovascular disease: a meta-analysis of randomized controlled trials. J Cardpulm Rehabil. 2006;26(3):131–9.
50. Kelley GA, Kelley KS. Impact of progressive resistance training on lipids and lipoproteins in adults: a meta-analysis of randomized controlled trials. Prev Med. 2009;48(1):9–19.
51. Chudyk A, Petrella RJ. Effects of exercise on cardiovascular risk factors in type 2 diabetes: a meta-analysis. Diabetes Care. 2011;34(5):1228–37.
52. Kessler HS, Sisson SB, Short KR. The potential for high-intensity interval training to reduce cardiometabolic disease risk. Sports Med. 2012;42(6):489–509.
53. Pan XH, Mahemuti A, Zhang XH, Wang YP, Hu P, Jiang JB, et al. Effect of tai chi exercise on blood lipid profiles: a meta-analysis of randomized controlled trials. J Zhejiang Univ Sci B. 2016;17(8):640–8.

# Impact of Exercise on Cardiovascular Risk Factors: Diabetes Mellitus

# 38

Sheri R. Colberg and David Niederseer

**Learning Objectives** Physical activity and exercise programs may be able to prevent type 2 diabetes, reverse prediabetes, and prevent or delay the onset of cardiovascular disease and other health complications associated with diabetes of any type. Readers should be able to:

1. Be aware of the detrimental effects of a sedentary lifestyle and physical inactivity both for the development and progression of type 2 diabetes.
2. Understand why increased physical activity is a key lifestyle component for gaining health benefits and preventing or delaying complications associated with diabetes.
3. List the types of exercise training that adults with diabetes should engage in regularly for prevention and management of diabetes and its complications.
4. Prescribe exercise programs for all individuals with diabetes that are both safe for them to do and effective for improving fitness and health.
5. Advise athletes with diabetes on how to manage diabetes in every day training and competition.

S. R. Colberg (✉)
Old Dominion University, Norfolk, VA, USA
e-mail: scolberg@odu.edu

D. Niederseer
Department of Cardiology, University Heart Center Zurich, University of Zurich, Zurich, Switzerland
e-mail: david.niederseer@usz.ch



A. Pressler, J. Niebauer (eds.), *Textbook of Sports and Exercise Cardiology*,
https://doi.org/10.1007/978-3-030-35374-2_38

## 38.1 Introduction

Comprehensive treatment of diabetes of any type frequently involves antihyperglycemic, antihypertensive, and lipid-lowering medications, especially in patients at risk for or with cardiovascular problems. Weight loss, dietary changes, and regular physical activity have been shown to reduce insulin resistance in individuals with type 2 diabetes and in those with type 1 who are also insulin resistant. The most important challenge faced by patients with diabetes is how to comply with and adhere to frequently complex treatment regimens, many of which include management of cardiovascular disease (CVD) risks along with blood glucose.

## 38.2 Overall Health and Fitness Benefits from Physical Activity in Patients with Diabetes

It has been shown in multiple studies that many health benefits can be gained by anyone with diabetes who engages in regular physical activity, including improved cardiorespiratory fitness, muscular strength, and muscular endurance. For example, the benefits of exercise for a patient with type 2 diabetes are even more substantial than for those without diabetes [1, 2]. Regular exercise participation results in the following for these individuals:

1. Enhanced cardiorespiratory fitness and greater muscular strength and endurance.
2. Improved blood glucose management (measured with A1C).
3. Greater insulin sensitivity, resulting in lower plasma insulin levels.
4. Reduced risk for CVD and its complications.
5. Lesser need for diabetes medications or lower doses required to manage glycemia.
6. Loss of body fat and easier maintenance of body weight.
7. Enhanced retention of muscle mass and lower risk of sarcopenia.
8. Improved overall health and quality of life, especially with comorbid health issues.
9. Prevention of or delay in the onset of type 2 diabetes in patients with prediabetes.

Many of the potential benefits of physical activity with respect to diabetes management result from enhancements in insulin sensitivity, which can be accomplished through both cardiorespiratory (aerobic) and resistance training. Enhanced cardiorespiratory fitness is also key for improving health outcomes and lowering the risk for premature mortality.

- In the Look AHEAD (Advances in Health in Diabetes) trial, change in cardiorespiratory fitness after 4 years of intensive lifestyle intervention was associated with improvements in glycemic control [3].

- Others have found that for each metabolic equivalent of task (MET) increase in aerobic capacity, mortality is decreased by 19% and 14% for Caucasian and African American men with type 2 diabetes, respectively [4].
- The Look AHEAD trial reported many other health benefits of such an intensive lifestyle intervention, such as improved glucose and lipid levels, less sleep apnea, lower liver fat, less depression, improved insulin sensitivity, less kidney disease, reduced need of diabetes medications, maintenance of physical mobility, improved quality of life, and lower costs [5].
- Regular physical activity participation heightens the action of insulin, which typically remains elevated for hours to days after each aerobic exercise training session [6].

While most of these benefits of exercise are also experienced by patients with type 1 diabetes, management of blood glucose during and after exercise can be more problematic due to the need to balance insulin levels with food intake [7]. Adjustment of insulin dosing and/or nutrition therapy is usually necessary to allow safe and effective participation and is an important management strategy in anyone who uses insulin [8, 9].

Particularly for patients who use insulin, it is the role of the clinician to:

- Encourage self-monitoring of blood glucose levels around physical activity;
- Make patients aware that hypoglycemia can occur during, immediately after, or many hours following cessation of activity;
- Teach patients that hyperglycemia can also result from activity under certain circumstances; knowledge of expected activity-related metabolic responses, as well as awareness of signs and symptoms and self-management, can minimize the risk;
- Help active individuals make appropriate insulin dose adjustments for various levels of exertion rather than solely focusing on nutritional changes to compensate.

Exercise increases glucose disposal and insulin sensitivity but can make maintaining glycemic balance a challenge when insulin is an additional variable.

## 38.3 Cardiovascular Health Benefits from Physical Activity in Patients with Diabetes

Most individuals with type 2 diabetes or prediabetes (and many with type 1 diabetes) are overweight and have an increased risk of developing CVD. Diabetes itself is considered a major CVD risk factor, along with other modifiable factors like insulin resistance, overweight/obesity, hypertension, dyslipidemia, physical inactivity, poor nutrition, psychosocial stress, and cigarette smoking.

Clinical trials have addressed potential beneficial outcomes associated with intentional weight loss on CVD and other metabolic considerations. For instance:

- The Look AHEAD clinical trial reported effects of intentional weight loss on cardiovascular morbidity and mortality in 5145 overweight or obese adults with type 2 diabetes followed for over 8 years. That trial found that an intensive lifestyle intervention aimed at achieving weight loss through dietary management and physical activity lowered body weight and enhanced cardiorespiratory fitness without having a differential effect on cardiovascular outcomes [5, 10].
- Individuals in that trial with the greatest weight loss and the most effective maintainers of such losses included regular participants in more total physical activity (usually moderate in intensity) and those who more tightly monitored their calorie intake over time [10].
- Others have suggested that a sustained weight loss of >5% appears necessary for beneficial effects on blood glucose (A1C), lipids, and blood pressure. Achieving this level of weight loss requires intense interventions, including energy restriction, regular physical activity, and frequent contact with health professionals [11].

Others have suggested that physical activity is more critical than weight loss in lowering cardiovascular mortality among those with diagnosed coronary artery disease (CAD), controlled for diabetes status.

- A recent, 30-year longitudinal study observed no mortality risk reductions associated with weight loss in individuals with diagnosed CAD, although mortality risk was lower with weight gain in individuals who were normal weight at baseline [12].
- The main variable that was associated with improved survival with known CAD was sustained participation in physical activity, low or high levels, during follow-up.

For adults with diabetes, one of the most critical benefits of physical activity is maximizing its cardiovascular benefits. Such benefits likely follow from better management of blood glucose levels via improved insulin sensitivity and reductions in inflammation [13–15].

- Low-level, systemic inflammation underlies many metabolic conditions, including obesity, insulin resistance, type 2 diabetes, hypertension, and vascular diseases.
- In individuals without diabetes, physical activity enhances sensitivity to insulin in a dose-dependent manner [16] and lowers inflammatory markers.
- Cardiac autonomic imbalance and inflammation occur early in diabetes and are interrelated; cardiac autonomic imbalance correlates with the adipose tissue-derived inflammation seen early in type 2 diabetes [17].
- Lower insulin sensitivity is associated with a more atherogenic lipid profile in both youths and adults with type 1 diabetes [18].
- Cellular uptake of glucose that lowers blood glucose typically results from physical activity undertaken by those with type 2 diabetes or prediabetes.

- For persons with type 1 diabetes, greater insulin sensitivity has little impact on the ability of pancreatic beta cells to make insulin, but regular training often lowers requirements for exogenous insulin [19].
- Healthy weight loss and maintenance of a lower body weight may be more pressing issues for individuals with type 2 diabetes and prediabetes, but excess body weight can occur in those with type 1 diabetes as well.
- Participation in regular physical activity can better manage blood glucose, body weight, and inflammatory markers in patients with diabetes or prediabetes.
- Physical activity participation is associated with a lower risk of premature all-cause and cardiovascular mortality in patients with type 1 diabetes, especially when it is more frequently undertaken and more vigorous in nature [20, 21].
- In patients with type 2 diabetes, engaging in lower intensity exercise improves endothelial function, suggesting that lower intensity exercise is not necessarily less cardioprotective than higher intensity training [22].

## 38.4 Risks Associated with Exercise in Patients with Diabetes

Most patients with diabetes can exercise safely and effectively. However, being active is not without risks in some cases [1]. Both patients and practitioners should be made aware of these risks so that exercise participation Is less likely to cause them to occur.

1. *Cardiovascular risks* of physical activity participation may include:
   - Cardiac dysfunction and dysrhythmias caused by subclinical or diagnosed ischemic heart disease (silent ischemia).
   - Myocardial infarction or stroke during activities.
   - Excessive increases or decreases in blood pressure or heart rate secondary to the presence of autonomic neuropathy.
   - Post-exercise and orthostatic hypotension due to autonomic neuropathy or medication use.
2. *Metabolic risks* are also present during activities:
   - Hypoglycemia resulting during or after exercise in patients taking insulin or select oral hypoglycemic agents (i.e., insulin secretagogues).
   - Exacerbation of hyperglycemia (in cases of insulin deficiency).
   - Dehydration and potential electrolyte imbalances, particularly when blood glucose levels have been elevated prior to activity.
3. *Musculoskeletal and traumatic risks* are generally the same for all individuals who are active, but may include others for those with diabetes:
   - Injuries, both acute (like ankle sprain) and overuse (such as tendinitis).
   - Foot ulcers (especially in the presence of peripheral neuropathy), which can develop from traumatized areas, blisters, calluses, and more.
   - Orthopedic injuries like Charcot foot or stress fractures related to peripheral neuropathy, the presence of which can affect stance, gait, and balance ability.

4. *Microvascular risks* are related to the presence of certain diabetes complications:
    - *Peripheral neuropathy*: Comprehensive foot care and daily monitoring are required to treat problems early to prevent greater foot damage, ulceration, and amputation.
    - *Retinopathy* (eye disease): Exercise that involves straining, jumping, jarring, head-down, or Valsalva-like maneuvers and vigorous activities are contraindicated in patients with unstable proliferative diabetic retinopathy due to the risk of retinal hemorrhages or detachment.
    - *Diabetic kidney disease*: Low- to moderate-intensity activities are safe (even during dialysis treatments), but high-intensity exercise may not be sustainable due to low fitness levels; also monitor for electrolyte imbalances.

## 38.5 Pre-Exercise Assessment and Exercise Testing of Patients with Diabetes

To maximize the benefits and minimize the risks associated with physical activity participation, appropriate screening of high-risk patients is essential. Furthermore, clinicians should emphasize adherence to programs and offer guidance to patients to enable them to improve glucose monitoring and lessen cardiovascular risks associated with being active.

Minimally, a patient's age and prior physical activity level should be considered when deciding on whether a pre-exercise evaluation is necessary and the extent of testing.

The presence of diabetes-related health complications or other comorbid conditions usually necessitates a more thorough patient evaluation prior to most exercise participation [1, 2, 23]. Patients should be assessed for conditions that might contraindicate certain types of activity or predispose them to injury, including:

- Uncontrolled hypertension
- Unstable diabetic proliferative retinopathy
- Autonomic neuropathy, especially cardiac autonomic neuropathy
- Severe peripheral neuropathy
- Presence of Charcot foot
- History of foot ulcers or amputation

Pre-exercise evaluation may include other important assessments, such as:

- Current and previous physical activity participation
- Review of current medications
- Physical, joint, or orthopedic limitations
- Signs and symptoms suggestive of other health complications
- Psychosocial situation

High-risk patients should be encouraged to start with short periods of low-intensity exercise and slowly increase intensity and duration. Start low and progress slowly.

In addition, clinicians should determine each individual patient's knowledge and understanding of diabetes and its management with activity, including medication interactions, dietary considerations, and exercise programming. This discussion should specifically include:

- Potential effects of insulin and other hypoglycemic agents on exercise responses
- Other medications taken, including side effects and potential drug interactions
- Importance of frequent self-monitoring of blood glucose levels with activity
- Impact of diet on exercise responses and treatment of hypoglycemia
- Progression of exercise programming based on current activity level and desired health and fitness outcomes

Is medical clearance or more extensive testing necessary for all patients with diabetes prior to participation in physical activity and exercise training? Not in all cases [1]. It depends on the training state of the individual and his or her planned physical activities, along with the presence or absence of known CAD or other cardiovascular risk factors and health complications. In general:

- Lower risk patients can usually begin engaging in low- to moderate-intensity physical activities like walking without obtaining medical clearance or undergoing additional testing, although regular medical checkups are advisable.
- For sedentary patients choosing to participate in these moderate activities, providers should use their clinical judgment in deciding whether to recommend further testing. If in doubt, a full clinical workup should be performed.
- Due to an increased incidence of asymptomatic CAD in patients with diabetes, however, obtaining medical clearance is advisable for previously sedentary individuals planning to undertake a vigorous exercise program (i.e., more intense than activities of daily living, including brisk walking).
- Higher risk individuals planning to undertake harder activities will likely benefit from being assessed more fully before starting. Providers should perform a careful history, assess cardiovascular risk factors, and be aware of the commonly atypical presentation of CAD in patients with diabetes.
- Graded exercise testing is not routinely recommended as its clinical utility for diagnosing CAD in asymptomatic patients remains controversial [1]. Providers should use their clinical judgment in deciding whether to recommend such testing.

Sedentary older individuals (≥40 years) with diabetes and anyone ≥30 years of age with a high cardiovascular risk should likely undergo medical screening and obtain medical clearance prior to performing vigorous-intensity exercise.

In some cases, conducting more extensive graded exercise testing can reveal cardiovascular abnormalities and increase the safety and effectiveness of prescribed exercise programs. The following guidelines [2] were established to help clinicians decide which patients may be candidates for more extensive, graded exercise stress testing and electrocardiogram (ECG) evaluation prior to starting physical activity training.

## 38.6 General Indications for Exercise Stress Testing in Patients with Diabetes [2]

1. Age > 40 years
2. Age > 30 years and any of the following:
   - Type 1 or 2 diabetes >10 years in duration
   - Hypertension
   - Cigarette smoking
   - Dyslipidemia
   - Proliferative or preproliferative retinopathy
   - Nephropathy including microalbuminuria
3. Any of the following, regardless of age:
   - Known or suspected coronary artery disease, cerebrovascular disease, or peripheral artery disease
   - Autonomic neuropathy
   - Advanced nephropathy with renal failure

If performed, graded exercise stress testing should evaluate the presence of ischemia, dysrhythmia, and abnormal blood pressure responses to exercise and recovery. Test results may provide more accurate information for the prescription of initial levels of exercise, along with corresponding training heart rates for specific activities, as well as identify any patient-specific precautions regarding exercise and physical activity.

Should clinicians order more intensive testing after an abnormal exercise stress test result?

- If a patient exhibits positive or nonspecific ECG changes during exercise or nonspecific ST and T wave changes at rest, follow-up diagnostic testing may be warranted.
- However, the DIAD (Detection of Ischemia in Asymptomatic Diabetes) trial involving 1123 individuals with type 2 diabetes and no symptoms of coronary artery disease found that screening with adenosine-stress radionuclide myocardial perfusion imaging for myocardial ischemia did not alter rates of cardiac events [24].
- The cost-effectiveness and diagnostic value of more intensive testing in all cases has not been investigated to date.

## 38.7 Benefits of Various Training Modalities for Patients with Diabetes

Individuals with diabetes will likely benefit from regularly engaging in more than one type of physical activity training. Some are more focused on improving cardiorespiratory fitness while others enhance muscular strength and endurance, flexibility, and/or balance ability.

1. *Aerobic and high-intensity interval training*:
   - Moderate intensity exercise totaling 150 min or more per week is associated with reduced morbidity and mortality in observational studies in all populations, including individuals with diabetes [25, 26].
   - Differences among training modalities have generally been trivial, with any type of regular exercise (or combinations of training) undertaken by adults with type 2 diabetes resulting in improved glucose tolerance, increased insulin sensitivity, and decreased A1C [27, 28].
   - For aerobic training, the total training volume (comprised of frequency, intensity, and duration) may have the greatest impact on glycemic control in adults with type 2 diabetes, with a greater volume producing a superior glucose lowering effect [29].
   - High-intensity interval training may benefit cardiorespiratory fitness in adults with diabetes but may cause a temporary elevation in blood glucose [30, 31].
   - Most adults with type 1 diabetes can safely engage in high-intensity interval training without significant deterioration in blood glucose management [32, 33].
2. *Resistance training:*
   - Resistance exercise does not differ from aerobic exercise in its safety or impact on CVD risk markers in adults with type 2 diabetes; thus, selecting one modality over the other may be less important than regularly engaging in either activity [34].
   - Weekly resistance training volume likely has an effect on glycemic management, however [29], with more training providing greater benefits.
   - Higher intensity, supervised resistance training results in lower A1C levels than unsupervised or similar, home-based training, at least in older adults with type 2 diabetes [35, 36].
   - Endurance strength training (lower resistance, higher repetitions) and hypertrophy strength training (higher resistance, fewer repetitions) may result in comparable effects on glycemic control, muscle mass, and strength in adults with diabetes [37].
   - Eccentric exercise might be as effective as concentric exercise, as a study showed equal to better results from walking downhill (eccentric) as compared to uphill [38].
   - Adults with type 1 diabetes may experience a lesser decline, or even an increase, in blood glucose levels during acute bouts of resistance exercise [33].

3. *Combined aerobic and resistance training:*
   - A combination of aerobic and resistance training lowers overall blood glucose levels more than either modality alone [19, 39, 40], but combined training studies have typically not controlled for calorie expenditure.
   - Whether glycemic benefits are the result of greater overall caloric usage [40] or are specific to the combination of aerobic and resistance training [19, 39] has not yet been fully resolved.
   - The exact regimen of resistance training undertaken appears less important than engaging in both types of training to gain improvements in glycemic control, cardiovascular risk factors, and body composition after 6 months of combined training in adults with type 2 diabetes [41].
4. *Balance and flexibility training*:
   - Reducing falls and falls risk is critical for aging populations, and falls are an even greater risk when diabetes is present [42].
   - All modes of balance training have been shown to be beneficial for lowering falls risk and may lessen mortality and morbidity associated with frequent or injurious falls in older individuals with diabetes [43, 44].
   - Similarly, flexibility training may also lower the risk of falling by improving range of motion around joints [45].
   - Flexibility training is recommended in addition to, not instead of, other recommended physical activities.
5. *Sedentary time and frequent activity breaks:*
   - Prolonged sedentary time is independently associated with deleterious health outcomes, such as onset of type 2 diabetes and all-cause mortality; however, such outcomes generally decrease with higher levels of physical activity [46].
   - Glycemic management postprandially and over a 24-h period is improved in adults with type 2 diabetes who take frequent activity breaks [47, 48].
   - All individuals with diabetes or prediabetes should be encouraged to be regularly physically active, including more daily physical movement and structured exercise, to improve their glycemic management, health, longevity, and quality of life.

## 38.8 Recommended Exercise Prescription for Patients with Diabetes

Exercise prescription for patients with diabetes or prediabetes must be individualized according to the following:

- Medication schedule
- Presence and severity of comorbid health complications
- Individual health and fitness goals
- Expected benefits and outcomes of the exercise program

The primary goals for patients participating in a training program may include the following:

**Table 38.1** Recommended physical activities for adults with diabetes

| | Aerobic | Resistance | Flexibility | Balance |
|---|---|---|---|---|
| Frequency | 3–7 day × week$^{-1}$ | A minimum of 2 nonconsecutive days × week$^{-1}$, but preferably 3 | ≥2–3 day × week$^{-1}$ | ≥2–3 day × week$^{-1}$ |
| Intensity | Moderate (40%–59% HRR, or 11–12 RPE, rating of perceived exertion, rating) to vigorous (60%–89% HRR or 14–17 RPE) | Moderate (50–69% of 1-repetition maximum, or 1-RM) to vigorous (70–85% of 1-RM) | Stretch to the point of tightness or slight discomfort | No prescribed intensity |
| Duration | At least 150–300 min × week$^{-1}$ of moderate intensity, or 75–150 min × week$^{-1}$ of vigorous intensity, or combination thereof; high-intensity interval training is a viable training mode as well as continuous training | At least 8–10 exercises with completion of 1–3 sets of 8–15 repetitions to near fatigue per set on every exercise | Hold static stretches for 10–30 s or move dynamically for that period; 2–4 repetitions of each exercise | No prescribed duration |
| Type | Prolonged, rhythmic activities using large muscle groups (*e.g.*, walking, cycling, swimming) or interval training | Resistance machines, resistance bands, free weights, use of body weight as resistance | Static and/or dynamic stretching | Single-leg stand, lower and core body exercises, balance training equipment, agility and neuromotor control exercises |

*HRR* Heart rate reserve, *1-RM* one-repetition maximum, *RPE* rating of perceived exertion

1. Improve management of blood glucose levels
2. Weight loss or weight maintenance
3. Delay or prevent onset of health complications of diabetes
4. Reduce cardiovascular risk
5. Enhance aerobic capacity, strength and endurance, flexibility, and/or balance
6. Heighten energy levels and well-being
7. Improve quality of life with fewer physical or mental limitations
8. Enhance mood, reduce anxiety, and manage depression

The components of an exercise prescription for patients with diabetes are essentially the same as those prescribed for all individuals, with minor exceptions.

Similar to guidelines for most healthy adults [49], it is recommended that adults with diabetes engage in the following types of physical activity [1, 2, 9, 50, 51], as summarized in Table 38.1 in more detail:

1. *Aerobic/cardiorespiratory training*:
   - Engage in moderate aerobic activities like walking for at least 150–300 min total weekly, 75–150 min of vigorous physical activity, or a combination thereof
   - Both high-intensity interval and continuous aerobic training are recommended forms of vigorous intensity exercise for individuals with diabetes [52].
   - It is recommended that individuals with diabetes allow no more than two consecutive days to lapse without activity (to keep insulin sensitivity heightened).
2. *Resistance training*:
   - At least 2, but preferably 3, nonconsecutive days per week
3. *Flexibility training*:
   - At least 2–3 days per week
4. *Balance/neuromotor training*:
   - At least 2–3 or more days per week (especially for all patients over 40 or with neuropathy of any type)
5. *Daily movement*:
   - Include more movement throughout each day; also break up prolonged sedentary time (every 20–30 min, if possible) by engaging in a few min of any activity

## 38.9 Exercise Training Considerations

In certain populations, physical activity training may be impacted by other health considerations related to the presence of diabetes. Patients should be advised of any training considerations relevant to their physical conditions, which include the following:

- Many individuals with diabetes or prediabetes are at high risk for or may already have CVD, whether diagnosed or undiagnosed.
- Due to low initial fitness levels, most individuals with type 2 diabetes may require at least 150 min × week.$^{-1}$ of moderate to vigorous aerobic exercise to achieve optimal CVD risk reduction [2].
- Vigorous aerobic exercise will increase cardiorespiratory fitness more effectively than lower intensity training, although the former may be complicated or even contraindicated by the presence of health-related complications.
- Higher intensity resistance training may be beneficial for optimization of skeletal muscle strength, insulin action and overall blood glucose management [36], although moderate resistance exercise may be equally effective in sedentary adults [53].
- Appropriate progression of resistance exercise is important to prevent injury as individuals with diabetes often have a more limited joint mobility due to the process of glycation of collagen [54].

- Beginning resistance training intensity should be moderate, involving 10–15 repetitions per set, with increases in weight or resistance undertaken with a lower number of repetitions [8–10] only after the target number of repetitions per set can consistently be exceeded. This increase in resistance can be followed by a greater number of sets and lastly by increased training frequency [49].
- During combined training, completing resistance training prior to aerobic training may lower the risk of hypoglycemia in individuals with type 1 diabetes [55, 56].
- Interspersing very short, high intensity intervals during moderate intensity aerobic exercise may be useful to lessen the decline in blood glucose during the early post-exercise recovery period in insulin users [57].
- Regardless of initial blood glucose levels, vigorous activity of any type may cause elevations in glucose due to an exaggerated release of counterregulatory hormones like epinephrine and glucagon [58]. In such cases, insulin users may need small doses of supplemental, short-acting insulin to lower post-exercise hyperglycemia.
- While flexibility training may be recommended for all individuals, it should not substitute for other activities (i.e., aerobic and resistance training), as flexibility training does not manage glucose control, body composition or insulin action.
- Complications may affect the appropriateness of some types of activities (e.g., those with unhealed foot ulcers should avoid weight-bearing and aquatic activities).
- Continuous glucose monitors can be very useful in detecting patterns in blood glucose across multiple days and evaluating immediate and delayed effects.

## 38.10 Exercise Training Precautions

Here are some general exercise safeguards for patients with diabetes to follow [1, 9]:

- Know the signs, symptoms, and management of hypoglycemia and hyperglycemia.
- Avoid vigorous exercise if blood glucose is already elevated.
- Hydrate adequately before, during, and after exercise.
- Use caution when exercising in the heat as temperature regulation may be impaired.
- Carry a personal identification specifying diabetes along with emergency contacts.
- Carry a mobile phone or have another means of reaching out in case of emergency.
- Instruct patients to prevent or treat early any trauma, even minor skin lacerations that may develop into serious health issues.
- Instruct patients to use appropriate socks, shoes, and sporting clothing to prevent trauma or injury.

Take appropriate precautions to avoid hypoglycemia or hyperglycemia during physical activity participation, especially when using insulin or oral insulin secretagogues:

- Check blood glucose frequently as responses may vary with each individual and activity session.
- When exercising in a supervised setting, check blood glucose prior to and after each exercise session, at least for the first few sessions, and document measurements.
- Continue having patients monitor more frequently whenever symptomatic or have experienced recent high or low blood glucose levels prior to exercise sessions.
- Always have a carbohydrate source available for rapid treatment of hypoglycemia, preferably glucose for fastest treatment.
- Insulin users should avoid exercising during peak insulin times by scheduling it 2 or more hours after meals for which insulin is taken.
- If exercising during insulin peaks, consider consuming a carbohydrate snack before or during exercise and/or decrease insulin or oral hypoglycemic dose of select medications before exercise.
- Longer-acting basal insulins (e.g., glargine, detemir, and NPH) are less likely to cause exercise-induced hypoglycemia [59].
- Overall doses of meal-time and basal insulins may need to be reduced to accommodate regular exercise training.
- With insulin pumps, insulin delivery during exercise can be markedly reduced by decreasing the basal rate or disconnecting the pump for short durations, depending on the intensity and duration of exercise.
- Reducing basal insulin delivery rates for up to 12 h post-exercise may be necessary to avoid later-onset hypoglycemia.
- Exercise undertaken later in the day may increase risk of nocturnal hypoglycemia, especially in insulin users.
- Hypoglycemia risk is higher during and immediately following exercise but can occur up to 12 h or more post-exercise, making food and/or medication adjustments necessary, mostly in insulin users [60].
- Other medications may mask or exacerbate exercise-related hypoglycemia, including beta-blockers, diuretics, calcium channel blockers, and warfarin.
- Exercise should be postponed when both hyperglycemia and ketones are evident. It is recommended that insulin users check for urine ketones when blood glucose levels are $\geq$250 mg • $dl^{-1}$ (13.9 mmol • $l^{-1}$) before starting to exercise [9].
- Autonomic neuropathy, long-standing type 1 diabetes, and recent antecedent hypoglycemia or exercise can contribute to impaired hormonal responses and hypoglycemia unawareness [61].
- In older patients with type 2 diabetes, the joint occurrence of hypoglycemia unawareness and deteriorated cognitive function is a critical factor that needs to be considered in their exercise blood glucose management [62].

## 38.11 Monitoring Blood Glucose Levels with Physical Activity

Monitoring blood glucose is vital for the long-term maintenance of glycemic management and is especially important during exercise given that beta-blocker therapy can mask the onset of hypoglycemia. Done during exercise, such monitoring may also provide positive feedback regarding the regulation or progression of the exercise prescription, which may result in greater subsequent long-term adherence to exercise. This is particularly important since exercise is a cornerstone of treatment for diabetes.

When patients with diabetes begin an exercise program, their blood glucose responses to exercise should be monitored closely. Monitoring and recording their levels before and after exercise is important because it may:

- Allow for early detection and prevention of hypoglycemia or hyperglycemia
- Help determine appropriate pre-exercise levels to lower risk of hypoglycemia or hyperglycemia
- Identify patients who can benefit from monitoring during and after exercise
- Provide information for modifying the exercise prescription
- Allow for better adjustment of diabetes regimens to manage all activities
- Motivate patients to remain more active to better manage their diabetes

## 38.12 Glycemic Impact of Exercise Timing

Timing of exercise is particularly important, especially in individuals taking insulin. Consider the following for patients using basal and/or bolus insulin:

- Changing insulin timing, reducing insulin doses, and/or increasing carbohydrate intake are effective strategies to prevent hypoglycemia and hyperglycemia during and after exercise [9, 63].
- Early morning exercise may result in elevations in blood glucose levels instead of the usual decrease with moderate activity [9, 64].
- Food intake must be considered with respect to the timing of exercise, particularly for anyone who takes insulin [9].

## 38.13 Exercising Safely with Diabetes-Related Health Complications

It is possible for patients to exercise safely and effectively with most diabetes-related health complications, assuming precautions are taken. In most cases, the potential benefits of being active outweigh the risks associated with the activity.

1. *Cardiovascular disease*:
    - It is generally safe for individuals with stable CVD to engage in various forms of physical exercise training, including resistance exercise.

- If angina occurs during physical activity, patients should keep their heart rate at least 10 beats per minute below its onset.
- Resistance and high-intensity aerobic exercise may improve coronary perfusion rather than restrict it due to a higher mean arterial pressure.
- Silent ischemia in patients with diabetes often goes undetected [65], and it may advisable to conduct annual cardiovascular risk factor assessments [2].

2. *Proliferative retinopathy and other eye diseases*:
   - Individuals with proliferative retinopathy at risk for vitreous hemorrhage can minimize this risk by avoiding activities that dramatically elevate blood pressure.
   - Patients with severe non-proliferative and proliferative diabetic retinopathy should avoid vigorous aerobic and resistance training, jumping, jarring, and head-down activities, and Valsalva (breath-holding) maneuvers.
   - If vision is impaired by cataracts, patients should use caution when exercising outdoors or to exercise using a sighted guide.
3. *Autonomic neuropathy*:
   - Autonomic neuropathy may cause a blunted blood pressure response, attenuated oxygen kinetics, and anhidrosis (i.e., water deprivation) during physical activities.
   - Monitor for signs and symptoms of silent ischemia, such as unusual shortness of breath or back pain, due to a reduced ability to perceive angina.
   - Monitor blood pressure before and after exercise to manage hypotension and hypertension associated with vigorous intensity exercise.
   - Heart rate and blood pressure responses to exercise may be blunted secondary to autonomic dysfunction; use ratings of perceived exertion (RPE) or heart rate reserve (HRR) to better assess exercise intensity [66].
4. *Peripheral neuropathy*:
   - Individuals with peripheral neuropathy need to take proper care of their feet to prevent foot ulcers and lower the risk of amputation [1].
   - Precautions should be taken to prevent blisters or other areas of trauma on the feet.
   - Feet should be kept dry with polyester or blend socks, and athletic footwear should fit well and contain silica gel or air midsoles.
   - All individuals should examine their feet daily to detect and treat problems early.
5. *Diabetic kidney disease*:
   - Exercise does not accelerate progression of kidney disease even though protein excretion may transiently increase after exercise.
   - Both aerobic and resistance training improve physical function and quality of life in individuals with kidney disease and should be encouraged to be active.
   - Exercise should begin at a low intensity and volume if a patient's aerobic capacity and muscle function are substantially reduced.

In summary, the exercise prescription for patients with diabetes should be tailored according to the timing of their medications, presence of diabetes complications, and individual exercise and glycemic goals. The benefits of regular physical activity participation go well beyond increasing insulin sensitivity and lowering blood glucose levels. A comprehensive exercise program performed consistently and progressively will help persons with diabetes manage the disease and improve their quality of life.

## 38.14 The Athletic Individual with Diabetes

While almost all adults with type 2 diabetes may be able to engage in exercise for preventive measures as outlined, in adolescents and adults with type 1 diabetes (and also some with type 2 diabetes), excelling in high-level competitive sports is possible.

Several aspects of glycemic management need specific attention in athletic individuals with diabetes, as illustrated in the Fig. 38.1 [50]:

- The type, order, timing, and duration of physical activities can impact blood glucose responses, and participation in aerobic, sprint, and resistance training can result in widely varying blood glucose responses [1, 9, 55].
- Exercise-related alterations in blood glucose levels can usually be managed effectively with appropriate diabetes regimen modifications.
- Insulin and food intake may require adjustments to prevent both hypoglycemia and hyperglycemia in individuals with diabetes before, during, and after activity [67].
- Hydration and electrolyte status, which can be affected by hyperglycemia and medications commonly prescribed for people with diabetes, also can affect performance.
- Boluses of mealtime insulin taken within 2–3 h of the onset of physical training may need to be reduced to prevent hypoglycemia, depending on the intensity and duration of the activity (Table 38.2).

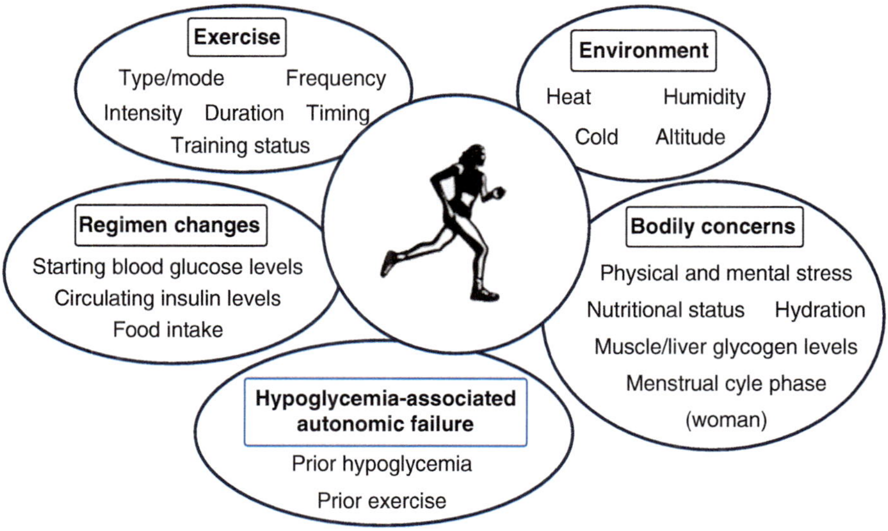


**Fig. 38.1** Multiple factors can influence the glycemic management of active individuals with diabetes (adapted from [50])

**Table 38.2** Recommended pre-exercise meal insulin bolus reductions for activities started within 90 min after administration (adapted from [50])

| Intensity of activity | Activity lasting 30 min | Activity lasting 60 min |
|---|---|---|
| Light aerobic (30–39% HRR) | −25% | −50% |
| Moderate aerobic (40–59% HRR) | −50% | −75% |
| Vigorous aerobic (60–89% HRR) | −75% | Not assessed |
| Maximal or near maximal (>89% HRR) | No reduction | Not assessed |

*HRR* heart rate reserve

- Athletic individuals with diabetes at any level of competition or sports participation can potentially be as successful as those without diabetes.
- Athletes and coaches should be aware of the impact of blood glucose levels and medications on hydration and electrolyte balance to make suitable adjustments to achieve optimal performance.
- Newer technologies like insulin pumps, continuous glucose monitors, and artificial pancreas (i.e., "closed loop" or "hybrid closed loop") systems, while somewhat limited at present in their accuracy and use, may assist some users in better managing their blood glucose levels for athletic endeavors.
- Insulin is prohibited under S4 of the WADA (World Anti-Doping Agency) Prohibited List – Hormone and Metabolic Modulators. All individuals with diabetes on insulin require a TUE (Therapeutic Use Exemption) to compete.
- Athletes with type 2 diabetes who are not on insulin do not require a TUE.

**Clinical Pearls** It is safe for most individuals with diabetes to begin an easy to moderate physical activity program, although in certain cases, pre-exercise physical assessment and exercise stress testing may be advisable, especially for sedentary, higher risk individuals desiring to engage in more vigorous activities.

- Exercise prescriptions should be tailored to meet the individual needs of patients with regards to their fitness, health, and blood glucose management goals.
- Most individuals with diabetes will benefit from self-monitoring of blood glucose when engaging in physical activities, as well as monitoring of other signs and symptoms associated with health complications.
- Athletic individuals with diabetes may engage in competitive sports at all levels if certain precautions (i.e., glucose monitoring, altered insulin regimens, individualized food intake) are made to manage glycemic levels.

## Case Study Wrap-Up

Case Vignette: A 54-year-old man presents for an assessment of his physical fitness. Two years ago, he experienced a non-ST-elevation myocardial infarction of the anterior wall, which necessitated placement of a drug-eluting stent in his left descending artery. He also reports that his GP told him that he has "elevated blood sugar levels" for which he received lifestyle advice. His family history is unremarkable for cardiovascular diseases and he reports no angina or other cardiovascular disorders. The patient smokes one pack of cigarettes per day (and has done so for 30 years). As for physical activity, he reports engaging in 30–45 min of jogging once a week. His present medications include 100 mg of acetylsalicylic acid, a beta-blocker (bisoprolol 5 mg 1–0-0), an angiotensin converting enzyme (ACE)-inhibitor (ramipril 2.5 mg 1–0-0), and a statin (simvastatin 20 mg 0–0-1).

On physical examination, his body mass index (BMI, 31.1 kg/m$^2$), waist circumference (105 cm), and blood pressure (145/95 mmHg) are elevated. Auscultation of heart and lungs reveal no pathologic findings and no signs of heart failure are noted. The ECG reveals a sinus rhythm with 65 beats per minute, normal indices, and no Q-waves. A maximal exercise stress test reveals a reduced exercise capacity (75% of age predicted, or 151 Watts), but it is negative for ischemia and other abnormalities.

Blood tests show a fasting plasma glucose of 6.6 mmol/l (119 mg/dl), HbA1c of 6.9%, and dyslipidemia despite use of a statin: total cholesterol, 7.0 mmol/l (270 mg/dl); low density lipoprotein (LDL)-cholesterol, 4.0 mmol/L (155 mg/dl); high density lipoprotein (HDL)-cholesterol, 2.2 mmol/l (85 mg/dl); and triglycerides, 1.7 mmol/l (148 mg/dl). Urinary analysis shows some microalbuminuria and glucosuria.

## Questions

1. In addition to optimization of his medications (change of statin, upped titration of ramipril, and addition of antidiabetic medications) and smoking cessation, what exercise advice would you give this patient?
2. Would you recommend blood glucose monitoring before, during and after exercise? What precisely do you recommend?
3. Would you perform a graded exercise stress test on this patient prior to his starting a more formal exercise program?
4. During routine exercise stress testing conducted on this patient, he becomes symptomatic with fatigue, dizziness, and a dry mouth. What is the most likely cause of his symptoms?

## Answers

1. All adults with diabetes are recommended to undertake at least 150 min per week of moderate to vigorous aerobic exercise training, although up to 300 min likely bestows additional health benefits. Given his underlying CVD (including a prior myocardial infarction and stent placement), his recommended intensity should be light to moderate, at least to start. He may choose to continue jogging (at a moderate pace) and include other types of aerobic training spread throughout the week, allowing no more than 2 days to lapse between bouts of activity. In addition, he should add in moderate resistance training exercises at least twice weekly (on nonconsecutive days) to enhance retention of his muscle mass. Engaging in flexibility exercises and balance training at least 2–3 days per week should also be recommended to someone his age

(see Table 38.1), along with staying more active overall on a daily basis and breaking up sedentary time with frequent bouts of activity.

At least initially, this patient's blood glucose should be monitored closely before, during and after exercise. Depending on which diabetes medications this patient is prescribed, monitoring blood glucose levels may remain important around exercise given that beta-blocker therapy can mask the onset of hypoglycemia. Done before and after exercise, such monitoring may also provide positive feedback regarding the glycemic benefits of regular exercise training, which may result in greater subsequent long-term adherence to his exercise training prescription. This is particularly important since exercise is a cornerstone for the management of all types of diabetes and its potential health complications.

2. Although routine monitoring around exercise is not recommended for all adults with type 2 diabetes (given that most have a low risk of developing exercise-related hypoglycemia), when such patients begin an exercise program, their blood glucose responses to exercise should be checked. Monitoring and recording blood glucose levels before and after exercise, at least initially, is important because it may:
   - Allow for early detection and prevention of hypoglycemia or hyperglycemia
   - Help determine appropriate pre-exercise blood glucose levels to lower risk of glycemic imbalances resulting from activities
   - Identify patients who may benefit from continued monitoring around exercise
   - Provide information for modifying prescribed exercise based on glycemic responses
   - Allow for better adjustment of diabetes regimens to manage all activities
   - Motivate patients to remain more active to better manage their diabetes
3. Likely yes, but it depends. Since this patient is already somewhat active, a stress test is only advisable if he plans to start new activities more vigorous than his current daily ones, which include weekly jogging (which he has been undertaking without any problems or symptoms arising). As stated, previously sedentary older individuals (≥ 40 years) with diabetes and anyone ≥30 years of age with a high cardiovascular risk should likely undergo medical screening and obtain medical clearance prior to performing vigorous intensity exercise. In addition, this patient does meet several criteria for a possible pre-participation exercise stress test, including his age, cigarette smoking, dyslipidemia, and known coronary artery disease (see section on "General Indications for Exercise Stress Testing in Patients with Diabetes").
4. Routine pre-session blood glucose measurement is 11.2 mmol/l (200 mg/dl), which compares well to his previous pre-session measurements. He starts to train on a cycle ergometer. After 10 min of ergometer training his heart rate starts to rise, although his workload is constantly decreasing from 75 to 45 W. The patient also reports feeling dizziness and a dry mouth. No ECG changes are evident, however. His immediate blood glucose is 19.4 mmol/l (350 mg/dl), indicating an increase in hyperglycemia in this patient. Some of his symptoms correspond to possible symptoms of hyperglycemia, which can include fatigue, hyperventilation, and dry mouth, along with polyphagia, polydipsia, polyuria, blurred vision, weight loss, poor wound healing, dry or itchy skin, impotence (male), recurrent infections such as vaginal yeast infections, groin rash, external ear infections (swimmer's ear), cardiac arrhythmias, stupor, and coma. Moreover, physical exhaustion causes glucose production in

the liver (glycogenesis and glycogenolysis) plus enhanced free fatty acid release by adipose tissue and reduced muscle uptake of glucose and, consequently, may contribute to hyperglycemia in exercising patients with diabetes.

After a few minutes of rest, the patient's symptoms resolve, but his blood glucose remains elevated at 19.4 mmol/l (342 mg/dl) 15 min later. A urinary analysis reveals moderate ketone bodies. When asked further, the patient reports having had a demanding week at his job and furthermore some domestic problems, resulting in significant insomnia during the prior week. To reduce his mental stress, he had exercised on a cycle ergometer for 2 h before this scheduled testing. He is instructed not to perform any exercise for the rest of the day and to continue to monitor his blood glucose levels frequently. The next day the patient's urine is rechecked and found to be free of ketones. His blood glucose is 9.6 mmol/l (174 mg/dl) and he reports feeling completely recovered after a day of rest. He reports that his GP has recommended that he start on diabetes medications immediately to lower his blood glucose levels and that he plans to do so.

## References

1. Colberg SR SR, Yardley JE, Riddell MC, Dunstan DW, Dempsey PC, Horton ES, Castorino K, Tate DF. Physical activity/exercise and diabetes: A position statement of the American Diabetes Association. Diabetes Care. 2016;39(11).
2. Colberg SR, Sigal RJ, Fernhall B, Regensteiner JG, Blissmer BJ, Rubin RR, et al. Exercise and type 2 diabetes: the American College of Sports Medicine and the American Diabetes Association: joint position statement. Diabetes Care. 2010;33(12):e147–67.
3. Jakicic JM, Egan CM, Fabricatore AN, Gaussoin SA, Glasser SP, Hesson LA, et al. Four-year change in cardiorespiratory fitness and influence on glycemic control in adults with type 2 diabetes in a randomized trial: the look AHEAD trial. Diabetes Care. 2013;36(5):1297–303. https://doi.org/10.2337/dc12-0712. Epub 2012 Dec 6
4. Kokkinos P, Myers J, Nylen E, Panagiotakos DB, Manolis A, Pittaras A, et al. Exercise capacity and all-cause mortality in African American and Caucasian men with type 2 diabetes. Diabetes Care. 2009;32(4):623–8.
5. Pi-Sunyer X. The look AHEAD trial: a review and discussion of its outcomes. Curr Nutr Rep. 2014;3(4):387–91.
6. Newsom SA, Everett AC, Hinko A, Horowitz JF. A single session of low-intensity exercise is sufficient to enhance insulin sensitivity into the next day in obese adults. Diabetes Care. 2013;36(9):2516–22.
7. Yardley JE, Hay J, Abou-Setta AM, Marks SD, McGavock J. A systematic review and meta-analysis of exercise interventions in adults with type 1 diabetes. Diabetes Res Clin Pract. 2014;106(3):393–400.
8. Ratjen I, Weber KS, Roden M, Herrmann ME, Mussig K. Type 1 diabetes mellitus and exercise in competitive athletes. Exp Clin Endocrinol Diabetes. 2015;123(7):419–22. https://doi.org/10.1055/s-0035-1545344. Epub 2015 Apr 8
9. Riddell MC, Gallen IW, Smart CE, Taplin CE, Adolfsson P, Lumb AN, et al. Exercise management in type 1 diabetes: a consensus statement. Lancet Diabetes Endocrinol. 2017;5(5):377–90. https://doi.org/10.1016/S2213-8587(17)30014-1. Epub 2017 Jan 24
10. Look AHEAD Research Group. Eight-year weight losses with an intensive lifestyle intervention: the look AHEAD study. Obesity (Silver Spring). 2014;22(1):5–13.
11. Franz MJ, Boucher JL, Rutten-Ramos S, VanWormer JJ. Lifestyle weight-loss intervention outcomes in overweight and obese adults with type 2 diabetes: a systematic review and meta-analysis of randomized clinical trials. J Acad Nutr Diet. 2015;115(9):1447–63. doi: 10.016/j.jand.2015.02.031. Epub Apr 29.

12. Moholdt T, Lavie CJ, Nauman J. Sustained Physical Activity, Not Weight Loss, Associated With Improved Survival in Coronary Heart Disease. J Am Coll Cardiol. 2018;71(10):1094–101. doi: 10.16/j.jacc.2018.01.011.
13. Nilsson A, Bergens O, Kadi F. Physical activity alters inflammation in older adults by different intensity levels. Med Sci Sports Exerc. 2018;16(10):0000000000001582.
14. Fuller KNZ, Summers CM, Valentine RJ. Effect of a single bout of aerobic exercise on high-fat meal-induced inflammation. Metabolism. 2017;71:144–152.(doi):https://doi.org/10.1016/j.metabol.2017.03.001. Epub Mar 8.
15. Rohling M, Herder C, Stemper T, Mussig K. Influence of acute and chronic exercise on glucose uptake. J Diabetes Res. 2016;2016:2868652.
16. Dube JJ, Allison KF, Rousson V, Goodpaster BH, Amati F. Exercise dose and insulin sensitivity: relevance for diabetes prevention. Med Sci Sports Exerc. 2012;44(5):793–9.
17. Lieb DC, Parson HK, Mamikunian G, Vinik AI. Cardiac autonomic imbalance in newly diagnosed and established diabetes is associated with markers of adipose tissue inflammation. Exp Diabetes Res. 2012;2012:878760.
18. Maahs DM, Nadeau K, Snell-Bergeon JK, Schauer I, Bergman B, West NA, et al. Association of insulin sensitivity to lipids across the lifespan in people with type 1 diabetes. Diabet Med. 2011;28(2):148–55.
19. D'Hooge R, Hellinckx T, Van Laethem C, Stegen S, De Schepper J, Van Aken S, et al. Influence of combined aerobic and resistance training on metabolic control, cardiovascular fitness and quality of life in adolescents with type 1 diabetes: a randomized controlled trial. Clin Rehabil. 2011;25(4):349–59.
20. Tikkanen-Dolenc H, Waden J, Forsblom C, Harjutsalo V, Thorn LM, Saraheimo M, et al. Physical Activity Reduces Risk of Premature Mortality in Patients With Type 1 Diabetes With and Without Kidney Disease. Diabetes Care. 2017;16(10):dc17–0615.
21. Tikkanen-Dolenc H, Waden J, Forsblom C, Harjutsalo V, Thorn LM, Saraheimo M, et al. Frequent and intensive physical activity reduces risk of cardiovascular events in type 1 diabetes. Diabetologia. 2017;60(3):574–80. https://doi.org/10.1007/s00125-016-4189-8. Epub 2016 Dec 24
22. Lee JH, Lee R, Hwang MH, Hamilton MT, Park Y. The effects of exercise on vascular endothelial function in type 2 diabetes: a systematic review and meta-analysis. Diabetol Metab Syndr. 2018;10:15.(doi):https://doi.org/10.1186/s13098-018-0316-7. eCollection 2018.
23. Riebe D, Franklin BA, Thompson PD, Garber CE, Whitfield GP, Magal M, et al. Updating ACSM's recommendations for exercise Preparticipation health screening. Med Sci Sports Exerc. 2015;47(11):2473–9.
24. Young LH, Wackers FJ, Chyun DA, Davey JA, Barrett EJ, Taillefer R, et al. Cardiac outcomes after screening for asymptomatic coronary artery disease in patients with type 2 diabetes: the DIAD study: a randomized controlled trial. JAMA. 2009;301(15):1547–55.
25. Physical Activity Guidelines Advisory Committee. 2018 Physical Activity Guidelines Advisory Committee Scientific Report. In: US Department of Health and Human Services, ed. Washington, D.C. 2018.
26. Kemps H, Kränkel N, Dörr M, Moholdt T, Wilhelm M, Paneni F, et al. Exercise training for patients with type 2 diabetes and cardiovascular disease: What to pursue and how to do it. A Position Paper of the European Association of Preventive Cardiology (EAPC). European Journal of Preventive Cardiology.0(0):2047487318820420.
27. Snowling NJ, Hopkins WG. Effects of different modes of exercise training on glucose control and risk factors for complications in type 2 diabetic patients: a meta-analysis. Diabetes Care. 2006;29(11):2518–27.
28. Umpierre D, Ribeiro PA, Kramer CK, Leitao CB, Zucatti AT, Azevedo MJ, et al. Physical activity advice only or structured exercise training and association with HbA1c levels in type 2 diabetes: a systematic review and meta-analysis. JAMA. 2011;305(17):1790–9.
29. Umpierre D, Ribeiro PA, Schaan BD, Ribeiro JP. Volume of supervised exercise training impacts glycaemic control in patients with type 2 diabetes: a systematic review with meta-regression analysis. Diabetologia. 2013;56(2):242–51.

30. Francois ME, Little JP. Effectiveness and safety of high-intensity interval training in patients with type 2 diabetes. Diabetes Spectr. 2015;28(1):39–44.
31. Gillen JB, Little JP, Punthakee Z, Tarnopolsky MA, Riddell MC, Gibala MJ. Acute high-intensity interval exercise reduces the postprandial glucose response and prevalence of hyperglycaemia in patients with type 2 diabetes. Diabetes Obes Metab. 2012;14(6):575–7.
32. Moser O, Tschakert G, Mueller A, Groeschl W, Pieber TR, Obermayer-Pietsch B, et al. Effects of high-intensity interval exercise versus moderate continuous exercise on glucose homeostasis and hormone response in patients with type 1 diabetes mellitus using novel ultra-long-acting insulin. PLoS One. 2015;10(8):e0136489.
33. Garcia-Garcia F, Kumareswaran K, Hovorka R, Hernando ME. Quantifying the acute changes in glucose with exercise in type 1 diabetes: a systematic review and meta-analysis. Sports Med. 2015;45(4):587–99.
34. Yang Z, Scott CA, Mao C, Tang J, Farmer AJ. Resistance exercise versus aerobic exercise for type 2 diabetes: a systematic review and meta-analysis. Sports Med. 2014;44(4):487–99.
35. Dunstan DW, Daly RM, Owen N, Jolley D, Vulikh E, Shaw J, et al. Home-based resistance training is not sufficient to maintain improved glycemic control following supervised training in older individuals with type 2 diabetes. Diabetes Care. 2005;28(1):3–9.
36. Dunstan DW, Daly RM, Owen N, Jolley D, De Courten M, Shaw J, et al. High-intensity resistance training improves glycemic control in older patients with type 2 diabetes. Diabetes Care. 2002;25(10):1729–36.
37. Egger A, Niederseer D, Diem G, Finkenzeller T, Ledl-Kurkowski E, Forstner R, et al. Different types of resistance training in type 2 diabetes mellitus: effects on glycaemic control, muscle mass and strength. Eur J Prev Cardiol. 2013;20(6):1051–60.
38. Zeppetzauer M, Drexel H, Vonbank A, Rein P, Aczel S, Saely CH. Eccentric endurance exercise economically improves metabolic and inflammatory risk factors. Eur J Prev Cardiol. 2013;20(4):577–84.
39. Church TS, Blair SN, Cocreham S, Johannsen N, Johnson W, Kramer K, et al. Effects of aerobic and resistance training on hemoglobin A1c levels in patients with type 2 diabetes: a randomized controlled trial. JAMA. 2010;304(20):2253–62.
40. Sigal RJ, Kenny GP, Boule NG, Wells GA, Prud'homme D, Fortier M, et al. Effects of aerobic training, resistance training, or both on glycemic control in type 2 diabetes: a randomized trial. Ann Intern Med. 2007;147(6):357–69.
41. Yang P, Swardfager W, Fernandes D, Laredo S, Tomlinson G, Oh PI, et al. Finding the Optimal volume and intensity of Resistance Training Exercise for Type 2 Diabetes: The FORTE Study, a Randomized Trial. Diabetes Res Clin Pract. 2017;130:98–107.(doi):https://doi.org/10.1016/j.diabres.2017.05.019.
42. Vinik AI, Vinik EJ, Colberg SR, Morrison S. Falls risk in older adults with type 2 diabetes. Clin Geriatr Med. 2015;31(1):89–99. viii
43. Morrison S, Simmons R, Colberg SR, Parson HK, Vinik AI. Supervised balance training and Wii fit-based exercises lower falls risk in older adults with type 2 diabetes. J Am Med Dir Assoc. 2017;27(17):004.
44. Morrison S, Colberg SR, Mariano M, Parson HK, Vinik AI. Balance training reduces falls risk in older individuals with type 2 diabetes. Diabetes Care. 2010;33(4):748–50.
45. Herriott MT, Colberg SR, Parson HK, Nunnold T, Vinik AI. Effects of 8 weeks of flexibility and resistance training in older adults with type 2 diabetes. Diabetes Care. 2004;27(12):2988–9.
46. Biswas A, Oh PI, Faulkner GE, Bajaj RR, Silver MA, Mitchell MS, et al. Sedentary time and its association with risk for disease incidence, mortality, and hospitalization in adults: a systematic review and meta-analysis. Ann Intern Med. 2015;162(2):123–32.
47. Larsen RN, Dempsey PC, Dillon F, Grace M, Kingwell BA, Owen N, et al. Does the type of activity "break" from prolonged sitting differentially impact on postprandial blood glucose reductions? An exploratory analysis. Appl Physiol Nutr Metab. 2017;42(8):897–900. https://doi.org/10.1139/apnm-2016-0642. Epub 2017 Mar 24
48. Dempsey PC, Larsen RN, Sethi P, Sacre JW, Straznicky NE, Cohen ND, et al. Benefits for type 2 diabetes of interrupting prolonged sitting with brief bouts of light walking or simple resistance activities. Diabetes Care. 2016;39(6):964–72.

49. Garber CE, Blissmer B, Deschenes MR, Franklin BA, Lamonte MJ, Lee IM, et al. American College of Sports Medicine position stand. Quantity and quality of exercise for developing and maintaining cardiorespiratory, musculoskeletal, and neuromotor fitness in apparently healthy adults: guidance for prescribing exercise. Med Sci Sports Exerc. 2011;43(7):1334–59.
50. Yardley JE, Colberg SR. Update on Management of Type 1 diabetes and type 2 diabetes in athletes. Curr Sports Med Rep. 2017;16(1):38–44.
51. Colberg SR, Sigal RJ. Prescribing exercise for individuals with type 2 diabetes: recommendations and precautions. Phys Sportsmed. 2011;39(2):13–26.
52. Karstoft K, Christensen CS, Pedersen BK, Solomon TP. The acute effects of interval- vs continuous-walking exercise on glycemic control in subjects with type 2 diabetes: a crossover, controlled study. J Clin Endocrinol Metab. 2014;99(9):3334–42.
53. Balducci S, Zanuso S, Cardelli P, Salvi L, Bazuro A, Pugliese L, et al. Effect of high- versus low-intensity supervised aerobic and resistance training on modifiable cardiovascular risk factors in type 2 diabetes; the Italian diabetes and exercise study (IDES). PLoS One. 2012;7(11):e49297.
54. Abate M, Schiavone C, Salini V, Andia I. Management of limited joint mobility in diabetic patients. Diabetes Metab Syndr Obes. 2013;6:197–207.
55. Yardley JE, Kenny GP, Perkins BA, Riddell MC, Balaa N, Malcolm J, et al. Resistance versus aerobic exercise: acute effects on glycemia in type 1 diabetes. Diabetes Care. 2013;36(3):537–42.
56. Yardley JE, Kenny GP, Perkins BA, Riddell MC, Malcolm J, Boulay P, et al. Effects of performing resistance exercise before versus after aerobic exercise on glycemia in type 1 diabetes. Diabetes Care. 2012;35(4):669–75.
57. Guelfi KJ, Ratnam N, Smythe GA, Jones TW, Fournier PA. Effect of intermittent high-intensity compared with continuous moderate exercise on glucose production and utilization in individuals with type 1 diabetes. Am J Physiol Endocrinol Metab. 2007;292(3):E865–70.
58. Sigal RJ, Fisher SJ, Halter JB, Vranic M, Marliss EB. Glucoregulation during and after intense exercise: effects of beta-adrenergic blockade in subjects with type 1 diabetes mellitus. J Clin Endocrinol Metab. 1999;84(11):3961–71.
59. Plockinger U, Topuz M, Riese B, Reuter T. Risk of exercise-induced hypoglycaemia in patients with type 2 diabetes on intensive insulin therapy: comparison of insulin glargine with NPH insulin as basal insulin supplement. Diabetes Res Clin Pract. 2008;81(3):290–5.
60. McMahon SK, Ferreira LD, Ratnam N, Davey RJ, Youngs LM, Davis EA, et al. Glucose requirements to maintain euglycemia after moderate-intensity afternoon exercise in adolescents with type 1 diabetes are increased in a biphasic manner. J Clin Endocrinol Metab. 2007;92(3):963–8.
61. Cryer PE. Hypoglycemia-associated autonomic failure in diabetes. Handb Clin Neurol. 2013;117:295–307.
62. Bremer JP, Jauch-Chara K, Hallschmid M, Schmid S, Schultes B. Hypoglycemia unawareness in older compared with middle-aged patients with type 2 diabetes. Diabetes Care. 2009;32(8):1513–7.
63. Chu L, Hamilton J, Riddell MC. Clinical management of the physically active patient with type 1 diabetes. Phys Sportsmed. 2011;39(2):64–77.
64. Poirier P, Tremblay A, Catellier C, Tancrede G, Garneau C, Nadeau A. Impact of time interval from the last meal on glucose response to exercise in subjects with type 2 diabetes. J Clin Endocrinol Metab. 2000;85(8):2860–4.
65. Wackers FJ, Young LH, Inzucchi SE, Chyun DA, Davey JA, Barrett EJ, et al. Detection of silent myocardial ischemia in asymptomatic diabetic subjects: the DIAD study. Diabetes Care. 2004;27(8):1954–61.
66. Colberg SR, Swain DP, Vinik AI. Use of heart rate reserve and rating of perceived exertion to prescribe exercise intensity in diabetic autonomic neuropathy. Diabetes Care. 2003;26(4):986–90.
67. Riddell MC, Zaharieva DP, Yavelberg L, Cinar A, Jamnik VK. Exercise and the Development of the Artificial Pancreas: One of the More Difficult Series of Hurdles. J Diabetes Sci Technol. 2015;9(6):1217–26. doi: 10.177/1932296815609370.

# Impact of Exercise on Cardiovascular Risk Factors: Obesity

# 39

Andrew Elagizi, Sergey Kachur, and Carl J. Lavie

**Learning Objectives**

1. Learn the vital importance of cardiorespiratory fitness (CRF) and its impact on mortality.
2. Understand the physiologic changes that occur with obesity and the associated increased cardiovascular risks.
3. Learn about the obesity mortality paradox; that being classified as "obese" alone does not necessarily equate to poor health as much as metabolic disturbances associated with obesity.
4. Understand the utility of cardiac rehabilitation in patients with cardiovascular disease.

## 39.1 Introduction

Worldwide obesity, as measured by the body mass index (BMI), has more than doubled between 1980 and 2014 and currently affects more than 10% of the global population. Obesity is a well-established risk factor for cardiovascular (CV) disease (CVD), and is the second leading cause of preventable death in developed countries, following tobacco use [1]. The American Heart Association (AHA) obesity guidelines recommend that physicians identify patients who meet clinical criteria for obesity using BMI $\geq 30$ kg/m$^2$ to identify adults who may be at elevated risk of mortality

A. Elagizi · S. Kachur
Department of Cardiovascular Diseases, John Ochsner Heart and Vascular Institute, New Orleans, LA, USA
e-mail: andrew.elagizi@ochsner.org

C. J. Lavie (✉)
John Ochsner Heart and Vascular Institute, Ochsner Clinical School–The University of Queensland School of Medicine, New Orleans, LA, USA
e-mail: clavie@ochsner.org



A. Pressler, J. Niebauer (eds.), *Textbook of Sports and Exercise Cardiology*,
https://doi.org/10.1007/978-3-030-35374-2_39

from all causes, because of the well documented increased morbidity and mortality in the obese population [2]. This increasing burden and obesity's role in the development of CVD has led the World Health Organization (WHO) to declare obesity as one of the nine target areas in fighting the global epidemic of non-communicable diseases. One of the major components of secondary prevention for CVD is exercise training (ET).

## 39.2 Current AHA Guidelines

The treatment of overweight and obesity allows patients to experience significant metabolic improvements that reduce their risk of CVD. Throughout this chapter, various tables are presented which summarize current recommendations from the AHA regarding obesity management, with a focus on evidence statements achieving a rating of high or moderate strength of evidence. The interested reader is encouraged to review the complete 2013 AHA guidelines for the management of overweight and obesity in adults [2].

## 39.3 Defining Obesity

### 39.3.1 WHO Definition of Obesity

The WHO defines overweight as a BMI $\geq$ 25 kg/m$^2$ and obesity as a BMI $\geq$ 30 kg/m$^2$, regardless of age, sex and race (Table 39.1) [3].

### 39.3.2 Calculating BMI

BMI is calculated as weight in kilograms divided by height in meters squared.

*BMI = weight (kg)/height (m$^2$)*

Therefore, BMI is merely a descriptor of an individual's weight relative to their height, however, it does not accurately describe body composition.

**Table 39.1** Weight classification according to Body Mass Index (BMI)

| Weight category | BMI |
|---|---|
| Underweight | <18.5 kg/m$^2$ |
| Normal weight | 18.5–24.9 kg/m$^2$ |
| Overweight | 25.0–29.9 kg/m$^2$ |
| **Obesity** | |
| Class I | 30.0–34.9 kg/m$^2$ |
| Class II | 35.0–39.9 kg/m$^2$ |
| Class III | 40.0–49.9 kg/m$^2$ |
| Class IV | 50.0–59.9 kg/m$^2$ |
| Class V | ≥60 kg/m$^2$ |

### 39.3.3 Criticism of BMI

The utility of BMI to assess obesity has been criticized for its inability to differentiate between fat, muscle and skeletal weight [1], therefore not being a precise measurement of adiposity.

- Having a normal BMI does not preclude an individual from having high levels of adipose tissue [4].
  - Patients who have normal BMI and high adiposity are known as "normal weight obese", who have been shown to have increased CVD and mortality risk [5, 6].
  - Those with increased muscle mass and shorter stature will have a higher BMI, and may be misclassified as overweight or obese, despite having low amounts of adipose tissue.

Therefore, BMI in the "normal" range may describe a person with high adiposity but a normal height-to-weight ratio, and falsely indicate good health status, and vice versa.

### 39.3.4 Clinical Utility of BMI

Because of the low cost and ease of use of the BMI calculation, despite its criticisms, BMI is still the most used anthropometric index in the literature and persists as a strong predictor of CVD mortality [7].

- BMI has been shown to be as clinically important or more important than total adiposity measured using accurate, complex and expensive methods, such as body fat percentage, fat mass index, fat-free mass and fat free mass index [8].

## 39.4 Etiology and Epidemiologic Trends

### 39.4.1 Etiology

It is widely accepted that increased body weight and overall adiposity are the result of a chronic positive energy balance (energy intake > energy expenditure) [9].

- However, the etiology of obesity can be multifactorial, including heritability [10].
  - Forms of monogenic obesity account for 2–4% of individuals with obesity, such as the autosomal dominant melanocortin-4 receptor gene mutation [11].
  - Autosomal recessively inherited leptin deficiency is the only form of monogenic obesity that can be treated causally via leptin replacement therapy [12].

### 39.4.2 Obesity Epidemic

The prevalence of overweight/obesity has reached epidemic proportions in Western countries, and is the second leading cause of preventable death following tobacco abuse [1].

- More than 78 million adults in the US were obese in 2009 and 2010 [13].
- The Global Burden of Disease obesity collaborators [14] analyzed data from 68.5 million persons between 1980 and 2015.
  - In 2015, a total of 107.7 million children and 603.7 million adults were obese.
    These statistics are magnified when realizing that approximately 90% of obese children will become obese adults [15].
    Due to increasing rates of childhood obesity in the USA, we may see the first generation which will be less healthy and have a shorter life expectancy than their parents [16].
  - Since 1980, the prevalence of obesity has doubled in >70 countries and has continuously increased in most others [14].
  - High BMI accounted for four million deaths globally, and over 2/3 of those deaths were due to CVD [14].

## 39.5 Physiologic Impact of Obesity (Fig. 39.1)

- Increasing adiposity leads to adipocyte hyperplasia, driven by recruitment of adipogenic progenitors and growth factors [17].
  - As obesity advances, hypertrophied adipocytes undergo apoptosis, cell necrosis and fibrosis, which further induce an inflammatory state and adipose tissue dysfunction [17].
    The inflammatory state is intensified by macrophage recruitment.
    These macrophages produce proinflammatory cytokines, inducible NO synthase, ROS and nitrogen intermediates and are thought to promote insulin resistance, metabolic syndrome or diabetes mellitus (DM) [17].

Increasing adiposity also has a negative impact on cardiac structure and function [18]:

1. Increased total and central blood volume.
2. Increased stroke volume.
3. Increased cardiac output.
4. Increased preload and left ventricular filling pressure.
5. Adverse impact on systolic, and especially diastolic dysfunction.

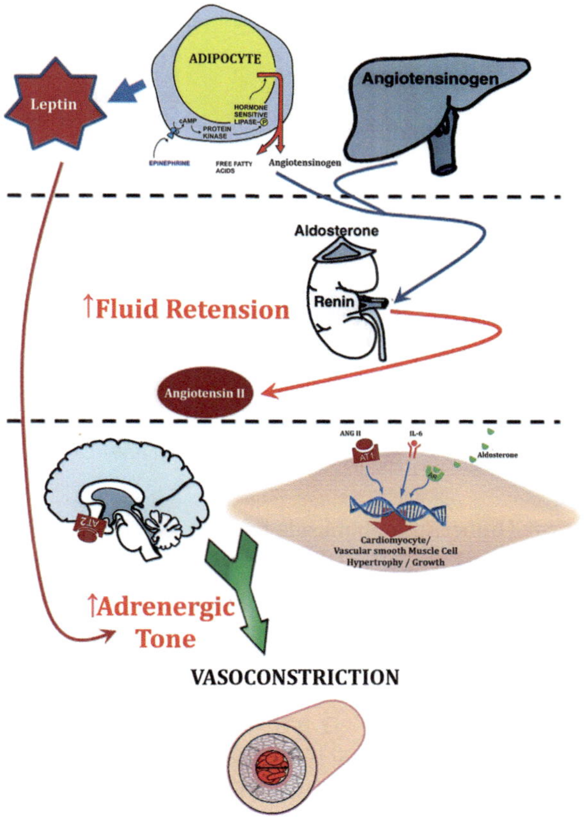


**Fig. 39.1** Physiologic impact of worsening obesity [30]

### 39.5.1 Mechanisms of Adipose-Associated Effects on CVD

The effects of adiposity on dysregulating homeostasis spans multiple organ systems, and increases the risks of renal disease, stroke, coronary heart disease (CHD), and mortality [19–22].

Adipose tissue causes cellular ischemia when accumulation out-strips available blood supply [23]. This helps initiate the release of adipokines and inflammatory factors such as C-reactive protein, Tumor necrosis factor (TNF), leptin, and adiponectin that trigger inflammation characteristic of atherosclerotic and hypertensive CVD [24].

- Weight-associated elevations in circulating blood volume cause a disproportionate increase in cardiac output that is related to an increase in free fatty acids (FFA) and sympathetic activity [25, 26].
- FFA increases sympathetic tone which inhibits sodium/potassium exchange pumps as well as sodium ATP pumps, leading to:

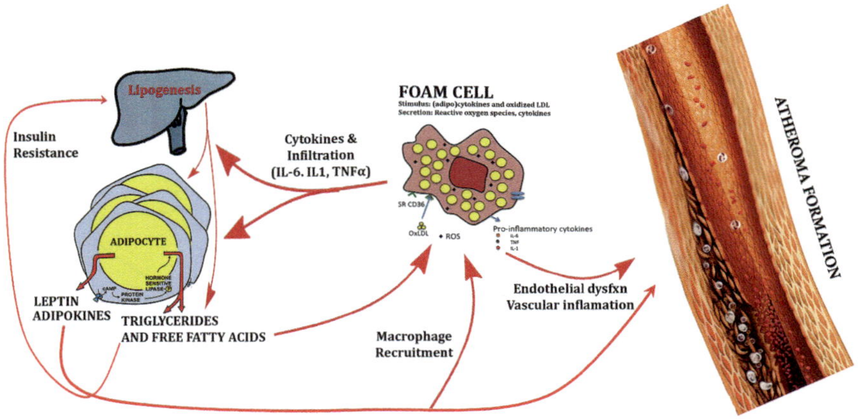


**Fig. 39.2** Obesity and hypertension [30]

  - Higher smooth muscle tonicity which causes higher peripheral resistance and blood pressure (BP) [27–29].
  - High sympathetic tone triggers excessive Renin-angiotensin-aldosterone system (RAAS) activation which leads to renal vasoconstriction and renin-dependent chronic hypertension (HTN) (Fig. 39.2).
- FFA increases infiltration of oxidized lipids in the artery wall, triggering a chronic inflammatory response with macrophage activation [31].
- Adipokines released from excess fat promote an inflammatory cascade
  - Activate cytokines that include IL-1β, IL-6, and nitric oxide (NO) synthase 2 [32, 33].
  - Stimulate macrophage infiltration into adipose and hepatic tissue.
  - Result in an inflammatory feedback loop, glucose dysregulation and ultimately potentiates dysfunction [34].
- The result is a feedback loop that stimulates additional FFA secretion, more adipokines, and worsening hyperglycemia that potentiate diabetes and atherosclerosis.
- Adiposity-related insulin resistance has been associated with reduced endothelial-dependent vasodilation [35, 36].
  - There is increasing evidence of endothelial dysfunction as a culprit in the oxygen imbalance of myocardial demand and supply that may lead to cardiac ischemia and infarction [37–39].

Dyslipidemia (decreases in high-density lipoprotein cholesterol (HDL-C), increases in low-density lipoprotein cholesterol (LDL-C)) is another mechanism of adiposity-related dysregulation; and is associated with FFA release, insulin resistance, and increased inflammation which lead to endothelial dysfunction [40].

- HDL-C protects against atherosclerosis by both removing excess cholesterol from macrophages and by downregulating adipokine secretion in fat tissue.
- Excess LDL-C promotes atherosclerosis through sub-endothelial deposition of LDL-C/apolipoprotein-B containing particles that stimulate macrophage-activity, phagocytosis, and foam cell formation.
  - This leads to increased oxidative stress and associated inflammation [41, 42].
- Oxidative stress is regulated by mechanisms that balance reactive oxygen species (ROS) production with ROS removal by anti-oxidant enzymes such as superoxide dismutase [43, 44].
  - Excessive ROS causes DNA damage, lipid oxidation, and protein denaturation.
- ROS likewise reduces vaso-reactivity by downregulating NO [45].
  - Lower NO levels lead to reduced vasodilation, impaired anti-coagulation, increased leukocyte adhesion, and smooth muscle proliferation [46].
  - The result is endothelial dysfunction and progression of CVD.

In summary, obesity promotes an inflammatory cascade through a combination of increased adrenergic tone, insulin resistance, and lipid dysregulation that accelerates inflammation and endothelial dysfunction leading to atherosclerotic diseases (Fig. 39.3) [47].

These changes lead to left ventricular hypertrophy and dysfunction, which becomes more pronounced with greater severity of obesity [1], and ultimately increases the incidence of heart failure (HF) and other CVD. Many of the physiologic effects of obesity can be reversed with purposeful weight loss [15]. Figure 39.4 illustrates mechanisms of CV risk related to obesity.

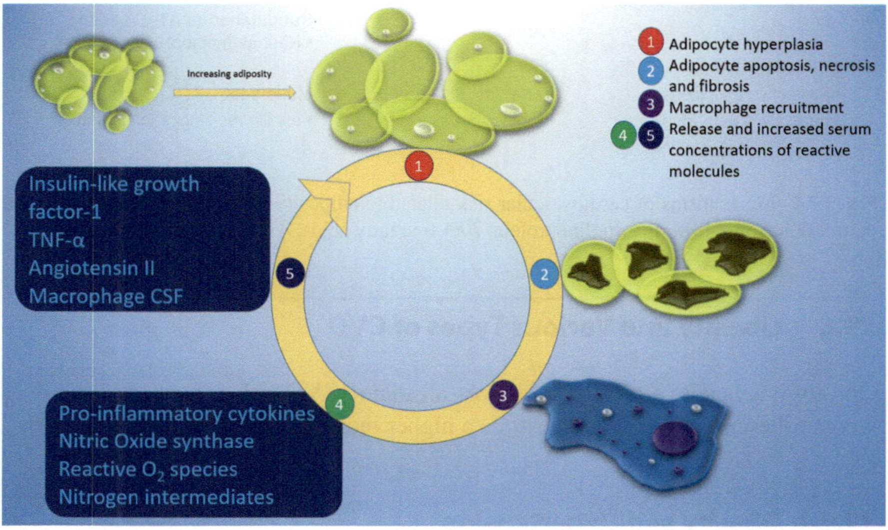


**Fig. 39.3** Obesity, inflammation, and atherosclerosis [30]

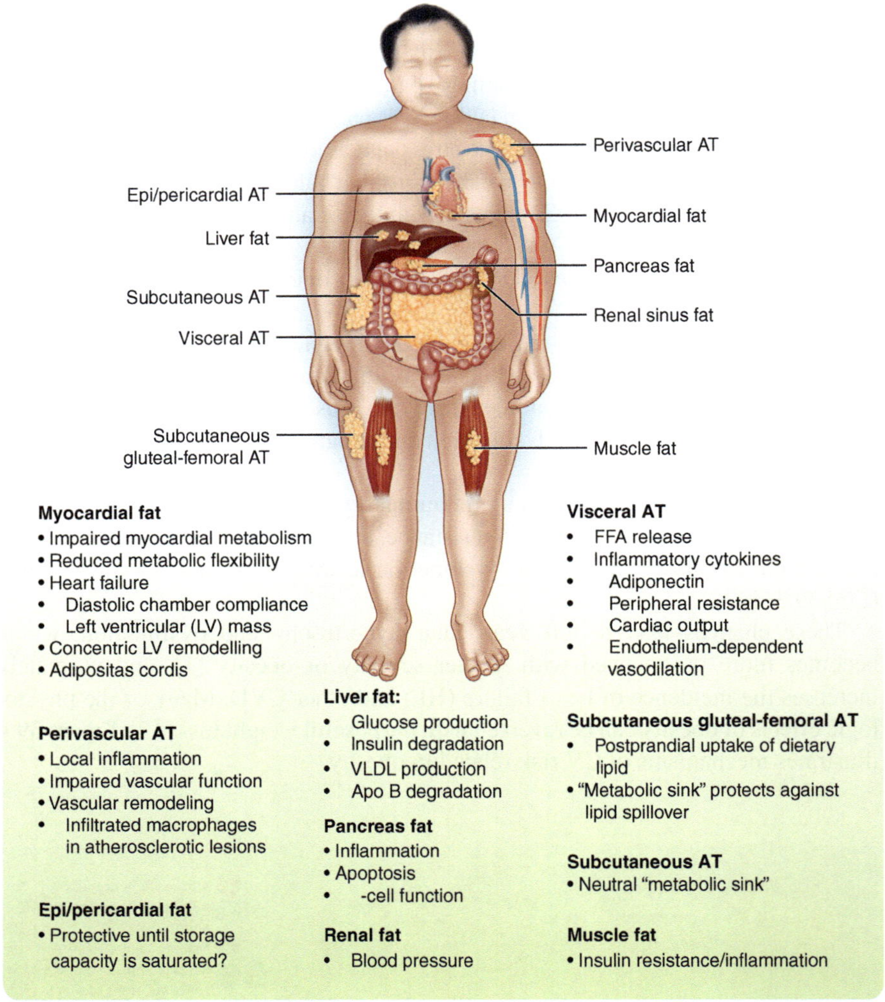


**Fig. 39.4** Mechanisms of cardiovascular risk related to adiposity in the obese (reproduced with permission from [48]). *Apo* apolipoprotein, *FFA* free fatty acids, *AT* adipose tissue

## 39.6 Obesity and Various Types of CVD

Obesity has negative effects on almost all major CVD risk factors, and the overweight/obese population demonstrate a higher incidence of almost all CVDs [1].

### 39.6.1 Obesity and Hypertension

Overweight/obesity is associated with increased risk of HTN (Table 39.2) via multiple mechanisms:

**Table 39.2** Weight loss and hypertension risk (adapted from [2])

| Evidence statement | Strength of evidence |
|---|---|
| In overweight/obese adults with increased CV risk (including HTN or DM2), there is a dose-response relationship between weight loss achieved up to 3 years by lifestyle intervention and lowering BP<br>• 5% weight loss results in mean systolic and diastolic BP reductions of 3 and 2 mmHg, respectively<br>• <5% weight loss has more modest and variable reductions in BP | High |
| Mean 5% weight loss achieved over 4 years by lifestyle intervention in overweight/obese adults with DM2 is associated with reduced antihypertensive medication prescriptions | Moderate |

**Table 39.3** Weight loss and Impact on cholesterol/lipid profiles (adapted from [2])

| Evidence statement | Strength of evidence |
|---|---|
| There is a dose-response relationship between weight loss and the improvement in lipid profile<br>• 3 kg weight loss leads to a mean triglyceride reduction of 15 mg/dl<br>• 5–8 kg weight loss lowers LDL-C approximately 5 mg/dl and increases HDL-C 2–3 mg/dl<br>• <3 kg weight loss has more modest and variable improvements | High |
| 5% weight loss achieved over 4 years in overweight/obese adults with DM2 is associated with reduced newly prescribed lipid-lowering medications | Moderate |
| Compared with placebo, Orlistat added to lifestyle intervention results in an average 3 kg greater weight loss and improved lipid profile | High |

- Obesity causes increases in renal sodium reabsorption, impairment in natriuresis and ultimately leads to extracellular volume expansion and elevated BP[15].
- Increased adiposity leads to RAAS activation and sympathetic system activation [17].
- The Physician's health study demonstrated approximately 8% increase risk of HTN per 1-unit increase in BMI [49].
- Weight loss can reverse some of the negative physiologic effects of obesity and reduce BP[1].
- The relationship between obesity and HTN has important prognostic implications considering the improved CVD outcomes with tight BP control in the SPRINT study [50].

### 39.6.2 Obesity and Dyslipidemia

Overweight/obesity increases CVD risk and leads to an unfavorable lipid profile (Table 39.3), such as increased fasting plasma triglycerides, higher LDL-C and lower HDL-C [49].

- Chylomicron remnants and LDL-C may migrate into the sub-endothelium and become trapped [51].

  - Remnants of chylomicrons and very low density lipoprotein are involved in the development of atherosclerosis [52].
- Treatment of obesity related dyslipidemia should focus on lifestyle changes including weight loss, physical activity (PA) and healthful diet.
  - PA has been shown to increase lipase activity which stimulates triglyceride lipolysis, possibly due to increased muscular lipase activity [51].

### 39.6.3 Obesity and Diabetes Mellitus

Globally, obesity is a bigger health crisis than hunger, and is the leading cause of death and disability around the world [53]. Obesity is also a major risk factor for diabetes mellitus (DM) and trends in the incidence and prevalence of DM have mirrored those of obesity (Table 39.4).

- Although historically thought to be an adult disease, increasing obesity prevalence among children and adolescents have resulted in increasing rates of DM among youth populations [53].
- It has been predicted that in 2030, DM will be prevalent in over 7.5% of the global population [16].
  - A direct relationship between DM and obesity has been demonstrated, and the pathogenesis is due to peripheral tissue insulin resistance [16].
- CVD is the leading cause of morbidity and mortality among individuals with DM, accounting for 68% of all DM deaths [54].
  - This excess risk of CHD in DM disproportionately affects women, such that DM completely eliminates or attenuates the CHD advantage of being female [53].
- For overweight and obese patients, a modest weight-loss goal of 5–10% can substantially reduce the risk of developing DM, and moderate-intensity PA such

**Table 39.4** Evidence for weight loss and risk of diabetes (adapted from [2])

| Evidence statement | Strength of evidence |
|---|---|
| Overweight/obese adults at risk for DM2, average weight loss of 2.5–5.5 kg can reduce the risk of DM2 by 30–60% | High |
| Overweight/obese adults with DM2, 2–5% weight loss with lifestyle intervention results in modest reductions in fasting plasma glucose (lowering hemoglobin A1c by 0.2% to 0.3%) | High |
| Overweight/obese adults who achieve greater weight loss at 1 year with lifestyle intervention have greater improvements in hemoglobin A1c. Weight loss of 5–10% is associated with hemoglobin A1c reductions of 0.6–1.0% | High |
| Overweight/obese adults with DM2 who lose more weight achieve greater reductions in plasma glucose concentrations (2–5% weight loss is achieved with clinically meaningful reductions of plasma glucose) | High |
| Overweight/obese adults with DM2 treated with orlistat with lifestyle intervention achieve 2–3 kg greater weight loss at 1 and 2 years than placebo with lifestyle intervention | High |

*DM* diabetes mellitus

as brisk walking for at least 150 min per week also plays an important role in reducing the risk of DM, even without weight loss [16].

### 39.6.4 Obesity and Heart Failure

Heart failure (HF) has been increasing in prevalence, alongside the increasing incidence of obesity. Despite therapeutic advances, morbidity and mortality after the onset of HF remain substantial [55].

- The Framingham study [55] demonstrated that every 1 kg/m$^2$ increase in BMI increased the risk of HF by 7% in women and 5% in men.
  - Approximately 11% cases of HF in men and 14% in women are attributable to obesity alone, and the contribution of obesity to the risk of HF has not been adequately recognized [55].

    The likelihood of HF increases as the duration of morbid obesity increases, up to a prevalence of almost 90% at 30 years [56].

    Elevated BMI was associated with an increased risk of HF, without evidence of a threshold, and this risk was evident in both sexes and not limited to those with extreme obesity [55].
- Kenchaiah et al. [55] suggested plausible mechanisms for increased HF in obesity:
  - Increased BMI is a risk factor for HTN, DM and dyslipidemia, all of which augment the risk for myocardial infarction (MI), an important antecedent of HF.

    In addition, HTN and DM independently increase the risk for HF.
  - Elevated BMI is associated with left ventricular remodeling and may account for the disproportionately greater prevalence of HF with preserved left ventricular function (compared to HF with reduced left ventricular function).
- It has been shown that the absence of HTN, DM and obesity at age 45 years and 55 years is associated with 73–86% lower risks for incident HF over the remaining life course compared to those with all 3 risk factors [57].
  - These data underscore the importance of preventing the development of risk factors in mid-life for decreasing the public health impact of HF.

### 39.6.5 Obesity and Coronary Heart Disease

The major effect of obesity on CHD risk is attributable to atherogenic dyslipidemia, metabolic syndrome and DM (Table 39.5) [1].

- According to the AHA, the current cut-points for overweight (BMI $\geq$ 25 kg/m$^2$) and obesity (BMI $\geq$ 30 kg/m$^2$) compared with normal weight are associated with elevated risk of combined fatal and nonfatal CHD [2].
  - The higher the BMI, the higher the risk of fatal and non-fatal CHD.

**Table 39.5** Current BMI cut-points with respect to coronary heart disease risk (adapted from [2])

| Evidence statement | Strength of evidence |
|---|---|
| The higher the BMI, the higher the risk of CHD, fatal and nonfatal CHD, ischemic and hemorrhagic stroke, fatal stroke, fatal and nonfatal CVD, risk of type 2 DM and all-cause mortality | Moderate |
| The current cut-points for overweight (BMI $\geq$ 25 kg/m$^2$) and obesity (BMI $\geq$ 30 kg/m$^2$) are associated with elevated risk of CHD and elevated risk of fatal CVD in men and women | Moderate |

*CHD* coronary heart disease, *CVD* cardiovascular disease, *DM* diabetes mellitus

- The INTERHEART study found that over 90% of the risk for acute MI is attributable to nine modifiable risk factors [58].
  - Dyslipidemia, the leading factor, could account for approximately 50% of the risk of developing acute MI.
- Although obese patients may have relatively normal LDL-C plasma levels, obese individuals typically have an increased proportion of smaller, denser and more atherogenic LDL-C particles [1], thus increasing their risk for atherosclerotic CVD.
- Obesity also increases CHD risk indirectly through its effect on related comorbidities, such as HTN, glucose intolerance, endothelial dysfunction and inflammation [53].
- The Nurse's health study found that obesity was associated with a nearly twofold higher risk of CHD even after adjustment for HTN, DM, dyslipidemia and family history, and this independent association between obesity and CHD was demonstrated in both men and women, even with small increases in BMI [53].

### 39.6.6 Obesity and Atrial Fibrillation

Atrial Fibrillation (AF) is the most common sustained arrhythmia with a projected prevalence that will rise from 5.2 million in 2010 to 12.1 million in 2030, driven primarily by our aging population [59]. Obesity is an independent risk factor for AF [60], and obese patients have been shown to have a 50% increased risk for developing AF [61].

- It has been shown that every 1-unit increase in BMI has been associated with an almost 4% increased risk of AF [62].
  - This increased prevalence of AF in obesity is multifactorial, and may be due to the increased prevalence of HTN, as well as increased left atrial size and volume [1].

    Obesity is also associated with left atrial enlargement, conduction slowing, conduction heterogeneity, increased interstitial fibrosis and myocardial lipidosis to result in increased spontaneous and induced AF [60].
- Obesity may also be a risk factor for progression of paroxysmal to persistent AF, which carries higher morbidity and mortality [9].

In summary, the available scientific evidence is clear that increasing obesity appears to have a causal effect on the development of various CVD risk factors and increasing the risk for various forms of CVD themselves, therefore leading to increased morbidity and mortality. Weight loss can improve outcomes, or even reverse some of these diseases.

## 39.7 Obesity and its Mortality Paradox

Despite the relationships of obesity with metabolic dysregulation and CVD presented earlier, there has been compelling evidence of survival benefits associated with obesity in populations with chronic disease; a phenomenon termed the obesity paradox.

- The obesity paradox has been found in individuals with both medically and surgically treated disease and extends to non-cardiac diseases, including renal and pulmonary diseases [63–66].
- The nadir of mortality occurs in the overweight group, with a U and/or reverse-J-shaped distribution of increasing mortality as BMI values diverge in the positive and negative direction (Fig. 39.5) [67–69].

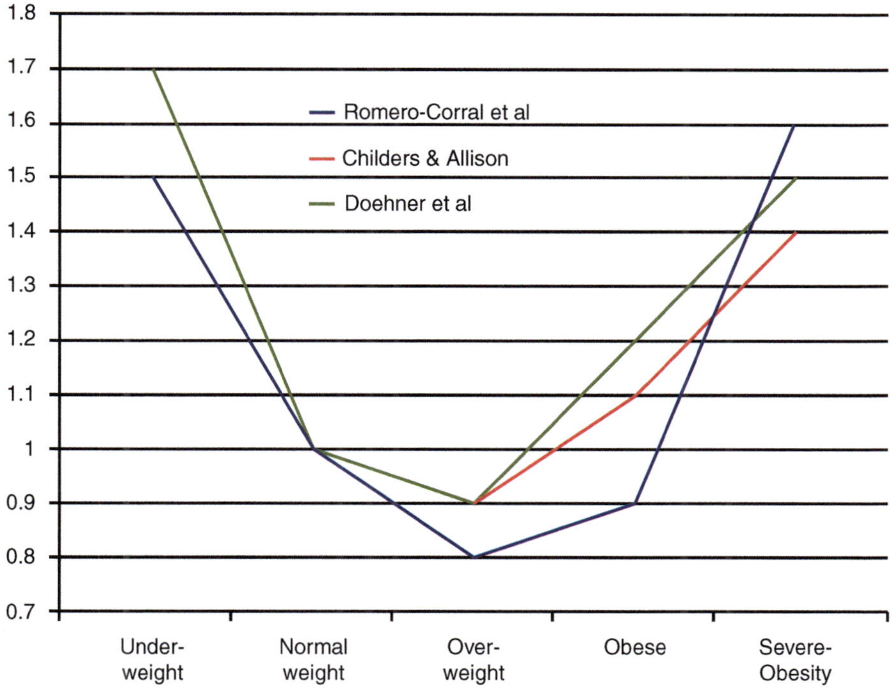


**Fig. 39.5** Obesity paradox by BMI in patients with CHD. Modelled relative risk from three studies of the obesity paradox, in each case normal weight is the comparison group. A U-shaped distribution is formed with the trough (lowest mortality risk) anchored in the overweight and obese groups. This visual representation does not denote the presence of absence of statistical significance (refs. are [65–67])

The reasons for the obesity paradox are thought to either come indirectly from increases in lean mass (LM) and earlier exposure to healthcare, or directly from body fat providing cytokine sequestration, or serving as a metabolic reservoir in those with severe chronic diseases with persistent catabolic states.

- Increases in LM associated with obesity have been found to have improved outcomes; the metabolically-healthy obese (MHO) [7].
- These benefits erode in the morbidly obese as increasing visceral adiposity increases the risk of developing metabolic syndrome and other precursors of CVD [70].
- Mortality benefits attributed to obesity have been found to be interrelated with cardiorespiratory fitness (CRF) [71–73].
  - When 10,000 patients divided into MHO and non-MHO groups were stratified by CRF, only those in the bottom 20th percentile for age and gender levels of CRF demonstrated an obesity paradox [74, 75].
- Cytokine sequestration is a possible protective mechanism due to increased production of soluble TNF receptors [76].
- Normal-weight individuals (whether healthy or chronically ill) have both low adiposity and lower LM. In this group weight loss often becomes the defining metric of outcomes.
  - When stratifying weight loss by fat loss, those with fat loss alone had a reduced risk of death by ~15%, while those with overall weight loss (including lean mass) had a ~35% higher mortality risk [77].
  - Stratifying weight loss by unintentional versus intentional weight loss also provides a basis for discriminating between outcomes:
    Intentional weight loss was associated with a 24% lower mortality compared with the mean while those with unintentional weight loss had a 31% higher mortality rate [78].
- Weight loss coupled with a fitness program has been associated with a significantly lower risk of combined CVD events and mortality regardless of baseline BMI [79].
- A study of associations with differing levels of BMI in chronic disease found that obese individuals had shorter overall survival but lived significantly longer with HF than those without obesity [80].

Based on current literature, the benefits of excess BMI on survival are greatest in the mildly obese and in those with obesity that is not complicated by CVD risk factors such as metabolic syndrome. Furthermore, the effects appear to be inversely related to the degree of CV fitness. In discussing the obesity paradox, it is perhaps most important to note that increasing CRF regardless of body mass has been shown to improve CV outcomes and longevity [81].

## 39.8 Cardiorespiratory Fitness

### 39.8.1 Definition

In 1923, Hill and Lupton [82] first described CRF as a plateau in oxygen uptake, above which further increases in exercise intensity produced no additional increase in oxygen uptake, representing the capacity of the circulatory-respiratory system.

### 39.8.2 Benefits of CRF

Besides being perhaps the strongest predictor for CVD and total mortality, CRF is also related to depression, dementia and various cancers [83]. In most cases, patients with major CHD risk factors (obesity, DM, HTN, etc.) and high CRF have lower mortality than patients without these risk factors but low CRF [83]. Thus, CRF seems to neutralize the negative impact of multiple traditional CVD risk factors [84].

### 39.8.3 Fat But Fit

Studies have shown that obese patients with higher levels of CRF ("fat but fit") have lower mortality than the non-fit, non-obese population [84–86]. These findings suggest that fitness is a more important predictor of CV health outcomes than BMI or adiposity alone.

- High levels of CRF largely neutralize the adverse effects of excess adiposity and other CVD risk factors [5, 84, 86].
  - It has been shown that overweight unfit individuals showed a significant mortality risk compared to normal weight fit individuals, while overweight individuals who were fit did not experience significant risk [85].

    Mortality in this study depended on the level of fitness, not BMI.
- Individuals who are unfit are at twice the risk of death compared to their fit counterparts, regardless of BMI [87].
- Differences in all-cause and CVD morbidity and mortality between MHO and normal weight individuals are largely explained by differences in CRF [88].
- CRF appears to have a stronger impact on CVD than individual risk factors, including obesity, such that efforts to improve CVD risk and outcomes in patients with obesity should focus not only on weight loss, but more importantly to increase fitness.
- Higher CRF level independently reduces mortality risk regardless of BMI [89].

- Studies have shown that the inverse association of BMI with mortality was nullified among patients with high fitness but persisted in those with low fitness [74].

### 39.8.4 Small Improvements in CRF Significantly Affect Mortality

According to available data, small improvements in CRF often translate into substantial benefits regarding overall health, morbidity and mortality [88].

- Each 1 metabolic equivalent (MET) increase in CRF has been associated with large (10–25%) improvements in survival [83].
- A meta-analysis by Kodama et al. [90] (n = 103,000) showed 13% and 15% reductions in CVD and all-cause mortality, respectively, per MET achieved.
  - Largest impact and health benefits were observed in the least fit groups of multiple studies, who improved their CRF.
- Therefore, not only do small improvements of CRF improve health outcomes, but they also seem to have the largest impact on the least fit individuals.

### 39.8.5 Optimal Exercise

- One large study, the Aerobics Center Longitudinal Study [91], followed 55,000 people (13,000 runners and 42,000 non-runners) over a mean of 15 years, and found that runners had 30% and 45% decreased all-cause and CVD mortality, respectively.
  - Those in the least intense ET program (<6 miles per week, 1–2 times per week, <51 min per week) had similar benefits to those with more intense training, and greater benefit than those in the highest intensity group.

    These results and other studies suggest that with running, the maximal effect on all-cause and CVD mortality occurs at low doses, well below the current major PA guidelines [92–94].
- These studies would suggest that low to moderate levels of PA/ET are associated with better outcomes than no exercise, as well as excess exercise, which can also have negative CV effects [95].

### 39.8.6 Physical Activity Guidelines

Exercise programs consistent with the minimum PA guidelines (150–300 min/week of moderate intensity PA or 75 min/week of vigorous intensity PA) are associated with CV health benefits (Table 39.6) [96].

- Patients seeking to lose weight without changing dietary habits require high PA levels (225–420 min/week of exercise).

**Table 39.6** Lifestyle Intervention (adapted from [2])

| Evidence statement | Strength of evidence |
|---|---|
| High intensity lifestyle intervention should include all 3 of the following: reduced-calorie diet (energy deficit ≥500 kcal/d), increased PA (≥150 min/week equal to ≥30 min/d most days of the week) and behavior therapy | High |
| Overweight/obese who participate in comprehensive lifestyle interventions consisting of all 3 components have average weight loss of up to 8 kg in 6 months of frequent on-site treatment | High |

*PA* physical activity

- For patients seeking to maintain weight loss, high levels of PA (200–300 min/week of moderate intensity PA) have been associated with improved weight maintenance compared to lower levels (<150 min/week).

As previously mentioned, various studies have demonstrated health benefits with PA levels well below those recommended in current PA guidelines. Therefore, current PA guidelines serve as a target PA level, rather than a minimum requirement.

### 39.8.7 CRF and Improved Outcomes in Various Types of Heart Disease

- In 2066 systolic HF patients followed up to 5 years, in patients with low CRF annual mortality was 8.2%, compared with 2.8% in those with high CRF ($p < 0.001$) [97].
- Multiple studies demonstrated a consistent dose-dependent inverse association between CRF and the risk of AF [60].
  - Higher CRF has been associated with greater arrhythmia-free survival in patients with existing AF.
- In patients with CHD, sustained PA has been associated with better survival than weight loss [98].

### 39.8.8 Advocacy for the Clinical Use of CRF

- CRF is one of the best predictors of health outcome, regardless of age, sex, ethnicity, body habitus, chronic disease risk factors or actual chronic disease [1].
- The evidence for CRF importance is so compelling that the AHA has advocated for the routine use of CRF as a vital sign [95].
- A policy statement from the AHA has suggested the need for a CRF database [83].

In summary, CRF appears to be the most important predictor of CV health and health outcomes. While there are clear health benefits from weight loss in those with obesity to reduce their overall CVD risk, the emphasis for treatment of patients with obesity should focus on increasing fitness, rather than weight loss alone.

## 39.9 Cardiac Rehabilitation and Cardiovascular Disease

Cardiovascular rehabilitation (CR) is a multi-disciplinary approach to develop and maintain an optimal level of physical, social, and psychological well-being in order to promote recovery from CV illness that has a Class I recommendation from both American and European cardiac societies [99, 100]. Beneficial CV effects include improving CHD risk factors; particularly exercise capacity, reversing cardiac remodeling, and favorably modifying metabolism and systemic oxygen transport. Major components of secondary prevention for CHD are formal CR and exercise training ET programs that have been shown to lower rates of recurrent MI, improve favorable ventricular remodeling, lower re-hospitalizations, and decrease mortality [101–104].

- Most CR programs have three phases that combine education, ongoing medical management, dietary modifications, lifestyle changes and structured ET to optimize recovery and decrease subsequent CVD morbidity and mortality.
  - Phase I: Inpatient enrollment: Education and early physical therapy with the goal of performing activities of daily living and transitions of care to outpatient CR facilities.
  - Phase II: Outpatient supervised exercise program that commonly consists of up to 12 weeks of supervised ET and aggressive risk factor reduction.

    Medical care includes patient assessment and aggressive risk factor management; the PA component consists of both education and supervision of a structured ET regimen with periodic reassessments [105].

    Efficacy is improved with psychosocial stress counseling and therapeutic education in cardioprotective lifestyle changes [106].
  - Phase III: Continuation of lifestyle changes learned in phase II, outside of a supervised healthcare setting with the goal of improving CVD outcomes, health-related quality of life, and mortality.
- CR programs have been shown to reduce mortality, morbidity, and hospital readmissions.
- CR currently has a class I recommendation for patients after an acute MI, heart failure, and coronary revascularization procedure [99, 100, 107].

Efforts at innovation in CR have focused on expanding the scope of education and support (adding structured psychosocial and lifestyle counseling), using mobile and home-based delivery, and innovating exercise protocols to improve outcomes [106, 108].

- Numerous studies have looked at high intensity interval training (HIIT) protocols versus the standard of moderate intensity continuous training (MICT).

- HIIT consists of short, high-intensity intervals (75–95% of maximal effort) interrupted by periods of rest [109].
- MICT involves continuous maintenance of workload at an intensity of 50–65% of the peak oxygen consumption or heart rate.
- HIIT regimens are superior in improving CRF when compared to MICT groups [110–113]:
  - Improvements in CV events found in HIIT groups over MICT participants can be attributed to improvements in CRF [114].

    Two recent randomized trials have found no significant differences in fitness and other parameters of health between HIIT and MICT protocols [115, 116].

    In both trials, there was loose adherence to protocol parameters, leading to overlap in metrics of intensity between the two groups, likely decreasing the resolving ability.
- Pre-surgical rehabilitation protocols (PREhabilitation) have shown better post-operative outcomes; reductions in hospital length of stay, time on mechanical ventilation, and lower medical complication rates have been found [117].

To date, studies of HIIT protocols suggest more benefits from higher intensity ET, and current AHA guidelines on PA have suggested duration of both moderate and high intensity exercises, but well controlled randomized controlled trials are needed to confirm these findings.

## 39.10 Impact of CR on the CVD Risk Factor Profile

- In one meta-analysis of CHD patients, total cholesterol and LDL-C levels were significantly decreased in patients in the comprehensive CR intervention, but not the ET-only group [118] .
- Another meta-analysis demonstrated reductions in total cholesterol and triglycerides, without improvements in LDL-C and HDL-C levels [119].
- A trend toward an improved lipid profile and BP was reported in another CR systematic review and meta-analysis, but the differences were not statistically significant [102].
- In randomized trials that prescribed and modulated medications within preventive and rehabilitative ET programs, significant reductions in LDL-C and systolic BP were noted. However, this was not the case in the ET-only interventions.
- In addition, one randomized trial that addressed ≥6 CVD risk factors during CR demonstrated a reduction in overall mortality, but no differences in overall mortality were present in more recent studies with adherence to guideline-directed medical therapies, that addressed fewer risk factors [106].

Based on available data, improvement in CHD risk factors observed with CR are closely linked to concomitant comprehensive medical management with ET-based programs, suggesting a critical role of risk factor modification in the secondary prevention of CHD.

## 39.11 Mortality Effects of CR

The benefits of regular PA on mortality in CHD patients has been examined in observational and case-control studies, establishing PA as one of the principal modifiers of mortality risk [58, 120].

- Early meta-analyses showed reductions in all-cause and CVD mortality of ~20–25% associated with CR [121, 122].
  - Represented middle-aged male post-MI survivors, with low proportions of women and elderly.
- Subsequent Cochrane reviews and newer meta-analyses showed reductions in mortality rates associated between 13–27% for all-cause and 26–36% for CVD mortality [102, 118, 119, 123].
- Over time, these benefits have decreased; a large meta-analysis of 25 randomized and non-randomized studies from 1995 onward showed continued mortality benefits [124].
  - However, a Cochrane review and meta-analysis of 63 randomized controlled trials between 1970 and 2014 showed that significant differences in all-cause mortality were absent (though CV mortality was still improved) [125].
    Subgroup analyses suggested that all-cause mortality becomes non-significant after 1995, and a meta-regression analysis demonstrated an overall gradual reduction in pooled total mortality over time.
- This was found in another meta-analysis spanning randomized controlled trials from 2010 to 2015 showing significant reductions in CVD, but not in all-cause mortality [106].
  - In a sub-group analysis of comprehensive CR programs, both all-cause and CVD mortality were significantly decreased.
- One possible explanation is that optimal medical therapy and advances in interventions likely play a major role in mortality benefit.
- Another is that mortality effects in later studies have been more realistic with the inclusion of more women and elderly in later trials.
- The van Halewijn study suggests that improved risk factor modification in comprehensive CR programs can make up for both demographic differences and therapeutic changes over time.
- Patient compliance with Phase II is one indicator of long-term retention of CR-associated lifestyle modification and is suggested to have a direct association with mortality benefits [126].

Given the current environment of shrinking healthcare funding, it will be crucial to identify the types of patients most likely to benefit from CR, as this will improve resource utilization in long-term management of CVD patients.

**Table 39.7** Dietary intervention (adapted from [2])

| Evidence statement | Strength of evidence |
|---|---|
| To achieve weight loss, an energy deficit is required, and techniques for reducing energy intake include:<br>• Energy intake target less than that required for an energy balance, usually 1200–1500 kcal/d for women and 1500–1800 kcal/d for men<br>• Estimation of individual energy requirements and prescription of an energy deficit of 500 kcal/d or 750 kcal/d or 30% energy deficit<br>• Restriction or elimination of particular food groups or provision of prescribed foods | High |

## 39.12 Weight Loss

Considering that obesity is generally attributed to an excess in energy consumption, to achieve weight loss, an energy deficit is required, which can be achieved by various dietary methods (Table 39.7). The AHA defines a comprehensive lifestyle intervention for weight loss and weight loss maintenance to include all 3 of the following: [2].

1. Prescription of a moderately reduced calorie diet.
2. A program of increased PA.
3. The use of behavioral strategies to facilitate adherence to diet and activity recommendations.
   - Comprehensive lifestyle programs typically prescribe increased aerobic PA (such as brisk walking) ≥150 min per week (equal to ≥30 min per day most days of the week) [2].
   - Higher levels of activity, approximately 200–300 min per week, are recommended to maintain lost weight or minimize long-term weight regain (>1 year) [2].

## 39.13 Conclusion

The increasing burden of obesity has taken a large toll on healthcare systems and the economy. Obesity is associated with many unfavorable physiologic changes that increase the risk for various types of CVD, which increase morbidity and mortality. Many of these diseases can be prevented, or even reversed with increased levels of PA/ET. The importance of CRF cannot be emphasized enough with respect to the role that it plays in maintaining health, in obese and non-obese persons alike. In fact, CRF is so important that, as discussed above, obese patients with higher CRF have been shown to have lower mortality than unfit non-obese adults, and the AHA has advocated for the use of CRF as a vital sign. Regarding obesity and CVD, although weight loss can be beneficial, increasing PA and CRF levels is of utmost importance.

**Clinical Pearls**

- Cardiorespiratory fitness (CRF) is perhaps the strongest predictor for CVD and total mortality, and the clinical emphasis for obese patients should be to increase fitness, rather than to lose weight.
- Increasing the level of CRF is not only beneficial for obesity, but for most lifestyle diseases.
- Obesity alone (as represented by high BMI) is not as important a predictor of health outcomes as the metabolic disturbances (HTN, DM, HLD, CVD) that some patients with obesity develop.

## Practice Questions

### Questions

1. An obese patient is undergoing routine clinical evaluation. The patient suffers from hypertension and diabetes mellitus, but in recent months has made lifestyle changes in an effort to improve his overall health. He has begun a regimen of brisk walking for 20 min, three days per week, and has started resistance training at the local gym for 40 min once per week (moderate intensity). He inquires if this is an effective regimen based on current physical activity guidelines, what is your response?
2. You are hired as a consultant for a clinic which has recently opened, which specializes in the primary prevention and treatment of cardiovascular diseases. The clinical manager requests your advice regarding cost-effective screening tools to combat the increasing obesity epidemic and cardiovascular diseases which are becoming more prevalent in the community. What advice can you give, based on the information in this chapter?
3. Two patients are evaluated at a follow-up visit, they both have New York Heart Association stage III congestive heart failure and have been hospitalized multiple times in the past year. Patient A is an obese male whose BMI has remained elevated at 30, despite multiple efforts to lose weight. Patient B is a formerly obese male whose BMI is now 18 (below normal) and states that he has been losing weight unintentionally. How would you classify these patients regarding their overall prognosis?

### Answers

1. This patient should be advised to increase his physical activity regimen to meet the current guidelines. The minimum physical activity guidelines include 150–300 min per week of moderate intensity physical activity or 75 min per week of

vigorous intensity activity which are associated with cardiovascular health benefits. This patient is only achieving 100 min per week of moderate intensity exercise, which does not meet the current guidelines.

2. The American Heart Association has advocated for the routine use of cardiorespiratory fitness as a vital sign in clinical practice, and this method has been adopted by large institutions, such as Kaiser Permanente, Intermountain Healthcare (Utah), and Greenville Health System (South Caroline). This is a vital marker of overall health that is much more important than measurements such as BMI alone, and can allow clinicians to more effectively select patients who require lifestyle modifications to improve their overall health and cardiovascular risk.
3. Patient B has a worse prognosis. There are multiple clinical teaching points in this question. First, unintentional weight loss is almost always a bad sign, typically representing some underlying disease process that is causing decreased appetite (e.g., abdominal congestion due to advancing heart failure) or stealing nutrition (e.g., rapidly advancing malignancy). Second, multiple hospitalizations are typically a sign of advancing disease, and both of these patients seem to be suffering from progressively worsening heart failure. Patient B who is obese and unable to lose weight would have the better prognosis according to the obesity paradox, possibly due to having increased metabolic reserve. Multiple studies have shown an obesity paradox in which obese patients tend to have better clinical outcomes compared to underweight (and sometimes normal weight) patients. Cachexia carries a devastating prognosis in many diseases, including heart failure.

## References


1. Lavie C, Arena R, Alpert M, Milani R, Ventura H. Management of cardiovascular diseases in patients with obesity. Nat Rev Cardiol. 2018;15(1):45–56. https://doi.org/10.1038/nrcardio.2017.108.
2. Jensen MD, Ryan DH, Apovian CM, et al. AHA/ACC/TOS guideline for the management of overweight and obesity in adults. J Am Coll Cardiol. 2013;63(25 Pt B):2985–3023. https://doi.org/10.1016/j.jacc.2013.11.004.
3. World Health Organization. Expert committee on physical status: the use and interpretation of anthropometric physical status. Geneva: World Health Organization; 1995.
4. Carbone S, Lavie CJ, Arena R. Obesity and heart failure: focus on the obesity paradox. Mayo Clin Proc. 2017;92(2):266–79. https://doi.org/10.1016/j.mayocp.2016.11.001.
5. Lavie CJ, McAuley PA, Church TS, Milani RV, Blair SN. Obesity and cardiovascular diseases: Implications regarding fitness, fatness, and severity in the obesity paradox. J Am Coll Cardiol. 2014;63(14):1345–54. https://doi.org/10.1016/j.jacc.2014.01.022.
6. Oliveros E, Somers VK, Sochor O, Goel K, Lopez-Jimenez F. The concept of normal weight obesity. Prog Cardiovasc Dis. 2014;56(4):426–33. https://doi.org/10.1016/j.pcad.2013.10.003.
7. Ortega FB, Lavie CJ, Blair SN. Obesity and cardiovascular disease. Circ Res. 2016;118(11):1752–70. https://doi.org/10.1161/CIRCRESAHA.115.306883.
8. Ortega FB, Sui X, Lavie CJ, Blair SN. Body mass index, the most widely used but also widely criticized index: would a criterion standard measure of total body fat be a better predictor of cardiovascular disease mortality? Mayo Clin Proc. 2016;91(4):443–55. https://doi.org/10.1016/j.mayocp.2016.01.008.

9. Lavie CJ, De Schutter A, Parto P, et al. Obesity and prevalence of cardiovascular diseases and prognosis-the obesity paradox updated. Prog Cardiovasc Dis. 2016;58(5):537–47. https://doi.org/10.1016/j.pcad.2016.01.008.
10. Nan C, Guo B, Warner C, et al. Heritability of body mass index in pre-adolescence, young adulthood and late adulthood. Eur J Epidemiol. 2012;27(4):247–53. https://doi.org/10.1007/s10654-012-9678-6.
11. Hebebrand J, Holm JC, Woodward E, et al. A proposal of the European association for the study of obesity to improve the ICD-11 diagnostic criteria for obesity based on the three dimensions etiology, degree of adiposity and health risk. Obes Facts. 2017;10(4):284–307. https://doi.org/10.1159/000479208.
12. Farooqi SI, O'Rahilly S. Human disorders of leptin action. J Endocrinol. 2014;223(1):T63–70. https://doi.org/10.1530/JOE-14-0480.
13. Ogden CL, Carroll MD, Kit BK, Flegal KM. Prevalence of obesity in the United States, 2009–2010. NCHS Data Brief. 2012;82:1–8.
14. Global Obesity Health Collaborators. Health effects of overweight and obesity in 195 Countries over 25 years. N Engl J Med. 2017;377(1):13–27. https://doi.org/10.1056/NEJMc1710026.
15. Parto P, Lavie CJ, Arena R, Bond S, Popovic D, Ventura HO. Body habitus in heart failure: understanding the mechanisms and clinical significance of the obesity paradox. Futur Cardiol. 2016;12(6):639–53. https://doi.org/10.2217/fca-2016-0029.
16. Riobo Servan P. Obesity and diabetes. Nutr Hosp. 2013;28(Suppl 5):138–43. https://doi.org/10.3305/nh.2013.28.sup5.6929.
17. Parto P, Lavie CJ. Obesity and cardiovascular diseases. Curr Probl Cardiol. 2017;42(11):376–94. https://doi.org/10.1016/j.cpcardiol.2017.04.004.
18. Lavie CJ, Sharma A, Alpert MA, et al. Update on obesity and obesity paradox in heart failure. Prog Cardiovasc Dis. 2016; https://doi.org/10.1016/j.pcad.2015.12.003.
19. Huang Y, Su L, Cai X, et al. Association of all-cause and cardiovascular mortality with prehypertension: a meta-analysis. Am Heart J. 2014;167(2):160–168.e1. https://doi.org/10.1016/j.ahj.2013.10.023.
20. Huang Y, Cai X, Li Y, et al. Prehypertension and the risk of stroke: a meta-analysis. Neurology. 2014;82(13):1153–61. https://doi.org/10.1212/WNL.0000000000000268.
21. Huang Y, Wang S, Cai X, et al. Prehypertension and incidence of cardiovascular disease: a meta-analysis. BMC Med. 2013;11(1) https://doi.org/10.1186/1741-7015-11-177.
22. Leiba A, Twig G, Vivante A, et al. Prehypertension among 2.19 million adolescents and future risk for end-stage renal disease. J Hypertens. 2017;35(6):1290–6. https://doi.org/10.1097/HJH.0000000000001295.
23. de Voorde J, Pauwels B, Boydens C, Decaluwé K. Adipocytokines in relation to cardiovascular disease. Metabolism. 2013;62(11):1513–21.
24. Visser M. Elevated C-reactive protein levels in overweight and obese adults. JAMA. 1999;282(22):2131. https://doi.org/10.1001/jama.282.22.2131.
25. Bell BB, Rahmouni K. Leptin as a mediator of obesity-induced hypertension. Curr Obes Rep. 2016;5(4):397–404. https://doi.org/10.1007/s13679-016-0231-x.
26. Alpert MA, Omran J, Mehra A, Ardhanari S. Impact of obesity and weight loss on cardiac performance and morphology in adults. Prog Cardiovasc Dis. 2013;56(4):391–400. https://doi.org/10.1016/j.pcad.2013.09.003.
27. Oishi K, Zheng B, Kuo JF. Inhibition of Na,K-ATPase and sodium pump by protein kinase C regulators sphingosine, lysophosphatidylcholine, and oleic acid. J Biol Chem. 1990;265(1):70–5.
28. Hall JE, Hildebrandt DA, Kuo J. Obesity hypertension: role of leptin and sympathetic nervous system. Am J Hypertens. 2001;14(6 Pt 2):103S–15S.
29. Stepniakowski KT, Goodfriend TL, Egan BM. Fatty acids enhance vascular alpha-adrenergic sensitivity. Hypertension. 1995;25(4 Pt 2):774–8.
30. Kachur S, Morera R, De Schutter A, Lavie CJ. Cardiovascular risk in patients with prehypertension and the metabolic syndrome. Curr Hypertens Rep. 2018;20(2):15. https://doi.org/10.1007/s11906-018-0801-2.

31. Libby P, Ridker PM, Hansson GK. Inflammation in Atherosclerosis. J Am Coll Cardiol. 2009;54(23):2129–38. https://doi.org/10.1016/j.jacc.2009.09.009.
32. Lumeng CN, Bodzin JL, Saltiel AR. Obesity induces a phenotypic switch in adipose tissue macrophage polarization. J Clin Invest. 2007;117(1):175–84. https://doi.org/10.1172/JCI29881.
33. Li P, Wang L, Liu C. Overweightness, obesity and arterial stiffness in healthy subjects: a systematic review and meta-analysis of literature studies. Postgrad Med. 2017;129(2):224–30. https://doi.org/10.1080/00325481.2017.1268903.
34. Samuel VT, Shulman GI. The pathogenesis of insulin resistance: integrating signaling pathways and substrate flux. J Clin Invest. 2016;126(1):12–22. https://doi.org/10.1172/jci77812.
35. Caballero AE. Endothelial dysfunction in obesity and insulin resistance: a road to diabetes and heart disease. Obes Res. 2003;11(11):1278–89. https://doi.org/10.1038/oby.2003.174.
36. Yang J, Park Y, Zhang H, et al. Role of MCP-1 in tumor necrosis factor-alpha-induced endothelial dysfunction in type 2 diabetic mice. Am J Physiol Heart Circ Physiol. 2009;297(4):H1208–16. https://doi.org/10.1152/ajpheart.00396.2009.
37. Tsao PS, Aoki N, Lefer DJ, Johnson G, Lefer AM. Time course of endothelial dysfunction and myocardial injury during myocardial ischemia and reperfusion in the cat. Circulation. 1990;82(4):1402–12.
38. Schächinger V, Britten MB, Zeiher AM. Prognostic impact of coronary vasodilator dysfunction on adverse long-term outcome of coronary heart disease. Circulation. 2000;101(16):1899–906.
39. Pepine CJ, Nichols WW. The pathophysiology of chronic ischemic heart disease. Clin Cardiol. 2007;30(2 Suppl 1):4–9. https://doi.org/10.1002/clc.20048.
40. Despres JP, Krauss RM. Obesity and lipoprotein metabolism. In: Handbook of obesity: etiology and pathophysiology. 2nd ed. New York: Marcel Dekker; 2004. p. 845–71.
41. Song G, Wu X, Zhang P, et al. High-density lipoprotein inhibits ox-LDL-induced adipokine secretion by upregulating SR-BI expression and suppressing ER Stress pathway. Sci Rep. 2016;6:30889. https://doi.org/10.1038/srep30889.
42. Tabas I, Williams KJ, Boren J. Subendothelial lipoprotein retention as the initiating process in atherosclerosis: update and therapeutic implications. Circulation. 2007;116(16):1832–44. https://doi.org/10.1161/CIRCULATIONAHA.106.676890.
43. Lee S, Park Y, Zuidema MY, Hannink M, Zhang C. Effects of interventions on oxidative stress and inflammation of cardiovascular diseases. World J Cardiol. 2011;3(1):18–24. https://doi.org/10.4330/wjc.v3.i1.18.
44. Lee S, Park Y, Dellsperger KC, Zhang C. Exercise training improves endothelial function via adiponectin-dependent and independent pathways in type 2 diabetic mice. Am J Physiol Heart Circ Physiol. 2011;301(2):H306–14. https://doi.org/10.1152/ajpheart.01306.2010.
45. Karasu C. Glycoxidative stress and cardiovascular complications in experimentally-induced diabetes: effects of antioxidant treatment. Open Cardiovasc Med J. 2010;4:240–56. https://doi.org/10.2174/1874192401004010240.
46. Besler C, Heinrich K, Rohrer L, et al. Mechanisms underlying adverse effects of HDL on eNOS-activating pathways in patients with coronary artery disease. J Clin Invest. 2011;121(7):2693–708. https://doi.org/10.1172/JCI42946.
47. Davignon J, Ganz P. Role of endothelial dysfunction in atherosclerosis. Circulation. 2004;109(23 Suppl 1):III27–32. https://doi.org/10.1161/01.CIR.0000131515.03336.f8.
48. Bastien M, Poirier P, Lemieux I, Després J-P. Overview of epidemiology and contribution of obesity to cardiovascular disease. Prog Cardiovasc Dis. 2013;56(4):369–81. https://doi.org/10.1016/j.pcad.2013.10.016.
49. Gelber RP, Gaziano JM, Manson JE, Buring JE, Sesso HD. A prospective study of body mass index and the risk of developing hypertension in men. Am J Hypertens. 2007;20(4):370–7. https://doi.org/10.1016/j.amjhyper.2006.10.011.
50. SPRINT Research Group. A randomized trial of intensive versus standard blood-pressure control. N Engl J Med. 2015;373(22):2103–16. https://doi.org/10.1056/NEJMoa1511939.
51. Klop B, Elte JWF, Cabezas MC. Dyslipidemia in obesity: mechanisms and potential targets. Nutrients. 2013;5(4):1218–40. https://doi.org/10.3390/nu5041218.

52. Cabezas MC, Erkelens DW. The direct way from gut to vessel wall: Atheroinitiation. Eur J Clin Investig. 1998;28(6):504–5. https://doi.org/10.1046/j.1365-2362.1998.00318.x.
53. Bhupathiraju SN, Hu FB. Epidemiology of obesity and diabetes and their cardiovascular complications. Circ Res. 2016;118(11):1723–35. https://doi.org/10.1161/CIRCRESAHA.115.306825.
54. Mozaffarian D, Benjamin E, Go A, et al. Heart disease and stroke statistics--2015 update: A report from the American Heart Association. Circulation. 2015;131(4):e29–322.
55. Kenchaiah S, Evans JC, Levy D, et al. Obesity and the risk of heart failure. N Engl J Med. 2002;347(5):305–13. https://doi.org/10.1056/NEJMoa020245.
56. Alpert MA, Terry BE, Mulekar M, et al. Cardiac morphology and left ventricular function in normotensive morbidly obese patients with and without congestive heart failure, and effect of weight loss. Am J Cardiol. 1997;80(6):736–40. https://doi.org/10.1016/S0002-9149(97)00505-5.
57. Ahmad FS, Ning H, Rich JD, Yancy CW, Lloyd-Jones DM, Wilkins JT. Hypertension, obesity, diabetes, and heart failure–free survival: the cardiovascular disease lifetime risk pooling project. JACC Hear Fail. 2016;4(12):911–9. https://doi.org/10.1016/j.jchf.2016.08.001.
58. Yusuf S, Hawken S, Ounpuu S, et al. Effect of potentially modifiable risk factors associated with myocardial infarction in 52 countries (the INTERHEART study): case control study. Lancet. 2004;364(9438):937–52. https://doi.org/10.1016/S0140-6736(04)17018-9.
59. Miller JD, Aronis KN, Chrispin J, et al. Obesity, exercise, obstructive sleep apnea, and modifiable atherosclerotic cardiovascular disease risk factors in atrial fibrillation. J Am Coll Cardiol. 2015;66(25):2899–906. https://doi.org/10.1016/j.jacc.2015.10.047.
60. Lavie CJ, Pandey A, Lau DH, Alpert MA, Sanders P. Obesity and atrial fibrillation prevalence, pathogenesis, and prognosis: effects of weight loss and exercise. J Am Coll Cardiol. 2017;70(16):2022–35. https://doi.org/10.1016/j.jacc.2017.09.002.
61. Wanahita N, Messerli FH, Bangalore S, Gami AS, Somers VK, Steinberg JS. Atrial fibrillation and obesity-results of a meta-analysis. Am Heart J. 2008;155(2):310–5. https://doi.org/10.1016/j.ahj.2007.10.004.
62. Wang TJ, Parise H, Levy D, et al. Obesity and the risk of new-onset atrial fibrillation. JAMA. 2004;292(20):2471–7. https://doi.org/10.1001/jama.292.20.2471.
63. Fonarow GC, Srikanthan P, Costanzo MR, Cintron GB, Lopatin M. ADHERE Scientific Advisory Committee and Investigators. An obesity paradox in acute heart failure: analysis of body mass index and inhospital mortality for 108,927 patients in the acute decompensated heart failure national registry. Am Heart J. 2007;153(1):74–81. https://doi.org/10.1016/j.ahj.2006.09.007.
64. Khaled S, Matahen R. Obesity paradox in heart failure patients – Female gender characteristics-KAMC single center experience. Egypt Hear J. 2017;69(3):209–13. https://doi.org/10.1016/j.ehj.2017.06.002.
65. Uretsky S, Messerli FH, Bangalore S, et al. Obesity paradox in patients with hypertension and coronary artery disease. Am J Med. 2007;120(10):863–70. https://doi.org/10.1016/j.amjmed.2007.05.011.
66. Stamou SC, Nussbaum M, Stiegel RM, et al. Effect of body mass index on outcomes after cardiac surgery: is there an obesity paradox? Ann Thorac Surg. 2011;91(1):42–7. https://doi.org/10.1016/j.athoracsur.2010.08.047.
67. Romero-Corral A, Montori VM, Somers VK, et al. Association of bodyweight with total mortality and with cardiovascular events in coronary artery disease: a systematic review of cohort studies. Lancet. 2006;368:666–78.
68. Childers DK, Allison DB. The 'obesity paradox': a parsimonious explanation for relations among obesity, mortality rate and aging? Int J Obes. 2010;34(8):1231–8. https://doi.org/10.1038/ijo.2010.71.
69. Doehner W, Clark A, Anker SD. The obesity paradox: weighing the benefit. Eur Heart J. 2010;31(2):146–8. https://doi.org/10.1093/eurheartj/ehp339.
70. Dhana K, Koolhaas CM, van Rossum EFC, et al. Metabolically healthy obesity and the risk of cardiovascular disease in the elderly population. PLoS One. 2016;11(4):e0154273. https://doi.org/10.1371/journal.pone.0154273.

71. Lavie CJ, De Schutter A, Milani RV. Healthy obese versus unhealthy lean: The obesity paradox. Nat Rev Endocrinol. 2015; https://doi.org/10.1038/nrendo.2014.165.
72. Katzmarzyk PT, Church TS, Blair SN. Cardiorespiratory fitness attenuates the effects of the metabolic syndrome on all-cause and cardiovascular disease mortality in men. Arch Intern Med. 2004;164(10):1092–7. https://doi.org/10.1001/archinte.164.10.1092.
73. Kokkinos P, Faselis C, Myers J, et al. Cardiorespiratory fitness and the paradoxical BMI-mortality risk association in male veterans. Mayo Clin Proc. 2014;89(6):754–62. https://doi.org/10.1016/j.mayocp.2014.01.029.
74. McAuley PA, Artero EG, Sui X, et al. The obesity paradox, cardiorespiratory fitness, and coronary heart disease. Mayo Clin Proc. 2012;87(5):443–51. https://doi.org/10.1016/j.mayocp.2012.01.013.
75. Ortega FB, Lee DC, Katzmarzyk PT, et al. The intriguing metabolically healthy but obese phenotype: cardiovascular prognosis and role of fitness. Eur Heart J. 2013;34(5):389–97. https://doi.org/10.1093/eurheartj/ehs174.
76. Mohamed-Ali V, Goodrick S, Bulmer K, Holly JM, Yudkin JS, Coppack SW. Production of soluble tumor necrosis factor receptors by human subcutaneous adipose tissue in vivo. Am J Physiol Endocrinol Metab. 1999;277(6 Pt 1):E971–5.
77. Allison DB, Zannolli R, Faith MS, et al. Weight loss increases and fat loss decreases all-cause mortality rate: results from two independent cohort studies. Int J Obes Relat Metab Disord. 1999;23(6):603–11.
78. Gregg EW, Gerzoff RB, Thompson TJ, Williamson DF. Intentional weight loss and death in overweight and obese U.S. adults 35 years of age and older. Ann Intern Med. 2003;138(5):383–9.
79. Sierra-Johnson J, Romero-Corral A, Somers VK, et al. Prognostic importance of weight loss in patients with coronary heart disease regardless of initial body mass index. Eur J Cardiovasc Prev Rehabil. 2008;15(3):336–40. https://doi.org/10.1097/HJR.0b013e3282f48348.
80. Ahmad FS, Ning H, Rich JD, Yancy CW, Lloyd-Jones DM, Wilkins JT. Hypertension, obesity, diabetes, and heart failure–free survival. JACC Heart Fail. 2016;4(12):911–9. https://doi.org/10.1016/j.jchf.2016.08.001.
81. Budoff MJ. Exercise capacity and biological age. Heart. 2016;102(6):415. https://doi.org/10.1136/heartjnl-2015-309008.
82. Hill AV, Lupton H. Muscular exercise, lactic acid, and the supply and utilization of oxygen. QJM. 1923;16(62):135–71. https://doi.org/10.1093/qjmed/os-16.62.135.
83. Kaminsky LA, Arena R, Beckie TM, et al. The importance of cardiorespiratory fitness in the United States: The need for a national registry: A policy statement from the American Heart Association. Circulation. 2013;127(5):652–62. https://doi.org/10.1161/CIR.0b013e31827ee100.
84. Oktay AA, Lavie CJ, Kokkinos PF, Parto P, Pandey A, Ventura HO. The interaction of cardiorespiratory fitness with obesity and the obesity paradox in cardiovascular disease. Prog Cardiovasc Dis. 2017;60(1):30–44. https://doi.org/10.1016/j.pcad.2017.05.005.
85. Barry VW, Baruth M, Beets MW, Durstine JL, Liu J, Blair SN. Fitness vs. fatness on all-cause mortality: A meta-analysis. Prog Cardiovasc Dis. 2014;56(4):382–90. https://doi.org/10.1016/j.pcad.2013.09.002.
86. Ortega FB, Ruiz JR, Labayen I, Lavie CJ, Blair SN. The Fat but Fit paradox: What we know and don't know about it. Br J Sports Med. 2017;52(3):151–3. https://doi.org/10.1136/bjsports-2016-097400.
87. Barry VW, Caputo JL, Kang M. The joint association of fitness and fatness on cardiovascular disease mortality: a meta-analysis. Prog Cardiovasc Dis. 2018;61(2):136–41. https://doi.org/10.1016/j.pcad.2018.07.004.
88. Ortega FB, Cadenas-Sanchez C, Migueles JH, et al. Role of physical activity and fitness in the characterization and prognosis of the metabolically healthy obesity phenotype: a systematic review and meta-analysis. Prog Cardiovasc Dis. 2018;61(2):190–205. https://doi.org/10.1016/j.pcad.2018.07.008.
89. Pedersen BK. Body mass index-independent effect of fitness and physical activity for all-cause mortality. Scand J Med Sci Sports. 2007;17(3):196–204. https://doi.org/10.1111/j.1600-0838.2006.00626.x.

90. Kodama S, Saito K, Tanaka S, et al. Cardiorespiratory fitness as a quantitative predictor of all-cause mortality and cardiovascular events in healthy men and women: a meta-analysis. JAMA. 2009;301(19):2024–35. https://doi.org/10.1001/jama.2009.681.
91. Lee DC, Pate RR, Lavie CJ, Sui X, Church TS, Blair SN. Leisure-time running reduces all-cause and cardiovascular mortality risk. J Am Coll Cardiol. 2014;64(5):472–81. https://doi.org/10.1016/j.jacc.2014.04.058.
92. Lavie CJ, Lee DC, Sui X, et al. Effects of running on chronic diseases and cardiovascular and all-cause mortality. Mayo Clin Proc. 2015;90(11):1541–52. https://doi.org/10.1016/j.mayocp.2015.08.001.
93. Lee DC, Lavie CJ, Sui X, Blair SN. Running and mortality: is more actually worse? Mayo Clin Proc. 2016;91(4):534–6. https://doi.org/10.1016/j.mayocp.2016.01.013.
94. chul LD, Brellenthin AG, Thompson PD, Sui X, Lee IM, Lavie CJ. Running as a key lifestyle medicine for longevity. Prog Cardiovasc Dis. 2017;60(1):45–55. https://doi.org/10.1016/j.pcad.2017.03.005.
95. Lavie CJ, Arena R, Swift DL, et al. Exercise and the cardiovascular system: Clinical science and cardiovascular outcomes. Circ Res. 2015;117(2):207–19. https://doi.org/10.1161/CIRCRESAHA.117.305205.
96. Piercy KL, Troiano RP, Ballard RM, et al. The physical activity guidelines for Americans. JAMA. 2018; https://doi.org/10.1001/jama.2018.14854.
97. Lavie CJ, Cahalin LP, Chase P, et al. Impact of cardiorespiratory fitness on the obesity paradox in patients with heart failure. Mayo Clin Proc. 2013;88(3):251–8. https://doi.org/10.1016/j.mayocp.2012.11.020.
98. Moholdt T, Lavie CJ, Nauman J. Sustained physical activity, not weight loss, associated with improved survival in coronary heart disease. J Am Coll Cardiol. 2018;71(10):1094–101. https://doi.org/10.1016/j.jacc.2018.01.011.
99. Amsterdam EA, Wenger NK, Brindis RG, et al. 2014 AHA/ACC guideline for the management of patients with non-ST-elevation acute coronary syndromes: executive summary: a report of the American College of Cardiology/American Heart Association task force on practice guidelines. Circulation. 2014;130(25):2354–94. https://doi.org/10.1161/CIR.0000000000000133.
100. Piepoli MF, Hoes AW, Agewall S, et al. 2016 European Guidelines on cardiovascular disease prevention in clinical practice: The sixth joint task force of the European society of cardiology and other societies on cardiovascular disease prevention in clinical practice. Eur Heart J. 2016;37(29):2315–81. https://doi.org/10.1093/eurheartj/ehw106.
101. Edelmann F, Gelbrich G, Düngen HD, et al. Exercise training improves exercise capacity and diastolic function in patients with heart failure with preserved ejection fraction: results of the Ex-DHF (Exercise training in Diastolic Heart Failure) pilot study. J Am Coll Cardiol. 2011;58(17):1780–91. https://doi.org/10.1016/j.jacc.2011.06.054.
102. Lawler PR, Filion KB, Eisenberg MJ. Efficacy of exercise-based cardiac rehabilitation post-myocardial infarction: a systematic review and meta-analysis of randomized controlled trials. Am Heart J. 2011;162(4):571–584.e2. https://doi.org/10.1016/j.ahj.2011.07.017.
103. Wisløff U, Støylen A, Loennechen JP, et al. Superior cardiovascular effect of aerobic interval training versus moderate continuous training in heart failure patients: a randomized study. Circulation. 2007;115(24):3086–94. https://doi.org/10.1161/CIRCULATIONAHA.106.675041.
104. Dunlay SM, Pack QR, Thomas RJ, Killian JM, Roger VL. Participation in cardiac rehabilitation, readmissions, and death after acute myocardial infarction. Am J Med. 2014;127(6):538–46. https://doi.org/10.1016/j.amjmed.2014.02.008.
105. Bethell HJ. Cardiac rehabilitation: from Hellerstein to the millennium. Int J Clin Pract. 2000;54(2):92–7.
106. van Halewijn G, Deckers J, Tay HY, van Domburg R, Kotseva K, Wood D. Lessons from contemporary trials of cardiovascular prevention and rehabilitation: a systematic review and meta-analysis. Int J Cardiol. 2017;232:294–303. https://doi.org/10.1016/j.ijcard.2016.12.125.

107. Hillis LD, Smith PK, Anderson JL, et al. 2011 ACCF/AHA guideline for coronary artery bypass graft surgery: executive summary: a report of the American college of cardiology foundation/American Heart Association task force on practice guidelines. J Thorac Cardiovasc Surg. 2012;143(1):4–34. https://doi.org/10.1016/j.jtcvs.2011.10.015.
108. Buckingham SA, Taylor RS, Jolly K, et al. Home-based versus centre-based cardiac rehabilitation: abridged Cochrane systematic review and meta-analysis. Open Heart. 2016;3(2):e000463. https://doi.org/10.1136/openhrt-2016-000463.
109. MacInnis MJ, Gibala MJ. Physiological adaptations to interval training and the role of exercise intensity. J Physiol. October 2016; https://doi.org/10.1113/JP273196.
110. Weston KS, Wisløff U, Coombes JS. High-intensity interval training in patients with lifestyle-induced cardiometabolic disease: a systematic review and meta-analysis. Br J Sports Med. 2014;48(16):1227–34. https://doi.org/10.1136/bjsports-2013-092576.
111. Milanović Z, Sporiš G, Weston M. Effectiveness of high-intensity interval training (HIT) and continuous endurance training for VO2max improvements: a systematic review and meta-analysis of controlled trials. Sports Med. 2015;45(10):1469–81. https://doi.org/10.1007/s40279-015-0365-0.
112. Rognmo Ø, Hetland E, Helgerud J, Hoff J, Slørdahl SA. High intensity aerobic interval exercise is superior to moderate intensity exercise for increasing aerobic capacity in patients with coronary artery disease. Eur J Cardiovasc Prev Rehabil. 2004;11(3):216–22.
113. Warburton DER, McKenzie DC, Haykowsky MJ, et al. Effectiveness of high-intensity interval training for the rehabilitation of patients with coronary artery disease. Am J Cardiol. 2005;95(9):1080–4. https://doi.org/10.1016/j.amjcard.2004.12.063.
114. Shiroma EJ, Sesso HD, Moorthy MV, Buring JE, Lee I-M. Do moderate-intensity and vigorous-intensity physical activities reduce mortality rates to the same extent? J Am Heart Assoc. 2014;3(5):e000802. https://doi.org/10.1161/JAHA.114.000802.
115. Ellingsen Ø, Halle M, Conraads V, et al. High-intensity interval training in patients with heart failure with reduced ejection fraction. Circulation. 2017;135(9):839–49. https://doi.org/10.1161/CIRCULATIONAHA.116.022924.
116. Conraads VM, Pattyn N, De Maeyer C, et al. Aerobic interval training and continuous training equally improve aerobic exercise capacity in patients with coronary artery disease: The SAINTEX-CAD study. Int J Cardiol. 2015;179:203–10. https://doi.org/10.1016/j.ijcard.2014.10.155.
117. Weston M, Weston KL, Prentis JM, Snowden CP. High-intensity interval training (HIT) for effective and time-efficient pre-surgical exercise interventions. Perioper Med. 2016;5(1) https://doi.org/10.1186/s13741-015-0026-8.
118. Jolliffe JA, Rees K, Taylor RS, Thompson D, Oldridge N, Ebrahim S. Exercise-based rehabilitation for coronary heart disease. Cochrane Database Syst Rev. 2000;4:CD001800. https://doi.org/10.1002/14651858.CD001800.
119. Taylor RS, Brown A, Ebrahim S, et al. Exercise-based rehabilitation for patients with coronary heart disease: systematic review and meta-analysis of randomized controlled trials. Am J Med. 2004;116(10):682–92. https://doi.org/10.1016/j.amjmed.2004.01.009.
120. Wannamethee SG, Shaper AG, Walker M. Physical activity and mortality in older men with diagnosed coronary heart disease. Circulation. 2000;102(12):1358–63.
121. Oldridge NB, Guyatt GH, Fischer ME, Rimm AA. Cardiac rehabilitation after myocardial infarction. Combined experience of randomized clinical trials. JAMA. 1988;260(7):945–50.
122. O'Connor GT, Buring JE, Yusuf S, et al. An overview of randomized trials of rehabilitation with exercise after myocardial infarction. Circulation. 1989;80(2):234–44.
123. Heran BS, Chen JM, Ebrahim S, et al. Exercise-based cardiac rehabilitation for coronary heart disease. Cochrane Database Syst Rev. 2011;7:CD001800. https://doi.org/10.1002/14651858.CD001800.pub2.
124. Rauch B, Davos CH, Doherty P, et al. The prognostic effect of cardiac rehabilitation in the era of acute revascularisation and statin therapy: A systematic review and meta-analysis of randomized and non-randomized studies – The Cardiac Rehabilitation Outcome Study (CROS). Eur J Prev Cardiol. 2016;23(18):1914–39. https://doi.org/10.1177/2047487316671181.

125. Anderson L, Oldridge N, Thompson DR, et al. Exercise-based cardiac rehabilitation for coronary heart disease. J Am Coll Cardiol. 2016;67(1):1–12. https://doi.org/10.1016/j.jacc.2015.10.044.
126. Hammill BG, Curtis LH, Schulman KA, Whellan DJ. Relationship between cardiac rehabilitation and long-term risks of death and myocardial infarction among elderly medicare beneficiaries. Circulation. 2010;121(1):63–70. https://doi.org/10.1161/CIRCULATIONAHA.109.876383.

# Exercise and Vascular Function

# 40

Nicolle Kränkel, Emeline van Craenenbroeck, and Volker Adams

**Learning Objectives**

After having read this chapter, you should be able to:

1. Explain how dysfunction and loss of the endothelial layer leads to a higher risk of cardiovascular events.
2. Explain how high LDL cholesterol levels modulate the development of atherosclerosis.
3. Explain how regular exercise affects the profile of circulating pro-and anti-inflammatory mediators.
4. Explain how exercise can modulate vascular stiffness and furthermore vascular function.
5. Name methodologies to investigate vascular function in a clinical/experimental setting.

N. Kränkel (✉)
Department of Cardiology, Charité–Universitätsmedizin Berlin, Berlin, Germany
e-mail: Nicolle.kraenkel@charite.de

E. van Craenenbroeck
Department of Cardiology, Antwerp University Hospital, Antwerpen, Belgium
e-mail: Emeline.Vancraenenbroeck@uantwerpen.be

V. Adams
Heart Center Dresden, Laboratory for Molecular and Experimental Cardiology, TU Dresden, Dresden, Germany
e-mail: Volker.adams@mailbox.tu-dresden.de





A. Pressler, J. Niebauer (eds.), *Textbook of Sports and Exercise Cardiology*,
https://doi.org/10.1007/978-3-030-35374-2_40

## 40.1 Introduction

The vascular system ensures delivery of nutrients and oxygen to the organs, drainage of toxic products and de-oxygenated blood from the organs, and inter-organ communication. While this prominent task at organ level is performed by the capillaries (below 10 μm in diameter), arteries and veins of increasing calibre perform different functions: the regulation of local blood flow to each organ or tissue, the adjustment of vessel diameter (which translates into pressure if blood volume remains constant) and the conductance of the flowing blood.

Two loops, the pulmonary and the systemic circulation, are powered by the pump work of the heart to drive re-oxygenation of the blood and to distribute re-oxygenized blood throughout the body.

The architecture of the whole vascular system, as well as the structure of the vascular wall at each level reflect these different tasks and also determine the typical symptoms of vascular dysfunction in the various cardiovascular diseases:

- **Capillaries**, where permeability needs to be high, but controlled, effect tissue oxygen and nutrient supply. These small vessels are more or less fenestrated—depending on the organ—and partially covered by pericytes on the abluminal side. Dysfunction and death of endothelial cells at this level of the vascular tree initially results in increased adhesion and extravasation of inflammatory cells and leakage of blood components into the surrounding tissue, aggravating the inflammatory response. Loss of microvessels due to endothelial cell death results in underperfusion of the limb or organ.
- At the next higher level, **resistance arteries** feature a small lumen and a well muscularised medial layer. Those vessels regulate blood flow at the organ level and are the main resistance vessels. Dysfunction and remodelling of these vessels results in hypertension and organ underperfusion.
- Walls of **large and medium-sized arteries** are multi-layered and well muscularised to convey stability as well as flexibility under the higher and alternating pressure conditions they are exposed to and furthermore prevent leakage of blood components. Especially haemodynamic flow patterns—velocity, laminar or turbulent flow—in combination with pressure-mediated strain and biochemical cues—e.g., inflammatory cytokines, fine particular matter—induce endothelial cell injury in larger arteries [1]. An inflammatory response is triggered, which leads to sub-endothelial deposition and modification of lipoproteins. Continued, unresolved inflammation furthermore drives atherosclerotic plaque growth and rupture, finally resulting in thrombogenic vessel occlusion [2, 3]. In the absence of atherosclerotic plaque rupture, thrombogenesis leading to coronary vessel occlusion may still occur due to loss of endothelial cells [4].
- **Veins** collect deoxygenated blood from the tissues and transport it back to the heart. Pressure is lower in the venous system, reflected by the thinner medial layer. In veins below hip level, valves prevent backflow. Skeletal muscle contractions—e.g., during walking—support venous function. Ageing and physical inactivity affect venous valve integrity, thereby allowing backflow of the blood into the lower

extremities and increasing venous pressure. In contrast to arterial thrombi, venous thrombus formation is not strongly associated with endothelial damage, but rather with a combination of enhanced pro-coagulant state and blood stasis. The specific flow conditions at the venous valves make them predilection sites of venous thrombus formation. Venous thrombi differ from arterial thrombi both in their distribution of fibrin and platelets as well as in their erythrocyte content.

The **three main layers** of the vascular wall (except capillaries) are (Fig. 40.1):

1. The **tunica intima**, containing the endothelium and the internal elastic membrane, providing an adhesion platform as well as survival signals for endothelial cells.
2. The **tunica media**, containing smooth muscle cells embedded in extracellular matrix to convey both stability and elasticity, and the external elastic membrane (arteries). The smooth muscle cell layer is thicker in the more highly pressurized arterial system than in the veins.
3. The **tunica adventitia**, containing fibroblasts, macrophages, and dendritic cells which conduct immune surveillance, *vasa vasorum*, which provide nutrient and oxygen supply, *nervi vasorum*, which convey contractile signals from the sympathetic nervous system, as well as perivascular adipose tissue, which can

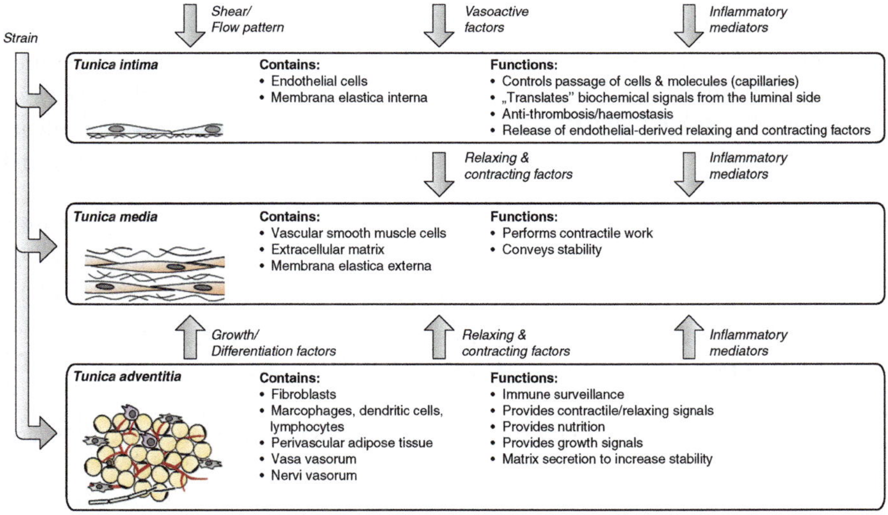


**Fig. 40.1** Schematic of a healthy arterial wall showing cell types and structures present and stimuli impacting upon vascular function. Physical forces, such as strain and shear stress are exerted by the pulse wave and blood flow patterns and impact directly or indirectly (via the endothelium) on smooth muscle cells and fibroblasts within the medial and adventitial layers. Circulating factors, including neuro-humoral mediators and lipoproteins, as well as circulating and cell-derived inflammatory mediators can act upon the endothelium or reach the media from the adventitial side (via vasa and nervi vasorum). The endothelium and perivascular adipose tissue process some of these signals, including vasoactive peptides and catecholamines

mediate and buffer sympathetic neurotransmitters and furthermore provides growth and inflammatory signals.

While the contractile activity of the medial smooth muscle cells realises the actual volume adjustments, the endothelium is a crucial regulator of smooth muscle cell contractile status (see also Box 40.1). Arterial smooth muscle cells also underlie regulation from the abluminal side: *nervi vasorum* deliver pro-contractile signals, *vasa vasorum* allow for the influx of leukocytes, and perivascular adipose tissue can provide growth and proliferation signals, in addition to mediating noradrenaline signals and regulating inflammatory status (Fig. 40.1) [5, 6].

**Box 40.1**

The term "Endothelial Dysfunction" refers to the loss of main functions of the endothelial layer:

- **Regulation of vascular tone:** The ability of the endothelium to balance vasoconstrictive with vasodilative mechanisms. Endothelial dysfunction results in a predominance of constrictive mechanisms.
- **Quiescence/selective permeability:** Dysfunctional endothelial cells exhibit a more inflammatory phenotype, including the synthesis of cytokines, expression of adhesion molecules, downregulation of intercellular junctions and loss of endothelial cells by detachment and apoptosis. This allows for lipoprotein deposition within the vascular wall and leukocyte recruitment resulting in vascular inflammation pertinent to atherosclerosis.
- **Anti-thrombotic activity:** In dysfunctional endothelium, pro-thrombotic effects predominate anti-thrombotic mechanisms, resulting in increased platelet adhesion and activation.

## 40.2 Mechanisms of Vascular Functional Regulation and its Dysregulation in Cardiovascular Disease

A number of physical and bio-chemical stimuli can regulate the function of the various vascular cells both acutely and chronically. Adaptations to non-injurious stimuli, such as adaptive intimal thickening due to increased flow or single occurrence of injurious stimuli, may not progress to atherosclerotic plaques, while repeated or chronic exposure to injurious signals and combination of multiple influencing factors results in dysregulated remodelling (Fig. 40.2).

Impaired functionality of the cells populating all vascular layers and beds can result in diverse clinical manifestations, including thrombosis with acute ischaemia of the heart, lung, brain, or limbs and chronic ischaemia of the skin, gut, or limbs.

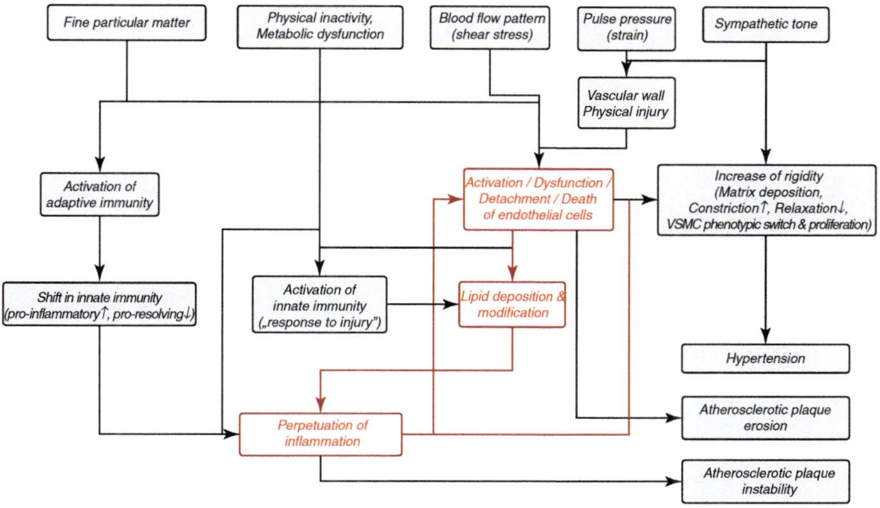


**Fig. 40.2** Main bio-chemical processes leading to vascular dysfunction in the persistent presence of physical and bio-chemical risk factors. At the centre, a triad of endothelial dysfunction, lipid deposition, and unresolved inflammation drives atherosclerotic plaque progression and instability as well as endothelial loss leading to plaque erosion—both can eventually initiate thrombotic coronary artery occlusion. Inflammatory mechanisms are also involved in a shift of endothelial-derived vasoactive factor release towards a more pro-contractile and less relax ative spectrum. Together with the mechanical strain affected by the pulse pressure and sympathetic tone, this leads to more contracted, stiffer resistance vessels and hypertension

### 40.2.1 Factors Regulating Vascular Tone

Under physiological conditions, the vascular endothelium and the perivascular adipose tissue, nerves and capillaries in the adventitia release a broad range of substances which induce relaxation or contraction in the medial smooth muscle cells momentarily (Table 40.1). Repeated mechanical injury and chronic exposure to certain bio-chemical factors such as

(a) Cytokines,
(b) Oxidative stress,
(c) Sympathetic messengers,
(d) Mediators of the renin-angiotensin-aldosterone system,
(e) Platelet-derived and coagulation factors

shift the balance of endothelial-derived relaxing-versus-contracting factors towards a pathological state [38, 39]. In addition, platelets, recruited to micro-injuries of the vascular wall and activated by loss of endothelial anti-thrombotic activity also are a source of vasoconstrictive factors, including serotonin and thromboxane [31].

**Table 40.1** Main factors and mechanisms affecting vascular smooth muscle cell tone

| Relaxing factors and mechanisms | Contracting factors and mechanisms |
|---|---|
| • **Nitric oxide** (NO) is released by endothelial cells in response to a number of stimuli. NO induces relaxation of the vascular smooth muscle cells in a cyclic adenosine monophosphate-dependent manner.<br>• **Prostacyclin** (prostaglandin I2; PGI2) induces smooth muscle cell relaxation via adenylate cyclase/cyclic adenosine monophosphate (cAMP) [7, 8], inhibits thromboxane $A_2$-induced platelet aggregation and vasoconstriction and influences the phenotype of vascular smooth muscle cells [9, 10]. Within the endothelial cell, prostacyclin conveys resistance to apoptosis [11].<br>• Even after inhibition of NO and prostacyclin-dependent pathways, one or more factors remain to mediate endothelial-dependent relaxation of smooth muscle cells [12]. This unknown factor or rather factors have been referred to as "**endothelium-derived hyperpolarizing factor**" (EDHF). Several candidates have been discussed, including epoxyeicosatrienoic acids (EETs) [13], potassium ions [14, 15], or a hydrogen sulfate leading to sulfhydration and thus activation of potassium channels [16], endocannabinoids [17] as well as C-type natriuretic peptide (CNP) [18].<br>• **Kinins** are mediators of the Kallikrein-Kinin-System. Bradykinin acts upon endothelial cells via G-protein coupled receptors, the most prominent being the kinin B2 receptor. Activation of the endothelial kinin B2 receptor leads to NO synthesis [19]. Bradykinin also induces cytoskeletal re-arrangement and loosening of tight junctions in endothelial cells, thereby increasing endothelial permeability.<br>• In general, **catecholamines** exert vasoconstrictive effects via α1-adrenergic receptors on vascular smooth muscle cells. However, α2-adrenergic receptors on endothelial cells can mediate the synthesis and release of NO and prostacyclin by endothelial cells, thus inducing smooth muscle cell relaxation [20, 21]. | • **Endothelin 1** (ET-1) is produced by vascular endothelial cells upon exposure to vasopressor hormones, platelet-derived factors, coagulation products, as well as cytokines and acts upon the smooth muscle cell endothelin receptors to induce contraction [22], albeit this mechanism is more relevant in pathological circumstances than in the physiological regulation of vascular tone [23]. ET-1 also causes a compensatory release of the vasodilators NO and prostacyclin [24].<br>• The Renin-Angiotensin-Aldosteron System (RAAS) produces a number of mediators with vasoactive properties, including **angiotensin II** and **aldosterone**. Both can bind to the angiotensin receptor 1 ($AT_1$) and initiate vasoconstriction [25] and pro-fibrotic mechanisms, including the deposition of collagen [26]. Aldosterone, via activating the vascular mineralocorticoid receptor, affects vascular tone regulation, thrombosis, inflammation, and vascular remodelling/fibrosis [27, 28]. In addition, angiotensin II and aldosterone can synergistically activate vasoconstriction, pro-inflammatory and pro-fibrotic mechanisms [29].<br>• **Vasopressin**, also termed anti-diuretic hormone, enhances water re-absorption in the distal tubule and collecting duct of the kidney via its V2 receptor. In addition, vasopressin acts via a second receptor – the V1 receptor – on vascular smooth muscle cells to increase vasoconstriction [30].<br>• Besides its role as a pro-coagulant factor, **thromboxane A2** also mediates endothelial-dependent contraction of arteries [31]. The endothelium-dependent contractions shown in hypertension, diabetes, atherogenesis, and other cardiovascular diseases have been significantly reduced by antagonism of cyclooxygenase, thromboxane synthase, or the thromboxane A2/prostanoid receptor.<br>• Sympathetic *nervi vasorum* release a number of vasoconstrictors, including **noradrenaline**, which induces contraction of vascular smooth muscle cells by binding to their $\alpha_1$ adrenergic receptors [32, 33] and **neuropeptide Y** [34, 35]. Noradrenaline may also derive from the perivascular adipose tissue [36, 37].<br>• **Serotonin** released from activated platelets induces contraction of vascular smooth muscle cells and potentiates the action of other vasoconstrictors (e.g. angiotensin II, noradrenaline). |

#### 40.2.1.1 Shear Stress and Strain

Blood vessels are permanently subjected to mechanical forces in the form of stretch, encompassing cyclic mechanical strain due to the pulsatile nature of blood flow, and shear stress. Blood pressure is the major determinant of vessel stretch. It creates radial and tangential forces affecting all cell types in the vessel. In comparison, fluid shear stress results from the friction of blood against the vessel wall, and it acts in parallel to the vessel surface. Accordingly, shear is sensed principally by endothelial cells, strategically located at the interface between the blood and the vessel wall. Several lines of evidence documented that mechanotransduction, a process converting physical forces into intracellular biochemical signals, is mediated by multiple mechanosensors [40]. Endothelial cells sense fluid shear stress by employing a wide repertoire of mechanosensors, including

(a) Junctional proteins (VE-cadherin, occludin) [41],
(b) Receptor kinases (vascular endothelial growth factor (VEGF) receptor 2 (VEGFR2) and others),
(c) Integrins,
(d) Focal adhesions (FAs) [42],
(e) G-proteins and G-protein coupled receptors (GPCRs) [43],
(f) Ion carriers (Piezo1) [44], and
(g) The glycocalyx.

Key molecules influenced by shear stress, which finally lead to changes in cell function, are endothelial nitric oxide synthase (eNOS) and enzymes regulating concentration of reactive oxygen species (ROS). With respect to shear stress we have to discriminate between unidirectional, laminar shear stress, in the range of 10–70 dyne/cm$^2$ in the arterial system which is atheroprotective, and turbulent/multidirectional shear at low or alternating velocities (<10 dyne/cm$^2$) which is implicated in the development of atherosclerotic lesions embedded in arterial bifurcations or tortuous arteries [40, 45]. Especially physiological shear stress induces the expression/activity of eNOS via several mechanisms including phosphorylation at specific sites (for review see [46, 47]) and increased expression via the activation of the transcription factor KLF2 [48, 49]. On the other hand, low shear results in vascular eNOS uncoupling (eNOS generates superoxide instead of nitric oxide) [50] and the inhibitory phosphorylation of eNOS at Thr495 via ERK1/2, thereby inhibiting eNOS function [51].

Cyclic strain has been shown to cause an increase in production of various vasoactive substances, including prostacyclin, ET-1, tPA, ROS, and monocyte chemotactic protein-1 (MCP-1) (Table 40.1) [52–54]. It also affects endothelial cell gene expression, and many transcription factors, including AP-1, cAMP response element binding protein (CREB), and NF-κB, are known to be involved in the cyclic strain-mediated regulation of gene expression [55, 56].

## 40.2.2 The Vascular Response to Injury—Unresolved Inflammation

Physical and/or bio-chemical micro-injuries to the endothelium and underlying vascular layers initiate a "**response to injury**" (see also Box 40.2), which involves the activation of platelets and the innate immune response. Persistence and repetition of injurious signals in individuals with high cardiovascular risk prevents the resolution of the inflammation, as would be typical for "healthy" wound healing.

**Box 40.2**

The ***response-to-injury*** concept describes atherosclerotic vascular disease initiation and progression as the result of a non-resolved, perpetuating inflammatory reaction, which does not result in wound healing, but in progressive and ultimately destructive vascular wall remodelling.

- Injuries are inflicted upon the endothelium by turbulent flow conditions – at sites of arterial bifurcations and curvatures [68]—in combination with mechanical strain exerted by the pulse wave [1] and toxic bio-chemical mediators, such as fine particular matter [69], oxygen and nitroso radicals and damage-associated molecular patterns.
- Acutely, these lead to inflammatory activation of endothelial cells—characterized by upregulation of adhesion molecules, downregulation of inter-endothelial cell junctions, enhanced motility and accelerated proliferation.
- As a result, permeability of the endothelial layer increases and low-density lipoproteins (LDL) and leukocytes can enter the sub-endothelial layer.
- Moreover, vasospasms—contraction of the smooth muscle cells—are induced by the endothelium early after vascular injury and activated platelets release pro-coagulant and pro-constrictive factors, including adenosine diphosphate (ADP), serotonin and thromboxane A2.
- Normally, wound healing would be induced by progression of the initial pro-inflammatory "defensive" M1-type macrophage response, which includes release of pro-oxidative and proteolytic enzymes, to a pro-resolving M2-type macrophage response, which employs efferocytosis and the release of "specialized pro-resolving mediators" [70].
- The continuous or repetitive presence of injurious stimuli in individuals with high cardiovascular risk prevents effective resolution of inflammation and tissue healing in favour of a continuous and/or constantly re-activated "defensive" M1 response.
- M1 macrophage response is supported by a $T_H1$-type adaptive immune response to antigens typical for metabolic dysfunction and injury (LDL, heat shock proteins) [71].
- Efferocytosis, crucial for the resolution of inflammation, becomes dysfunctional in prolonged atherosclerosis [72].

#### 40.2.2.1 Lipoproteins

The plasma lipoproteins transport cholesterol and triglycerides between the liver and tissues, where they may be used for synthesis of cellular organelles and hormones and serve as substrates in energy metabolism.

- High levels of **low-density lipoproteins (LDL)** in plasma are indicative of high amounts of cholesterol being transported from the liver towards the organs and are considered pro-atherosclerotic.
- High plasma levels of **high-density lipoproteins (HDL)** indicate a high flux of cholesterol from the tissues and organs towards the liver—a process called "reverse cholesterol transport". This is considered anti-atherosclerotic.

LDL binding to endothelial cells, smooth muscle cells and macrophages within the vascular wall leads to shuttling of cholesterol into the recipient cell. High intra-cellular cholesterol levels usually leads to down-regulation of the LDL receptor, preventing further cholesterol uptake. However, LDL can be oxidized and otherwise modified extracellularly and then bind to a different set of receptors, the so-called scavenger receptors [57], which are not downregulated at high intracellular cholesterol levels. Oxidized LDL therefore induces foam cell formation in vascular smooth muscle cells and macrophages. In endothelial cells, oxidized LDL induces the upregulation of adhesion molecules, which enhances the recruitment of leukocytes, downregulation of the cholesterol transporter ABCA1 and apoptosis [58, 59]. Oxidized LDL shifts the spectrum of endothelial-derived mediators controlling smooth muscle cell function away from the relaxant nitric oxide towards the vasoconstricting factor endothelin [60, 61].

HDL may stimulate outflow of cholesterol from the vascular wall and thus mediate regression of intravascular lipid deposits—at least in animal models [62]. In humans, targeting HDL in anti-atherosclerotic therapy has not been successful [63]. The reasons for this are likely complex, and include the modification of HDL in patients with cardiovascular or chronic kidney disease that reverses its anti-atherosclerotic and endothelial-protective action [64–67].

#### 40.2.2.2 Inflammation

Increased endothelial permeability allows for plasma lipoproteins to enter the sub-endothelial vascular wall, where they are retained by the extracellular matrix and prone to modification by macrophage-derived oxidative enzymes. Ingestion of oxidized LDL and attempted ingestion of cholesterol crystals by macrophages results in activation of inflammasome signalling and subsequent release of inflammatory cytokines such as interleukin-1β, foam cell generation, and macrophage death, giving rise to the lipid-rich necrotic core. Foamy macrophages cannot effectively perform efferocytosis, thus resolution of inflammation cannot be mounted, and vascular inflammation persists. The accumulation of cell debris and mediators released from dying cells—macrophages and smooth muscle cells—curbs macrophage infiltration and activation. In addition, LDL can be recognised as an antigen by CD4+ $T_H1$ cells, which promote macrophage polarisation towards the pro-inflammatory M1 phenotype [4, 71]. Effector molecules released from activated innate immune cells also include growth factors and proteases, which mediate intra-plaque angiogenesis and haemorrhage [73], smooth muscle cell proliferation and migration, as well as fibrous cap thinning and ultimately rupture—depending on their localization.

In contrast to plaque rupture, thrombus formation can also be initiated by erosion of the endothelial layer covering the culprit lesion [74].

### 40.2.3 Status of Pro−/Anti-oxidative Mechanisms

Homeostatic concentrations of reactive oxygen species (ROS) are an important factor in health and disease. A problem occurs when ROS bioavailability overtakes the antioxidant defences. In this situation, ROS act as destructive agents by affecting proteins, lipids and DNA, finally leading to cellular damage, tissue injury and inflammation. Vascular oxidative stress is the leading cause of cardiovascular diseases since it leads to vasoconstriction, vascular remodelling and fibrosis [77–79].

A variety of important ROS-producing systems are present in the vascular wall, including NADPH oxidase, xanthine oxidase, enzymes of the mitochondrial respiratory chain, and a dysfunctional, uncoupled eNOS [78, 80]. The major ROS produced in response to several stimuli, e.g. hyperlipidaemia or hypertension, is the superoxide anion ($O2^{\cdot -}$) that quickly reacts with nitric oxide (NO) to form peroxynitrite ($ONOO^{-}$), which decreases NO bioavailability and induces endothelial dysfunction [81–83]. Besides endothelial cells also vascular smooth muscle cells and invading and activated innate immune cells can be a source of ROS [84]. Various stimuli like increased cyclic stretch can promote ROS generation via up-regulation of lysyl oxidase (LOX) and NADPH oxidase. Activation of LOX is associated with enhanced oxidative stress that promotes p38MAPK activation, elastin structural alterations, and vascular stiffness thereby contributing to vascular abnormalities in hypertension [85]. As mentioned above increased ROS can also be attributed to a reduction in anti-oxidant defence. In the vascular wall, the primary antioxidant defence systems to neutralize ROS production are enzymatic detoxifiers such as

(a) Superoxide dismutases (MnSOD, CuZnSOD, EcSOD),
(b) Catalase,
(c) Glutathione peroxidase,
(d) Paraoxonase,
(e) Thioredoxin peroxidase, and
(f) Haeme oxygenases [86].

In addition, the transcription factor nuclear factor erythroid-2 related factor 2 (Nrf2) has also been shown to play a key role in establishing a cellular anti-oxidant defence mechanism against oxidative stress [87, 88] and is considered an important therapeutic target to manage vascular dysfunction [89].

### 40.2.4 Calcification

Besides the deposition of lipids and influx of inflammatory cells, deposition of calcium in the intimal and medial layers is a feature of atherosclerotic plaques.

- In larger elastic arteries, medial calcification leads to increased rigidity, thus increasing pulse wave velocity and pulse pressure, as well as systolic blood pressure.
- In arterioles, calcification can lead to organ ischaemia, e.g. in the skin and gut.
- Small vessel calcification occurs more frequently in patients of advanced age, diabetes and renal disease.

Beginning intimal calcification is associated with apoptotic smooth muscle cells and macrophages in lipid pools and early necrotic cores [75]. Subsequently, sheets of calcific deposit develop in proximity of and within the necrotic core. Microcalcification due to apoptotic smooth muscle cells and macrophages has also been observed in thin cap fibroatheromas, but a causative role of calcification and plaque rupture is still under discussion [75]. Microcalcifications then grow to form larger speckled and fragmented calcifications, especially in the deeper regions of the necrotic core. If calcified plates fracture, they may protrude into the lumen and initiate thrombus formation.

While a wide variety of factors—associated with genetic risk, ageing, oestrogen status and kidney function—might be implicated in the initiation of calcification of the intima and media in the different vascular beds, initial formation of micro-deposits by apoptotic smooth muscle cells and macrophages, as well as de-differentiation of smooth muscle cells into an osteoblast-like phenotype may be common processes.

While coronary calcification predicts generic risk of acute events, it does not characterize vulnerable lesions [76]. Instead, a number of observations indicate that calcium rather confers stability to plaques [75]. There may, however be a difference between the impact of smaller versus larger micro-calcifications on plaque stability [76].

## 40.3 Effect of Exercise on the Regulation and Dysregulation of Vascular Function

Physical activity over a sufficiently long-time course and with sufficient intensity elicits a number of systemic effects, ensuring adaptation of energy metabolism, thermal regulation and organ perfusion.

If repeated, skeletal muscle and vascular adaptations ensure improved effectivity of muscle work.

Factors mediating the effects of exercise on the vascular system include

(a) Physical forces of strain and shear,
(b) Sympathetic nerve activity,

(c) Systemic adaptation of energy metabolism (including the liver, adipose tissues and the skeletal muscle itself), as well as
(d) Anabolic factors released by the skeletal muscle.

In primary prevention, these mechanisms counteract the aforementioned processes contributing to increased cardiovascular risk: metabolic dysfunction, venous stasis and a shift towards more vasoconstrictive endothelium-mediated signalling.

### 40.3.1 Strain and Shear Stress

Increased shear stress during exercise improves vascular homeostasis by both, decreasing ROS and increasing NO bioavailability in the endothelium. In experimental [90–92] and in human studies [93–95] exercise training resulted in an activation of eNOS and a reduction of ROS, finally elevating NO bioavailability and subsequently endothelial function.

Determining the intensity and specific type of exercise that yields the optimal cardiovascular benefit is an area of still ongoing research. Already in 2003, Goto and colleagues investigated the optimal intensity to improve vascular function by assigning healthy adults to a mild (25% $VO_2$max), a medium (50% $VO_2$max) or high intensity (75% $VO_2$max) training regime for 12 weeks [96]. He clearly documented that only the medium exercise training group exhibited beneficial effects on vascular function. The authors speculated that in the high intensity exercise training group a threshold was surpassed where already an increased amount of ROS was generated, thereby reducing NO bioavailability. Together with results from other studies [97, 98] it is suggested that prolonged periods of intense exercise may cause excessive ROS generation, thereby negatively influencing vascular function. With respect to the question whether continuous exercise at moderate intensity (MCT) or high intensity interval training (HIIT) is superior for improving vascular function, the debate is still ongoing. Stimulated by the observation of Wisloff and colleagues in 2007 that in heart failure patients HIIT seems to be superior with respect to improved endothelial function several studies were initiated to compare both training modalities. Unfortunately, the results of Wisloff and colleagues could not be confirmed in larger clinical trials (see also Chap. 47) [99, 100].

Besides directly modulating NO bioavailability by increasing eNOS activation or expression, laminar shear stress is able to prevent inflammation-related alterations in eNOS levels and prostacyclin/thromboxane ratio [101].

### 40.3.2 Vasoactive Peptides and Hormones, Including Neurohumoral Activation

While the spectrum of endothelial-derived vasoactive factors shifts towards a more constrictive repertoire with age, in obesity, hypertension and with physical inactivity, these changes can be prevented, and even partially reversed, by habitual physical activity and participation in exercise programmes. In addition to a decline of plasma levels of vasoconstrictors, such as endothelin or noradrenalin, with regular exercise, also the sensitivity to those ligands partially declines, as seen for the $ET_A$ receptor [102]. This effect—known as functional sympatholysis in acute exercise—describes the ability to reduce the vasoconstrictive effects of noradrenaline in the active skeletal muscle and allowing for vasorelaxant effects to prevail in acute exercise, most likely through receptor desensitisation [103]. As discussed above, regular exercise increases nitric oxide synthesis, mainly through flow-dependent mechanisms, mediating vasorelaxation. In addition to the endothelium, also erythrocytes may release vasodilators while unloading oxygen from haemoglobin [104–107].

Underlying pathology, gene polymorphisms and exercise parameters, including duration and intensity, may mediate the effect, with higher intensities and durations usually achieving greater effects [102, 108, 109]. However, effects have already been shown with rather light exercises [110, 111], supporting a "something is better than nothing" approach.

Exercise training and habitual physical activity modulate the balance between vasodilating and vasoconstricting factors:

- **NO/ET-1 balance:** NO and ET-1 feedback on each other's synthesis and signalling. Habitual physical activity and participation in exercise training programmes are able to limit the age and morbidity-associated decline in NO and increase in ET-1 synthesis and can revert these pathological dysregulations.
  - Both, plasma levels [112, 113], and $ET_A$ receptor signalling are reduced by regular aerobic exercise in overweight and obese adults [102].
  - Several exercise programmes have been effective, including aerobic endurance and combined resistance/endurance exercise in men [112, 114, 115], young adolescent obese pre-hypertensive girls [116, 117] and post-menopausal hypertensive women [118].
  - While endothelin-related gene polymorphisms influenced the development of arterial stiffness over time, regular aerobic exercise attenuated arterial stiffening independently of endothelin-related genotype in a 10 year longitudinal study [119].
  - Exercise duration and intensity appear to impact on effect size, with longer duration and greater intensity, potentially mediated by $ET_A$ receptor function [108, 109, 112].
  - Yet, inactivity-mediated rises in ET-1 plasma levels could already be prevented by short resistance activities [110].
  - Animal experiments further point to enhanced kinin-mediated vasorelaxation after exercise training [120, 121].
- **Prostacyclin/thromboxane balance:** Both are downstream mediators of arachidonic acid, whose synthesis is controlled by cyclooxygenases.
  - Ageing, physical inactivity and hypertension have been reported to shift the balance towards the vasoconstrictor thromboxane.

  - This can be reversed by exercise training in normal and hypertensive participants [122].
  - Both, moderate continuous and high-intensity, high-amount exercise have been shown to be effective, with no comparative studies available [113].
  - There might, however, be an effect of intensity or extent of the underlying morbidity, as a 12-week treadmill training did not change thromboxane levels in a cohort of patients with peripheral artery disease [123], despite improvements in pain-free walking distance.
- **Sympathetic vasoconstrictors:** Sympathetic nerve activity is usually increased in cardiovascular disease. Exercise training can reduce or normalize sympathetic drive [124, 125].
  - Noradrenaline levels have been observed to decrease by water-based exercise in patients with resistant hypertension [111].
  - Exercise intensity might affect the extent of benefit conveyed, as HIIT achieved greater reductions in ET-1 plasma levels than equal-volume MCT in young women with high familial risk of hypertension [126].
  - A lack of decrease in plasma noradrenaline levels during a 3-month exercise programme was a strong predictor of cardiac mortality in patients with chronic heart failure [127].
- **Angiotensin II:** According to a recent meta-analysis, plasma levels of angiotensin II decrease with exercise [128].
  - In patients with stable coronary artery disease exercise resulted in downregulation of the AT1 receptor, accompanied by a reduction in angiotensin II-dependent vasoconstriction [94].
  - Exercise effects may be stronger in pathologic dysregulation of the renin-angiotensin-aldosterone system, as no differences in forearm vasoconstriction in response to angiotensin II were observed between elite athletic and sedentary healthy men, and exercise did not reduce plasma angiotensin II or aldosterone levels in healthy [129, 130].

### 40.3.3 Vascular Remodelling

The vascular layout is constantly re-organized, including the formation and stabilisation of new vessels (see also Box 40.3), the change in lumen diameter and wall architecture of existing vessels, as well as their regression. These processes are driven by blood flow and shear stress-dependent mechanisms as well as by hypoxia-dependent and -independent growth factors. Inflammatory cells take on a crucial role in the organisation and (de-) stabilisation of newly forming vascular networks [131]. In physiological angiogenesis, macrophages can localise to vessel branch points, promote vascular anastomosis and suppress tip cell sprouting, thus stabilising the newly formed anastomosis [131, 132]. In pathological angiogenesis, macrophages release proteases, which degrade extracellular matrix and modulate cytokine and growth factor activity, thereby leading to a less well-organised and less stable capillary network. Release of growth factors, such as the TGF-β, also contributes to increased rigidity of muscular arteries [133].

- Both, the number of capillaries per muscle fibre, as well as the vascular wall architecture are modulated by exercise training [134–137], reflecting an increased potential for nutrient and oxygen supply, as well as an increased conductance higher up in the vascular tree [138, 139].
- Of note, increased perfusion results from a combination of vasodilation, neovascularization, and (flow-mediated) stabilisation of neovessels as well as existing ones.
- Vascular adaptation to regular exercise is heterogeneous, with the muscles exercised and the type, duration and intensity of exercise impacting on the extent and contribution of each influencing process [140].

Sprouting angiogenesis in exercise training has been associated with an initial upregulation of hypoxia-inducible signalling, followed by a downregulation of the HIF-1 pathway upon regular exercise training, which likely contributes to stability of the newly formed vessels [141, 142]. Hypoxia-dependent and -independent growth factors, involved in exercise-mediated angiogenesis and vascular stabilisation, include vascular endothelial growth factor (VEGF) and angiopoietins, as well as the insulin-like growth factor 1 (IGF-1) [143–147]. In mice and men, also PDGF-levels in skeletal muscle were increased, supporting a stabilisation of microvessels [148, 149].

The pro-angiogenic effect of exercise is not limited to the exercising skeletal muscle:

- Increased angiogenesis of adipose tissue by exercise was associated to a reduction of pro-inflammatory cells and mediators in subcutaneous adipose tissue of overweight and obese adults [150].
- Differences were observed for insulin-resistant individuals, which showed an impaired angiogenesis response in adipose tissue, albeit an angiogenic response in the skeletal muscle was achieved [144].
- Increased coronary collateral flow was observed in patients with coronary artery disease after moderate- and high-intensity exercise training, albeit this might rely on a combination of pro-angiogenic and vasodilative mechanisms [151].

Habitual physical activity is associated with lower arterial stiffness [152, 153], and exercise interventions have shown a reduction of arterial stiffness [154]. TGF-β increase with ageing and ageing-associated arterial stiffening were reduced by aerobic exercise in both, mice and men [154]. TGF-β can increase oxidative stress in fibroblasts and increase collagen I deposition [154]. The data agree with human observations of increased oxidative stress being associated to large elastic artery compliance in habitually exercising versus sedentary postmenopausal women [155].

**Box 40.3**
Blood vessels can form and remodel by three main processes:

- **Angiogenesis** refers to the sprouting of a new capillary branch from an existing blood vessel. The main angiogenesis-inducing signal is tissue hypoxia. Depending on local distribution of angiogenic (growth factor) signals, the initially quiescent endothelial cells establish a hierarchy of "tip" and "stalk" cells. The tip cell protrudes filopodia, releases proteolytic enzymes to degrade the basement membrane and invades the tissue towards the angiogenic stimulus [156]. Signalling from the tip cell back towards the stalk cell limits filopodia formation in stalk cells and supports their proliferation, migratory behaviour to follow the tip cell-initiated sprout and lumen establishment. When meeting with another sprout, tip cells of both sprouts fuse to establish an anastomosis [132]. Flow- and macrophage-mediated mechanisms organise and stabilise newly formed anastomoses [131, 157].
- **Vasculogenesis** describes the de novo formation of blood vessels from angiogenic progenitor cells in situ. This process mainly takes place during embryogenesis [158]. Despite initial reports of adult vasculogenesis, strong supporting data are rare [159].
- **Arteriogenesis** denotes the remodelling of an existing arteriole, including the increase of lumen diameter and wall cellularity [160]. The main stimulus inducing arteriogenesis is flow.

## 40.3.4 Dysregulated and Dysfunctional Lipoproteins

In various primary prevention cohorts, exercise induced a modest, but clear and statistically significant increase in plasma HDL [113, 128, 161–163].

- Subjects with a higher initial plasma total cholesterol level and those who were less obese obtained a greater benefit from the exercise intervention [161].
  - Moreover, the effect size depended on exercise duration in endurance protocols—with the recommended duration of 30 min per day not being sufficient—but was not associated with exercise frequency or intensity [161].
- In patients with metabolic syndrome (MetS), HDL increase was only achieved in combined endurance/resistance training [164].
  - In addition, there was an indication that higher exercise intensities might achieve greater effects for HDL increase in MetS patients, but data directly comparing exercise modalities are scarce and it is therefore currently not possible to identify an "optimal" exercise intensity [164].

In patients with cardiovascular diseases or chronic kidney disease, the HDL particle is remodelled, resulting in a loss of anti-atherogenic or even a gain of pro-atherogenic properties [64, 65, 165].

- Endurance exercise was able to improve vascular effects of HDL, including endothelial cell NO synthesis [165].

Reduction of LDL by exercise intervention is less clear and appears to be tied to exercise-induced weight loss [166]. The effect of exercise on plasma LDL levels is likely modulated by a number of factors, such as underlying pathology and exercise modalities [128, 162–164, 166, 167]. Exercise volume might therefore have a larger impact on LDL reduction than exercise intensity [162]. LDL particle size and oxidation might provide additional insight into LDL pro-atherogenic effects, as small, dense LDL particles are associated with higher coronary artery stenosis [168] and oxidized LDL, more than unmodified LDL, exerts pro-atherogenic effects within the vascular wall and in platelet aggregation [58, 59].

- Exercise training with high volumes and at high intensities reduced the amount of small LDL particles and increased average size of LDL particles [162].
- Exercise training also appears to reduce LDL oxidation [169–172] and the susceptibility of platelets to oxidized LDL [173].
- Reduction of oxidized LDL might depend on exercise volume, similar to the findings reported for total LDL [162, 174].

The lipoprotein(a) (Lp(a)) is a sub-species of LDL, carrying the apolipoprotein (a) [apo(a)] and apoB. Lp(a) is a pro-atherogenic and anti-fibrinolytic factor [175]. Plasma concentrations of Lp(a) are mainly controlled through gene expression of the apo(a) and are highly heritable.

- Lp(a) levels have been reported to not change with exercise [176–178], while only one study reported a decrease of Lp(a) in exercising patients with chronic heart failure [179].

### 40.3.5 Status of Inflammatory Activation

Endurance training at low-to-moderate intensity has repeatedly been reported to lower levels of inflammatory markers, including C-reactive protein (CRP) [180–183], IL-18 [182], IL-1β [184] and IL-8 [185], while increasing IL-10 [182]. Effects of resistance training on the inflammatory profile varies, with a reduction in CRP, but controversial data for changes in IL-6 and TNF-α [186, 187].

- High-volume high-intensity exercise proved effective in men [113].
- A number of mechanisms are considered responsible for the anti-inflammatory effect of regular exercise training, including the reduction of adiposity as well as a range of anti-inflammatory and anabolic mediators released from the active skeletal muscle (referred to as "myokines" or "exerkines") [188].
- Especially in obese subjects, inflammation of the adipose tissue feeds into increased systemic levels of inflammatory cytokines. Reduction of body fat due to the higher energy expenditure reduces the pro-inflammatory activation of adipose tissue macrophages [188, 189]. This notion is in line with the observation

that exercise-mediated reduction in inflammatory status is more pronounced when it is associated with weight loss [190].
- In addition, exercise induces the release of adiponectin from adipose tissue, which harbours anti-inflammatory characteristics besides acting as a vasodilator [191–193].

The active skeletal muscle produces and releases a range of factors with systemic activity, chief among them is interleukin-6 (IL-6) [194, 195]. IL-6 in turn, can reduce the production of TNF-α and IL-1β [196, 197] and induce the release of IL-10 [198]. In line with this, exercise training can induce local reductions in TNF-α and IL-1β, even if these are not reflected by reduced plasma levels [199]. Nevertheless, the change in local cytokine levels might account for a systemic shift in the innate immunity towards a more pro-resolving phenotype [200, 201] and this would be in line with the observation of reduced toll-like receptor-4 expression on monocytes [202–205]. In addition, the regulatory arm of the adaptive immunity is upregulated by exercise [206, 207], supporting anti-inflammatory and pro-resolving mechanisms.

- A large number of studies have investigated anti-inflammatory effects of exercise, and while most support a lowering of inflammatory status, others could not find significant changes [190, 205, 208–211].
- Those data indicate a dependence on parameters such as underlying morbidities, especially metabolic and cardiovascular status, gender and exercise parameters.

### 40.3.6 Calcification

In endurance athletes with a life-long exercise volume > 2000 MET-min/week, a high coronary artery calcium score was observed (see also Chap. 32) [212]. In runners with atherosclerotic plaques, higher prevalence of purely calcified plaques and a lower prevalence of mixed plaques was reported in the most active as compared to the least active participants, indicating a more stable plaque phenotype [213, 214]. Life-long exercise might also exert different effects on calcification on men as compared to women [215]. In female marathon runners, coronary plaque load and calcium was lower than in sedentary women of comparable age and age was deemed the most relevant parameter for plaque formation in female athletes [216].

Overall, these results are usually interpreted as improvement of plaque stability with high life-long exercise volume [214].

Data on the effect of exercise training in patients with high cardiovascular risk are scarce.

- In patients with chronic kidney disease, exercise training led to a reduction of serum alkaline phosphatase (ALP), a putative risk factor for vascular calcification [217].
- In contrast, in obese patients, a 6-month walking-based training did reduce pulse wave velocity, but not osteoprotegerin, TRAIL or hsCRP. The authors therefore speculated that effects mainly were due to improved smooth muscle cell relaxation [218].

## 40.4 Methodology: Assessment of Vascular Function

### 40.4.1 Assessment of Vascular Endothelial Function: Coronary Versus Peripheral

Early studies focussed on **coronary** endothelial function and measured coronary artery diameter before and after administration of acetylcholine or other vasodilating stimuli. After the development of flow-sensitive wires, coronary flow reserve (CFR), defined as the ratio of coronary blood flow after the vasodilating stimulus over blood flow at rest, could be calculated. Invasive intracoronary measurement is considered the gold standard for CFR, but recently transthoracic echocardiography and position emission tomography (PET) have also been validated (Table 40.2).

For assessment of **peripheral** endothelial function, older studies used invasive venous occlusion plethysmography of the forearm. A vasodilating drug is directly infused in the brachial artery, and the rate of forearm swelling is recorded during venous occlusion. This technique has however largely been replaced by non-invasive techniques such as flow mediated dilatation (FMD) and peripheral arterial tonometry (PAT). The rationale for this technique is the fact that healthy arteries dilate in response to hyperaemia or pharmacologic stimuli via release of NO, whereas diseased arteries display reduced or absent endothelium-dependent vasodilatation.

An overview of available techniques is given in Table 40.2.

### 40.4.2 Non-invasive Assessment of Vascular Endothelial Function in Clinical Practice: FMD and PAT

Peripheral endothelial function can be easily measured in patients, and two different non-invasive techniques dominate the literature (Fig. 40.3).

#### 40.4.2.1 Flow-Mediated Dilation (FMD)

FMD uses high-resolution ultrasound to measure brachial (or radial) artery diameter before cuff occlusion and after cuff release at the distal vascular bed (the forearm). The increase in shear stress resulting from the distal reactive hyperaemia following cuff release, elicits a NO-dependent vasodilation. FMD is usually reported as percent increase in brachial artery diameter. It is an internationally standardised measurement for which several guidelines have been issued [229, 230].

1. FMD measures the response to shear stress in *conduit* vessels, which is *largely NO dependent.*
2. Possible drawbacks are
   (a) Strong operator-dependency of the technique
   (b) Steep learning curve
   (c) Lack of correction for systemic effects.

**Table 40.2** Techniques assessing endothelial function *in vivo* in patients

| Technique | Imaging modality | Invasive | Radiation | Vascular bed | Macro/micro | Measured parameter | Measurement | Operator dependent | Key reference |
|---|---|---|---|---|---|---|---|---|---|
| *Coronary vasculature* | | | | | | | | | |
| Coronary vasodilatation | Angiography | + | + | Coronary | Macro | % dilatation (mm) of left anterior descending artery | Manual | + | [219] |
| Coronary flow reserve | Intracoronary Doppler flow wire | + | + | Coronary | Micro | Ratio of hyperaemic flow vs baseline flow | Automatic | – | [220] |
| Coronary flow reserve | Ultrasound | – | – | Coronary | Micro | Ratio of hyperaemic flow vs baseline flow | Manual | + | [221] |
| Coronary flow reserve | Positron emission tomography | – | + | Coronary | Micro | Ratio of hyperaemic flow vs baseline flow | Semi-automatic | + | [222] |
| Coronary vasodilatation | Magnetic resonance imaging | – | – | Coronary | Macro | % dilatation (mm) of left anterior descending artery | Manual | + | [223] |
| *Forearm vasculature* | | | | | | | | | |
| Laser Doppler flowmetry | Laser Doppler | – | – | Skin | Micro | Skin erythrocyte flux | Automatic | – | [224] |
| Venous occlusion plethysmography | – | + | – | Forearm | Micro | Blood flow (ml/min/100 mL of forearm volume) | Automatic | – | [225] |
| Flow mediated dilatation | Ultrasound | – | – | Forearm | Macro | % dilatation of brachial artery | Semi-automatic | + | [226] |
| Peripheral arterial tonometry | – | – | – | Index finger | Micro | Ratio of hyperaemic signal vs baseline signal: reactive hyperaemia index | Automatic | – | [227] |
| *Leg vasculature* | | | | | | | | | |
| Flow mediated dilatation | Magnetic resonance imaging | – | – | Leg | Macro | % change in femoral artery area | Manual | – | [228] |

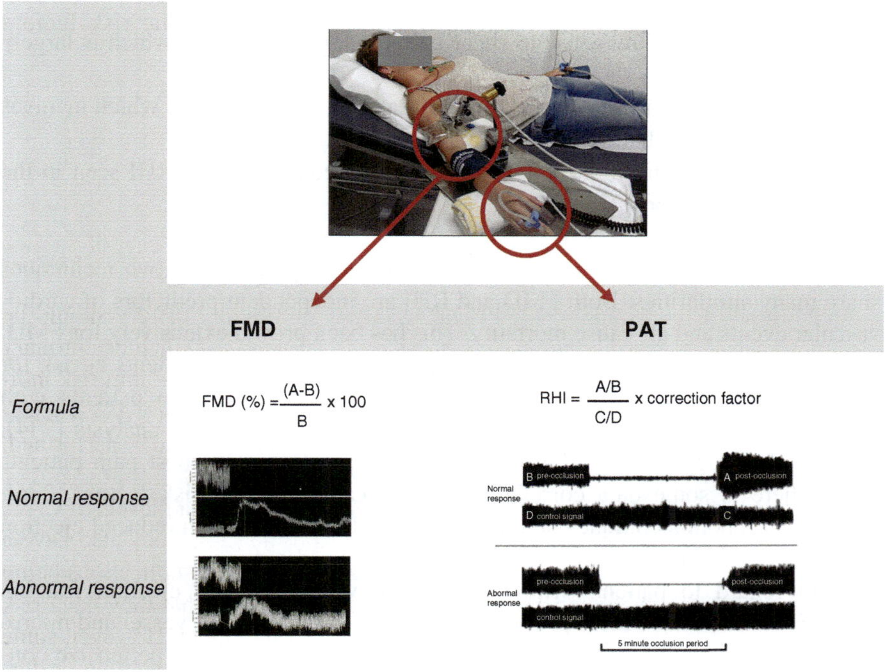


**Fig. 40.3** Non-invasive clinical assessment of vascular endothelial function using both *Flow-mediated dilation* (**FMD**) and *Peripheral arterial tonometry* (**PAT**) in the same patient, including the calculation of the particular parameter as well as an illustration of normal and abnormal responses (see text for detailed description)

### 40.4.2.2 Peripheral Arterial Tonometry (PAT)

PAT, commercialised in the EndoPAT® device (Itamar Medical, Israel), detects plethysmographic pressure changes in the finger tips caused by the arterial pulse and translates this to a peripheral arterial tone. Again, forearm occlusion and release are used to elicit a reactive hyperaemia. Measurements on the contralateral arm are used to control for concurrent changes in vascular tone, e.g. sympathetic activation [230]. Usually, PAT measurements are reported as reactive hyperemia index (RHI), the ratio of baseline to hyperemic peripheral arterial tone. It is an operator-independent technique using computerised analysis.

1. RHI measures the response to shear stress in the *micovasculature*, which is *not merely NO-dependent* [231].
2. A possible drawback is the price of the single-use finger probes.

#### 40.4.2.3 Comparison of FMD and PAT

- FMD measures the response to shear stress in *conduit* vessels, which is largely NO dependent.
- RHI, however, measures *microvascular* dilatation to shear stress, which involves other vascular mediators in addition to NO [232].
- This could explain the lack of correlation between FMD and RHI seen in the Framingham cohort [233].

Despite this functional difference, clinical data regarding the two techniques share many similarities. Both FMD and RHI are independent predictors of cardiovascular events and all-cause mortality. This has been proven extensively for FMD, in cohorts ranging from an unselected general population over patients at risk for cardiovascular disease (hypertension, chronic kidney disease) to patients with established cardiovascular disease, as described in a recent meta-analysis [234]. Besides one study linking RHI to cardiovascular outcome in chest pain patients [235], there is some data correlating RHI to cardiovascular risk factors [236]. Furthermore, both techniques predict survival in HF patients with reduced ejection fraction [236, 237].

With regard to patients with heart failure with preserved ejection fraction (HFpEF), it has been widely proven that they have both, conduit vessel and microvascular endothelial dysfunction, when compared to healthy or hypertensive controls (see Chap. 46) [238].

### 40.4.3 Effects of Physical Activity on Vascular Endothelial Function

As expected from above-mentioned molecular and cellular mechanisms, FMD and RHI are improved by physical activity, both in patients with cardiovascular risk factors (*primary prevention*) and in patients with established cardiovascular disease (*secondary prevention*):

- In asymptomatic patients with cardiovascular risk factors [239, 240].
- In coronary artery disease patients. A training program improves endothelial function as measured invasively or by FMD [100]. In one study, RHI did not change after training despite a significant improvement in FMD, possibly reflecting diverging effects on conduit vessel and microvascular function [241].
- In heart failure with reduced ejection fraction (HFrEF) patients, peripheral endothelial function (as measured invasively or by FMD) is improved by exercise training (see Chap. 47) [242].
- In heart failure with preserved ejection fraction (HFpEF) patients, Kitzman et al. failed to demonstrate an improvement of endothelial function, using brachial artery FMD as endothelial function measurement [243]. Studies on RHI as outcome measure are currently ongoing (OptimEx-Clin) [244].

In conclusion, FMD and RHI are measures of conduit vessel endothelial function and microvascular endothelial function, respectively. Although they share a prognostic value for cardiovascular events and mortality in diverse populations, the differences between both techniques are reflected in conflicting evidence of the beneficial effects of exercise in patients with cardiovascular disease.

**Clinical Pearls**

- Exercise is an essential stimulus for the maintenance of vascular health. Repeated episodic bouts of exercise induce functional adaptation of the arteries and, ultimately, structural arterial remodelling.
- These physiological adaptations in response to exercise training result in clear clinical benefits regarding the development of atherosclerosis and the occurrence of cardiovascular disease, including myocardial infarction and heart failure.

The magnitude of the effects on vascular function and structure are dependent on the type of training and are modulated by exercise-induced inflammation and oxidative stress.

## Review

### Questions

1. Which is the most prominent factor regulating vasodilation?
   (a) Bioavailability of nitric oxide (NO)
   (b) Degradation of extracellular matrix by matrix metalloproteases
   (c) Expression of ROS generating enzymes and subsequently the concentration of ROS.
   (d) The level of ATP generated by the mitochondria
2. Increased plasma levels of LDL cholesterol and low plasma levels of HDL cholesterol are associated with increased cardiovascular risk. How can regular exercise training affect HDL and LDL levels? Which exercise parameters (type, duration, intensity, frequency) impact on the outcome? Which patients benefit most?
   (a) HDL levels are increased by endurance exercise with longer exercise durations improving the effect.
   (b) Lipoprotein(a) is decreased by high-intensity training in non-diabetic individuals.
   (c) LDL is increased by combined endurance/resistance exercise.
   (d) LDL levels are reduced by high-intensity interval endurance exercise in MetS.
   (e) HDL levels are only increased in exercise interventions when the weight remains stable.

3. What is the underlying mechanism for vasodilation in response to cuff occlusion/release in healthy arteries?
   (a) Shear stress-induced NO production through mechanosensors in the endothelial cell
   (b) Accumulated ROS, generated during occlusion, suddenly flood the artery.
   (c) Temperature increase due to restored blood flow.
   (d) Hypoxia-induced signalling from the occluded region.
   (e) Oxygen-induced spike in NO production after the cuff has been released.

## Answers

1. (a) Bioavailability of nitric oxide (NO)
2. (a) HDL levels are increased by endurance exercise with longer exercise durations improving the effect.
3. (a) Shear stress-induced NO production through mechanosensors in the endothelial cell

## References


1. Franck G, Even G, Gautier A, Salinas M, Loste A, Procopio E, et al. Haemodynamic stress-induced breaches of the arterial intima trigger inflammation and drive atherogenesis. Eur Heart J. 2018;40(11):928–37.
2. Ross R. AtherosclerosisDOUBLEHYPHENan inflammatory disease. N Engl J Med. 1999;340(2):115–26.
3. Frostegard J, Ulfgren AK, Nyberg P, Hedin U, Swedenborg J, Andersson U, et al. Cytokine expression in advanced human atherosclerotic plaques: dominance of pro-inflammatory (Th1) and macrophage-stimulating cytokines. Atherosclerosis. 1999;145(1):33–43.
4. Kanwar SS, Stone GW, Singh M, Virmani R, Olin J, Akasaka T, et al. Acute coronary syndromes without coronary plaque rupture. Nat Rev Cardiol. 2016;13(5):257–65.
5. Gutterman DD. Adventitia-dependent influences on vascular function. Am J Phys. 1999;277(4):H1265–72.
6. Rey FE, Pagano PJ. The reactive adventitia: fibroblast oxidase in vascular function. Arterioscler Thromb Vasc Biol. 2002;22(12):1962–71.
7. Kukovetz WR, Holzmann S, Wurm A, Poch G. Prostacyclin increases cAMP in coronary arteries. J Cyclic Nucleotide Res. 1979;5(6):469–76.
8. Dusting GJ, Moncada S, Vane JR. Prostacyclin (PGX) is the endogenous metabolite responsible for relaxation of coronary arteries induced by arachindonic acid. Prostaglandins. 1977;13(1):3–15.
9. Tsai MC, Chen L, Zhou J, Tang Z, Hsu TF, Wang Y, et al. Shear stress induces synthetic-to-contractile phenotypic modulation in smooth muscle cells via peroxisome proliferator-activated receptor alpha/delta activations by prostacyclin released by sheared endothelial cells. Circ Res. 2009;105(5):471–80.
10. Moncada S, Higgs EA, Vane JR. Human arterial and venous tissues generate prostacyclin (prostaglandin x), a potent inhibitor of platelet aggregation. Lancet. 1977;1(8001):18–20.
11. Liou JY, Lee S, Ghelani D, Matijevic-Aleksic N, Wu KK. Protection of endothelial survival by peroxisome proliferator-activated receptor-delta mediated 14-3-3 upregulation. Arterioscler Thromb Vasc Biol. 2006;26(7):1481–7.

12. Luksha L, Agewall S, Kublickiene K. Endothelium-derived hyperpolarizing factor in vascular physiology and cardiovascular disease. Atherosclerosis. 2009;202(2):330–44.
13. Campbell WB, Gebremedhin D, Pratt PF, Harder DR. Identification of epoxyeicosatrienoic acids as endothelium-derived hyperpolarizing factors. Circ Res. 1996;78(3):415–23.
14. Edwards G, Dora KA, Gardener MJ, Garland CJ, Weston AH. K+ is an endothelium-derived hyperpolarizing factor in rat arteries. Nature. 1998;396(6708):269–72.
15. Feletou M, Vanhoutte PM. Endothelium-dependent hyperpolarization of vascular smooth muscle cells. Acta Pharmacol Sin. 2000;21(1):1–18.
16. Mustafa AK, Sikka G, Gazi SK, Steppan J, Jung SM, Bhunia AK, et al. Hydrogen sulfide as endothelium-derived hyperpolarizing factor sulfhydrates potassium channels. Circ Res. 2011;109(11):1259–68.
17. Randall MD, Alexander SP, Bennett T, Boyd EA, Fry JR, Gardiner SM, et al. An endogenous cannabinoid as an endothelium-derived vasorelaxant. Biochem Biophys Res Commun. 1996;229(1):114–20.
18. Chauhan SD, Nilsson H, Ahluwalia A, Hobbs AJ. Release of C-type natriuretic peptide accounts for the biological activity of endothelium-derived hyperpolarizing factor. Proc Natl Acad Sci U S A. 2003;100(3):1426–31.
19. Toda N, Bian K, Akiba T, Okamura T. Heterogeneity in mechanisms of bradykinin action in canine isolated blood vessels. Eur J Pharmacol. 1987;135(3):321–9. https://doi.org/10.1016/0014-2999(87)90681-9.
20. Boer C, Scheffer GJ, de Lange JJ, Westerhof N, Sipkema P. Alpha-1-adrenoceptor stimulation induces nitric oxide release in rat pulmonary arteries. J Vasc Res. 1999;36(1):79–81.
21. Zschauer AO, Sielczak MW, Smith DA, Wanner A. Norepinephrine-induced contraction of isolated rabbit bronchial artery: role of alpha 1- and alpha 2-adrenoceptor activation. J Appl Physiol (1985). 1997;82(6):1918–25.
22. Seo B, Oemar BS, Siebenmann R, von Segesser L, Luscher TF. Both ETA and ETB receptors mediate contraction to endothelin-1 in human blood vessels. Circulation. 1994;89(3):1203–8.
23. De Mey JG, Vanhoutte PM. End o' the line revisited: moving on from nitric oxide to CGRP. Life Sci. 2014;118(2):120–8.
24. Zellers TM, McCormick J, Wu Y. Interaction among ET-1, endothelium-derived nitric oxide, and prostacyclin in pulmonary arteries and veins. Am J Phys. 1994;267(1 Pt 2):H139–47.
25. Yamada M, Kushibiki M, Osanai T, Tomita H, Okumura K. Vasoconstrictor effect of aldosterone via angiotensin II type 1 (AT1) receptor: possible role of AT1 receptor dimerization. Cardiovasc Res. 2008;79(1):169–78.
26. Ruperez M, Lorenzo O, Blanco-Colio LM, Esteban V, Egido J, Ruiz-Ortega M. Connective tissue growth factor is a mediator of angiotensin II-induced fibrosis. Circulation. 2003;108(12):1499–505.
27. Biwer LA, Wallingford MC, Jaffe IZ. Vascular mineralocorticoid receptor: evolutionary mediator of wound healing turned harmful by our modern lifestyle. Am J Hypertens. 2019;32(2):123–34.
28. Zhu CJ, Wang QQ, Zhou JL, Liu HZ, Hua F, Yang HZ, et al. The mineralocorticoid receptor-p38MAPK-NFkappaB or ERK-Sp1 signal pathways mediate aldosterone-stimulated inflammatory and profibrotic responses in rat vascular smooth muscle cells. Acta Pharmacol Sin. 2012;33(7):873–8.
29. Rautureau Y, Paradis P, Schiffrin EL. Cross-talk between aldosterone and angiotensin signaling in vascular smooth muscle cells. Steroids. 2011;76(9):834–9.
30. Vanner S, Jiang MM, Brooks VL, Surprenant A. Characterization of vasopressin actions in isolated submucosal arterioles of the intestinal microcirculation. Circ Res. 1990;67(4):1017–26.
31. Golino P, Ashton JH, Buja LM, Rosolowsky M, Taylor AL, McNatt J, et al. Local platelet activation causes vasoconstriction of large epicardial canine coronary arteries in vivo. Thromboxane A2 and serotonin are possible mediators. Circulation. 1989;79(1):154–66.

32. Marin EP, Jozsef L, Di Lorenzo A, Held KF, Luciano AK, Melendez J, et al. The protein acyl transferase ZDHHC21 modulates alpha1 adrenergic receptor function and regulates hemodynamics. Arterioscler Thromb Vasc Biol. 2016;36(2):370–9.
33. Hjemdahl P, Belfrage E, Daleskog M. Vascular and metabolic effects of circulating epinephrine and norepinephrine. Concentration-effect study in dogs. J Clin Invest. 1979;64(5):1221–8.
34. Ekblad E, Edvinsson L, Wahlestedt C, Uddman R, Hakanson R, Sundler F. Neuropeptide Y co-exists and co-operates with noradrenaline in perivascular nerve fibers. Regul Pept. 1984;8(3):225–35.
35. Rosano GMC, Tousoulis D, McFadden E, Clarke J, Davies GJ, Kaski JC. Effects of neuropeptide Y on coronary artery vasomotion in patients with microvascular angina. Int J Cardiol. 2017;238:123–7.
36. Ayala-Lopez N, Watts SW. New actions of an old friend: perivascular adipose tissue's adrenergic mechanisms. Br J Pharmacol. 2017;174(20):3454–65.
37. Ayala-Lopez N, Martini M, Jackson WF, Darios E, Burnett R, Seitz B, et al. Perivascular adipose tissue contains functional catecholamines. Pharmacol Res Perspect. 2014;2(3):e00041.
38. Touyz RM, Schiffrin EL. Signal transduction mechanisms mediating the physiological and pathophysiological actions of angiotensin II in vascular smooth muscle cells. Pharmacol Rev. 2000;52(4):639–72.
39. Endemann DH, Schiffrin EL. Endothelial dysfunction. J Am Soc Nephrol. 2004;15(8): 1983–92.
40. Chistiakov DA, Orekhov AN, Bobryshev YV. Effects of shear stress on endothelial cells: go with the flow. Acta Physiol (Oxf). 2017;219(2):382–408.
41. Rampersad SN, Wudwud A, Hubert F, Maurice DH. Adaptive phenotypic modulation of human arterial endothelial cells to fluid shear stress-encoded signals: modulation by phosphodiesterase 4D-VE-cadherin signalling. Cell Signal. 2016;28(7):741–8.
42. Russell-Puleri S, Dela Paz NG, Adams D, Chattopadhyay M, Cancel L, Ebong E, et al. Fluid shear stress induces upregulation of COX-2 and PGI2 release in endothelial cells via a pathway involving PECAM-1, PI3K, FAK, and p38. Am J Physiol Heart Circ Physiol. 2017;312(3):H485–h500.
43. Dela Paz NG, Melchior B, Frangos JA. Shear stress induces Galphaq/11 activation independently of G protein-coupled receptor activation in endothelial cells. Am J Physiol Cell Physiol. 2017;312(4):C428–c37.
44. John L, Ko NL, Gokin A, Gokina N, Mandala M, Osol G. The Piezo1 cation channel mediates uterine artery shear stress mechanotransduction and vasodilation during rat pregnancy. Am J Physiol Heart Circ Physiol. 2018;315(4):H1019–h26.
45. Green J, Yurdagul A Jr, McInnis MC, Albert P, Orr AW. Flow patterns regulate hyperglycemia-induced subendothelial matrix remodeling during early atherogenesis. Atherosclerosis. 2014;232(2):277–84.
46. Gielen S, Sandri M, Erbs S, Adams V. Exercise-induced modulation of endothelial nitric oxide production. Curr Pharm Biotechnol. 2011;12(9):1375–84.
47. Fleming I. Molecular mechanisms underlying the activation of eNOS. Pflugers Arch. 2010;459(6):793–806.
48. Boon RA, Horrevoets AJ. Key transcriptional regulators of the vasoprotective effects of shear stress. Hamostaseologie. 2009;29(1):39–40. 1–3
49. Wang W, Ha CH, Jhun BS, Wong C, Jain MK, Jin ZG. Fluid shear stress stimulates phosphorylation-dependent nuclear export of HDAC5 and mediates expression of KLF2 and eNOS. Blood. 2010;115(14):2971–9.
50. Zhang JX, Qu XL, Chu P, Xie DJ, Zhu LL, Chao YL, et al. Low shear stress induces vascular eNOS uncoupling via autophagy-mediated eNOS phosphorylation. Biochim Biophys Acta, Mol Cell Res. 2018;1865(5):709–20.

51. Kong X, Qu X, Li B, Wang Z, Chao Y, Jiang X, et al. Modulation of low shear stress-induced eNOS multisite phosphorylation and nitric oxide production via protein kinase and ERK1/2 signaling. Mol Med Rep. 2017;15(2):908–14.
52. Hishikawa K, Luscher TF. Pulsatile stretch stimulates superoxide production in human aortic endothelial cells. Circulation. 1997;96(10):3610–6.
53. Howard AB, Alexander RW, Nerem RM, Griendling KK, Taylor WR. Cyclic strain induces an oxidative stress in endothelial cells. Am J Phys. 1997;272(2 Pt 1):C421–7.
54. Iba T, Shin T, Sonoda T, Rosales O, Sumpio BE. Stimulation of endothelial secretion of tissue-type plasminogen activator by repetitive stretch. J Surg Res. 1991;50(5):457–60.
55. Du W, Mills I, Sumpio BE. Cyclic strain causes heterogeneous induction of transcription factors, AP-1, CRE binding protein and NF-kB, in endothelial cells: species and vascular bed diversity. J Biomech. 1995;28(12):1485–91.
56. Wung BS, Cheng JJ, Chao YJ, Hsieh HJ, Wang DL. Modulation of Ras/Raf/extracellular signal-regulated kinase pathway by reactive oxygen species is involved in cyclic strain-induced early growth response-1 gene expression in endothelial cells. Circ Res. 1999;84(7):804–12.
57. Kunjathoor VV, Febbraio M, Podrez EA, Moore KJ, Andersson L, Koehn S, et al. Scavenger receptors class A-I/II and CD36 are the principal receptors responsible for the uptake of modified low density lipoprotein leading to lipid loading in macrophages. J Biol Chem. 2002;277(51):49982–8.
58. Sata M, Walsh K. Oxidized LDL activates fas-mediated endothelial cell apoptosis. J Clin Invest. 1998;102(9):1682–9.
59. Li D, Mehta JL. Oxidized LDL, a critical factor in atherogenesis. Cardiovasc Res. 2005;68(3):353–4.
60. Myers PR, Wright TF, Tanner MA, Ostlund RE Jr. The effects of native LDL and oxidized LDL on EDRF bioactivity and nitric oxide production in vascular endothelium. J Lab Clin Med. 1994;124(5):672–83.
61. Dong Y, Wu Y, Wu M, Wang S, Zhang J, Xie Z, et al. Activation of protease calpain by oxidized and glycated LDL increases the degradation of endothelial nitric oxide synthase. J Cell Mol Med. 2009;13(9A):2899–910.
62. Badimon JJ, Badimon L, Fuster V. Regression of atherosclerotic lesions by high density lipoprotein plasma fraction in the cholesterol-fed rabbit. J Clin Invest. 1990;85(4):1234–41.
63. Karalis I, Jukema JW. HDL mimetics infusion and regression of atherosclerosis: is it still considered a valid therapeutic option? Curr Cardiol Rep. 2018;20(8):66.
64. O'Neill F, Riwanto M, Charakida M, Colin S, Manz J, McLoughlin E, et al. Structural and functional changes in HDL with low grade and chronic inflammation. Int J Cardiol. 2015;188:111–6.
65. Riwanto M, Rohrer L, Roschitzki B, Besler C, Mocharla P, Mueller M, et al. Altered activation of endothelial anti- and proapoptotic pathways by high-density lipoprotein from patients with coronary artery disease: role of high-density lipoprotein-proteome remodeling. Circulation. 2013;127(8):891–904.
66. Shroff R, Speer T, Colin S, Charakida M, Zewinger S, Staels B, et al. HDL in children with CKD promotes endothelial dysfunction and an abnormal vascular phenotype. J Am Soc Nephrol. 2014;25(11):2658–68.
67. Speer T, Rohrer L, Blyszczuk P, Shroff R, Kuschnerus K, Krankel N, et al. Abnormal high-density lipoprotein induces endothelial dysfunction via activation of Toll-like receptor-2. Immunity. 2013;38(4):754–68.
68. Kwak BR, Back M, Bochaton-Piallat ML, Caligiuri G, Daemen MJ, Davies PF, et al. Biomechanical factors in atherosclerosis: mechanisms and clinical implications. Eur Heart J. 2014;35(43):3013–20, 20a-20d.
69. Araujo JA, Nel AE. Particulate matter and atherosclerosis: role of particle size, composition and oxidative stress. Part Fibre Toxicol. 2009;6:24.

70. Fredman G, Hellmann J, Proto JD, Kuriakose G, Colas RA, Dorweiler B, et al. An imbalance between specialized pro-resolving lipid mediators and pro-inflammatory leukotrienes promotes instability of atherosclerotic plaques. Nat Commun. 2016;7:12859.
71. Stemme S, Faber B, Holm J, Wiklund O, Witztum JL, Hansson GK. T lymphocytes from human atherosclerotic plaques recognize oxidized low density lipoprotein. Proc Natl Acad Sci U S A. 1995;92(9):3893–7.
72. Kojima Y, Weissman IL, Leeper NJ. The role of efferocytosis in atherosclerosis. Circulation. 2017;135(5):476–89.
73. Kolodgie FD, Gold HK, Burke AP, Fowler DR, Kruth HS, Weber DK, et al. Intraplaque hemorrhage and progression of coronary atheroma. N Engl J Med. 2003;349(24):2316–25.
74. Burke AP, Farb A, Malcom GT, Liang YH, Smialek J, Virmani R. Coronary risk factors and plaque morphology in men with coronary disease who died suddenly. N Engl J Med. 1997;336(18):1276–82.
75. Otsuka F, Sakakura K, Yahagi K, Joner M, Virmani R. Has our understanding of calcification in human coronary atherosclerosis progressed? Arterioscler Thromb Vasc Biol. 2014;34(4):724–36.
76. Kelly-Arnold A, Maldonado N, Laudier D, Aikawa E, Cardoso L, Weinbaum S. Revised microcalcification hypothesis for fibrous cap rupture in human coronary arteries. Proc Natl Acad Sci U S A. 2013;110(26):10741–6.
77. Forstermann U, Xia N, Li H. Roles of vascular oxidative stress and nitric oxide in the pathogenesis of atherosclerosis. Circ Res. 2017;120(4):713–35.
78. Li H, Horke S, Forstermann U. Vascular oxidative stress, nitric oxide and atherosclerosis. Atherosclerosis. 2014;237(1):208–19.
79. Sena CM, Leandro A, Azul L, Seica R, Perry G. Vascular oxidative stress: impact and therapeutic approaches. Front Physiol. 2018;9:1668.
80. Stocker R, Keaney JF Jr. Role of oxidative modifications in atherosclerosis. Physiol Rev. 2004;84(4):1381–478.
81. Kanaan GN, Harper ME. Cellular redox dysfunction in the development of cardiovascular diseases. Biochim Biophys Acta Gen Subj. 2017;1861(11 Pt A):2822–9.
82. Fukai T, Ushio-Fukai M. Superoxide dismutases: role in redox signaling, vascular function, and diseases. Antioxid Redox Signal. 2011;15(6):1583–606.
83. Forstermann U. Nitric oxide and oxidative stress in vascular disease. Pflugers Arch. 2010;459(6):923–39.
84. Lim S, Park S. Role of vascular smooth muscle cell in the inflammation of atherosclerosis. BMB Rep. 2014;47(1):1–7.
85. Martinez-Revelles S, Garcia-Redondo AB, Avendano MS, Varona S, Palao T, Orriols M, et al. Lysyl oxidase induces vascular oxidative stress and contributes to arterial stiffness and abnormal elastin structure in hypertension: role of p38MAPK. Antioxid Redox Signal. 2017;27(7):379–97.
86. Santilli F, D'Ardes D, Davi G. Oxidative stress in chronic vascular disease: From prediction to prevention. Vasc Pharmacol. 2015;74:23–37.
87. Bryan HK, Olayanju A, Goldring CE, Park BK. The Nrf2 cell defence pathway: Keap1-dependent and -independent mechanisms of regulation. Biochem Pharmacol. 2013;85(6):705–17.
88. Lee C. Collaborative power of Nrf2 and PPARgamma activators against metabolic and drug-induced oxidative injury. Oxidative Med Cell Longev. 2017;2017:1378175.
89. Forstermann U. Oxidative stress in vascular disease: causes, defense mechanisms and potential therapies. Nat Clin Pract Cardiovasc Med. 2008;5(6):338–49.
90. Schmederer Z, Rolim N, Bowen TS, Linke A, Wisloff U, Adams V, et al. Endothelial function is disturbed in a hypertensive diabetic animal model of HFpEF: Moderate continuous vs. high intensity interval training. Int J Cardiol. 2018;273:147–54.
91. Couto GK, Paula SM, Gomes-Santos IL, Negrao CE, Rossoni LV. Exercise training induces eNOS coupling and restores relaxation in coronary arteries of heart failure rats. Am J Physiol Heart Circ Physiol. 2018;314(4):H878–h87.

92. Medeiros RF, Gaique TG, Bento-Bernardes T, Motta NA, Brito FC, Fernandes-Santos C, et al. Aerobic training prevents oxidative profile and improves nitric oxide and vascular reactivity in rats with cardiometabolic alteration. J Appl Physiol (1985). 2016;121(1):289–98.
93. Sandri M, Viehmann M, Adams V, Rabald K, Mangner N, Hollriegel R, et al. Chronic heart failure and aging - effects of exercise training on endothelial function and mechanisms of endothelial regeneration: Results from the Leipzig exercise intervention in chronic heart failure and aging (LEICA) study. Eur J Prev Cardiol. 2016;23(4):349–58.
94. Adams V, Linke A, Krankel N, Erbs S, Gielen S, Mobius-Winkler S, et al. Impact of regular physical activity on the NAD(P)H oxidase and angiotensin receptor system in patients with coronary artery disease. Circulation. 2005;111(5):555–62.
95. Hambrecht R, Adams V, Erbs S, Linke A, Krankel N, Shu Y, et al. Regular physical activity improves endothelial function in patients with coronary artery disease by increasing phosphorylation of endothelial nitric oxide synthase. Circulation. 2003;107(25):3152–8.
96. Goto C, Higashi Y, Kimura M, Noma K, Hara K, Nakagawa K, et al. Effect of different intensities of exercise on endothelium-dependent vasodilation in humans: role of endothelium-dependent nitric oxide and oxidative stress. Circulation. 2003;108(5):530–5.
97. Bergholm R, Makimattila S, Valkonen M, Liu ML, Lahdenpera S, Taskinen MR, et al. Intense physical training decreases circulating antioxidants and endothelium-dependent vasodilatation in vivo. Atherosclerosis. 1999;145(2):341–9.
98. Hoch AZ, Lynch SL, Jurva JW, Schimke JE, Gutterman DD. Folic acid supplementation improves vascular function in amenorrheic runners. Clin J Sport Med. 2010;20(3):205–10.
99. Ellingsen O, Halle M, Conraads V, Stoylen A, Dalen H, Delagardelle C, et al. High-intensity interval training in patients with heart failure with reduced ejection fraction. Circulation. 2017;135(9):839–49.
100. Conraads VM, Pattyn N, De Maeyer C, Beckers PJ, Coeckelberghs E, Cornelissen VA, et al. Aerobic interval training and continuous training equally improve aerobic exercise capacity in patients with coronary artery disease: the SAINTEX-CAD study. Int J Cardiol. 2015;179:203–10.
101. Grimm H, Kretzschmar J, Cook MD, Brown MD. The effects of exercise, aspirin, and celecoxib in an atherogenic environment. Med Sci Sports Exerc. 2018;50(10):2033–9.
102. Dow CA, Stauffer BL, Brunjes DL, Greiner JJ, DeSouza CA. Regular aerobic exercise reduces endothelin-1-mediated vasoconstrictor tone in overweight and obese adults. Exp Physiol. 2017;102(9):1133–42.
103. Mortensen SP, Gonzalez-Alonso J, Nielsen JJ, Saltin B, Hellsten Y. Muscle interstitial ATP and norepinephrine concentrations in the human leg during exercise and ATP infusion. J Appl Physiol. 2009;107(6):1757–62.
104. Pawloski JR, Hess DT, Stamler JS. Export by red blood cells of nitric oxide bioactivity. Nature. 2001;409(6820):622–6.
105. Cosby K, Partovi KS, Crawford JH, Patel RP, Reiter CD, Martyr S, et al. Nitrite reduction to nitric oxide by deoxyhemoglobin vasodilates the human circulation. Nat Med. 2003;9(12):1498–505.
106. Jagger JE, Bateman RM, Ellsworth ML, Ellis CG. Role of erythrocyte in regulating local O2 delivery mediated by hemoglobin oxygenation. Am J Physiol Heart Circ Physiol. 2001;280(6):H2833–9.
107. Ellsworth ML, Sprague RS. Regulation of blood flow distribution in skeletal muscle: role of erythrocyte-released ATP. J Physiol. 2012;590(20):4985–91.
108. Merkus D, Sorop O, Houweling B, Boomsma F, van den Meiracker AH, Duncker DJ. NO and prostanoids blunt endothelin-mediated coronary vasoconstrictor influence in exercising swine. Am J Physiol Heart Circ Physiol. 2006;291(5):H2075–81.
109. Merkus D, Houweling B, Mirza A, Boomsma F, van den Meiracker AH, Duncker DJ. Contribution of endothelin and its receptors to the regulation of vascular tone during exercise is different in the systemic, coronary and pulmonary circulation. Cardiovasc Res. 2003;59(3):745–54.

110. Climie RE, Wheeler MJ, Grace M, Lambert E, Cohen N, Owen N, et al. Simple intermittent resistance activity mitigates the detrimental effect of prolonged unbroken sitting on arterial function in overweight and obese adults. J Appl Physiol (1985). 2018;125:6.
111. Cruz LG, Bocchi EA, Grassi G, Guimaraes GV. Neurohumoral and endothelial responses to heated water-based exercise in resistant hypertensive patients. Circ J. 2017;81(3):339–45.
112. Davis PG, Ferguson MA, Alderson NL, Pate RR, Bodary PF, Durstine JL. Effect of exercise duration on plasma endothelin-1 concentration. J Sports Med Phys Fitness. 2005;45(3):419–23.
113. Santilli F, Vazzana N, Iodice P, Lattanzio S, Liani R, Bellomo RG, et al. Effects of high-amount-high-intensity exercise on in vivo platelet activation: modulation by lipid peroxidation and AGE/RAGE axis. Thromb Haemost. 2013;110(6):1232–40.
114. Nyberg M, Mortensen SP, Hellsten Y. Physical activity opposes the age-related increase in skeletal muscle and plasma endothelin-1 levels and normalizes plasma endothelin-1 levels in individuals with essential hypertension. Acta Physiol (Oxf). 2013;207(3):524–35.
115. Izadi MR, Ghardashi Afousi A, Asvadi Fard M, Babaee Bigi MA. High-intensity interval training lowers blood pressure and improves apelin and NOx plasma levels in older treated hypertensive individuals. J Physiol Biochem. 2018;74(1):47–55.
116. Son WM, Sung KD, Bharath LP, Choi KJ, Park SY. Combined exercise training reduces blood pressure, arterial stiffness, and insulin resistance in obese prehypertensive adolescent girls. Clin Exp Hypertens. 2017;39(6):546–52.
117. Sung KD, Pekas EJ, Scott SD, Son WM, Park SY. The effects of a 12-week jump rope exercise program on abdominal adiposity, vasoactive substances, inflammation, and vascular function in adolescent girls with prehypertension. Eur J Appl Physiol. 2019;119(2):577–85.
118. Son WM, Sung KD, Cho JM, Park SY. Combined exercise reduces arterial stiffness, blood pressure, and blood markers for cardiovascular risk in postmenopausal women with hypertension. Menopause. 2017;24(3):262–8.
119. Sugawara J, Tomoto T, Noda N, Matsukura S, Tsukagoshi K, Hayashi K, et al. Effects of endothelin-related gene polymorphisms and aerobic exercise habit on age-related arterial stiffening: a 10-yr longitudinal study. J Appl Physiol. 2018;124(2):312–20.
120. Silva JA Jr, Santana ET, Manchini MT, Antonio EL, Bocalini DS, Krieger JE, et al. Exercise training can prevent cardiac hypertrophy induced by sympathetic hyperactivity with modulation of kallikrein-kinin pathway and angiogenesis. PLoS One. 2014;9(3):e91017.
121. Mombouli JV, Nakashima M, Hamra M, Vanhoutte PM. Endothelium-dependent relaxation and hyperpolarization evoked by bradykinin in canine coronary arteries: enhancement by exercise-training. Br J Pharmacol. 1996;117(3):413–8.
122. Hellsten Y, Jensen L, Thaning P, Nyberg M, Mortensen S. Impaired formation of vasodilators in peripheral tissue in essential hypertension is normalized by exercise training: role of adenosine and prostacyclin. J Hypertens. 2012;30(10):2007–14.
123. Januszek R, Mika P, Nowobilski R, Maga P, Nizankowski R. The improvement of walking abilities and endothelial function after the supervised training treadmill program (STTP) in patients with peripheral artery disease (PAD) is not related to prostacyclin and thromboxane release. Int J Cardiol. 2016;222:813–8.
124. Fraga R, Franco FG, Roveda F, de Matos LN, Braga AM, Rondon MU, et al. Exercise training reduces sympathetic nerve activity in heart failure patients treated with carvedilol. Eur J Heart Fail. 2007;9(6–7):630–6.
125. Roveda F, Middlekauff HR, Rondon MU, Reis SF, Souza M, Nastari L, et al. The effects of exercise training on sympathetic neural activation in advanced heart failure: a randomized controlled trial. J Am Coll Cardiol. 2003;42(5):854–60.
126. Ciolac EG, Bocchi EA, Bortolotto LA, Carvalho VO, Greve JM, Guimaraes GV. Effects of high-intensity aerobic interval training vs. moderate exercise on hemodynamic, metabolic and neuro-humoral abnormalities of young normotensive women at high familial risk for hypertension. Hypertens Res. 2010;33(8):836–43.

127. Rengo G, Pagano G, Parisi V, Femminella GD, de Lucia C, Liccardo D, et al. Changes of plasma norepinephrine and serum N-terminal pro-brain natriuretic peptide after exercise training predict survival in patients with heart failure. Int J Cardiol. 2014;171(3):384–9.
128. Lin X, Zhang X, Guo J, Roberts CK, McKenzie S, Wu WC, et al. Effects of exercise training on cardiorespiratory fitness and biomarkers of cardiometabolic health: a systematic review and meta-analysis of randomized controlled trials. J Am Heart Assoc. 2015;4(7):e002014.
129. Kingwell BA, Tran B, Cameron JD, Jennings GL, Dart AM. Enhanced vasodilation to acetylcholine in athletes is associated with lower plasma cholesterol. Am J Phys. 1996;270(6 Pt 2):H2008–13.
130. Goessler K, Polito M, Cornelissen VA. Effect of exercise training on the renin-angiotensin-aldosterone system in healthy individuals: a systematic review and meta-analysis. Hypertens Res. 2016;39(3):119–26.
131. Fantin A, Vieira JM, Gestri G, Denti L, Schwarz Q, Prykhozhij S, et al. Tissue macrophages act as cellular chaperones for vascular anastomosis downstream of VEGF-mediated endothelial tip cell induction. Blood. 2010;116(5):829–40.
132. Tammela T, Zarkada G, Nurmi H, Jakobsson L, Heinolainen K, Tvorogov D, et al. VEGFR-3 controls tip to stalk conversion at vessel fusion sites by reinforcing Notch signalling. Nat Cell Biol. 2011;13(10):1202–13.
133. Smith JD, Bryant SR, Couper LL, Vary CP, Gotwals PJ, Koteliansky VE, et al. Soluble transforming growth factor-beta type II receptor inhibits negative remodeling, fibroblast transdifferentiation, and intimal lesion formation but not endothelial growth. Circ Res. 1999;84(10):1212–22.
134. Lithell H, Krotkiewski M, Kiens B, Wroblewski Z, Holm G, Stromblad G, et al. Non-response of muscle capillary density and lipoprotein-lipase activity to regular training in diabetic patients. Diabetes Res. 1985;2(1):17–21.
135. Williamson JR, Hoffmann PL, Kohrt WM, Spina RJ, Coggan AR, Holloszy O. Endurance exercise training decreases capillary basement membrane width in older nondiabetic and diabetic adults. J Appl Physiol. 1996;80(3):747–53.
136. Gando Y, Yamamoto K, Kawano H, Murakami H, Ohmori Y, Kawakami R, et al. Attenuated age-related carotid arterial remodeling in adults with a high level of cardiorespiratory fitness. J Atheroscler Thromb. 2011;18(3):248–54.
137. Wagner H, Fischer H, Degerblad M, Alvarsson M, Gustafsson T. Improvement of insulin sensitivity in response to exercise training in type 2 diabetes mellitus is associated with vascular endothelial growth factor A expression. Diab Vasc Dis Res. 2016;13(5):361–6.
138. Martin WH 3rd, Ogawa T, Kohrt WM, Malley MT, Korte E, Kieffer PS, et al. Effects of aging, gender, and physical training on peripheral vascular function. Circulation. 1991;84(2):654–64.
139. Spurway NC, Ekblom B, Noakes TD, Wagner PD. What limits [V(.)]O(2max)? A symposium held at the BASES Conference, 6 September 2010. J Sports Sci. 2012;30(6):517–31.
140. Laughlin MH. Physical activity-induced remodeling of vasculature in skeletal muscle: role in treatment of type 2 diabetes. J Appl Physiol. 2016;120(1):1–16.
141. Lindholm ME, Rundqvist H. Skeletal muscle hypoxia-inducible factor-1 and exercise. Exp Physiol. 2016;101(1):28–32.
142. Kon M, Ohiwa N, Honda A, Matsubayashi T, Ikeda T, Akimoto T, et al. Effects of systemic hypoxia on human muscular adaptations to resistance exercise training. Physiol Rep. 2014;2(6):e12033.
143. Hoier B, Hellsten Y. Exercise-induced capillary growth in human skeletal muscle and the dynamics of VEGF. Microcirculation. 2014;21(4):301–14.
144. Walton RG, Finlin BS, Mula J, Long DE, Zhu B, Fry CS, et al. Insulin-resistant subjects have normal angiogenic response to aerobic exercise training in skeletal muscle, but not in adipose tissue. Physiol Rep. 2015;3(6):e12415.

145. Gavin TP, Drew JL, Kubik CJ, Pofahl WE, Hickner RC. Acute resistance exercise increases skeletal muscle angiogenic growth factor expression. Acta Physiol (Oxf). 2007;191(2):139–46.
146. Timmons JA, Jansson E, Fischer H, Gustafsson T, Greenhaff PL, Ridden J, et al. Modulation of extracellular matrix genes reflects the magnitude of physiological adaptation to aerobic exercise training in humans. BMC Biol. 2005;3:19.
147. Eleuteri E, Mezzani A, Di Stefano A, Vallese D, Gnemmi I, Delle Donne L, et al. Aerobic training and angiogenesis activation in patients with stable chronic heart failure: a preliminary report. Biomarkers. 2013;18(5):418–24.
148. Lee HJ. Exercise training regulates angiogenic gene expression in white adipose tissue. J Exerc Rehabil. 2018;14(1):16–23.
149. Trenerry MK, Della Gatta PA, Larsen AE, Garnham AP, Cameron-Smith D. Impact of resistance exercise training on interleukin-6 and JAK/STAT in young men. Muscle Nerve. 2011;43(3):385–92.
150. Van Pelt DW, Guth LM, Horowitz JF. Aerobic exercise elevates markers of angiogenesis and macrophage IL-6 gene expression in the subcutaneous adipose tissue of overweight-to-obese adults. J Appl Physiol. 2017;123(5):1150–9.
151. Mobius-Winkler S, Uhlemann M, Adams V, Sandri M, Erbs S, Lenk K, et al. Coronary collateral growth induced by physical exercise: results of the impact of intensive exercise training on coronary collateral circulation in patients with stable coronary artery disease (EXCITE) trial. Circulation. 2016;133(15):1438–48. discussion 48
152. Tarumi T, Gonzales MM, Fallow B, Nualnim N, Pyron M, Tanaka H, et al. Central artery stiffness, neuropsychological function, and cerebral perfusion in sedentary and endurance-trained middle-aged adults. J Hypertens. 2013;31(12):2400–9.
153. Tanaka H, DeSouza CA, Seals DR. Absence of age-related increase in central arterial stiffness in physically active women. Arterioscler Thromb Vasc Biol. 1998;18(1):127–32.
154. Fleenor BS, Marshall KD, Durrant JR, Lesniewski LA, Seals DR. Arterial stiffening with ageing is associated with transforming growth factor-beta1-related changes in adventitial collagen: reversal by aerobic exercise. J Physiol. 2010;588(Pt 20):3971–82.
155. Moreau KL, Gavin KM, Plum AE, Seals DR. Oxidative stress explains differences in large elastic artery compliance between sedentary and habitually exercising postmenopausal women. Menopause. 2006;13(6):951–8.
156. Gerhardt H, Golding M, Fruttiger M, Ruhrberg C, Lundkvist A, Abramsson A, et al. VEGF guides angiogenic sprouting utilizing endothelial tip cell filopodia. J Cell Biol. 2003;161(6):1163–77.
157. Franco CA, Jones ML, Bernabeu MO, Geudens I, Mathivet T, Rosa A, et al. Dynamic endothelial cell rearrangements drive developmental vessel regression. PLoS Biol. 2015;13(4):e1002125.
158. Risau W, Flamme I. Vasculogenesis. Annu Rev Cell Dev Biol. 1995;11:73–91.
159. Purhonen S, Palm J, Rossi D, Kaskenpaa N, Rajantie I, Yla-Herttuala S, et al. Bone marrow-derived circulating endothelial precursors do not contribute to vascular endothelium and are not needed for tumor growth. Proc Natl Acad Sci U S A. 2008;105(18):6620–5.
160. Heil M, Eitenmuller I, Schmitz-Rixen T, Schaper W. Arteriogenesis versus angiogenesis: similarities and differences. J Cell Mol Med. 2006;10(1):45–55.
161. Kodama S, Tanaka S, Saito K, Shu M, Sone Y, Onitake F, et al. Effect of aerobic exercise training on serum levels of high-density lipoprotein cholesterol: a meta-analysis. Arch Intern Med. 2007;167(10):999–1008.
162. Kraus WE, Houmard JA, Duscha BD, Knetzger KJ, Wharton MB, McCartney JS, et al. Effects of the amount and intensity of exercise on plasma lipoproteins. N Engl J Med. 2002;347(19):1483–92.
163. Kelley GA, Kelley KS. Impact of progressive resistance training on lipids and lipoproteins in adults: a meta-analysis of randomized controlled trials. Prev Med. 2009;48(1):9–19.
164. Ostman C, Smart NA, Morcos D, Duller A, Ridley W, Jewiss D. The effect of exercise training on clinical outcomes in patients with the metabolic syndrome: a systematic review and meta-analysis. Cardiovasc Diabetol. 2017;16(1):110.

165. Adams V, Besler C, Fischer T, Riwanto M, Noack F, Hollriegel R, et al. Exercise training in patients with chronic heart failure promotes restoration of high-density lipoprotein functional properties. Circ Res. 2013;113(12):1345–55.
166. Kelley GA, Kelley KS, Vu TZ. Aerobic exercise, lipids and lipoproteins in overweight and obese adults: a meta-analysis of randomized controlled trials. Int J Obes. 2005;29(8):881–93.
167. Gordon B, Chen S, Durstine JL. The effects of exercise training on the traditional lipid profile and beyond. Curr Sports Med Rep. 2014;13(4):253–9.
168. Toft-Petersen AP, Tilsted HH, Aaroe J, Rasmussen K, Christensen T, Griffin BA, et al. Small dense LDL particlesDOUBLEHYPHENa predictor of coronary artery disease evaluated by invasive and CT-based techniques: a case-control study. Lipids Health Dis. 2011;10:21.
169. Ziegler S, Schaller G, Mittermayer F, Pleiner J, Mihaly J, Niessner A, et al. Exercise training improves low-density lipoprotein oxidability in untrained subjects with coronary artery disease. Arch Phys Med Rehabil. 2006;87(2):265–9.
170. Schjerve IE, Tyldum GA, Tjonna AE, Stolen T, Loennechen JP, Hansen HE, et al. Both aerobic endurance and strength training programmes improve cardiovascular health in obese adults. Clin Sci. 2008;115(9):283–93.
171. Thomas TR, Warner SO, Dellsperger KC, Hinton PS, Whaley-Connell AT, Rector RS, et al. Exercise and the metabolic syndrome with weight regain. J Appl Physiol. 2010;109(1):3–10.
172. Ficker ES, Maranhao RC, Chacra AP, Neves VC, Negrao CE, Martins VC, et al. Exercise training accelerates the removal from plasma of LDL-like nanoemulsion in moderately hypercholesterolemic subjects. Atherosclerosis. 2010;212(1):230–6.
173. Wang JS, Chow SE, Chen JK, Wong MK. Effect of exercise training on oxidized LDL-mediated platelet function in rats. Thromb Haemost. 2000;83(3):503–8.
174. Tiainen S, Kiviniemi A, Hautala A, Huikuri H, Ukkola O, Tokola K, et al. Effects of a two-year home-based exercise training program on oxidized LDL and HDL lipids in coronary artery disease patients with and without type-2 diabetes. Antioxidants (Basel). 2018;7(10):E144.
175. Nordestgaard BG, Chapman MJ, Ray K, Boren J, Andreotti F, Watts GF, et al. Lipoprotein(a) as a cardiovascular risk factor: current status. Eur Heart J. 2010;31(23):2844–53.
176. Mankowitz K, Seip R, Semenkovich CF, Daugherty A, Schonfeld G. Short-term interruption of training affects both fasting and post-prandial lipoproteins. Atherosclerosis. 1992;95(2–3):181–9.
177. Hubinger L, Mackinnon LT, Lepre F. Lipoprotein(a) [Lp(a)] levels in middle-aged male runners and sedentary controls. Med Sci Sports Exerc. 1995;27(4):490–6.
178. Thomas TR, Ziogas G, Harris WS. Influence of fitness status on very-low-density lipoprotein subfractions and lipoprotein(a) in men and women. Metabolism. 1997;46(10):1178–83.
179. Tsarouhas K, Tsitsimpikou C, Haliassos A, Georgoulias P, Koutsioras I, Kouretas D, et al. Study of insulin resistance, TNF-alpha, total antioxidant capacity and lipid profile in patients with chronic heart failure under exercise. In Vivo. 2011;25(6):1031–7.
180. Tisi PV, Hulse M, Chulakadabba A, Gosling P, Shearman CP. Exercise training for intermittent claudication: does it adversely affect biochemical markers of the exercise-induced inflammatory response? Eur J Vasc Endovasc Surg. 1997;14(5):344–50.
181. Walther C, Mobius-Winkler S, Linke A, Bruegel M, Thiery J, Schuler G, et al. Regular exercise training compared with percutaneous intervention leads to a reduction of inflammatory markers and cardiovascular events in patients with coronary artery disease. Eur J Cardiovasc Prev Rehabil. 2008;15(1):107–12.
182. Kadoglou NP, Iliadis F, Angelopoulou N, Perrea D, Ampatzidis G, Liapis CD, et al. The anti-inflammatory effects of exercise training in patients with type 2 diabetes mellitus. Eur J Cardiovasc Prev Rehabil. 2007;14(6):837–43.
183. Campbell PT, Campbell KL, Wener MH, Wood BL, Potter JD, McTiernan A, et al. A year-long exercise intervention decreases CRP among obese postmenopausal women. Med Sci Sports Exerc. 2009;41(8):1533–9.
184. Goldhammer E, Tanchilevitch A, Maor I, Beniamini Y, Rosenschein U, Sagiv M. Exercise training modulates cytokines activity in coronary heart disease patients. Int J Cardiol. 2005;100(1):93–9.

185. Troseid M, Lappegard KT, Claudi T, Damas JK, Morkrid L, Brendberg R, et al. Exercise reduces plasma levels of the chemokines MCP-1 and IL-8 in subjects with the metabolic syndrome. Eur Heart J. 2004;25(4):349–55.
186. Sardeli AV, Tomeleri CM, Cyrino ES, Fernhall B, Cavaglieri CR, Chacon-Mikahil MPT. Effect of resistance training on inflammatory markers of older adults: A meta-analysis. Exp Gerontol. 2018;111:188–96.
187. Macedo Santiago LA, Neto LGL, Borges Pereira G, Leite RD, Mostarda CT, de Oliveira Brito Monzani J, et al. Effects of resistance training on immunoinflammatory response, TNF-alpha gene expression, and body composition in elderly women. J Aging Res. 2018;2018:1467025.
188. Pedersen BK, Akerstrom TC, Nielsen AR, Fischer CP. Role of myokines in exercise and metabolism. J Appl Physiol. 2007;103(3):1093–8.
189. Kawanishi N, Yano H, Yokogawa Y, Suzuki K. Exercise training inhibits inflammation in adipose tissue via both suppression of macrophage infiltration and acceleration of phenotypic switching from M1 to M2 macrophages in high-fat-diet-induced obese mice. Exerc Immunol Rev. 2010;16:105–18.
190. Lavie CJ, Milani RV, Artham SM, Patel DA, Ventura HO. The obesity paradox, weight loss, and coronary disease. Am J Med. 2009;122(12):1106–14.
191. Mujumdar PP, Duerksen-Hughes PJ, Firek AF, Hessinger DA. Long-term, progressive, aerobic training increases adiponectin in middle-aged, overweight, untrained males and females. Scand J Clin Lab Invest. 2011;71(2):101–7.
192. Yu Z, Ye X, Wang J, Qi Q, Franco OH, Rennie KL, et al. Associations of physical activity with inflammatory factors, adipocytokines, and metabolic syndrome in middle-aged and older Chinese people. Circulation. 2009;119(23):2969–77.
193. Hui X, Lam KS, Vanhoutte PM, Xu A. Adiponectin and cardiovascular health: an update. Br J Pharmacol. 2012;165(3):574–90.
194. Pedersen BK, Steensberg A, Fischer C, Keller C, Keller P, Plomgaard P, et al. Searching for the exercise factor: is IL-6 a candidate? J Muscle Res Cell Motil. 2003;24(2–3):113–9.
195. Steensberg A, van Hall G, Osada T, Sacchetti M, Saltin B, Klarlund PB. Production of interleukin-6 in contracting human skeletal muscles can account for the exercise-induced increase in plasma interleukin-6. J Physiol. 2000;529(Pt 1):237–42.
196. Pedersen BK, Steensberg A, Keller P, Keller C, Fischer C, Hiscock N, et al. Muscle-derived interleukin-6: lipolytic, anti-inflammatory and immune regulatory effects. Pflugers Arch. 2003;446(1):9–16.
197. Schindler R, Mancilla J, Endres S, Ghorbani R, Clark SC, Dinarello CA. Correlations and interactions in the production of interleukin-6 (IL-6), IL-1, and tumor necrosis factor (TNF) in human blood mononuclear cells: IL-6 suppresses IL-1 and TNF. Blood. 1990;75(1):40–7.
198. Steensberg A, Fischer CP, Keller C, Moller K, Pedersen BK. IL-6 enhances plasma IL-1ra, IL-10, and cortisol in humans. Am J Physiol Endocrinol Metab. 2003;285(2):E433–7.
199. Gielen S, Adams V, Mobius-Winkler S, Linke A, Erbs S, Yu J, et al. Anti-inflammatory effects of exercise training in the skeletal muscle of patients with chronic heart failure. J Am Coll Cardiol. 2003;42(5):861–8.
200. Timmerman KL, Flynn MG, Coen PM, Markofski MM, Pence BD. Exercise training-induced lowering of inflammatory (CD14+CD16+) monocytes: a role in the anti-inflammatory influence of exercise? J Leukoc Biol. 2008;84(5):1271–8.
201. Yakeu G, Butcher L, Isa S, Webb R, Roberts AW, Thomas AW, et al. Low-intensity exercise enhances expression of markers of alternative activation in circulating leukocytes: roles of PPARgamma and Th2 cytokines. Atherosclerosis. 2010;212(2):668–73.
202. McFarlin BK, Flynn MG, Campbell WW, Craig BA, Robinson JP, Stewart LK, et al. Physical activity status, but not age, influences inflammatory biomarkers and toll-like receptor 4. J Gerontol A Biol Sci Med Sci. 2006;61(4):388–93.
203. Stewart LK, Flynn MG, Campbell WW, Craig BA, Robinson JP, McFarlin BK, et al. Influence of exercise training and age on CD14+ cell-surface expression of toll-like receptor 2 and 4. Brain Behav Immun. 2005;19(5):389–97.

204. McFarlin BK, Flynn MG, Campbell WW, Stewart LK, Timmerman KL. TLR4 is lower in resistance-trained older women and related to inflammatory cytokines. Med Sci Sports Exerc. 2004;36(11):1876–83.
205. Lambert CP, Wright NR, Finck BN, Villareal DT. Exercise but not diet-induced weight loss decreases skeletal muscle inflammatory gene expression in frail obese elderly persons. J Appl Physiol (1985). 2008;105(2):473–8.
206. Handzlik MK, Shaw AJ, Dungey M, Bishop NC, Gleeson M. The influence of exercise training status on antigen-stimulated IL-10 production in whole blood culture and numbers of circulating regulatory T cells. Eur J Appl Physiol. 2013;113(7):1839–48.
207. Rehm K, Sunesara I, Marshall GD. Increased circulating anti-inflammatory cells in marathon-trained runners. Int J Sports Med. 2015;36(10):832–6.
208. Sallam N, Laher I. Exercise modulates oxidative stress and inflammation in aging and cardiovascular diseases. Oxidative Med Cell Longev. 2016;2016:7239639.
209. Sloan RP, Shapiro PA, McKinley PS, Bartels M, Shimbo D, Lauriola V, et al. Aerobic exercise training and inducible inflammation: results of a randomized controlled trial in healthy, young adults. J Am Heart Assoc. 2018;7(17):e010201.
210. Barry JC, Simtchouk S, Durrer C, Jung ME, Mui AL, Little JP. Short-term exercise training reduces anti-inflammatory action of interleukin-10 in adults with obesity. Cytokine. 2018;111:460–9.
211. Stensvold D, Slordahl SA, Wisloff U. Effect of exercise training on inflammation status among people with metabolic syndrome. Metab Syndr Relat Disord. 2012;10(4):267–72.
212. Aengevaeren VL, Mosterd A, Braber TL, Prakken NHJ, Doevendans PA, Grobbee DE, et al. Relationship between lifelong exercise volume and coronary atherosclerosis in athletes. Circulation. 2017;136(2):138–48.
213. Merghani A, Maestrini V, Rosmini S, Cox AT, Dhutia H, Bastiaenan R, et al. Prevalence of subclinical coronary artery disease in masters endurance athletes with a low atherosclerotic risk profile. Circulation. 2017;136(2):126–37.
214. Merghani A, Maestrini V, Rosmini S, Cox AT, Dhutia H, Bastiaenan R, et al. Response by Merghani et al to letters regarding article, "prevalence of subclinical coronary artery disease in masters endurance athletes with a low atherosclerotic risk profile". Circulation. 2018;137(5):541–2.
215. Schmermund A. Letter by schmermund regarding article, "prevalence of subclinical coronary artery disease in masters endurance athletes with a low atherosclerotic risk profile". Circulation. 2018;137(5):539–40.
216. Roberts WO, Schwartz RS, Kraus SM, Schwartz JG, Peichel G, Garberich RF, et al. Long-term marathon running is associated with low coronary plaque formation in women. Med Sci Sports Exerc. 2017;49(4):641–5.
217. Wilund KR, Tomayko EJ, Wu PT, Ryong Chung H, Vallurupalli S, Lakshminarayanan B, et al. Intradialytic exercise training reduces oxidative stress and epicardial fat: a pilot study. Nephrol Dial Transplant. 2010;25(8):2695–701.
218. Davenport C, Kenny H, Ashley DT, O'Sullivan EP, Smith D, O'Gorman DJ. The effect of exercise on osteoprotegerin and TNF-related apoptosis-inducing ligand in obese patients. Eur J Clin Investig. 2012;42(11):1173–9.
219. Ludmer PL, Selwyn AP, Shook TL, Wayne RR, Mudge GH, Alexander RW, et al. Paradoxical vasoconstriction induced by acetylcholine in atherosclerotic coronary arteries. N Engl J Med. 1986;315(17):1046–51.
220. Wilson RF, Laughlin DE, Ackell PH, Chilian WM, Holida MD, Hartley CJ, et al. Transluminal, subselective measurement of coronary artery blood flow velocity and vasodilator reserve in man. Circulation. 1985;72(1):82–92.
221. Caiati C, Montaldo C, Zedda N, Montisci R, Ruscazio M, Lai G, et al. Validation of a new noninvasive method (contrast-enhanced transthoracic second harmonic echo Doppler) for the evaluation of coronary flow reserve: comparison with intracoronary Doppler flow wire. J Am Coll Cardiol. 1999;34(4):1193–200.

222. Dayanikli F, Grambow D, Muzik O, Mosca L, Rubenfire M, Schwaiger M. Early detection of abnormal coronary flow reserve in asymptomatic men at high risk for coronary artery disease using positron emission tomography. Circulation. 1994;90(2):808–17.
223. Terashima M, Meyer CH, Keeffe BG, Putz EJ, de la Pena-Almaguer E, Yang PC, et al. Noninvasive assessment of coronary vasodilation using magnetic resonance angiography. J Am Coll Cardiol. 2005;45(1):104–10.
224. Gush RJ, King TA. Discrimination of capillary and arterio-venular blood flow in skin by laser Doppler flowmetry. Med Biol Eng Comput. 1991;29(4):387–92.
225. Panza JA, Quyyumi AA, Brush JE Jr, Epstein SE. Abnormal endothelium-dependent vascular relaxation in patients with essential hypertension. N Engl J Med. 1990;323(1):22–7.
226. Celermajer DS, Sorensen KE, Gooch VM, Spiegelhalter DJ, Miller OI, Sullivan ID, et al. Non-invasive detection of endothelial dysfunction in children and adults at risk of atherosclerosis. Lancet. 1992;340(8828):1111–5.
227. Bonetti PO, Pumper GM, Higano ST, Holmes DR Jr, Kuvin JT, Lerman A. Noninvasive identification of patients with early coronary atherosclerosis by assessment of digital reactive hyperemia. J Am Coll Cardiol. 2004;44(11):2137–41.
228. Alexander MR, Kitzman DW, Khaliq S, Darty SN, Hamilton CA, Herrington DM, et al. Determination of femoral artery endothelial function by phase contrast magnetic resonance imaging. Am J Cardiol. 2001;88(9):1070–4.
229. Corretti MC, Anderson TJ, Benjamin EJ, Celermajer D, Charbonneau F, Creager MA, et al. Guidelines for the ultrasound assessment of endothelial-dependent flow-mediated vasodilation of the brachial artery: a report of the International brachial artery reactivity task force. J Am Coll Cardiol. 2002;39(2):257–65.
230. Thijssen DH, Black MA, Pyke KE, Padilla J, Atkinson G, Harris RA, et al. Assessment of flow-mediated dilation in humans: a methodological and physiological guideline. Am J Physiol Heart Circ Physiol. 2011;300(1):H2–12.
231. Hedetoft M, Olsen NV. Evaluation of endothelial function by peripheral arterial tonometry and relation with the nitric oxide pathway. Nitric Oxide. 2014;42:1–8.
232. Hamburg NM, Benjamin EJ. Assessment of endothelial function using digital pulse amplitude tonometry. Trends Cardiovasc Med. 2009;19(1):6–11.
233. Hamburg NM, Palmisano J, Larson MG, Sullivan LM, Lehman BT, Vasan RS, et al. Relation of brachial and digital measures of vascular function in the community: the Framingham heart study. Hypertension. 2011;57(3):390–6.
234. Xu Y, Arora RC, Hiebert BM, Lerner B, Szwajcer A, McDonald K, et al. Non-invasive endothelial function testing and the risk of adverse outcomes: a systematic review and meta-analysis. Eur Heart J Cardiovasc Imaging. 2014;15(7):736–46.
235. Rubinshtein R, Kuvin JT, Soffler M, Lennon RJ, Lavi S, Nelson RE, et al. Assessment of endothelial function by non-invasive peripheral arterial tonometry predicts late cardiovascular adverse events. Eur Heart J. 2010;31(9):1142–8.
236. Hamburg NM, Keyes MJ, Larson MG, Vasan RS, Schnabel R, Pryde MM, et al. Cross-sectional relations of digital vascular function to cardiovascular risk factors in the Framingham Heart Study. Circulation. 2008;117(19):2467–74.
237. Matsue Y, Suzuki M, Nagahori W, Ohno M, Matsumura A, Hashimoto Y, et al. Endothelial dysfunction measured by peripheral arterial tonometry predicts prognosis in patients with heart failure with preserved ejection fraction. Int J Cardiol. 2013;168(1):36–40.
238. Marechaux S, Samson R, van Belle E, Breyne J, de Monte J, Dedrie C, et al. Vascular and microvascular endothelial function in heart failure with preserved ejection fraction. J Card Fail. 2016;22(1):3–11.
239. Higashi Y, Sasaki S, Sasaki N, Nakagawa K, Ueda T, Yoshimizu A, et al. Daily aerobic exercise improves reactive hyperemia in patients with essential hypertension. Hypertension. 1999;33(1 Pt 2):591–7.
240. Lavrencic A, Salobir BG, Keber I. Physical training improves flow-mediated dilation in patients with the polymetabolic syndrome. Arterioscler Thromb Vasc Biol. 2000;20(2):551–5.

241. Cornelissen VA, Onkelinx S, Goetschalckx K, Thomaes T, Janssens S, Fagard R, et al. Exercise-based cardiac rehabilitation improves endothelial function assessed by flow-mediated dilation but not by pulse amplitude tonometry. Eur J Prev Cardiol. 2014;21(1):39–48.
242. Linke A, Schoene N, Gielen S, Hofer J, Erbs S, Schuler G, et al. Endothelial dysfunction in patients with chronic heart failure: systemic effects of lower-limb exercise training. J Am Coll Cardiol. 2001;37(2):392–7.
243. Kitzman DW, Brubaker PH, Herrington DM, Morgan TM, Stewart KP, Hundley WG, et al. Effect of endurance exercise training on endothelial function and arterial stiffness in older patients with heart failure and preserved ejection fraction: a randomized, controlled, single-blind trial. J Am Coll Cardiol. 2013;62(7):584–92.
244. Suchy C, Massen L, Rognmo O, Van Craenenbroeck EM, Beckers P, Kraigher-Krainer E, et al. Optimising exercise training in prevention and treatment of diastolic heart failure (OptimEx-CLIN): rationale and design of a prospective, randomised, controlled trial. Eur J Prev Cardiol. 2014;21(2 Suppl):18–25.

# The Optimal Dose of Exercise

# 41

Thijs M. H. Eijsvogels and Aaron L. Baggish

**Learning Objectives**

1. Become familiar with methods to assess physical activity and exercise characteristics.
2. Become familiar with the WHO physical activity recommendations.
3. Understand the dose-response relationship between physical activity or exercise and health outcomes.
4. Understand the minimal and optimal exercise dose to yield health benefits.
5. Be able to differentiate between different aspects of the 'too much exercise' hypothesis.
6. Be able to prescribe exercise as medicine in clinical practice.

## 41.1 Introduction

Habitual physical activity (PA) and exercise training (EX) are part of a healthy lifestyle. Regular performance of physical activities is known to reduce the risk of chronic diseases including, but not limited to, cardiovascular morbidity and mortality, neurological diseases, type 2 diabetes, pulmonary diseases, musculoskeletal disorders and several types of cancer (i.e. bladder, breast, colon, endometrium, esophagus, kidney, stomach, and lung) [1]. Exercise prescription is an important

T. M. H. Eijsvogels
Department of Physiology, Radboud Institute for Health Sciences, Radboud University Medical Center, Nijmegen, The Netherlands
e-mail: Thijs.Eijsvogels@Radboudumc.nl

A. L. Baggish (✉)
Cardiovascular Performance Program, Division of Cardiology, Massachusetts General Hospital, Boston, MA, USA
e-mail: abaggish@partners.org





A. Pressler, J. Niebauer (eds.), *Textbook of Sports and Exercise Cardiology*,
https://doi.org/10.1007/978-3-030-35374-2_41

component of primary and secondary prevention strategies [2]. Nevertheless, the prevalence of physical inactivity remains high across the globe, and initiatives to increase the amount of physical activity in the general population have only little or temporal effects. This chapter will provide an overview of the dose-response relationship between PA/EX and associated health outcomes. The minimal, optimal and potential harmful dose of exercise to induce risk reductions in all-cause and cardiovascular mortality will be addressed.

## 41.2 Physical Activity Definitions and Measurements

### 41.2.1 Physical Activity Versus Exercise

- PA is defined as any bodily movement resulting from the contraction of skeletal muscle that increases energy expenditure above the basal level.
- EX, as a subcategory of PA, is defined as any planned and structured action with the objective of improving or maintaining physical fitness or health and/or achieving athletic goals.
- EX involves a combination of isometric (static) and isotonic (dynamic) stress, which serves as the basis for the physiological classification of competitive sports (see Chap. 1) [3, 4].
- EX is most commonly divided into the broad subgroups of aerobic/endurance (i.e., running, walking) and resistance (i.e., weight lifting) activity, although many sport and EX modalities integrate both physiological disciplines.

### 41.2.2 Subjective Versus Objective Measurements

PA and EX characteristics can be assessed using **objective** and **subjective** measurement tools. An appropriate measurement tool should be chosen to ensure the accuracy and validity of data collection, and may depend on the group size, age, disabilities, budget and PA characteristic of interest.

- **Subjective** measurements rely on a person's recall and personal perception of PA and their involvement in it. Examples of subjective measurements are recall surveys, questionnaires, logbooks and journals.
  - Benefits of subjective methods are its low costs, low participant burden, can easily be applied in large numbers, and can collect data from all dimensions of activities.
  - Subjective methods are vulnerable to recall bias, cannot be applied to young children or cognitive impaired individuals, whereas over- or under reporting can easily occur due to socially desirable responses. The use of validated methods and clear instructions are therefore preferred in clinical and research settings.
- **Objective measurements** make use of direct observations or an electronic instrument to determine the amount of PA and EX training. Examples of

objective measurements are *pedometers*, *accelerometers*, *global positioning system (GPS)-enabled devices* and *direct observation*. Benefits and limitations of objective measurements strongly depend on the measurement tool of choice:
- *Pedometers* are cheap, small, non-invasive and easy to use devices that can be used in large groups of individuals. The pedometer records the daily number of steps taken, but does not provide insight on the frequency, intensity or duration of activities. Also, types of activities other than walking, jogging or running, are typically not accurately recorded by a pedometer.
- *Accelerometers* are small, non-invasive devices that can record movement for several consecutive days to weeks, with low participant burden. Some types of accelerometers have the possibility to provide real-time feedback. Limitations of accelerometers are its relatively high costs, the possibility of developing skin reactivity, people may forget to wear them, and controversy about analytic techniques data processing.
- *GPS-enabled devices* are increasingly commonly used to measure PA and EX. These devices include smart phones with location services and wrist mounted units that are often coupled with heart rate monitoring technology. GPS data permits accurate determination of distance covered and thus pace during outdoor activities and serves as the gold standard for this purpose. GPS-enabled devices are not currently suitable for monitoring of indoor PA or EX.
- *Direct observation* allows collection of data from all PA dimensions, but also its context. Nevertheless, this type of data collection and analysis is intrusive, highly labour intensive, and presence of an observer may cause changes in behavioural activities.

### 41.2.3 Exercise Intensity

EX intensity can be quantified in **absolute** terms as the metabolic cost of an EX session or in **relative** terms as the performance of a given activity as a function of the percentage of measurable maximal capacity.

- **Absolute** measures of EX intensity include kilocalories per unit of time (1 l $O_2$ consumption = 5 kcal) or assessment of the Metabolic Equivalent of Task score (METs, 1 MET = 3.5 mL $O_2$ consumption/kg·min = quiet sitting).
  - A limitation of absolute intensity metrics is their innate inability to account for the large variability in fitness that exists across individuals. For example, EX intensity of 5 METs may simultaneously represent a peak EX effort for a patient with advanced CVD and a relatively easy effort for a competitive athlete.
  - Indexes of relative EX intensity account for differences in individual fitness levels by defining intensity as a percentage of some peak or maximal physiological parameters (i.e. heart rate and oxygen consumption). Accordingly, a relative intensity of 75% peak oxygen consumption ($\dot{V}O_2$) may translate into

a treadmill walk at 3 mph for a patient with advanced CVD and a treadmill run at 8 mph for a competitive athlete.

- The use of **relative** EX intensity is common in clinical practice for the generation of EX prescription and in high-quality observational and interventional EX studies.
  - Relative EX intensity metrics may be preferable to absolute intensity metrics when they can be applied with rigor.
  - However, effective application of a relative intensity metric requires accurate determination of a peak value for the metric of choice, which typically involves some form of laboratory- or field-based EX assessment. This is typically a resource-intensive process that may not be feasible for large population-based studies.
  - Although the use of equations or predictive algorithms for metrics such as peak heart rate have been developed, the application of these tools is associated with considerable inaccuracy.

### 41.2.4 Calculation of Exercise Dose

Quantification of EX exposure is typically accomplished with the concept of EX dose, which can be calculated as the product of the **duration**, **frequency**, and **intensity** of EX.

- **Duration** reflects the amount of time accrued in a single EX session and, for aerobic/endurance EX, is most often characterized as minutes or hours.
- **Frequency** captures the number of EX sessions over more extended periods (i.e., days, weeks, or months). The product of these 2 parameters reflect the total amount of time spent in EX over a given period.
- When EX is measured in terms of
  - *Absolute* **intensity**, this translates to total dose expressed as kilocalories per week, MET-hours per week, or MET-minutes per week. These values are commonly used in epidemiological studies of EX dose because they can be extrapolated from self-reported activity patterns.
  - *Relative* **intensity**, total dose is instead expressed as time per week spent in light/moderate/vigorous EX. These terms may be patient-friendlier but, as noted above, require some knowledge of an individual patient's physiology and EX capacity.
- Peak oxygen consumption ($\dot{V}O_2$) and exercise capacity (Watt) can be measured in a cardiopulmonary exercise test with breath-by-breath analyses of $\dot{V}O_2$ and $\dot{V}CO_2$ for accurate quantification of relative intensity (see Chap. 44).

## 41.3 Physical Activity Recommendations

### 41.3.1 Historical Perspectives

Survival of the human species has depended on routine PA for thousands of our years. Access to food and water required us to move on a regular basis. We therefore evolved the capacity to walk and to run, oftentimes over long distances, and our survival depended on our ability to do so.

During so-called ‘persistence hunts’, distances more than 30 km were regularly covered [5]. In contrast to this intermittent but substantial exertion, it is believed that hunters were predominantly physically inactive during the remainder of the day [6]. This inactive behavior reduced their energy expenditure and was essential to maintain a proper balance between energy intake and expenditure.

The concept that regular PA could also promote health and longevity was first recognized by Hippocrates (460–377 B.C.):

- “All parts of the body, if used in moderation and exercised in labours to which each is accustomed, become thereby healthy and well developed and age slowly; but if they are unused and left idle, they become liable to disease, defective in growth and age quickly”.

Henschen [7] and Darling [8] were the first visionary investigators to recognize the impact of EX training on cardiac remodeling. Both researchers described independently and nearly simultaneously observations of enlarged cardiac silhouettes among Nordic skiers and rowers, respectively.

The first scientific evidence for health benefits of an active lifestyle were published by Morris and colleagues in 1953. They reported lower rates of coronary heart disease among the conductors of London’s double-decker buses who spent their working time walking up and down aisles and double-decker staircases, had approximately half the rate of coronary heart disease of substantially more sedentary streetcar drivers [9]. These findings were reinforced in a second study in which they found a lower incidence of coronary heart disease among English postmen compared with telephone operators working at the same company [9].

Many subsequent epidemiological studies confirmed the inverse relationship between PA and cardiovascular diseases [10–12], but none have proven causation because all such studies are observational.

- To date, there are no randomized clinical trials directly testing whether PA prevents CVD.
- Such a study would require an enormous sample size and study duration because of subject crossover among those volunteering for an “EX study” and because the progressively lower rates of primary CVD in the general population would reduce CVD endpoints.

Powell et al. [13] evaluated the possibly causative relationship between PA and cardiovascular disease using the same criteria used to document a causative relationship between cigarette smoking and health [14], a relationship also lacking a randomized, controlled clinical trial. They demonstrated that the relationship between PA and CVD

1. Was strong,
2. Was consistent among studies,
3. Had a graded risk reduction with increasing EX volumes, and
4. Was coherent with clinical studies showing a putatively beneficial effect of EX on CVD risk factors [13].

They concluded that increasing PA was causally related to lower rates of CVD despite the absence of the classical clinical trial.

### 41.3.2 Physical Activity Guidelines

Writing groups of the American College of Sports Medicine and the Centers for Disease Control [15], the National Institutes of Health [16], and the US Department of Health and Human Services (HHS) [17] concluded between 1990 and 2000 that routine moderate-intensity EX was an effective means to reduce the overall risk of chronic disease. The consistent recommendation across these initial guidelines was that all people should engage in at least 30 min of moderate-intensity EX on most, preferably all, days of the week. Similar recommendations were developed in many other countries, including EU nations, Australia, Canada, and Brazil.

The current "Global Recommendations on Physical Activity for Health"of the World Health Organization (WHO) address three age groups: **5–17** years old, **18–64** years old and **65 years** old and above. These age groups were selected taking into consideration the nature and availability of the scientific evidence relevant to the prevention of noncommunicable diseases through PA [18].

1. For *children and young people*, PA includes play, games, sports, transportation, chores, recreation, physical education, or planned EX, in the context of family, school, and community activities. In order to improve cardiorespiratory and muscular fitness, bone health, and cardiovascular and metabolic health biomarkers, it is recommended that children and youth aged **5–17**:
   (a) Accumulate at least 60 min of moderate- to vigorous-intensity PA daily.
   (b) Amounts of PA greater than 60 min provide additional health benefits.
   (c) Most of the daily PA should be aerobic. Vigorous-intensity activities should be incorporated, including those that strengthen muscle and bone, at least three times per week.
2. In adults aged **18–64**, PA includes leisure time PA (for example: walking, dancing, gardening, hiking, swimming), transportation (e.g. walking or cycling), occupational (i.e. work), household chores, play, games, sports or planned EX, in the context of daily, family, and community activities. In order to improve cardiorespiratory and muscular fitness, bone health, reduce the risk of NCDs and depression:
   (a) Adults aged 18–64 should do at least 150 min of moderate-intensity aerobic PA throughout the week or do at least 75 min of vigorous-intensity aerobic PA throughout the week or an equivalent combination of moderate- and vigorous-intensity activity.
   (b) Aerobic activity should be performed in bouts of at least 10 min duration.
   (c) For additional health benefits, adults should increase their moderate-intensity aerobic PA to 300 min per week or engage in 150 min of vigorous-intensity aerobic PA per week, or an equivalent combination of moderate- and vigorous-intensity activity.

   (d) Muscle-strengthening activities should be done involving major muscle groups on 2 or more days a week.

3. In *adults* aged **65** years and above, PA includes leisure time PA (for example: walking, dancing, gardening, hiking, swimming), transportation (e.g. walking or cycling), occupational (if the individual is still engaged in work), household chores, play, games, sports or planned EX, in the context of daily, family, and community activities. In order to improve cardiorespiratory and muscular fitness, bone and functional health, reduce the risk of NCDs, depression and cognitive decline:
   (a) Older adults should do at least 150 min of moderate-intensity aerobic PA throughout the week or do at least 75 min of vigorous-intensity aerobic PA throughout the week or an equivalent combination of moderate- and vigorous-intensity activity.
   (b) Aerobic activity should be performed in bouts of at least 10 min duration.
   (c) For additional health benefits, older adults should increase their moderate-intensity aerobic PA to 300 min per week or engage in 150 min of vigorous-intensity aerobic PA per week, or an equivalent combination of moderate-and vigorous-intensity activity.
   (d) Older adults, with poor mobility, should perform PA to enhance balance and prevent falls on 3 or more days per week.
   (e) Muscle-strengthening activities, involving major muscle groups, should be done on 2 or more days a week.
   (f) When older adults cannot do the recommended amounts of PA due to health conditions, they should be as physically active as their abilities and conditions allow.

### 41.3.3 Dose-Response Relationship

The association between EX or PA volumes and health outcome is most frequently described as a curvilinear relationship (Fig. 41.1) [20]. The nature of this relationship indicates that a change from being sedentary to a mild or moderately active lifestyle yields relatively large health benefits with substantial risk reductions for adverse outcomes.

- A similar increase in PA dosage in a more active individual produces smaller risk reductions.
- Very active individuals who will further increase their weekly EX dosage are unlikely to experience any additional health benefit.
- Calculations reveal that compared with an essentially sedentary lifestyle (<0.5 h/week of moderate to vigorous EX), 1.5 h of moderate- to vigorous-intensity EX is associated with a 20% risk reduction in mortality [21]. To attain an additional 20% risk reduction (for a total of 40% risk reduction in mortality), an additional 5.5 h of moderate to vigorous EX was required for a total of 7 h/wk.
- Although increasing EX doses were associated with diminishing returns, there was no EX dose at which more did not yield progressive benefit.

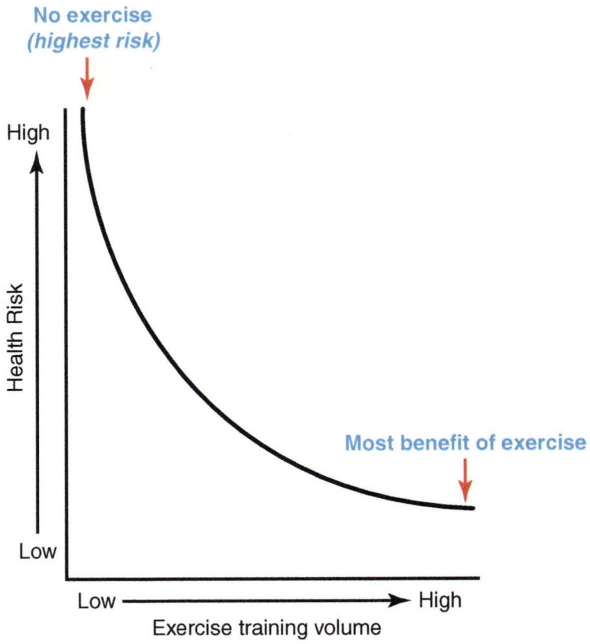


**Fig. 41.1** Conceptual overview of the dose–response association between physical activity volume and health outcomes (adapted from [19])

## 41.4 Minimal Effective Exercise Dose

### 41.4.1 Targeting Sedentary Behaviour

Sedentary behaviour refers to any waking activity characterized by an energy expenditure ≤1.5 metabolic equivalents and a sitting or reclining posture. In general, this means that any time a person is sitting or lying down, they are engaging in sedentary behaviour.

A worldwide trend of increased sedentary behaviour is observed, which can largely be ascribed due to technological 'progression' that allow individuals to be physically inactive throughout the majority of the day.

- The concerns about the increasing prevalence of a physically inactive lifestyle were summarized at the cover of the 2012 *Lancet* physical activity series as
  - "Pandemic, with far-reaching health, economic, environmental, and social consequences" [22], followed by
  - "Bold actions are needed to make active living a more desired, affordable, and accessible choice for all population groups" [23] in the 2016 series.

Physical inactivity is estimated to cause 6% of the global burden of disease from coronary heart disease, 7% of type 2 diabetes, 10% of breast and colon cancer, and 9% of premature mortality, equivalent to about five million inactivity-related deaths per year [24]. A meta-analysis reported that increased sedentary time was associated with

(a) All-cause mortality (HR: 1.24, 95% CI: 1.09–1.41)
(b) Cardiovascular disease incidence (HR: 1.14, 95% CI: 1.002–1.73),
(c) Cardiovascular mortality (HR: 1.18, 95% CI: 1.11–1.26),
(d) Cancer incidence (HR: 1.13, 95% CI 1.05–1.21),
(e) Cancer mortality (HR: 1.17, 95% CI: 1.11–1.24), and
(f) Type 2 diabetes incidence (HR: 1.91, 95% CI: 1.64–2.22) [25].

Accumulating evidence suggests that the detrimental health effects of sedentary time are independent from physical activity behavior, in particular among the most inactive group [25–27].

Ekelund *et al.* performed a meta-analyses to explore the joint associations of sitting time and physical activity with all-cause mortality among 1,005,791 individuals (Fig. 41.2) [28].

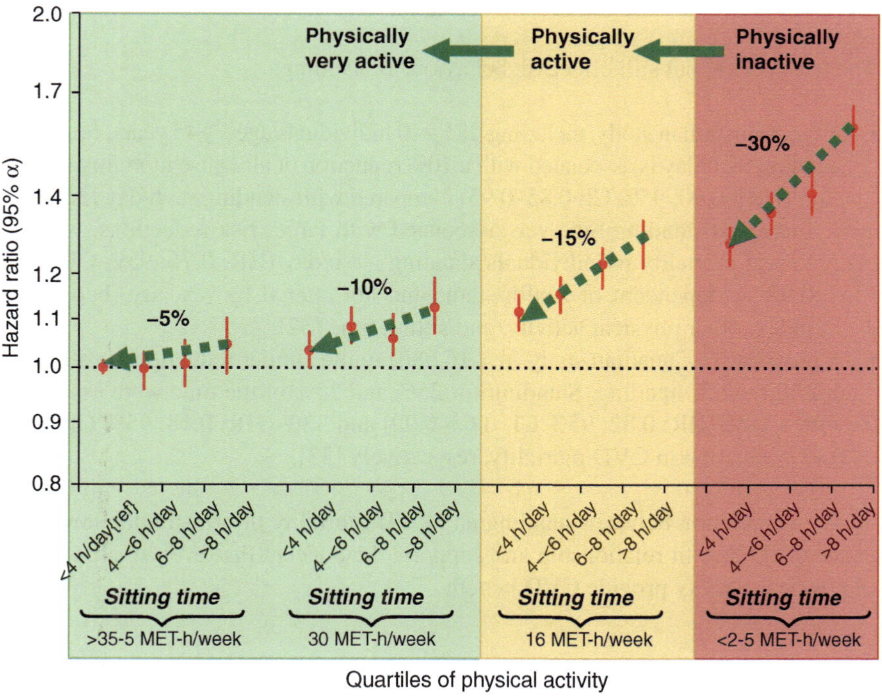


**Fig. 41.2** The joint association of sitting time and physical activity volumes on all-cause mortality. Data are presented for physically inactive individuals (<2.5 MET-h/week; red box), active individuals meeting the upper end of the WHO recommendations (16 MET-h/week; yellow box), and very active individuals performing physical activity for ≥2.5 times the WHO recommendations (> 30 MET-h/week; green box). Increasing volumes of physical activity (red → yellow → green) are associated with a lower mortality risk. Similarly, green dashed arrows highlight that a decrease of sitting time is associated with a mortality risk reduction within each activity quartile (adapted from [28])

- High volumes of sitting time were associated with higher mortality risks within each physical activity quartile.
- Both, increasing levels of habitual physical activity and reducing the time spend sitting, resulted in a lower mortality risk, even for individuals performing exercise volumes above the WHO recommendations, although at a much lower magnitude of effect than individuals engaging in low levels of physical activity (Fig. 41.2) [28].

These observations highlight the need for effective interventions aimed at reducing prolonged sitting time, particularly among individuals that don't engage very high levels of physical activity. Breaking up sitting time with short (1–5 min) bouts of light-intensity EX or PA are shown to improve cardiovascular health [29] and glucose homeostasis [30], and replacement of sitting time effectively reduces all-cause mortality [31].

### 41.4.2 Health Benefits of Standing

The least active, but still effective, behaviour is standing:

- A large Australian study, including 221,240 individuals aged ≥45 years, found that standing >2 h/day is associated with a 10% reduction of all-cause mortality (hazard ratio [HR]: 0.90; 95% CI: 0.85–0.95) compared with standing <2 h/day [32].
  - Increased standing time was associated with larger risk reductions, with the lowest mortality in individuals standing ≥8 h/day (HR: 0.76; 95% CI: 0.69–0.95), independent of health status and not altered by sex, age, body mass index, other physical activity, and sitting time [32].
- A prospective Canadian study (n = 16,586) found similar reductions in all-cause mortality with standing. Standing for 25% and 75% of the time were associated with a 18% (HR: 0.82; 95% CI: 0.68–0.99) and 32% (HR: 0.68; 95% CI: 0.50–0.92) reduction in CVD mortality, respectively [33].

The association between standing and CVD mortality informs on the lower end of the CVD benefit relationship and supports the concept that even small amounts of physical activity provide CVD benefit.

### 41.4.3 Physical Activity

PA and EX volumes below the WHO recommendations can also yield substantial health benefits given the curvilinear dose-response association between PA/EX and health outcomes (Fig. 41.1):

- Low volumes of vigorous-intensity EX, such as running for 51 min/week (i.e. 68% of WHO recommendations), lowered CVD mortality with 55% (HR: 0.45; 95% CI: 0.31–0.66) and all-cause mortality with 30% (HR: 0.70; 95% CI: 0.58–0.85) compared with no running [34].

- Low volumes of moderate-intensity EX, such as walking for 92 min/week (61% of WHO recommendations), lowered CVD mortality with 19% (HR: 0.81; 95% CI:0.71–0.93) and all-cause mortality with 14% (HR: 0.86; 95% CI: 0.81–0.91) compared with inactive individuals [35].
- A meta-analysis including data from 661,137 American and European men and women explored the dose-response association between moderate- to vigorous-intensity PA and health outcomes. Individuals performing volumes of leisure time PA below the WHO recommendations had a 20% reduction in CVD mortality (HR: 0.80; 95% CI: 0.77–0.84) and all-cause mortality (HR: 0.80; 95% CI: 0.78–0.82) compared with physically inactive controls [36].

Thus, low volumes of EX and PA can substantially reduce the risk for all-cause and CVD mortality, with the greatest health benefits at high-intensity EX and PA. As lack of time is a critical barrier for many individuals to engage in physical activity, these results also show that even the busiest individuals can benefit from regular "exercise snacks". In clinical practice, this translates into the important concept that it is the least active individuals who stand to benefit the most from even the smallest increments in EX and PA.

## 41.5 Optimal Exercise Dose

The "optimal" dose of EX or PA depends upon the desired outcome. The amount of EX needed to maximize longevity (i.e. to extend the life span) lies far below the amount needed to perform successfully at the elite and sub-elite levels of competitive sport.

- The optimal dose of EX or PA to maximize longevity remains incompletely understood.
- However, compelling aggregate data from many studies indicate that 2–2.5 h of moderate intensity EX or PA appears to be the minimal amount required for significant effect on longevity [17].
- Comparatively limited data examining the impact of habitual EX or PA doses that exceed this level do not suggest further incremental longevity benefit at higher levels.
- However, and of paramount importance, there are no data to suggest that high doses of habitual EX or PA lead to any attenuation or reduction of the longevity benefit conferred by 2–2.5 h per week of moderate intensity activity among healthy people without underlying cardiovascular disease as suggested by most guidelines.

Cardiac risk factor profile attenuation (i.e. reductions in blood pressure, improvements in plasma lipoprotein profiles, etc.) can be achieved with habitual EX or PA with dose response relationships that vary by specific risk factors:

- EX or PA aimed at targeting *plasma lipoproteins* appear to be most effective when they reach or exceed levels suggested by PA guidelines (see Chap. 38).
  - Across the plasma lipoprotein sub-types, EX has the most profound effect on high density lipoprotein with increases in the order of 2.5 mg/dL attributable to EX interventions with doses approximating PA guidelines [37], and more robust responses observed during higher levels of EX such as marathon training [38].
- EX training studies routinely document reductions in both systolic *blood pressure* (Δ~3–5 mmHg), and diastolic blood pressure (Δ~2–4 mmHg) [39–42].
  - The magnitude of reduction appears to be determined in part by pre-EX blood pressure with overtly hypertensive patient deriving greater benefit (see Chap. 37).
  - However, available data do not permit determination of an optimal dose response relationship between EX and blood pressure reduction and the impact of high versus moderate intensity EX is unknown.
- EX at any dose, particular when introduced among previously sedentary people and when coupled with control of caloric intake, stimulates weight loss (see Chap. 40) [43, 44].
  - However, long-term maintenance of this weight loss and/or maintenance of ideal body weight typically requires doses of EX that exceed PA guidelines by twofold–threefold [45].

Recent data suggest incremental benefit when high intensity EX replaces or is added to moderate intensity EX [46]. However, there are currently inadequate aggregate data to facilitate a definitive comparison of moderate intensity versus high intensity EX as related to longevity and cardiac risk factor attenuation. At present, both EX intensities appear to be safe and comparably effective across both primary and secondary cardiovascular disease prevention populations.

## 41.6 Can One Exercise Too Much?

Concern about "too much exercise" dates back to the initial descriptions of EX-induced cardiac remodelling in the late 1800s and remains an area of active controversy and investigation [7] and Darling [8]. Longevity studies of young elite endurance and team-sport athletes suggest a legacy effect that translates into later life reductions in healthcare system utilization [47], and improved mortality [48]. Age-related changes of cardiac structure and function including impaired diastolic function and reductions in left ventricular chamber volume may be prevented or reversed by high levels of EX during later life [38, 49].

However, vigorous EX increases the short term risk of myocardial infarction and sudden death irrespective of fitness level [50, 51], and recent data suggest that high levels of EX may increase the risk of certain forms of cardiovascular pathology (see also Chap. 32) [52]:

- Atrial tachyarrhythmia, most commonly ***atrial fibrillation***, may be considered a form of "overuse pathology" among high-level exercisers and competitive athletes [53, 54].
  - Numerous observational studies suggest an increased prevalence of atrial fibrillation among master athletes compared to sedentary age and gender matched controls.
  - Atrial fibrillation appears to be more common among aging male than female athletes and risk of incident atrial fibrillation appears to adhere to a direct EX intensity and EX volume dose relationship [55].
- Several reports document non-ischemic ***myocardial fibrosis*** among trained master athletes [56–58].
  - Hemodynamic mechanism related to interventricular dependence and systemic blood pressure responses to EX have been proposed.
  - To date, no data link this phenotype to any clinically relevant phenotype such as malignant arrhythmia or sudden death.
- EX confers favourable changes across atherosclerotic risk factors and reduces mortality from coronary heart disease. However, several recent observation cross sectional studies report higher levels of ***atherosclerosis***, as defined by cardiac CT imaging, among trained athletes than other similar less active people [59, 60].
  - Sub-clinical atherosclerosis among trained athletes appears to be largely calcific disease with minimal luminal impingement.
  - While it has been proposed that this may paradoxically have a stabilizing and thus protective effect [61], outcomes data defining the prognostic and mechanistic relevance of coronary calcium in high-level exercisers is lacking.

## 41.7 Physical Activity Prescription in Clinical Practice

PA and EX habits should be assessed by clinicians during all medical encounters and may represent a useful "vital sign" [62]. We advocate careful documentation of PA and EX habits for all patients.

Assessment of PA permits clinicians to categorize patients into one of three groups based on their assessment of PA and EX habits (Fig. 41.3):

1. Patients who routinely **fail to meet** PA guidelines
2. Patients who routinely **meet** PA guidelines
3. Patients who routinely **exceed** PA guidelines
   1. Patients who routinely **fail to meet** PA guidelines present the greatest clinical opportunity for positive impact. These patients deserve education about the benefits of increased PA, an assessment of perceived and/or objective barriers to PA, and the development of an EX prescription tailored to address these barriers.
   2. Patients who routinely **meet** PA guidelines deserve praise and reinforcement. Changes in habits over time that result in failure to meet PA guidelines

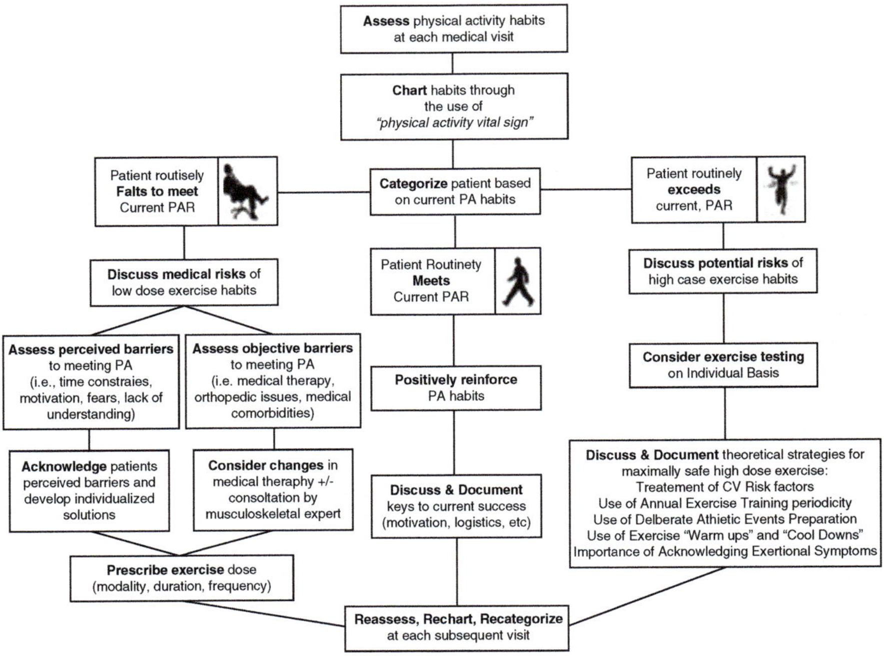


**Fig. 41.3** Integration of exercise dose in clinical practice. Algorithmic approach to the assessment and management of patients in clinical practice based on habitual physical activity (PA) and exercise dose exposure. PAR indicates physical activity recommendation (reproduced with permission from [63])

provides a valuable opportunity to detect incident disease or address potentially unhealthy lifestyle changes.

3. Patients who routinely **exceed** PA guidelines should not be discouraged from lifestyle due to concerns of overuse-pathology based on the available contemporary literature. Such patients benefit most from a discussion about "safe EX" practices and a clear acknowledgement about some element of scientific uncertainty about the impact of long-term high levels of EX.

## Clinical Pearls

- Exercise exposure or exercise "dose" is calculated as the product of the exercise duration, frequency, and intensity. This approach can be used rigorously in both research and clinical settings.
- The relationship between habitual physical activity and/or structured exercise and health outcomes is curvilinear. Thus, the greatest opportunity for improving health outcomes by the implementation of an exercise prescription lies with patients that begin with a truly sedentary baseline.
- While several forms of cardiac pathology including atrial fibrillation, sub-clinical myocardial fibrosis, and sub-clinical coronary artery calcification appear to be

enriched among aging competitive athletes, there is no established optimal exercise dose. Clinical recommendations to reduce exercise dose among aging athletes may at time be appropriate, must be individualized, and are best approached using a shared decision-making process.

## Review

### Questions

1. A 62-year old man with multiple risk factors for atherosclerotic disease inquires about the efficacy of a moderate intensity exercise program for risk attenuation. Of the following independent determinants of cardiac risk: (1) hypertension, (2) dyslipidemia, (3) obesity, and (4) coronary artery calcium, which has **NOT** been shown to respond favorably to the initiation of routine moderate intensity aerobic exercise?
2. The greatest absolute improvement in health outcomes, specifically longevity, conferred by an increase in exercise dose or habitual physical activity will occur among which of the following patients:
   (a) A sedentary office worker who begins a 30 min daily walking program,
   (b) A routine exerciser who meets physical activity recommendations and decides to increase from 150 to 300 min weekly of aerobic activity, or
   (c) An accomplished triathlete who decides to train for an Ironman-distance triathlon and thereby increases their training load from 10 to 20 h weekly?

### Answers

1. Routine moderate to high intensity aerobic exercise leads to modest but clinically relevant reductions in systolic blood pressure, improvements in plasma lipoprotein profiles, and weight loss. Coronary artery calcium, an independent determinant of prognosis, has not been shown to diminish in response to exercise. Several small cross-sectional studies among masters athletes and high active people actually suggest that extended exposure to high levels of exercise may increase coronary calcium burden. The prognostic significance of coronary artery calcium among masters athletes and high active people remains unknown.
2. The correct answer is the sedentary office worker who begins a 30-min daily walking program. The association between exercise dose and/or habitual physical activity and health outcomes adheres to a curvilinear relationship. The nature of this relationship indicates that a change from being completely sedentary to adopting an even minimally active lifestyle affords the greatest improvements in health outcomes.

## References


1. Pedersen BK, Saltin B. Exercise as medicine - evidence for prescribing exercise as therapy in 26 different chronic diseases. Scand J Med Sci Sports. 2015;25(Suppl 3):1–72.
2. Eijsvogels TM, Thompson PD. Exercise is medicine: at any dose? JAMA. 2015;314(18):1915–6.
3. Levine BD, Baggish AL, Kovacs RJ, Link MS, Maron MS, Eligibility MJH. Disqualification recommendations for competitive athletes with cardiovascular abnormalities: task force 1: classification of sports: dynamic, static, and impact: a scientific statement from the American heart association and American college of cardiology. J Am Coll Cardiol. 2015;66(21):2350–5.
4. Pelliccia A, Caselli S, Sharma S, Basso C, Bax JJ, Corrado D, et al. European Association of preventive cardiology (EAPC) and European association of cardiovascular imaging (EACVI) joint position statement: recommendations for the indication and interpretation of cardiovascular imaging in the evaluation of the athlete's heart. Eur Heart J. 2018;39(21):1949–69.
5. Liebenberg L. Persistence hunting by modern hunter-gatherers. Curr Anthropol. 2006;47:1017–26.
6. Lieberman DE. Is exercise really medicine? An evolutionary perspective. Curr Sports Med Rep. 2015;14(4):313–9.
7. Henschen S. Skidlauf und Skidwettlauf. EInde medizinische Sportstudie. Mitt Med Klin Upsala. 1899;2:15–8.
8. Darling EA. The effects of training. A study of the Harvard University Crews. Boston Med Surg J. 1899;CXLI:229–33.
9. Morris JN, Heady JA, Raffle PA, Roberts CG, Parks JW. Coronary heart-disease and physical activity of work. Lancet. 1953;265(6796):1111–20; concl.
10. Paffenbarger RS Jr, Hyde RT, Wing AL, Hsieh CC. Physical activity, all-cause mortality, and longevity of college alumni. N Engl J Med. 1986;314(10):605–13.
11. Paffenbarger RS Jr, Laughlin ME, Gima AS, Black RA. Work activity of longshoremen as related to death from coronary heart disease and stroke. N Engl J Med. 1970;282(20):1109–14.
12. Paffenbarger RS Jr, Wing AL, Hyde RT. Physical activity as an index of heart attack risk in college alumni. Am J Epidemiol. 1978;108(3):161–75.
13. Powell KE, Thompson PD, Caspersen CJ, Kendrick JS. Physical activity and the incidence of coronary heart disease. Annu Rev Public Health. 1987;8:253–87.
14. Public ACttSGot. Health service. Smoking and health. Washington D.C: U.S. Department of Health, Education, And Welfare; 1964.
15. Pate RR, Pratt M, Blair SN, Haskell WL, Macera CA, Bouchard C, et al. Physical activity and public health. A recommendation from the centers for disease control and prevention and the American College of Sports Medicine. JAMA. 1995;273(5):402–7.
16. Physical activity and cardiovascular health. NIH consensus development panel on physical activity and cardiovascular health. JAMA. 1996;276(3):241–6.
17. Services USDoHaH. Physical activity and health: a report of the surgeon general. Atlanta, GA: U.S. Department of health and human services, centers for disease control and prevention, national center for chronic disease prevention and Health Promotion; 1996.
18. WHO. Global recommendations on physical activity for health. Available from: http://www.who.int/dietphysicalactivity/factsheet_recommendations/en/.
19. Eijsvogels TMH, Thompson PD, Franklin B. The 'extreme exercise hypothesis': recent findings and cardiovascular health implications. Curr Treat Options Cardiovasc Med. 2018;20(10):84. In press
20. Powell KE, Paluch AE, Blair SN. Physical activity for health: What kind? How much? How intense? On top of what? Annu Rev Public Health. 2011;32:349–65.
21. Physical Activity Guidelines Advisory Committee. Physical activity guidelines advisory committee report. Washington DC: U.S.: Department of Health and Human Services; 2008.
22. Lancet Physical Activity Series Working G. Physical activity. Lancet. 2012;380(9838):219.

23. Lancet Physical Activity Series 2 Executive C, Lancet Sedentary Behaviour Working G. Physical activity 2016: progress and challenges. Lancet. 2016;388:10051.
24. Lee IM, Shiroma EJ, Lobelo F, Puska P, Blair SN, Katzmarzyk PT, et al. Effect of physical inactivity on major non-communicable diseases worldwide: an analysis of burden of disease and life expectancy. Lancet. 2012;380(9838):219–29.
25. Biswas A, Oh PI, Faulkner GE, Bajaj RR, Silver MA, Mitchell MS, et al. Sedentary time and its association with risk for disease incidence, mortality, and hospitalization in adults: a systematic review and meta-analysis. Ann Intern Med. 2015;162(2):123–32.
26. van der Ploeg HP, Chey T, Korda RJ, Banks E, Bauman A. Sitting time and all-cause mortality risk in 222 497 Australian adults. Arch Intern Med. 2012;172(6):494–500.
27. Chomistek AK, Manson JE, Stefanick ML, Lu B, Sands-Lincoln M, Going SB, et al. Relationship of sedentary behavior and physical activity to incident cardiovascular disease: results from the Women's Health Initiative. J Am Coll Cardiol. 2013;61(23):2346–54.
28. Ekelund U, Steene-Johannessen J, Brown WJ, Fagerland MW, Owen N, Powell KE, et al. Does physical activity attenuate, or even eliminate, the detrimental association of sitting time with mortality? A harmonised meta-analysis of data from more than 1 million men and women. Lancet. 2016;388(10051):1302–10.
29. Healy GN, Dunstan DW, Salmon J, Cerin E, Shaw JE, Zimmet PZ, et al. Breaks in sedentary time: beneficial associations with metabolic risk. Diabetes Care. 2008;31(4):661–6.
30. Dunstan DW, Kingwell BA, Larsen R, Healy GN, Cerin E, Hamilton MT, et al. Breaking up prolonged sitting reduces postprandial glucose and insulin responses. Diabetes Care. 2012;35(5):976–83.
31. Matthews CE, Moore SC, Sampson J, Blair A, Xiao Q, Keadle SK, et al. Mortality benefits for replacing sitting time with different physical activities. Med Sci Sports Exerc. 2015;47(9):1833–40.
32. van der Ploeg HP, Chey T, Ding D, Chau JY, Stamatakis E, Bauman AE. Standing time and all-cause mortality in a large cohort of Australian adults. Prev Med. 2014;69:187–91.
33. Katzmarzyk PT. Standing and mortality in a prospective cohort of Canadian adults. Med Sci Sports Exerc. 2014;46(5):940–6.
34. Lee DC, Pate RR, Lavie CJ, Sui X, Church TS, Blair SN. Leisure-time running reduces all-cause and cardiovascular mortality risk. J Am Coll Cardiol. 2014;64(5):472–81.
35. Wen CP, Wai JP, Tsai MK, Yang YC, Cheng TY, Lee MC, et al. Minimum amount of physical activity for reduced mortality and extended life expectancy: a prospective cohort study. Lancet. 2011;378(9798):1244–53.
36. Arem H, Moore SC, Patel A, Hartge P, Berrington de Gonzalez A, Visvanathan K, et al. Leisure time physical activity and mortality: a detailed pooled analysis of the dose-response relationship. JAMA Intern Med. 2015;175(6):959–67.
37. Kodama S, Tanaka S, Saito K, Shu M, Sone Y, Onitake F, et al. Effect of aerobic exercise training on serum levels of high-density lipoprotein cholesterol: a meta-analysis. Arch Intern Med. 2007;167(10):999–1008.
38. Zilinski JL, Contursi ME, Isaacs SK, Deluca JR, Lewis GD, Weiner RB, et al. Myocardial adaptations to recreational marathon training among middle-aged men. Circ Cardiovasc Imaging. 2015;8(2):e002487.
39. Fagard RH. Exercise characteristics and the blood pressure response to dynamic physical training. Med Sci Sports Exerc. 2001;33(6 Suppl):S484–92. discussion S93-4.
40. Cornelissen VA, Fagard RH. Effects of endurance training on blood pressure, blood pressure-regulating mechanisms, and cardiovascular risk factors. Hypertension. 2005;46(4):667–75.
41. Whelton SP, Chin A, Xin X, He J. Effect of aerobic exercise on blood pressure: a meta-analysis of randomized, controlled trials. Ann Intern Med. 2002;136(7):493–503.
42. Kelley G, Tran ZV. Aerobic exercise and normotensive adults: a meta-analysis. Med Sci Sports Exerc. 1995;27(10):1371–7.
43. Slentz CA, Aiken LB, Houmard JA, Bales CW, Johnson JL, Tanner CJ, et al. Inactivity, exercise, and visceral fat. STRRIDE: a randomized, controlled study of exercise intensity and amount. J Appl Physiol (1985). 2005;99(4):1613–8.

44. Irwin ML, Yasui Y, Ulrich CM, Bowen D, Rudolph RE, Schwartz RS, et al. Effect of exercise on total and intra-abdominal body fat in postmenopausal women: a randomized controlled trial. JAMA. 2003;289(3):323–30.
45. Ades PA, Savage PD, Toth MJ, Harvey-Berino J, Schneider DJ, Bunn JY, et al. High-calorie-expenditure exercise: a new approach to cardiac rehabilitation for overweight coronary patients. Circulation. 2009;119(20):2671–8.
46. Gebel K, Ding D, Chey T, Stamatakis E, Brown WJ, Bauman AE. Effect of moderate to vigorous physical activity on all-cause mortality in middle-aged and older Australians. JAMA Intern Med. 2015;175(6):970–7.
47. Kujala UM, Sarna S, Kaprio J, Koskenvuo M. Hospital care in later life among former world-class Finnish athletes. JAMA. 1996;276(3):216–20.
48. Kontro TK, Sarna S, Kaprio J, Kujala UM. Mortality and health-related habits in 900 Finnish former elite athletes and their brothers. Br J Sports Med. 2018;52(2):89–95.
49. Howden EJ, Sarma S, Lawley JS, Opondo M, Cornwell W, Stoller D, et al. Reversing the cardiac effects of sedentary aging in middle age-a randomized controlled trial: implications for heart failure prevention. Circulation. 2018;137(15):1549–60.
50. Albert CM, Mittleman MA, Chae CU, Lee IM, Hennekens CH, Manson JE. Triggering of sudden death from cardiac causes by vigorous exertion. N Engl J Med. 2000;343(19):1355–61.
51. Siscovick DS, Weiss NS, Fletcher RH, Lasky T. The incidence of primary cardiac arrest during vigorous exercise. N Engl J Med. 1984;311(14):874–7.
52. Eijsvogels TM, Fernandez AB, Thompson PD. Are there deleterious cardiac effects of acute and chronic endurance exercise? Physiol Rev. 2016;96(1):99–125.
53. Sorokin AV, Araujo CG, Zweibel S, Thompson PD. Atrial fibrillation in endurance-trained athletes. Br J Sports Med. 2011;45(3):185–8.
54. Abdulla J, Nielsen JR. Is the risk of atrial fibrillation higher in athletes than in the general population? A systematic review and meta-analysis. Europace. 2009;11(9):1156–9.
55. Andersen K, Farahmand B, Ahlbom A, Held C, Ljunghall S, Michaelsson K, et al. Risk of arrhythmias in 52 755 long-distance cross-country skiers: a cohort study. Eur Heart J. 2013;34(47):3624–31.
56. Wilson M, O'Hanlon R, Prasad S, Deighan A, Macmillan P, Oxborough D, et al. Diverse patterns of myocardial fibrosis in lifelong, veteran endurance athletes. J Appl Physiol. 2011;110(6):1622–6.
57. La Gerche A, Burns AT, Mooney DJ, Inder WJ, Taylor AJ, Bogaert J, et al. Exercise-induced right ventricular dysfunction and structural remodelling in endurance athletes. Eur Heart J. 2012;33(8):998–1006.
58. Breuckmann F, Mohlenkamp S, Nassenstein K, Lehmann N, Ladd S, Schmermund A, et al. Myocardial late gadolinium enhancement: prevalence, pattern, and prognostic relevance in marathon runners. Radiology. 2009;251(1):50–7.
59. Aengevaeren VL, Mosterd A, Braber TL, Prakken NHJ, Doevendans PA, Grobbee DE, et al. Relationship between lifelong exercise volume and coronary atherosclerosis in athletes. Circulation. 2017;136(2):138–48.
60. Merghani A, Maestrini V, Rosmini S, Cox AT, Dhutia H, Bastiaenan R, et al. Prevalence of subclinical coronary artery disease in masters endurance athletes with a low atherosclerotic risk profile. Circulation. 2017;136(2):126–37.
61. Baggish AL, Levine BD. Coronary artery calcification among endurance athletes: hearts of stone. Circulation. 2017;136(2):149–51.
62. Sallis RE, Baggish AL, Franklin BA, Whitehead JR. The call for a physical activity vital sign in clinical practice. Am J Med. 2016;129(9):903–5.
63. Wasfy MM, Baggish AL. Exercise dose in clinical practice. Circulation. 2016;133(23):2297–313.

# Part IV

# Exercise in Secondary Prevention and Cardiac Rehabilitation

# Modalities of Exercise Training in Cardiac Rehabilitation

42

Luc Vanhees and Dominique Hansen

**Learning Objectives**

1. To understand the FITT principles in exercise programming for patients with cardiovascular disease.
2. To understand in depth the role and effect of strength training, and how different modalities may affect acute exercise responses.
3. To understand in depth the role and effect of endurance training, and how different modalities may affect acute exercise responses.
4. To understand how to maximise the medical safety of exercise training and what strategies are available to optimise the patients' adherence to exercise prescriptions.

## 42.1 General Concepts of Exercise Prescription (FITT Principles)

Recommendations for prescription of exercise and sports require a basic knowledge of physiological responses to exercise, along with an understanding of concepts and characteristics of physical activity, exercise interventions and sports. In this section we will briefly discuss the components of exercise, and the so-called "**FITT**" concept:

L. Vanhees (✉)
Department of Rehabilitation Sciences, Research group Rehabilitation for internal disorders, University of Leuven, Leuven, Belgium
e-mail: luc.vanhees@kuleuven.be

D. Hansen
Heart Centre Hasselt, Jessa Hospital, BIOMED (Biomedical Research Institute) and REVAL (Rehabilitation Research Centre), Hasselt University, Hasselt, Belgium
e-mail: dominique.hansen@uhasselt.be



A. Pressler, J. Niebauer (eds.), *Textbook of Sports and Exercise Cardiology*,
https://doi.org/10.1007/978-3-030-35374-2_42

- **F**requency
- **I**ntensity
- **T**ype
- **T**ime (duration of sessions and duration of programme).

In terms of the type of exercise, this involves the exercise mode:

- Type of muscular work
- Type of exercise intervention and is included as an important characteristic of exercise.

Although exercise and physical activity (PA) are often used interchangeably, it is important to recognize that guidelines tend to separate the two.

- PA has been defined as any bodily movement produced by the skeletal muscle that results in energy expenditure.
- Exercise or exercise training, on the other hand, is considered a subcategory of PA and is, by definition, PA that is planned, structured, repetitive, and purposeful in the sense that improvement or maintenance of one or more components of physical fitness (PF) is the objective [1].

The health-related fitness of a person can be expressed by five major components:

1. A *morphological* component (body mass relative to height, body composition, subcutaneous fat distribution, abdominal visceral fat, bone density and flexibility);
2. A *muscular* component (power or explosive strength, isometric strength, muscular endurance);
3. A *motor* component (agility, balance, coordination, speed of movement);
4. A *cardiorespiratory* component (endurance or submaximal exercise capacity, maximal aerobic power, heart function, lung function, blood pressure); and
5. A *metabolic* component (glucose tolerance, insulin sensitivity, lipid and lipoprotein metabolism, substrate oxidation characteristics).

Traditionally, different types of exercise are classified in binary terms as **endurance** or **resistance** (strength) sports or exercise. However, this is a little oversimplified. Further classifications of exercise are metabolically related (*aerobic* versus *anaerobic* exercise) or those related to muscle: isotonic, isometric or isokinetic muscular work. Another classification is dynamic versus static exercise.

- *Aerobic* exercise refers to activity performed at an intensity that allows metabolism of stored energy to occur mainly through the use of oxygen. It involves large muscle groups in dynamic activities, resulting in substantial increases in heart rate and energy expenditure. Examples of aerobic exercise include cycling, running, and swimming performed at low to moderate intensity [2].

- In contrast, *anaerobic* exercise refers to movement performed at an increasingly high intensity unsustainable by $O_2$ alone or requiring metabolism of stored energy to be processed largely without oxygen (i.e. energy is predominantly provided by anaerobic glycolysis and stored phosphocreatine). A sustained isometric muscle action which is not working maximally but nevertheless does not depend upon oxygen during the muscle contraction is also an example of anaerobic exercise. Another example of this type of activity is intermittent high-intensity exercise [3, 4].

Because no muscular exercise occurs entirely in the absence of oxygen, the term "anaerobic" has been controversial and terms such as "oxygen independent glycolysis" are preferred by some researchers.

## 42.2 Exercise Modes in Strength Training

As explained in the first part of this chapter, specific exercise modalities are recommended during strength training in cardiovascular rehabilitation. However, within strength training many different combinations of exercise modalities can be made. In this part of the chapter, the impact of these different exercise modalities is discussed in greater detail.

### 42.2.1 Volume of Recruited Muscles: Small vs. Large Muscle Groups

According to clinical guidelines [3, 5], it is recommended to mainly target large muscle groups during strength training in order to elicit greater improvements in muscle mass, bone mineral density and exercise tolerance, and to induce a greater metabolic effect (e.g. glycaemic control) [6, 7]. In principle, the following muscle groups should thus be targeted during strength training:

(a) M. quadriceps femoris,
(b) Hamstrings,
(c) Calf muscles,
(d) Abdominal muscles,
(e) Back muscles,
(f) Shoulder muscles, and
(g) M. biceps brachii.

It is generally known that the larger the activated muscle bulk is during strength training, the greater the impact will be on blood pressure, heart rate and blood lactate concentrations (increments should be anticipated) [8]. However, also intermuscular coordination, balance and the prevention of falls is of key importance, especially in older patients (>70 years) with cardiovascular disease [9–11]. In general, strength training of the large weight-baring muscles (legs and trunk) will already lead to significant reductions in this fall risk [12]. However, in order to further maximize the impact of exercise intervention on fall risk in these individuals, it is important to also exercise the smaller muscles that are relevant to balance. In this regard, for example, also M. tibialis anterior should undergo strength training, and balance exercises should be incorporated which are, in fact, functional strengthening exercises for (very) small muscle groups (including at the hips and spine) [12].

In final, due to a median sternotomy (e.g. during CABG) and/or fear avoidance to use the upper extremities, significant muscle wasting in the arms can occur [13]. In such event, the arms muscles, which are smaller muscle groups, should receive strength training, but in a medically safe manner.

As a result,

- Clinicians should assess muscle strength at entry of cardiovascular rehabilitation, to detect muscle weakness and modify the exercise program accordingly.
- In this regard, large muscle groups must be trained.
- However, also balance should be assessed in older patients (>70 years) to include specific exercises to prevent falls.

### 42.2.2 Volume of Strength Training

In order to maximize the clinical benefits of strength training, it is important to expose the patient to a sufficient volume of strength training. This can be done by

1. Increasing the number of sets/muscle groups and/or.
2. Increasing the number of exercises or muscle groups.

It has been shown that a larger number of sets per muscle group (e.g. one vs. three sets) elicits significantly greater improvements in muscle strength and mass in cardiac rehabilitation [14]. As a result, it is generally recommended that at least three sets per muscle group should be applied. Even if at least three sets per muscle group are applied during strength training, the impact of this type of exercise intervention can be maximized by increasing the number of exercises or muscle groups. Obviously, by targeting more muscle groups by strength training, greater increments in muscle mass and bone mineral density may be anticipated. However, also glycaemic control is affected far better by increasing the number of muscle groups, and it seems that 21 sets (three sets multiplied by seven muscle groups) is mandatory if improvements in glycaemic control are ambitioned [15].

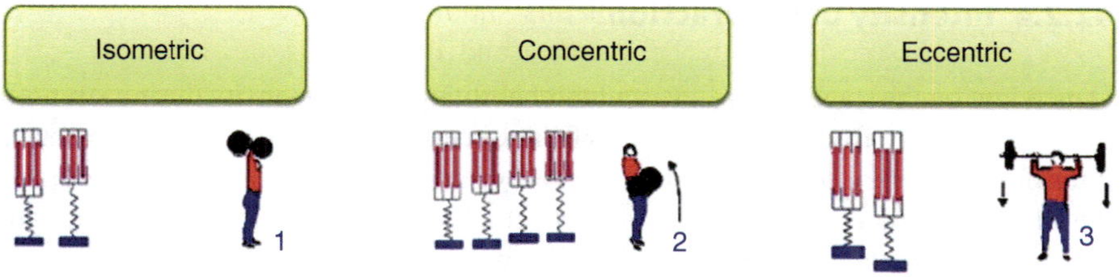


**Fig. 42.1** Different types of strength training (see text for more details)

### 42.2.3 Type of Contraction: Isometric/Isotonic/Isokinetic/Eccentric

It is important to understand the distinction between *dynamic concentric* and *eccentric* or *isometric* muscle strength training (Fig. 42.1).

- During *concentric* strength training the externally applied load can be overcome, leading to muscular shortening, while during
- *Eccentric* strength training the externally applied load is too high to sustain so that during muscular contraction this muscle prolongs.
- When the joint velocity is controlled/standardized during muscular contraction, *isokinetic* muscle training is applied.
- When no movements are allowed in the joint during muscular contraction, *isometric* muscle training is applied.

In general, isokinetic muscle strength training is not applied regularly in cardiovascular rehabilitation, as this would require strength training on a dynamometer, which is time-consuming and very costly. Isometric strength is also applied rarely in cardiovascular rehabilitation because this type of strength training is not functional and/or may induce the Valsalva manoeuvre (see below). As a result, what is or can most commonly used in cardiovascular rehabilitation is concentric or eccentric strength training. At the moment it is assumed that, when matched for either maximum load or work, similar increases in muscle size is found between concentric and eccentric strength training [16]. On the other hand, eccentric strength training allows the muscle to be exposed to greater loads. In this particular situation, greater increments in muscle strength are then noticed (vs. concentric strength training), at least in healthy subjects [17, 18]. This remains to be studied in greater detail in patients with cardiovascular disease. Interestingly, the application of eccentric strength training seems to lead to smaller increments in blood pressure and heart rate, when compared with concentric strength training, at least in healthy individuals [19]. The latter also remains to be studied in patients with cardiovascular disease.

### 42.2.4 Intensity of Contraction

Dependent on the stage of cardiovascular rehabilitation, the intensity during strength training can vary from 30 up to 70% of one-repetition maximum, in which lower intensities are often proposed [5]. However, when increments in muscle mass and muscle strength are ambitioned, which is actually the impetus for adding strength training to endurance training, it has been shown in many studies that higher intensities of strength training (>65% of one-repetition maximum) should be selected [20].

One of the most important reasons to avoid strength training at higher intensities could be the **Valsalva manoeuvre** (see also Chap. 37):

- The Valsalva manoeuvre is a forced expiration against a closed glottis, which leads to an increase in intrathoracic pressure, and a potential reduction in cardiac output due to a decreased venous return (from which syncope may result).
- After the termination of this compressed breathing a large increase in venous return may be provoked and thus an increased cardiac output (through a constricted arterial vascular system).
- This may lead to sharp increments in blood pressure and myocardial oxygen demand.

Therefore, patients should pay attention to their breathing while executing strength exercises. However, when such Valsalva manoeuvre is avoided (by exhaling during muscular contraction), high-intense resistance training (high load, low number of repetitions) in fact induces smaller increments in blood pressure, heart rate and cardiac output as opposed to low-intense resistance training (low load, high number of repetitions) [21–24], which is in contrast to common belief.

### 42.2.5 Endurance vs. Strength Training

The elicited physiological and clinical adaptations as a result of **endurance** vs. **strength** exercise training are very different:

- As a result of **endurance** exercise training, skeletal muscle mitochondrial biogenesis is activated after phosphorylation of 5′ adenosine monophosphate-activated protein kinase (AMPK), which in effect will lead to enhanced muscle respiration capacity to resynthesize ATP.
  - In addition, muscle fibre type shifts may be induced (in favour of type 1 muscle fibre) next to enhanced capillarisation.
  - From these molecular changes, improvements in endurance capacity and skeletal muscle fat oxidation capacity are the key adaptations.
  - Moreover, in the heart hypertrophy of the left ventricle, together with increments in left-ventricular cavity, can be induced by long-term exposure to endurance training.

- **Strength** training, on the other hand, induces completely different molecular and clinical adaptations.
  - As result of strength training, skeletal muscle ribosomal biogenesis is induced after activation of mammalian target of rapamycin (mTOR), which in effect will lead to muscle hypertrophy to be able to generate greater muscle tension/strength.
  - In addition, muscle fibre type shifts may be induced (in favour of type 2b muscle fibre).
  - From these molecular changes, improvements in muscle strength and mass are the key adaptations.
  - Moreover, in the heart more pronounced hypertrophy of the left ventricle, but without increments in left-ventricular cavity, can be induced by long-term exposure to strength training.

In final, recent studies have shown that these different molecular cascades, as activated by different types of exercise, can interfere with each other [25–26]. Whether this would also lead to suboptimal clinical benefits of exercise intervention in patients with cardiovascular disease, remains to be studied in greater detail [25, 26].

## 42.3 Exercise Modes in Aerobic (Endurance) Training

The most common modes of aerobic exercise are walking, jogging, cycling, and swimming, which, when carried out at moderate intensity, represent good examples of aerobic activity. To achieve an effective and safe exercise training response, the appropriate intensity, duration, and frequency should be chosen.

### 42.3.1 Exercise Intensity

Submaximal prolonged walking, jogging, cycling, and swimming are representative types of exercise that are usually termed aerobic or endurance. Of all the basic elements of exercise prescription, exercise intensity is generally considered to be the most critical for the development of aerobic fitness and to have the most favorable impact on risk factors [27, 28].

- Absolute intensity refers to the rate of energy expenditure during exercise and is usually expressed in kcal/min or metabolic equivalent tasks (METs) [2, 29].
- Relative exercise intensity refers to a fraction of an individual's maximal power (load) that is maintained during exercise and is usually prescribed as a percentage of maximal aerobic capacity ($VO_2max$) on the basis of a cardiopulmonary exercise test [29].

- Training intensity can also be expressed as a percentage of maximal heart rate (HRmax) recorded during an exercise test [30] or predicted on the basis of the equation [HRmax = 220 − age] [31]. The use of prediction equations for HRmax are not recommended, because there is a large standard deviation around the regression line between age and HRmax [32].
- Alternatively, exercise intensity can be expressed relative to a percentage of a person's HR reserve (HRR) which uses a percentage of the difference between HRmax and resting HR and adds it to the resting HR (Karvonen's formula) [33].

There are caveats to the use of HR for prescribing and evaluating exercise intensity in persons using beta-blocking medications [34]. Ideally, the HR derived for training should only be used if functional capacity was determined (the exercise test was performed) while taking the medication.

Intensity is also commonly monitored using the rate of perceived exertion scale (Fig. 42.2) or "talk test" (see Chap. 1) or "breathing rule" ('to be able to talk while exercising'; [32]), or arterialized blood lactate concentrations [1, 17–19] (Table 42.1).

**Fig. 42.2** Borg scale for ratings of perceived exertion

| No. | Subjective intensity / effort |
|---|---|
| 6 | No exertion at all |
| 7 | Extremely light |
| 8 | |
| 9 | Very light |
| 10 | |
| 11 | Light |
| 12 | |
| 13 | Somewhat hard |
| 14 | |
| 15 | Hard (heavy) |
| 16 | |
| 17 | Very hard |
| 18 | |
| 19 | Extremely hard |
| 20 | Maximal exertion |

### 42.3.2 Exercise Training Zones

According to the Greek physician Galen (180 AD), not all movement constitutes exercise; vigorous movement is required, which is indicated by a marked alteration in respiration [35]. Nowadays it is accepted that in order to enhance cardiorespiratory fitness, exercise should be sufficiently intense to "overload" the aerobic system.

- Aerobic fitness is improved when exercise intensity is above the aerobic threshold [36] and within an aerobic training zone, the boundaries of which are indicated in the Table 42.1.
- The first aerobic threshold, measured by gas exchange or by blood lactate levels, is indicative of everyday activities and presumably corresponds to 2 mmol/l lactate, while
- the second anaerobic threshold emerges from more intense aerobic activities which usually leads to a blood lactate accumulation of 4 mmol/l [36, 37].

For both primary and secondary cardiovascular disease prevention, the target intensity is usually recommended to be close to the second anaerobic threshold [30, 38]. Subsequent to the aerobic threshold is the anaerobic training zone (Table 42.1) [28, 36, 37]. Cardiorespiratory endurance is also effectively improved when a training stimulus is applied within this zone (6–10 mmol/l lactate or between 14 and 20 on the rate of perceived exertion scale), but this intensity of exercise is more appropriate for athletic purposes [36, 37].

### 42.3.3 Training Volume

Exercise intensity is inversely related to exercise time. Their product (in kcal or kJ) defines the volume of each training unit which in turn multiplied by frequency

**Table 42.1** Relationship among indices of exercise intensity and training zones

| Intensity | Lactate (mmol/l) | METs | $VO_2$max (%) | HRR (%) | HRmax (%) | RPE scale | Training zone |
|---|---|---|---|---|---|---|---|
| Low intensity, light effort | 2–3 | 2–4 | 28–39 | 30–39 | 45–54 | 10–11 | Aerobic |
| Moderate intensity, moderate effort | 4–5 | 4–6 | 40–59 | 40–59 | 55–69 | 12–13 | Aerobic |
| High intensity, vigorous effort | 6–8 | 6–8 | 60–79 | 60–84 | 70–89 | 14–16 | Lactate, aerobic, anaerobic |
| Very hard effort | 8–10 | 8–10 | >80 | >84 | >89 | 17–19 | Lactate, aerobic, anaerobic |

*METs* Metabolic equivalent of tasks, *HRR* Heart rate reserve, *HRmax* maximum heart rate, *RPE* Borg rating of perceived exertion (6–20 scale (Fig. 42.2))

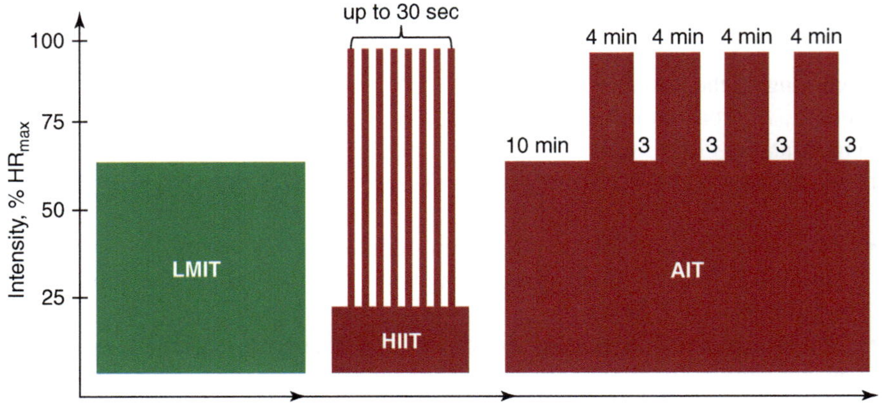


**Fig. 42.3** Schematic depiction of different exercise protocols applying either low-to-moderate intensity continuous training (LMIT) or high-intensity interval exercise. The latter can be performed in different ways according to the length and intensities of both the high-intensity intervals and the moderate recovery phases in-between. The term "HIIT" does not refer to a specific protocol but rather to the application of high-intensity intervals at all, whereas AIT (Aerobic Interval Training) refers to the 4 × 4 min protocol that has been used in many studies in recent years

provides an estimate of the energy expenditure of the training bout or session. The frequency of training sessions and the duration of the training period provide total energy expenditure of a training programme. Training volume should increase weekly either by 2.5% in intensity [4] or 2 min duration [39], although rate of progression should be individualized according to the biological adaptation of the individual. Training adaptation is also influenced by genetics [40] and environmental factors, such as hydration, heat, cold, and altitude [41–43].

### 42.3.4 Mode of Training

Aerobic exercise training can either be **continuous** or **interval**. In order to improve endurance capacity, clinicians can opt for continuous low-to-moderate intense exercise training (LMIT) or high-intensity interval training (HIIT). These types of exercise are very different from each other in terms of programming.

- HIIT is characterised by peaks of high-intense exercise (often at 80–100% of peak heart rate, between 30 s and 4 min) interspersed by exercises at a low intensity (40–60% of peak heart rate, between 1 and 4 min) (see Fig. 42.3 for examples) [44].
- During LMIT these exercise peaks and periods of cooling down are absent, and often the sessions are longer as opposed to HIIT sessions.

The rationale to use HIIT is to prevent a full cardiorespiratory adaptation to high-intense exercise, despite the fact that the skeletal muscle is stimulated maximally.

As a result, this type of exercise training is very interesting for patients with significant cardiac (e.g. heart failure) or pulmonary (e.g. COPD) limitations. Indeed, it is now widely established that this type of exercise training is feasible [45], although the exercise peak may not last too long in order to prevent these cardiorespiratory compensations.

The latter is currently the most difficult aspect in HIIT application: there is at the moment no formal consensus

1. How long and high the exercise peak should be,
2. How long and low the cooling down exercise should be,
3. How many peaks should be executed each training session.

It is very likely that the patient phenotype will dictate what is possible and desirable (physical fitness, age, medical history, heart function, lung function, muscle strength, etc.), next to the goals of the exercise intervention [44]. The clinical effectiveness of HIIT in patients with cardiovascular disease has received great interest in the last decade.

- From a recent meta-analysis, it was concluded that HIIT resulted in a higher increase in peak oxygen uptake compared with LMIT in patients with coronary artery disease or chronic heart failure with reduced ejection fraction.
- Moreover, a larger increase of the first ventilatory threshold and peak heart rate was observed after HIIT in all these patients, while other cardiorespiratory parameters, cardiovascular risk factors, and quality of life were equally affected [45].

It thus follows that HIIT can be considered more often in cardiovascular rehabilitation, but it remains to be studied which HIIT protocols are best applicable.

## 42.4 Attractiveness of PA and Training Programmes

To maximise the adherence of home-based physical activity and exercise training in patients with cardiovascular disease, it is also important to maximise the attractiveness of these exercises. In many centres the long-term adherence rates to exercise recommendations, even after completion of ambulatory cardiac rehabilitation, can be low [46, 47]. To increase the attractiveness of cardiovascular rehabilitation, various strategies are optional, such as:

(a) Allowing the patient to self-select the type of exercise,
(b) Organise group exercise sessions and/or
(c) Offer digital technologies.

To start with, the rehabilitation unit should be inviting and appealing to patients: this should be a facility with music and/or screens on the background, with lots of light from outdoor (or preferentially with big windows), in which communicative and helpful personnel/clinicians assist the patients, and with comfortable/appealing training systems. Clinicians should realize that exercise training on stationary devices can be very boring, particularly when large volumes of exercise must be achieved, so maximal efforts should be made to adhere to this suggestion. In this regard, mixing or varying with exercise modes can also be helpful to break-up prolonged or high effort/difficult exercises. Moreover, the application of virtual reality during exercise and exergaming is being studied in cardiovascular rehabilitation at the moment, with some promising effects on patient satisfaction and exercise adherence [48, 49].

During this ambulatory rehabilitation, it is important to address which types of exercise are favoured by the patient, or what types of exercises are ambitioned to execute after the phase 2 rehabilitation program, and to try to accustom the program accordingly. However, allowing the patients to fully self-select the type, volume and intensity of exercises should not be considered as the standard, as smaller clinical benefits of exercise intervention can be observed, probably due to insufficient exercise intensities and volumes, but also improperly selected exercise modes [50]. Therefore, specific exercise advices from qualified clinicians remain mandatory.

- Offering exercise training in groups (with peers) is highly warranted: this will lead to a significantly greater exercise adherence, both during phase two rehabilitation programs as well as in maintenance programs.

Finally, in order to optimise exercise adherence as well as the clinical effectiveness of cardiovascular rehabilitation both in the short and long term, the application of telemonitoring and telerehabilitation seems highly effective [50, 51]. Such intervention allows the patient the get daily feedback on their physical activity intensity and/or volume, and how to exercise or progress the exercises. In addition, such intervention also provides monitoring of physiological parameters to optimise medical safety of exercise training.

**Clinical Pearls**

- To maximise the clinical effectiveness, but maintain medical safety of exercise intervention, clinicians should carefully select the FITT components in exercise prescription: Frequency, Intensity, Type and Time.
- Dynamic strength training at moderate intensity should be prescribed to many patients with cardiovascular disease (risk) (based on indication and phenotype), but the effects of isometric strength remains to be studied in greater detail.
- Next to the classical moderate-intense endurance training, clinicians can opt for high-intensity interval training (HIIT) as this training type leads to favourable changes in physical fitness and cardiovascular risk factors.
- Next to selecting exercise modalities to optimise health in individuals, it is also of key importance to maximise the attractiveness of exercise intervention to support long-term therapy adherence.

## Review

## Questions

1. What are the 5 major components of health-related fitness?
2. How should we classify the different characteristics of exercise?
3. How can the intensity of aerobic exercise be individually determined?
4. In what effects are endurance and strength training different from each other?

## Answers

1. Major components of health related fitness are (1) a morphological component (body mass relative to height, body composition, subcutaneous fat distribution, abdominal visceral fat, bone density and flexibility); (2) a muscular component (power or explosive strength, isometric strength, muscular endurance); (3) a motor component (agility, balance, coordination, speed of movement); (4) a cardiorespiratory component (endurance or submaximal exercise capacity, maximal aerobic power, heart function, lung function, blood pressure); and (5) a metabolic component (glucose tolerance, insulin sensitivity, lipid and lipoprotein metabolism, substrate oxidation characteristics).
2. The FITT$^{++}$ principles are Frequency, Intensity, Type, Time (or duration) and Mode$^{(+)}$ and Attractiveness$^{(+)}$ of exercise.
3. After performing a maximal exercise test (until exhaustion or until symptoms), maximal heart rate, maximal load or capacity and ventilatory or lactic thresholds can be used to determine the individual intensity of aerobic exercise.
4. As a result of endurance exercise training, skeletal muscle mitochondrial biogenesis is activated after phosphorylation of 5′ adenosine monophosphate-activated protein kinase (AMPK), which in effect will lead to enhanced muscle respiration capacity to resynthesize ATP. In addition, muscle fibre type shifts may be induced (in favour of type 1 muscle fibre) next to enhanced capillarisation. From these molecular changes, improvements in endurance capacity and skeletal muscle fat oxidation capacity are the key adaptations. Finally, in the heart hypertrophy of the left ventricle, together with increments in left-ventricular cavity, can be induced by long-term exposure to endurance training.

   Strength training, on the other hand, induces completely different molecular and clinical adaptations. As result of strength training, skeletal muscle ribosomal biogenesis is induced after activation of mammalian target of rapamycin (mTOR), which in effect will lead to muscle hypertrophy to be able to generate greater muscle tension/strength. In addition, muscle fibre type shifts may be induced (in favour of type 2b muscle fibre). From these molecular changes, improvements in muscle strength and mass are the key adaptations. Moreover, in the heart more pronounced hypertrophy of the left ventricle, but without increments in left-ventricular cavity, can be induced by long-term exposure to strength training.

## References


1. Caspersen CJ, Powell KE, Christensen GM. Physical activity, exercise, and physical fitness: definitions and distinctions for health-related research. Public Health Rep. 1985;100(2):126–31.
2. Vanhees L, Rauch B, Piepoli M, van Buuren F, Takken T, Börjesson M, Bjarnason-Wehrens B, Doherty P, Dugmore D, Halle M, Writing Group, EACPR. Importance of characteristics and modalities of physical activity and exercise in the management of cardiovascular health in individuals with cardiovascular disease (Part III). Eur J Prev Cardiol. 2012;19:1333–56.
3. Vanhees L, Geladas N, Hansen D, Kouidi E, Niebauer J, Reiner Z, Cornelissen V, Adamopoulos S, Prescott E, Börjesson M. EACPR writing group. Importance of characteristics and modalities of physical activity and exercise in the management of cardiovascular health in individuals with cardiovascular risk factors: recommendations from the EACPR. Part II. Eur J Prev Cardiol. 2012;19(5):1005–33.
4. Warburton DE, Nicol CW, Bredin SS. Health benefits of physical activity: the evidence. CMAJ. 2006;174(6):801–9.
5. Piepoli M, Corra U, Benzer W, Bjarnason-Wehrens B, Dendale P, Gaita D, McGee H, Mendes M, Niebauer J, Zwisler AD, Schmid JP, Cardiac Rehabilitation Section of the European Association of Cardiovascular Prevention and Rehabilitation. Secondary prevention through cardiac rehabilitation: from knowledge to implementation. A position paper from the Cardiac Rehabilitation Section of the European Association of Cardiovascular Prevention and Rehabilitation. Eur J Cardiovasc Prev Rehabil. 2010;17:1–17.
6. Marzolini S, Candelaria H, Oh P. Prevalence and impact of musculoskeletal comorbidities in cardiac rehabilitation. J Cardiopulm Rehabil Prev. 2010;30:391–400.
7. Yamamoto S, Hotta K, Ota E, Mori R, Matsunaga A. Effects of resistance training on muscle strength, exercise capacity, and mobility in middle-aged and elderly patients with coronary artery disease: A meta-analysis. J Cardiol. 2016;68:125–34.
8. Matos-Santos L, Farinatti P, Borges J, Massaferri R, Monteiro W. Cardiovascular responses to resistance exercise performed with large and small muscle mass. Int J Sports Med. 2017;38(12):883–9.
9. Gillespie LD, Gillespie WJ, Robertson MC, Lamb SE, Cumming RG, Rowe BH. Interventions for preventing falls in elderly people. Cochrane Database Syst Rev. 2003;4:CD000340.
10. Latham NK, Bennett DA, Stretton CM, Anderson CS. Systematic review of progressive resistance strength training in older adults. J Gerontol A Biol Sci Med Sci. 2004;59:48–61.
11. Latham N, Anderson C, Bennett D, Stretton C. Progressive resistance strength training for physical disability in older people. Cochrane Database Syst Rev. 2003;2:CD002759.
12. Lee SH, Kim HS. Exercise interventions for preventing falls among older people in care facilities: a meta-analysis. Worldviews Evid-Based Nurs. 2017;14(1):74–80.
13. Hansen D, Linsen L, Verboven K, Hendrikx M, Rummens JL, van Erum M, Eijnde BO, Dendale P. Magnitude of muscle wasting early after on-pump coronary artery bypass graft surgery and exploration of aetiology. Exp Physiol. 2015;100(7):818–28.
14. Marzolini S, Oh PI, Thomas SG, Goodman JM. Aerobic and resistance training in coronary disease: single versus multiple sets. Med Sci Sports Exerc. 2008;40(9):1557–64.
15. Ishiguro H, Kodama S, Horikawa C, Fujihara K, Hirose AS, Hirasawa R, Yachi Y, Ohara N, Shimano H, Hanyu O, Sone H. In search of the ideal resistance training program to improve glycemic control and its indication for patients with type 2 diabetes mellitus: a systematic review and meta-analysis. Sports Med. 2016;46(1):67–77.
16. Franchi MV, Reeves ND, Narici MV. Skeletal muscle remodeling in response to eccentric vs. concentric loading: morphological, molecular, and metabolic adaptations. Front Physiol. 2017;8:447.
17. Roig M, O'Brien K, Kirk G, Murray R, McKinnon P, Shadgan B, Reid WD. The effects of eccentric versus concentric resistance training on muscle strength and mass in healthy adults: a systematic review with meta-analysis. Br J Sports Med. 2009;43(8):556–68.

18. Schoenfeld BJ, Ogborn DI, Vigotsky AD, Franchi MV, Krieger JW. Hypertrophic effects of concentric vs. eccentric muscle actions: a systematic review and meta-analysis. J Strength Cond Res. 2017;31(9):2599–608.
19. Agarwal M, Singh S, Narayan J, Pandey S, Tiwari S, Sharma P. Cardiovascular response and serum interleukin-6 level in concentric Vs. eccentric exercise. J Clin Diagn Res. 2017;11(4):CC04–8.
20. Raymond MJ, Bramley-Tzerefos RE, Jeffs KJ, Winter A, Holland AE. Systematic review of high-intensity progressive resistance strength training of the lower limb compared with other intensities of strength training in older adults. Arch Phys Med Rehabil. 2013;94(8):1458–72.
21. Lamotte M, Niset G, van de Borne P. The effect of different intensity modalities of resistance training on beat-to-beat blood pressure in cardiac patients. Eur J Cardiovasc Prev Rehabil. 2005;12(1):12–7.
22. Nery SS, Gomides RS, da Silva GV, et al. Intra-arterial blood pressure response in hypertensive subjects during low- and high-intensity resistance exercise. Clinics. 2010;65(3):271–7.
23. de Sousa NM, Magosso RF, Dipp T, et al. Continuous blood pressure response at different intensities in leg press exercise. Eur J Prev Cardiol. 2014;21(11):1324–31.
24. Gjøvaag TF, Mirtaheri P, Simon K, et al. Hemodynamic responses to resistance exercise in patients with coronary artery disease. Med Sci Sports Exerc. 2016;48(4):581–8.
25. Murlasits Z, Kneffel Z, Thalib L. The physiological effects of concurrent strength and endurance training sequence: A systematic review and meta-analysis. J Sports Sci. 2018;36(11):1212–9.
26. Fyfe JJ, Loenneke JP. Interpreting adaptation to concurrent compared with single-mode exercise training: some methodological considerations. Sports Med. 2018;48(2):289–97.
27. Schjerve IE, Tyldum GA, Tjønna AE, Stølen T, Loennechen JP, Hansen HE, et al. Both aerobic endurance and strength training programmes improve cardiovascular health in obese adults. Clin Sci. 2008;115(9):283–93.
28. Tjønna AE, Stølen TO, Bye A, Volden M, Slørdahl SA, Odegard R, et al. Aerobic interval training reduces cardiovascular risk factors more than a multitreatment approach in overweight adolescents. Clin Sci. 2009;116(4):317–26.
29. Shephard RJ, Balady GJ. Exercise as cardiovascular therapy. Circulation. 1999;99(7):963–72.
30. Lavie CJ, Thomas RJ, Squires RW, Allison TG, Milani RV. Exercise training and cardiac rehabilitation in primary and secondary prevention of coronary heart disease. Mayo Clin Proc. 2009;84(4):373–83.
31. Franckowiak SC, Dobrosielski DA, Reilley SM, Walston JD, Andersen RE. Maximal heart rate prediction in adults that are overweight or obese. J Strength Cond Res. 2010;25(5):1407–12.
32. Vanhees L, Stevens A. Exercise intensity: a matter of measuring or of talking? J Cardpulm Rehabil. 2006;26(2):78–9.
33. Myers J, Hadley D, Oswald U, Bruner K, Kottman W, Hsu L, et al. Effects of exercise training on heart rate recovery in patients with chronic heart failure. Am Heart J. 2007;153(6):1056–63.
34. Tabet JY, Meurin P, Ben Driss A, Thabut G, Weber H, Renaud N, et al. Determination of exercise training heart rate in patients on beta-blockers after myocardial infarction. Eur J Cardiovasc Prev Rehabil. 2006;13(4):538–43.
35. Berryman JW. The tradition of the 'six things non-natural': exercise and medicine from Hippocrates through ante-bellum America. Exerc Sport Sci Rev. 1989;17:515–59.
36. Binder RK, Wonisch M, Corra U, Cohen-Solal A, Vanhees L, Saner H, et al. Methodological approach to the first and second lactate threshold in incremental cardiopulmonary exercise testing. Eur J Cardiovasc Prev Rehabil. 2008;15(6):726–34.
37. Faude O, Kindermann W, Meyer T. Lactate threshold concepts: how valid are they? Sports Med. 2009;39(6):469–90.
38. Milani RV, Lavie CJ, Mehra MR, Ventura HO. Understanding the basics of cardiopulmonary exercise testing. Mayo Clin Proc. 2006;81(12):1603–11.
39. Glowacki SP, Martin SE, Maurer A, Baek W, Green JS, Crouse SF. Effects of resistance, endurance, and concurrent exercise on training outcomes in men. Med Sci Sports Exerc. 2004;36(12):2119–27.

40. Gonzalez NC, Kirkton SD, Howlett RA, Britton SL, Koch LG, Wagner HE, et al. Continued divergence in VO2max of rats artificially selected for running endurance is mediated by greater convective blood O2 delivery. J Appl Physiol. 2006;101(5):1288–96.
41. Glass RI, Zack MM Jr. Increase in deaths from ischaemic heart-disease after blizzards. Lancet. 1979;1(8114):485–7.
42. Pandolf KB, Cafarelli E, Noble BJ, Metz KF. Hyperthermia: effect on exercise prescription. Arch Phys Med Rehabil. 1975;56(12):524–6.
43. Hammoudeh AJ, Haft JI. Coronary-plaque rupture in acute coronary syndromes triggered by snow shoveling. N Engl J Med. 1996;335(26):2001–2.
44. Ribeiro PAB, Boidin M, Juneau M, Nigam A, Gayda M. High-intensity interval training in patients with coronary heart disease: Prescription models and perspectives. Ann Phys Rehabil Med. 2017;60(1):50–7.
45. Pattyn N, Beulque R, Cornelissen V. Aerobic interval vs. continuous training in patients with coronary artery disease or heart failure: an updated systematic review and meta-analysis with a focus on secondary outcomes. Sports Med. 2018;48(5):1189–205.
46. Oosenbrug E, Marinho RP, Zhang J, Marzolini S, Colella TJ, Pakosh M, Grace SL. sex differences in cardiac rehabilitation adherence: a meta-analysis. Can J Cardiol. 2016;32(11):1316–24.
47. Ruano-Ravina A, Pena-Gil C, Abu-Assi E, Raposeiras S, van 't Hof A, Meindersma E, Bossano Prescott EI, González-Juanatey JR. Participation and adherence to cardiac rehabilitation programs. A systematic review. Int J Cardiol. 2016;223:436–43.
48. Volmer J, Burkert M, Krumm H, Abodahab A, Dinklage P, Feltmann M, Kröger C, Panta P, Schäfer F, Scheidt D, Sellung M, Singerhoff H, Steingrefer C, Schmidt T, Hoffmann JD, Willemsen D, Reiss N. Enhancing long-term motivation of cardiac patients by applying exergaming in rehabilitation training. Stud Health Technol Inform. 2017;237:183–7.
49. Chuang TY, Sung WH, Chang HA, Wang RY. Effect of a virtual reality-enhanced exercise protocol after coronary artery bypass grafting. Phys Ther. 2006;86(10):1369–77.
50. Kim C, Youn JE, Choi HE. The effect of a self exercise program in cardiac rehabilitation for patients with coronary artery disease. Ann Rehabil Med. 2011;35(3):381–7.
51. Frederix I, Vanhees L, Dendale P, Goetschalckx K. A review of telerehabilitation for cardiac patients. J Telemed Telecare. 2015;21(1):45–53.

# Cardiopulmonary Exercise Testing and Prescription of Exercise

# 43

Jeffrey Wilcox Christle and Ross Arena

**Learning Objectives**

1. Recognize individuals who would benefit from exercise prescription using CPET.
2. Understand the benefits of precise exercise prescription for cardiovascular exercise.
3. Recognize the components of CPET which may be used for exercise prescription and how to identify them.
4. Understand how to apply multiple CPET-metrics to guidelines-based exercise prescription.

## 43.1 Introduction

Prior to beginning an exercise program, all patients with cardiovascular disease (CVD) require a comprehensive clinical evaluation, including treatment of underlying pathophysiologic processes that have not been addressed, optimal pharmacologic therapy, and risk stratification. Cardiorespiratory fitness (CRF) is now established as a vital sign and should be assessed at every clinical encounter for risk stratification and exercise prescription [1–3]. Exercise prescription itself is a complex endeavor which combines several factors that have been traditionally encapsulated into the FITT principle [4, 5]. FITT stands for Frequency, Intensity, Time and Type. Frequency, Time and Type are illustrated by the questions

J. W. Christle (✉)
Division of Cardiovascular Medicine, Department of Medicine, Falk Cardiovascular Research Center, Stanford Sports Cardiology, Stanford University, Stanford, CA, USA
e-mail: christle@stanford.edu

R. Arena
Department of Physical Therapy, College of Applied Health Sciences, University of Illinois at Chicago, Chicago, IL, USA
e-mail: raarena@uic.edu





A. Pressler, J. Niebauer (eds.), *Textbook of Sports and Exercise Cardiology*,
https://doi.org/10.1007/978-3-030-35374-2_43

(a) "How often?",
(b) "What mode of exercise?", and
(c) "How long?"

which can be answered based on individual goals and established guidelines, largely without the need for exercise testing [6]. Intensity, which is related to the question, "How hard should I exercise?", has clear dependencies on the other FITT metrics but is much harder to define without knowledge of an individual's exercise capacity. There are several methods available to prescribe exercise intensity, including talk tests, rating of perceived exertion (RPE), prediction formulas, submaximal exercise testing, standard maximal exercise testing and the subject of this chapter, Cardiopulmonary Exercise Testing (CPET) [5, 7–15].

Although not a widely used modality for exercise prescription, CPET is clearly the most precise and effective tool for this purpose. Table 43.1 lists a selection of reviewed articles which have applied CPET to exercise prescription.

- In fact, CPET is indicated by the American College of Sports Medicine (ACSM), American Heart Association (AHA), American Thoracic Society (ATS), American College of Chest Physicians (ACCP), European Society of Cardiology (ESC) and European Association of Preventive Cardiology (EAPC) for exercise prescription for cardiac/pulmonary rehabilitation, CVD, pulmonary disease and as a gold standard for general exercise prescription [16–22].

Through the precise detection of individuals' effort through the monitoring of ventilation and respiratory gases, CPET makes it possible to report peak measures of heart rate (HR), oxygen consumption ($VO_2$) and RPE, the major tools of exercise prescription. Furthermore, HR and $VO_2$ reserve, as well as ventilatory equivalents (minute ventilation (VE)/$VO_2$ and VE/carbon dioxide production ($VCO_2$)) and thresholds can be detected, increasing the precision of a personalized exercise prescription [20]. Cost and a higher level of technical specialization have limited CPET to use within research, clinical and elite athletic environments, but technological advances have begun to reduce the costs of equipment and a larger number of clinicians and sport scientists are becoming trained in the performance and interpretation of these tests [5, 21–24]. With these known limitations, the advantages of using CPET for individualized exercise prescription are paramount, and although most of the data available is from clinical populations, the recent FRIEND (Fitness Registry and Importance of Exercise National Database) project has added a great deal of normative exercise data to the literature [25–29]. This project has also reinforced the importance of precise assessment of CRF as a vital sign for all individuals [30, 31]. As advances in the field allow for more widespread use of CPET, there is a great need to establish standards and guidelines for exercise prescription using CPET that are feasible for clinical and non-clinical exercise professionals.

Furthermore, the utility of CPET goes beyond initial prescription but is also a valuable tool for the assessment of the physical response to exercise, one of the greatest challenges in preventive health [32]. Without measuring cardiopulmonary

**Table 43.1** Summary of selected studies of applying CPET to exercise prescription

| Author | Year | # Subjects | Comparator | Intervention | Main findings |
|---|---|---|---|---|---|
| Mann et al. [16] | 2013 | Review | Relative peak $VO_2$ Relative peak HR | Relative $VO_2R$ Relative HRR Thresholds | Exercise prescribed relative to VT1 and VT2 produce less variation in metabolic responses and time to exhaustion at a constant exercise intensity. Thresholds determined from single incremental tests cannot be assumed to be accurate in all individuals without verification trials. |
| Weatherwax et al. [17] | 2018 | 9 men 30 women | 3 d/wk for 12 wk exercise based on HRR | 3 d/wk for 12 wk exercise based on Thresholds | Relative $VO_2max$ increased ($p < .05$) from 24.3 ± 4.6 to 26.0 ± 4.2 $mlO_2•kg^{-1}•min^{-1}$ and 29.2 ± 7.5 to 32.8 ± 8.6 $mlO_2•kg^{-1}•min^{-1}$ for the HRR and VT groups. 100% VT and 60% HRR categorized as responders, respectively. |
| Da Cunha et al. [18] | 2011 | Review. All studies between 1966 and 2010 (15 studies) | | Experimental studies published between 1966 and 2010, which investigated the relationships between the %HRR, % $VO_2max$ and % $VO_2R$. | %HRR-%$VO_2max$ relationship using a ramp protocol leads to strong relationship with measured $VO_2$ and avoids problems with high variance in resting $VO_2$. $VO_2$ should be directly determined using recommended guidelines. |
| Díaz-Buschmann et al. [19] | 2014 | 102 patients on a beta-blocker and 39 not treated with negative chronotropic effect drugs | None | None | Prescribed exercise intensity should be within VT1 and VT2, so that the efficacy and safety is guaranteed. HR methods result in a large proportion of individuals exercising at intensities above VT2 |

responses to exercise, there are few non-clinical methods to measure the effect that an exercise program is having on health, fitness and ultimately prognosis (i.e., no change or an improvement in CRF). Other indirect markers of health and fitness (e.g., body weight, body fat, resting HR) have been used as indirect health related effects of endurance exercise but have significant limitations.

- The combination of exercise prescription using initial CPET testing and regular (e.g., annual) assessment of the training response with CPET is a superior way to offer individuals a precise evidence-based prescription of intensity and an accurate assessment of the effect of that prescription.
- Regular assessment of an aerobic exercise prescription offers the clinician/instructor specific data to adjust the exercise prescription and substantial feedback for the individual that may motivate and increase the chances of success [33, 34].

## 43.2 Populations Who May Benefit from CPET for Exercise Prescription

Although several statements have been published on the usefulness of CPET, current standards have primarily limited the use of CPET to clinical populations [35–39]. Those with pulmonary and/or CVD comprise most patients who perform CPET as part of clinical care. When CPET is performed, the data is primarily used for diagnostic and prognostic assessments as opposed to exercise prescription.

All individuals would benefit from CPET for the purposes of risk stratification and exercise prescription, however administrative constraints and local availability limit CPET as a realistic option for many [36].

## 43.3 Pre-prescription Evaluation

- All individuals should be screened for signs and symptoms of cardiovascular and pulmonary diseases before performing CPET.
- Individuals who report symptoms, especially chest pain, shortness of breath and/or lightheadedness, with or without exercise induction, should be thoroughly prescreened. These symptoms may be used to set safe upper limits for exercise intensity (Table 43.2).

**Table 43.2** Signs and symptoms below which an upper limit for exercise intensity should be set[a] (adapted from [4])

| |
|---|
| • Onset of angina or other symptoms of cardiovascular insufficiency |
| • Plateau or decrease in systolic blood pressure, systolic blood pressure of >250 mmHg or diastolic blood pressure of >115 mmHg |
| • ‡1.0 mm ST-segment depression, horizontal or downsloping |
| • Radionuclide evidence of left ventricular dysfunction or onset of moderate to severe wall motion abnormalities during exertion |
| • Increased frequency of ventricular dysrhythmias |
| • Other significant ECG disturbances (e.g., 2- or 3-degree atrioventricular block, atrial fibrillation, supraventricular tachycardia, complex ventricular ectopy, etc.) |
| • Other signs/symptoms of intolerance to exercise |

[a]The exercise heart rate generally should be at least 10 bpm below the heart rate associated with any of the referenced criteria. Other variables (e.g., the corresponding systolic blood pressure response and perceived exertion), however, also should be considered when establishing exercise intensity

- Medical history should include any/all medical diagnoses, previous physical examination findings, history of symptoms, recent hospitalizations and illnesses, orthopedic problems, medication and drug use, exercise history, work history and family history [5].
- Physical examination should include body weight, HR and rhythm, blood pressure, auscultation of the heart and lungs, palpitation of cardiac pulse, carotid, abdominal and femoral arteries, evaluation of the abdomen and lower extremities, evaluation of tendon xanthoma and skin xanthelasma, neurological examination, and inspection of the lower extremities, especially in patients with Diabetes Mellitus [5].

## 43.4 General Principles of Exercise Prescription Using CPET

- All individuals could potentially benefit from exercise therapy and secondary prevention.
- The FITT tenets (Frequency, Intensity, Time and Type) are effective in creating and monitoring an exercise prescription (Table 43.3)
  - Frequency: How often (e.g., days per week).
  - Intensity: How difficult (e.g., with RPE scale and/or target HR range).
  - Type: Which mode of exercise is appropriate?
  - Time: How long of a duration (e.g., 150 min per week, 30 min per session)
- When creating an exercise prescription, always consider that individuals tend to adhere when they have control over these variables (e.g., can choose the type of exercise).
- When creating an endurance exercise prescription, studies have shown that the addition of resistance exercises can improve overall health and fitness, improve health-related quality of life and increase success with long term weight control.

**Table 43.3** Example of components of the clinical exercise prescription

| |
|---|
| • Type |
| O Endurance, dynamic exercise |
| O Light resistance training (high repetition, low resistance) |
| O Avoid isometric, body-building type activities |
| • Intensity |
| O Below second ventilatory threshold |
| O Target work rate corresponding to 50–70% of peak $VO_2$ |
| O Rating of perceived exertion (Borg 6–20 scale) approximately 12–14 |
| O Heart rate reserve 60–80% of maximum |
| • Duration |
| O May need to start at only 10–20 min/sessions |
| O Work up to 30–40 min/sessions |
| • Frequency |
| O 3–5 times/week |

- When using exercise testing to create physiologically comprehensive exercise prescriptions, individualized ramp testing should be used. This type of testing will add precision by accurately identifying ventilatory thresholds when present.
- To assess effort, CPET should be done to maximum effort reflected by a peak respiratory exchange ratio (RER) of at least 1.00 and ideally >1.10. Other measures that complement the assessment of exercise effort include peak HR (>85%) and RPE (>16).

## 43.5 Choosing Appropriate Intensities Using CPET

- CPET is a very specific and effective mode for selecting intensities for an exercise prescription. It is mode-specific (i.e., the HR ranges, workloads and $VO_2$ at ventilatory threshold (VT) are only applicable for the mode of testing).
- Most patients will profit substantially from exercise at moderate to high intensities, which can be established through different measures (12–14 on a classic RPE scale or 40–60% $VO_2R$/HRR; see also Chap. 44).
- To establish HR targets for exercise prescription, the range of corresponding HR between the first and second ventilatory thresholds have been observed to reflect steady state [17, 40, 41].
- Applying a threshold prescription such as the American Council on Exercise 3-zone method may lead to higher overall intensities compared to other methods, which may explain observations of improved CRF outcomes using these thresholds [40, 41].
- Detection of $VO_2$ at VT1 and especially VT2 can be challenging; If possible having two clinicians independently assess VT is recommended [21].
- In monitoring a threshold-based exercise prescription, initial exercise sessions should be performed at intensities closer to VT1, but should progress towards VT2, with a target of performing 30–40 min at close to but under VT2. Once this goal is reached, a new exercise assessment with CPET would ideally be performed for adjustment of the prescription.
- When using formulas to establish HR targets for exercise prescription, most patients will benefit from "reserve" formulas, in which the range (i.e. peak-resting) of $VO_2$ or HR are combined with published intensity recommendations (Table 43.4).
- In lieu of ventilatory data, exercise testing can still provide accurate rest and maximal HR for exercise prescription based on heart rate reserve (HRR).

**Table 43.4** Standards for prescribing exercise intensity (adapted from [4])

| Intensity | %HRR or %$VO_2$R | %peak HR | %peak $VO_2$ | RPE [6–15, 35, 36, 42–44] |
|---|---|---|---|---|
| Very light | <30 | <57 | <37 | <9 |
| Light | 30 < 40 | 57 < 64 | 37 < 45 | 9 < 11 |
| Moderate | 40 < 60 | 64 < 76 | 45 < 64 | 11 < 14 |
| Vigorous | 60 < 90 | 76 < 96 | 64 < 91 | 14 < 17 |
| Near max to maximal | >90 | >96 | >91 | >17 |

*HRR* Heart rate reserve, *$VO_2R$* Oxygen uptake reserve, *RPE* Rating of perceived exertion (based on a scale of 6–20)

## 43.6 Specific Metrics for the Establishment of Exercise Intensity

### 43.6.1 Ratings of Perceived Exertion

1. RPE used as the traditional 6–20 scale or 0–10 scale (Table 43.5) is a simple and accurate method for individuals to assess personal exercise intensity during graded exercise (Chap. 44) [46].
2. RPE has been shown to correlate very well to other more established measures of exercise intensity [15].

### 43.6.2 Heart Rate

1. HR is the most common measure for establishing and monitoring endurance exercise.
2. Several methods of exercise prescription using HR exist, with HRR being the most established and universal.
3. Example of the HRR method for moderate endurance exercise prescription from exercise test data: rest HR = 70 bpm, peak HR = 150 bpm, target intensity 60% HRR:
   (a) 150 (peak HR) − 70 (rest HR) = 80 (HRR)
   (b) 80 (HRR) × 0.6 (60%) = 48 bpm
   (c) 48 bpm + 70 bpm (rest HR) = 118 bpm (Target HR)
4. Note: HRR method has been used without testing by using a prediction formula (e.g. 220-age) instead of actual peak HR. Importantly, prediction formulas produce very crude estimates of peak HR in healthy and CVD populations and should only be used in cases where the measurement of peak HR is not possible

**Table 43.5** Borg's scales of pain and perceived exertion [45]

| Borg CR-10 Scale | | Borg RPE Scale | |
|---|---|---|---|
| 0 | Nothing at all | 6 | |
| 0.5 | Just noticeable | 7 | Extremely light |
| 1 | Very weak | 8 | |
| 2 | Weak | 9 | Very light |
| 3 | Moderate | 10 | |
| 4 | Somewhat strong | 11 | Fairly light |
| 5 | Strong | 12 | |
| 6 | | 13 | Somewhat hard |
| 7 | Very Strong | 14 | |
| 8 | | 15 | Hard (heavy) |
| 9 | | 16 | |
| 10 | Extremely Strong | 17 | Very hard |
| • | Maximal | 18 | |
| | | 19 | Extremely hard |
| | | 20 | |

[47–49]. For example, in using estimates of peak HR, arrhythmias, arterial hypertension, myocardial ischemia etc. go undetected. Therefore, the use of HR prediction formulas is not recommended for patients with established or suspected CVD.

### 43.6.3 Ventilatory Gas Exchange

1. Peak $VO_2$ is the gold standard for accurate measurement of exercise capacity and is a key CRF metric.
2. $VO_2$ is not practical for regular monitoring of endurance exercise.
3. Peak $VO_2$ is the gold standard for assessing the effect of regular exercise on CRF through CPET.

### 43.6.4 First Ventilatory Threshold (VT1)

1. The first VT is a well-established marker of fitness and health and change in VT1 is a strong indicator of response to training and detraining.
2. Detection and agreement between experienced reviewers for VT1 is good but is highly protocol dependent. Differences in protocol (Bruce vs Balke vs Ramp; see Chap. 11), method of determination (V-slope vs ventilatory equivalents method) and reviewer are all important considerations in assessing $VO_2$ at VT1 [50–53].
3. The VT1 can be detected by the V-slope method, which identifies the point at which the relationship between $VCO_2$ and $VO_2$ significantly increases due to a sudden increase of $CO_2$ due to lactic acid buffering (Panel 5). The lowest nadir of the relationship between VE and $VO_2$ (Panel 6) also identifies the VT1 with good reliability (Figs. 43.1 and 43.2) [54].

### 43.6.5 Second Ventilatory Threshold (VT2)

1. Whereas the VT1 has a large amount of data supporting its significance, the VT2 is much more difficult to detect and its value is uncertain. Is has been suggested that graphical methods, interobserver variability and type of protocol may all influence the ability to detect VT2 [55].
2. Beyond protocol type, method of determination and reviewer, the presence of VT2 can also be affected by effort and non-cardiovascular limitations to exercise, and many patients with low exercise tolerance (e.g. in severe CHF) do not reach VT2 [56].
3. The VT2, although not always detectable, may be identified through inspection of the relationship between VE and $VCO_2$ over time (Panel 6).

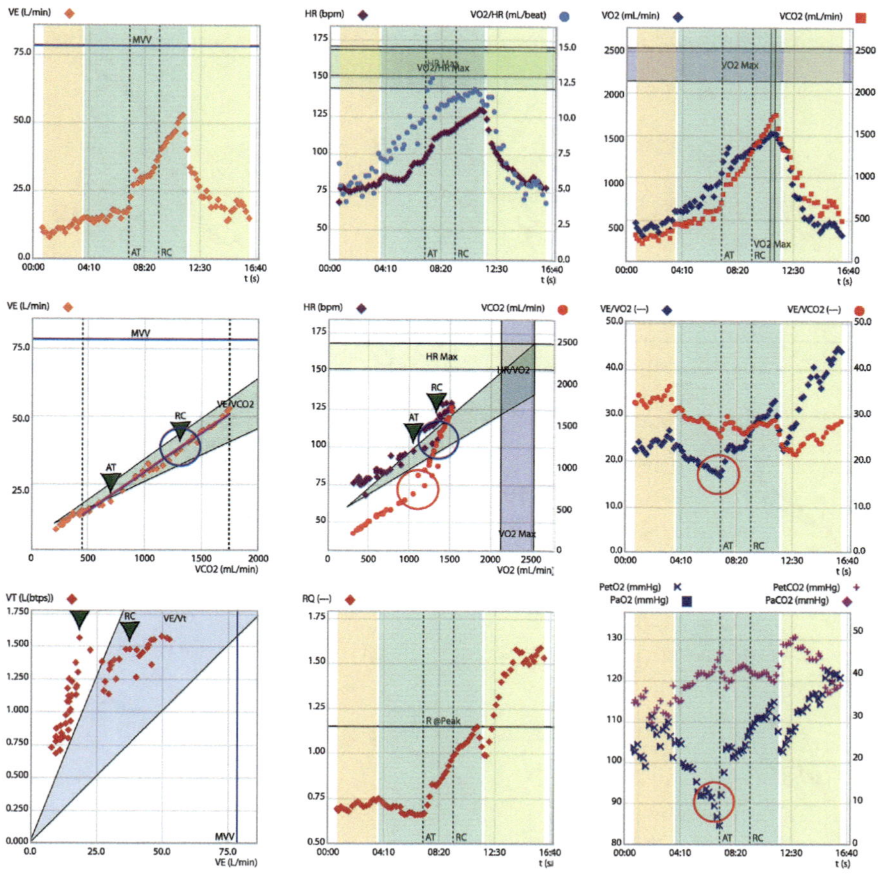

**Fig. 43.1** A real-life example of a cardiopulmonary exercise test for a patient referred for exercise testing. The red circles indicate the location of the VT1 in panel 5 (change in slope of $VCO_2/VO_2$), panel 6 (lowest point of $VE/VO_2$ slope) and panel 9 (nadir of $VE/VO_2$ slope and a leveling off of $VE/VCO_2$). The blue circles indicate the location of VT2 in panel 4 (break in linearity in $VE/VCO_2$), panel 5 (second change in slope of $VCO_2/VO_2$). Target HR for moderate (steady state) ambulatory endurance exercise were determined to be between 97 and 117 bpm, corresponding to 68–87% of peak $VO_2$ (Graphics from Omnia, Cosmed, Rome, Italy)

(a) Visually it is located at the lowest nadir of the $VE/VCO_2$ relationship; it is the point at which VE begins to increase significantly relative to $VCO_2$ (which can also be visualized in the same panel as the $VE/VCO_2$ slope (Panel 4) [54].

(b) This relationship has been identified as the "respiratory compensation point (RCP)" which represents a point of exercise intensity at which metabolic acidosis overwhelms bicarbonate buffering capacity leading to marked hyperventilation (i.e., overbreathing due to hypercapnia) (Figs. 43.1 and 43.2).

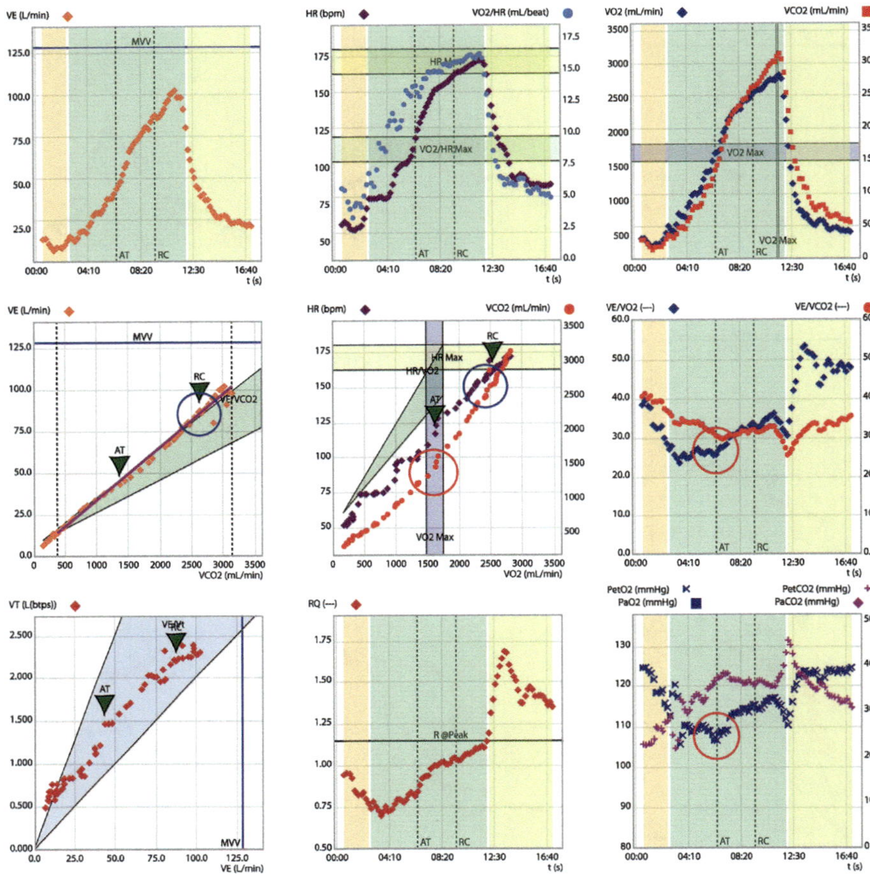


**Fig. 43.2** A real-life example of a cardiopulmonary exercise test for a patient referred for exercise testing. The red circles indicate the location of the VT1 in panel 5 (change in slope of $VCO_2/VO_2$), panel 6 (lowest point of $VE/VO_2$ slope) and panel 9 (nadir of $VE/VO_2$ slope and a leveling off of $VE/VCO_2$). The blue circles indicate the location of VT2 in panel 4 (break in linearity in $VE/VCO_2$), panel 5 (second change in slope of $VCO_2/VO_2$). Based on VT1 and VT2, target HR for moderate (steady state) ambulatory endurance exercise were determined to be 117–164 bpm

## 43.7 Exercise Prescription After Cardiac Transplantation

- Patients post heart transplantation (HTx) tend to improve exercise capacity to a greater extent than with patients in end-stage heart failure (see also Chap. 49) [57–59].
- Prescription for post HTx are largely the same as with CVD (see above) with the exception that patients post HTx are denervated, which results in the HR response to exercise being driven by catecholamines from the adrenal glands, resulting in higher resting HR and slower chronotropic response, especially at the beginning

of an exercise bout, reduced peak HR and slower HR recovery upon cessation of exercise. This necessitates a longer warm-up and cool-down period than in other CVD populations.

- Patients post HTx have been shown to improve HR response for some time after HTx, suggesting that at least partially reinnervation is possible. This phenomenon and its relevance are poorly understood but may have importance in the future for exercise prescription in this group.
- Although it has been suggested that patients after HTx may benefit more from higher intensity exercise, this has not been thoroughly studied and guidelines for exercise post HTx have not been recently updated [60–62].
- Current guidelines, a lack of large RCTs and the need for long periods of warm-up and cool down due to denervation combined lead to the recommendation for moderate exercise intensity and somewhat longer duration than other cardiac conditions.
- Specific guidelines for patients with LVAD do not exist, but the use of CPET to establish exercise capacity and appropriate intensities is recommended (see Chap. 49). In lieu of CPET, a 6-min walking test would be appropriate for this population [16, 20, 45].
- For patients with LVAD, it is recommended to begin exercise programming at or below the VT2. If patients are able to reach a peak $VO_2 > 14$ $mlO_2\ kg^{-1}\ min^{-1}$ or 6-min walking distance >300 m, a higher relative exercise intensity may be performed [20, 45].
- While the AHA Guidelines on Exercise Testing reviewed the applications of the test in a wide variety of cardiovascular and related conditions HTx is not mentioned [39]. Likewise, exercise testing is not mentioned in the AHA/American College of Cardiology (ACC) Practice Guidelines on Vascular Disease [18].

## 43.8 Summary

The role of CPET in prescribing exercise has been limited by cost and technical and interpretive ability to clinical populations and elite athletes. However, technological advances in CPET equipment and an increasing number of health professionals with the prerequisite skills are changing the paradigm. Evidence supporting the clinical value of CRF as a valuable vital sign has increased interest in broadening the use of CPET to a larger more diverse population. Using ventilatory expired gas measures, in conjunction with HR and subjective symptoms to prescribe endurance exercise and follow individuals has significant advantages. These include accounting for the individual respiratory and metabolic exercise response using a combination of HRR, $VO_2R$ and VT for exercise prescription. In cases where VT1 and VT2 are present and measurable, HR at these thresholds may be used to guide the exercise prescription. In cases where one or both VT are not measurable, HR at % $VO_2R$ may be used as an alternate using established guidelines. In general, using % peak HR or % predicted peak HR is not recommended, but serves as an alternative when resources are limited. Any methods for exercise prescription should be supplemented with perceived exertion as a subjective measure that individuals may use when objective data is not available.

**Clinical Pearls**

- Alongside the assessment of cardiorespiratory fitness, guideline-based exercise prescription should be applied to all clinical visits.
- When applicable, applying mixed methods including the individual's preference for mode should be applied to clinical exercise prescription. This includes percent of heart rate reserve, consideration of ventilatory thresholds and ratings of perceived exertion.
- The F.I.T.T. principles of Frequency, Intensity, Timing and Type should always be applied to clinical exercise prescription regardless of mode of assessment. To be effective, these principles should be adjusted to match the individual's symptoms, lifestyle and preferences.
- All clinical exercise prescriptions should be followed up with cardiorespiratory fitness assessment—ideally with cardiopulmonary exercise testing—after at least 12 weeks of regular endurance exercise.

## 43.9 Review

### Questions

1. Of the following options, how should the limits for steady state endurance exercise be determined from CPET for a patient who has symptoms of angina (chest pain)?
   (a) 40–60% of $VO_2R$
   (b) VT1-VT2
   (c) VT1-Onset of Angina
   (d) VT1- RPE 16
   (e) Patients with angina should not perform endurance exercise until resolution of symptoms
2. The first ventilatory threshold is identified as:
   (a) V-slope method
   (b) The lowest nadir of the relationship between VE and $VO_2$
   (c) The point at which the relationship between $VCO_2$ and $VO_2$ significantly increases due to a sudden increase of $VCO_2$ due to lactic acid buffering
   (d) a and b only
   (e) All of the above
3. Based on current exercise prescription guidelines, vigorous exercise is defined as:
   (a) 60 < 90% HRR/$VO_2R$, 76 < 96% peak HR, 64 < 91% peak $VO_2$, RPE 14 < 17
   (b) 40–60% HRR/$VO_2R$, 57 < 64% peak HR, 37 < 45% peak $VO_2$, RPE 11 < 14
   (c) >90% HRR/$VO_2R$, >96% peak HR, >91% peak $VO_2$, RPE >17
   (d) VT1 < VT2
   (e) >VT2

## Answers

1. **c)**—VT1-Onset of Angina. Of the options, only "VT1 - onset of angina" is reasonable for a patient who has exercise induced angina. Although the upper limit of steady state is defined by the guidelines as 60% of VO2R, VT2 and RPE 16, the presence of angina defines the upper limit for those who are symptomatic. Furthermore, patients who have exercise induced angina can increase their angina threshold by performing endurance exercise and should be encouraged to do so.
2. **e)**—all of the above. The first ventilatory threshold may be defined by all these listed methods, but clinicians are encouraged to apply all of them when visually inspecting CPET reports. The V-Slope method identifies a point at which carbon dioxide production increases over-proportional to oxygen uptake; The lowest nadir of the relationship between VE and $VO_2$ reflects a point at which ventilation increases over-proportional to oxygen uptake, reflecting the increased ventilatory demand due to increased carbon dioxide production; The relationship between VCO2 and VO2 is illustrated by the other two methods, representing an increased ventilatory drive driven by the increase in CO2 production and buffering of lactic acid.
3. **a)**—60 < 90% HRR/$VO_2$R, 76 < 96% peak HR, 64 < 91% peak $VO_2$, RPE 14 < 17. Vigorous exercise is exercise at a high intensity and is commonly used in exercise prescription for those individuals who show moderate to high cardiorespiratory fitness. Option "b" is a mixture of light and moderate intensities, option "c" is defined as near max to maximal, which is seldom used for clinical exercise prescription, and options "d" and "e" represent moderate and near maximal, respectively, but using ventilatory thresholds for reference.

## References


1. Kaminsky LA, Arena R, Ellingsen Ø, Harber MP, Myers J, Ozemek C, Ross R. Cardiorespiratory fitness and cardiovascular disease–The past, present, and future. Prog Cardiovasc Dis. 2019; https://doi.org/10.1016/j.pcad.2019.01.002.
2. Addoh O, Edwards MK, Loprinzi PD. Considerations for the inclusion of cardiorespiratory fitness as a vital sign in the clinical setting. Prev Med. 2017;96:85–6.
3. Ross R, Blair SN, Arena R, et al. Importance of assessing cardiorespiratory fitness in clinical practice: a case for fitness as a clinical vital sign: a scientific statement from the American heart association. Circulation. 2016;134:e653–99.
4. American College of Sports Medicine. ACSM's resource manual for guidelines for exercise testing and prescription, 7th edition. Philidelphia; Lippincott Williams & Wilkins; 2012.
5. American College of Sports Medicine. ACSM's guidelines for exercise testing and prescription, 10th edition. Philidelphia; Lippincott Williams & Wilkins; 2017.
6. American College of Sports Medicine. ACSM's guidelines for exercise testing and prescription, 9th edition. Philidelphia; Lippincott Williams & Wilkins; 2013.
7. Persinger R, Foster C, Gibson M, Fater DCW, Porcari JP. Consistency of the talk test for exercise prescription. Med Sci Sports Exerc. 2004;36:1632–6.
8. Birk TJ, Birk CA. Use of ratings of perceived exertion for exercise prescription. Sports Med. 1987;4:1–8.

9. Garnacho-Castaño MV, Domínguez R, Muñoz González A, Feliu-Ruano R, Serra-Payá N, Maté-Muñoz JL. Exercise prescription using the borg rating of perceived exertion to improve fitness. Int J Sports Med. 2018;39:115–23.
10. Borg GA. Psychophysical bases of perceived exertion. Med Sci Sports Exerc. 1982;14:377–81.
11. Camarda SR de A, Tebexreni AS, Páfaro CN, Sasai FB, Tambeiro VL, Juliano Y, de Barros Neto TL. Comparison of maximal heart rate using the prediction equations proposed by Karvonen and Tanaka. Arq Bras Cardiol. 2008;91:311–4.
12. Nikolic G. Submaximal exercise testing early after myocardial infarction. Heart. 1985;53:471.
13. Oliveira MF, Zanussi G, Sprovieri B, Lobo DML, Mastrocolla LE, Umeda IIK, Sperandio PA. Alternatives to aerobic exercise prescription in patients with chronic heart failure. Arq Bras Cardiol. 2016;106:97–104.
14. Gloeckl R, Teschler S, Jarosch I, Christle JW, Hitzl W, Kenn K. Comparison of two- and six-minute walk tests in detecting oxygen desaturation in patients with severe chronic obstructive pulmonary disease - A randomized crossover trial. Chron Respir Dis. 2016; https://doi.org/10.1177/1479972316636991.
15. Scherr J, Wolfarth B, Christle JW, Pressler A, Wagenpfeil S, Halle M. Associations between Borg's rating of perceived exertion and physiological measures of exercise intensity. Eur J Appl Physiol. 2013;113:147–55.
16. American Association of Cardiovascular & Pulmonary Rehabilitation. Guidelines for cardiac rehabilitation and secondary prevention programs: Human Kinetics; 2004.
17. Weatherwax RM, Harris NK, Kilding AE, Dalleck LC. Incidence of VO2max Responders to Personalized vs Standardized Exercise Prescription. Med Sci Sports Exerc. 2018; https://doi.org/10.1249/MSS.0000000000001842.
18. Garbi M, Allen C (2017) Faculty of 1000 revaluation for 2017 AHA/ACC focused update of the 2014 AHA/ACC guideline for the management of patients with valvular heart disease: A report of the american college of cardiology/American Heart Association task force on clinical practice guidelines. F1000 - Post-publication peer review of the biomedical literature. doi: https://doi.org/10.3410/f.727426955.793533368
19. Díaz-Buschmann I, Jaureguizar KV, Calero MJ, Aquino RS. Programming exercise intensity in patients on beta-blocker treatment: the importance of choosing an appropriate method. Eur J Prev Cardiol. 2014;21(12):1474–80.
20. Mezzani A, Hamm LF, Jones AM, et al. Aerobic exercise intensity assessment and prescription in cardiac rehabilitation: a joint position statement of the European association for cardiovascular prevention and rehabilitation, the American association of cardiovascular and pulmonary rehabilitation and the Canadian association of cardiac rehabilitation. Eur J Prev Cardiol. 2013;20:442–67.
21. Binder RK, Wonisch M, Corra U, Cohen-Solal A, Vanhees L, Saner H, Schmid J-P. Methodological approach to the first and second lactate threshold in incremental cardiopulmonary exercise testing. Eur J Cardiovasc Prev Rehabil. 2008;15:726–34.
22. Skinner JS. Exercise testing and exercise prescription for special cases: theoretical basis and clinical application: Lippincott Williams & Wilkins; 2005.
23. Winter UJ, Wassermann K, Treese N, Höpp W. Computerized cardiopulmonary exercise testing: Springer Science & Business Media; 2012.
24. Agostoni P, Guazzi M (2002) Evolving role of cardiopulmonary exercise testing in heart failure and cardiac transplantation. In: Progress in Respiratory Research. pp. 99–108.
25. Kaminsky LA, Imboden MT, Arena R, Myers J. Reference standards for cardiorespiratory fitness measured with cardiopulmonary exercise testing using cycle ergometry: data from the fitness registry and the importance of exercise national database (FRIEND) registry. Mayo Clin Proc. 2017;92:228–33.
26. Kaminsky LA, Harber MP, Imboden MT, Arena R, Myers J. Peak ventilation reference standards from exercise testing: from the FRIEND registry. Med Sci Sports Exerc. 2018;50:2603–8.
27. de Souza E, Silva CG, Kaminsky LA, Arena R, Christle JW, Araújo CGS, Lima RM, Ashley EA, Myers J. A reference equation for maximal aerobic power for treadmill and cycle ergometer exercise testing: Analysis from the FRIEND registry. Eur J Prev Cardiol. 2018;25:742–50.

28. Sabbahi A, Arena R, Kaminsky LA, Myers J, Phillips SA. Peak blood pressure responses during maximum cardiopulmonary exercise testing: reference standards from FRIEND (Fitness registry and the importance of exercise: a national database). Hypertension. 2018;71:229–36.
29. Kokkinos P, Kaminsky LA, Arena R, Zhang J, Myers J. A new generalized cycle ergometry equation for predicting maximal oxygen uptake: the fitness registry and the importance of exercise national database (FRIEND). Eur J Prev Cardiol. 2018;25:1077–82.
30. Kaminsky LA, Myers J, Arena R. Determining cardiorespiratory fitness with precision: compendium of findings from the FRIEND registry. Prog Cardiovasc Dis. 2018; https://doi.org/10.1016/j.pcad.2018.10.003.
31. Moneghetti KJ, Hock J, Kaminsky L, et al. Applying current normative data to prognosis in heart failure: The Fitness Registry and the Importance of Exercise National Database (FRIEND). Int J Cardiol. 2018;263:75–9.
32. American College of Sports Medicine. ACSM's clinical exercise physiology: Lippincott Williams & Wilkins; 2019.
33. Mouratidis A, Vansteenkiste M, Lens W, Sideridis G. The motivating role of positive feedback in sport and physical education: evidence for a motivational model. J Sport Exerc Psychol. 2008;30:240–68.
34. Roberts GC, Treasure D. Advances in motivation in sport and exercise: Human Kinetics; 2018.
35. Ross RM. ATS/ACCP statement on cardiopulmonary exercise testing. Am J Respir Crit Care Med. 2003;167:1451. author reply 1451.
36. Balady GJ, Arena R, Sietsema K, et al. Clinician's Guide to cardiopulmonary exercise testing in adults: a scientific statement from the American Heart Association. Circulation. 2010;122:191–225.
37. Guazzi M, Adams V, Conraads V, et al. EACPR/AHA scientific statement. Clinical recommendations for cardiopulmonary exercise testing data assessment in specific patient populations. Circulation. 2012;126:2261–74.
38. Piepoli MF, Corrà U, Agostoni PG, Belardinelli R, Cohen-Solal A, Hambrecht R, Vanhees L, Task Force of the Italian Working Group on Cardiac Rehabilitation and Prevention (Gruppo Italiano di Cardiologia Riabilitativa e Prevenzione, GICR), Working Group on Cardiac Rehabilitation and Exercise Physiology of the European Society of Cardiology. Statement on cardiopulmonary exercise testing in chronic heart failure due to left ventricular dysfunction: recommendations for performance and interpretation Part II: How to perform cardiopulmonary exercise testing in chronic heart failure. Eur J Cardiovasc Prev Rehabil. 2006;13:300–11.
39. Fletcher GF, Ades PA, Kligfield P, et al. Exercise standards for testing and training: a scientific statement from the American Heart Association. Circulation. 2013;128:873–934.
40. Wolpern AE, Burgos DJ, Janot JM, Dalleck LC. Is a threshold-based model a superior method to the relative percent concept for establishing individual exercise intensity? a randomized controlled trial. BMC Sports Sci Med Rehabil. 2015;7:16.
41. American Council on Exercise (2010) ACE personal trainer manual: the ultimate resource for fitness professionals (Fourth Edition). Coaches Choice.
42. Guazzi M, Arena R, Halle M, Piepoli MF, Myers J, Lavie CJ. 2016 focused update: clinical recommendations for cardiopulmonary exercise testing data assessment in specific patient populations. Circulation. 2016;133:e694–711.
43. Kaminsky LA, Brubaker PH, Guazzi M, Lavie CJ, Montoye AHK, Sanderson BK, Savage PD. Assessing physical activity as a core component in cardiac rehabilitation: a position statement of the American association of cardiovascular and pulmonary rehabilitation. J Cardiopulm Rehabil Prev. 2016;36:217–29.
44. Mezzani A, Agostoni P, Cohen-Solal A, et al. Standards for the use of cardiopulmonary exercise testing for the functional evaluation of cardiac patients: a report from the exercise physiology section of the European association for cardiovascular prevention and rehabilitation. Eur J Cardiovasc Prev Rehabil. 2009;16:249–67.
45. Adamopoulos S, Corrà U, Laoutaris ID, et al. Exercise training in patients with ventricular assist devices: a review of the evidence and practical advice. A position paper from the

Committee on Exercise Physiology and Training and the Committee of Advanced Heart Failure of the Heart Failure Association of the European Society of Cardiology. Eur J Heart Fail. 2019;21:3–13.
46. Whaley MH, Brubaker PH, Kaminsky LA, Miller CR. Validity of rating of perceived exertion during graded exercise testing in apparently healthy adults and cardiac patients. J Cardpulm Rehabil. 1997;17:261–7.
47. Gellish RL, Goslin BR, Olson RE, McDonald A, Russi GD, Moudgil VK. Longitudinal modeling of the relationship between age and maximal heart rate. Med Sci Sports Exerc. 2007;39:822–9.
48. Sarzynski MA, Rankinen T, Earnest CP, Leon AS, Rao DC, Skinner JS, Bouchard C. Measured maximal heart rates compared to commonly used age-based prediction equations in the Heritage Family Study. Am J Hum Biol. 2013;25:695–701.
49. Brawner CA, Ehrman JK, Schairer JR, Cao JJ, Keteyian SJ. Predicting maximum heart rate among patients with coronary heart disease receiving beta-adrenergic blockade therapy. Am Heart J. 2004;148:910–4.
50. Shimizu M, Myers J, Buchanan N, Walsh D, Kraemer M, McAuley P, Froelicher VF. The ventilatory threshold: method, protocol, and evaluator agreement. Am Heart J. 1991;122:509–16.
51. Myers J, Ashley E. Dangerous curves. A perspective on exercise, lactate, and the anaerobic threshold. Chest. 1997;111:787–95.
52. Myers J, Goldsmith RL, Keteyian SJ, Brawner CA, Brazil DA, Aldred H, Ehrman JK, Burkhoff D. The ventilatory anaerobic threshold in heart failure: a multicenter evaluation of reliability. J Card Fail. 2010;16:76–83.
53. Vainshelboim B, Rao S, Chan K, Lima RM, Ashley EA, Myers J. A comparison of methods for determining the ventilatory threshold: implications for surgical risk stratification. Can J Anaesth. 2017;64:634–42.
54. Wasserman K, Mcilroy MB. Detecting the threshold of anaerobic metabolism in cardiac patients during exercise. Am J Cardiol. 1964;14:844–52.
55. Cohen-Solal A, Zannad F, Kayanakis JG, Gueret P, Aupetit JF, Kolsky H. Multicentre study of the determination of peak oxygen uptake and ventilatory threshold during bicycle exercise in chronic heart failure. Comparison of graphical methods, interobserver variability and influence of the exercise protocol. The VO2 French Study Group. Eur Heart J. 1991;12:1055–63.
56. Opasich C, Pinna GD, Bobbio M, et al. Peak exercise oxygen consumption in chronic heart failure: toward efficient use in the individual patient. J Am Coll Cardiol. 1998;31:766–75.
57. Kobashigawa JA, Leaf DA, Lee N, et al. A controlled trial of exercise rehabilitation after heart transplantation. N Engl J Med. 1999;340:272–7.
58. Bachmann JM, Shah AS, Duncan MS, et al. Cardiac rehabilitation and readmissions after heart transplantation. J Heart Lung Transplant. 2018;37:467–76.
59. Janaudis-Ferreira T, Mathur S, Konidis S, Tansey CM, Beaurepaire C. Outcomes in randomized controlled trials of exercise interventions in solid organ transplant. World J Transplant. 2016;6:774–89.
60. Pokan R, Von Duvillard SP, Ludwig J, Rohrer A, Hofmann P, Wonisch M, Smekal G, Schmid P, Pacher R, Bachl N. Effect of high-volume and -intensity endurance training in heart transplant recipients. Med Sci Sports Exerc. 2004;36:2011–6.
61. Hermann TS, Dall CH, Christensen SB, Goetze JP, Prescott E, Gustafsson F. Effect of high intensity exercise on peak oxygen uptake and endothelial function in long-term heart transplant recipients. Am J Transplant. 2011;11:536–41.
62. Christensen SB, Dall CH, Prescott E, Pedersen SS, Gustafsson F. A high-intensity exercise program improves exercise capacity, self-perceived health, anxiety and depression in heart transplant recipients: A randomized, controlled trial. J Heart Lung Transplant. 2012;31:106–7.

# Exercise in Specific Diseases: Coronary Artery Disease

# 44

Mats Börjesson, Josef Niebauer, and Mikael Dellborg

**Learning Objectives**

1. Recognize the importance of cardiovascular risk factors for the varying comprehensiveness of pre-participation examination.
2. Appreciate that given the wealth of evidence supporting the benefits of physical activity and exercise for primary and secondary prevention of CAD, individuals should be permitted to participate in competitive sport whenever medically justifiable.
3. Recognize that recommendations on participation in competitive sports largely depend on the patient's individual risk.
4. Understand the safety but also the caveats of exercise testing and training in patients with CAD.

M. Börjesson (✉)
Department of Neuroscience and Physiology, Sahlgrenska Academy and Center for Health and Perfoamce, Gothenburg University and Sahlgrenska University Hospital/Ostra, Gothenburg, Sweden
e-mail: mats.brjesson@telia.com

J. Niebauer
University Institute of Sports Medicine, Prevention and Rehabilitation, Paracelsus Medical University, Salzburg, Austria
e-mail: j.niebauer@salk.at

M. Dellborg
Department of Molecular and Clinical Medicine, Institute of Medicine, Sahlgrenska Academy, University of Gothenburg and Sahlgrenska University Hospital/Ostra, Gothenburg, Sweden
e-mail: mikael.dellborg@gu.se



A. Pressler, J. Niebauer (eds.), *Textbook of Sports and Exercise Cardiology*,
https://doi.org/10.1007/978-3-030-35374-2_44

## 44.1 Introduction

Coronary artery disease (CAD) is a progressive disease, typically starting early in life in asymptomatic individuals as accumulation of lipids and inflammatory cells in the arterial vessel wall [1]. Early signs of vascular aortic disease can be found in sudden death victims of traffic incidents even in their 20s [2]. The disease usually progresses over many years and individuals may remain asymptomatic (i.e. subclinical CAD). CAD is a major cause of premature death and is strongly associated with cardiovascular morbidity and mortality, i.e. myocardial infarction, stroke, and sudden death [3].

The CAD prevalence is currently decreasing in incidence in the Western World but still remains the leading cause of deaths overall. In other parts of the world the incidence continues to increase [4]. These differences are to a small extent attributable to differences in health care provision, but varying levels of lifestyle related risk factors, such as hypertension, obesity, dyslipidemia and diabetes mellitus type 2, smoking and physical inactivity are playing a major role [5] with many of the mentioned risk factors strongly related to reduced levels of physical activity.

Regular physical activity (PA) has positive effects on multiple risk factors for CAD [6], including:

(a) Arterial hypertension
(b) Obesity
(c) Dyslipidemia
(d) Insulin resistance/diabetes mellitus type 2
(e) Endothelial dysfunction
(f) Thrombogenicity
(g) Arrhythmias

- **Aerobic PA 30 min/day, 5 days/week at least at medium intensity is therefore universally recommended for health, by cardiac and other major organizations** [7].

Unfortunately, PA levels and associated aerobic fitness have decreased in the last 20–30 years in modern societies [8, 9], making efforts to increase PA an utmost priority for future health care.

In contrast, it is also known that high-intensity PA, such as sporting activity, may at least temporarily increase the risk of sudden cardiac events [10], while regular PA has been shown to attenuate this risk-increment [11]. There has been a worldwide increase in sports endurance events, targeting athletes of all ages. Around 800 city marathons are arranged globally every year with several thousand participants in most. As a result, more older individuals including individuals at risk are taking part in high-intensity sporting activities. In general terms, this may be very positive but must also be acknowledged, since high-intensity PA may act as a trigger for SCD, especially in susceptible individuals with an underlying cardiovascular abnormality [12].

For young athletes (<35 years) with no underlying cardiovascular disease, the risk of SCD is extremely low, while in athletes over 35 years, in particular athletes with a high-risk profile for CAD, or even established CAD, the risk associated with high-intensive activity may be substantial. The major cause of SCD in master athletes (>35 years) is, indeed, CAD [13]. Already from the age of 25, CAD may be the most common cause of SCD [14], while in even younger athletes the cause is most often congenital/inherited disease [14].

The risk of SCD in master athletes has been estimated from studies on endurance races, such as marathons, where the mean age of participants varies between 35 and 45 in most races. Overall, the risk of SCA during marathon running is around 1/50,000 [15]. Importantly, cardiac arrest during exercise has a better outcome than usual, since subjects tend to be younger, events are usually witnessed, CPR is most often started immediately, AEDs are readily available and arrhythmias are more frequently shockable [16].

Possibly, the mechanisms for SCA may be different in exercise-related arrest, although this has not yet been shown [13]. Proposed mechanisms of arrest in athletes with underlying CAD include plaque rupture, demand ischemia during activity in stable CAD and endothelial erosion [17, 18].

As the risk of SCA is higher, recommendations for cardiovascular evaluation of older individuals aiming to participate in leisure-time or competitive sports [19], as well as for those with risk factors for or with established CAD [20], has been established.

## 44.2 Evaluation of Individuals with Risk Factors for CAD

### 44.2.1 Risk Stratification

- As CAD is a progressive disease, with the atherosclerotic process starting from young age, the main risk factors of CAD are age and sex. These risk factors are non-midifiable.
- These are complemented by modifiable risk factors, such as arterial hypertension, dyslipidemia, insulin resistance/diabetes mellitus type 2, smoking and physical inactivity [7]. See respective chapters in this book for the specific details of each risk factor.

Age is a major determinant of CAD. The majority of individuals with subclinical CAD are symptom-free and unaware of their disease. Importantly, more and older runners are participating in endurance events [21].

By using the traditional risk factors, individuals may be risk stratified for the risk of cerebrovascular (CVD) death in the coming 10 years (or if extrapolated to 60 years of age), according to the ESC SCORE [7]. The SCORE can thereby act as an indirect assessment (proxy) of the level of CAD. The risk factors included are

(a) Age,
(b) Sex,
(c) Blood pressure,
(d) Smoking status, and
(e) Cholesterol-level.

In addition, diabetes mellitus, physical inactivity and family history should be taken into consideration. Other possible predictors of future CVD include coronary artery calcium (CAC), which will add to the predictive power in medium risk individuals, according to SCORE or Framingham [22]. However, using CAC, a selection of patients suitable for additional risk stratification by CAC should be performed, ideally using traditional risk factors [23].

Interestingly, older master endurance athletes show higher mean levels of CAC, compared to non-athletes, with the same risk factor profile [24]. They also have a higher degree of stable plaques [25], with the long-term clinical implications being unknown at present (see Chap. 32). Individuals may be aware that they have risk factors for CAD and are currently seeing a physician for treatment. However, some individuals may be detected during pre-competition evaluations, screening or during physical exercise testing.

Pre-race evaluation of master athletes (>35 years of age) has been advocated by the ESC since 2011 [19], using initial self-assessment prior to enrollment to the race, with a few simple questions, such as the 7 questions of the revised Physical activity readiness questionnaire (PAR-Q; see Chap. 7) [26]. If anyone tick yes on any of these questions, they are recommended to seek a physician for formal risk stratification, as described here.

For athletes or patients with risk factors for CAD wanting to engage in leisure-time sports or equivalent exercise, recommendations for risk stratification have been published by the ESC [20].

In summary,

- Pre-participation assessment is recommended for leisure time and master athletes, aiming for participation in sports. The level of examination is dependent on the risk profile and evidence of CAD.
- The traditional risk factor profile of the European-SCORE (or American Framingham) is recommended for initial risk stratification of individuals with risk factors for CAD [19, 20].
- In medium-risk individuals, additional risk stratification with CAC-score may be advocated.

### 44.2.2 Evaluation

The current evaluation of individuals with risk factors for CAD, should take into account [20]:

1. The individual risk profile (see above)
2. The intended level of physical activity
3. The habitual exercise level.

For sedentary individuals or active individuals having a positive self-assessment and wanting to engage in at least medium-intensity activity, maximal exercise testing should be performed if individuals have [20]:

- A high-risk profile (SCORE > 5% risk of CVD-death in the coming 10 years),
- Symptoms, indicating CAD (chest pain, syncope etc),
- Abnormal findings on physical examination, or
- Abnormalities on resting-ECG (arrhythmias, ischemia).

The first step of further evaluation in individuals with a higher risk profile, is the maximal exercise test, using a cycle ergometer or a treadmill (see Chap. 11). Then according to the result of the exercise-test, or a similar stress-image test, further evaluations are performed.

1. If the maximal exercise test is normal, no additional tests are mandatory and no restriction for sports is advised. Risk factors should be treated and followed-up according to standards (see respective chapters).
2. If the exercise test is abnormal (Box 44.1), showing signs of myocardial ischemia, a CT or coronary angiogram should be performed to rule out/confirm the presence of clinically relevant CAD (see confirmed CAD below).
3. If the exercise test shows borderline results or is interpretable, additional stress testing must be performed. For example, stress-echo, CMR/PET/SPECT could all be used, depending on local availability and expertise (see Chap. 33).

**Box 44.1 Abnormalities of a Maximal Exercise Test**

- Signs of ischemia on ECG: ST-depression >1 mm, descending or horizontal and/or
- Ventricular arrhythmias
- Abnormal BP response (BP decreasing during activity)
- Low exercise capacity
- Symptoms of possible ischemia (angina, dyspnea, syncope, pallor, cyanosis)

- **In summary, if an athlete has a high-risk profile but a normal, truly maximal exercise test, no restrictions apply for any competitive sport.**

## 44.3 Individuals with Confirmed CAD [20]

Assessment of athletes with established CAD for eligibility to participate in competitive sports is done with the assumption that they have to be able to compete without limitations. Because, in sports very-high intensity levels are generally achieved, regardless of what the original intention of the athlete may be. When giving advice for participation in leisure time and amateur sports, a measure of control of the intensity and duration of the exercise load can be expected.

- Besides the level of competition, the specific type of sport should be considered (Fig. 44.1 and Chap. 1). Some sports may be more prone to induce myocardial ischemia than others, due to the differing intensity and duration of the event/game.

In advising patient-athletes with CAD to engage in competitive sports, as well as in high-intensity leisure time and amateur sports, we need to carefully calculate and balance the documented benefits of exercise programs with the potential risk for adverse events. But, given the wealth of evidence supporting the benefits of physical activity and exercise for primary and secondary prevention of CAD, individuals should rarely be restricted from competitive sport. This is only reasonable when a substantial risk of adverse events or disease progression is present.

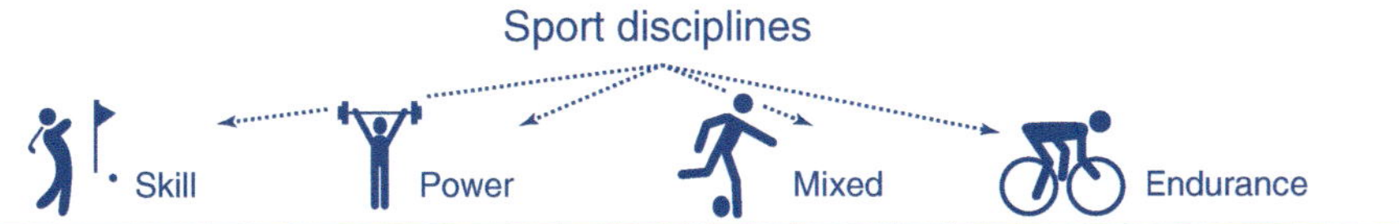


| | | | | | | | |
|---|---|---|---|---|---|---|---|
| Isometric | +/- | Isometric | +++/++++ | Isometric | ++/+++ | Isometric | ++/+++ |
| Isotonic | +/- | Isotonic | +/++ | Isotonic | ++/+++ | Isotonic | +++/++++ |
| Cardiac remodeling | +/- | Cardiac remodeling | +/++ | Cardiac remodeling | ++/+++ | Cardiac remodeling | ++++ |

- Golf
- Archery
- Sailing
- Table Tennis
- Equestrian
- Karate
- Shooting/Rifle
- Curling
- Sled disciplines
- Ski Jumping

- Weight lifting
- Wrestling / Judo
- Boxing
- Short distance running
- Shot-putting
- Discus / Javelin
- Artistic gymnastics
- Bobsleigh
- Short-track kating
- Alpine skiing
- Snowboarding

- Soccer
- Basketball
- Volleyball
- Water polo
- Badminton
- Tennis
- Fencing
- Handball
- Rugby
- Hockey / Ice-hockey

- Cycling
- Rowing
- Mid/long distance swimming
- Mid/long distance running
- Canoeing
- Triathlon
- Pentathlon
- X-country skiing
- Biathlon
- Long distance skating

**Fig. 44.1** Simplified classification of the most common Olympic sport disciplines, according to the relative isometric and isotonic components of exercise and resulting cardiovascular adaptation (see also Chap. 1, depicted here again to facilitate reading of the chapter; adapted from [27])

Indeed, leisure time physical activity is only contraindicated in extreme circumstances. Conversely, individual exercise prescription to all individuals with risk factors for CAD and patient-athletes with manifest CAD should be part of clinical routine.

CAD in a previously healthy individuals is typically suspected based on a history of anginal symptoms and on traditional risk factors being present. Importantly, most athletes with risk factors for and/or underlying CAD may be asymptomatic and may only be detected during pre-race or pre-competition medical evaluation, cardiac screening and/or functional physical exercise testing.

### 44.3.1 Evaluation of Athletes with CAD [20]

In patient-athletes with an earlier clinical CAD event or a CT-scan or coronary-angiography demonstrating CAD, advice relative to sport participation may be given only after individual assessment. Recommendations on eligibility for competitive sports should be based on:

1. Presence or absence of exercise-induced myocardial ischemia or exercise induced arrhythmia
2. Presence or absence of evidence of myocardial dysfunction
3. Type and level of sport competition
4. Individual fitness
5. Cardiovascular risk factor profile

After diagnostic testing, patient-athletes with proven CAD may be stratified as follows:

- *Low probability* for adverse cardiac events during exercise (all the following must apply) [20]:
  - Absence of critical coronary stenoses (i.e., <70%) of major coronary arteries or <50% of left main stem on coronary angiography
  - Ejection fraction ≥50% on echocardiography, CMR or angiography (and no wall motion abnormalities)
  - Normal, age-adjusted exercise capacity and absence of inducible ischemia on maximal exercise testing
  - Absence of major ventricular tachyarrhythmias at rest and during maximal stress testing
- *High probability* for adverse cardiac events during exercise (at least one of the following must apply) [20]:
  - Presence of critical (>70%) coronary stenosis of a major coronary artery or (>50%) left main stem on coronary angiography
  - Ejection fraction <50% on echocardiography (or other tests)

- Exercise-induced ischemia (>0.1 mV ST depression (horizontal or down-sloping in 2 chest leads) or ST elevation >0.1 mV (in a non–Q-wave lead and excluding aortic valve replacement)) or new left bundle branch block at low exercise intensity or immediately post-exercise.
- Dyspnea at low exercise intensity (angina equivalent)
- Relevant ventricular tachyarrhythmias (i.e., non-sustained ventricular tachycardia (NSVT), polymorphic or very frequent ventricular extra beats (VEBs), at any time
- Dizziness or syncope on exertion
- High degree of myocardial scarring on CMR imaging

Revascularization may be primarily considered if ischemia is present during functional testing despite adequate treatment. If the patient-athlete wants to participate in competitive sports, revascularization should also be preferred. During maximal exercise the risks of myocardial ischemia and cardiac events are increased due to the high myocardial oxygen consumption attained and to neuro-hormonal activation. Antianginal medications such as beta-blockers may also be less well tolerated in athletes.

If despite revascularization and/or adequate medical treatment ischemia cannot be completely resolved, the patient-athlete is restricted from competitive sport and advised to enter leisure-time sports activities only. Such activities are associated with less physical demands and lower intensity, so that ischemia may more likely be avoided.

### 44.3.2 Recommendations [20]

- **Patient-athletes with clinically proven CAD and considered to be at low-risk for cardiac events may be selectively advised to participate in competitive sports but restrictions may apply on an individual basis for certain sports with the highest CV demand (such as extreme power and endurance disciplines, see** Fig. 44.1)**. Older patient-athletes with CAD may also be restricted since they have a high risk of SCD during endurance events.**
- **Patient-athletes with clinically proven CAD, defined as high risk, should receive appropriate management and be restricted from competitive sport. In patient-athletes with CAD and significant ischemia during exercise, as in all patients, anti-ischemic therapy needs to be optimized. In case of inducible ischemia, revascularization is strongly suggested.**

## 44.4 Exercise-Prescription and Follow-up

### 44.4.1 Exercise Prescription for All

Even after a cardiac event, regular PA conveys positive effects on health. Cardiac rehabilitation post-MI has been shown to decrease cardiovascular mortality [28] as well as increasing aerobic fitness substantially [29].

Also, little PA may be beneficial. Recent data from the Swedish national registry SWEDEHEART showed that not being physically inactive was associated with reduced risk of mortality and readmission [30], and increased PA during the first year post-MI, was associated with halved mortality in the following 4.5 years [31].

Similarly, in different studies, for example by Williams et al., the risk of deaths in patients with an earlier cardiac event, was substantially decreasing with increasing activity, up to a daily activity of 7 km jogging, above which level the risk increased [12].The relationship between exercise intensity/duration and risk is often described as a u- or j-shaped curve, with the lowest and highest levels of PA being associated with the highest risk [32].

In any individual, including athletes who have been revascularized due to CAD, exercise is encouraged, initially as part of a cardiac rehabilitation program as recommended by the ESC [7], followed by lifelong PA.

Methods to increase PA in the long-term, i.e. also after cardiac rehabilitation, are much needed. Lifestyle behavioral change including increased PA is an essential part of secondary prevention of CAD [7], however difficult to achieve. In recent years, various methods and attempts to introduce and implement "exercise on prescription"-models have been tried, showing varying efficacy. In a systematic review of the Swedish model for physical activity on prescription (PAP), this method was shown to increase the level of PA in patients being insufficiently active [33].

For everyone with CAD, including post-MI, individual exercise prescription is advocated. Exercise should be prescribed, starting from low intensity activity, gradually progressing to higher intensities and/or duration of activity (see Chap. 44) [20].

### 44.4.2 Exercise for Competitive Patient-Athletes

Previously, patients with established CAD, including post-MI and/or post-PCI, were restricted from competitive sports [34]. However, the latest recommendations from both the US [35] and Europe [20] have become more liberal and now allow participation even in competitive sports to a larger extent. Also, for healthy competitive athletes the same principles of progressively increasing physical activity in terms of intensity and duration on their return to sports apply:

- The period between exercise rehabilitation and return to normal sporting activity is dependent upon the extent of myocardial injury and remodeling.
- Progress of rehabilitation efforts should be serially assessed e.g. for symptoms.
- Adherence to individual exercise recommendations must be ensured.
- Contact sport must be avoided in case of increased risk of bleeding, e.g. while on dual antiplatelet therapy.
- Correct warm-up/cool-down procedures should be followed.

In summary, athletes considered as "low-risk" (see above) for cardiac events post-MI and/or post-PCI are recommended a minimum of 3 months structured and progressive rehabilitation before (resumed) participation in competitive sports [20].

### 44.4.3 Follow-up

Periodical, at least annual, follow-ups of athletes with CAD are recommended. These follow-ups should include:

- Risk factor management by lifestyle and medications according to guidelines [7].
- Any (emerging) symptom should be evaluated.
- Repeated exercise-testing could be used for risk stratification and/or modified exercise prescription, particularly if changes in symptoms or risk factor profile occur.

**Clinical Pearls**

- Physical inactivity is one of the strongest prognosticators for all-cause as well as cardiovascular morbidity and mortality.
- Physical activity or even better exercise training is a class I level A intervention for primary and secondary prevention, not only for cardiovascular but many other diseases.
- Aerobic physical activity of at least 30–60 min/day on 3–7 days/week at moderate (to high) intensity is universally recommended. Health benefits can certainly be expected if training is performed for up to 300 min/week.
- Pre-participation assessment is recommended not only for competitive athletes but also for leisure time and master athletes. The level of examination is dependent on the risk profile and evidence of CAD.
- In case of a high-risk cardiovascular profile in an otherwise healthy subject with a normal, truly maximal exercise test, no restrictions apply for any competitive sport.
- Patient-athletes at "low-risk" for cardiac events post-MI and/or post-PCI are recommended a minimum of 3 months structured and progressive rehabilitation before participation in competitive sports.
- Patient-athletes with clinically proven CAD at a low-risk for cardiac events may be selectively advised to participate in competitive sports.
- Patient-athletes with clinically proven CAD at a high risk for cardiac events, are restricted from competitive sport.
- Patients-athletes with ischemia are no different than non-athlete patients and therefore need to be treated according to guidelines, i.e. anti-ischemic therapy has to be started or optimized and where appropriate revascularization has to be performed.

## Case Presentations

### Case 1

Glenn is a 63-year old man, formerly manual worker but these days mostly office work. He seeks medical advice since he has entered into a betting contest with his son: Glenn has pledged to enter, and finish, a local 21 km half marathon race next spring. He refers to himself as interested in sports, with an active interest in sports, in particular soccer. He also played in a national low-level league in his youth.

Before starting practice for the race, his wife has insisted on a medical check-up and you agree to see him.

Glenn is modestly overweight with a BMI of 29.5, waist circumference is 105 cm, sitting blood pressure is 160/90, LDL-cholesterol of 3.2 mmol/l (123 mg/dl), total cholesterol is 6.1 mmol/l (235 mg/dl), fasting glucose is at the upper limit of normal, ECG at rest shows normal sinus rhythm without ST-changes. Glenn smoked for about 10 years but stopped at 30 years of age. His wife complains that he snores a lot and for this reason they do not share the same bedroom anymore. He has no symptoms on exercise, his two older brothers are healthy, his father suffered from stroke at 72 years of age and his mother is healthy at 91. Upon questioning, it becomes evident that he has done little exercise during at least the last 10–15 years.

So what do we need to consider?

- What is he intending to do? 21 km half marathon, which is a substantial effort
- What is his level of fitness? We don't really know but probably quite low.
- What are his risk factors and his 10-year risk? According to the SCORE diagram his risk is about 10% for fatal CVD within the next 10 years, thus he is not in a low-risk category.

## Questions

1. Do we need additional workup?
2. Do we need to do more?
3. What would our advice be to Glenn?

## Answers

1. Yes, a truly maximal exercise test should be performed. This was done and was completely normal; he reached a maximum load of 155 W (slightly below average for age/sex/weight), maximum heart rate of 158, no chest pain, no arrhythmias, adequate evolution of blood pressure, no ST-changes.
2. We need to address his risk factors i.e. re-check his blood pressure, give dietary advice for cholesterol, advice on weight loss. Given the normal exercise test, no further evaluation is required.
3. He needs to start regular exercise, should start on a modest level since his fitness is also modest. If he can successfully train regularly there is no reason to prohibit him from entering the 21 km race, in the coming spring.

## Case 2

Björn is a 46-year-old man, never smoked, regular physical activity, in particular greatly into cycling. He frequently participates in competitive bicycle races. When doing a 120 km 1-day race in the French alps, he developed chest pain during a long climb. He managed to finish the race but then sought medical attention. An ECG showed inferior ST-depression and troponin was elevated. A coronary angiogram revealed a subtotal occlusion of the proximal right coronary artery, due to a thrombus at the site of a ruptured plaque. Residual stenosis was less than 50% and no angioplasty was therefore done. He was given a statin, ACE inhibitor, dual antiplatelet treatment and discharged from hospital. He comes to see you after 4 weeks, is about to return to work full time and is anxious to go back to training.

At this visit he is in good general condition, reports no chest pain, his blood pressure is 120/70 mmHg, LDL cholesterol is 1.9 mmol/l (73 mg/dl), glucose normal, BMI 24, ECG shows sinus rhythm, 48/min, inferiorly negative T-waves.

So what do we need to consider?

- He is a patient with stable coronary artery disease, survived an MI, and his risk factors are under control.
- What does he intend to do? He wants to go back to competitive cycling on a high to extreme level of effort.
- What is his level of fitness? Probably quite good although he hasn't been training for the last month.
- What are his risk factors? He has a 50% residual stenosis, is free from angina, has no palpitations, and his risk factors are rather well controlled.

### Questions

1. Do we need additional workup?
2. What would your advice be to Björn?

### Answers

1. We need to know how his left ventricular function is and how he performs on a maximum exercise test. One may also consider adding an isotope to the exercise test or re-do the angiogram. An echocardiogram was done at the visit, which showed slight inferior hypokinesia, overall good left ventricular function with an EF of 55%, normal valvular function. A maximum exercise test was done the following day, showing good exercise capacity with a maximum load of 250 W, maximum heart rate of 172/min, no signs of ischemia, no arrhythmias and no symptoms.
2. He is now free to go back to training and may go back to competitive cycling but has to understand that as a MI survivor his risk of further cardiac events including cardiac death will be increased both at rest and during exercise.

## References

1. Palmefors H, DuttaRoy S, Rundqvist B, Borjesson M. The effect of physical activity or exercise on key biomarkers in atherosclerosis–a systematic review. Atherosclerosis. 2014;235(1):150–61.
2. Strong JP, Malcolm GT, McMahan CA, Tracy RE, Newman WP, Herderick EE, et al. Prevalence and extent of atherosclerosis in adolescents and young adults: implications for prevention from the pathobiological determinants of atherosclerosis in youth study. JAMA. 1999;281:727–35.

3. Montalescot G, Sechtem U, Achenbach S, Andreotti F, Arden C, Budaj A, et al. 2013 ESC guidelines on the management of stable coronary artery disease. Eur Heart J. 2013;34:2949–3003.
4. GBD 2013 Mortality and Causes of Death Collaborators. Global, regional, and national age-sex specific all-cause and cause-specific mortality for 240 causes of death, 1990–2013: a systematic analysis for the global burden of disease study 2013. Lancet. 2015;385:117–71.
5. Anand SS, Islan S, Rosengren A, Franzosi MG, Steyn K, Yusufali AH, et al. Risk factors for myocardial infarction in women and men: insights from the INTERHEART study. Eur Heart J. 2008;29:932–40.
6. Blair SN, Morris JN. Healthy hearts and the beneficial effect of being physically active. Ann Epidemiol. 2009;19:253–6.
7. Piepoli M, Hoes A, Agewall S, Albus C, Brotons C, Catapano A, et al. 2016 European guidelines on cardiovascular disease prevention in clinical practice: The sixth joint task force of the European Society of Cardiology and other socities on cardiovascular disease prevention in clinical practice. Eur Heart J. 2016;37:2315–81.
8. Ng SW, Popkin BM. Time use and physical activity: a shift away from movement across the globe. Obes Rev. 2012;13(8):659–80.
9. Ekblom-Bak E, Ekblom O, Andersson G, Wallin P, Soderling J, Hemmingsson E, et al. Decline in cardiorespiratory fitness in the Swedish working force between 1995 and 2017. Scand J Med Sci Sports. 2018;29(2):232–9.
10. Albert CM, Mittleman MA, Chae CU, Lee IM, Hennekens CH, Manson JE. Triggering of sudden death from cardiac causes by vigorous exertion. N Engl J Med. 2000;343:1355–61.
11. Mittleman MA, Maclure M, Tofler GH, Sherwood JB, Goldberg RJ, Muller JE. Triggering of acute myocardial infarction by heavy physical exertion. Protection against triggering by regular exercise. N Engl J Med. 1993;329:1677–83.
12. Williams PT, Thompson PD. Increased cardiovascular disease mortality associated with excessive exercise in heart attack survivors. Mayo Clin Proc. 2014;89:1187–94.
13. Gerardin B, Collet JP, Mustafic H, Bellemain-Appaix A, Benamer H, Monsegu J, et al. Registry on acute cardiovascular events during endurance running races: the prospective RACE Paris registry. Eur Heart J. 2016;37:2531–41.
14. Meyer L, B S, C F, C M, K H, M E, et al. Incidence, cases and survival trends from cardiovascular-related sudden cardiac arrest in children and young adults 0 to 35 years of age: a 30-year review. Circulation. 2012;126:1363–72.
15. Kim JH, Malhotra R, Chiampas G, d´Hemecourt P, Troyanos C, Cianca J, et al. Cardiac arrest during long-distance running races. Race associated cardiac arrest event registry (RACER) study group. N Engl J Med. 2012;366:130–40.
16. Frisk-Torell M, Stromsoe A, Zagerholm E, Herlitz J, Claesson A, Svensson L, et al. Higher survival rates in exercise-related out-of-hospital cardiac arrests, compared to non-exercise related- a study from the Swedish register of cardiopulmonary resuscitation. Eur J Prev Cardiol. 2017;24:1673–9.
17. Thompson PD, Franklin BA, Balady GJ, Blair SN, Corrado D, EstesIII NAM, et al. Exercise and acute cardiovascular events. Placing the risks into perspective. A scientific statement from the American Heart Association council on nutrition, physical activity, and metabolism and the council on clinical cardiology. Circulation. 2007;115:2358–68.
18. Quillard T, Franck G, Mawson T, Folco E, Libby P. Mechanisms of erosion of atherosclerotic plaques. Curr Opin Lipidol. 2017;28:434–41.
19. Börjesson M, Urhausen A, Kouidi E, Dugmore D, Sharma S, Halle M, et al. Cardiovascular evaluation of middle-aged/senior individuals engaged in leisure-time sport activities: position stand from the section of exercise physiology and sports cardiology of the European Association of Cardiovascular Prevention and Rehabilitation. Eur J Cardiovasc Prev Rehabil. 2011;18:446–58.
20. Borjesson M, Dellborg M, Niebauer J, LaGerche A, Schmied C, Solberg EE, et al. Recommendations for participation in leisure-time or competitive sports in athletes-patients with coronary artery disease-A position statement from the sports cardiology section of the European association of preventive cardiology (EAPC). Eur Heart J. 2019;40:13–8.

21. Aagaard P, Sahlén A, Braunschweig F. Performance trends and cardiac biomarkers in a 30-km cross-country race, 1993–2007. Med Sci Sports Exerc. 2012;44:894–9.
22. Greenland P, LaBree L, Axzen SP, Doherty TM, Detrano RC. Coronary artery calcium score combined with Framingham score for risk prediction in asymptomatic individuals. JAMA. 2004;291:563.
23. Saad M, Pothineni NV, Thomas J, Parikh R, Kovelamundi S, Elsayed D, et al. Coronary artery calcium scoring in young adults: evidence and challenges. Curr Cardiol Rep. 2018;20:10.
24. Mohlenkamp S, Lehmann N, Breuckmann F, Brocker-Preuss M, Nassenstein K, Halle M, et al. Running: the risk of coronary events : prevalence and prognostic relevance of coronary atherosclerosis in marathon runners. Eur Heart J. 2008;29(15):1903–10.
25. Aengevaeren VL, Mosterd A, Braber TL, Prakken NHJ, Doevendans PA, Grobbee DE, et al. Relationship between lifelong exercise volume and coronary atherosclerosis in athletes. Circulation. 2017;136:138–48.
26. Balady GJ, Chaitman B, Driscoll D, Foster C, Froelicher E, Gordon N, et al. Recommendations for cardiovascular screening, staffing, and emergency policies at health/fitness facilities. Circulation. 1998;97:2283–93.
27. Pelliccia A, Adami PE, Quattrini F, Squeo MR, Caselli S, Verdile L, et al. Are Olympic athletes free from cardiovascular diseases? Systematic investigation in 2352 participants from Athens 2004 to Sotchi 2014. Br J Sports Med. 2017;51(4):238–43.
28. Anderson L, Thompson DR, Oldridge N, Zwisler AD, Rees K, Martin N, et al. Exercise-based cardiac rehabilitation for coronary heart disease. Cochrane Database Syst Rev. 2016;1(Jan 5):CD001800.
29. Mitchell BL, Lock MJ, Davison K, Parfitt G, Buckley JP, Eston RG. What is the effect of aerobic exercise intensity on cardiorespiratory fitness in those undergoing cardiac rehabilitation? A systematic review with meta-analysis. Br J Sports Med. 2018;53(21):1341–51. epub ahead of print
30. Ek A, Ekblom O, Hambraeus K, Cider A, Kallings LV, Borjesson M. Physical inactivity and smoking after myocardial infarction as predictors for readmission and survival- Results from the SWEDEHEART-registry. Clin Res Cardiol. 2018;108(3):324–32.
31. Ekblom O, Ek A, Cider A, Hambraeus K, Borjesson M. Increased physical activity post-myocardial infarction is related to reduced mortality-results from the Swedeheart registry. J Am Heart Assoc. 2018;7:e010108.
32. Mons U, Hahmann H, Brenner H. A reverese J-shaped association of leisure-time physical activity prognosis in patients with stable coronary heart disease: evidence from a large cohort with repeated measurements. Heart. 2014;100:1043–9.
33. Onerup A, Arvidsson D, Blomqvist A, Daxberg E-L, Jivegard L, Jonsdottir IH, et al. Physical activity on prescription in accordance with the Swedish model increases physical activity: a systematic review. Br J Sports Med. 2018;53(6):383–8.
34. Pelliccia A, Fagard R, Bjornstad HH, Anastassakis A, Arbustini E, Assanelli D, et al. Recommendations for competitive sports participation in athletes with cardiovascular disease: a consensus document from the study group of sports cardiology of the working group of cardiac rehabilitation and exercise physiology and the working group of myocardial and pericardial diseases of the European society of cardiology. Eur Heart J. 2005;26(14):1422–45.
35. Thompson P, Myerburg R, Levine B, Udelson J, Kovacs R. Eligibility and disqualification recommendations for competitive athletes with cardiovascular abnormalities: task force 8: coronary artery disease. A scientific statement from the American Heart Association and the American College of Cardiology. Circulation. 2015;132:e310–4.

# Exercise in Specific Diseases: Heart Failure with Preserved Ejection Fraction

45

Bharathi Upadhya, Frank Edelmann, and Dalane W. Kitzman

**Learning Objectives**

1. Clinical importance of exercise intolerance in HFpEF.
2. Pathophysiology of exercise intolerance in HFpEF patients.
3. Role of Aging, Frailty and Comorbidities.
4. Mechanisms of the Improvement of Exercise intolerance with Exercise Training in HFpEF.
5. Exercise prescription for prevention and management of HFpEF.
6. Exercise Training Modalities in HFpEF.

## 45.1 Introduction

Heart failure (HF) with preserved ejection fraction (HFpEF) is the most common form of HF in patients older than 65 years [1]; among older women, > 80% of new cases of HF are HFpEF [2]. In contrast to HF with reduced ejection fraction (HFrEF), the prevalence of HFpEF is increasing and its prognosis is not improving,

B. Upadhya
Cardiovascular Medicine Section, Department of Internal Medicine, Wake Forest School of Medicine, Winston-Salem, NC, USA
e-mail: bupadhya@wakehealth.edu

F. Edelmann
Department of Internal Medicine and Cardiology, Charité Universitätsmedizin Berlin, Campus Virchow Klinikum, Berlin, Germany
e-mail: frank.edelmann@charite.de

D. W. Kitzman (✉)
Kermit Glenn Phillips II Chair in Cardiovascular Medicine, Cardiovascular Medicine Section, Department of Internal Medicine, Wake Forest School of Medicine, Winston-Salem, NC, USA
e-mail: dkitzman@wakehealth.edu



A. Pressler, J. Niebauer (eds.), *Textbook of Sports and Exercise Cardiology*, https://doi.org/10.1007/978-3-030-35374-2_45

which may be due to the combination of aging of the population and increasing rates of obesity [3]. The health and economic impact of HFpEF is at least as great as that of HFrEF, with almost similar severity of acute hospitalization rates, and substantial mortality [3, 4]. Despite the importance of HFpEF, and in stark contrast to HFrEF where there is a broad range of proven, effective therapies, our understanding of HFpEF pathophysiology is incomplete and optimal treatment remains uncertain. Pharmacologic management of HFpEF is a challenge due to the heterogeneity of the disease, and clinical studies continue to add to a growing body of knowledge surrounding its treatment modalities. Several recent studies have evaluated exercise training (ET) as a therapeutic management strategy in patients with HFpEF. Although these studies were not designed to address clinical endpoints, such as HF hospitalizations and mortality, they showed that ET is a safe and effective intervention to improve exercise capacity as measured by peak exercise oxygen uptake (peak $VO_2$) and health related quality of life (HRQOL) in clinically stable HF patients.

In this chapter, we will discuss the current understanding of the pathophysiology of exercise intolerance, pathophysiology of exercise intolerance including the systemic nature of HFpEF and its role in development and worsening of exercise intolerance, results from completed ET trials in HFpEF, mechanisms of benefit, and future directions.

## 45.2 Pathophysiology of Exercise Intolerance in HFpEF Patients

A cardinal feature of HFpEF is exercise intolerance even when well compensated, measured objectively as peak $VO_2$ that results in decreased HRQOL [5–8]. In addition, exercise intolerance is often used as an end point or outcome measure for therapeutic trials. According to the Fick equation, $VO_2$ is equal to the product of cardiac output (CO) and arterial–venous oxygen content difference (A-$VO_2$ Diff). This results in the following Fick equation:

$$VO_2 = CO \times A - VO_2\,\text{Diff} = \left[\text{heart rate}(HR) \times \text{stroke volume}(SV)\right] \times A - VO_2\,\text{Diff}.$$

In assessing the capacity to augment $VO_2$ in HFpEF, it is important to consider relative increases in each of the 3 components of $VO_2$ (HR, SV, and A-$VO_2$ Diff.)

## 45.3 Central Contributions to Exercise Intolerance

### 45.3.1 Diastolic and Systolic Limitations

One of the most commonly cited mechanisms of HFpEF has been left ventricle (LV) diastolic dysfunction consisting of abnormal LV active relaxation and increased LV passive stiffness contributing to the cardiac limitations in exercise capacity [9]. Increased diastolic stiffness can prevent the increase in LV end-diastolic volume that normally accompanies exercise, resulting in a limited ability to use the Frank-Starling mechanism to increased SV, despite greater filling pressures which have been reported in several studies [10–15]. Studies have shown that HFpEF patients have multiple functional abnormalities in diastole:

(a) Prolonged rate of LV pressure decay during isovolumic relaxation,
(b) Impaired mitral annular longitudinal motion,
(c) Impaired LV 'untwisting' that occurs during early diastole, and
(d) Increased passive diastolic stiffness [9, 11, 16–21].

These abnormalities have been observed to be more pronounced during the stress of exercise, such that the LV fills at the expense of left atrial (LA) hypertension [11, 18–21].

- Nonetheless, recently in a pilot study, combining early transmitral inflow velocity to early diastolic mitral annulus velocity ratio (E/e') [LV filling pressure index] with tricuspid regurgitation velocity > 2.8 m/s during exercise provided a significant increase in the sensitivity to detect patients with HFpEF during exercise and an increase of E/e' was significantly linked to worse peak $VO_2$ [22].
- In addition, Borlaug et al. showed an upward and leftward shift of the end-diastolic pressure-volume relationship in HFpEF, attributing increased filling pressures to intrinsic ventricular stiffness and reduced diastolic filling time at higher HRs [18].

Data from multiple sources indicate that even in well-characterized, symptomatic HFpEF, many patients do not have echo-Doppler indexes of severe diastolic dysfunction, at least at rest, or that differ greatly from that expected based on age and comorbidities [23, 24]. Moreover, many patients have significant measurable diastolic dysfunction, yet remain asymptomatic and without HF [25]. In addition, noninvasive measures interpreted as diastolic dysfunction are prevalent in asymptomatic persons, particularly the elderly [26, 27]. Most HFpEF trials have measured diastolic function or other cardiovascular (CV) measures at rest and not during exercise where symptoms become manifest.

- A recent trial of well characterized HFpEF patients showed that only 8% of patients had LV hypertrophy at baseline and 50% had significant or severe diastolic function at rest [28].
- Similarly, Maurer and colleagues found no significantly increased LV mass in older HFpEF patients compared to controls with hypertension but not HF [29, 30].
- In addition, the degree of fibrosis in HFpEF patients appears modest [31].
- Similarly a cross-sectional analysis from the prospective cohort programme Prevalence and Clinical Course of Diastolic Dysfunction and HF (DIAST-CHF) study revealed that classical risk factors for HF and neuroendocrine activation

are independently associated with sub-maximal exercise capacity, while diastolic function parameters obtained at rest were not [32].

These data have led to reconsideration of the initial hypothesis of HTN-induced LV hypertrophy, diastolic function, and cardiac fibrosis as the primary underlying pathophysiological mechanisms of HFpEF and led to broadening to include consideration of other potential contributing factors. As a result of this progress in our pathophysiological understanding, this disorder underwent a name change from the plausible term "diastolic HF" to the broader term "HFpEF" and henceforth HFpEF has become acknowledged as a distinct clinical syndrome [33, 34].

More recently, impaired systolic reserve function and abnormal LV-central vascular coupling have also been implicated in causing impaired exercise capacity in HFpEF [16]. Combined ventricular-vascular stiffening means that small changes in LV filling volumes can induce wide swings in arterial blood pressure and thus increase cardiac work with little increase in SV [16, 35]. The inability to vasodilate, to accommodate increased boluses of blood without increases in pressure, together with previously described limitations in systolic reserve, leads to dynamic limitations in ventricular-vascular coupling with exercise in patients with HFpEF [20, 36].

- This was demonstrated by Tartiere-Kesri et al., who showed a steep increase in proximal afterload after moderate exercise that is underestimated at rest and is associated with unfavorable ventricular- arterial coupling and exercise intolerance [37].
- Some reports indicated that HFpEF patients can have blunted increases in EF, contractility and longitudinal systolic shortening velocities during exercise [7, 20, 38, 39].
- HFpEF patients were found to have reduced longitudinal and circumferential strain by speckle tracking compared to age and gender matched hypertensive patients with diastolic dysfunction but without clinical HF [40].

### 45.3.2 Heart Rate

Decreased HR response also significantly contributes to the reduced CO at peak exercise and thus to reduced peak exercise $VO_2$.

- Chronotropic incompetence, the inability of HR to increase adequately during physical exertion, has been observed in greater than 25% of patients with HFpEF and found to be associated with their exercise intolerance [7, 38, 41–43].

Despite the overall consensus that peak HR is depressed in HFpEF, this effect may not be causal. Studies have reported that significant reductions in the rate of HR increase during exercise were primary contributors to reduced peak cardiac index and maximal exercise $VO_2$ [7] Indeed, chronotropic reserve is depressed in HFpEF even when compared with older, age-matched controls, independently from rate-lowering medication use. Additionally, autonomic dysfunction may be a contributing factor, as HR recovery is abnormal and baroreflex sensitivity impaired in HFpEF [41].

### 45.3.3 Left Atrial Structure and Function

Patients with HFpEF have impaired LA reservoir, conduit and pump function. Recently, it appeared that the LA is not simply being a passive marker of disease severity—it is an active component of the HFpEF syndrome.

- Indeed, it has been noted that in HFpEF patients, reduced LA strain (indicative of intrinsic LA mechanical dysfunction) is a major driver of both elevated pulmonary vascular resistance and decreased peak $VO_2$ on cardiopulmonary exercise testing [44].
- Recently, von Roeder et al. found that cardiac magnetic resonance myocardial feature tracking-derived LA conduit strain is significantly impaired in HFpEF and associated with exercise intolerance [45]. They showed that the abnormal LA conduit function is a distinct feature of HFpEF, independent of LV stiffness and relaxation—thus arguing that LA conduit function reflects intrinsic LA pathology, not completely explained by ventricular pathology [45].

In addition, many of the clinical risk factors associated with HFpEF—obesity, hypertension, diabetes—may directly contribute to LA fibrosis through inflammation and oxidative stress [46]. Furthermore, atrial dyssynchrony is common in HFpEF [47]. These factors likely contribute to the development of new onset or progression of atrial arrhythmias, a frequent complication of HFpEF.

### 45.3.4 Right Ventricular (RV) Dysfunction, Pulmonary Vascular Disease

Pulmonary vascular disease is common in patients with HFpEF, particularly during exercise and predicts increased mortality in HFpEF [48, 49]. In addition, pulmonary pressure increases with aging and is correlated with ventricular-vascular stiffening, both common risk factors for HFpEF [50]. Furthermore, the pulmonary pressure decreases more precipitously with acute vasodilator therapy in HFpEF than in HFrEF, suggesting increased RV end-systolic elastance [51]. A large percentage of patients have co-existing pulmonary disease that can worsen pulmonary hypertension [52].

Recent studies have also shown that a significant number of patients display RV dysfunction and patients with this phenotype suffer from high morbidity and mortality [53–55]. It has been noted that HFpEF patients showed a substantial decline in RV function and even greater degree of RV dilation over a time and these changes in the right heart structure and systolic function greatly exceeding corresponding changes in the left side of the heart [56].

## 45.4 Peripheral Mechanisms of Exercise Intolerance in HFpEF

### 45.4.1 Impaired Arterial Function

In healthy older adults, the 11-fold increase in blood flow to the active muscles during peak cycle exercise is caused by sympathetic-mediated redistribution of blood from non-exercising regions to the working muscles coupled with metabolic-mediated vasodilation in the exercising muscles [57, 58]. Impaired $O_2$ extraction during exercise can be the result of abnormal diffusive $O_2$ transport, diminished $O_2$ utilization, or both. Decreased diffusive $O_2$ transport can result from abnormalities in either the macrovascular or microvascular beds. Changes in arterial function may result in inefficient distribution of CO to the active muscles and contribute to exercise intolerance in patients with HFpEF [59].

- Both aortic distensibility and carotid artery distensibility are severely reduced in elderly HFpEF patients and correlate with their degree of exercise intolerance and objectively measured peak exercise $VO_2$ [60, 61].
- In addition, reductions in both exercise and post-exercise leg blood flow and leg venous conductance have been reported in these patients [62].

Similarly, impaired peripheral arterial endothelial function may result in impaired exercise blood flow reserve in patients with HFpEF.

- Using phase-contrast magnetic resonance imaging (superficial femoral artery), Hundley, *et al.* showed that resting and flow-mediated increases in leg blood flow in elderly HFpEF patients are not significantly impaired and were similar to those of age-matched healthy subjects [63].
- Haykowsky *et al.* using high resolution brachial artery ultrasound to assess flow-mediated dilation found no reduction in endothelial function in HFpEF patients who were free of clinically significant vascular disease [64].

However, flow-mediated vasodilation in large conduit arteries (e.g., femoral) may differ from that observed in the microvasculature.

- Microvascular endothelial dysfunction (measured by digital artery tonometry) was impaired in HFpEF, correlated with reduced exercise capacity 38 and was an independent predictor of poorer prognosis, mainly readmission, in patients with HfpEF [65].
- Recently in an autopsy-based study, Mohammed *et al*, showed reduced microvascular density in HFpEF patients which was independent of coronary artery disease and hypertension and appeared to account for the increased fibrosis [24].

This supports an over-arching hypothesis for HFpEF pathogenesis as originally proposed by Paulus: a systemic pro-inflammatory state that results in systemic arterial and microvascular dysfunction [66].

A consequence of the blunted microvascular reserve is that it may be associated with decreased diffusive oxygen transport to the active muscle, which would reduce exercise tolerance. Indeed, peripheral endothelial dysfunction might impair matching of perfusion to regional demand in skeletal muscle microcirculation.

Perhaps a greater factor in the impaired $O_2$ extraction during exercise is abnormal $O_2$ utilization by exercising skeletal muscle.

### 45.4.2 Role of Skeletal Muscle in Exercise Intolerance

Emerging evidence demonstrates that peripheral "non-cardiac" factors are important determinants of reduced peak $VO_2$ in HFpEF [67, 68].

- Haykowsky et al. found that the change in A-$VO_2$ Diff. from rest to peak exercise was an independent predictor of the reduced peak $VO_2$ in elderly HFpEF patients (Fig. 45.1) [67].

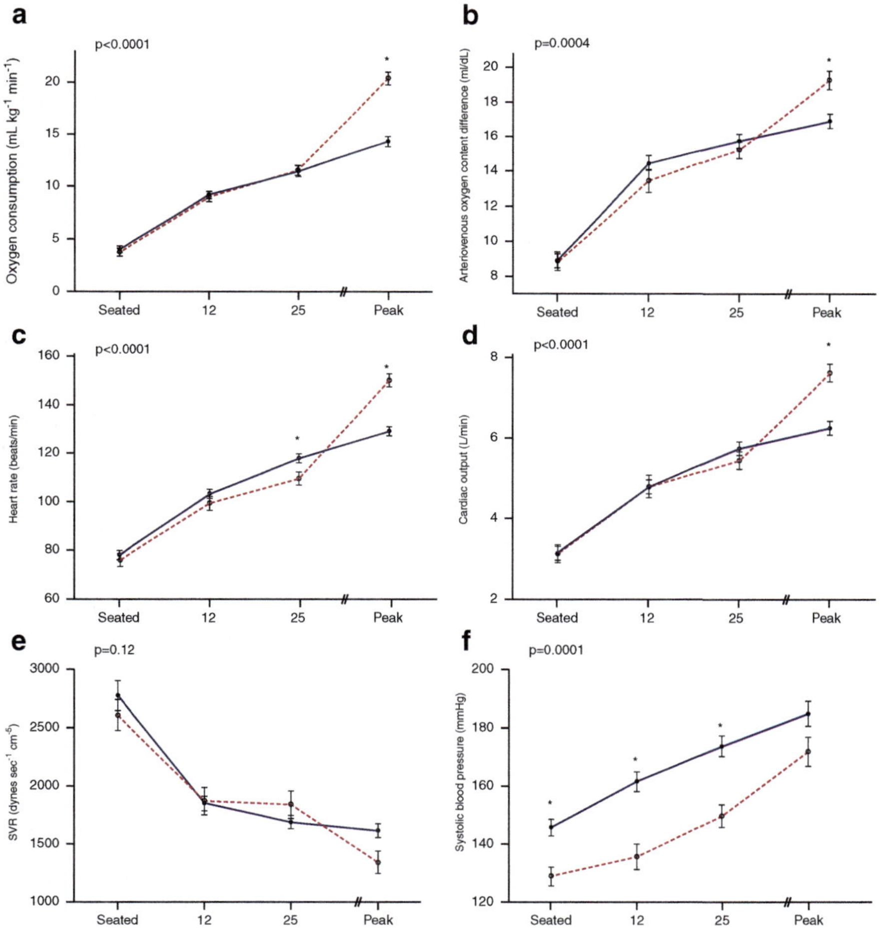


**Fig. 45.1** Comparison between HFpEF Patients and healthy controls at rest, 12 W, 25 W, and peak Exercise. (**a**) Oxygen consumption, (**b**) arteriovenous oxygen content difference, (**c**) heart rate, (**d**) cardiac output, (**e**) systemic vascular resistance (SVR), and (**f**) systolic blood pressure. All variables adjusted for sex ($*p < 0.05$). The p value at the upper left of each panel represents the group-by-intensity interaction. Red dashed lines represent healthy controls (HC) and blue solid lines represent patients with heart failure with preserved ejection fraction (HFpEF) (reproduced with permission from JACC [67])

- Similarly, Dhakal et al. showed that directly measured A-$VO_2$ Diff. was the major determinant of exercise capacity in HFpEF, and impaired peripheral $O_2$ extraction was the predominant limiting factor to exercise capacity in 40% of patients with HFpEF [68].
- Haykowsky and colleagues further extended their results by using dual energy x-ray absorptiometry and found that percent body fat and percent leg fat were significantly increased, whereas percent body lean and leg lean mass were significantly reduced and the slope of the relation of peak $VO_2$ with percent leg lean mass was markedly reduced in the older HFpEF versus healthy control group [69].

These data suggest that poor "quality" of skeletal muscle may contribute to the reduced peak $VO_2$ found in older HFpEF patients. These investigators stretched these results by directly characterizing thigh muscle composition using phase-contrast MRI, which showed abnormal fat infiltration into the thigh skeletal muscle and that this was associated with reduced peak exercise $VO_2$ in HFpEF [70]. Both intermuscular adipose area and intermuscular adipose to skeletal muscle area were independent predictors of peak $VO_2$ in HFpEF, suggesting it is not only the loss of lean body mass, but the quality of muscle that determines peak $VO_2$ [70]. Importantly, skeletal muscle atrophy and increased intermuscular adipose tissue detected in HFpEF can be seen also in a variety of other conditions including aging [71].

- Kitzman and Haykowsky also showed that older HFpEF patients had a shift in skeletal muscle fiber type distribution with a reduced percentage of slow twitch type I fibers and reduced type I-to-type-II fiber ratio and reduced capillary-to-fiber ratio [72].
  - Furthermore, both the capillary-to-fiber ratio and percentage of type I fibers were significant, independent predictors of peak $VO_2$.
  - Indeed, this finding of nearly 50% lower capillary density in thigh muscles nicely parallels with a recent report showing microvascular rarefaction in cardiac muscle [24].
  - They further found that older patients with HFpEF also had abnormal skeletal muscle oxidative capacity, mitochondrial content, and mitochondrial fusion and that contributed to their severe exercise intolerance [73].
- Indeed, Bhella et al. [74], using phosphate-31 magnetic resonance spectroscopy during and after performing static leg lifts, showed impaired skeletal muscle oxidative metabolism in patients with HFpEF.

These evidences support that patients with HFpEF have multiple skeletal muscle abnormalities which impair oxygen uptake and utilization and contribute greatly to exercise intolerance. In addition to this, it is known that aging results in alterations in skeletal muscle, including a reduction in the relative number of type II fibers [75] and in capillary density [76], and that these are associated with a decline in physical performance. The loss of skeletal muscle and age-related alterations in skeletal muscle are major factors in the age-associated decline in peak $VO_2$ [77–79].

## 45.5 Impact of Aging, Frailty and Comorbidities on Exercise Intolerance in HFpEF

Aging is associated with a progressive decline in exercise capacity and decreased physiological reserve in CV function as well as in most other organ systems. There are a number of normal age-related changes in CV structure and function such as

(a) Increased arterial stiffening,
(b) Increased myocardial stiffness,
(c) Decreased diastolic myocardial relaxation,
(d) Increased LV mass,
(e) Decreased peak contractility,
(f) Reduced myocardial and vascular responsiveness to β-adrenergic stimulation,
(g) Decreased coronary flow reserve, and
(h) Decreased mitochondrial response to increased demand for adenosine triphosphate production)

that are likely relevant to the development of HfpEF [80]. Aging is also associated with a decline in a variety of neural, hormonal and environmental trophic signals; this can lead to loss of muscle mass and mass-specific strength, characteristic changes in body composition, including decreases in lean body mass and muscle strength, and increases in adiposity –vulnerable for sarcopenic obesity [81]. In addition, aging is linked with a systemic pro inflammatory state, and accompanied by increased levels of cytokines, that may lead to a functional decline in multiple organs even in the absence of a specific disease [82]. These normal age-related changes result in decreased CV reserve which contributes, along with reduced skeletal muscle mass and function, to an approximately 1%/year decline in maximal peak $VO_2$.

Older adults hospitalized with a primary diagnosis of HF often have multiple non-cardiac comorbidities (5.5 on average) and high proportions are frail [83, 84]. The adverse impacts of aging, frailty and comorbidities on functional capacity and clinical outcomes are cumulative and synergistic [84]. Muscle atrophy leads to a reduction in metabolic rate both at rest and during physical activity, thus further aggravating the sedentary state, all of which can cause obesity.

- Indeed, approximately 85% of elderly HFpEF patients are overweight or obese, and the HFpEF epidemic has largely paralleled the obesity epidemic [46, 85].

Adiposity-induced inflammation has wide-ranging adverse effects, including endothelial dysfunction, capillary rarefaction, and mitochondrial dysfunction in both the cardiac and systemic vascular beds [46]. A recent study demonstrated that body mass index was a key contributor to symptoms of breathlessness in patients with HFpEF [86]. Furthermore, aging and obesity are well established, risk factors for both HFpEF and several common respiratory diseases [like chronic obstructive lung disease (COPD)].

- In fact, nearly two-thirds of HFpEF patients have COPD [1, 52, 83].
- In addition, even in the absence of formal COPD diagnosis, patients with HFpEF have multiple pulmonary abnormalities and may contribute to their poor outcomes [87–89].
- Likewise, obstructive sleep apnea is common in individuals with HFpEF, with a prevalence of 69–81%, and is independently associated with a worse prognosis, even when HF therapy is optimal [90].

These multiple non-cardiac comorbidities not only contribute to the pathophysiology of HFpEF, but are also strong contributors to exercise intolerance in individuals with chronic HFpEF and to the high rate of clinical events, including hospitalizations and death [83].

Aging and the aforementioned comorbidities may initiate and/or aggravate chronic systemic inflammation that may affect myocardial remodeling and dysfunction in HFpEF through a signaling cascade, which begins with coronary microvascular endothelial dysfunction as shown in Fig. 45.2 [66, 91]. This reduces myocardial nitric oxide (NO) bioavailability and leads to low protein kinase G activity in

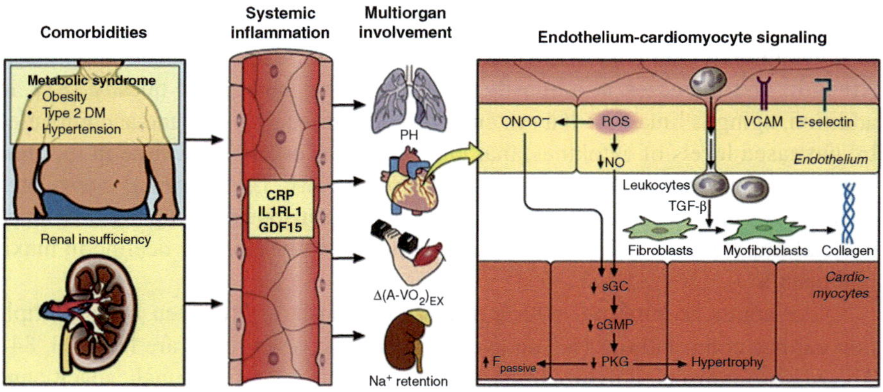


**Fig. 45.2** Systemic and myocardial signaling in heart failure with preserved ejection fraction (HFpEF). Comorbidities induce systemic inflammation, evident from elevated plasma levels of inflammatory biomarkers such as soluble interleukin 1 receptor-like 1 (IL1RL1), C-reactive protein (CRP), and growth differentiation factor 15 (GDF15). Chronic inflammation affects the lungs, myocardium, skeletal muscle, and kidneys, leading to diverse HFpEF phenotypes with variable involvement of pulmonary hypertension (PH), myocardial remodeling, deficient skeletal muscle oxygen extraction during exercise ($\Delta(A\text{-}VO_2)_{EX}$), and renal sodium (Na+) retention. Myocardial remodeling and dysfunction begin with coronary endothelial microvascular inflammation manifest from endothelial expression of adhesion molecules such as vascular cell adhesion molecule (VCAM) and E-selectin. Expression of adhesion molecules attracts infiltrating leukocytes secreting transforming growth factor beta (TGF-$\beta$), which converts fibroblasts to myofibroblasts with enhanced interstitial collagen deposition. Endothelial inflammation also results in the presence of reactive oxygen species (ROS), lack of nitric oxide (NO) bioavailability, and production of peroxynitrite (ONOO–). This reduces soluble guanylate cyclase (sGC) activity, cyclic guanosine monophosphate (cGMP) content, and the favorable effects of protein kinase G (PKG) on cardiomyocyte stiffness and hypertrophy (reproduced with permission from Circulation [142])

cardiomyocytes, which become stiff and hypertrophied, and these abnormalities also promote microvascular rarefaction and dysfunction in cardiac and skeletal muscle [24, 66, 70, 92].

Given such a multi-factorial, complex milieu, it's not surprising that drugs and interventions aimed primarily at a central hemodynamics repeatedly failed to strongly impact overall outcomes in HFpEF [93–99]. Given these considerations, what kinds of novel interventions are promising? So far nonpharmacological therapies, including disease management, ET, and caloric restriction weight loss in obese individuals, have been shown to be effective in improving exercise function in HFpEF function [14, 100–108].

- Interestingly, Edelmann and his group showed that higher amount of physical activity (PA) [as assessed by a self-report questionnaire] are related to higher submaximal exercise capacity and HRQOL.
  - Regarding maximal exercise capacity, only high-intensity PA showed significant association in HFpEF patients [109].

## 45.6 Exercise Training in HFpEF

Aerobic ET has been shown to increase peak $VO_2$ by 2.1–3.0 ml/kg/min and HRQOL in patients with HFpEF [14, 100–108], and has become an accepted adjunct therapy for these patients [110]. To date, several randomized controlled trials have examined the efficacy of ET to improve peak $VO_2$, 6 min walk distance (6MWD), and HRQOL in patients with HFpEF (Table 45.1) [103–108, 111–113].

- In a preliminary study, Gary et al. [113] showed that a 12-week walking and education program improved aerobic endurance and HRQOL in women HFpEF patients compared to controls. However, the major limitation in this study was the investigator who administered all tests familiar of group assignment that can pose a possibility of bias.
- The first medically supervised randomized controlled, single blinded trial of ET in HFpEF reported by Kitzman and colleagues found increased peak $VO_2$, ventilatory anaerobic threshold, 6 WMD, and HRQOL scores [107].
- These results were confirmed in a subsequent multicenter, randomized trial of 3 months of combined ET and strength training in HFpEF patients led by Edelmann et al. [106].
- Similarly, Kitzman et al. showed that among older obese patients with chronic, stable HFpEF, intentional weight loss via calorie restriction diet significantly improved the exercise capacity to a degree similar to ET. The combination of calorie restriction and ET produced a robust increase in exercise capacity (+2.5 mL/kg/min $VO_2$, substantially greater than the accepted clinically meaningful increase of 1.0 mL/kg/min, Fig. 45.3) [103].
- In a pilot study, 4 week of high-intensity interval training (HIIT) significantly improved peak $VO_2$ in HFpEF patients [105].

**Table 45.1** Overview of clinical Trials on exercise therapy in HFpEF

| First author/ trial (Ref.#) | Intervention | HFpEF patient type | LVEF | Primary endpoint | Trial result |
|---|---|---|---|---|---|
| Gary et al. [113] | Exercise training (n = 32) | Aged 67 ± 11, all females, NYHA class II/III diastolic HF, h/o ECHO –DD or diastolic HF, LVEF ≥45% | 54 ± 73% (Mean ± SD) | 6 MWD | [a]Improved 6MWD [a]Quality-of-life and depression scores |
| PARIS / Kitzman et al. [107] | Exercise training (n = 53) | Aged 70 ± 6 years, 87% female, ambulatory HF patients with NYHA class II-III symptoms, LVEF ≥50% | 61 ± 5% (Mean ± SD) | Peak $VO_2$ | [a]Improved peak and submaximal exercise capacity This benefit was not associated with any measurable change in resting LV structure or function |
| PARIS II / Haykowsky et al. [112] | Exercise training (n = 40) | Aged 69 ± 6 years,82% female, ambulatory HF patients with NYHA class II-III symptoms, LVEF ≥50% | 61 ± 5% (Mean ± SD) | Peak $VO_2$ | [a]Improved peak $VO_2$. Arterial-venous oxygen difference was primary contributor to improved peak $VO_2$ |
| Kitzman et al. [111] | Exercise training (n = 63) | Aged 70 ± 7 years, 76% female, ambulatory HF patients with NYHA class II-III symptoms, LVEF ≥50% | 58 ± 6 (Mean ± SD) | Peak $VO_2$, 6MWD | [a]Improved peak $VO_2$ without altering endothelial function |
| SECRET-1 / Kitzman et al. [103] | Caloric restriction and exercise training (n = 100) | Aged 67 ± 5 years, 41% female, ambulatory HF patients with NYHA class II-III symptoms LVEF ≥50% | 61 ± 6% (Mean ± SD) | Peak $VO_2$ and Quality of Life | [a]Increased peak $VO_2$ and the effects may be additive [a]Quality of life by KCCQ was improved, and benefit was greatest for caloric restriction |
| Ex-DHF trial Edelmann et al. [106] | Exercise training (n = 64) | Aged 65 ± 7 years,56% female symptomatic, ambulatory NYHA II/III symptoms, echo-DD, LVEF ≥50% | 68 ± 7% (Mean ± SD) | Peak $VO_2$ | [a]Improved exercise capacity and quality of life scores life by KCCQ This benefit was associated with atrial reverse remodeling and improved LV diastolic function |

**Table 45.1** (continued)

| First author/ trial (Ref.#) | Intervention | HFpEF patient type | LVEF | Primary endpoint | Trial result |
|---|---|---|---|---|---|
| Smart et al. [108] | Exercise training (n = 25) | Aged 64 ± 8 years, 48% female, well compensated HF, LVEF >45% | 57 ± 10% (Mean ± SD) | Peak $VO_2$ | Improved Peak $VO_2$<br>No significant changes in diastolic, systolic function, Quality-of-life life by KCCQ and depression scores |
| Fu et al. [104] | Exercise training (n = 30) | Aged 61 ± 3 years, 33% female, NYHA class II/III HF, LVEF ≥50% with episodes of acute pulmonary edema. | 58 ± 2% (Mean ± SD) | Peak $VO_2$ | Improved Peak $VO_2$<br>Improved diastolic function with reduction of the E/e' ratio<br>Improved quality of life scores |
| Angadi et al. [105] | Exercise training (n = 9) | Aged 69 ± 6 years, 11% female, NYHA class II/III HF, ECHO-DD, LVEF ≥50% | 65 ± 5% (Mean ± SD) | Peak $VO_2$ | Improved Peak $VO_2$<br>Improved diastolic dysfunction |
| Alves et al. [122] | Exercise training (n = 31) | Aged 63 ± 11 years, 29% female, admission with clinical signs of HF | 56 ± 3% (Mean ± SD) | Exercise tolerance (METS), LVEF and E/e" | [a]Improved exercise tolerance, cardiac systolic and diastolic function |

*HFpEF* heart failure with preserved ejection fraction, *LVEF* left ventricular ejection fraction, *n* number of participants, *NYHA* New York heart association, *HF* heart failure, *ECHO* echocardiographically assessed, *DD* diastolic dysfunction, *SD* standard deviation, *MWD* minute walk distance, $VO_2$ oxygen consumption, *KCCQ* Kansas City Cardiomyopathy Questionnaire, *E* Mitral early diastolic velocity, *e'* mitral annular velocity
[a]Significant improvement

A critical question in these studies is the mechanisms underlying the training-related improvement in exercise capacity. In addition, none of these trials supported a long-term exercise intervention to properly evaluate the impact of ET on clinical outcome measures in HFpEF. The Ex-DHF trial will be the first multicenter trial to assess the long-term effects of a supervised ET program on different outcome measures in patients with HFpEF [114]. Sub-studies of the Ex-DHF trial will also assess the effects of ET on inflammatory markers, metabolic parameters, collagen turnover, as well as on vascular function and ventriculo–arterial coupling, and novel non-standard echocardiographic parameters of systolic and diastolic function [114, 115].

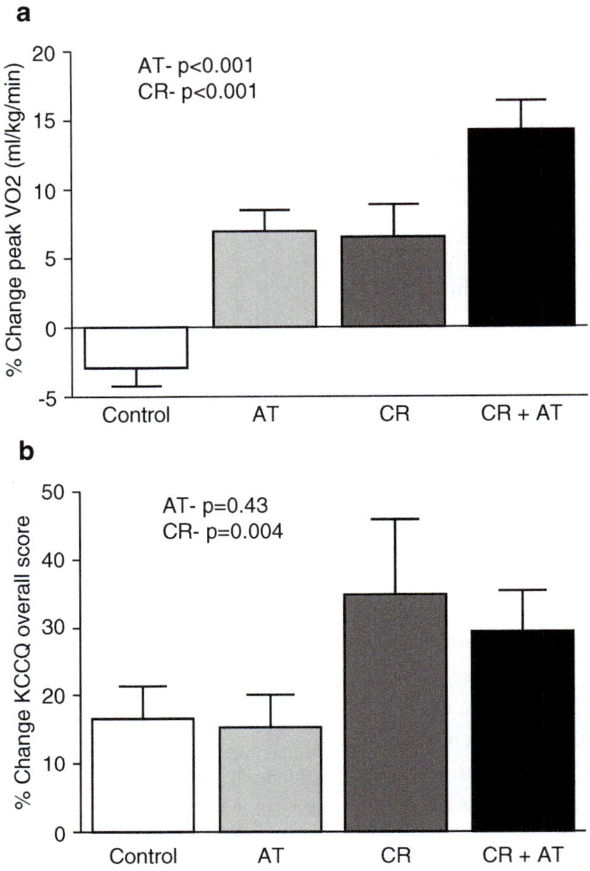


**Fig. 45.3** Effects of a 20-week caloric restriction diet on exercise capacity and quality of life in HFpEF. Data displayed are percent changes ± standard error at the 20-week follow-up relative to baseline by randomized group for peak $VO_2$ (mL $kg^{-1} \cdot min^{-1}$, **a**), and Kansas City Cardiomyopathy Questionnaire (KCCQ) overall score (Quality of Life Score; **b**). P values represent effects for AT and CR (reproduced with permission from JAMA [103]). *AT* aerobic exercise training, *CR* caloric restriction diet

### 45.6.1 Mechanisms of the Improvement of Exercise Intolerance with Exercise Training in HFpEF

Understanding the mechanisms of training-related improvements in exercise intolerance allows the opportunity to enhance the effectiveness of a new therapy. This needs careful measurements, not only of peak exercise $VO_2$, but also of its determinants, CO and A-$VO_2$ Diff. before and after an intervention [116]. These factors should be measured simultaneously during exercise along with peak $VO_2$, and it is feasible with a number of techniques that have been developed [38, 67, 116, 117]. The several reported mechanistic studies of ET in HFrEF indicated that training-related improvements in peak $VO_2$ result from favorable changes in cardiac, peripheral vascular, and skeletal muscle function that increase oxygen delivery to and utilization by the active muscles [117–119]. However, the underlying mechanisms responsible for improvements in peak $VO_2$ appear to differ between HFrEF and HfpEF [14].

### 45.6.2 Exercise Training and Peripheral, Non-cardiac Factors

- Haykowsky et al. showed that 84% of the improvement in $VO_2$ after 16 weeks of ET was attributed to increases in peak A-$VO_2$diff [112].
- This result was confirmed by Fu et al. who found that the ET mediated increase in peak $VO_2$ was secondary to the increased $AVO_2$ Diff. as peak HR, stroke volume index and cardiac index were unchanged after training [104].
- In fact, Bhella et al. recently reported that elderly HFpEF patients have baseline impaired skeletal muscle oxidative metabolism, which can be favorably shifted by ET to more efficient muscle $O_2$ utilization [111].

Thus, these data suggest that peripheral mechanisms, such as improved skeletal muscle perfusion and metabolism, likely play a major role in the adaptation to ET in HFpEF.

### 45.6.3 Exercise Training and Vascular Function

A small number of studies have investigated the effect of ET on vascular function in HfpEF:

- The studies done by Kitzman et al. showed improvements in peak $VO_2$, despite no change in indices of arterial stiffness, or conduit artery flow-mediated vasodilation [103, 111].
- Similarly, 4 weeks of HIIT showed no change in brachial artery flow mediated arterial dilation in HFpEF.

This indicates that improvements in large arterial function were not responsible for the ET-related improvement in peak $VO_2$ [105]. Similarly, ET had no influence on NO parameters in HFpEF patients [120].

### 45.6.4 Exercise Training and Cardiac Function

Central effects of ET in HFpEF have been minimal in the few studies to date.

- Edelmann et al. showed that a combination of moderate-intensity aerobic ET and resistance training (RT) resulted in an improvement in resting diastolic function in patients with HFpEF, as evidenced by a significant reduction in resting LA volume and E/e′ ratio and procollagen type 1 levels and the improvement in peak $VO_2$ was related to the decrease in E/e’ ratio [106].
- In another study they showed that combined endurance/RT over 6 months resulted in improvement in peak $VO_2$ and diastolic function in both patients with diastolic dysfunction without HF and with clinical HfpEF [121].

- Similarly, Alves et al. reported that 6 months of moderate-intensity aerobic interval training improved resting LV ejection fraction and diastolic function in HFpEF [122].
- Likewise, a pilot study showed HIIT improved diastolic dysfunction grade.
- Although these non-invasive measures suggested that ET may improve LV filling pressure, Fujimoto et al. showed no evidence of a beneficial effect of ET on the diastolic properties (LV compliance -assessed by invasive measurements) of LV in the HFpEF elderly patients [123].
- In addition, a meta–analysis showed ET in patients with HFpEF is associated with an improvement in $VO_2$ and HRQOL without significant changes in LV systolic (assessed by ejection fraction) or diastolic function (assessed by E/A ratio and early deceleration time) [14, 100].
- Furthermore, a study showed that despite of higher PA resulted in improved peak $VO_2$ in HFpEF patients, no association was seen with PA and echocardiographic parameters of diastolic function [109].

Taken together, these data suggest that the majority of ET-related improvements in exercise capacity may be related to microvascular and/or skeletal muscle adaptations that increase diffusive oxygen transport and/or utilization by the active muscles [124, 125]. Given the strong contribution of peripheral factors towards improvement in peak $VO_2$ in patients with HFpEF, future studies are warranted to examine the role of ET to improve skeletal muscle morphology and oxidative capacity [126].

In addition, pleiotropic stimulus of ET leaves room for mechanistic considerations regarding the beneficial effect of ET in HFpEF including anti-inflammation.

- In a *post hoc* analysis of the Ex-DHF-P trial, ET associated with increased levels of endogenous ghrelin which is a growth hormone-releasing peptide and which has been mainly attributed to the metabolic system and changes in body composition [115]. Ghrelin was found to inhibit apoptosis of cardiomyocytes and endothelial cells in vitro and has favorable effect on neuro hormonal activation, sarcopenic obesity [127, 128].
- Recently, in an exploratory post-hoc analysis, ET improved the energy metabolism in HFpEF, and exercise-induced improvements of exercise and ventilatory capacity as well as ventricular dysfunction were associated with several of these metabolic changes [129].
  - In addition, they identified heterogeneous metabolic responses to the same ET in HFpEF patients independent of improvements in cardiorespiratory, ventilatory and echocardiographic parameters [129].

## 45.7 Exercise Training Modalities in HFpEF

Exercise intervention trials for clinically stable patients with HFpEF and HFrEF have primarily focused on continuous moderate-intensity aerobic training (MICT) [130]. In five of HFpEF studies, MICT was performed 3–5 days per week for

1–5 months. This exercise prescription is in line with the American Heart Association exercise guidelines for overall CV health [131]. RT was included as an adjunctive modality to standard aerobic ET in 1 trial of HFpEF (Edelmann et al.) [106]. Although they described it as a pilot, they successfully tested the key outcome of exercise capacity, showing a 2.6 ml/kg/min (16%) increase in peak $VO_2$. Edelmann and his group are currently conducting the largest randomized multicenter trial to determine the benefit of supervised ET (combination of both endurance and RT, based on the Ex-DHF pilot study) on a clinical composite outcome score in HFpEF patients [114].

There has been recent interest in the role of HIIT, on improving peak $VO_2$ in individuals with clinically stable HF. Only two randomized controlled trials have assessed the efficacy of HIIT on $VO_2$ in patients with HFpEF [104, 105]. These studies incorporated HIIT, consisting of 4–5 intervals performed at 80–95% peak HR for 2–4 min interspersed with 2–3 min of active recovery, for 1–3 months [104, 105].

- Angadi et al. was the first study to show that short duration (4 weeks) HIIT yielded a significant increase in peak $VO_2$ (+1.8 ml/kg/min, $p = 0.04$), with no significant changes reported following MICT.
- Fu and colleagues measured peak $VO_2$ and its determinants before and after 12 weeks of HIIT in patients with HFpEF. Peak $VO_2$ was significantly elevated after HIIT and the increase in peak $VO_2$ observed in patients with HFpEF was secondary to enhanced peak exercise A-$VO_2$diff.

In summary, HIIT is a potent short–term training, characterized by brief, intermittent bursts of vigorous aerobic exercise interspersed with periods of low-intensity active recovery (see Chap. 44). However, the magnitude of improvement (mean change: +2.2 ml/kg/min peak $VO_2$) is similar to the improvements observed following MICT (mean change: +1.9 ml/kg/min peak $VO_2$).101 Furthermore, to date the safety and efficacy of HIIT in patients with HFpEF has not been studied. A large, multicenter randomized controlled ET trial (OptimEx-CLIN study) is currently ongoing to establish whether 12 months of HIIT is superior to MICT for improving peak $VO_2$ in patients with HFpEF [132]. Another trial is looking at the effect of 12-weeks HIIT on a bicycle ergometer in HFpEF patients on peak $VO_2$, cardiac and arterial function and HRQOL (NCT03184311).

## 45.8 Early Rehabilitation After Hospitalization for Acute Decompensated HF

Studies of ET in HF have focused almost exclusively on chronic, stable HF patients. The current literature regarding the safety and efficacy of ET that specifically target patients hospitalized HF is limited to observational data or small randomized trial, both of which showed benefit [133, 134].

- Recently, the REHAB-HF prospective, multicenter pilot clinical trial evaluated novel rehabilitation intervention in hospitalized, older HF patients.
  - The study successfully randomized 27 patients ≥60 years of age hospitalized with acute decompensated HF (both HFrEF and HFpEF) to either a novel multidomain physical rehabilitation intervention or attention control.
  - The study showed that a novel, tailored, progressive, multidomain physical rehabilitation is feasible in older patients with acute decompensated HF who have high rates of frailty and comorbidities and has the potential to improve physical function and reduce rehospitalization rates [135].

Based on these preliminary findings, the multicenter prospective randomized controlled trial REHAB –HF will determine if a tailored, structured, progressive multi-domain physical rehabilitation intervention addressing deficits in physical function and reduces rehospitalizations compared to attention control in older patients hospitalized with ADHF [136, 137]. Similarly, another trial is designed to provide evidence for the clinical efficacy and safety of a multidisciplinary disease management program in recently hospitalized HFpEF patients [138].

## 45.9 Exercise Prescription Recommendations for HFpEF

- A supervised maximal exercise test with monitoring for ischemia should be performed before HFpEF patients beginning an ET program.
- Exercise protocols used in clinical trials primarily included aerobic-type activities such as walking, stationary cycling, or rowing [139].
- The ET program for stable HFpEF patients should consist of continuous large muscle mass endurance exercise performed at an intensity between 40% and 80% peak $VO_2$ (40–70% heart rate reserve or Borg rate of perceived exertion between 10 and 14 out of 20; see Chap. 44) for 20–60 min per session, 3–5 days per week [139].
- The duration and frequency of effort should be uptitrated before intensity is increased.
- Once patients demonstrate a tolerance of aerobic training levels, RT activities should be considered, ranging from 40 to 60% of maximal strength for 1 set, 2–3 days per week [139].

After supervised setting with direct supervision and monitoring, depending on individual progress, patients usually should be able to be transitioned to a home exercise maintenance training program. Recently, digital training and decision support system exercise prescription was developed by the European Association of Preventive Cardiology (the Exercise Prescription in Everyday Practice and Rehabilitative Training (EXPERT) tool), and this may contribute to overcoming barriers in exercise implementation in common CV diseases [140].

## 45.10 Safety and Adherence Issues in Exercise Training in HFpEF

HFpEF patients are often older, deconditioned, and have many comorbidities; so widespread implementation of formal cardiac rehabilitation and home-based ET in this population presents special challenges. The safety of ET was reported in the four randomized exercise intervention trials. No adverse events occurred with any of these trials [106, 107, 113, 122]. Of note, 20% of the combined aerobic and strength-trained patients reported mild musculoskeletal discomfort during exercise. This indicates well-screened HFpEF patients can safely perform physical training in a partially supervised or supervised setting.

The major clinical hindrance for the use of ET as a therapeutic option in the HF population is how to get individuals to initiate and maintain an ET program. Despite a well-organized and resourced effort to optimize adherence in HF-ACTION, only ~40% of patients in the intervention arm achieved the target of 90 min of exercise/week at 3 months [130]. In order to maximize the constructive effects of regular exercise in individuals with HF, more information about the psychosocial, behavioral factors and social barriers for adherence to ET must be acquired, thus, identifying vulnerable individuals who are at risk for non-adherence. In addition, novel interventions to improve adherence are critically needed.

In February 2014, the Centers for Medicare and Medicaid Services (CMS) approved coverage for cardiac rehabilitation for selected patients with chronic HF. The criteria match the HF-ACTION inclusion criteria, with stable medications for at least 6 weeks and LVEF ≤35%. This generally excludes patients with recent hospitalization as well as all of those with HFpEF [141]. This lack of coverage can be a major barrier to formal cardiac rehab in older HFpEF patients.

## 45.11 Conclusion

HFpEF is the most common form of HF, nearly unique to older adults, and is a true geriatric syndrome. An evolving paradigm suggests that HFpEF is complex and multifactorial, probably systemic, and clinically heterogeneous and has a multifactorial pathophysiology, underlying age-related changes, frequent multiple chronic comorbidities, and multiorgan involvement. Individuals with HFpEF have severe exercise intolerance that is due, in part, to impaired cardiac, vascular, and skeletal muscle function that results in decreased oxygen delivery or utilization by the active muscles. The few randomized controlled exercise intervention trials performed to date show that physical training (aerobic training alone or combined with strength training) is a safe and effective intervention to increase aerobic capacity and endurance and HRQOL in HFpEF patients. In addition, these studies have shown that exercise intolerance can improve significantly in the absence of improvements in exercise CO, indicating a role of peripheral, non-cardiac adaptations. However, the optimal modality (or combinations of modalities) of ET remains unknown in HFpEF

[142]. In addition, the lack of CMS coverage can be a major barrier to formal cardiac rehab in older HFpEF patients. Unfortunately, insistence upon demonstration of mortality improvement before approving reimbursement overlooks the valuable and clearly demonstrated benefits on function and HRQOL.

**Clinical Pearls**
- HFpEF is uncommon in younger persons but highly prevalent in older adults, particularly women aged 80 and older, in whom it comprises nearly 100% of new HF cases.
- HFpEF is a chronic systemic debilitating syndrome associated with increased risk for hospitalization, death and poor HRQOL with garden-variety of HFpEF phenotypes.
- Many patients go undiagnosed for years, thus always think of HFpEF in a dyspneic elderly patient.
- HFpEF is more than just diastolic dysfunction.
- Prevent HFpEF before it even occurs.
- HFpEF needs multidisciplinary care.
- Exercise training is a safe and effective intervention to improve exercise intolerance and HRQOL in clinically stable HFpEF patients.
- Endurance training alone or combined with RT is an effective therapy to improve exercise intolerance in HFpEF patients.
- Given the persistent failure to demonstrate mortality benefits with pharmacologic interventions in patients with HFpEF, ET represent an important practical intervention for such patients with otherwise limited options.

## Review

## Questions

1. Select the correct answer(s): Exercise training in HFpEF patients is associated with improvements in
   (a) Peak oxygen consumption
   (b) Mortality
   (c) Reduced hospitalization
   (d) Reduced number of heart failure episodes
2. Select the correct answer(s): The mechanisms of improvement of exercise intolerance in HFpEF are uncertain. Evidence is strongest for
   (a) Improvement in oxygen extraction by skeletal muscle
   (b) Improvement in diastolic function
   (c) Improvement in vascular function
   (d) Improvement in pulmonary hypertension
3. A 68-year old lady presents with shortness of breath on exertion that began 6 months earlier and has since then gradually worsened. When walking on level ground, she does well, but any hill causes dyspnea. She has a history of

hypertension but no history of hyperlipidemia, diabetes, tobacco abuse, or family history of early coronary artery disease. No prior sign of coronary artery disease, no medication. Her BP is 160/80 mmHg, HR 78/min, BMI 36 kg/m$^2$. Clinically, she has peripheral edema; increased JVD elevated 10 cm above the right atrium. Cardiac examination is normal. ECG: sinus rhythm with no significant ST/T changes. **Echocardiography:** LVEF 55% with normal valves and normal left and right ventricular size and function; no regional wall motion abnormalities; normal wall thickness. **Stress Test:** ability to walk for 5 min on Bruce protocol (80% of predicted functional aerobic capacity), blood pressure increased to 190/98 mmHg; stopped test because of dyspnea; negative electrocardiographic findings for ischemia. Which one of the following actions would be least appropriate for this patient?

(a) Initiate treatment with an ACEI for blood pressure.
(b) Initiate treatment with a diuretic agent to resolve her congestion and peripheral edema.
(c) Recommend a regular exercise program, telling her to start low and increase gradually.
(d) Encourage her to lose weight.
(e) Refer her to coronary angiography.

## Answers

1. **A**: Exercise training has been shown to increase peak oxygen consumption and health related quality of life scores in patients with HFpEF in many randomized trials and has become an accepted adjunct therapy for these patients. So far, no exercise training studies have looked at clinical endpoints.
2. **A**: Randomized trials and meta-analyses showed that the majority of the improvement in oxygen consumption after exercise training was attributed to increases in peak arterio-venous oxygen difference, suggesting peripheral mechanisms, such as improved skeletal muscle perfusion and metabolism, thus likely playing a major role in the adaptation to exercise training in HFpEF. Central effects of exercise training in HFpEF have been minimal in the few studies to date.
3. **E**: This clinical vignette describes an obese HFpEF patient with volume overload on clinical examination and poorly controlled hypertension. So, she will need diuretics for symptomatic relief and ACE-I for blood pressure control. Exercise is indicated in all patients with HFpEF. Her symptoms are not related to ischemia; hence referring to coronary angiography is not an optimal option.

## References

1. Kitzman DW, Gardin JM, Gottdiener JS, et al. Importance of heart failure with preserved systolic function in patients > or = 65 years of age. CHS research group. Cardiovascular health study. Am J Cardiol. 2001;87:413–9.

2. Aurigemma GP, Gottdiener JS, Shemanski L, Gardin JM, Kitzman DW. Predictive value of systolic and diastolic function for incident congestive heart failure in the elderly: the cardiovacular health study. J Am Coll Cardiol. 2001;37:1042–8.
3. Owan TE, Hodge DO, Herges RM, Jacobsen SJ, Roger VL, Redfield MM. Trends in prevalence and outcome of heart failure with preserved ejection fraction. N Engl J Med. 2006;355:251–9.
4. Dunlay SM, Redfield MM, Weston SA, et al. Hospitalizations after heart failure diagnosis: a community perspective. J Am Coll Cardiol. 2009;54:1695–702.
5. Kitzman DW, Little WC, Brubaker PH, et al. Pathophysiological characterization of isolated diastolic heart failure in comparison to systolic heart failure. JAMA. 2002;288:2144–50.
6. Maeder MT, Thompson BR, Brunner-La Rocca HP, Kaye DM. Hemodynamic basis of exercise limitation in patients with heart failure and normal ejection fraction. J Am Coll Cardiol. 2010;56:855–63.
7. Borlaug BA, Melenovsky V, Russell SD, et al. Impaired chronotropic and vasodilator reserves limit exercise capacity in patients with heart failure and a preserved ejection fraction. Circulation. 2006;114:2138–47.
8. Guazzi M, Adams V, Conraads V, et al. Clinical recommendations for cardiopulmonary exercise testing data assessment in specific patient populations. Circulation. 2012;126:2261–74.
9. Zile MR, Baicu CF, Gaasch WH. Diastolic heart failure--abnormalities in active relaxation and passive stiffness of the left ventricle. N Engl J Med. 2004;350:1953–9.
10. Little WC, Kitzman DW, Cheng CP. Diastolic dysfunction as a cause of exercise intolerance. Heart Fail Rev. 2000;5:301–6.
11. Kitzman DW, Higginbotham MB, Cobb FR, Sheikh KH, Sullivan M. Exercise intolerance in patients with heart failure and preserved left ventricular systolic function: failure of the Frank-Starling mechanism. J Am Coll Cardiol. 1991;17:1065–72.
12. Westermann D, Kasner M, Steendijk P, et al. Role of left ventricular stiffness in heart failure with normal ejection fraction. Circulation. 2008;117:2051–60.
13. Wolsk E, Kaye D, Komtebedde J, et al. Central and peripheral determinants of exercise capacity in heart failure patients with preserved ejection fraction. JACC Heart Fail. 2019;7(4):321–32.
14. Pandey A, Parashar A, Kumbhani DJ, et al. Exercise training in patients with heart failure and preserved ejection fraction: meta-analysis of randomized control trials. Circ Heart Fail. 2015;8:33–40.
15. Howden EJ, Sarma S, Lawley JS, et al. Reversing the cardiac effects of sedentary aging in middle age - a randomized controlled trial: implications for heart failure prevention. Circulation. 2018;137:1549–60.
16. Kawaguchi M, Hay I, Fetics B, Kass DA. Combined ventricular systolic and arterial stiffening in patients with heart failure and preserved ejection fraction. Circulation. 2003;107:714–20.
17. Wachter R, Schmidt-Schweda S, Westermann D, et al. Blunted frequency-dependent upregulation of cardiac output is related to impaired relaxation in diastolic heart failure. Eur Heart J. 2009;30:3027–36.
18. Borlaug BA, Jaber WA, Ommen SR, Lam CSP, Redfield MM, Nishimura RA. Diastolic relaxation and compliance reserve during dynamic exercise in heart failure with preserved ejection fraction. Heart. 2011;97(12):964–9.
19. Tan YT, Wenzelburger F, Lee E, et al. The pathophysiology of heart failure with normal ejection fraction: exercise echocardiography reveals complex abnormalities of both systolic and diastolic ventricular function involving torsion, untwist, and longitudinal motion. J Am Coll Cardiol. 2009;54:36–46.
20. Phan TT, Abozguia K, Nallur Shivu G, et al. Heart failure with preserved ejection fraction is characterized by dynamic impairment of active relaxation and contraction of the left ventricle on exercise and associated with myocardial energy deficiency. J Am Coll Cardiol. 2009;54:402–9.

21. Ohara T, Niebel C, Stewart K, et al. Loss of adrenergic augmentation of diastolic intra-LV pressure difference in patients with diastolic dysfunction: evaluation by color M-mode echocardiography. JACC Cardiovasc Imaging. 2012;5:861–70.
22. Belyavskiy E, Morris DA, Url-Michitsch M, et al. Diastolic stress test echocardiography in patients with suspected heart failure with preserved ejection fraction: a pilot study. ESC Heart Fail. 2019;6:146–53.
23. Kitzman DW, Upadhya B, Vasu S. What the dead can teach the living: the systemic nature of heart failure with preserved ejection fraction. Circulation. 2015;131:522–4.
24. Mohammed SF, Hussain S, Mirzoyev SA, Edwards WD, Maleszewski JJ, Redfield MM. Coronary microvascular rarefaction and myocardial fibrosis in heart failure with preserved ejection fraction. Circulation. 2015;131:550–9.
25. Redfield MM, Jacobsen SJ, Burnett JC Jr, Mahoney DW, Bailey KR, Rodeheffer RJ. Burden of systolic and diastolic ventricular dysfunction in the community: appreciating the scope of the heart failure epidemic. JAMA. 2003;289:194–202.
26. Zile MR, Gottdiener JS, Hetzel SJ, et al. Prevalence and Significance of Alterations in Cardiac Structure and Function in Patients With Heart Failure and a Preserved Ejection Fraction. Circulation. 2011;124:2491–501.
27. Lam CS, Roger VL, Rodeheffer RJ, et al. Cardiac structure and ventricular-vascular function in persons with heart failure and preserved ejection fraction from Olmsted County, Minnesota. Circulation. 2007;115:1982–90.
28. Solomon S, Zile M, Pieske B, et al. The angiotensin receptor neprilysin inhibitor LCZ696 in heart failure with preserved ejection fraction: a phase 2 double-blind randomised controlled trial. Lancet. 2012;380:1387–95.
29. Maurer MS, Burkhoff D, Fried LP, Gottdiener J, King DL, Kitzman DW. Ventricular structure and function in hypertensive participants with heart failure and a normal ejection fraction: the cardiovascular health study. J Am Coll Cardiol. 2007;49:972–81.
30. Solomon SD, Verma A, Desai A, et al. Effect of intensive versus standard blood pressure lowering on diastolic function in patients with uncontrolled hypertension and diastolic dysfunction. Hypertension. 2010;55:241–8.
31. Su MY, Lin LY, Tseng YH, et al. CMR-verified diffuse myocardial fibrosis is associated with diastolic dysfunction in HFpEF. JACC Cardiovasc Imaging. 2014;7:991–7.
32. Stahrenberg R, Duvinage A, Mende M, et al. Determinants of submaximal exercise capacity in patients at risk for heart failure with preserved ejection fraction-results from the DIAST-CHF study. ESC Heart Fail. 2015;2:76–84.
33. Hunt SA, Abraham WT, Chin MH, et al. 2009 focused update incorporated into the ACC/AHA 2005 guidelines for the diagnosis and management of heart failure in adults: a report of the American college of cardiology foundation/American heart association task force on practice guidelines developed in collaboration with the International society for heart and lung transplantation. J Am Coll Cardiol. 2009;53:e1–90.
34. Redfield MM, Kitzman DW. Heart failure: a rose by another name? Congest Heart Fail. 2006;12:166–8.
35. Gandhi SK, Powers JC, Nomeir AM, et al. The pathogenesis of acute pulmonary edema associated with hypertension. N Engl J Med. 2001;344:17–22.
36. Borlaug BA, Nishimura RA, Sorajja P, Lam CSP, Redfield MM. Exercise hemodynamics enhance diagnosis of early heart failure with preserved ejection fraction. Circ Heart Fail. 2010;3:588–95.
37. Tartiere-Kesri L, Tartiere JM, Logeart D, Beauvais F, Cohen SA. Increased proximal arterial stiffness and cardiac response with moderate exercise in patients with heart failure and preserved ejection fraction. J Am Coll Cardiol. 2012;59:455–61.
38. Borlaug BA, Olson TP, Lam CSP, et al. Global cardiovascular reserve dysfunction in heart failure with preserved ejection fraction. J Am Coll Cardiol. 2010;56:845–54.
39. Ennezat PV, Lefetz Y, Marechaux S, et al. Left ventricular abnormal response during dynamic exercise in patients with heart failure and preserved left ventricular ejection fraction at rest. J Card Fail. 2008;14:475–80.

40. Kraigher-Krainer E, Shah AM, Gupta DK, et al. Impaired systolic function by strain imaging in heart failure with preserved ejection fraction. J Am Coll Cardiol. 2014;63:446–56.
41. Phan T, Shivu G, Weaver R, Ahmed I, Frenneaux M. Impaired heart rate recovery and chronotropic incompetence in patients with heart failure with preserved ejection fraction. Circ Heart Fail. 2010;3:29–34.
42. Brubaker PH, Joo KC, Stewart KP, Fray B, Moore B, Kitzman DW. Chronotropic incompetence and its contribution to exercise intolerance in older heart failure patients. J Cardpulm Rehabil. 2006;26:86–9.
43. Edelmann F, Gelbrich G, Duvinage A, et al. Differential interaction of clinical characteristics with key functional parameters in heart failure with preserved ejection fraction - results of the Aldo-DHF trial. Int J Cardiol. 2013;169:408–17.
44. Freed BH, Daruwalla V, Cheng JY, et al. Prognostic utility and clinical significance of cardiac mechanics in heart failure with preserved ejection fraction: importance of left atrial strain. Circ Cardiovasc Imaging. 2016;9:e003754.
45. von Roeder M, Rommel KP, Kowallick JT, et al. Influence of left atrial function on exercise capacity and left ventricular function in patients with heart failure and preserved ejection fraction. Circ Cardiovasc Imaging. 2017;10:e005467.
46. Kitzman DW, Shah SJ. The HFpEF obesity phenotype: the elephant in the room. J Am Coll Cardiol. 2016;68:200–3.
47. Eicher JC, Laurent G, Mathe A, et al. Atrial dyssynchrony syndrome: an overlooked phenomenon and a potential cause of 'diastolic' heart failure. Eur J Heart Fail. 2012;14:248–58.
48. Lam CSP, Roger VL, Rodeheffer RJ, Borlaug BA, Enders FT, Redfield MM. Pulmonary hypertension in heart failure with preserved ejection fraction: a community-based study. J Am Coll Cardiol. 2009;53:1119–26.
49. Guazzi M, Borlaug B. Pulmonary hypertension due to left heart disease. Circulation. 2012;126:975–90.
50. Lam C, Borlaug B, Kane G, Enders F, Rodeheffer R, Redfield M. Age-associated increases in pulmonary artery systolic pressure in the general population. Circulation. 2009;119:2663–70.
51. Schwartzenberg S, Redfield MM, From AM, Sorajja P, Nishimura RA, Borlaug BA. Effects of vasodilation in heart failure with preserved or reduced ejection fraction: implications of distinct pathophysiologies on response to therapy. J Am Coll Cardiol. 2012;59:442–51.
52. Hawkins NM, Petrie MC, Jhund PS, Chalmers GW, Dunn FG, McMurray JJ. Heart failure and chronic obstructive pulmonary disease: diagnostic pitfalls and epidemiology. Eur J Heart Fail. 2009;11:130–9.
53. Melenovsky V, Hwang S, Lin G, Redfield M, Borlaug B. Right heart dysfunction in heart failure with preserved ejection fraction. Eur Heart J. 2014;35:3452–62.
54. Mohammed SF, Hussain I, Abou Ezzeddine OF, et al. Right ventricular function in heart failure with preserved ejection fraction: a community-based study. Circulation. 2014;130:2310–20.
55. Gorter TM, Hoendermis ES, van Veldhuisen DJ, et al. Right ventricular dysfunction in heart failure with preserved ejection fraction: a systematic review and meta-analysis. Eur J Heart Fail. 2016;18:1472–87.
56. Obokata M, Reddy YNV, Melenovsky V, Pislaru S, Borlaug BA. Deterioration in right ventricular structure and function over time in patients with heart failure and preserved ejection fraction. Eur Heart J. 2018;40(8):689–97.
57. Beere PA, Kitzman DW, Morey MC, Higginbotham MB, et al. Circulation. 1991;84:II–186.
58. Katz SD, Zheng H. Peripheral limitations of maximal aerobic capacity in patients with chronic heart failure. J Nucl Cardiol. 2002;9:215–25.
59. Haykowsky M, Brubaker P, Kitzman D. Role of physical training in heart failure with preserved ejection fraction. Curr Heart Fail Rep. 2012;9:101–6.
60. Hundley WG, Kitzman DW, Morgan TM, et al. Cardiac cycle-dependent changes in aortic area and aortic distensibility are reduced in older patients with isolated diastolic heart failure and correlate with exercise intolerance. J Am Coll Cardiol. 2001;38:796–802.

61. Kitzman DW, Herrington DM, Brubaker P, Moore J, Eggebeen J, Haykowsky MJ. Carotid arterial stiffness and its relationship to exercise intolerance in older patients with heart failure and preserved ejection fraction. Hypertension. 2013;61:112–9.
62. Puntawangkoon C, Kitzman D, Kritchevsky S, et al. Reduced peripheral arterial blood flow with preserved cardiac output during submaximal bicycle exercise in elderly heart failure. J Cardiovasc Magn Reson. 2009;11:48.
63. Hundley WG, Bayram E, Hamilton CA, et al. Leg flow-mediated arterial dilation in elderly patients with heart failure and normal left ventricular ejection fraction. Am J Physiol Heart Circ Physiol. 2007;292:H1427–34.
64. Haykowsky MJ, Herrington DM, Brubaker PH, Morgan TM, Hundley WG, Kitzman DW. Relationship of flow mediated arterial; dilation and exercise capacity in older patients with heart failure and preserved ejection fraction. J Gerontol A Biol Sci Med Sci. 2013;68:161–7.
65. Matsue Y, Suzuki M, Nagahori W, et al. Endothelial dysfunction measured by peripheral arterial tonometry predicts prognosis in patients with heart failure with preserved ejection fraction. Int J Cardiol. 2013;168:36–40.
66. Paulus W, Tschope C. A novel paradigm for heart failure with preserved ejection fraction: comorbidities drive myocardial dysfunction and remodeling through coronary microvascular endothelial inflammation. J Am Coll Cardiol. 2013;62:263–71.
67. Haykowsky MJ, Brubaker PH, John JM, Stewart KP, Morgan TM, Kitzman DW. Determinants of exercise intolerance in elderly heart failure patients with preserved ejection fraction. J Am Coll Cardiol. 2011;58:265–74.
68. Dhakal BP, Malhotra R, Murphy RM, et al. Mechanisms of exercise intolerance in heart failure with preserved ejection fraction: the role of abnormal peripheral oxygen extraction. Circ Heart Fail. 2015;8:286–94.
69. Haykowsky MJ, Brubaker PH, Morgan TM, Kritchevsky SB, Eggebeen J, Kitzman DW. Impaired aerobic capacity and physical functional performance in older heart failure patients with preserved ejection fraction: role of lean body mass. J Gerontol A Biol Sci Med Sci. 2013;68:968–75.
70. Haykowsky M, Kouba EJ, Brubaker PH, Nicklas BJ, Eggebeen J, Kitzman DW. Skeletal muscle composition and its relation to exercise intolerance in older patients with heart failure and preserved ejection fraction. Am J Cardiol. 2014;113:1211–6.
71. Delmonico M, Harris T, Visser M, et al. Longitudinal study of muscle strength, quality, and adipose tissue infiltration. Am J Clin Nutr. 2009;90:1579–85.
72. Kitzman DW, Nicklas B, Kraus WE, et al. Skeletal muscle abnormalities and exercise intolerance in older patients with heart failure and preserved ejection fraction. Am J Physiol Heart Circ Physiol. 2014;306:H1364–70.
73. Molina AJ, Bharadwaj MS, Van Horn C, et al. Skeletal muscle mitochondrial content, oxidative capacity, and Mfn2 expression are reduced in older patients with heart failure and preserved ejection fraction and are related to exercise intolerance. JACC Heart Fail. 2016;4:636–45.
74. Bhella PS, Prasad A, Heinicke K, et al. Abnormal haemodynamic response to exercise in heart failure with preserved ejection fraction. Eur J Heart Fail. 2011;13:1296–304.
75. Larsson L, Sjodin B, Karlsson J. Histochemical and biochemical changes in human skeletal muscle with age in sedentary males, age 22-65 years. Acta Physiol Scand. 1978;103:31–9.
76. Coggan AR, Spina RJ, King DS. Histochemical and enzymatic comparison of the gastrocnemius muscle of young and elderly men and women. J Gerontol. 1992;47:B71–6.
77. Franssen F, Wouters E, Schols A. The contribution of starvation, deconditioning and ageing to the observed alterations in peripheral skeletal muscle in chronic organ diseases. Clin Nutr. 2002;21:1–14.
78. Coats A, Clark A, Piepoli M, Volterrani M, Poole-Wilson P. Symptoms and quality of life in heart failure: the muscle hypothesis. Br Heart J. 1994;72:S39.
79. Middlekauff HR. Making the case for skeletal myopathy as the major limitation of exercise capacity in heart failure. Circ Heart Fail. 2010;3:537–46.

80. Rich MW, Kitzman DW. Heart failure in octogenarians: a fundamentally different disease. Am J Geriatr Cardiol. 2000;9:97–104.
81. Upadhya B, Haykowsky MJ, Eggebeen J, Kitzman DW. Sarcopenic obesity and the pathogenesis of exercise intolerance in heart failure with preserved ejection fraction. Curr Heart Fail Rep. 2015;12:205–14.
82. Franceschi C, Bonafe M, Valensin S, et al. Inflamm-aging: An evolutionary perspective on immunosenescence. Ann N Y Acad Sci. 2000;908:244–54.
83. Ather S, Chan W, Bozkurt B, et al. Impact of noncardiac comorbidities on morbidity and mortality in a predominantly male population with heart failure and preserved versus reduced ejection fraction. J Am Coll Cardiol. 2012;59:998–1005.
84. Murad K, Kitzman D. Frailty and multiple comorbidities in the elderly patient with heart failure: implications for management. Heart Fail Rev. 2011;17:581–8.
85. Ndumele CE, Coresh J, Lazo M, et al. Obesity, subclinical myocardial injury, and incident heart failure. JACC Heart Fail. 2014;2:600–7.
86. Dalos D, Mascherbauer J, Zotter-Tufaro C, et al. NYHA functional class is associated with diastolic pulmonary pressure and predicts outcome in patients with heart failure and preserved ejection fraction. J Am Coll Cardiol. 2016;68:189–99.
87. Kitzman DW, Guazzi M. Impaired alveolar capillary membrane diffusion: a recently recognized contributor to exertional dyspnea in heart failure with preserved ejection fraction. JACC Heart Fail. 2016;4:499–501.
88. Andrea R, Lopez-Giraldo A, Falces C, et al. Lung function abnormalities are highly frequent in patients with heart failure and preserved ejection fraction. Heart Lung Circ. 2014;23:273–9.
89. Borlaug BA, Olson TP. The lungs in heart failure: not an innocent bystander. JACC Heart Fail. 2016;4:450–2.
90. Bitter T, Faber L, Hering D, Langer C, Horstkotte D, Oldenburg O. Sleep-disordered breathing in heart failure with normal left ventricular ejection fraction. Eur J Heart Fail. 2009;11:602–8.
91. Franssen C, Chen S, Unger A, et al. Myocardial microvascular inflammatory endothelial activation in heart failure with preserved ejection fraction. JACC Heart Fail. 2015;4:312–24.
92. Dhakal BP, Malhotra R, Murphy RM, et al. Mechanisms of exercise intolerance in heart hailure with preserved ejection fraction: the role of abnormal peripheral oxygen extraction. Circ Heart Fail. 2015;8:286–94.
93. Massie BM, Carson PE, McMurray JJ, et al. Irbesartan in patients with heart failure and preserved ejection fraction. N Engl J Med. 2008;359:2456–67.
94. Edelmann F, Aldo-DHF investigators. Effect of spironolactone on diastolic function and exercise capacity in patients with heart failure with preserved ejection fraction: The aldo-dhf randomized controlled trial. JAMA. 2013;309:781–91.
95. Pitt B, Pfeffer M, Assmann S, et al. Spironolactone for heart failure with preserved ejection fraction. N Engl J Med. 2014;370:1383–92.
96. Yusuf S, Pfeffer MA, Swedberg K, et al. Effects of candesartan in patients with chronic heart failure and preserved left-ventricular ejection fraction: the CHARM-Preserved Trial. Lancet. 2003;362:777–81.
97. Kitzman DW, Hundley WG, Brubaker P, Stewart K, Little WC. A randomized, controlled, double-blinded trial of enalapril in older patients with heart failure and preserved ejection fraction; effects on exercise tolerance, and arterial distensibility. Circ Heart Fail. 2010;3:477–85.
98. Cleland JG, Tendera M, Adamus J, et al. Perindopril for elderly people with chronic heart failure: the PEP-CHF study. The PEP investigators [see comments]. Eur J Heart Fail. 1999;1:211–7.
99. Upadhya B, Hundley WG, Brubaker PH, Morgan TM, Stewart KP, Kitzman DW. Effect of Spironolactone on exercise tolerance and arterial function in older adults with heart failure with preserved ejection fraction. J Am Geriatr Soc. 2017;65:2374–82.
100. Taylor RS, Davies EJ, Dalal HM, et al. Effects of exercise training for heart failure with preserved ejection fraction: A systematic review and meta-analysis of comparative studies. Int J Cardiol. 2012;162:6–13.

101. Tucker WJ, Nelson MD, Beaudry RI, et al. Impact of exercise training on peak oxygen uptake and its determinants in heart failure with preserved ejection fraction. Card Fail Rev. 2016;2:95–101.
102. Tucker WJ, Lijauco CC, Hearon CM Jr, et al. Mechanisms of the improvement in peak VO2 with exercise training in heart failure with reduced or preserved ejection fraction. Heart Lung Circ. 2018;27:9–21.
103. Kitzman DW, Brubaker P, Morgan T, et al. Effect of caloric restriction or aerobic exercise training on peak oxygen consumption and quality of life in obese older patients with heart failure with preserved ejection fraction: a randomised clinical trial. JAMA. 2016;315:36–46.
104. Fu TC, Yang NI, Wang CH, et al. Aerobic interval training elicits different hemodynamic adaptations between heart failure patients with preserved and reduced ejection fraction. Am J Phys Med Rehabil. 2016;95:15–27.
105. Angadi SS, Mookadam F, Lee CD, Tucker WJ, Haykowsky MJ, Gaesser GA. High-intensity interval training vs. moderate-intensity continuous exercise training in heart failure with preserved ejection fraction: A pilot study. J Appl Physiol. 2014;95:15–27.
106. Edelmann F, Gelbrich G, Dungen H, et al. Exercise training improves exercise capacity and diastolic function in patients with heart failure with preserved ejection fraction: results of the Ex-DHF (Exercise training in diastolic heart failure) pilot study. J Am Coll Cardiol. 2011;58:1780–91.
107. Kitzman DW, Brubaker PH, Morgan TM, Stewart KP, Little WC. Exercise training in older patients with heart failure and preserved ejection fraction. Circ Heart Fail. 2010;3:659–67.
108. Smart NA, Haluska B, Jeffriess L, Leung D. Exercise training in heart failure with preserved systolic function: A randomized controlled trial of the effects on cardiac function and functional capacity. Congest Heart Fail. 2012;18:295–301.
109. Bobenko A, Bartels I, Munch M, et al. Amount or intensity? Potential targets of exercise interventions in patients with heart failure with preserved ejection fraction. ESC Heart Fail. 2018;5:53–62.
110. Heart Failure Society of America. Executive summary: HFSA 2010 comprehensive heart failure practice guideline. J Card Fail. 2010;16:475–539.
111. Kitzman DW, Brubaker PH, Herrington DM, et al. Effect of endurance exercise training on endothelial function and arterial stiffness in older patients with heart failure and preserved ejection fraction: A randomized, controlled, single-blind trial. J Am Coll Cardiol. 2013;62:584–92.
112. Haykowsky MJ, Brubaker PH, Stewart KP, Morgan TM, Eggebeen J, Kitzman DW. Effect of endurance training on the determinants of peak exercise oxygen consumption in elderly patients with stable compensated heart failure and preserved ejection fraction. J Am Coll Cardiol. 2012;60:120–8.
113. Gary RA, Sueta CA, Dougherty M, et al. Home-based exercise improves functional performance and quality of life in women with diastolic heart failure. Heart Lung. 2004;33:210–8.
114. Edelmann F, Bobenko A, Gelbrich G, et al. Exercise training in Diastolic Heart Failure (Ex-DHF): rationale and design of a multicentre, prospective, randomized, controlled, parallel group trial. Eur J Heart Fail. 2017;19:1067–74.
115. Trippel TD, Holzendorf V, Halle M, et al. Ghrelin and hormonal markers under exercise training in patients with heart failure with preserved ejection fraction: results from the Ex-DHF pilot study. ESC Heart Fail. 2017;4:56–65.
116. Kitzman DW. Understanding results of trials in heart failure with preserved ejection fraction: remembering forgotten lessons and enduring principles. J Am Coll Cardiol. 2011;57:1687–9.
117. Sullivan M, Higginbotham MB, Cobb FR. Exercise training in patients with severe left ventricular dysfunction. Hemodynamic and metabolic effects. Circulation. 1988;78:506–15.
118. Coats A. Exercise training for heart failure: coming of age. Circulation. 1999;99:1138–40.
119. Hambrecht R, Gielen S, Linke A, et al. Effects of exercise training on left ventricular function and peripheral resistance in patients with chronic heart failure. JAMA. 2000;283:3095–101.

120. Baldassarri F, Schwedhelm E, Atzler D, et al. Relationship between exercise intervention and NO pathway in patients with heart failure with preserved ejection fraction. Biomarkers. 2018;23:540–50.
121. Nolte K, Schwarz S, Gelbrich G, et al. Effects of long-term endurance and resistance training on diastolic function, exercise capacity, and quality of life in asymptomatic diastolic dysfunction vs. heart failure with preserved ejection fraction. ESC Heart Fail. 2014;1:59–74.
122. Alves AJ, Ribeiro F, Goldhammer E, et al. Exercise training improves diastolic function in heart failure patients. Med Sci Sports Exerc. 2012;44:776–85.
123. Fujimoto N, Prasad A, Hastings JL, et al. Cardiovascular effects of 1 year of progressive endurance exercise training in patients with heart failure with preserved ejection fraction. Am Heart J. 2012;164:869–77.
124. Erbs S, Hollriegel R, Linke A, et al. Exercise training in patients with advanced chronic heart failure (NYHA IIIb) promotes restoration of peripheral vasomotor function, induction of endogenous regeneration, and improvement of left ventricular function. Circ Heart Fail. 2010;3:486–94.
125. Esposito F, Reese V, Shabetai R, Wagner PD, Richardson RS. Isolated Quadriceps Training Increases Maximal Exercise Capacity in Chronic Heart Failure: The Role of Skeletal Muscle Convective and Diffusive Oxygen Transport. J Am Coll Cardiol. 2011;58:1353–62.
126. Fleg JL, Cooper LS, Borlaug BA, et al. Exercise training as therapy for heart failure: current status and future directions. Circ Heart Fail. 2015;8:209–20.
127. Baldanzi G, Filigheddu N, Cutrupi S, et al. Ghrelin and des-acyl ghrelin inhibit cell death in cardiomyocytes and endothelial cells through ERK1/2 and PI 3-kinase/AKT. J Cell Biol. 2002;159:1029–37.
128. Mao Y, Tokudome T, Kishimoto I, et al. Endogenous ghrelin attenuates pressure overload-induced cardiac hypertrophy via a cholinergic anti-inflammatory pathway. Hypertension. 2015;65:1238–44.
129. Bahls M, Friedrich N, Pietzner M, et al. Heterogeneous metabolic response to exercise training in heart failure with preserved ejection fraction. J Clin Med. 2019;8(5):E591. (In press)
130. O'Connor CM, Whellan DJ, Lee KL, et al. Efficacy and safety of exercise training in patients with chronic heart failure: HF-ACTION randomized controlled trial. JAMA. 2009;301:1439–50.
131. Haskell WL, Lee I, Pate RR, Powell KE, Blair SN, Franklin BA. Physical activity and public health: Updated recommendation for adults from the American College of Sports Medicine and the American Heart Association. Circulation. 2007;116:1081–3.
132. Suchy C, Massen L, Rognmo O, et al. Optimising exercise training in prevention and treatment of diastolic heart failure (OptimEx-CLIN): rationale and design of a prospective, randomised, controlled trial. Eur J Prev Cardiol. 2014;21:18–25.
133. Scrutinio D, Passantino A, Catanzaro R, et al. Inpatient cardiac rehabilitation soon after hospitalization for acute decompensated heart failure: a propensity score study. J Cardiopulm Rehabil Prev. 2012;32:71–7.
134. Babu AS, Maiya AG, George MM, Padmakumar R, Guddattu V. Effects of combined early in-patient cardiac rehabilitation and structured home-based program on function among patients with congestive heart failure: a randomized controlled trial. Heart Views. 2011;12:99–103.
135. Reeves GR, Whellan DJ, O'Connor CM, et al. A novel rehabilitation intervention for older patients with acute decompensated heart failure: The REHAB-HF Pilot Study. JACC Heart Fail. 2016;5:359–66.
136. Reeves GR, Whellan DJ, Duncan P, et al. Rehabilitation therapy in older acute heart failure patients (REHAB-HF) trial: design and rationale. Am Heart J. 2016;185:130–9.
137. Warraich HJ, Kitzman DW, Whellan DJ, et al. Physical function, frailty, cognition, depression, and quality of life in hospitalized adults GëÑ60 years with acute decompensated heart failure with preserved versus reduced ejection fraction. Circ Heart Fail. 2018;11:e005254.
138. Koifman E, Grossman E, Elis A, et al. Multidisciplinary rehabilitation program in recently hospitalized patients with heart failure and preserved ejection fraction: Rationale and design of a randomized controlled trial. Am Heart J. 2014;168:830–7.

139. Piepoli MF, Conraads V, Corrá U, et al. Exercise training in heart failure: from theory to practice. A consensus document of the heart failure association and the European association for cardiovascular prevention and rehabilitation. Eur J Heart Fail. 2011;13:347–57.
140. Hansen D, Dendale P, Coninx K, et al. The European association of preventive cardiology exercise prescription in everyday practice and rehabilitative training (EXPERT) tool: a digital training and decision support system for optimized exercise prescription in cardiovascular disease. Concept, definitions and construction methodology. Eur J Prev Cardiol. 2017;24:1017–31.
141. Centers for Medicare and Medicaid Services. Physician fee schedule. National Payment Amount File. Available at: http://www.cms.gov/Medicare/Medicare-Fee-for-Service-Payment/PhysicianFeeSched/index.html. Accessed 29 May 2013.
142. Shah SJ, Kitzman DW, Borlaug BA, et al. Phenotype-specific treatment of heart failure with preserved ejection fraction: a multiorgan roadmap. Circulation. 2016;134:73–90.

# Exercise in Specific Diseases: Heart Failure with Reduced Ejection Fraction

# 46

Verena Heinicke, Wesley J. Tucker, Mark J. Haykowsky, and Martin Halle

**Learning Objectives**

1. Become familiar with the definition, classification, terminology and diagnosis of heart failure.
2. Understand the association between physical activity and HF with reduced ejection fraction.
3. Become familiar with the most relevant interventional studies, which show the different beneficial effects of exercising in HF patients with reduced ejection fraction.
4. Be able to give practical recommendations for HF patients for endurance and resistance training.

## 46.1 Definition of Heart Failure (HF)

HF is a clinical syndrome, which is defined by clinical symptoms and functional or structural cardiac abnormalities [1, 2] that result in reduced cardiac output and/or increased intracardiac filling pressures [2]. Typical symptoms and clinical signs [1, 2] are

V. Heinicke · M. Halle (✉)
Department of Prevention, Sports Medicine and Sports Cardiology, University hospital 'Klinikum rechts der Isar', Technical University of Munich, DZHK (German Center for Cardiovascular Research), Munich, Germany
e-mail: verena.heinicke@mri.tum.de; martin.halle@mri.tum.de

W. J. Tucker
College of Nursing and Health Innovation, University of Texas, Arlington, TX, USA
e-mail: wesley.tucker@uta.edu

M. J. Haykowsky
University of Alberta, Edmonton, Alberta, Canada
e-mail: mhaykows@ualberta.ca



A. Pressler, J. Niebauer (eds.), *Textbook of Sports and Exercise Cardiology*,
https://doi.org/10.1007/978-3-030-35374-2_46

- Shortness of breath (at rest and/or on exertion)
- Orthopnoea
- Paroxysmal nocturnal dyspnoe
- Reduced exercise tolerance
- Fatigue
- Ankle swelling, Peripheral oedema
- Pulmonary congestion
- Increased jugular venous pressure
- Hepatojugular reflux, gastroenterological symptoms
- Third Heart Sound, galopp rhythm, tachycardia
- Laterally displaced apical impulse

## 46.2 Terminology

HF is categorised based on left ventricular ejection fraction (LVEF) as [2]:

1. HF with *reduced* Ejection Fraction (HFrEF):
   (a) Symptoms and/or clinical signs
   (b) LVEF: <40%
2. HF with *mid-range* Ejection Fraction (HFmrEF):
   (a) Symptoms and/or clinical signs
   (b) LVEF: 40–49%
   (c) Increased levels of natriuretic peptides (BNP > 35 pg/ml and/or NT-proBNP >125 pg/ml)
   (d) + ≥ 1 criterion:
      - relevant structural heart disease (left ventricular hypertrophy (LVH) and/or left atrial enlargement (LAE)
      - diastolic dysfunction
3. HF with *preserved* Ejection Fraction (HFpEF):
   (a) Symptoms and/or clinical signs
   (b) LVEF ≥50%
   (c) Increased levels of natriuretic peptides (BNP > 35 pg/ml and/or NT-proBNP >125 pg/ml)
   (d) + ≥ 1 criterion
      - relevant structural heart disease (LVH and/or LAE).
      - diastolic dysfunction

Of note, signs may not be present in an early stage or in patients under diuretical medication. Even individuals with mid-range or reduced LVEF may have very few symptoms dependent on peripheral training adaptations.

## 46.3 Time Course

- New-onset HF: new symptoms ± signs and functional and/or structural cardiac abnormalities

  - Acute (e.g. patients with acute myocardial infarction, myocarditis or Takotsubo cardiomyopathy)
  - Sub-acute (e.g. patients with DCM, valvular heart disease)
- Chronic HF: having HF for a longer period of time
- Stable HF: patients under medical therapy, who have unchanged symptoms and signs ≥1 month
- Decompensated HF: worsening of symptoms and signs often leading to hospitalization
  - Acute
  - Sub-acute
- Congestive HF: volume overload

## 46.4 Classification

According to the American College of Cardiology Foundation (ACCF) and the American Heart Association (AHA), HF is classified into stages A-D [3]. This classification comprises the development and progression of heart disease:

- Stage A: HF risk factors
- Stage B: HF risk factors, LV remodeling, yet no signs or symptoms of HF
- Stages C and D: patients fulfilling criteria of HF

The traditional New York Heart Association (NYHA) functional classification defines four clinical stages I–IV) based upon exercise capacity and clinical symptoms [4].

Both classifications can be used together.

## 46.5 Epidemiology

- Prevalence of heart failure: ~ 1–2% of the population in developed countries [5]
- Incidence of heart failure: 5–10 per 1000 persons per year [5]
- Risk factor age:
  - US epidemiological study, prevalence [6]: age 45–54 years: 0.7%; 55–64 years 1.3%, 65–74 years 1.5%, >75 years: 8.4%
  - European study (Rotterdam study), prevalence: age 55–64 years 0.9%; ≥85 years 17.4%
  - At age 55 years, lifetime risk for HF is 33% for men and 29% for women [5].

## 46.6 Aetiology

HF is not equivalent to either cardiomyopathy or LV dysfunction. There are many possible causes and diseases leading to the syndrome of HF, including both cardiac and non-cardiac aetiologies.

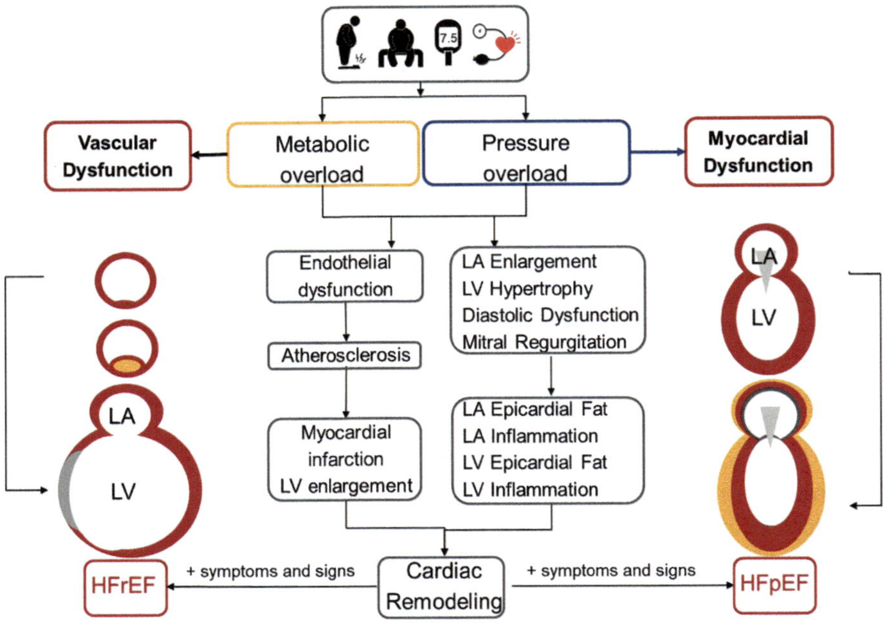


**Fig. 46.1** Pathophysiology of HFrEF and HFpEF by metabolic overload and pressure overload [8]. *LA* left atrium, *LV* left ventricle

- Coronary artery disease is the most common cause for HF in the Western world [7].
  - Metabolic and pressure overload are leading to arteriosclerosis, myocardial infarction and cardiac remodelling (Fig. 46.1).
- Pressure overload, especially hypertensive disease often predisposes to HFpEF by cardiac remodelling (Fig. 46.1).

## 46.7 Diagnosis

The diagnosis of HF in patients with typical signs and symptoms should be based on physical examination, medical history, ECG, laboratory testing and echocardiography [2].

## 46.8 Physical Activity and the Risk of Heart Failure

There is a dose–response relationship between physical activity and the risk of developing HF [9]. A recent large meta-analysis of prospective cohort studies analysed the effect of the amount of physical activity (PA) on incidence of heart failure:

- N = 12 prospective cohort studies with 370,460 participants were included (53.5% women, studies from U.S.A. and Europe)
- During median follow-up of 13 years, there were 20,203 HF events.

- PA was categorised into
  - Inactive
  - Light PA
  - Moderate PA
  - High PA
- Reduced risks of HF compared to inactive category were observed for
  - Light PA: risk reduction of 15% (pooled Hazard ratio (HR) 0.85; 95% Confidence Interval (CI) 0.79–0.92; $I^2 = 3.4\%$)
  - Moderate PA: risk reduction of 22% (pooled HR 0.78; 95% CI 0.75–0.82; $I^2 = 20.3\%$)
  - High PA: risk reduction of 30% (pooled HR 0.70; 95% CI 0.67–0.73; $I^2 = 36.4\%$)
- A dose-response effect was observed:
  - Minimum guideline-recommended PA level is ≈500 MET∗min/wk.
  - Meeting the guideline PA was associated with a modest risk reduction of 10% compared to no activity.
  - Meeting the recommended amount of PA twice (≈1000 MET∗min/wk) or even 4 times per week (≈2000 MET∗min/wk) reduced risk by 19% and 35%, respectively.
- Findings were consistent in the subgroups of men and women, ages below or above 55 years, and between European and US American studies.

## 46.9 Therapy

The goals of an adequate HF therapy include

(a) Improving prognosis and reducing mortality
(b) Preventing hospitalization
(c) Symptom relief
(d) Improving exercise capacity
(e) Improving Quality of Life

### 46.9.1 Pharmacological Therapy

Every patient must be on optimal medical therapy. All other treatment options—including exercise—should be seen as additive to best pharmacological therapy in HFrEF patients. Angiotensin-converting enzyme inhibitors (ACE-I), Antiotensin Receptor antagonists or blockers (ARBs) and beta-blockers are the basis for every HFrEF patient, except when there are contraindications or not tolerated.

- ACE-I, ARBs [10–14] and beta-blockers [15–19] reduce mortality and morbidity.
- These substances should be increased to the highest tolerated (symptoms such as dizziness, but not blood pressure values) dosage.

If LVEF is ≤35% and symptoms still exist, a mineralocorticoid receptor antagonist (MRA) is recommended for all patients without contraindications. MRA also reduce mortality and hospitalization [20, 21]. If patients are still symptomatic with either ACE-I or ARB, a beta-blocker, and a MRA there are other pharmacological treatment approaches:

- Angiotensin receptor—neprilysin inhibitor (ARNI, Valsartan plus sacubitril) showed superiority to enalapril [22], so that replacement of ACE-I or ARB ARNI is recommended if tolerated.
- Ivabradine, an $I_f$-channel inhibitor, reduces mortality and hospitalization for HF [23] and should be considered in patients with sinus rhythm and HF ≥ 70/min.
- If in sinus rhythm QRS duration is ≥130 ms with LBBB morphology and LVEF remains ≤35% despite optimal medical therapy, cardiac resynchronization therapy (CRT) is recommended [2].
- Diuretics should also be used to relieve symptoms and reduce congestive symptoms [2].

### 46.9.2 Exercise as Therapy

Exercise in HF patients has a class IA recommendation [2]

(a) to improve exercise capacity
(b) to improve symptoms
(c) to decrease rehospitalization rates

Several RCTs and meta-analyses have evaluated the effect of exercise interventions on mortality, hospitalization, and Quality of Life, of which the following are the most relevant:

#### 46.9.2.1 The HF-ACTION Trial

The HF-ACTION trial [24] is a large, multicentre (82 centers in the US, Canada, and France), prospective, randomized controlled study, which was initiated with the aim to clarify, whether exercise improves survival in HF patients with reduced ejection fraction.

- 2331 patients with LVEF <35% and with NYHA classification II-IV were included (median age 59 years, 72% males).
- Exercise intervention: During the first 3 months patients exercised 3×/week for a total of 36 supervised training sessions. Thereafter, patients were asked to exercise for 40 min/day, 5×/week at an exercise intensity of 60–70% of heart rate reserve (HRR). The usual care/control group received educational materials which included guidelines from ACC/AHA for PA: being active 30 min/day on most days of the week with moderate intensity.
- The median follow-up was 30.1 months.

This study showed only a non-significant reduction in the primary end point (all-cause mortality and all-cause hospitalization) in the exercise group compared to the usual care group (HR 0.93 [95% CI, 0.84–1.02]; p = 0.13).

- However, after adjusting for HF etiology and for four strongly predictive factors (LVEF, history of atrial fibrillation, baseline exercise capacity, and depression score) exercising was associated with a significant 11% reduction for all-cause mortality and hospitalization and a significant 15% reduction for cardiovascular mortality and HF hospitalization.
- Exercise training in stable HF patients was safe with little to no adverse events associated with this treatment modality.
- $VO_2$peak increased significantly at 3 and 12 months following exercise training. However, the median increase in $VO_2$peak was lower than observed in previous smaller studies.

Study limitations included high patient dissatisfaction within the usual care group and poor adherence to exercise training (particularly with regard to the prescribed exercise training intensity). Specifically, over 50% of the patients in the usual care control group were unsatisfied with not being randomized to exercise training. In addition, over 33% of patients randomized to the exercise training group did not meet their required exercise intervention targets.

The conclusions of this trial were as follows:

- A structured aerobic exercise training program to improve morbidity and mortality in patients with HFrEF is feasible.
- When adjusted for highly predictive risk factors, exercise training resulted in a significantly reduced mortality.
- As a typical limitation pertaining to exercise training interventions, the adherence rate was low.

#### 46.9.2.2 Cochrane Review

This review [25] summarizes the results of 33 randomized, controlled interventional trials with cardiac rehabilitation programmes in HF patients. Primarily patients with HFrEF were included. HFpEF patients were evaluated in only four studies. In total, 4740 HF patients were analyzed, of which 87% were men.

Three main findings of the meta-analysis were important:

- There were no short-term effects (duration of studies up to 1 year) on mortality between training groups and usual care groups, but a trend towards improvement of survival with long-term exercise training (n = 6 studies with >1 year of follow-up) compared to controls (relative risk (RR) = 0.88; 95% CI 0.75–1.02, fixed-effect analysis).
- A clinically important 25% and 39% reduction in all-cause and HF hospitalizations with exercise training was observed compared to usual care controls, respectively.
- Quality of life was improved significantly through exercise programmes.

Findings were independent of age and HF stage, and similar efficacy was observed across genders.

In summary, these findings highlight the beneficial impact of exercise training on clinical outcomes such long-term mortality, hospitalizations, and quality of life in patients with HFrEF and support its recommendation as an adjuvant therapy in this patient population.

### 46.9.3 Effect on Exercise Capacity

Several randomized, controlled exercise intervention trials (RCTs) have shown that different kinds of training protocols can improve exercise capacity in HFrEF patients [24, 26, 27]:

- The largest trial is still the HF-ACTION trial—using a training protocol with moderate to vigorous intensity with 60–70% of heart rate reserve (HRR; see Chap. 44). In this study, a significant but modest increase of 0.7 ml/kg/min in $VO_2$peak was seen after 1 year of training, compared to 0.1 ml/kg/min improvement in the control group.
- A meta-analysis by Ismail et al. [26] showed larger improvements in $VO_2$peak in exercise interventional trials applying higher intensities (improvements always compared to control groups):
  - High intensity training programmes: +3.33 ml/kg/min
  - Vigorous intensity training programmes: +2.27 ml/kg/min
  - Moderate intensity training programmes: +2.17 ml/kg/min
  - Light intensity training programmes: + 1.04 ml/kg/min (not significant)

The greatest limitation of the study was that only a few studies with high and low intensity training programmes have been performed so far.

- The first randomized controlled exercise intervention trial using a high intensity interval training protocol was published in 2007 [28]:
  - 27 patients with HFrEF (median LVEF 29%) were included.
  - Training protocols (3×/week over 12 weeks) were:

    AIT: Aerobic interval training group with high intensities: brisk walking, jogging or cycling for 4 min at an intensity of 90–95% of peak heart rate, with 3 min of active recovery between each phase at moderate intensity, including warm-up and cool-down sessions, lasting a total of 38 min.

    MCT: Moderate intensity continuous training: walking or cycling at 70–75% of peak heart rate for a total of 47 min each session.

    Control group receiving a recommendation for regular exercise
  - AIT was associated with a superior 46% improvement in $VO_2$peak (from 13.0 ± 1.6 to 19.0 ± 2.1 ml/kg/min) compared to an increase of 14% with MCT. There was no change in exercise capacity in the control group.

- The SMARTEX-HF [29] trial applied an identical study protocol, but included a much larger sample size with 261 HFrEF patients (LVEF ≤ 35% and NYHA class II-III):
  - This study showed a clinically important increase in exercise capacity (secondary endpoint) following the structured exercise training programme after 12 weeks, but did not confirm a significant difference between the AIT and MCT groups.
  - Nonetheless, both the AIT and MCT groups were superior to the control group with respect to a small but significant increase in $VO_2$peak.
  - However, at 1-year follow-up these improvements were not maintained in either exercise group.
  - Clinically important: both training regimes were safe.
  - Limitation of the study: 51% of the AIT patients trained at a lower intensity than intended, whereas 80% of the MCT patients trained at higher than intended intensities, resulting in a less than anticipated between-group difference in training intensities.
- A recent meta-analysis [27] comparing AIT to MCT included a sub-analysis on isocaloric exercise protocols, as the same duration with different intensities leads to a greater energy expenditure with higher intensities. AIT is slightly more time-efficient as less time is needed to achieve the same energy expenditure as elicited by MCT protocols.
  - This meta-analysis included 13 studies and 411 HFrEF patients and showed a superior improvement of 1.35 ml/kg/min for $VO_2$peak with high-intensity training protocols compared to moderate intensity training.
  - However, after performing a sub-analysis that included only isocaloric exercise protocols, these differences were no longer present.

### 46.9.4 Effect on Cardiac Function

The ability of exercise training to attenuate pathological cardiac remodeling is still unclear. A recently published meta-analysis by Tucker et al. [30] showed that structured exercise training improved left ventricular function in patients with HFrEF:

- 18 randomized, controlled exercise intervention trials with HFrEF patients were included in this meta-analysis.
- MCT showed a median improvement of 3.79% in LVEF, with even better results occurring after training programmes of longer duration (≥6 months; 6.3% increase in LVEF). In comparison, shorter training programmes (<6 months) resulted in a 2.3% increase in LVEF (all results compared to non-exercising controls).
- High intensity interval training also led to significant improvements in LVEF compared to controls. However, high intensity interval training was not superior to MCT.

### 46.9.5 Safety

HFrEF is a severe chronic disease, and therapy should not increase the risk for disease deterioration, non-cardiac side effects or even mortality.

- The largest HF exercise intervention trial to date, the above-mentioned HF-ACTION study, showed that exercise is a safe supportive therapy; adverse events did not differ between groups.
- These findings are supported by many other similar studies [26, 27] independent of the intensities performed in the training groups.
- Moderate and high intensity training are associated with very low risks of exercise-related adverse events.

## 46.10 Practical Recommendations for Exercise Training

A structured exercise training program should be considered as an efficacious adjunct to optimal pharmacological therapy and a healthy lifestyle which also includes daily PA. A supervised setting is generally recommended for HF patients, at least in the initial phases of therapy and particularly in patients with severe deconditioning. Patients should get a structured exercise training programme with individual training intensity recommendations that are tailored and adapted to their current health status and their exercise preferences.

### 46.10.1 Medical Examinations

Before starting exercise the following examinations should be done to rule out contraindications:

- Medical history
- Clinical examination
- ECG
- Echocardiography
- Exercise ECG
- Cardiopulmonary exercise testing (CPET) if available (see Chap. 45), in order to
  - Rule out other cardiac or pulmonal causes of dyspnoe
  - Determine exercise capacity ($VO_2$peak) and ventilatory efficiency (VE/VCO2)
  - Determine ventilatory thresholds (VT1 and VT2)

CPET is considered the gold standard for exercise prescription.

### 46.10.2 Contraindications

Beside the general contraindications for exercising (e.g. first days after myocardial infarction, myocarditis, uncontrolled hypertension, severe aortic stenosis etc.) be aware of heart failure specific contraindications [31]:

- Haemodynamic instable patients should not exercise and are not allowed for exercise testing.
- Patients must be aware of typical heart failure symptoms which show decompensation of HF:
  - gaining weight
  - worsening of dyspnoe
  - reduced exercise capacity

  Medical consultation is needed before exercising!

### 46.10.3 Clinical Conditions of the Patient

The following recommendations of a structured exercise training below are for patients with clinically stable heart failure. Decompensated patients should first be recompensated by intensified medical therapy and kept stable for at least 4–6 weeks before (re-)starting an exercise training programme. Nonetheless, it is important to note that decompensated HF patients also benefit from an adapted training programme constantly adapted to the clinical status of the patient [31], such as:

(a) Respiratory training
(b) Increasing mobilization e.g. walking
(c) Muscle mass strength training (e.g. short bouts of low weights, isometric)

### 46.10.4 Individualized Recommendations for Intensity

Intensity recommendations should be given by targeted heart rate (beats per min) or power (watts). The gold standard used for this purpose is CPET (Fig. 46.2), where the training intensity is usually prescribed relative to $VO_2$peak or at/between VT1 and VT2. As CPET is not always available in clinical practice there are alternative ways to provide intensity recommendations (see Chap. 44):

- percentage of heart rate reserve (%HRR = difference between the resting and peak HR)

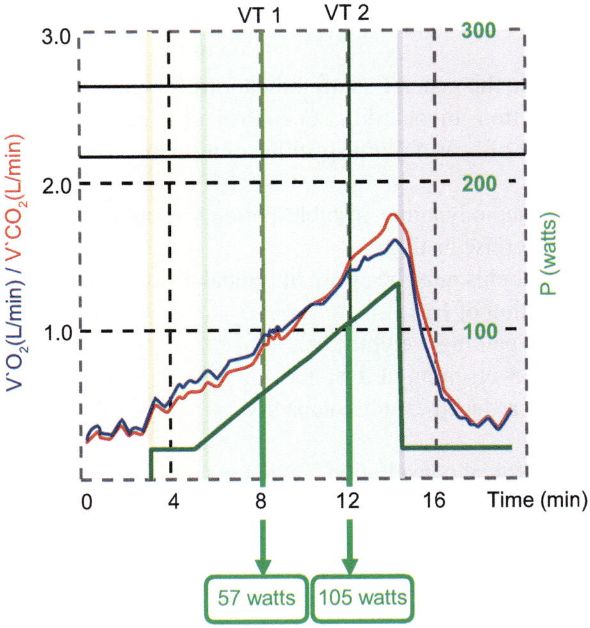


**Fig. 46.2** Cardiopulmonary exercise testing of a 52-year old HFrEF patient with reduced exercise capacity (medication with a beta-blocker): $VO_2$peak 19.5 ml/kg/min at 132 watts with maximal heart rate (HR) of 108 bpm. Training intensities: 50% $VO_2$peak: HR 72 bpm, 60% $VO_2$peak: HR 79 bpm, 70% $VO_2$peak: HR 88 bpm, 80% $VO_2$peak: HR 95 bpm and 90% $VO_2$peak HF 100 bpm. The power (watts) at VT1 and VT2 is marked in green

- rate of perceived exertion (RPE)
- percentage of maximal heart rate (%HRmax); this is however not applicable in patients treated with beta blockers or with chronotropic incompetence

RPE is of particular relevance to patients with atrial fibrillation, where HR-based calculations of intensity are usually not applicable.

## 46.10.5 Training Recommendations for Aerobic Training

### 46.10.5.1 Training Intensity

Moderate exercise training programme is the most widely investigated training schedule which is safe and leads to improvements in exercise capacity. Therefore, it should be considered as the primary intensity for exercise prescription in HF patients. High intensity exercise may also be considered in addition the moderate exercise intensity sessions.

- During the initial phase of an exercise programme, patients should start with low to moderate intensities—adpated to individual health status—and should increase intensity over time.
  - The programme should start at 40–50% $VO_2$peak and gradually increase to higher intensities during the following weeks and months.
  - In HF patients with very low $VO_2$peak, i.e. <14 ml/kg/min, or chronotropic incompetence, percentage $VO_2$peak or %HRmax will result in recommended intensities equalling resting values. In these cases, other measures such as HRR should be applied.

- In the long-term, besides the stability of the health status of the patient, the exercise preference and motivation of the patient is a major determinant for including a high intensity training programme into a basic moderate intensity programme.
- If patients are not satisfied with the training programme, adherence will decrease over time.

#### 46.10.5.2 Training Duration

Duration should be adapted to the current health status of the patient; as little as 5 min per session can be enough in the beginning for HF patients with severely reduced exercise capacity.

- If so, patients may even benefit from several short sessions of exercise per day, e.g. 5 min exercise bouts, 3×/day
- Duration of sessions should be increased over time.
- Always increase duration before intensity.
- Very short bouts of higher intensity exercise e.g. 30 s or short bouts of resistance training providing sufficient recovery time post exercise will induce beneficial peripheral effects while sparing central myocardial strain. During very short bouts of resistance exercise Valsalva manoeuvre should be performed briefly to reduce net-intrathoracic pressure.
- After several weeks of exercise training, training sessions should last at least 20 min, with longer durations being more beneficial.

#### 46.10.5.3 Training Frequency

HF patients benefit from regular physical activity. A minimum of three training sessions per week should thus be performed. Optimally daily training sessions are advised. Especially when starting exercise training, the highest benefit can be derived from daily activities with short durations, but performed several times a day.

#### 46.10.5.4 Continuous vs. Interval Training

- Continuous aerobic exercise training is characterised by the same intensity throughout the training session, usually at a moderate intensity (Fig. 46.3).

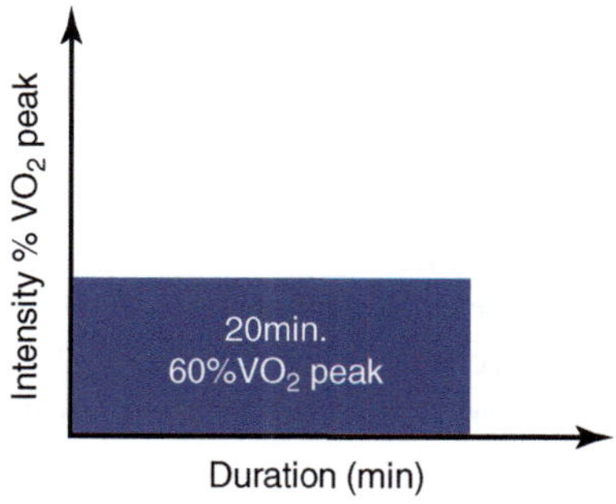


**Fig. 46.3** Schematic depiction of a moderate continous training programme

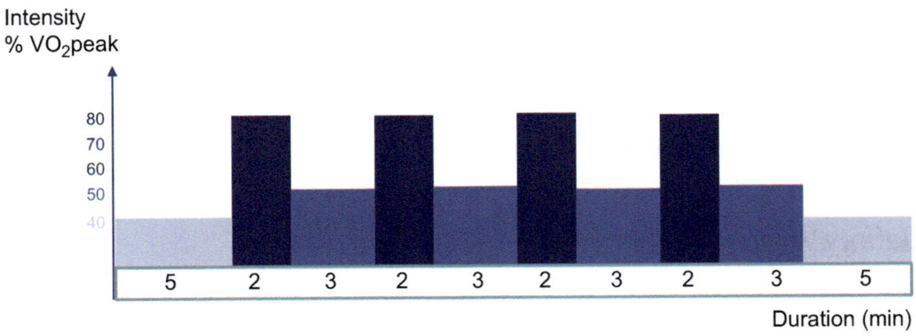


**Fig. 46.4** Schematic depiction of an interval training programme

- High interval exercise training (Fig. 46.4) is characterised by bouts of higher (even submaximal) intensity exercise interspersed with periods of lower intensity exercise (mostly active recovery).
  - Generally, intervals can be performed at moderate or higher, intensities in stable patients with mild HF symptoms.
  - For HFrEF submaximal intensity (typically 85–95% of peak HR) seems to be optimal, as previous studies have demonstrated that maximal intensity during intervals may not be feasible. Higher intensity interval training should best be performed between 75% and 85% peak HR or $VO_2$peak, as this is feasible in most patients.
  - To date, no optimal duration of intervals has clearly been defined, but 4 min at very high intensity seem to be too long for HFrEF patients; thus, adapted to the individual patient, intervals of shorter duration at least at the beginning (30 s to 1 min) extending intervals to 2–3 min are more realistic.
  - When starting very short high intensity intervals, symptoms of patients should be closely monitored.
  - Exercise intensity has to be monitored by heart rate monitors.
  - Patients should be instructed on self-assessing deterioration of heart failure symptoms including daily weighing.

#### 46.10.5.5 Type of Endurance Training

In the beginning, the best choices for endurance training are treadmill or cycle ergometers in a supervised setting. Training programmes can easily be controlled by HR and power displayed on these devices or by heart rate monitors. Long-term exercise training programme prescription should be in line with the preferences of the patient to increase adherence. Aerobic sports such as

(a) Walking,
(b) Nordic Walking,
(c) Cycling,
(d) Cross-Country Skiing at a walking speed primarily with classical style (skating limited to very trained and stable HF patients)

are also viable options for HF patients. Swimming is not primarily recommended as the first choice for endurance sports as it increases venous return to the failing heart and poses a problem in patients with ICD (malfunction or therapeutic shock). Most importantly, continuous monitoring of HR during exercise training is definitely recommended for HF patients to ensure that they are meeting the required exercise intensity goals of the programme.

#### 46.10.5.6 Recommendations for Resistance Training

There are many reasons for implementing resistance training in HF exercise therapy:

- Sarcopenia is often diagnosed in this patient group.
- Ageing is associated with a physiological decline in muscle mass.
- Reductions in muscle mass and muscle quality contribute to reductions in exercise capacity in HF patients.

Due to the superiority of endurance training programmes to increase exercise capacity and improve left ventricular function, aerobic endurance training represents the main recommended exercise modality for patients with HFrEF [31]. Nonetheless,

- Resistance training should be performed in addition to, but not instead of endurance training [31].
- Resistance training should optimally be started in a supervised setting.

To determine the optimal intensity for resistance training, the commonly used 1-repetition maximum test is not recommended in HF patients. Intensity should be controlled using the Borg rating scale with a maximum rating of perceived exertion (RPE) of 15 used for HF patients with moderate risk [32]. For maximal safety, workload must always be adapted to clinical conditions of the patient:

- Patients with severe HF should start the training with small muscle groups with very low workload and enough time to recover.
  - Training with elastic bands might also be an option.
- Usually resistance training includes three steps [31]:
  - Starting period: Learning the exercises in the correct way, so that patients are confident with the particular movements. Muscular coordination is the primary target. Training with very low workload is initiated.
  - Intoducing dynamic resistance training: High amount of repetitions at low workloads (8–10 per min).
  - Increasing work-load: Aiming at increasing muscle mass by training at moderate to higher intensities.

Each step must always be introduced on an individual basis.

Frequency of resistance training is usually 2–3×/week for longer duration e.g. 30 min, but can be included in the daily routine with short sessions.

#### 46.10.5.7 Respiratory Training

Inspiratory muscle training can also be seen as an additional training mode to increase exercise capacity and quality of life [33]. In particular, HF patients with inspiratory muscle weakness may benefit from this type of training, but overall recommendations are lower than for exercise training.

- Training recommendation: 20–30 min per day, 3–5 days a week for a minimum of 8 weeks [31].

#### 46.10.5.8 Patients with Implantable Cardioverter-Defibrillator (ICD)

HFrEF patients with an ICD benefit from a structured training programme for improving exercise capacity and quality of life [34, 35]. Thus, ICD patients should be encouraged to start training.

- Training must begin in a supervised setting.
- Target heart rate is typically 20 bpm lower than VT detection rate.

  See Chap. 52 for more details.

**Clinical Pearls**

- Pharmacological treatment reduces mortality and morbidity. Thus, every HFrEF patient must be on optimal pharmacological therapy.
- A structured exercise training programme should be started as soon as possible in newly diagnosed but stable HF patients.
- Exercise training
  - Improves exercise capacity
  - Improves Quality of Life
  - Reduces (re-)hospitalization rates
  - Is safe
- Aerobic endurance training is the most commonly recommended form of exercise training in heart failure.
- This type of training should always be started with short duration and moderate intensity—adapted to the clinical status of the patient. First, duration should be increased, then intensity.
- Both moderate intensity continuous and high intensity interval training are suitable and efficacious training modes; however, high intensity interval training can be introduced in addition to moderate intensity training when moderate intensities have been well tolerated.
- Recommendation for long-term exercise training: exercise at least 20 min with moderate to high intensity on most days of the week.
- Resistance training should be implemented in addition to endurance training.
- Contraindications must be considered and patients should be regularly re-evaluated (first half year every 3 months, thereafter every 6–12 months depending on the individual patient).

## Review

### Questions

1. A 65-year old patient with newly diagnosed HF with reduced ejection fraction asks you for training recommendations. He was told by his doctor in hospital that regular exercise can improve fitness and HF symptoms. So instead of taking the pills, which were also recommended by the doctor he wants to start exercising. What's your advice for the patient?
2. The patient wants to know if he can start directly with the training program or if he has to do any additional testing. He was discharged from hospital 3 weeks ago and feels much better after being recompensated.
3. After the examinations you discuss the results with the patient. There are no contraindications starting physical exercise. The $VO_2$peak of 17 ml/kg/min shows a deconditioned physical status of the patient. The patient tells you that he has never done any sports in his life, but now he wants to start exercising to get fitter. A friend of him—also a HF patient—exercises every day a so called "high intensity training". As a HIT takes less time than a moderate endurance training he would like to start tomorrow with that type of training. What's your advice?

### Answers

1. A structured exercise program improves fitness, reduce HF symptoms and improves left ventricular function in patients with HFrEF. Even mortality may be reduced in the longer term. Therefore you confirm the beneficial effects of regular physical exercise in HFrEF patients. But physical activity is always a supportive therapy and should be performed in addition to the medical therapy only. The patient should definitely continue taking the recommended HF medication and should thereafter start a structured training program.
2. As it is the first appointment of the patient in your clinic you will need medical information and perform medical examinations to rule out any contraindication for physical activity and to be able to give individual training recommendations. Beside medical history you will perform a clinical examination, an ECG and an echocardiography. In addition cardiopulmonary exercise testing will have to be performed by the patient in order to determine abnormalities under exercise as well as values of maximal exercise capacity for individual training recommendations.
3. In general a moderate aerobic training as well as a high intensity training is possible for HFrEF patients when contraindication are excluded. But for the beginning of an exercise program HFrEF patients should always start with low or moderate intensity adapted to the individual fitness level. For very deconditioned patients—like your HFrEF patient—who has never done any kind of sports before, a daily activity of 5–10 min of low intensity is enough for the beginning. This amount of activity may also be done twice or even more frequently per day.

In the next weeks first the duration of exercise should be increased, later the intensity. Overall a HIT is not recommended for the next weeks, but may be possible when physical performance increases over time without a deterioration of HF symptoms. For deconditioned patients a supervised setting is recommended.

## References


1. Yancy CW, Jessup M, Bozkurt B, Butler J, Casey DE Jr, Drazner MH, et al. 2013 ACCF/AHA guideline for the management of heart failure: executive summary: a report of the American College of Cardiology Foundation/American Heart Association task force on practice guidelines. Circulation. 2013;128(16):1810–52.
2. Ponikowski P, Voors AA, Anker SD, Bueno H, Cleland JGF, Coats AJS, et al. 2016 ESC Guidelines for the diagnosis and treatment of acute and chronic heart failure: the task force for the diagnosis and treatment of acute and chronic heart failure of the European Society of Cardiology (ESC) developed with the special contribution of the Heart Failure Association (HFA) of the ESC. Eur Heart J. 2016;37(27):2129–200.
3. Hunt SA, Abraham WT, Chin MH, Feldman AM, Francis GS, Ganiats TG, et al. 2009 focused update incorporated into the ACC/AHA 2005 guidelines for the diagnosis and management of heart failure in adults: a report of the American College of Cardiology Foundation/American Heart Association task force on practice guidelines: developed in collaboration with the International Society for Heart and Lung Transplantation. Circulation. 2009;119(14):e391–479.
4. Association TCCotNYH. Nomenclature and criteria for diagnosis of diseases of the heart and great vessels. 9th ed. Boston, MA: Little & Brown; 1994.
5. Mosterd A, Hoes AW. Clinical epidemiology of heart failure. Heart. 2007;93(9):1137–46.
6. Redfield MM, Jacobsen SJ, Burnett JC Jr, Mahoney DW, Bailey KR, Rodeheffer RJ. Burden of systolic and diastolic ventricular dysfunction in the community: appreciating the scope of the heart failure epidemic. JAMA. 2003;289(2):194–202.
7. Lip GY, Gibbs CR, Beevers DG. ABC of heart failure: aetiology. BMJ. 2000;320(7227):104–7.
8. Schindler MJ, Adams V, Halle M. Exercise in heart failure-what is the optimal dose to improve pathophysiology and exercise capacity? Curr Heart Fail Rep. 2019;16(4):98–107.
9. Pandey A, Garg S, Khunger M, Darden D, Ayers C, Kumbhani DJ, et al. Dose-response relationship between physical activity and risk of heart failure: a meta-analysis. Circulation. 2015;132(19):1786–94.
10. Investigators S, Yusuf S, Pitt B, Davis CE, Hood WB, Cohn JN. Effect of enalapril on survival in patients with reduced left ventricular ejection fractions and congestive heart failure. N Engl J Med. 1991;325(5):293–302.
11. Investigators S, Yusuf S, Pitt B, Davis CE, Hood WB Jr, Cohn JN. Effect of enalapril on mortality and the development of heart failure in asymptomatic patients with reduced left ventricular ejection fractions. N Engl J Med. 1992;327(10):685–91.
12. Packer M, Poole-Wilson PA, Armstrong PW, Cleland JG, Horowitz JD, Massie BM, et al. Comparative effects of low and high doses of the angiotensin-converting enzyme inhibitor, lisinopril, on morbidity and mortality in chronic heart failure. ATLAS Study Group. Circulation. 1999;100(23):2312–8.
13. Garg R, Yusuf S. Overview of randomized trials of angiotensin-converting enzyme inhibitors on mortality and morbidity in patients with heart failure. Collaborative group on ACE inhibitor trials. JAMA. 1995;273(18):1450–6.
14. Group CTS. Effects of enalapril on mortality in severe congestive heart failure. Results of the cooperative north Scandinavian Enalapril survival study (CONSENSUS). N Engl J Med. 1987;316(23):1429–35.

15. Effect of metoprolol CR/XL in chronic heart failure: Metoprolol CR/XL randomised intervention trial in congestive heart failure (MERIT-HF). Lancet. 1999;353(9169):2001–7.
16. The cardiac insufficiency bisoprolol study II (CIBIS-II): a randomised trial. Lancet. 1999;353(9146):9–13.
17. Hjalmarson A, Goldstein S, Fagerberg B, Wedel H, Waagstein F, Kjekshus J, et al. Effects of controlled-release metoprolol on total mortality, hospitalizations, and well-being in patients with heart failure: the metoprolol CR/XL randomized intervention trial in congestive heart failure (MERIT-HF). MERIT-HF study group. JAMA. 2000;283(10):1295–302.
18. Packer M, Coats AJ, Fowler MB, Katus HA, Krum H, Mohacsi P, et al. Effect of carvedilol on survival in severe chronic heart failure. N Engl J Med. 2001;344(22):1651–8.
19. Flather MD, Shibata MC, Coats AJ, Van Veldhuisen DJ, Parkhomenko A, Borbola J, et al. Randomized trial to determine the effect of nebivolol on mortality and cardiovascular hospital admission in elderly patients with heart failure (SENIORS). Eur Heart J. 2005;26(3):215–25.
20. Zannad F, McMurray JJ, Krum H, van Veldhuisen DJ, Swedberg K, Shi H, et al. Eplerenone in patients with systolic heart failure and mild symptoms. N Engl J Med. 2011;364(1):11–21.
21. Pitt B, Zannad F, Remme WJ, Cody R, Castaigne A, Perez A, et al. The effect of spironolactone on morbidity and mortality in patients with severe heart failure. Randomized Aldactone Evaluation Study Investigators. N Engl J Med. 1999;341(10):709–17.
22. McMurray JJ, Packer M, Desai AS, Gong J, Lefkowitz MP, Rizkala AR, et al. Angiotensin-neprilysin inhibition versus enalapril in heart failure. N Engl J Med. 2014;371(11):993–1004.
23. Swedberg K, Komajda M, Bohm M, Borer JS, Ford I, Dubost-Brama A, et al. Ivabradine and outcomes in chronic heart failure (SHIFT): a randomised placebo-controlled study. Lancet. 2010;376(9744):875–85.
24. O'Connor CM, Whellan DJ, Lee KL, Keteyian SJ, Cooper LS, Ellis SJ, et al. Efficacy and safety of exercise training in patients with chronic heart failure: HF-ACTION randomized controlled trial. JAMA. 2009;301(14):1439–50.
25. Taylor RS, Sagar VA, Davies EJ, Briscoe S, Coats AJ, Dalal H, et al. Exercise-based rehabilitation for heart failure. Cochrane Database Syst Rev. 2014;(4):CD003331.
26. Ismail H, McFarlane JR, Nojoumian AH, Dieberg G, Smart NA. Clinical outcomes and cardiovascular responses to different exercise training intensities in patients with heart failure: a systematic review and meta-analysis. JACC Heart Fail. 2013;1(6):514–22.
27. Gomes Neto M, Duraes AR, Conceicao LSR, Saquetto MB, Ellingsen O, Carvalho VO. High intensity interval training versus moderate intensity continuous training on exercise capacity and quality of life in patients with heart failure with reduced ejection fraction: a systematic review and meta-analysis. Int J Cardiol. 2018;261:134–41.
28. Wisloff U, Stoylen A, Loennechen JP, Bruvold M, Rognmo O, Haram PM, et al. Superior cardiovascular effect of aerobic interval training versus moderate continuous training in heart failure patients: a randomized study. Circulation. 2007;115(24):3086–94.
29. Ellingsen O, Halle M, Conraads V, Stoylen A, Dalen H, Delagardelle C, et al. High-intensity interval training in patients with heart failure with reduced ejection fraction. Circulation. 2017;135(9):839–49.
30. Tucker WJ, Beaudry RI, Liang Y, Clark AM, Tomczak CR, Nelson MD, et al. Meta-analysis of exercise training on left ventricular ejection fraction in heart failure with reduced ejection fraction: a 10-year update. Prog Cardiovasc Dis. 2019;62(2):163–71.
31. Piepoli MF, Conraads V, Corra U, Dickstein K, Francis DP, Jaarsma T, et al. Exercise training in heart failure: from theory to practice. A consensus document of the heart failure association and the European Association for Cardiovascular Prevention and Rehabilitation. Eur J Heart Fail. 2011;13(4):347–57.
32. Pollock ML, Franklin BA, Balady GJ, Chaitman BL, Fleg JL, Fletcher B, et al. AHA science advisory. Resistance exercise in individuals with and without cardiovascular disease: benefits, rationale, safety, and prescription: an advisory from the committee on exercise, rehabilitation,

and prevention, council on clinical cardiology, American Heart Association; position paper endorsed by the American College of Sports Medicine. Circulation. 2000;101(7):828–33.
33. Ribeiro JP, Chiappa GR, Neder JA, Frankenstein L. Respiratory muscle function and exercise intolerance in heart failure. Curr Heart Fail Rep. 2009;6(2):95–101.
34. Davids JS, McPherson CA, Earley C, Batsford WP, Lampert R. Benefits of cardiac rehabilitation in patients with implantable cardioverter-defibrillators: a patient survey. Arch Phys Med Rehabil. 2005;86(10):1924–8.
35. Dougherty CM, Glenny RW, Burr RL, Flo GL, Kudenchuk PJ. Prospective randomized trial of moderately strenuous aerobic exercise after an implantable cardioverter defibrillator. Circulation. 2015;131(21):1835–42.

# Exercise in Specific Diseases: Heart Transplantation and Left Ventricular Assist Device

# 47

Birna Bjarnason-Wehrens, Thomas Schmidt, and Nils Reiss

**Learning Objectives**

1. Understand the importance of HTX and LVAD implantation within the therapy of terminal HF.
2. Be able to perform an adequate evaluation of functional or cardiopulmonary exercise capacity in HTX and LVAD patients.
3. Acquire knowledge about the clinical condition, special hemodynamic principles and exercise physiology of HTX and LVAD patients.
4. Gain an overview on the effectiveness of exercise-based interventions in HTX and LVAD patients and become familiar with the current recommendations for exercise training.
5. Acquire knowledge about special safety aspects for functional and exercise training in LVAD patients.

## 47.1 Surgical Therapy Options in Patients with Advanced and Terminal Heart Failure

In the western world, heart failure (HF) affects approx. 1–2% of the adult population. The prevalence rises continually after the age of 50 years, and in 75-year olds is over 8% [1, 2]. Within HF, advanced and terminal stages account for

B. Bjarnason-Wehrens (✉)
Department of Preventive and Rehabilitative Sport and Exercise Medicine, Institute for Cardiology and Sports Medicine, German Sports University Cologne, Cologne, Germany
e-mail: bjarnason@dshs-koeln.de

T. Schmidt · N. Reiss
Institute for Cardiovascular Research, Schüchtermann-Klinik Bad Rothenfelde, Bad Rothenfelde, Germany
e-mail: tschmidt@schuechtermann-klinik.de; nreiss@schuechtermann-klinik.de



A. Pressler, J. Niebauer (eds.), *Textbook of Sports and Exercise Cardiology*,
https://doi.org/10.1007/978-3-030-35374-2_47

6–25% of patients, with a significantly increasing tendency [3]. This increase is due to different factors:

- On the one hand, the population is becoming older, and the prevalence of chronic HF increases continually with age.
- On the other hand, mortality during the early stages of chronic HF is drastically decreasing, due to considerably improved treatment options (e.g. drug therapy, electrotherapy, interventional procedures) [1, 4].

For the treatment of advanced and terminal HF, orthotopic heart transplantation (HTX) was long considered the gold standard [5]. HTX leads to a significant improvement in the physical capacity of patients, and thus also to a considerable increase in their quality of life. The survival rates are currently around 85%, 70% and 50% after 1, 5 and 10 years, respectively [6]. The lack of donor organs today, however, means that HTX is now unfortunately only an option for a minority of HF patients, with the gap between organ availability and patients requiring treatment increasing. For a long time there were hardly any other options for the treatment of advanced and terminal HF which had a beneficial prognosis except HTX, but over the past two decades enormous progress has been made in the development of so-called mechanical circulatory support systems (MCS), to the extent that they are now considered an alternative to HTX [7]. In most cases the used MCS systems are left ventricular assist devices (LVAD) [8], and the number of LVAD systems implanted now even exceeds the number of HTX performed by quite a margin [9–12] (Fig. 47.1).

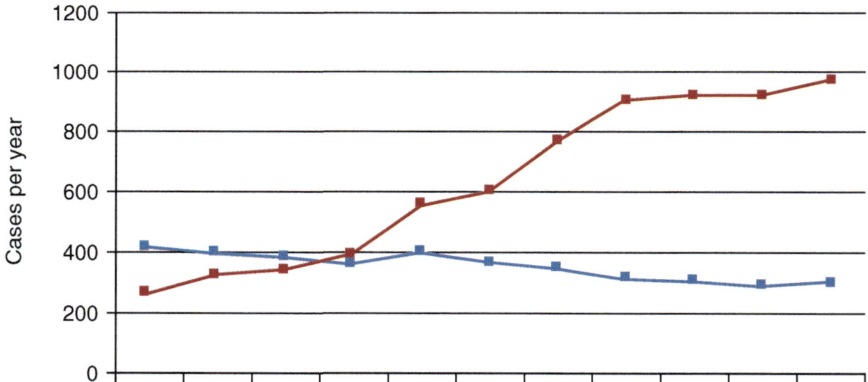


| | 2006 | 2007 | 2008 | 2009 | 2010 | 2011 | 2012 | 2013 | 2014 | 2015 | 2016 |
|---|---|---|---|---|---|---|---|---|---|---|---|
| HTX | 412 | 394 | 382 | 363 | 393 | 366 | 345 | 313 | 304 | 286 | 297 |
| LVAD | 260 | 324 | 340 | 390 | 555 | 601 | 766 | 898 | 915 | 915 | 965 |

**Fig. 47.1** Surgical treatment of advanced and terminal HF; development in Germany since 2006 [9–12]. *HF* heart failure, *HTX* heart transplantation, *LVAD*, left ventricular assist device

- The prevalence of advanced and terminal HF has increased considerably over the past few years.
- Treatment options with beneficial prognoses are HTX and LVAD implantation.
- Due to the lack of donor organs, the number of LVAD implanted now considerably exceeds the number of HTX.

So-called paracorporeal systems were already being used for circulation support more than 40 years ago [13, 14]. Back then, the pump chambers were on the abdominal wall, and the drive system was the size of a fridge. These systems could be used for right-heart, left-heart or biventricular support. Two mechanical valves determined the direction of blood flow. A sensor detected when the pump was filled with blood and signalled to the drive system to eject the blood out of the pump and into the circulation of the patient. Clinical experience showed that an effective stroke volume (SV) of up to 65 ml could be achieved, as well as a cardiac output (CO) of 4–7 l/min, with a heart rate (HR) of approximately 70–100/min. This technology was used successfully for years [14]. During this time, it was also discovered, however, that biventricular cardiac support is not always necessary: usually isolated left-ventricular support is sufficient. And this was the starting point for the further development of LVAD.

The second-generation systems were intracorporeal rotation pumps with axial flow [14, 15]. The size of these rotation pumps was small compared to that of the previous pulsatile systems. The pumps also no longer worked with pulsatile, but with continuous blood flow, were driven by a rotating impeller and employed very high rotational speeds (e.g. 15,000 rotations per minute for the HeartMate 2 (Abbott Laboratories, IL, USA)). This made blood flow of up to 8–10 l/min theoretically possible. A further essential difference to the first generation of pulsatile systems was the absence of flow-regulating valves and compliance chambers (Windkessel effect) [14]. Moreover, these devices were much quieter than the pulsatile systems. For the first time, patients could be rapidly mobilised. And they made it possible for patients to be discharged to their home environment, increasing their quality of life significantly [16].

The latest, third-generation LVADs are miniaturised centrifugal pumps which are implanted. Like the pumps of the second generation, they are not pulsatile, but ensure continuous blood flow. This time, however, flow is not axial, but centrifugal [15, 17–19], with in- and outflow cannulas arranged at 90°. Also, they run at a lower speed (1800–9000 rotations per minute, depending on the model). The main representatives of this new group are HVAD [20, 21] (Medtronic Inc., MN, USA) (Fig. 47.2) and HeartMate3 [19] (Abbott Laboratories, IL, USA).

In these systems, the small size of the pump facilitates implantation within the pericardium without the necessary creation of an additional cavity for the device itself. The outflow graft is usually connected to the ascending aorta. The pump is

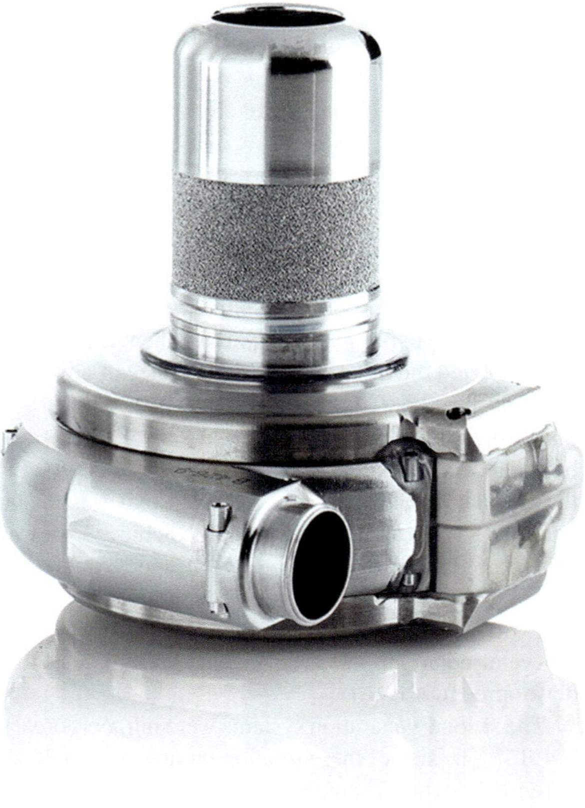

**Fig. 47.2** State-of-the-art LVAD continuous flow pumps exemplified by the HVAD system from Medtronic Inc. [21]. *HVAD* HeartWare ventricular assist device, *LVAD* left ventricular assist device

connected via a relatively thin driveline, tunnelled through the abdominal muscles, to an external controller which takes care of device management and power supply [18, 19, 22] (Fig. 47.3).

- In the past, paracorporeal systems generated a pulsatile flow via a pneumatically driven pump and supported both ventricles.
- Nowadays, implantation of an LVAD is sufficient in most cases.
- State-of-the-art LVADs are intracorporeal, continuous-flow pumps which operate at a pre-set and fixed rotational speed.
- Device management and power supply are taken care of by an external controller which is connected to the LVAD via a so-called driveline through the abdominal wall.

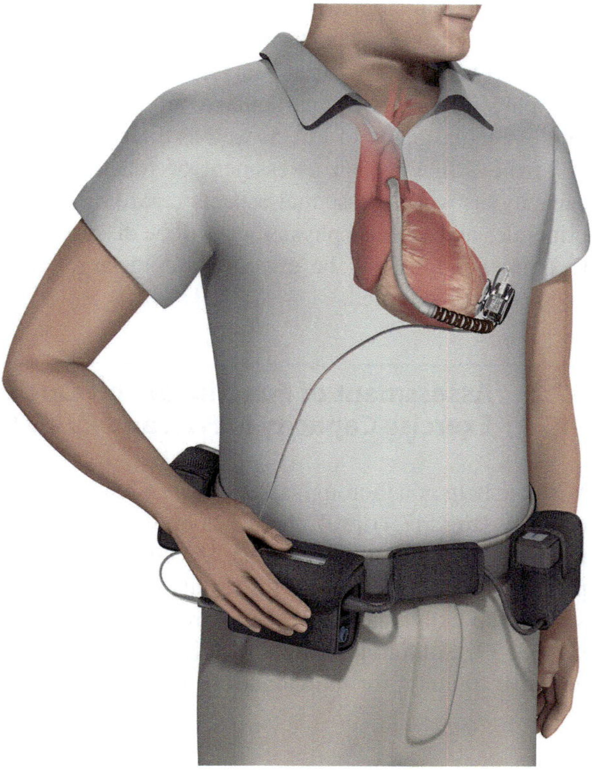

**Fig. 47.3** Internal and external system components of the LVAD systems used today, exemplified by the HVAD system from Medtronic Inc. [22]. *HVAD* HeartWare ventricular assist device, *LVAD* left ventricular assist device

Due to technical developments over the past few years, the survival rates following LVAD implantation are now very good and, at least in the first years, comparable with results following HTX. The probability of survival following LVAD implantation in patient collectives comparable with HTX patients is currently 85% in the first year, 77% in the second and 59% in the fifth year [8, 23]. Good results are also being achieved in the long term, significantly superior to those of drug therapy [24, 25], although long-term survival following HTX is still better (38% after 15 years, sometimes even 20–30 years) [6, 26, 27]. Nevertheless, encouraged by the good results after LVAD implantation and justified by the increasing number of patients requiring treatment, as well as the evident shortage of donors, the status of LVAD therapy is rising all the time. Whereas in the past these systems were only implanted temporarily, either until a possible recovery of the myocardium (bridge to recovery) or until HTX (bridge to transplant), today they are increasingly being used as a long-term solution (destination therapy) [28, 29].

- In the initial period following LVAD implantation, survival is good, comparable to HTX.
- Over the long-term course, HTX is superior to LVAD implantation.
- LVADs are now largely implanted as destination therapy, that is as a permanent solution until the end of life.

Two different surgical procedures are thus currently available for the long-term therapy of advanced and terminal HF, differing considerably in their impact on patients. Over the long-term course, the attainment and maintenance of an acceptable physical capacity is particularly important for both patient groups in order to improve their quality of life, as well as their participation in everyday activities.

In the following, an assessment of functional and cardiopulmonary exercise capacity, as well as essential aspects regarding clinical condition, haemodynamic principles and exercise physiology will be discussed for both target groups. Finally, recommendations will be given regarding target-group-specific exercise training and peculiarities noted.

## 47.2 Assessment of Functional and Cardiopulmonary Exercise Capacity in HTX and LVAD Patients

With the help of a thorough assessment of functional and cardiopulmonary exercise capacity (Fig. 47.4) [30], the cardiopulmonary, metabolic and muscular exercise tolerance of HF patients can be objectively determined [31, 32]. In both HTX patients and LVAD patients, the results serve to evaluate the patient's condition, to stratify the individual risks, and to provide information aiding a long-term prognosis [33–39]. A thorough assessment is a prerequisite for the contentual planning of effective training, for individual control of exercise levels and for follow-up. The

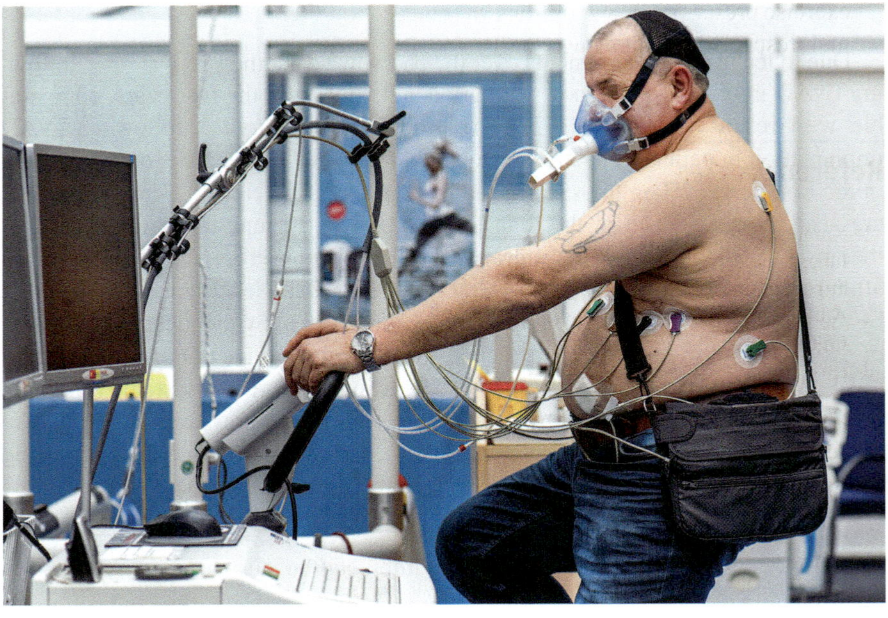

**Fig. 47.4** LVAD patient during cardiopulmonary exercise testing on bicycle ergometer [30]. *LVAD* left ventricular assist device

diagnostic measures make equal sense within the framework of rehabilitation measures, ambulatory follow-up programmes or for patients who would like to pursue sports activities.

Table 47.1 lists possible assessment procedures for the testing of functional and cardiopulmonary exercise capacity in HTX and LVAD patients [31, 32, 40–43], whereby the individual situation of a patient is always crucial to the exercise type and protocol. In addition, performance-limiting comorbidities, particularly those of an internal, neurological or orthopaedic nature, should be ascertained and documented.

In addition to objective parameters, the subjective exercise tolerance of patients should also and in particular be ascertained in order to train adequate perception and to prepare patients for the challenges of everyday life [34, 39]. In addition to the

**Table 47.1** Possible assessments for testing of functional and cardiopulmonary exercise capacity in HTX and LVAD patients [31, 32, 39–42]

| | Test | Test protocol | Measurement parameters |
|---|---|---|---|
| Functional assessment | 6-min walking test | ATS standard with/without aids | Distance, RPE, usage of aids, number/duration of recovery periods, reason for stopping |
| | Timed up and go test[a] | Standard with/without aids | Time, usage of aids, certainty of movement, mobility classification |
| Ergometry | CPET on bicycle | 1. Ramp (5–10 watt/min)<br>2. WHO step (25 watt/2 min)<br>3. In patients with good exercise tolerance, higher increases/steps are also thinkable | ECG, HR, Watt, RPE, exercise duration, reason for stopping, $VO_2$, $VE/VCO_2$ slope, RER, lactate, oxygen saturation, values at VAT |
| | CPET on treadmill[b] | Select protocol with constant low speed and increase load by increasing elevation | ECG, HR, elevation, RPE, exercise duration, reason for stopping, $VO_2$, $VE/VCO_2$ slope, RER, lactate, oxygen saturation, values at VAT |
| | IGR on bicycle | 4-minute step protocol at different exercise levels | ECG, HR, Watt, RPE, $VO_2$, CO, $avDO_2$, RER, lactate, oxygen saturation, systolic blood pressure, cardiac index, LVAD flow |
| Strength assessment | Handgrip strength test | Standard one-arm for both, right and left hand | Newton |
| | Knee extension | Standard one-leg for both, right and left leg | Newton |

*ATS* American Thoracic Society, *$avDO_2$* arteriovenous oxygen difference, *CO* cardiac output, *CPET* cardiopulmonary exercise test, *CR* cardiac rehabilitation, *ECG* electrocardiogram, *HR* heart rate, *HTX* heart transplantation, *IGR* inert gas rebreathing, *RER* respiratory exchange ratio, *RPE* rated perceived exertion, *LVAD* left ventricular assist device, *VAT* ventilator anaerobic threshold, *$VE/VCO_2$* slope, relation between ventilation and carbon dioxide production, *$VO_2$* oxygen uptake, *WHO* World Health Organization

[a]Only in patients with 6-min walking distance below 200 m and using aids

[b]Only for patients without balance disorders

assessments proposed in the Table 47.1, specific sports related diagnostics are also conceivable for patients with sporty ambitions.

When conducting assessments, the peculiarities and limitations specific to HTX or LVAD implantation must be taken into account. The published counterindications for HF patients must be observed during all tests [44].

LVAD patients have some additional system-relevant abort criteria, such as device alarms, LVAD flow less than 3 l/min, haemorrhaging (e.g. nosebleeds) or oxygen saturation below 90% [45]. Relevant safety standards must be observed at all times (see below).

- Assessment of functional and cardiopulmonary exercise capacity is recommended.
- In addition to objective parameters, subjective exercise tolerance should also and in particular be ascertained and trained.
- When assessing LVAD patients, specific safety standards and system-relevant abort criteria must be observed at all times.

## 47.3 Heart Transplantation

### 47.3.1 Clinical Condition, Haemodynamic Principles and Exercise Physiology

#### 47.3.1.1 Clinical Condition

Compared to life with advanced or terminal HF, HTX brings a significant improvement in functional status, quality of life and ultimately survival in patients who are usually still quite young (average age on transplantation approximately 50 years) [26, 46]. Clinical condition following HTX is influenced by the individual anamnesis of the patient, the altered haemodynamics of the transplanted heart, sequelae from the life-prolonging immunosuppression and potentially severe complications. The most frequent complications in heart transplant recipients include

(a) infections (esp. respiratory system),
(b) cardiac allograft vasculopathy (CAV),
(c) renal failure,
(d) rejection and, in the long term,
(e) cancer [46].

An early diagnosis of CAV is extremely important with regard to exercise training since a denervated heart gives no warning symptoms such as perceptible pectanginous pain (silent ischaemia) [47]. The patient is thus unwittingly in danger of overexertion, with the potential consequence of arrhythmia, heart attack or even sudden cardiac death.

In addition to the potential complications listed here, transplanted patients are also restricted by damage suffered prior to transplantation:

- For example, persistent damage of the pulmonary capillary bed can be observed in many patients with a long history of HF.
- Furthermore, inactivity, sometimes for years, will often have led to a deconditioning of the peripheral muscles [48–50].
  - The result is a shift in muscle fibre composition from type I to types IIa and IIb.
  - Following HTX, the muscle fibre cross-section usually does increase again, but the proportion of type I muscle fibres remains reduced [51–53].
- This is also encouraged by the immunosuppressive medication (calcineurin inhibitors, corticosteroids), which causes a reduction in the oxidative function of the skeletal muscle fibres.
- The administration of corticosteroids and potential physical inactivity additionally lead also to a decrease in bone density [54].

Despite the changes to heart, lungs and motor apparatus described here, as well as the potential occurrence of complications, physical exercise capacity rises significantly following HTX, albeit being still below the values of a control group of the same age without heart disease [55]. The results from CPET usually reveals peak oxygen consumptions (peak $VO_2$) of approximately 16–20 ml/kg/min, corresponding to around 50–70% of predicted values [56]. In individual patients significantly better values can be achieved: in the normal range or even in the range for high-performance athletes [57]. These patients are the exception, however, and were usually active sportsmen and women prior to HTX.

With regard to symptoms, most patients are in NYHA class I following HTX, so that approximately 90% of patients are unrestricted in their activity [58]. The average six-minute walking distance (6MWD) achieved is usually 500 m or more (>85% of predicted), meaning that patients are well suited to everyday life [59–61].

- Complications can occur following HTX, such as infections, CAV, renal failure, rejection and cancer.
- Peak exercise values are usually approximately 50–70% of predicted. Individual values may be better.
- Patient symptoms improve significantly to NYHA class 1, concomitant with good functional capacity at >85% of predicted.

In the following, we shall discuss haemodynamic principles and exercise physiology.

#### 47.3.1.2 Haemodynamic Principles and Exercise Physiology

HTX leads to key haemodynamic changes (Fig. 47.5) [47]. The most frequently used surgical techniques for HTX are standard excision of the heart with biatrial

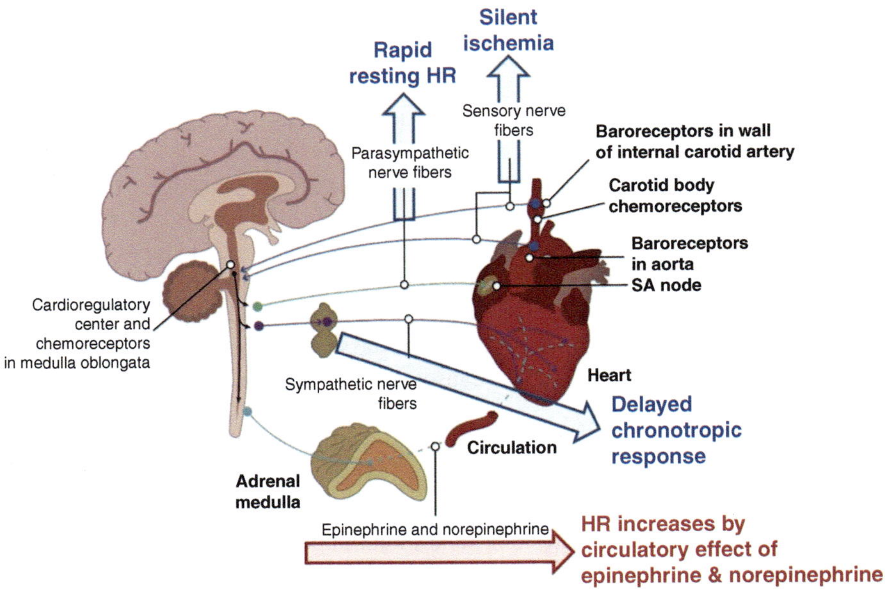


**Fig. 47.5** Physiological changes at rest and during exercise in patients after heart transplantation. Blue arrows indicate blockage of the nerve fibres, red arrow indicates residual effect of circulatory catecholamines (reprinted with kind permission from The Korean Circulation Journal [47]). *HR* heart rate, *SA* sinoatrial

anastomosis, and the bicaval technique with resection in the region of both venae cavae [62, 63]. Both techniques lead to a denervation of sympathetic and parasympathetic nerve fibres. This denervation is responsible for numerous physiological phenomena in heart transplant patients [47, 64, 65], both at rest and under exercise conditions, e.g.:

- high resting HR (approximately 95 bpm),
- delayed increase in HR under exercise conditions (chronotropic incompetence),
- delayed achievement of resting HR in the recovery phase following physical exercise,
- significantly restricted HR variability.

Denervation leads to an emptying of the catecholamine storage of the myocardium, in turn leading to a dependence of the donor organ on circulating catecholamines (epinephrine, norepinephrine) [47, 64]. Due to an increased sensitivity to circulating catecholamines, the consequence can be an increased occurrence of arrhythmia. The administration of betablockers to HTX patients is, however, counterindicated since their exercise tolerance level is significantly reduced.

In order to compensate chronotropic incompetence in conjunction with physical exertion, the donor heart must increase its SV via the Frank Starling mechanism, so that CO can be adapted at least partially to the level of exertion. In many patients, however (particularly initially), a decreased compliance of the left ventricle can be observed (diastolic dysfunction) [66, 67]. The consequence is increased enddiastolic pressure in the left chamber, despite reduced enddiastolic volume. This in turn hinders the Frank Starling mechanism, accompanied by a non-optimal adaptation of SV under exercise conditions [68]. Overall, the CO remains reduced, both at rest and under exercise conditions, and only a slight increase in systolic blood pressure can be generated [69–71].

Partial reinnervation following HTX is fundamentally possible and also has a clinical impact on exercise capacity. Overall, 40–70% of patients display cardiac reinnervation over the long-term course. Corresponding changes in the sympathetic nerve fibres can be observed very early on (after approx. 6 months), and later in the parasympathetic nerve fibres (after more than 1 to 3 years) [65]. However, despite long-term compensation mechanisms the overall result is still inferior to nerve fibres in subjects without heart disease [65].

- HTX leads to denervation of parasympathetic and sympathetic nerve fibres in the myocardium.
- This denervation in turn leads to a changed HR pattern at rest and under exercise conditions, whereby peak exercise values remain restricted.
- Over the long-term course, partial reinnervation is possible and has a positive clinical impact.

## 47.4 Exercise Training

### 47.4.1 Efficacy of Exercise-Based Interventions

Results from a smaller retrospective study provide first hints of a protective effect of exercise-based rehabilitation immediately after transplantation [72]. They showed a significant association between the number of completed rehabilitation units in the first 90 days after HTX and survival rates (hazard ratio, 0.90, 95% CI, 0.82–0.97, $p = 0.007$) [72]. In the meantime, the efficacy of exercise-based rehabilitation on physical performance (peak $VO_2$, MD 2.49 ml/kg/min, 95% CI, 1.63–3.36) has been confirmed by a meta-analysis of 9 studies including 284 patients [73]. Only one of the studies evaluated documented adverse events.

The ability of moderate aerobic endurance training (60–80% peak $VO_2$) to improve exercise capacity in HTX patients has been confirmed by meta-analyses and systematic reviews including a few smaller studies [56, 74, 75]. Other documented positive effects of moderate aerobic endurance training (60–80% peak $VO_2$) are:

- increase in peak HR,
- improvement in the oxidative capacity of skeletal muscle [76],
- improvement in blood pressure [77],
- improvement in endothelial function [78–80],
- improvement in quality of life [81–84].

Randomized controlled trials have confirmed the feasibility of high-intensity interval training (30/60 seconds at 90–100% peak $VO_2$; 4x4 min 90% peak HR or 80–90% peak $VO_2$) in HTX patients >1 year after transplantation. These studies show that interval training can be considered in the long-term care (> 1 year after HTX) with positive improvements in:

- peak $VO_2$ [85–88],
- muscular endurance [85],
- endothelial function [89],
- quality of life [90],
- reduced anxiety and depression [90],

The results of a randomized crossover study show a low superiority of the interval training method (60% -70% peak $VO_2$ vs. > 80% peak $VO_2$) in terms of improvement in exercise capacity and quality of life [91, 92]. However, the impact of exercise on the progression of CAV needs further investigation [56, 93].

Moderate resistance training (50% of 1 repetition maximum (RM)) improves muscle strength [74] and counteracts the negative effects of immunosuppressive therapy on muscle and bone metabolism [50, 94–96].

There are currently no studies showing a favourable long-term effect of any type of exercise intervention on the prognosis and clinical course of HTX patients [97, 98].

- Participation in exercise-based cardiac rehabilitation can provide protective effects.
- Both moderate aerobic endurance training and high-intensity interval training reveal positive effects on exercise capacity, quality of life and peripheral adaptions.
- Moderate resistance training can counteract the negative effects of immunosuppressive therapy on muscle and bone metabolism.
- To date no studies are available on the long-term effects of exercise-based interventions.

### 47.4.2 Recommendations for Exercise Training

After HTX, haemodynamically stable patients should participate in medically supervised exercise-based measures, and all training measures should be continued in the long term [97, 99, 100].

Before the onset of exercise training, as well as at regular intervals, an ischaemia diagnosis is recommended to rule out the possibility of CAV (silent ischaemia). The CPET results cannot be used for this purpose due to low sensitivity [101].

The planning and execution of exercise training must always be adapted to the individual clinical condition. Attention should be paid to signs of possible rejection episodes (e.g. low exercise tolerance, shortness of breath, oedemas). During such episodes, the exercise intensity must be clearly reduced. Any cortisone bolus therapy should lead to interruption of exercise training [100]. Likewise, restrictions linked to treatment of concomitant cancer must be taken into account.

For all patients: a sophisticated fluid balance must be sought to ensure optimal hemodynamic performance.

### 47.4.3 Aerobic Endurance Training

- After heart transplantation, patients should be introduced as early as possible (second to third week postoperatively) to individually adapted, supervised and monitored aerobic endurance training [97, 99, 100].
- From the third postoperative week, a stepwise stress test with small increments of 5–15 watts should be performed to assess exercise tolerance and possible exercise intensity [48, 65].
- Aerobic exercise training should be started at low intensity (<50% of the peak $VO_2$ or 10% below the ventilatory threshold) [99].
- Exercise intensity should be determined using the Borg scale (RPE 11–14) and/or the respiratory rate ("Speech Rule"), which means that the respiratory rate should permit conversation [99, 100]. Due to chronotropic incompetence, the use of HR to determine exercise intensity is inadequate.
- Exercise intensity can also be defined as up to 50% of the maximum load (watt) achieved during CPET [99, 100].
- Clinically stable patients with good exercise tolerance should gradually be brought up to a more intensive aerobic endurance training (60–80% of peak $VO_2$) in the long term, possibly also in the form of high-intensity interval training (> 80% of peak $VO_2$) [56].

## 47.5 Resistance Training

- Moderate and individually dosed resistance training (50–60% of 1 RM) should be integrated into the exercise regime postoperatively as soon as possible [97, 99, 100].
- In particular, individually dosed resistance training is suitable for counteracting catabolic side-effects of immunosuppressive therapy and the loss of muscle mass, muscle strength and bone density caused preoperatively by HF and inactivity.
- All measures performed shortly after HTX should be gentle on the sternum.

- Aerobic endurance training and resistance training are recommended.
- Before the onset of exercise training, an ischaemia diagnosis should be performed.
- During exercise training, attention should be paid to possible signs of rejection episodes.
- Due to chronotropic incompetence, training should be controlled using the Borg scale or via percentage of peak $VO_2$, of the $VO_2$ reserve or peak load.
- Resistance training soon after HTX should be gentle on the sternum due to sternotomy.

## 47.6 LVAD Implantation

### 47.6.1 Clinical Condition, Haemodynamic Principles and Exercise Physiology

#### 47.6.1.1 Clinical Condition

LVAD patients are usually older (approx. 60 years on implantation) than HTX patients [102, 103] and/or display corresponding counterindications for transplantation. Depending on their individual disease course and possible concomitant diseases, their clinical condition can differ considerably [34, 104]. Possible comorbidities in LVAD patients are e.g.

(a) renal failure,
(b) atrial fibrillation,
(c) diabetes mellitus,
(d) respiratory diseases,
(e) neurological problems,
(f) orthopaedic problems,
(g) sarcopaenia,
(h) obesity or
(i) psychiatric problems [29, 104–108].

In addition, in connection with the LVAD therapy, severe complications such as bleeding, thromboembolic events, driveline infections or right HF can occur [8, 28], having a considerable influence on clinical condition.

Overall, however, after LVAD implantation patients experience a considerable increase both in quality of life and in NYHA symptoms (80% of patients after implantation are in NYHA class 1–2) [16, 109]. The patients are capable of increasing their daily life activities significantly, even though in the long term their performance remains below that of healthy subjects [110].

Maximum exercise capacity remains considerably restricted after implantation, with a peak $VO_2$ of 10–13 ml/kg/min (approximately 40–45% of predicted), and over time hardly improves (up to approximately 50% of predicted) [111–116]. In contrast to peak exercise values, the achieved functional performance can be evaluated as better than could be expected from the peak $VO_2$ [117]. In the six-minute walking test (6MWT), for example, patients frequently achieve values between 350 and 400 m (70% of predicted) [33, 109, 115], which can sometimes even be increased further over the long-term course (~450 m, 80% of predicted) [116]. Likewise, after implantation improvements in muscle strength and in the musculoskeletal prerequisites (fibre composition, fibre thickness, oxidative function, hormonal signal chain) can be observed [118]. It is conspicuous that (without dietary intervention) a significant weight increase can be observed in the patients over the long-term course, with a tendency towards obesity. This is most likely to be attributable to lifestyle causes [116, 119].

- LVAD patients are a heterogeneous patient collective which can differ considerably in clinical condition.
- The most frequent complications are bleeding, thromboembolic events, driveline infections or right HF.
- The peak exercise values remain restricted, at 50% of predicted.
- The functional performance is much better, at 80% of predicted.
- Without dietary intervention, a long-term significant weight gain can be observed in many patients, with a tendency towards obesity.

The reasons why the peak exercise values remain so significantly restricted and the submaximum values are, in contrast, considerably better, must be seen as lying in the special haemodynamic situation following LVAD implantation.

#### 47.6.1.2 Haemodynamic Principles and Exercise Physiology

In LVAD patients, the native left ventricle and the assist device usually both contribute to the total CO. At rest, the predominant proportion of the blood volume flows over the pump, which in this situation strongly relieves the left ventricle [40, 120, 121]. With increasing physical exercise, the venous return increases and the result is an increased supply of blood in the left ventricle [122]. Dependently on the achieved intraventricular pressure and the contractile residual function of the myocardium, in most patients an additional blood volume can be ejected via the aortic valve. The result is a special haemodynamic situation with two parallel circulations [40, 120, 121] (Fig. 47.6) [123].

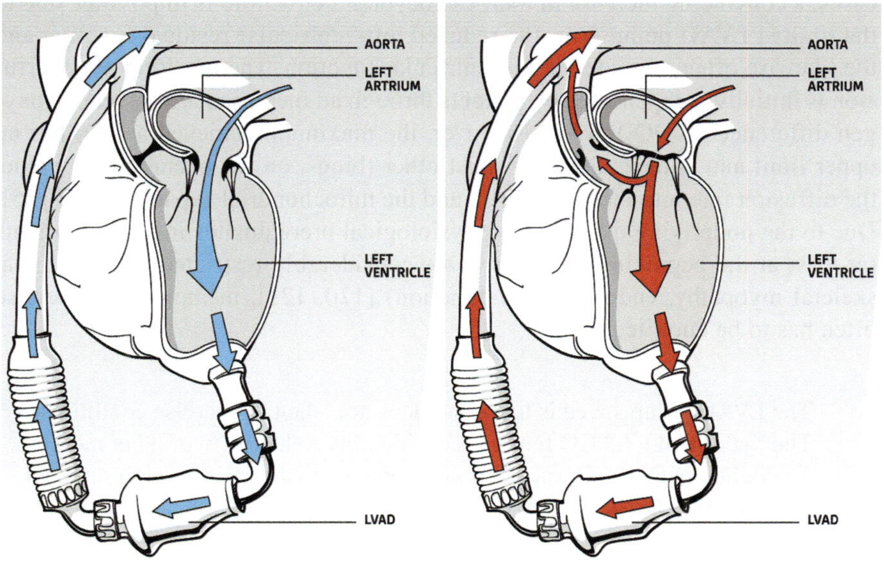


**Fig. 47.6** Special haemodynamic situation in LVAD patients. Left: at rest, the largest proportion of the total CO flows from the left ventricle via the LVAD into the aorta. Right: under exercise conditions most patients eject additional blood volume via the aortic valve. Two parallel circulations result [123]. *CO* cardiac output, *LVAD* left ventricular assist device

The regular function of the aortic valve is also significant for the haemodynamic prerequisites. Following LVAD implantation, many patients develop at least mild to moderate aortic valve insufficiency over the long-term course [124, 125]. The reasons for this are not yet fully researched and probably complex. However, in the presence of aortic valve insufficiency a retrograde circulation (blind circulation) can sometimes occur, resulting in a further reduction in effective total CO [125].

- In LVAD patients, both pump flow and native ejection via the aortic valve contribute to total CO under exercise conditions.
- Aortic valve insufficiency is common in LVAD therapy over the long-term course and can cause retrograde circulation.

In LVAD patients, due to the underlying disease or the corresponding medication, a chronotropic incompetence can often be observed [121, 126, 127]. Likewise, the pump speed in LVAD patients is fixed and does not alter under exercise conditions. Nevertheless, pump flow can increase to a certain level under exercise conditions through a change in pressure gradient (changes in preload and afterload) [40, 120, 121]. Crucial for the patient is the composite amount of blood which can be transported through the two parallel outputs. The total CO at rest is approximately 4 to 6 l/min and increases up to twofold under maximum exertion [128–134]. The large part of this increase takes place under submaximal exertion and considerably decreases with increasing exertion [134]. In most cases, a convincing increase in total CO beyond the twofold is impossible due to the limited LVAD pump flow, the reduced left-ventricular residual function and the likewise often restricted right-ventricular function. The resulting hypoperfusion is initially compensated by patients through an increased arteriovenous oxygen difference ($avDO_2$) [134]. However, the maximum achieved $avDO_2$ has an upper limit and is dependent, amongst other things, on the haemoglobin value, the diffusion rate into the muscle cell and the mitochondrial capacity [122, 135]. Due to the underlying disease, the physiological prerequisites in LVAD patients (at least at the beginning of therapy) are considerably restricted (e.g. anaemia, skeletal myopathy, endothelial dysfunction) [120, 121], meaning that exercise often has to be curtailed.

- The LVAD pump speed is fixed and does not adapt to exercise conditions.
- The maximum total CO remains considerably reduced (twofold at most).
- The deficit in total CO can be compensated up to a certain level through an increase in $avDO_2$.

## 47.7 Exercise Training

### 47.7.1 Safety Aspects During Exercise

All therapists involved in functional and exercise training (physicians, exercise therapists, physiotherapists) should have profound knowledge of the special needs of LVAD patients and the relevant safety aspects. Based on current guidelines [34], regular refresher courses on device management and emergency measures should be offered to all staff involved. In case of adverse events, a centre-specific emergency chain must be in place in order to care for patients as quickly and efficiently as possible. Concerning equipment, all system-relevant replacement parts (e.g. charged batteries, controllers, charging stations) should be in stock [34, 39].

Before initiating functional and/or exercise therapy, patients must be in a clinically and haemodynamically stable condition. Exclusion criteria are [34, 39, 45, 136]:

- low volume status with orthostatic reaction,
- bleeding,
- signs of systemic infection,
- ventricular arrhythmias and/or technical LVAD problems.

Before carrying out any functional or exercise-based measures, the following safety aspects must be strictly observed:

- checking of the batteries,
- monitoring of the driveline length and location,
- choice and control of mounting of the controller and batteries (the use of safari jackets has been positively tried and tested).

While performing functional and/or exercise-based measures, the following termination criteria must be observed:

- pump flow reduction <3 l/min,
- inadequate increase in the energy requirement of the pump in watts (note for thrombus formation!),
- oxygen saturation < 90% (pulse oxymeter),
- bleeding (e.g. nosebleeds)

Special care is required in the exercise selection and choice of training equipment. While performing functional and exercise-based activities, rapid shifts in body position should always be avoided (e.g. from sitting to standing with rapid blood volume displacement) due to blood volume shifts and the risk of suction events. All activities that could lead to an uncontrolled, inadequate load on the system or activities which involve an increased risk of bleeding must be strictly avoided (water sports, contact sports, competitive game forms, etc.) [34, 39]. In patients with a fresh sternotomy, special caution is required when exercising the upper extremities in the first 3 months, due to possible instability of the sternum. In addition to the LVAD-specific aspects, the general recommendations for HF patients also apply [137].

- All involved therapists should be trained device-specifically and receive regular refresher courses.
- In case of adverse events, a centre-specific emergency chain must be in place.
- All activities which lead to an uncontrolled inadequate loading of the system or an increased risk of bleeding must be strictly avoided.

### 47.7.2 Efficacy of Exercise-Based Interventions

Results from previous studies do not permit a reliable estimation of the safety [45, 138–142] and effectiveness of exercise-based measures after LVAD implantation. Only a few retrospective analyses [81, 104, 113, 143], controlled or comparative studies [119] and very small randomized, controlled trials [144–146] report on experiences and results, and this on the basis of a very heterogeneous patient population. However, these studies provide evidence that LVAD patients benefit from individualised and adapted endurance exercise training [81, 104, 113, 119, 144–146], at least in the short term. The results show that

(a) improvement in physical capacity [144, 146],
(b) functional performance [144, 146],
(c) quality of life [144, 145] and
(d) pulmonary capacity [144]

can be achieved. Long-term effects of exercise-based measures are not yet available [34, 120, 121, 139].

- Results from a recent meta-analysis [141] and a systematic review [140] confirm the positive effect of exercise-based rehabilitation on
  - peak $VO_2$ (WMD: 3.0 ml/kg/min; 95% CI 0.64–5.35, $p < 0.001$, SMD = 0.736, 95% CI 0.32–1.15, $p = 0.001$),
  - 6MWD (WMD: 60.06 m, 95% CI: 22.61–97.50 $p = 0.002$),
  - quality of life (SMD = 1.58, 95% CI 0.97–2.20, $p < 0.001$).
- In four studies, individualised low-dose resistance training was implemented [104, 113, 145, 146]. The authors confirm the effectiveness and the feasibility of highly individualised low-dose resistance training. This training mode is well tolerated and accepted by the patients.

- Beyond special training contents, a recently published study [147] reports the positive effect of structured rehabilitation programmes on 1-year hospitalisation (23% lower risk) and 1-year mortality (47% lower risk) in LVAD patients.

In summary, taking into account the overall experience gained in chronic HF patients, [99, 137] the results permit cautious recommendations for exercise training after LVAD implantation [34, 45, 148, 149].

- To date, few studies on exercise-based interventions have been published.
- Through aerobic endurance training and low-dose resistance training, short-term follow-up effects on physical capacity, functional performance, quality of life and pulmonary capacity could be achieved.
- Results regarding long-term effects are not yet available.

### 47.7.3 Recommendations for Exercise Training

After LVAD implantation, haemodynamically stable patients should participate in medically supervised exercise-based measures [34, 136]. In patients with a newly implanted LVAD system, the onset of functional or exercise-based measures should be primarily guided by the individual clinical conditions and the disease progression. Usually LVAD patients require a high degree of individualised and controlled measures, which are often only available in a single care setting [34].

The supervision should be carried out by experienced, well-trained therapists who are familiar with management of the LVAD systems used, the general safety aspects and the special emergency management [34]. The safety aspects listed below must be strictly observed.

## 47.8 Aerobic Endurance Training

The basis of exercise therapy in LVAD patients should be an individually adapted, mild to moderate continuous aerobic endurance training.

- Alternatively, aerobic interval training with short moderate load phases (20–30 s) alternating with recovery phases twice the length (40–60 s) can be performed.
- Initial aerobic endurance training should be performed on a cycle ergometer with monitoring.
- In addition to training on a cycle ergometer, other endurance exercise forms, esp. individualised walking programmes with or without walking aids should be integrated.
  - If tolerated, a walking programme can be repeated several times per day.
  - Treadmill training should initially be avoided due to safety aspects.

- Due to the lack of a pulse, a control of exercise intensity based on heart rate cannot be carried out in the usual manner. Therefore, the use of subjective parameters like Borg-Scale (RPE, rated, perceived exertion) is recommended:
  - A value ≤13 RPE (somewhat hard) can be used as orientation.
  - With good exercise tolerance, the intensity of the exercise load can be increased up to a value of ≤15 RPE (hard/heavy) [34, 45].
- The respiratory rate can also be used to assess exercise intensity via the so-called "Speech Rule", which means that the respiratory rate should permit conversation.
- If CPET was performed, the intensity of ergometer training with permanent exertion can be ascertained as a percentage of the peak $VO_2$ (40–60%), of the $VO_2$ reserve (30–50%) or of the peak load (40–50%) [99, 145, 150]. For interval training, it is possible to start with low intensities (40–50% of the peak load), as exercise tolerance increases, intensive exertion of 75–85% of the peak load can become the target [150].

## 47.9 Resistance Training

An individually adapted resistance training of low to moderate intensity with a low isometric component can be considered as a supplement to (but not as a substitute for) endurance training.

- Special care is required in the exercise selection and choice of training equipment.
- Using a strength training machine can be an advantage because it limits the range of motion and the amplitude of movement, thereby reducing the risk of inadequate exercise performance, with the associated risk of unintentional loading of the driveline.
- The focus of resistance training should be on training the lower limb muscles since they are crucial for carrying the burden of everyday life and are particularly affected by deconditioning.
- A careful individualised introduction of every patient is mandatory.
- Resistance training should be started with a very low intensity (equivalent to <30% of 1RM) and then gradually be adjusted as patient exercise capacity improves.
  - The load should be effortless to perform without evasive movements and/or compressed breathing.
  - As an orientation, the Borg scale can be used (<13 RPE with good load tolerance gradual increase also <15 RPE) [34, 99, 137].
- In the initial state, exercises for the abdominal and back muscles must be avoided. Caution is also required in all exercises for the muscles of the upper extremities and the shoulder girdle, especially in sternotomised patients. In the long term, these exercise forms should also be carefully considered.
- If necessary, respiratory training should be carried out (see Chap. 48).

- Aerobic endurance training and low-dose resistance training are recommended.
- Aerobic endurance training should initially be performed on a cycle ergometer with monitoring.
- Individual training control should be performed using the Borg scale or via percentage of peak $VO_2$, of the $VO_2$ reserve or peak load.
- Resistance training should focus on the lower extremities.
- During resistance training, caution is required in all exercises for the muscles of the upper extremities and the shoulder girdle, especially in sternotomised patients.

## 47.10 Outlook

All recommendations listed here are based on the status quo of current operating techniques, medications and technical systems. When reading and implementing them, the impact of possible future technical developments, changes in drugs and/or new study results must be taken into account.

Within the framework of HTX therapy, future developments are conceivable in immunosuppressive medication, concomitant with impacts on the clinical condition of the patient. Likewise, the increased use of rate-responsive pacemakers is conceivable in order to minimise the consequences of chronotropic incompetence [69]. In the long term, xenotransplantations are also conceivable [47].

The current focus in LVAD therapy research is on the development of a transcutaneous energy transfer and the development of so-called smart pumps. A safe and reliable transcutaneous energy transfer would mean elimination of the driveline, accompanied by enormous advantages regarding general freedom of movement and the possibility of being able to pursue underwater activities. Likewise, severe problems involving infections of the driveline exit site could be prevented [151].

Smart pumps are LVAD systems equipped with sensors which no longer have fixed speed, but which can adapt pump speed to suit the degree of exertion and the cardiac filling status [152]. Current studies show that here, at least in the submaximum region, increases in exercise tolerance can be achieved [153].

In the future, further randomised and controlled studies should be performed in both HTX and LVAD patients in order to be able to evaluate the long-term effects of different exercise interventions with regard to their effectivity and safety.

**Clinical Pearls**

- For patients with terminal HF, the treatments options with beneficial prognoses are HTX and LVAD implantation, with the number of implanted LVADs now considerably exceeding the number of HTX.

- State-of-the-art LVADs are intracorporeal, continuous-flow pumps which operate at a pre-set and fixed rotational speed. The device management and power supply are taken care of by an external controller which is connected to the LVAD via a so-called driveline through the abdominal wall.
- Following HTX and LVAD implantation, specific complications are common and must be attended. Both patient groups are affected by a special hemodynamic situation (HTX: cardiac denervation causing a changed HR pattern; LVAD: fixed pump speed and parallel circulation through LVAD and aortic valve), with HTX patients usually achieving better cardiopulmonary exercise capacity and fewer symptoms than LVAD patients.
- Assessment of functional and cardiopulmonary exercise capacity is recommended in both patient groups, taking into account specific safety aspects.
- Following HTX and LVAD implantation, haemodynamically stable patients should participate in medically supervised exercise-based measures, and all training measures should be continued in the long term. In particular, endurance and strength training should be performed with special regards to the individual status of the patients and specific safety aspects.
- Due to altered HR patterns (HTX patients) or the lack of a pulse wave (LVAD patients) the training control should be carried out primary via Borg-Scale, breathing intensity or percentage of the peak $VO_2$, $VO_2$ reserve or peak workload.

## Review

### Questions

1. Which of the following statements is true regarding the hemodynamic situation and regulation after LVAD implantation?
   (a) Under exercise conditions the LVAD pump speed will automatically adapt to the increased HR to ensure enhanced pump flow.
   (b) Aortic valve insufficiency after LVAD implantation is always asymptomatic and can be ignored because of the supporting function of LVAD.
   (c) Because of the underlying disease LVAD patients have usually good physiological prerequisites for achieving optimal $avDO_2$.
   (d) In LVAD patients, both pump flow and native ejection via the aortic valve can contribute to total CO under exercise conditions.
   (e) In LVAD patients with chronotropic incompetency, there is the possibility to adapt the pump speed manually to improve peripheral perfusion under exercise conditions.
2. Which of the following statements is true regarding the hemodynamic situation and regulation after HTX?
   (a) Only the bicaval technique with resection in the region of both venae cavae lead to a denervation of sympathetic and parasympathetic nerve fibres. Standard excision of the heart with biatrial anastomosis preserves nervation of the sinus node leading to a physiologic HR pattern of the myocardium.

   (b) After an HTX the resting HR is usually lowered due to the lack of sympathetic stimulation of the sinus node.
   (c) Over the long-term course, 15–30% of patients display cardiac reinnervation resulting in a normal HR pattern compared to patients without heart diseases.
   (d) After an HTX circulating epinephrine and norepinephrine play an important role for the HR adaption under exercise conditions.
   (e) Over the long-term course, partial reinnervation is possible in 40–70% of patients. First compensation mechanisms are related to parasympathetic nerve fibres (approximately 6 month after HTX) followed by sympathetic reinnervation (after more than 1–3 years)
3. Which of the following statements is true regarding exercise training in patients after HTX and/or LVAD implantation?
   (a) Moderate resistance training can counteract the negative effects of immunosuppressive therapy on muscle and bone metabolism in patients after LVAD implantation.
   (b) Silent ischaemia displays a significant risk for exercise training in patients after HTX. Therefore, an ischaemia diagnosis is recommended before the onset of exercise training.
   (c) Training control for patients after HTX or LVAD implantation can be carried out most appropriately by HR. Values below 130 bpm are considered safe and correspond to a value ≤13 at the Borg scale ("somewhat hard").
   (d) For patients after HTX or LVAD implantation especially various floor exercises (gymnastics, resistance training, mobilization) are suitable to improve body awareness and strength in the first 3 month after operation.
   (e) For LVAD patients the replacement parts (e.g. charged batteries, controllers, charging stations) should be in stock and they can be used across the different LVAD models through standardization of the appropriate interfaces.

## Answers

1. Question 1
   (a) is not correct as pump speed is currently still fixed and will not adapt to other parameters for safety reasons.
   (b) is not correct as aortic valve insufficiency can cause retrograde circulation from the LVAD to the left ventricle resulting in a further reduction in effective total CO.
   (c) is not correct as peripheral factors such as capillarization, diffusion rate into the muscle cell or mitochondrial capacity are usually reduced in patients with HF.
   (d) **is the correct answer. In LVAD patients, at rest the predominant proportion of total CO flows over the pump. With increasing physical exercise, in most of the patients an additional blood volume can be ejected via the aortic valve.**

   (e) is not correct as pump speed is currently still fixed. An LVAD monitor is required to adjust the pump speed manually. LVAD monitors are not given to patients, but only to authorized medical stuff.
2. Question 2
   (a) is not correct as both techniques are leading to denervation of parasympathetic and sympathetic nerve fibres in the myocardium accompanied by an altered HR pattern.
   (b) is not correct as resting HR is usually elevated (approximately 95 bpm) due to the lack of parasympathetic control.
   (c) is not correct as 40–70% of patients display cardiac reinnervation over the long-term course. However, the overall results are still inferior compared to subjects without heart disease.
   (d) **is the correct answer. Denervation leads to an emptying of the catecholamine storage of the myocardium, in turn leading to a dependence of the donor organ on circulating catecholamines.**
   (e) is not correct as first nerval compensation mechanisms will usually affect the sympathetic fibres (approximately 6 month after HTX) followed by parasympathetic reinnervation (after more than 1–3 years).
3. Question 3
   (a) is not correct. LVAD patients usually do not take immunosuppressive medications, but oral anticoagulants. For HTX patients, however, this statement would be true.
   (b) **is the correct answer. CAV represents a common complication after HTX and should be negated before the onset of exercise training since a denervated heart gives no warning symptoms (silent ischaemia)**
   (c) is not correct for both groups. Due to changed HR patterns (HTX patients) or the lack of pulse wave (LVAD patients) the training control should be carried out primary via the Borg scale, breathing intensity or percentage of the peak $VO_2$, $VO_2$ reserve or peak load.
   (d) is not correct. For patients after median sternotomy all exercise measures should be gentle to the sternum, at least in the first months. In addition, for LVAD patients rapid changes of the body position should always be avoided due to blood volume shifts and the risk for suction events. Also, for the LVAD system and the driveline it is important that all activities that could lead to an uncontrolled, inadequate load on the system must be strictly avoided. Therefore, the use of a strength training machine can be an advantage because it limits the range of motion and the amplitude of movement with reducing the risk of unintentional loading of the driveline.
   (e) is not correct as for the different LVAD systems also different replacement parts are required.

## References

1. Mosterd A, Hoes AW. Clinical epidemiology of heart failure. Heart. 2007;93(9):1137–46.
2. Redfield MM, Jacobsen SJ, Burnett JC, Mahoney DW, Bailey KR, Rodeheffer RJ. Burden of systolic and diastolic ventricular dysfunction in the community: appreciating the scope of the heart failure epidemic. JAMA. 2003;289(2):194–202.
3. Roger VL, Weston SA, Redfield MM, Hellermann-Homan JP, Killian J, Yawn BP, et al. Trends in heart failure incidence and survival in a community-based population. JAMA. 2004;292(3):344–50.
4. Yancy CW, Jessup M, Bozkurt B, Butler J, Casey DE, Drazner MH, et al. 2013 ACCF/AHA guideline for the management of heart failure: A report of the American College of Cardiology Foundation/American Heart Association Task Force on Practice Guidelines. J Am Coll Cardiol. 2013;62(16):e147–239.
5. Stehlik J, Kobashigawa J, Hunt SA, Reichenspurner H, Kirklin JK. Honoring 50 years of clinical heart transplantation in circulation: in-depth state-of-the-art review. Circulation. 2018;137(1):71–87.
6. Lund LH, Edwards LB, Kucheryavaya AY, Benden C, Dipchand AI, Goldfarb S, et al. The registry of the International Society for Heart and Lung Transplantation: thirty-second official adult heart transplantation report—; focus theme: early graft failure. J Heart Lung Transplant. 2015;34(10):1244–54.
7. Stewart GC, Givertz MM. Mechanical circulatory support for advanced heart failure: patients and technology in evolution. Circulation. 2012;125(10):1304–15.
8. Kirklin JK, Pagani FD, Kormos RL, Stevenson LW, Blume ED, Myers SL, et al. Eighth annual INTERMACS report: special focus on framing the impact of adverse events. J Heart Lung Transplant. 2017;36(10):1080–6.
9. Beckmann A, Meyer R, Lewandowski J, Frie M, Markewitz A, Harringer W. German heart surgery report 2017: the annual updated registry of the German society for thoracic and cardiovascular surgery. Thorac Cardiovasc Surg. 2018;66(8):608–21.
10. Beckmann A, Funkat A-K, Lewandowski J, Frie M, Ernst M, Hekmat K, et al. German heart surgery report 2015: the annual updated registry of the German society for thoracic and cardiovascular surgery. Thorac Cardiovasc Surg. 2016;64(6):462–74.
11. Eurotransplant. Transplants in Germany, by year, by donor type, by organ type: statistics. eurotransplant.org: 2212P_Germany: 17.03.2016: counting recipient transplants by organ type; 2016.
12. Eurotransplant. Heart transplants in Germany, by year, by donor type, by organ combination: statistics.eurotransplant.org: 2052P_Germany_heart: 09.04.2018: counting recipient transplants; 2018.
13. DeBakey ME. Left ventricular bypass pump for cardiac assistance. Am J Cardiol. 1971;27(1):3–11.
14. Birks EJ. Left ventricular assist devices. Heart. 2010;96(1):63–71.
15. Patel CB, Alexander KM, Rogers JG. Mechanical circulatory support for advanced heart failure. Curr Treat Options Cardiovasc Med. 2010;12(6):549–65.
16. Maciver J, Ross HJ. Quality of life and left ventricular assist device support. Circulation. 2012;126(7):866–74.
17. Moazami N, Fukamachi K, Kobayashi M, Smedira NG, Hoercher KJ, Massiello A, et al. Axial and centrifugal continuous-flow rotary pumps: a translation from pump mechanics to clinical practice. J Heart Lung Transplant. 2013;32(1):1–11.
18. Larose JA, Tamez D, Ashenuga M, Reyes C. Design concepts and principle of operation of the HeartWare ventricular assist system. ASAIO J. 2010;56(4):285–9.

19. Netuka I, Sood P, Pya Y, Zimpfer D, Krabatsch T, Garbade J, et al. Fully magnetically levitated left ventricular assist system for treating advanced HF: a multicenter study. J Am Coll Cardiol. 2015;66(23):2579–89.
20. Wieselthaler GM, O Driscoll G, Jansz P, Khaghani A, Strueber M. Initial clinical experience with a novel left ventricular assist device with a magnetically levitated rotor in a multi-institutional trial. J Heart Lung Transplant. 2010;29(11):1218–25.
21. Medtronic Inc. HVAD® Pump; 2018 [cited 2018 Dec 18]. https://www.heartware.com/sites/default/files/fields/library/hvad-pump_0.jpg.
22. Medtronic Inc. Implanted HVAD® Pump; 2018. https://www.heartware.com/sites/default/files/fields/library/carrying_case-high.jpg.
23. Schmitto JD, Zimpfer D, Fiane AE, Larbalestier R, Tsui S, Jansz P, et al. Long-term support of patients receiving a left ventricular assist device for advanced heart failure: a follow-up analysis of the registry to evaluate the HeartWare left ventricular assist system. Eur J Cardiothorac Surg. 2016;50(5):834–8.
24. Hanke JS, Rojas SV, Mahr C, Schmidt A-F, Zoch A, Dogan G, et al. Five-year results of patients supported by HeartMate II: outcomes and adverse events. Eur J Cardiothorac Surg. 2018;53(2):422–7.
25. Gosev I, Kiernan MS, Eckman P, Soleimani B, Kilic A, Uriel N, et al. Long-term survival in patients receiving a continuous-flow left ventricular assist device. Ann Thorac Surg. 2018;105(3):696–701.
26. Rizvi S-SA, Luc JGY, Choi JH, Phan K, Moncho Escrivà E, Patel S, et al. Outcomes and survival following heart retransplantation for cardiac allograft failure: a systematic review and meta-analysis. Ann Cardiothoracic Surg. 2018;7(1):12–8.
27. Alraies MC, Eckman P. Adult heart transplant: indications and outcomes. J Thorac Dis. 2014;6(8):1120–8.
28. Kirklin JK, Naftel DC, Pagani FD, Kormos RL, Stevenson LW, Blume ED, et al. Seventh INTERMACS annual report: 15,000 patients and counting. J Heart Lung Transplant. 2015;34(12):1495–504.
29. Pinney SP, Anyanwu AC, Lala A, Teuteberg JJ, Uriel N, Mehra MR. Left ventricular assist devices for lifelong support. J Am Coll Cardiol. 2017;69(23):2845–61.
30. Schüchtermann-Schiller'sche Kliniken Bad Rothenfelde GmbH & Co. KG. LVAD-patient during cardiopulmonary exercise testing; 2017.
31. Malhotra R, Bakken K, D'Elia E, Lewis GD. Cardiopulmonary exercise testing in heart failure. JACC Heart Fail. 2016;4(8):607–16.
32. Crespo-Leiro MG, Metra M, Lund LH, Milicic D, Costanzo MR, Filippatos G, et al. Advanced heart failure: a position statement of the heart failure Association of the European Society of cardiology. Eur Heart J. 2018;20(11):1505–35.
33. Hasin T, Topilsky Y, Kremers WK, Boilson BA, Schirger JA, Edwards BS, et al. Usefulness of the six-minute walk test after continuous axial flow left ventricular device implantation to predict survival. Am J Cardiol. 2012;110(9):1322–8.
34. Willemsen D, Cordes C, Bjarnason-Wehrens B, Knoglinger E, Langheim E, Marx R, et al. Rehabilitation standards for follow-up treatment and rehabilitation of patients with ventricular assist device (VAD). Clin Res Cardiol Suppl. 2016;11(Suppl 1):2–49.
35. Tsai H-Y, Tsai W-J, Kuo L-Y, Lin Y-S, Chen B-Y, Lin W-H, et al. Oxygen consumption at anaerobic threshold predicts cardiac events after heart transplantation. Transplant Proc. 2018;50(9):2742–6.
36. Mathur S, Janaudis-Ferreira T, Wickerson L, Singer LG, Patcai J, Rozenberg D, et al. Meeting report: consensus recommendations for a research agenda in exercise in solid organ transplantation. Am J Transplant. 2014;14(10):2235–45.
37. Raichlin E, Selim A, Zolty R, Burdorf A, Siddique A, Moulton MJ, et al. Cardiopulmonary stress test one year after HTx predicts the development of CAV. J Heart Lung Transplant. 2017;36(4):S296.
38. Yardley M, Havik OE, Grov I, Relbo A, Gullestad L, Nytrøen K. Peak oxygen uptake and self-reported physical health are strong predictors of long-term survival after heart transplantation. Clin Transpl. 2016;30(2):161–9.

39. Reiss N, Schmidt T, Langheim E, Bjarnason-Wehrens B, Marx R, Sindermann JR et al. Inpatient cardiac rehabilitation of LVAD patients-updated recommendations from the working group of the German Society for prevention and rehabilitation of cardiovascular diseases. Thorac Cardiovasc Surg. 2019. https://doi.org/10.1055/s-0039-1691837. [Epub ahead of print].
40. Reiss N, Schmidt T, Workowski A, Willemsen D, Schmitto JD, Haverich A, et al. Physical capacity in LVAD patients: hemodynamic principles, diagnostic tools and training control. Int J Artif Organs. 2016;39(9):451–9.
41. Reiss N, Schmidt T, Mommertz S, Feldmann C, Schmitto JD. Inert gas rebreathing - helpful tool in the management of left ventricular assist device patients. Perfusion. 2018;33(5):335–8.
42. Guazzi M, Arena R, Halle M, Piepoli MF, Myers J, Lavie CJ. 2016 focused update: clinical recommendations for cardiopulmonary exercise testing data assessment in specific patient populations. Eur Heart J. 2018;39(14):1144–61.
43. Pollentier B, Irons SL, Benedetto CM, Dibenedetto A-M, Loton D, Seyler RD, et al. Examination of the six minute walk test to determine functional capacity in people with chronic heart failure: a systematic review. Cardiopulm Phys Ther J. 2010;21(1):13–21.
44. Corrà U, Piepoli MF, Adamopoulos S, Agostoni P, Coats AJS, Conraads V, et al. Cardiopulmonary exercise testing in systolic heart failure in 2014: the evolving prognostic role: a position paper from the committee on exercise physiology and training of the heart failure association of the ESC. Eur J Heart Fail. 2014;16(9):929–41.
45. Scheiderer R, Belden C, Schwab D, Haney C, Paz J. Exercise guidelines for inpatients following ventricular assist device placement: a systematic review of the literature. Cardiopulm Phys Ther J. 2013;24(2):35–42.
46. Lund LH, Khush KK, Cherikh WS, Goldfarb S, Kucheryavaya AY, Levvey BJ, et al. The registry of the International Society for Heart and Lung Transplantation: thirty-fourth adult heart transplantation report-2017; focus theme: allograft ischemic time. J Heart Lung Transplant. 2017;36(10):1037–46.
47. Kim IC, Youn JC, Kobashigawa JA. The past, present and future of heart transplantation. Korean Circ J. 2018;48(7):565–90.
48. Kavanagh T, Mertens DJ, Shephard RJ, Beyene J, Kennedy J, Campbell R, et al. Long-term cardiorespiratory results of exercise training following cardiac transplantation. Am J Cardiol. 2003;91(2):190–4.
49. Zoll J, N'Guessan B, Ribera F, Lampert E, Fortin D, Veksler V, et al. Preserved response of mitochondrial function to short-term endurance training in skeletal muscle of heart transplant recipients. J Am Coll Cardiol. 2003;42(1):126–32.
50. Braith RW, Magyari PM, Pierce GL, Edwards DG, Hill JA, White LJ, et al. Effect of resistance exercise on skeletal muscle myopathy in heart transplant recipients. Am J Cardiol. 2005;95(10):1192–8.
51. Bussières LM, Pflugfelder PW, Taylor AW, Noble EG, Kostuk WJ. Changes in skeletal muscle morphology and biochemistry after cardiac transplantation. Am J Cardiol. 1997;79(5):630–4.
52. Stratton JR, Kemp GJ, Daly RC, Yacoub M, Rajagopalan B. Effects of cardiac transplantation on bioenergetic abnormalities of skeletal muscle in congestive heart failure. Circulation. 1994;89(4):1624–31.
53. Lampert E, Mettauer B, HOPPELER H, Charloux A, Charpentier A, Lonsdorfer J. Structure of skeletal muscle in heart transplant recipients. J Am Coll Cardiol. 1996;28(4):980–4.
54. Henderson NK, Sambrook PN, Kelly PJ, Macdonald P, Keogh AM, Spratt P, et al. Bone mineral loss and recovery after cardiac transplantation. Lancet. 1995;346(8979):905.
55. Givertz MM, Hartley LH, Colucci WS. Long-term sequential changes in exercise capacity and chronotropic responsiveness after cardiac transplantation. Circulation. 1997;96(1):232–7.
56. Nytrøen K, Gullestad L. Exercise after heart transplantation: an overview. World J Transplant. 2013;3(4):78–90.
57. Haykowsky MJ, Halle M, Baggish A. Upper limits of aerobic power and performance in heart transplant recipients: legacy effect of prior endurance training. Circulation. 2018;137(7):650–2.
58. Anyanwu A, Treasure T. Prognosis after heart transplantation: transplants alone cannot be the solution for end stage heart failure. BMJ. 2003;326(7388):509–10.

59. Kelly RL, Walsh JR, Paratz JD, Yerkovich ST, McKenzie SC, Morris NR. Quadriceps muscle strength and body mass index are associated with estimates of physical activity postheart transplantation. Transplantation. 2019;103(6):1253–9.
60. Chen S-Y, Lu P-C, Lan C, Chou N-K, Chen Y-S, Lai J-S, et al. Six-minute walk test among heart transplant recipients. Transplant Proc. 2014;46(3):929–33.
61. Doutreleau S, Di Marco P, Talha S, Charloux A, Piquard F, Geny B. Can the six-minute walk test predict peak oxygen uptake in men with heart transplant? Arch Phys Med Rehabil. 2009;90(1):51–7.
62. John R, Liao K. Orthotopic heart transplantation. Oper Tech Thorac Cardiovasc Surg. 2010;15(2):138–46.
63. Jungschleger JGM, Boldyrev SY, Kaleda VI, Dark JH. Standard orthotopic heart transplantation. Ann Cardiothoracic Surg. 2018;7(1):169–71.
64. Kobashigawa J, Olymbios M. Physiology of the transplanted heart. In: Kobashigawa J, editor. Clinical guide to heart transplantation. Cham: Springer International Publishing; 2017. p. 81–93.
65. Awad M, Czer LSC, Hou M, Golshani SS, Goltche M, de Robertis M et al. Early denervation and later reinnervation of the heart following cardiac transplantation: a review. J Am Heart Assoc. 2016; 5(11).
66. Tallaj JA, Kirklin JK, Brown RN, Rayburn BK, Bourge RC, Benza RL, et al. Post-heart transplant diastolic dysfunction is a risk factor for mortality. J Am Coll Cardiol. 2007;50(11):1064–9.
67. Paulus WJ, Bronzwaer JG, Felice H, Kishan N, Wellens F. Deficient acceleration of left ventricular relaxation during exercise after heart transplantation. Circulation. 1992;86(4):1175–85.
68. Kao AC, van Trigt P, Shaeffer-McCall GS, Shaw JP, Kuzil BB, Page RD, et al. Central and peripheral limitations to upright exercise in untrained cardiac transplant recipients. Circulation. 1994;89(6):2605–15.
69. Braith RW, Clapp L, Brown T, Brown C, Schofield R, Mills RM, et al. Rate-responsive pacing improves exercise tolerance in heart transplant recipients: a pilot study. J Cardpulm Rehabil. 2000;20(6):377–82.
70. Braith RW, Wood CE, Limacher MC, Pollock ML, Lowenthal DT, Phillips MI, et al. Abnormal neuroendocrine responses during exercise in heart transplant recipients. Circulation. 1992;86(5):1453–63.
71. Pflugfelder PW, Purves PD, McKenzie FN, Kostuk WJ. Cardiac dynamics during supine exercise in cyclosporine-treated orthotopic heart transplant recipients: assessment by radionuclide angiography. J Am Coll Cardiol. 1987;10(2):336–41.
72. Rosenbaum AN, Kremers WK, Schirger JA, Thomas RJ, Squires RW, Allison TG, et al. Association between early cardiac rehabilitation and long-term survival in cardiac transplant recipients. Mayo Clin Proc. 2016;91(2):149–56.
73. Anderson L, Nguyen TT, Dall CH, Burgess L, Bridges C, Taylor RS. Exercise-based cardiac rehabilitation in heart transplant recipients. Cochrane Database Syst Rev. 2017;4:CD012264.
74. Hsieh P-L, Wu Y-T, Chao W-J. Effects of exercise training in heart transplant recipients: a meta-analysis. Cardiology. 2011;120(1):27–35.
75. Didsbury M, McGee RG, Tong A, Craig JC, Chapman JR, Chadban S, et al. Exercise training in solid organ transplant recipients: a systematic review and meta-analysis. Transplantation. 2013;95(5):679–87.
76. Tegtbur U, Busse MW, Jung K, Pethig K, Haverich A. Time course of physical reconditioning during exercise rehabilitation late after heart transplantation. J Heart Lung Transplant. 2005;24(3):270–4.
77. Pascoalino LN, Ciolac EG, Tavares AC, Castro RE, Ayub-Ferreira SM, Bacal F, et al. Exercise training improves ambulatory blood pressure but not arterial stiffness in heart transplant recipients. J Heart Lung Transplant. 2015;34(5):693–700.
78. Schmidt A, Pleiner J, Bayerle-Eder M, Wiesinger GF, Rödler S, Quittan M, et al. Regular physical exercise improves endothelial function in heart transplant recipients. Clin Transpl. 2002;16(2):137–43.

79. Braith RW, Schofield RS, Hill JA, Casey DP, Pierce GL. Exercise training attenuates progressive decline in brachial artery reactivity in heart transplant recipients. J Heart Lung Transplant. 2008;27(1):52–9.
80. Pierce GL, Schofield RS, Casey DP, Hamlin SA, Hill JA, Braith RW. Effects of exercise training on forearm and calf vasodilation and proinflammatory markers in recent heart transplant recipients: a pilot study. Eur J Cardiovas Prev Rehabil. 2008;15(1):10–8.
81. Karapolat H, Engin C, Eroglu M, Yagdi T, Zoghi M, Nalbantgil S, et al. Efficacy of the cardiac rehabilitation program in patients with end-stage heart failure, heart transplant patients, and left ventricular assist device recipients. Transplant Proc. 2013;45(9):3381–5.
82. Tegtbur U, Busse MW, Jung K, Markofsky A, Machold H, Brinkmeier U, et al. Phase III rehabilitation after heart transplantation. Z Kardiol. 2003;92(11):908–15.
83. Wu Y-T, Chien C-L, Chou N-K, Wang S-S, Lai J-S, Wu Y-W. Efficacy of a home-based exercise program for orthotopic heart transplant recipients. Cardiology. 2008;111(2):87–93.
84. Kugler C, Malehsa D, Tegtbur U, Guetzlaff E, Meyer AL, Bara C, et al. Health-related quality of life and exercise tolerance in recipients of heart transplants and left ventricular assist devices: a prospective, comparative study. J Heart Lung Transplant. 2011;30(2):204–10.
85. Nytrøen K, Rustad LA, Aukrust P, Ueland T, Hallén J, Holm I, et al. High-intensity interval training improves peak oxygen uptake and muscular exercise capacity in heart transplant recipients. Am J Transplant. 2012;12(11):3134–42.
86. Rustad LA, Nytrøen K, Amundsen BH, Gullestad L, Aakhus S. One year of high-intensity interval training improves exercise capacity, but not left ventricular function in stable heart transplant recipients: a randomised controlled trial. Eur J Prev Cardiol. 2014;21(2):181–91.
87. Monk-Hansen T, Dall CH, Christensen SB, Snoer M, Gustafsson F, Rasmusen H, et al. Interval training does not modulate diastolic function in heart transplant recipients. Scand Cardiovasc J. 2014;48(2):91–8.
88. Nytrøen K, Rustad LA, Erikstad I, Aukrust P, Ueland T, Lekva T, et al. Effect of high-intensity interval training on progression of cardiac allograft vasculopathy. J Heart Lung Transplant. 2013;32(11):1073–80.
89. Hermann TS, Dall CH, Christensen SB, Goetze JP, Prescott E, Gustafsson F. Effect of high intensity exercise on peak oxygen uptake and endothelial function in long-term heart transplant recipients. Am J Transplant. 2011;11(3):536–41.
90. Christensen SB, Dall CH, Prescott E, Pedersen SS, Gustafsson F. A high-intensity exercise program improves exercise capacity, self-perceived health, anxiety and depression in heart transplant recipients: a randomized, controlled trial. J Heart Lung Transplant. 2012;31(1):106–7.
91. Dall CH, Snoer M, Christensen S, Monk-Hansen T, Frederiksen M, Gustafsson F, et al. Effect of high-intensity training versus moderate training on peak oxygen uptake and chronotropic response in heart transplant recipients: a randomized crossover trial. Am J Transplant. 2014;14(10):2391–9.
92. Dall CH, Gustafsson F, Christensen SB, Dela F, Langberg H, Prescott E. Effect of moderate- versus high-intensity exercise on vascular function, biomarkers and quality of life in heart transplant recipients: a randomized, crossover trial. J Heart Lung Transplant. 2015;34(8):1033–41.
93. DeCampli WM. Of mice and men ... does exercise decrease progression of transplant coronary vasculopathy? J Thorac Cardiovasc Surg. 2015;149(1):337–9.
94. Braith RW, Mills RM, Welsch MA, Keller JW, Pollock ML. Resistance exercise training restores bone mineral density in heart transplant recipients. J Am Coll Cardiol. 1996;28(6):1471–7.
95. Braith RW, Welsch MA, Mills RM, Keller JW, Pollock ML. Resistance exercise prevents glucocorticoid-induced myopathy in heart transplant recipients. Med Sci Sports Exerc. 1998;30(4):483–9.
96. Braith RW, Magyari PM, Fulton MN, Aranda J, Walker T, Hill JA. Resistance exercise training and alendronate reverse glucocorticoid-induced osteoporosis in heart transplant recipients. J Heart Lung Transplant. 2003;22(10):1082–90.

97. Costanzo MR, Dipchand A, Starling R, Anderson A, Chan M, Desai S, et al. The International Society of Heart and Lung Transplantation Guidelines for the care of heart transplant recipients. J Heart Lung Transplant. 2010;29(8):914–56.
98. Yardley M, Gullestad L, Bendz B, Bjørkelund E, Rolid K, Arora S et al. Long-term effects of high-intensity interval training in heart transplant recipients: a 5-year follow-up study of a randomized controlled trial. Clin Transpl. 2017;31(1).
99. Vanhees L, Rauch B, Piepoli M, van Buuren F, Takken T, Börjesson M, et al. Importance of characteristics and modalities of physical activity and exercise in the management of cardiovascular health in individuals with cardiovascular disease (part III). Eur J Prev Cardiol. 2012;19(6):1333–56.
100. Squires RW. Exercise therapy for cardiac transplant recipients. Prog Cardiovasc Dis. 2011;53(6):429–36.
101. Ehrman JK, Keteyian SJ, Levine AB, Rhoads KL, Elder LR, Levine TB, et al. Exercise stress tests after cardiac transplantation. Am J Cardiol. 1993;71(15):1372–3.
102. Mehra MR, Goldstein DJ, Uriel N, Cleveland JC, Yuzefpolskaya M, Salerno C, et al. Two-year outcomes with a magnetically levitated cardiac pump in heart failure. N Engl J Med. 2018;378(15):1386–95.
103. Gustafsson F, Rogers JG. Left ventricular assist device therapy in advanced heart failure: patient selection and outcomes. Eur J Heart Fail. 2017;19(5):595–602.
104. Hildebrandt A, Willemsen D, Reiss N, Bartsch P, Schmidt T, Bjarnason-Wehrens B. Characteristics, therapeutic needs, and scope of patients with a continuous-flow left ventricular device entering cardiac rehabilitation: a RETROSPECTIVE ANALYSIS. J Cardiopulm Rehabil Prev. 2019;39(2):91–6.
105. Hernandez RE, Singh SK, Hoang DT, Ali SW, Elayda MA, Mallidi HR, et al. Present-day hospital readmissions after left ventricular assist device implantation: a large single-center study. Tex Heart Inst J. 2015;42(5):419–29.
106. McCarthy FH, Kobrin D, Rame JE, Groeneveld PW, McDermott KM, Atluri P, et al. Increasing Frequency of Left Ventricular Assist Device Exchanges in the United States. Ann Thorac Surg. 2015;100(5):1660–4; discussion 1665
107. Kerrigan DJ, Williams CT, Ehrman JK, Bronsteen K, Saval MA, Schairer JR, et al. Muscular strength and cardiorespiratory fitness are associated with health status in patients with recently implanted continuous-flow LVADs. J Cardiopulm Rehabil Prev. 2013;33(6):396–400.
108. Chung CJ, Wu C, Jones M, Kato TS, Dam TT, Givens RC, et al. Reduced handgrip strength as a marker of frailty predicts clinical outcomes in patients with heart failure undergoing ventricular assist device placement. J Card Fail. 2014;20(5):310–5.
109. Rogers JG, Aaronson KD, Boyle AJ, Russell SD, Milano CA, Pagani FD, et al. Continuous flow left ventricular assist device improves functional capacity and quality of life of advanced heart failure patients. J Am Coll Cardiol. 2010;55(17):1826–34.
110. Granegger M, Schlöglhofer T, Ober H, Zimpfer D, Schima H, Moscato F. Daily life activity in patients with left ventricular assist devices. Int J Artif Organs. 2016;39(1):22–7.
111. Leibner ES, Cysyk J, Eleuteri K, El-Banayosy A, Boehmer JP, Pae WE. Changes in the functional status measures of heart failure patients with mechanical assist devices. ASAIO J. 2013;59(2):117–22.
112. Compostella L, Russo N, Setzu T, Compostella C, Bellotto F. Exercise performance of chronic heart failure patients in the early period of support by an axial-flow left ventricular assist device as destination therapy. Artif Organs. 2014;38(5):366–73.
113. Marko C, Danzinger G, Käferbäck M, Lackner T, Müller R, Zimpfer D, et al. Safety and efficacy of cardiac rehabilitation for patients with continuous flow left ventricular assist devices. Eur J Prev Cardiol. 2015;22(11):1378–84.
114. Marko C, Xhelili E, Lackner T, Zimpfer D, Schima H, Moscato F. Exercise performance during the first two years after left ventricular assist device implantation. ASAIO J. 2017;63(4):408–13.
115. Schmidt T, Bjarnason-Wehrens B, Bartsch P, Deniz E, Schmitto J, Schulte-Eistrup S, et al. Exercise capacity and functional performance in heart failure patients supported by a left ventricular assist device at discharge from inpatient rehabilitation. Artif Organs. 2018;42(1):22–30.

116. Schmidt T, Bjarnason-Wehrens B, Mommertz S, Schulte-Eistrup S, Willemsen D, Sindermann J, et al. Development of exercise-related values in heart failure patients supported with a left ventricular assist device. Int J Artif Organs. 2019;42(4):201–6.
117. Nahumi N, Morrison KA, Garan AR, Uriel N, Jorde UP. Peak exercise capacity is a poor indicator of functional capacity for patients supported by a continuous-flow left ventricular assist device. J Heart Lung Transplant. 2014;33(2):213–5.
118. Khawaja T, Chokshi A, Ji R, Kato TS, Xu K, Zizola C, et al. Ventricular assist device implantation improves skeletal muscle function, oxidative capacity, and growth hormone/insulin-like growth factor-1 axis signaling in patients with advanced heart failure. J Cachexia Sarcopenia Msucle. 2014;5(4):297–305.
119. Kugler C, Malehsa D, Schrader E, Tegtbur U, Guetzlaff E, Haverich A, et al. A multimodal intervention in management of left ventricular assist device outpatients: dietary counselling, controlled exercise and psychosocial support. Eur J Cardiothorac Surg. 2012;42(6):1026–32.
120. Jung MH, Gustafsson F. Exercise in heart failure patients supported with a left ventricular assist device. J Heart Lung Transplant. 2015;34(4):489–96.
121. Loyaga-Rendon RY, Plaisance EP, Arena R, Shah K. Exercise physiology, testing, and training in patients supported by a left ventricular assist device. J Heart Lung Transplant. 2015;34(8):1005–16.
122. Joyner MJ, Casey DP. Regulation of increased blood flow (hyperemia) to muscles during exercise: a hierarchy of competing physiological needs. Physiol Rev. 2015;95(2):549–601.
123. Schüchtermann-Schiller'sche Kliniken Bad Rothenfelde GmbH & Co. KG. Special haemodynamic situation in LVAD patients; 2015.
124. Bouabdallaoui N, El-Hamamsy I, Pham M, Giraldeau G, Parent M-C, Carrier M, et al. Aortic regurgitation in patients with a left ventricular assist device: a contemporary review. J Heart Lung Transplant. 2018;37(11):1289–97.
125. Truby LK, Garan AR, Givens RC, Wayda B, Takeda K, Yuzefpolskaya M, et al. Aortic insufficiency during contemporary left ventricular assist device support: analysis of the INTERMACS Registry. JACC Heart Fail. 2018;6(11):951–60.
126. Dimopoulos S, Diakos N, Tseliou E, Tasoulis A, Mpouchla A, Manetos C, et al. Chronotropic incompetence and abnormal heart rate recovery early after left ventricular assist device implantation. Pacing Clin Electrophysiol. 2011;34(12):1607–14.
127. Grosman-Rimon L, Lalonde SD, Sieh N, Pakosh M, Rao V, Oh P, et al. Exercise rehabilitation in ventricular assist device recipients: a meta-analysis of effects on physiological and clinical outcomes. Heart Fail Rev. 2019;24(1):55–67.
128. Andersen M, Gustafsson F, Madsen PL, Brassard P, Jensen AS, Secher N, et al. Hemodynamic stress echocardiography in patients supported with a continuous-flow left ventricular assist device. JACC Cardiovasc Imaging. 2010;3(8):854–9.
129. Jakovljevic DG, Birks EJ, George RS, Trenell MI, Seferovic PM, Yacoub MH, et al. Relationship between peak cardiac pumping capability and selected exercise-derived prognostic indicators in patients treated with left ventricular assist devices. Eur J Heart Fail. 2011;13(9):992–9.
130. Jacquet L, Vancaenegem O, Pasquet A, Matte P, Poncelet A, Price J, et al. Exercise capacity in patients supported with rotary blood pumps is improved by a spontaneous increase of pump flow at constant pump speed and by a rise in native cardiac output. Artif Organs. 2011;35(7):682–90.
131. Brassard P, Jensen AS, Nordsborg N, Gustafsson F, Møller JE, Hassager C, et al. Central and peripheral blood flow during exercise with a continuous-flow left ventricular assist device: constant versus increasing pump speed: a pilot study. Circ Heart Fail. 2011;4(5):554–60.
132. Muthiah K, Robson D, Prichard R, Walker R, Gupta S, Keogh AM, et al. Effect of exercise and pump speed modulation on invasive hemodynamics in patients with centrifugal continuous-flow left ventricular assist devices. J Heart Lung Transplant. 2015;34(4):522–9.

133. Vignati C, Apostolo A, Cattadori G, Farina S, Del Torto A, Scuri S, et al. Lvad pump speed increase is associated with increased peak exercise cardiac output and vo2, postponed anaerobic threshold and improved ventilatory efficiency. Int J Cardiol. 2017;230:28–32.
134. Schmidt T, Bjarnason-Wehrens B, Mommertz S, Hannig M, Schulte-Eistrup S, Willemsen D, et al. Changes in total cardiac output and oxygen extraction during exercise in patients supported with an HVAD left ventricular assist device. Artif Organs. 2018;42(7):686–94.
135. Brooks GA, Fahey TD, Baldwin KM. Exercise physiology: human bioenergetics and its applications. 4th ed. Boston: McGraw-Hill; 2005.
136. Adamopoulos S, Corrà U, Laoutaris ID, Pistono M, Agostoni PG, Coats AJS, et al. Exercise training in patients with ventricular assist devices: a review of the evidence and practical advice. A position paper from the committee on exercise physiology and training and the Committee of Advanced Heart Failure of the heart failure Association of the European Society of cardiology. Eur J Heart Fail. 2019;21(1):3–13.
137. Piepoli MF, Conraads V, Corrà U, Dickstein K, Francis DP, Jaarsma T, et al. Exercise training in heart failure: from theory to practice. A consensus document of the heart failure association and the European Association for Cardiovascular Prevention and Rehabilitation. Eur J Heart Fail. 2011;13(4):347–57.
138. Alsara O, Perez-Terzic C, Squires RW, Dandamudi S, Miranda WR, Park SJ, et al. Is exercise training safe and beneficial in patients receiving left ventricular assist device therapy? J Cardiopulm Rehabil Prev. 2014;34(4):233–40.
139. Compostella L, Russo N, Setzu T, Bottio T, Compostella C, Tarzia V, et al. A practical review for cardiac rehabilitation professionals of continuous-flow left ventricular assist devices: historical and current perspectives. J Cardiopulm Rehabil Prev. 2015;35(5):301–11.
140. Ganga HV, Leung A, Jantz J, Choudhary G, Stabile L, Levine DJ, et al. Supervised exercise training versus usual care in ambulatory patients with left ventricular assist devices: a systematic review. PLoS One. 2017;12(3):e0174323.
141. Mahfood Haddad T, Saurav A, Smer A, Azzouz MS, Akinapelli A, Williams MA, et al. Cardiac rehabilitation in patients with left ventricular assist device: a SYSTEMATIC REVIEW AND META-ANALYSIS. J Cardiopulm Rehabil Prev. 2017;37(6):390–6.
142. Yamamoto S, Hotta K, Ota E, Matsunaga A, Mori R. Exercise-based cardiac rehabilitation for people with implantable ventricular assist devices. Cochrane Database Syst Rev. 2018;9:CD012222.
143. English ML, Speed J. Effectiveness of acute inpatient rehabilitation after left ventricular assist device placement. Am J Phys Med Rehabil. 2013;92(7):621–6.
144. Laoutaris ID, Dritsas A, Adamopoulos S, Manginas A, Gouziouta A, Kallistratos MS, et al. Benefits of physical training on exercise capacity, inspiratory muscle function, and quality of life in patients with ventricular assist devices long-term postimplantation. Eur J Cardiovas Prev Rehabil. 2011;18(1):33–40.
145. Hayes K, Leet AS, Bradley SJ, Holland AE. Effects of exercise training on exercise capacity and quality of life in patients with a left ventricular assist device: a preliminary randomized controlled trial. J Heart Lung Transplant. 2012;31(7):729–34.
146. Kerrigan DJ, Williams CT, Ehrman JK, Saval MA, Bronsteen K, Schairer JR, et al. Cardiac rehabilitation improves functional capacity and patient-reported health status in patients with continuous-flow left ventricular assist devices: The Rehab-VAD randomized controlled trial. JACC Heart Fail. 2014;2(6):653–9.
147. Bachmann JM, Duncan MS, Shah AS, Greevy RA, Lindenfeld J, Keteyian SJ, et al. Association of cardiac rehabilitation with decreased hospitalizations and mortality after ventricular assist device implantation. JACC Heart Fail. 2018;6(2):130–9.
148. Feldman D, Pamboukian SV, Teuteberg JJ, Birks E, Lietz K, Moore SA, et al. The 2013 International Society for Heart and Lung Transplantation guidelines for mechanical circulatory support: executive summary. J Heart Lung Transplant. 2013;32(2):157–87.
149. Wells CL. Physical therapist management of patients with ventricular assist devices: key considerations for the acute care physical therapist. Phys Ther. 2013;93(2):266–78.

150. Ellingsen Ø, Halle M, Conraads V, Støylen A, Dalen H, Delagardelle C, et al. High-intensity interval training in patients with heart failure with reduced ejection fraction. Circulation. 2017;135(9):839–49.
151. Bleszynski PA, Luc JGY, Schade P, PhilLips SJ, Tchantchaleishvili V. Current state and future perspectives of energy sources for totally implantable cardiac devices. ASAIO J. 2016;62(6):639–45.
152. Grinstein J, Rodgers D, Kalantari S, Sayer G, Kim GH, Sarswat N, et al. HVAD waveform analysis as a noninvasive marker of pulmonary capillary wedge pressure: a first step toward the development of a smart left ventricular assist device pump. ASAIO J. 2018;64(1):10–5.
153. Schmidt T, Bjarnason-Wehrens B, Schulte-Eistrup S, Reiss N. Effects of pump speed changes on exercise capacity in patients supported with a left ventricular assist device-an overview. J Thorac Dis. 2018;10(Suppl 15):S1802–10.

# Exercise in Specific Diseases: Valvular Heart Disease

# 48

Elena Cavarretta and Axel Pressler

**Learning Objectives**

1. Potential impact of exercise training on molecular pathways involving e.g. reactive oxygen in the development of valvular heart disease.
2. Useful or even required pre-exercise clinical evaluations such as exercise testing or the assessment of predictive markers during stress echocardiography.
3. Clinical and hemodynamic effects of exercise interventions in different types of valvular heart disease, both prior to and after surgical valve replacement.
4. Effects of cardiac rehabilitation and exercise training in patients after transcatheter aortic valve implantation.

## 48.1 Introduction

The prevalence of any type of valvular heart disease (VHD) increases with age, reaching an overall proportion of 11.7% in individuals >75 years of age [1]. In the Western countries, this is mainly caused by degenerative processes of the leaflets or the apparatus while a small proportion of young and middle-aged individuals suffer from congenital valve diseases such as bicuspid aortic valve. The relationship between exercise and VHD is more complex compared with coronary artery disease or heart failure, as moderate to severe VHD represents a relative or even absolute contraindication to physical exhaustion. On the other hand, exercise is also urgently

E. Cavarretta
Department of Medical-Surgical Sciences and Biotechnologies, Sapienza University of Rome, Rome, Italy

Mediterranea Cardiocentro, Naples, Italy
e-mail: elena.cavarretta@uniroma1.it

A. Pressler (✉)
Private Center of Sports & Exercise Cardiology, Munich, Germany
e-mail: axel.pressler@kardiologie-mit-herz.de



A. Pressler, J. Niebauer (eds.), *Textbook of Sports and Exercise Cardiology*,
https://doi.org/10.1007/978-3-030-35374-2_48

required to maintain a healthy lifestyle and to counteract sedentary behavior and sitting time. From a clinical perspective, patients with VHD, at least following surgery, have routinely been included in cardiac rehabilitation programs since many years. In contrast, scientific evidence referring to this particular population is surprisingly scarce but nevertheless promising according to recent research, particularly after minimally invasive valvular surgery and percutaneous approaches, as outlined below.

## 48.2 Evidence from Preclinical Studies

The biological systems respond to physiological stressors such as physical exercise, showing a bell-shaped or an inverted-U curve. At both lateral end-points of this curve are the extremes, as both inactivity and over-training may result in an unfavorably altered pathophysiological function; in contrast, in the middle (or the median) of the relationship the benefit is highest. Reactive oxygen species (ROS) such as

(a) superoxide ($O_2^-$),
(b) hydroxyl radical (•OH),
(c) hydrogen peroxide ($H_2O_2$), and
(d) peroxynitrite ($ONOO^-$)

also represent important stressors. ROS can also exert both positive or negative effects on the body, and an imbalance between ROS and antioxidant defense is involved in the aging process and in various cardiovascular pathologies [2].

The relationship between oxidative stress and exercise is regulated by the same U-shaped curve, because exercise can also have a negative or positive impact on oxidative stress, based on intensity, duration, frequency and type of exercise as well as on the basic training level [3]. The correlation between exercise and ROS has mostly been studied in atherosclerosis, hypertension and vascular disease, where moderate physical activity has been shown to reduce oxidative stress and to increase superoxide dismutase (SOD) activity to counteract a reduction in endothelial function, independently from blood pressure [4].

- Degenerative aortic valve (AV) disease shares common features with atherosclerosis, including
  - clinical risk factors (i.e., inactivity, high-fat high-carbohydrate diet)
  - molecular-cellular mechanisms (i.e., valvular/vascular endothelial disruption, enhanced oxidative stress, calcification), and both can be classified as fibrocalcific diseases [5].
- Regular exercise training (ET) prevents the progression of atherosclerotic lesions, improves endothelial function, reduces neointimal growth and oxidative stress [6] (Chap. 41), and Matsumoto et al. [7] demonstrated that ET prevents the

development of AV sclerosis in a low-density lipoprotein receptor-deficient mouse model, due to
  - a reduction in oxidative stress and inflammation,
  - an inhibition of the osteogenic pathway, and
  - a preservation of endothelial integrity.
- A few years later, the same group failed to demonstrate that a change in diet or regular ET attenuated AV calcification *once the process is initiated*, in the same animal model [8].
- Oxidative modifications have been linked also to bioprosthetic valve degeneration [9, 10]; in particular, the amount of oxidized amino acid formation seems to be a more significant determinant of implant duration, compared to the amount of calcium. These promising results indicating a protective role of exercise need, however, to be further confirmed in this setting.
- Moderate ET is also beneficial
  - in a mouse model of Marfan syndrome, in terms of reduced aortic root dilation, while histological damages, in particular elastic lamina ruptures, were not increased in the ET group [11], and
  - in a rat model of chronic aortic regurgitation, where moderate aerobic ET can help to reduce LV dilation and hypertrophy, thus improving LV diastolic function [12].

The changes induced by ET include "remodeling" of the myocardial energy metabolism, comparable to beta-blocker effects [13].

## 48.3 Exercise in Patients with Valvular Heart Disease

There are no prospective studies evaluating the outcome of VHD patients participating in ET programs of longer duration compared to sedentary counterparts. Long-term follow-up studies of subjects with VHD and recommendations based on expert consensus can help guiding the management of these patients [14, 15].

- In case of asymptomatic subjects with VHD engaging in competitive sports participation, there are only few restrictions (see also Chap. 17) [16].
- On the contrary, subjects with moderate to severe VHD are generally discouraged from more vigorous exercise regimens, due to the detrimental effects of increased hemodynamic load combined with adrenergic surges on the heart that can cause clinical consequences such as
  - reduced functional capacity,
  - syncope,
  - myocardial ischemia,
  - onset or worsening of supraventricular and/or ventricular arrhythmias, and
  - sudden death

- The presence of one or more of the following markers represents a clear contraindication for ET, and the indication for surgery must be carefully considered in these patients:
  - exercise-induced symptoms
  - history of syncope
  - family history of sudden death
  - sustained and non-sustained arrhythmias
- Exercise testing is recommended
  - to objectively evaluate symptom status,
  - to evaluate exercise capacity (in terms of exercise duration, peak oxygen consumption ($VO_2$ peak) or age- and gender-predicted metabolic equivalents (METs))
  - to identify exercise-induced arrhythmias
- The use of exercise echocardiography can be useful to add prognostic risk markers (see below), which are specific for aortic or mitral valve disease, and to assess left ventricular (LV) contractile reserve.

## 48.3.1 Exercise in Mitral Valve Disease

### 48.3.1.1 Mitral Stenosis (MS)

The acute effects of exercise in the presence of MS are related to the increase in heart rate, which can be particularly significant in the presence of atrial fibrillation and elevation of transmitral gradients with elevated left atrial pressure. Systolic pulmonary artery pressure (sPAP) also markedly increases, thus patients are limited by dyspnea and fatigue [17]. Studies that evaluated the effects of chronic exercise training in patients with MS and that aimed to identify the optimal intensity of ET are lacking.

- A case report on a 38-year old male, affected by severe MS complicated by pulmonary hypertension, practicing isometric and isotonic exercise for 20 years has been described [18].

Thus, whether ET can be regarded as a non-pharmacological intervention to increase exercise tolerance in these patients needs to be confirmed. Similarities in the pathophysiology of MS and heart failure do exist (increase in left atrial pressure leading to pulmonary hypertension and neurohormonal activation) and may suggest a potential benefit of ET in terms of improved exercise tolerance [18].

If a mismatch between clinical symptoms and severity of MS as assessed by resting echocardiography is observed, stress echocardiography is indicated to evaluate hemodynamic changes during exercise and to provoke symptoms. Stress echocardiography is also useful to evaluate the impact of ET or pregnancy on the hemodynamic severity of MS [19]. Table 48.1 summarizes the principal parameters considered important in the evaluation of MS before initiation of ET.

**Table 48.1** Predictive parameters evaluated during stress echocardiography

| Parameter | Variation during stress echo | Reference |
|---|---|---|
| Transmitral mean pressure gradient | MS is severe if mean gradient increases<br>>15 mmHg at peak physical exercise<br>>18 mmHg during dobutamine infusion | [20] |
| Mitral valve resistance | A drop in MV resistance <21.5 dynes •s/cm$^5$ at peak dobutamine infusion identifies hemodynamically significant mild-to-moderate MS | [21] |
| Systolic pulmonary artery pressure | A sPAP elevation >60 mmHg or a rapid increase in sPAP (>90% increase at second step of exercise) are highly predictive of exercise-induced dyspnea | [22] |

*MS* mitral stenosis, *MV* mitral valve, *sPAP* systolic pulmonary artery pressure

#### 48.3.1.2 Mitral Valve Prolapse (MVP) with Mitral Regurgitation (MR)

In women affected by MVP, a 12-week aerobic training program (3 times a week, heart rate between 60% and 85% of maximum, with intensity levels increasing over time) improved symptoms, functional capacity and well-being, and reduced anxiety, atypical chest pain and fatigue related to MVP syndrome [23]. Unfortunately, these promising results have not been tested in a larger cohort or in a randomized trial.

Patients, predominantly women, may develop MVP syndrome with symptoms unrelated to MR severity that have been explained by a hypersensitivity to adrenergic stimulation and a β1-adrenergic receptor polymorphism [24], and they might benefit of a dedicated ET programme.

- Absolute contraindications for exercise training are:
  - severe MR,
  - arrhythmias (sustained or non-sustained ventricular tachycardia) independent of MR severity,
  - history of syncope, and
  - family history of sudden cardiac death that has been associated with MVP
- Arrhythmic patients are more frequently [25]
  - female
  - with MVP bi-leaflet involvement,
  - with ventricular arrhythmias of LV origin
  - with repolarization abnormalities on inferior leads at resting ECG
  - with mitral annulus disjunction and presence of LV fibrosis at cardiac magnetic resonance imaging
- Exercise echocardiography in asymptomatic MVP patients prior to ET is very useful to identify predictors of adverse long-term outcomes, specifically [26]
  - impaired exercise capacity (<85% of age- and sex-predicted METs),
  - impaired heart rate recovery,
  - exercise-induced atrial fibrillation or complex ventricular arrhythmias,
  - impaired LV contractile reserve, and
  - increase in sPAP >60 mmHg.
- In contrast, dobutamine stress echocardiography has no role in the evaluation of MR dynamics because its effects are not physiologic [19].

#### 48.3.1.3 Secondary Mitral Regurgitation

In the presence of secondary or functional MR, the indication for ET should be geared to the concomitant myocardial pathology (ischemic heart disease or cardiomyopathy). During exercise echocardiography, a decrease in MR severity, often related to the recruitment of LV basal contractile reserve, is a marker of a better outcome under appropriate medical therapy; it may thus benefit from a dedicated rehabilitative ET for heart failure [19].

### 48.3.2 Exercise in Aortic Valve Disease

#### 48.3.2.1 Aortic Stenosis (AS)

In asymptomatic patients with AS, it is still unclear if ET may be helpful or even harmful in increasing LV hypertrophy and provoke exercise-induced symptoms that may eventually lead to sudden death. Therefore, careful evaluation with exercise testing and echocardiography is required before entering a supervised, limited ET program to counteract deconditioning. Exercise testing is particularly useful to assess “truly” asymptomatic patients and to rule-out concomitant coronary artery disease (CAD), due to the fact that AS and CAD basically share the same risk factors.

Parameters associated with an adverse outcome are [27, 28].

(a) exercise-induced symptoms (angina, dyspnea, dizziness or syncope),
(b) increase >18 mmHg of the mean transvalvular gradient during exercise echocardiography,
(c) exercise-induced hypotension.

In patients affected by AS with severe LV hypertrophy, isometric exercise increases LV end-diastolic pressure and decreases the isovolumic relaxation rate. During recovery, only the patients with associated CAD maintain a significant alteration of both parameters and should be further evaluated [29].

#### 48.3.2.2 Aortic Regurgitation (AR)

Despite the LV pressure and volume overload in the presence of chronic AR leading to a progressive LV dilation, many patients remain asymptomatic until LV systolic function declines significantly because the marked LV dilation can maintain a normal LV stroke volume.

- In AR patients, exercise capacity may be markedly reduced due to a reduced preload reserve and can predict post-operative outcome after aortic valve replacement [30].
- At peak effort in the presence of severe AR in asymptomatic patients with normal LV systolic function, there is a reduction of the regurgitation fraction, thus of the severity of AR [31, 32].

- This can be related both to the exercise-induced tachycardia that reduces the diastolic period and to the reduction of peripheral resistance reducing the retrograde flow and improving diastolic function.
- This can explain why patients with severe AR can still enjoy physical activity and may show a better exercise tolerance.
- Despite the LV enlargement induced by ET, the LV end-diastolic diameter usually remains <60 mm in the physiological athletes' heart [33].
  - Further LV enlargement should be carefully evaluated to rule-out a pathological LV dilation.
  - Indexing to body surface area can be useful to correctly evaluate the degree of dilation.
- Long-term effects of ET in AR have not been studied in human, but only in rats.
- Exercise stress testing or echocardiography is particularly useful to assess the presence of symptoms and to establish the baseline level of exercise capacity, but not to re-grade the severity of AR, due to the reduction of AR during exercise [34].
  - In particular, at peak effort, the presence of resting LV and RV systolic dysfunction (evaluated by global longitudinal strain), associated with exercise RV dysfunction evaluated by tricuspid annular plane systolic excursion (TAPSE) are independent predictors of future aortic valve surgery [35].

#### 48.3.2.3 Frailty, Exercise and Aortic Valve Disease

Frailty is a geriatric syndrome, defined as a reduced capability to recover from pathological or iatrogenic stressors due to multi-dimensional aging-related impairments [36, 37]. The extent of frailty is not purely related to the quantification of comorbidities or disabilities, because patients with the same comorbidities may have different degrees of frailty or no frailty at all. At present, multidomain frailty scales have been proposed (e.g., 5-meter gait speed ≥6 s, Fried's phenotype frailty index, frailty index based on the deficit accumulation mode, FRAIL scale, Edmonton frailty scale etc.), but there is a lack of consensus in frailty assessment, thus hampering a systematic evaluation of frailty in clinical practice [38].

- Frailty is particularly important in the stratification of operative risk and recovery time in older patients referred for aortic valve surgery.
- Among different frailty scales, a 4-item essential frailty toolset (EFT) has been specifically tested in patients undergoing transcatheter aortic valve implantation (TAVI) [36].
  - EFT is a 0–5 scale composed by 4 items (Table 48.2) [36].
  - This simple and quick to perform frailty assessment was found to be the most robust predictor of outcomes in a large cohort of patients undergoing aortic valve replacement, in comparison with other frailty scales tested [36].

**Table 48.2** 4-Item essential frailty toolset (EFT)

| Parameter | Discriminator | Points |
|---|---|---|
| Five chair rises | <15 s | 0 point |
| | ≥15 s | 1 point |
| | Not able to perform | 2 points |
| Cognitive impairment | No | 0 point |
| | Yes | 1 point |
| Hemoglobin | >13 g/dl in males<br>>12 g/dl in females | 0 point |
| | <13 g/dl in males<br><12 g/dl in females | 1 point |
| Serum albumin | >3.5 g/dl | 0 point |
| | <3.5 g/dl | 1 point |

This score ranges from 0 (least frail) to 5 (most frail), it is very helpful to identify vulnerable older adults who are at high risk of mortality for any cause 1-year after transcatheter or surgical aortic valve replacement (adapted from [36])

Regular ET is the only effective strategy to prevent frailty, improve sarcopenia and physical function, and contrast cognitive deterioration. In older adults, ET increases aerobic endurance capacity and muscular strength, thus reproducing the beneficial effects observed in younger individuals [38].

- In an exploratory study, a home-based preoperative rehabilitation ("prehab") has been proposed in frail patients undergoing valve surgery with the aim to improve physical function and reduce hospital length [39].
  - Exercise prescription should be individually tailored to each patient, modulating balance and strength exercise with progressive levels, and the patients should exercise for 3 weeks before scheduled surgery [39].
  - A larger randomized study is required to confirm potential benefits or prehab.
- Pre-operative frailty assessment using a clinical frailty scale is of particularly relevance since it can identify patients who are less likely to attend and complete CR after valve surgery [40].

## 48.4 Exercise After Valve Replacement

### 48.4.1 Exercise After Open-Heart Valve Surgery

The benefits of cardiac rehabilitation (CR) after surgical or percutaneous coronary revascularization have been extensively demonstrated (Chap. 46). The observed improvements

(a) in cardiovascular fitness,
(b) in the overall response to exercise with reduced heart rates and blood pressure,
(c) in counteracting depression and anxiety, and
(d) in improved health-related quality of life

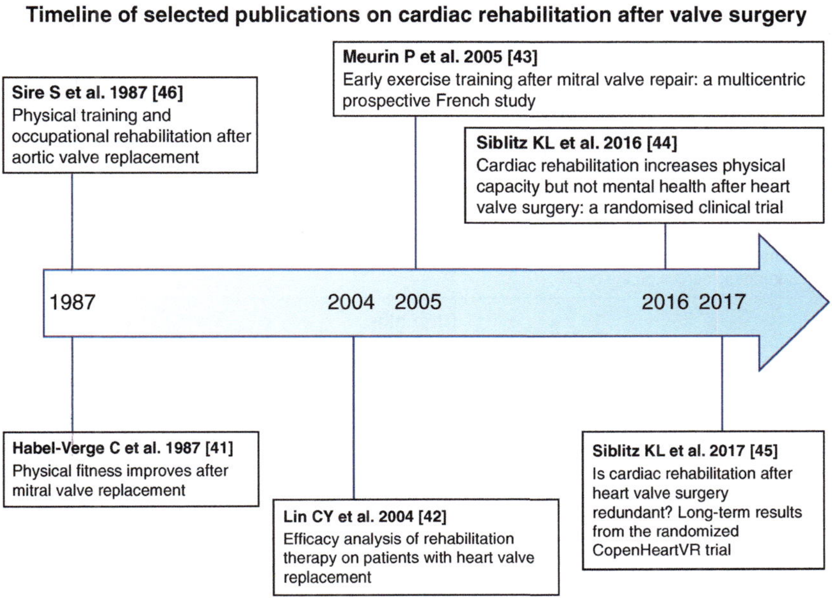


**Fig. 48.1** Timeline of published articles on cardiac rehabilitation after heart valve surgery

represent attractive therapeutic goals also after valve surgery. ET is particularly interesting in post-surgical VHD patients after years of restriction from regular physical activity (Fig. 48.1).

- Moreover, immediately after open-heart surgery the fitness is particularly impaired due to:
  - the surgical procedure itself, as i.e. the sternotomy,
  - the effects of cardio-pulmonary by-pass,
  - the post-operative anemia and inflammation
  - the inactivity during the intensive care and in-hospital stay
- Post-operative ET is also particularly appealing
  - in young individuals who aim to return to work and exercise early after surgery;
  - in frail older people to counteract deconditioning and maintain their physical integrity and independency

Surprisingly, only very few studies are available demonstrating the effects of ET in VHD patients following cardiac surgery (Fig. 48.2), although their results are promising in showing a consistent increase in exercise capacity ranging from 25% to 38% [41–46].

- The largest CR trial performed in VHD patients after cardiac surgery showed the improvement in cardiovascular fitness by demonstrating an increase in $VO_2$peak,

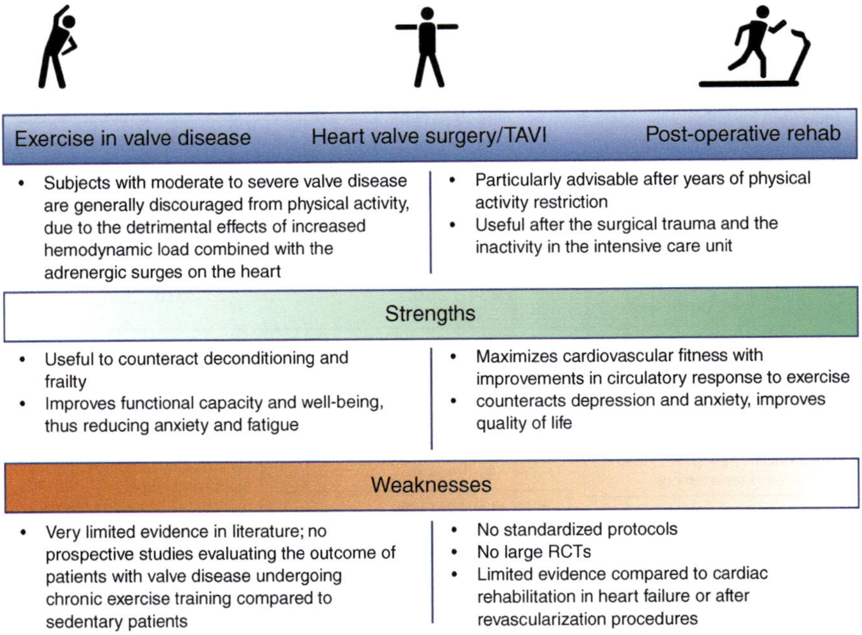


**Fig. 48.2** Central illustration: Strengths and weaknesses of exercise training in heart valve disease according to the current evidence. *RCTs* randomized controlled trials

but not in the mental health score as evaluated by the SF-36 questionnaire. Exercise-based CR should be offered to patients after valve surgery, but it must be planned individually to meet the patients' individual needs [44].

- A recent meta-analysis on this topic concluded that the actual body of evidence does not allow any reliable conclusions about the effectiveness, and future large trials are urgently warranted [47].
- While CR for heart failure and after coronary revascularization is considered to be cost-effective [48], cost-effectiveness for exercise-based CR after valve surgery has not been fully demonstrated [49].

## 48.4.2 Exercise-Based Cardiac Rehabilitation

In low-risk patients, CR with aerobic exercise can be started early (2–3 weeks) after surgery, without safety concerns and difference in adverse events rate [50]. Especially after minimally invasive cardiac surgery, as mini-thoracotomy or robotic approach, CR is encouraged early after surgery, because of the reduced surgical trauma and the absence of sternotomy.

- Before enrolling in a CR program, patients should undergo
  - clinical assessment of post-operative functional status
  - echocardiography with a complete assessment of hemodynamic status

  - exercise testing or even better cardio-pulmonary exercise testing to assess exercise capacity and cardiovascular fitness
  - ECG Holter monitoring to identify potential arrhythmias
- Exercise prescription should be individualized and must take into account [51–53]
  - Age of the patient
  - Weight
  - Previous level of physical activity
  - Frailty status
  - Hemodynamic status
  - Exercise capacity
  - Wound healing
  - Eventual physical impairments
- Exercise prescription should specify:
  - type of exercise (endurance/strength)
  - intensity (e.g., 50–80% of exercise capacity)
  - duration (20–60 min)
  - frequency (3 to 5 times per week)
  - modality (walking, cycling, treadmill etc.) (Chap. 44)

### 48.4.3 Exercise After Percutaneous Valve Replacement

Among the percutaneous approaches that have emerged in recent years as alternatives to open valve surgery, particularly TAVI has gained enormous attraction. Since its first application in a human only in the year 2002 [54], it has rapidly evolved as the alternative of choice for aortic valve replacement in elderly, multimorbid patients who would otherwise have an inappropriately high perioperative mortality risk [55]. During only one decade, supported by a steady progress in valve types and technologies, TAVI has now been expanded also to patients with moderate or even low risk, and large studies have shown that the long-term outcomes of this procedure can be regarded as being at least equal to open valve surgery [56, 57].

Thus, a completely "new" target population of VHD patients requiring tailored CR and ET programs has evolved in only very few years who, due to their often high degrees of deconditioning and their multimorbid nature, are expected to particularly benefit from the common advantages of such interventions [58]. This has been reflected in research by a growing number of observational and randomized studies on the effects of CR and ET in patients after TAVI, as compared to counterparts undergoing open surgery or as an independent target group:

- Early observational studies have evaluated the effect of short-term inpatient CR programs in patients after TAVI [59–61].
  - These studies have almost consistently shown improvements in e.g. 6-min walking distances and in parameters of physical and cognitive function, albeit less pronounced compared to mostly younger and less frail patients after open surgery.

  - Of note, it should be kept in mind that the TAVI procedure itself already results in rather quick improvements in some of these outcomes, but it is likely that ET may contribute to enhance and maintain these effects over time.
- The results of these mostly small studies were confirmed in a meta-analysis primarily showing overall improvements in the 6-min walking distance and the Barthel Index as a measure of frailty [62], but the overall number of included patients was still rather low (n = 292), and the interventions included were still very heterogeneous, limiting definitive conclusions on the effect of particular types of intervention at this point of time.
- In another recent observational study, the effects of participating in either cardiac, geriatric or in no inpatient rehabilitation on mortality 6 months after the procedure were analyzed in a large cohort of 1017 TAVI patients [63]. Interestingly, only patients participating in CR showed a lower mid-term mortality.
- In the randomized controlled SPORT:TAVI pilot trial, 30 patients early after a TAVI procedure were assigned to either an ET group undergoing supervised, combined low-to-moderate endurance and strength training over 8 weeks or to a non-exercising control group [64].
  - The ET intervention resulted in significant improvements in submaximal and maximal exercise capacity, muscular strength and components of quality of life, and this study included also nonagenarians, indicating that also very old patients may still benefit from structured post-interventional programs.
  - In a long-term follow-up of this study (24 ± 6 months after the procedure), at least the initial improvements in submaximal endurance exercise capacity were maintained [65], indicating an at least partly sustained effect of initial interventional approaches.
  - Due to a lack of adverse effects including prosthesis function, this study also showed that ET can be regarded as a safe treatment modality even in very old, frail and multimorbid patients, providing they are still physically able to use bicylces or strength training machines, at least at low intensities.

From a practical perspective, the intensity of exercise training in the latter study has been adapted from recommendations valid for heart failure patients of patients after heart transplantation (see Chaps. 44, 48 and 51 for details on this). Precisely, regarding aerobic exercise, patients started with 2 sessions per week at an intensity level of 30–50% $VO_2$peak and a duration of 10–20 min, followed by a gradual increase over time of duration and intensity up to 30–40 min 3 times per week at 50–70% $VO_2$peak. Regarding strength training performed twice weekly, intensity was calculated from the initial assessments of the 1-repetition maximum (1-RM; Chap. 44) and started with one set of 8–10 repetitions at 30–50% 1-RM. Intensity increased over time, depending on the individual improvements, to 3 sets with 10–15 repetitions each at 40–60% 1-RM.

Regarding other percutaneous valve replacement procedures such as MitraClip, transcatheter mitral or tricuspid valve replacement, currently no data on the effects of CR and/or ET is yet available, although a technical and clinical development similar to TAVI regarding the application of these procedures can be expected in the very near future. Currently these procedures are still only evaluated as a procedural alternative to open surgery in small populations, apart from the MitraClip procedure which can be regarded as clinically established. Since these interventions are almost exclusively performed in very high risk, multimorbid patients (similar to the first TAVI experiences), a comparable effect of individually tailored ET interventions is likely to be expected, thus studies are required and recommended.

## 48.5 Conclusion

Evidence on the effects of ET interventions in VHD patients is surprisingly scarce, and well-designed studies focusing on this particular population are still urgently warranted. Although degenerative VHD shares many common pathophysiological features with atherosclerotic vascular disease it is still not known whether regular physical activity or ET may delay (or even prevent) the natural course of the disease. Nonetheless, the available data indicates promising preliminary effects through the application of ET interventions either alone or as part of multi-modal CR programs. These programs resulted in improvements in exercise capacity, cardiorespiratory fitness, muscular strength, flexibility and overall quality of life. Recent studies have shown that also elderly, frail and multimorbid patients may benefit from ET interventions, which is of particular relevance with regard to the rapid increase of patients undergoing percutaneous interventions such as TAVI. Prior to surgery or percutaneous intervention, individually prescribed exercise training holds promise to counteract muscular deconditioning, to reduce anxiety and fatigue and to reduce frailty. However, larger trials are also warranted pertaining to this particular issue to confirm these preliminary data.

**Clinical Pearls**

- Compared to other cardiac diseases such as heart failure or coronary artery disease the evidence on exercise training interventions in valvular heart disease is surprisingly scarce, but available data indicate similar beneficial effects on clinical outcomes
- Exercise training may also have a protective function on a molecular level in favorably modifying pathophysiological features of valve degeneration
- A decrease of the severity of aortic or mitral regurgitation may occur during exercise and indicates improved outcomes
- The potential impact of exercise training on the natural history of valvular heart disease prior to surgical or percutaneous interventions remains to be elucidated
- The available data indicates beneficial effects of increased physical activity, exercise training and cardiac rehabilitation programs on cardiorespiratory fitness, muscular strength and quality of life in valvular heart disease, particularly also after transcatheter aortic valve implantation

# Review

## Questions

1. A 66-year-old male patient is referred to your outpatient clinic for the evaluation of continued eligibility to perform regular and partly intensive exercise after a moderate aortic stenosis had been incidentally diagnosed during a preventive examination. His non-indexed valve orifice area was 1.1 $cm^2$ due to valve calcification, but even during more intense activities such as mountain-biking (which he loves to perform) no symptoms had occurred so far. What would be your next steps and your final advice?
2. When performing exercise stress echocardiography in valvular heart disease, which of the following markers indicate an increased risk of symptoms or adverse outcomes during intensive exercise (more than one answer is correct)?
   (a) Increase of pressure gradient over mitral valve of 10 mmHg at peak exercise
   (b) Increase of pressure gradient over mitral valve of 20 mmHg at peak exercise
   (c) Increase of systolic pulmonary artery pressure of 30 mmHg at peak exercise
   (d) Increase of systolic pulmonary artery pressure of 70 mmHg at peak exercise
   (e) Increase of systolic pulmonary artery pressure of >90% of the baseline value early during exercise
3. A 91-year-old female patient has undergone transcatheter aortic valve implantation 1 week earlier and is now referred to a 3-week inpatient cardiac rehabilitation program. What would be your assessments and how would you start an exercise program?

## Answers

1. Prior to any exercise recommendation, an extensive work-up of medical history, risk factors and concomitant diseases such as coronary artery disease (CAD) is required, involving cardiopulmonary exercise testing to evaluate ECG and blood pressure responses during exercise and stress echocardiography to assess the pressure gradient. Coronary angiography may also be indicated in case of signs of ischemia to rule out additional CAD and to invasively assess the severity of aortic stenosis in case of equivocal findings during echocardiography. If the aortic stenosis remains the sole finding, the decision on participating in intensive sport such as mountain-biking depends on the presence of symptoms and signs of ischemia due to relatively reduced coronary blood supply. If an ischemia threshold is detectable by ECG, the patient should be advised to remain at least 10 bpm below this threshold which might preclude more intense efforts. In case of completely unremarkable findings the patient may be cleared for exercise at

higher intensities but should be advised to carefully observe symptoms during exercise and to undergo echocardiography and exercise testing follow-ups every 6 months.

2. The correct answers are (b), (c) and (e). These values indicate severe mitral valve stenosis and that exercise-induced dyspnea may readily be explained by hemodynamic compromises induced by valvular heart disease.
3. In this patient, assessments depend on the presence of any physical disabilities. Usually an evaluation of functional capacity should be performed at the beginning of a CR intervention. If possible, this patient should thus at least undergo a 6-min walking test; moreover, assessment of frailty status using one of the established methods (see text for details) and a questionnaire on health-related quality of life would be reasonable. If the patient is able to use a bicycle adequately, cardiopulmonary exercise testing should be performed in order to provide baseline parameters and to calculate exercise intensities from peak oxygen uptake. The program should then start with sessions of 10–20 min daily or even less, at an intensity of 30–50% $VO_2$peak or according to subjective exhaustion if not available, which often means very low, but still effective workloads of only about 20–30 Watts. A gradual increase in duration and intensity during CR should be aimed at. Strength training should also be conducted twice a week at very low intensities, e.g. 30–50% of the 1-repetition maximum, and consist of 1–2 sets with 10–15 repetitions. Although CR starts very early after the intervention there is no evidence that this might cause any harm to the newly implanted prosthesis.

## References


1. Benjamin EJ, Virani SS, Callaway CW, Chamberlain AM, Chang AR, Cheng S, et al. Heart disease and stroke statistics-2018 update: a report from the American Heart Association. Circulation. 2018;137(12):e67–e492.
2. Radak Z, Ishihara K, Tekus E, Varga C, Posa A, Balogh L, et al. Exercise, oxidants, and antioxidants change the shape of the bell-shaped hormesis curve. Redox Biol. 2017;12:285–90.
3. Cavarretta E, Peruzzi M, Frati G, Sciarretta S. When enough is more than enough: the hidden side of the cardiac effects of intense physical exercise. Int J Cardiol. 2018;258:224–5.
4. Guers JJ, Kasecky-Lardner L, Farquhar WB, Edwards DG, Lennon SL. Voluntary wheel running prevents salt-induced endothelial dysfunction: role of oxidative stress. J Appl Physiol (1985). 2019;126(2):502–10.
5. Ruiz JL, Hutcheson JD, Aikawa E. Cardiovascular calcification: current controversies and novel concepts. Cardiovasc Pathol. 2015;24(4):207–12.
6. Szostak J, Laurant P. The forgotten face of regular physical exercise: a 'natural' anti-atherogenic activity. Clin Sci (Lond). 2011;121(3):91–106.
7. Matsumoto Y, Adams V, Jacob S, Mangner N, Schuler G, Linke A. Regular exercise training prevents aortic valve disease in low-density lipoprotein-receptor-deficient mice. Circulation. 2010;121(6):759–67.
8. Schlotter F, Matsumoto Y, Mangner N, Schuler G, Linke A, Adams V. Regular exercise or changing diet does not influence aortic valve disease progression in LDLR deficient mice. PLoS One. 2012;7(5):e37298.
9. Christian AJ, Lin H, Alferiev IS, Connolly JM, Ferrari G, Hazen SL, et al. The susceptibility of bioprosthetic heart valve leaflets to oxidation. Biomaterials. 2014;35(7):2097–102.

10. Lee S, Levy RJ, Christian AJ, Hazen SL, Frick NE, Lai EK, et al. Calcification and oxidative modifications are associated with progressive bioprosthetic heart valve dysfunction. J Am Heart Assoc. 2017;6(5)
11. Mas-Stachurska A, Siegert AM, Batlle M, Gorbenko Del Blanco D, Meirelles T, Rubies C, et al. Cardiovascular benefits of moderate exercise training in Marfan syndrome: insights from an animal model. J Am Heart Assoc. 2017;6(9)
12. Lachance D, Champetier S, Plante E, Bouchard-Thomassin AA, Roussel E, Couet J, et al. Effects of exercise in volume overload: insights from a model of aortic regurgitation. Med Sci Sports Exerc. 2009;41(6):1230–8.
13. Lachance D, Dhahri W, Drolet MC, Roussel E, Gascon S, Sarrhini O, et al. Endurance training or beta-blockade can partially block the energy metabolism remodeling taking place in experimental chronic left ventricle volume overload. BMC Cardiovasc Disord. 2014;14:190.
14. Desai MY, Grigioni F, Di Eusanio M, Saccocci M, Taramasso M, Maisano F, et al. Outcomes in degenerative mitral regurgitation: current state-of-the art and future directions. Prog Cardiovasc Dis. 2017;60(3):370–85.
15. Genereux P, Stone GW, O'Gara PT, Marquis-Gravel G, Redfors B, Giustino G, et al. Natural history, diagnostic approaches, and therapeutic strategies for patients with asymptomatic severe aortic stenosis. J Am Coll Cardiol. 2016;67(19):2263–88.
16. Pelliccia A, Fagard R, Bjornstad HH, Anastassakis A, Arbustini E, Assanelli D, et al. Recommendations for competitive sports participation in athletes with cardiovascular disease: a consensus document from the study Group of Sports Cardiology of the Working Group of Cardiac Rehabilitation and Exercise Physiology and the Working Group of Myocardial and Pericardial Diseases of the European Society of Cardiology. Eur Heart J. 2005;26(14):1422–45.
17. Lev EI, Sagie A, Vaturi M, Sela N, Battler A, Shapira Y. Value of exercise echocardiography in rheumatic mitral stenosis with and without significant mitral regurgitation. Am J Cardiol. 2004;93(8):1060–3.
18. Altunbas G, Sari I, Davutoglu V. Potential benefits of exercise training in rheumatic severe mitral valve stenosis in a heavy trainer. Int J Cardiol. 2016;220:575–6.
19. Raissi SR, Kinno M, Rigolin VH. Stress echocardiography: the role in assessing valvular heart disease. Curr Cardiovasc Imaging Rep. 2018;11:33.
20. Reis G, Motta MS, Barbosa MM, Esteves WA, Souza SF, Bocchi EA. Dobutamine stress echocardiography for noninvasive assessment and risk stratification of patients with rheumatic mitral stenosis. J Am Coll Cardiol. 2004;43(3):393–401.
21. Roshdy HS, Meshrif AM, El D II. Value of the mitral valve resistance in evaluation of symptomatic patients with mild and moderate mitral stenosis—a dobutamine stress echocardiographic study. Echocardiography. 2014;31(3):347–52.
22. Brochet E, Detaint D, Fondard O, Tazi-Mezalek A, Messika-Zeitoun D, Iung B, et al. Early hemodynamic changes versus peak values: what is more useful to predict occurrence of dyspnea during stress echocardiography in patients with asymptomatic mitral stenosis? J Am Soc Echocardiogr. 2011;24(4):392–8.
23. Scordo KA. Effects of aerobic exercise training on symptomatic women with mitral valve prolapse. Am J Cardiol. 1991;67(9):863–8.
24. Theofilogiannakos EK, Boudoulas KD, Gawronski BE, Langaee TY, Dardas PS, Ninios V, et al. Floppy mitral valve/mitral valve prolapse syndrome: beta-adrenergic receptor polymorphism may contribute to the pathogenesis of symptoms. J Cardiol. 2015;65(5):434–8.
25. Basso C, Perazzolo Marra M, Rizzo S, De Lazzari M, Giorgi B, Cipriani A, et al. Arrhythmic mitral valve prolapse and sudden cardiac death. Circulation. 2015;132(7):556–66.
26. Naji P, Griffin BP, Asfahan F, Barr T, Rodriguez LL, Grimm R, et al. Predictors of long-term outcomes in patients with significant myxomatous mitral regurgitation undergoing exercise echocardiography. Circulation. 2014;129(12):1310–9.
27. Lancellotti P, Lebois F, Simon M, Tombeux C, Chauvel C, Pierard LA. Prognostic importance of quantitative exercise Doppler echocardiography in asymptomatic valvular aortic stenosis. Circulation. 2005;112(9 Suppl):I377–82.

28. Marechaux S, Hachicha Z, Bellouin A, Dumesnil JG, Meimoun P, Pasquet A, et al. Usefulness of exercise-stress echocardiography for risk stratification of true asymptomatic patients with aortic valve stenosis. Eur Heart J. 2010;31(11):1390–7.
29. Gabay J, Donato M, Pascua A, Gelpi RJ, Grinfeld L. Effects of isometric exercise on the diastolic function in patients with severe aortic stenosis with or without coronary lesion. Int J Cardiol. 2005;104(1):52–8.
30. Bonow RO, Picone AL, McIntosh CL, Jones M, Rosing DR, Maron BJ, et al. Survival and functional results after valve replacement for aortic regurgitation from 1976 to 1983: impact of preoperative left ventricular function. Circulation. 1985;72(6):1244–56.
31. Forteza Alberti JF, Noris Mora M, Carrillo Lopez A, Pericas P, Pasamar Marquez L, Calderon Montero FJ, et al. Changes in the severity of aortic regurgitation at peak effort during exercise. Int J Cardiol. 2017;228:145–8.
32. Stern H, Calavrezos L, Meierhofer C, Steinlechner E, Muller J, Hager A, et al. Physical exercise reduces aortic regurgitation: exercise magnetic resonance imaging. JACC Cardiovasc Imaging. 2014;7(3):314–5.
33. Pelliccia A, Culasso F, Di Paolo FM, Maron BJ. Physiologic left ventricular cavity dilatation in elite athletes. Ann Intern Med. 1999;130(1):23–31.
34. Popovic ZB, Desai MY, Griffin BP. Decision making with imaging in asymptomatic aortic regurgitation. JACC Cardiovasc Imaging. 2018;11(10):1499–513.
35. Kusunose K, Agarwal S, Marwick TH, Griffin BP, Popovic ZB. Decision making in asymptomatic aortic regurgitation in the era of guidelines: incremental values of resting and exercise cardiac dysfunction. Circ Cardiovasc Imaging. 2014;7(2):352–62.
36. Afilalo J, Lauck S, Kim DH, Lefevre T, Piazza N, Lachapelle K, et al. Frailty in older adults undergoing aortic valve replacement: the FRAILTY-AVR study. J Am Coll Cardiol. 2017;70(6):689–700.
37. Rodriguez-Manas L, Feart C, Mann G, Vina J, Chatterji S, Chodzko-Zajko W, et al. Searching for an operational definition of frailty: a Delphi method based consensus statement: the frailty operative definition-consensus conference project. J Gerontol A Biol Sci Med Sci. 2013;68(1):62–7.
38. Vigorito C, Abreu A, Ambrosetti M, Belardinelli R, Corra U, Cupples M, et al. Frailty and cardiac rehabilitation: a call to action from the EAPC cardiac rehabilitation section. Eur J Prev Cardiol. 2017;24(6):577–90.
39. Waite I, Deshpande R, Baghai M, Massey T, Wendler O, Greenwood S. Home-based preoperative rehabilitation (prehab) to improve physical function and reduce hospital length of stay for frail patients undergoing coronary artery bypass graft and valve surgery. J Cardiothorac Surg. 2017;12(1):91.
40. Kimber DE, Kehler DS, Lytwyn J, Boreskie KF, Jung P, Alexander B, et al. Pre-operative frailty status is associated with cardiac rehabilitation completion: a retrospective cohort study. J Clin Med. 2018;7(12)
41. Habel-Verge C, Landry F, Desaulniers D, Dagenais GR, Moisan A, Cote L, et al. Physical fitness improves after mitral valve replacement. CMAJ. 1987;136(2):142–7.
42. Lin CY, He Z, Chen J, Yang B, Gu JX. Efficacy analysis of rehabilitation therapy on patients with heart valve replacement. Chin J Clin Rehab. 2004;8(3):426–7.
43. Meurin P, Iliou MC, Ben Driss A, Pierre B, Corone S, Cristofini P, et al. Early exercise training after mitral valve repair: a multicentric prospective French study. Chest. 2005;128(3):1638–44.
44. Sibilitz KL, Berg SK, Rasmussen TB, Risom SS, Thygesen LC, Tang L, et al. Cardiac rehabilitation increases physical capacity but not mental health after heart valve surgery: a randomised clinical trial. Heart. 2016;102(24):1995–2003.
45. Sibilitz KL, Berg SK, Tang L, Thygesen LC, Hansen TB, Risom SS, et al. Is cardiac rehabilitation after heart valve surgery redundant? Long-term results from the randomized CopenHeartVR trial. Eur Heart J. 2017;38(suppl_1):517.
46. Sire S. Physical training and occupational rehabilitation after aortic valve replacement. Eur Heart J. 1987;8(11):1215–20.

47. Blokzijl F, Dieperink W, Keus F, Reneman MF, Mariani MA, van der Horst IC. Cardiac rehabilitation for patients having cardiac surgery: a systematic review. J Cardiovasc Surg. 2018;59(6):817–29.
48. Shields GE, Wells A, Doherty P, Heagerty A, Buck D, Davies LM. Cost-effectiveness of cardiac rehabilitation: a systematic review. Heart. 2018;104(17):1403–10.
49. Hansen TB, Zwisler AD, Berg SK, Sibilitz KL, Thygesen LC, Kjellberg J, et al. Cost-utility analysis of cardiac rehabilitation after conventional heart valve surgery versus usual care. Eur J Prev Cardiol. 2017;24(7):698–707.
50. Doyle MP, Indraratna P, Tardo DT, Peeceeyen SC, Peoples GE. Safety and efficacy of aerobic exercise commenced early after cardiac surgery: a systematic review and meta-analysis. Eur J Prev Cardiol. 2019;26(1):36–45.
51. Gohlke-Barwolf C, Gohlke H, Samek L, Peters K, Betz P, Eschenbruch E, et al. Exercise tolerance and working capacity after valve replacement. J Heart Valve Dis. 1992;1(2):189–95.
52. Nilsson H, Nylander E, Borg S, Tamas E, Hedman K. Cardiopulmonary exercise testing for evaluation of a randomized exercise training intervention following aortic valve replacement. Clin Physiol Funct Imaging. 2019;39(1):103–10.
53. Vitale G, Sarullo S, Vassallo L, Di Franco A, Mandala G, Marazia S, et al. Prognostic value of the 6-min walk test after open-heart valve surgery: EXPERIENCE OF A CARDIOVASCULAR REHABILITATION PROGRAM. J Cardiopulm Rehabil Prev. 2018;38(5):304–8.
54. Cribier A, Eltchaninoff H, Bash A, Borenstein N, Tron C, Bauer F, et al. Percutaneous transcatheter implantation of an aortic valve prosthesis for calcific aortic stenosis: first human case description. Circulation. 2002;106(24):3006–8.
55. Agarwal S, Tuzcu EM, Krishnaswamy A, Schoenhagen P, Stewart WJ, Svensson LG, et al. Transcatheter aortic valve replacement: current perspectives and future implications. Heart. 2015;101(3):169–77.
56. Mack MJ, Leon MB, Thourani VH, Makkar R, Kodali SK, Russo M, et al. Transcatheter aortic-valve replacement with a balloon-expandable valve in low-risk patients. N Engl J Med. 2019;380(18):1695–705.
57. Popma JJ, Deeb GM, Yakubov SJ, Mumtaz M, Gada H, O'Hair D, et al. Transcatheter aortic-valve replacement with a self-expanding valve in low-risk patients. N Engl J Med. 2019;380(18):1706–15.
58. Pressler A. Cardiac rehabilitation after transcatheter aortic valve implantation: growing needs in a growing population. Eur J Prev Cardiol. 2017;24(7):685–7.
59. Fauchere I, Weber D, Maier W, Altwegg L, Luscher TF, Grunenfelder J, et al. Rehabilitation after TAVI compared to surgical aortic valve replacement. Int J Cardiol. 2014;173(3):564–6.
60. Russo N, Compostella L, Tarantini G, Setzu T, Napodano M, Bottio T, et al. Cardiac rehabilitation after transcatheter versus surgical prosthetic valve implantation for aortic stenosis in the elderly. Eur J Prev Cardiol. 2014;21(11):1341–8.
61. Voller H, Salzwedel A, Nitardy A, Buhlert H, Treszl A, Wegscheider K. Effect of cardiac rehabilitation on functional and emotional status in patients after transcatheter aortic-valve implantation. Eur J Prev Cardiol. 2015;22(5):568–74.
62. Ribeiro GS, Melo RD, Deresz LF, Dal Lago P, Pontes MR, Karsten M. Cardiac rehabilitation programme after transcatheter aortic valve implantation versus surgical aortic valve replacement: systematic review and meta-analysis. Eur J Prev Cardiol. 2017;24(7):688–97.
63. Butter C, Gross J, Haase-Fielitz A, Sims H, Deutsch C, Bramlage P, et al. Impact of rehabilitation on outcomes after TAVI: a preliminary study. J Clin Med. 2018;7(10)
64. Pressler A, Christle JW, Lechner B, Grabs V, Haller B, Hettich I, et al. Exercise training improves exercise capacity and quality of life after transcatheter aortic valve implantation: a randomized pilot trial. Am Heart J. 2016;182:44–53.
65. Pressler A, Forschner L, Hummel J, Haller B, Christle JW, Halle M. Long-term effect of exercise training in patients after transcatheter aortic valve implantation: follow-up of the SPORT:TAVI randomised pilot study. Eur J Prev Cardiol. 2018;25(8):794–801.

# Exercise in Specific Diseases: Atrial Fibrillation

# 49

Roman Laszlo and Matthias Wilhelm

**Learning Objectives**
This chapter conveys the knowledge

1. On exercise as a protective or risk factor for atrial fibrillation.
2. On the pathophysiology of atrial fibrillation in non-athletes and the impact on exercise performance.
3. On special features of exercise testing and training recommendations in patients with atrial fibrillation.
4. On sports eligibility for non-athletes and special considerations regarding oral anticoagulation.
5. On the effects of cardiac rehabilitation in patients with atrial fibrillation.
6. On current gaps in evidence.

## 49.1 Introduction

Atrial fibrillation (AF) is the most common arrhythmia in adult age with a clear age-dependent prevalence [1]. As cardiovascular diseases—which often represent clinical AF risk factors—in general increase in our ageing population [2], an also increasing number of AF cases with a significant impact on health economics can be expected in the future [3].

R. Laszlo
Division of Sports and Rehabilitation Medicine, Center of Medicine, Ulm University Hospital, Ulm, Germany
e-mail: roman.laszlo@uni-ulm.de

M. Wilhelm (✉)
Department of Cardiology, Interdisciplinary Centre for Sports & Exercise Medicine, Inselspital, University Hospital of Bern, Bern University, Bern, Switzerland
e-mail: matthias.wilhelm@insel.ch



A. Pressler, J. Niebauer (eds.), *Textbook of Sports and Exercise Cardiology*,
https://doi.org/10.1007/978-3-030-35374-2_49

AF is characterized by an uncoordinated intra-atrial conduction propagation resulting in an atrial heart rate of 400–600 beats/min and irregular atrioventricular conduction. In surface ECG, an absolute arrhythmia with fibrillation waves, which often do not contrast with isoelectric baseline, can be found. Clinically, several types of AF (e.g. paroxysmal, short/long-standing persistent, permanent) can be distinguished [1].

Exercise can be either protective or a risk factor for AF. Thus, exercise recommendations have to be personalized, reflecting individual risk factors, comorbidities, abilities and attitude towards sports and exercise [4].

## 49.2 Pathophysiology

### 49.2.1 Clinical Risk Factors

Besides "classic" [5] risk factors (age, smoking, diabetes, left ventricular hypertrophy, hypertension, previous myocardial infarction, congestive heart failure, valvular heart disease), several "new" [6] risk factors including obesity, sleep apnoea, alcohol abuse and other intoxications, sedentary lifestyle but also excessive sports practice, latent hypertension, genetic factors and inflammation, have gained scientific attention during the last years. Specifically, recent research has highlighted the potential beneficial effects of lifestyle and risk factor management for AF as an „upstream"non-invasive therapy [7].

### 49.2.2 Molecular Mechanisms

AF pathophysiology is complex [8] and also depends on the above-mentioned respective type of AF. In brief, Moe's multiple wavelet theory [9] describes so-called "micro-reentry" as electrophysiological correlate of AF. This means that multiple fibrillation waves circulate simultaneously within the atrium whereby AF is more "stable" the larger the available "excitable mass" is (i.e. left atrial size) [9]. According to the seminal studies of Haissaguerre et al. [10], paroxysmal AF is induced by ectopic electrical activity within the pulmonary veins, which can be modulated by autonomic tone [11] and intraatrial pressure [12]. Increased vagal tone and intraatrial pressure, as well as LA size accompany the development of the athlete's heart [13] and therefore may also play a role in AF pathophysiology in athletes (see below and Chap. 34) [14, 15]. For the first time, Wijffels et al. described (atrial) tachycardia-induced changes of the atrium, so-called "atrial remodeling" (AR) in 1995 [16]. Tachycardia-dependent AR represents an adaptive mechanism starting after AF onset which includes electrophysiological, mechanical and structural alterations of the atrium [8]. Structural alterations favour AF (re-) initiation and propagation so that finally, AF can sustain itself ("AF begets AF") resulting in persistent AF. Interestingly, many clinical AF risk factors induce AR similar to tachycardia-induced AR for their part in turn explaining their respective role as AF risk factor [8].

Figure 49.1 summarizes clinical parameters and molecular mechanisms/changes in the atrial tissue which finally favour AF occurrence and maintenance [17].

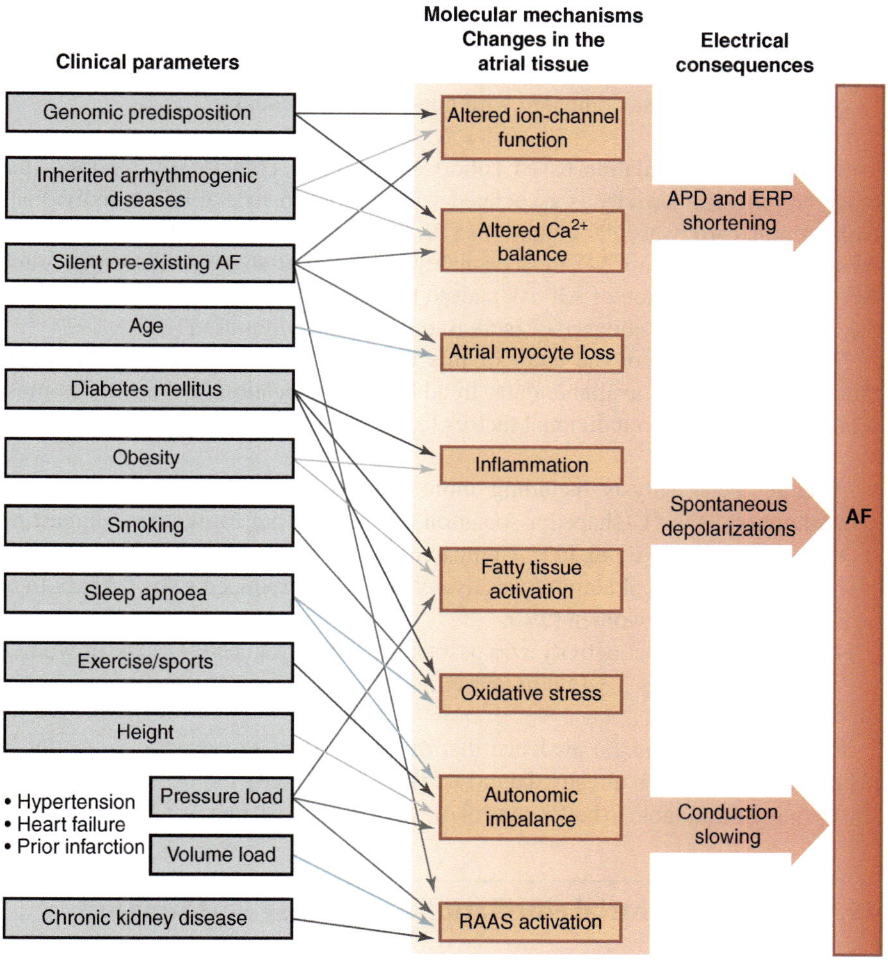


**Fig. 49.1** Hypothetical network of the clinical conditions and mechanisms associated with AF (reproduced with permission from [17], Nature Reviews Cardiology, http://creativecommons.org/licenses/by/4.0/)

## 49.3 Fitness, Exercise and Risk of Atrial Fibrillation in Non-athletes

At the epidemiological level, in a large cohort study with >64,000 older subjects (55 ± 13 years) who underwent exercise testing, an inverse relationship between cardiorespiratory fitness and incident AF was observed [18]:

- Each additional MET achieved during treadmill testing was associated with a 7% lower incidence of AF during a mean follow-up of 5.4 years, after adjustment for confounders.
- The magnitude of the inverse association between CRF and incident AF was greater among obese compared with non-obese individuals.

Several large population-based cohort studies have consistently reported that moderate physical activity is associated with a reduced risk of AF in individuals with specific cardiovascular conditions [19, 20]. In summary, together with data of AF in athletes (see Chap. 34), most probably there is an U-shaped relation of PA and AF risk with a reduction of AF risk caused by light/moderate PA and a progressive risk increase as a consequence of increased PA intensity/duration [21].

However, location of the nadir of this U-shaped association cannot be determined from currently available data. In addition, the location of the nadir is most probably dependent on individual factors (e.g. CV risk factors) [15].

- A large meta-analysis including more than 656.000 subjects supported the assumption of the U-shaped association for men but not for woman, suggesting a gender-specific AF risk [22]. Compared to a sedentary lifestyle
  - moderate physical activity was associated with a reduced risk of AF, both in men (19%) and women (9%).
  - vigorous physical activity was associated with a reduced AF risk in women (28%) but with a 3.3-fold increased AF risk in men.

Finally, there is clinical evidence that moderate exercise seems to be useful in patients who have been already diagnosed with AF whereby the benefits may be, at least in part, attributable to better control of "classic" AF risk factors [23] (see below).

## 49.4 Impact of Atrial Fibrillation on Exercise Performance

In large AF cohorts, more than half of all patients experience a reduction of exercise capacity, and suffer from dyspnea or early fatigue [24]. However, there is substantial inter-individual and intra-individual heterogeneity in type and severity of AF symptoms. The mechanistic link between AF and exercise intolerance is complicated by the fact that AF often occurs in the presence of heart disease like heart failure or valvular dysfunction, that exhibit similar symptoms.

Exercise performance depends on oxygen uptake, transportation and delivery to the working muscles. The cardiac output plays a crucial role for oxygen transportation (see Chap. 3). Both, underlying heart disease and AF may compromise cardiac output [24].

- AF contributes to decreased LV filling by fast heart rates, and loss of atrial contraction and atrioventricular synchrony.
- AF contributes to decreased LV systolic function by fast and/or irregular heart rate and tachycardia-induced cardiomyopathy.

In the absence of an underlying heart disease, patients with long-standing persistent AF may have a preserved exercise capacity, since loss of atrial function may partly be compensated by a higher maximal heart rate [25]. However, restoration and maintenance of sinus rhythm (SR) has been shown to improve exercise capacity and quality of life, compared to baseline values [26, 27].

- In an AF cardioversion cohort, patients with stable SR or SR with recurrent AF episodes had a 12–20% better exercise tolerance, representing an increase of 1.5–2.0 MET after 1 year of follow-up [27].
- In cohorts of patients with heart failure with preserved, mid-range or reduced ejection fraction, the presence of AF was associated with a lower exercise capacity (11–20%, or 0.5–0.9 METs) and a poorer prognosis [28–32].

## 49.5 Effects of Exercise Training on Burden of Atrial Fibrillation

In non-athletes with non-permanent AF, limited evidence suggests that exercise training may reduce the burden of AF and symptom severity, partly explained by beneficial effects on CV risk factor profile and atrial remodeling:

- A small randomized controlled trial (51 patients) compared a 12-week supervised aerobic interval training (AIT, four 4-min intervals at 85–95% of peak heart rate, three times a week) with a control group continuing their regular exercise habits [33].
  - AIT reduced the burden of AF (8.1–4.8%), AF symptom frequency and severity.
  - AIT improved cardiorespiratory fitness (+ 0.9 MET), left atrial and ventricular function, lipid levels, and quality of life.
- Another 12-week randomized controlled trial (76 patients) allocated patients to either low intensity or high intensity exercise training (50% and 80% of maximal perceived exertion, respectively, two weekly 60 min sessions).
  - After a 14-month follow-up, there were no group difference for burden of AF and fitness gain [34].

- A long-term observational study recruited 308 overweight patients (BMI ≥ 27 kg/m$^2$) from an arrhythmia clinic to participate in a structured risk factor management program. Face-to-face counseling was used for initiating and reinforcing graded exercise therapy along with weight reduction. Tailored exercise training recommendations were given (3 to 5 sessions per week, low to moderate intensity, <85% of peak heart rate, 60–200 min per week, aerobic and strength training) [35]. Patients who gained ≥2 METs participated in more scheduled visits (83% vs. 39%) and exhibited a larger weight loss (−12.0 ± 8.8 vs. −3.0 ± 7.6 kg). A fitness gain of ≥2 METs was associated with
  - a higher 5-year freedom of AF (37% vs. 13% in patients who lost <10% of weight, and 76% vs. 44% in patients who lost ≥10% of weight);
  - a better blood pressure control, lower proportion of diabetes mellitus, improved lipid profiles, and lower markers of inflammation;
  - a lower number of prescribed blood pressure and anti-arrhythmic drugs;
  - a lower atrial volume, favorable left ventricular geometry, and better diastolic function;
  - an improved quality of life.
- In chronic heart failure with reduced ejection fraction, the presence of AF is generally associated with older age, reduced exercise capacity and higher overall rate of clinical events. The largest training study in this population (HF-ACTION, 2331 patients; see Chap. 48) included 382 patients (17%) with documented AF at baseline [32]. Over a median follow-up of 2.6 years, heart failure patients with AF
  - exhibited similar benefits of exercise training for clinical outcomes, functional status and quality of life;
  - had no increased burden of AF events.

## 49.6 Sports Eligibility of Non-athletes with Atrial Fibrillation

### 49.6.1 Exercise Testing

Before engaging in exercise or sports, patients with AF require a clinical evaluation, optimal therapy for rate or rhythm control, risk stratification, and treatment of underlying causes like hypertension or heart failure. A maximum exercise testing should be performed [36, 37].

(a) to study the adequacy of rate control across a full spectrum of activity in patients with persistent or permanent AF
(b) to rule out exercise-induced myocardial ischemia or ventricular arrhythmias
(c) to study QRS duration if class Ic antiarrhythmic drug therapy is initiated (QRS width should not exceed 50%)
(d) to study the blood pressure profile during exercise
(e) to determine maximal exercise capacity
(f) to determine training zones.

A routine exercise protocol on a bicycle or treadmill can be used, based on availability and patient's preference (see also Chaps. 11 and 45) [36].

- Optimal test duration is 8–12 min, and protocols should be adapted accordingly.
- For determination of training zones ramp protocols are preferred over stage protocols.
- Incremental cardiopulmonary exercise testing (CPET; see Chap. 45) may be considered for determination of ventilatory thresholds, differentiation of exertional dyspnea in AF, and in special populations (e.g. heart failure)

No standard method for assessment of heart rate control has been established to guide management of AF patients. Criteria for rate control vary with patient age but usually involve achieving ventricular rates between 90 and 115 bpm during moderate exercise [37]. CPET allows the display of heart rate in relation to oxygen-uptake and helps in the judgement, whether a heart rate is appropriate for a given workload. See Fig. 49.1 for an example.

## 49.7 Oral Anticoagulation

At least in 80% of all AF patients, oral anticoagulation (OAC) is indicated according to current guidelines [1, 38]. Nevertheless, especially older patients are often highly undersupplied concerning OAC [39]. Despite the clear positive evidence of physical activity (PA) in cardiac rehabilitation of AF patients as depicted in this chapter, patients receiving OAC seem to avoid PA due to the fear of bleeding [40]. In addition, the risk of falling often represents a doctor's argument against OAC especially in geriatric patients [41].

- Indeed, in the elderly, falls often occurred during sports participation in a large cohort study of Mertz et al. [42].
  - However, the relative risk of falling was—at least in male subjects—negatively correlated with baseline fitness and PA level [42].

There are only few data concerning bleeding complications during cardiac rehabilitation indicating that cardiac rehabilitation of patients receiving OAC is most probably safe, especially when physical training is performed on stationary cycle ergometers [43]. Concerning the association of bleeding complications and everyday activities, there is evidence that a higher PA level goes along with a reduced risk of severe bleeding in patients receiving OAC [40, 44]. Notably, all depicted findings were mostly gained in subjects receiving warfarin derivatives but not NOACs [43].

Summarized, recreational sports participation of subjects receiving OAC should be an individual decision including overall clinical situation but also sport disciplines (Fig. 49.2).

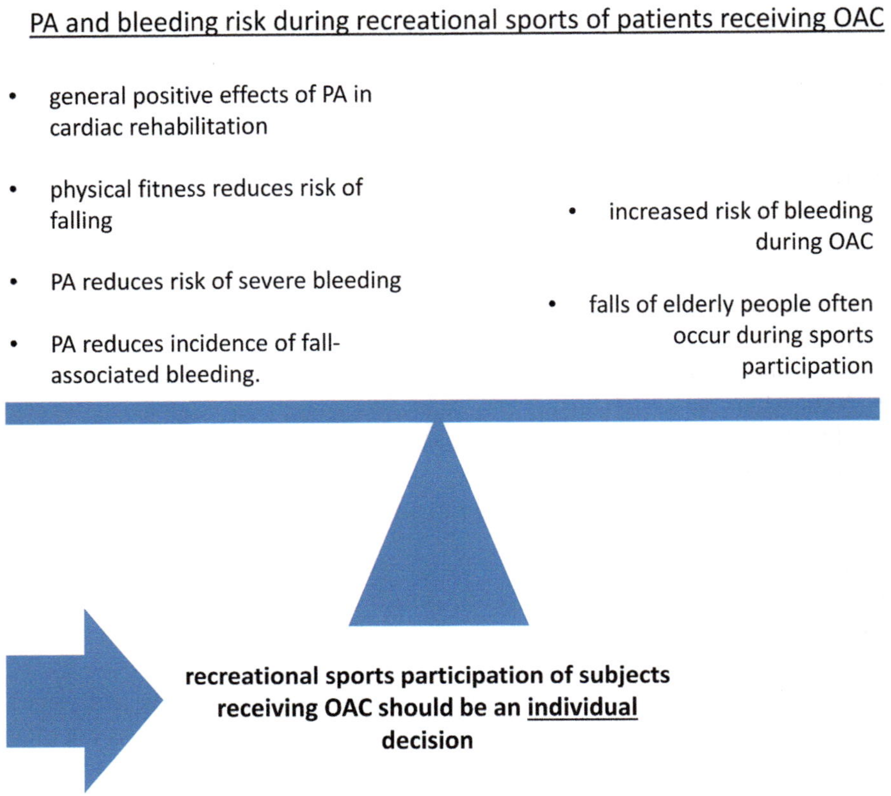


**Fig. 49.2** Risks and benefits of physical activity (PA) in patients receiving oral anticoagulation (OAC)

### 49.7.1 Training Recommendations

General exercise training recommendations apply also for patients with AF (see also Chap. 44). Non-athletes may also participate in leisure-time sports and non-elite competitions (see Chap. 34).

- For cardiovascular health and disease prevention, at least 150 min per week of moderate intensity or 75 min per week of vigorous intensity aerobic PA or equivalent combination thereof are recommended [45, 46].
- Moderate-to-vigorous aerobic exercise is recommended for supervised training programs and is feasible for most patients with AF [47].
- Aerobic interval training has been shown to improve AF burden, exercise capacity and quality of life, compared to unstructured exercise in selected patients with non-permanent AF, but long-term studies are lacking [33].
- Participation in leisure-time sports and non-elite competitions is possible, if heart rate during exercise is well controlled, there are no contraindications due to an underlying heart disease and bleeding risk of antithrombotic therapy is considered in the context of the specific sport discipline (see above) [48].

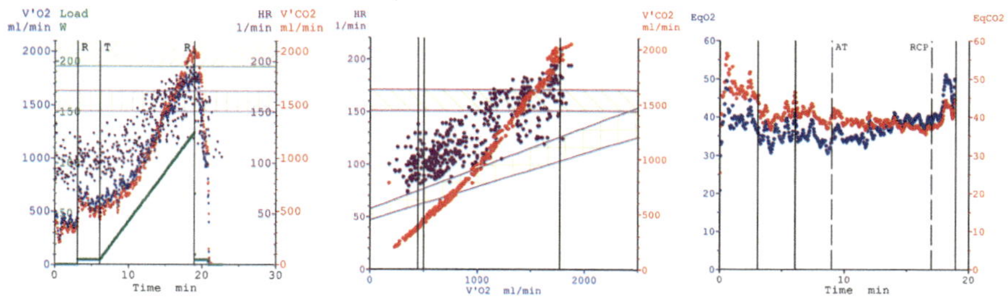


**Fig. 49.3** Exercise test of a 59-year-old patient with long-standing persistent AF, valvular and coronary heart disease, 1 month after aortic valve replacement, before starting a CR program. Left panel: Incremental ramp protocol showing a moderately reduced exercise capacity (55% of predicted). The scattered heart rate profile during exercise reflects the irregularity of AF. Middle panel: Display of heart rate in relation to oxygen uptake. At all time points, heart rate is higher than the reference range, and peak heart rate exceeded the predicted maximum, illustrating suboptimal rate control of AF. Right panel: Equivalents (Eq) for oxygen and carbon dioxide over time. Determination of the aerobic (first ventilatory) threshold (AT) and the respiratory compensation point (RCP, second ventilatory threshold). Workload at AT and RCP were 51 W and 111 W, respectively. The low workload at the first threshold reflects muscular deconditioning after valve surgery

Functional evaluation through exercise testing prior to starting an aerobic training program is recommended, and ramp incremental CPET, when available, is the gold standard for a physiologically comprehensive exercise intensity assessment and prescription. This may allow a shift from a 'range-based' to a 'threshold-based' aerobic exercise intensity prescription, which could maximize the benefits of training [47]. The highly variable chronotropic response at submaximal levels of exercise render heart rate of little utility for aerobic training prescription in AF patients. Training zones can be determined by using

(a) watt or treadmill speed/inclination at the ventilatory thresholds;
(b) percentage of peak watt or treadmill speed/inclination;
(c) values of the rating of perceived exertion (RPE) Borg scale;
(d) a combination of watt or treadmill speed/elevation with RPE.

Figure 49.3 illustrates the definition of training zones based on ventilatory thresholds.

## 49.8 Integrating Atrial Fibrillation Patients in Cardiac Rehabilitation Programs

Cardiac rehabilitation (CR) is recommended as a secondary prevention strategy for patients with chronic cardiovascular diseases like coronary artery disease, heart failure and peripheral artery occlusive disease [49]. Specific recommendations for PA counselling and exercise training during CR have been published (see also Chaps. 43 and 44) [50].

- In large randomized controlled trials comparing rate and rhythm control strategies for AF, approximately 30% of patients would qualify for a CR program, based on their underlying cardiac disease, mainly coronary artery disease [51, 52].
- However, in large observational studies the prevalence of AF in current CR programs is as low as 7–13% [53].
- The EURObservational Research Program on Atrial Fibrillation (EORP-AF) has demonstrated that only 21.7% of enrolled AF patients were regularly active, and 38.9% reported no PA. Regular exercise was associated with a lower risk of cardiovascular and all-cause mortality [54].

CR programs may have the potential to increase the level of PA among patients with AF to improve prognosis in addition to exercise capacity and quality of life. However, at present, clinical guidelines for the management of AF do not include referral to CR. However, they already recommend an integrated management of patients with AF, including patient education and empowerment, CV risk factor management and lifestyle changes [45]. Comprehensive CR programs would help to implement guideline recommendations. A recent position paper highlights the potential of CR for the prevention of AF in patients with risk factors [55].

Figure 49.4 illustrates the heat rate during an exercise training session of a patient with valvular heart disease and long-standing persistent AF during his CR program.

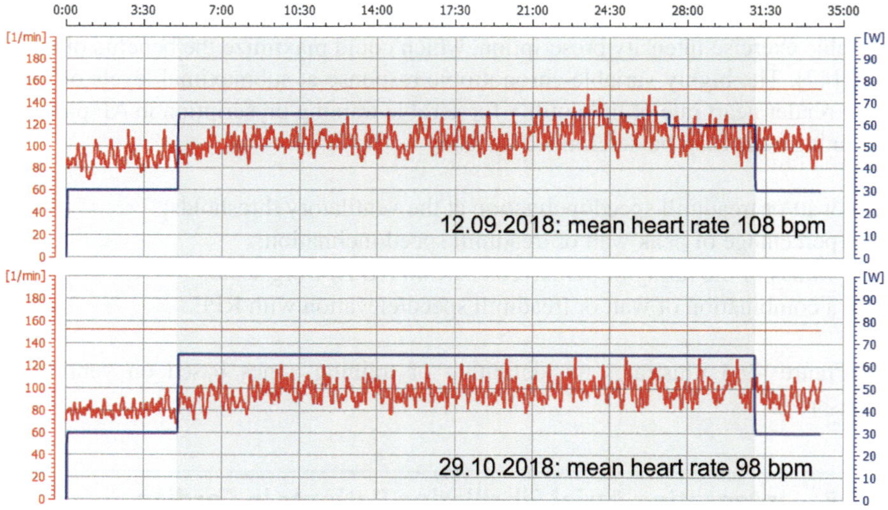


**Fig. 49.4** Two training sessions with a constant workload on a bicycle, 1 month after entering a CR program (same patient as in Fig. 49.1). The optimal training zone was determined from the ventilatory thresholds of the CPET (between 51 and 111 W). The betablocker dose was unchanged in this period (metoprolol 75 mg bid). Upper panel: Heart rate during warm-up exceeded 110 bpm and increased slightly during the training at 65 W, with peaks above 150 bpm, accompanied by patient's discomfort. Workload had to be reduced toward the end of the training to 60 W. Lower panel: Heart-rate remained below 100 bpm during warm-up. The workload of 65 W was tolerated over the whole training session at a lower average heart rate

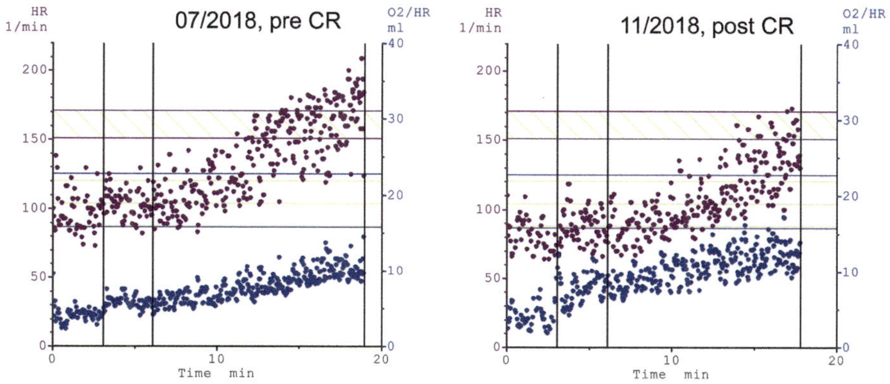


**Fig. 49.5** Heart rate profiles during a cardiopulmonary exercise test pre and post a 12-week CR program (same patient as in Figs. 49.1 and 49.2). Besides the exercise intervention, the betablocker dose was increased (from metoprolol 50 mg bid to 100 mg bid). Left panel: Resting heart rate exceeded 100 bpm and increased to values over the reference range for peak heart rate. The oxygen pulse ($O_2$/HR), a surrogate marker for left ventricular stroke volume, did not reach the reference range. Right panel: Improved heart rate profile with a resting heart rate below 100 bpm and a peak heart rate within the reference range. Improvement of the oxygen pulse

Figure 49.5 shows heart rate and oxygen pulse of the patient's cardiopulmonary exercise test at the beginning and end of the CR program.

Currently, only two systematic reviews have assessed the benefits and harms of exercise-based CR in adults with AF [56, 57].

- A small meta-analysis included only data from randomized controlled trials (6 studies, 421 participants) and found that CR increased exercise capacity, but had no clinically relevant impact on quality of life [57].
- A large meta-analysis included both observational and randomized controlled trials (12 studies, 4822 participants) and found limited evidence supporting the use of CR in AF patients to improve cardiometabolic health indicators and aerobic and functional capacity but conflicting data on quality of live and mental health [56].

## 49.9 Gaps in Evidence

The current evidence of the benefits of exercise training in the heterogeneous population of AF patients is restricted to observational studies and small randomized trials with low to moderate quality. Most trials focused on moderate intensity endurance exercise.

- The impact on mortality or serious adverse events remains to be established.
- The positive effect on exercise capacity did not translate into a relevant effect on health-related quality of life and needs to be re-examined in adequately powered trials.

- Large, multicenter trials of comprehensive CR, including risk-factor management, patient education and empowerment, in addition to exercise training are lacking.
- Data on strength training and long-term effects of aerobic interval training are lacking.
- The value of individualized training recommendation and specific training modalities needs to be assessed.

**Clinical Pearls**

- Most probably there is a U-shaped relation of PA and AF risk with a reduction of AF risk caused by light to moderate PA and a progressive risk increase as a consequence of increased PA intensity/duration.
- Exercise tolerance is often decreased in patients with AF but can be improved with exercise training.
- General exercise training recommendations apply also for patients with AF.
- Bleeding risk of AF patients under oral anticoagulation has to be considered for sports and exercise recommendations.

## Chapter Review Questions

### Questions

1. A 62-year-old obese patient (BMI 31.2 kg/m$^2$) with persistent AF is referred for exercise training recommendations prior to an AF ablation procedure. The patient is taking metoprolol 50 mg bid. A cardiopulmonary exercise test is being performed. What to look out for?
2. A 29-year-old female patient with newly diagnosed "lone" paroxysmal AF and a hitherto life-long history of recreational sports is somewhat uncertain about the cause of her disease and fears that sports has made its own contribution for disease development. As the absence of cardiac risk factors led to the diagnosis "lone" AF: which factors should particularly be considered during sports-cardiological work-up of the patient?

### Answers

1. Heart rate and blood pressure should be controlled throughout the whole activity spectrum. The ECG should show no signs of exercise-induced myocardial ischemia or ventricular arrhythmias. Maximum exercise capacity and ventilatory thresholds should be used for tailored training recommendations.
2. During work-up of the master athlete, special attention should be paid on "new" risk factors like obesity, sleep apnoea, family history of AF, inflammatory diseases. Intake of doping-relevant substances should be taken into account and also alcohol abuse (there is evidence that sports participation may

contribute to increased alcohol consumption in all age groups [58–61] or other addictive drugs. Finally, endocrinological disorders (especially thyroid) should be ruled out.

## References


1. Kirchhof P, Benussi S, Kotecha D, Ahlsson A, Atar D, Casadei B, et al. 2016 ESC guidelines for the management of atrial fibrillation developed in collaboration with EACTS. Europace. 2016;18(11):1609–78.
2. Timmis A, Townsend N, Gale C, Grobbee R, Maniadakis N, Flather M, et al. European Society of Cardiology: cardiovascular disease statistics 2017. Eur Heart J. 2018;39(7):508–79.
3. Le Heuzey JY, Paziaud O, Piot O, Said MA, Copie X, Lavergne T, et al. Cost of care distribution in atrial fibrillation patients: the COCAF study. Am Heart J. 2004;147(1):121–6.
4. Myrstad M, Malmo V, Ulimoen SR, Tveit A, Loennechen JP. Exercise in individuals with atrial fibrillation. Clin Res Cardiol. 2019;108(4):347–54.
5. Benjamin EJ, Levy D, Vaziri SM, et al. Independent risk factors for atrial fibrillation in a population-based cohort: the Framingham Heart Study. JAMA. 1994;271:840–4.
6. Schoonderwoerd BA, Smit MD, Pen L, Van Gelder IC. New risk factors for atrial fibrillation: causes of 'not-so-lone atrial fibrillation'. Europace. 2008;10(6):668–73.
7. Lau DH, Nattel S, Kalman JM, Sanders P. Modifiable risk factors and atrial fibrillation. Circulation. 2017;136(6):583–96.
8. Schotten U, Verheule S, Kirchhof P, Goette A. Pathophysiological mechanisms of atrial fibrillation: a translational appraisal. Physiol Rev. 2011;91(1):265–325.
9. Allessie MA, Lammers WJ, Bonke FI, Hollen J, Zipes DP, Jalife J. Experimental evaluation of Moe's multiple wavelet hypothesis of atrial fibrillation. In: Zipes DP, Jalife J, editors. Cardiac electrophysiology and arrhythmias. New York: Grune & Stratton; 1985. p. 265–75.
10. Haissaguerre M, Jais P, Shah DC, Takahashi A, Hocini M, Quiniou G, et al. Spontaneous initiation of atrial fibrillation by ectopic beats originating in the pulmonary veins. N Engl J Med. 1998;339(10):659–66.
11. Tai CT, Chiou CW, Wen ZC, Hsieh MH, Tsai CF, Lin WS, et al. Effect of phenylephrine on focal atrial fibrillation originating in the pulmonary veins and superior vena cava. J Am Coll Cardiol. 2000;36(3):788–93.
12. Kalifa J, Jalife J, Zaitsev AV, Bagwe S, Warren M, Moreno J, Berenfeld O, Nattel S. Intra-atrial pressure increases rate and organization of waves emanating from the superior pulmonary veins during atrial fibrillation. Circulation. 2003;108:668–71.
13. Beaudry R, Haykowsky MJ, Baggish A, La Gerche A. A modern definition of the Athlete's heart-for research and the clinic. Cardiol Clin. 2016;34(4):507–14.
14. Wilhelm M. Atrial fibrillation in endurance athletes. Eur J Prev Cardiol. 2014;21(8):1040–8.
15. Laszlo R, Steinacker JM. Atrial fibrillation and physical activity: an overview. Herz. 2016;41(2):131–7.
16. Wijffels MC, Kirchhof CJ, Dorland R, Allessie MA. Atrial fibrillation begets atrial fibrillation. A study in awake chronically instrumented goats. Circulation. 1995;92(7):1954–68.
17. Fabritz L, Guasch E, Antoniades C, Bardinet I, Benninger G, Betts TR, et al. Expert consensus document: defining the major health modifiers causing atrial fibrillation: a roadmap to underpin personalized prevention and treatment. Nat Rev Cardiol. 2016;13(4):230–7.
18. Qureshi WT, Alirhayim Z, Blaha MJ, Juraschek SP, Keteyian SJ, Brawner CA, et al. Cardiorespiratory fitness and risk of incident atrial fibrillation: results from the Henry ford exercise testing (FIT) project. Circulation. 2015;131(21):1827–34.
19. Ofman P, Khawaja O, Rahilly-Tierney CR, Peralta A, Hoffmeister P, Reynolds MR, et al. Regular physical activity and risk of atrial fibrillation: a systematic review and meta-analysis. Circ Arrhythm Electrophysiol. 2013;6(2):252–6.

20. Morseth B, Lochen ML, Ariansen I, Myrstad M, Thelle DS. The ambiguity of physical activity, exercise and atrial fibrillation. Eur J Prev Cardiol. 2018;25(6):624–36.
21. La Gerche A, Schmied CM. Atrial fibrillation in athletes and the interplay between exercise and health. Eur Heart J. 2013;34(47):3599–602.
22. Mohanty S, Mohanty P, Tamaki M, Natale V, Gianni C, Trivedi C, et al. Differential association of exercise intensity with risk of atrial fibrillation in men and women: evidence from a meta-analysis. J Cardiovasc Electrophysiol. 2016;27(9):1021–9.
23. Pathak RK, Middeldorp ME, Lau DH, Mehta AB, Mahajan R, Twomey D, et al. Aggressive risk factor reduction study for atrial fibrillation and implications for the outcome of ablation: the ARREST-AF cohort study. J Am Coll Cardiol. 2014;64(21):2222–31.
24. Rienstra M, Lubitz SA, Mahida S, Magnani JW, Fontes JD, Sinner MF, et al. Symptoms and functional status of patients with atrial fibrillation: state of the art and future research opportunities. Circulation. 2012;125(23):2933–43.
25. Atwood JE, Myers J, Sullivan M, Forbes S, Friis R, Pewen W, et al. Maximal exercise testing and gas exchange in patients with chronic atrial fibrillation. J Am Coll Cardiol. 1988;11(3):508–13.
26. Singh SN, Tang XC, Singh BN, Dorian P, Reda DJ, Harris CL, et al. Quality of life and exercise performance in patients in sinus rhythm versus persistent atrial fibrillation: a veterans affairs cooperative studies program substudy. J Am Coll Cardiol. 2006;48(4):721–30.
27. Atwood JE, Myers JN, Tang XC, Reda DJ, Singh SN, Singh BN. Exercise capacity in atrial fibrillation: a substudy of the Sotalol-amiodarone atrial fibrillation efficacy trial (SAFE-T). Am Heart J. 2007;153(4):566–72.
28. Elshazly MB, Senn T, Wu Y, Lindsay B, Saliba W, Wazni O, et al. Impact of atrial fibrillation on exercise capacity and mortality in heart failure with preserved ejection fraction: insights from cardiopulmonary stress testing. J Am Heart Assoc. 2017;6(11).
29. Kaye DM, Silvestry FE, Gustafsson F, Cleland JG, van Veldhuisen DJ, Ponikowski P, et al. Impact of atrial fibrillation on rest and exercise haemodynamics in heart failure with mid-range and preserved ejection fraction. Eur J Heart Fail. 2017;19(12):1690–7.
30. Lam CS, Rienstra M, Tay WT, Liu LC, Hummel YM, van der Meer P, et al. Atrial fibrillation in heart failure with preserved ejection fraction: association with exercise capacity, left ventricular filling pressures, natriuretic peptides, and left atrial volume. JACC Heart Fail. 2017;5(2):92–8.
31. Pardaens K, Van Cleemput J, Vanhaecke J, Fagard RH. Atrial fibrillation is associated with a lower exercise capacity in male chronic heart failure patients. Heart. 1997;78(6):564–8.
32. Luo N, Merrill P, Parikh KS, Whellan DJ, Pina IL, Fiuzat M, et al. Exercise training in patients with chronic heart failure and atrial fibrillation. J Am Coll Cardiol. 2017;69(13):1683–91.
33. Malmo V, Nes BM, Amundsen BH, Tjonna AE, Stoylen A, Rossvoll O, et al. Aerobic interval training reduces the burden of atrial fibrillation in the short term: a randomized trial. Circulation. 2016;133(5):466–73.
34. Skielboe AK, Bandholm TQ, Hakmann S, Mourier M, Kallemose T, Dixen U. Cardiovascular exercise and burden of arrhythmia in patients with atrial fibrillation - a randomized controlled trial. PLoS One. 2017;12(2):e0170060.
35. Pathak RK, Elliott A, Middeldorp ME, Meredith M, Mehta AB, Mahajan R, et al. Impact of CARDIOrespiratory FITness on arrhythmia recurrence in obese individuals with atrial fibrillation: the CARDIO-FIT study. J Am Coll Cardiol. 2015;66(9):985–96.
36. Fletcher GF, Ades PA, Kligfield P, Arena R, Balady GJ, Bittner VA, et al. Exercise standards for testing and training: a scientific statement from the American Heart Association. Circulation. 2013;128(8):873–934.
37. Morise AP. Exercise testing in nonatherosclerotic heart disease: hypertrophic cardiomyopathy, valvular heart disease, and arrhythmias. Circulation. 2011;123(2):216–25.
38. Friberg L, Bergfeldt L. Atrial fibrillation prevalence revisited. J Intern Med. 2013;274(5):461–8.
39. Wilke T, Groth A, Mueller S, Pfannkuche M, Verheyen F, Linder R, et al. Oral anticoagulation use by patients with atrial fibrillation in Germany. Adherence to guidelines, causes of

anticoagulation under-use and its clinical outcomes, based on claims-data of 183,448 patients. Thromb Haemost. 2012;107(6):1053–65.
40. Frey PM, Mean M, Limacher A, Jaeger K, Beer HJ, Frauchiger B, et al. Physical activity and risk of bleeding in elderly patients taking anticoagulants. J Thromb Haemost. 2015;13(2):197–205.
41. Gosch M, Roller RE, Bohmdorfer B, Benvenuti-Falger U, Iglseder B, Lechleitner M, et al. Management and therapy of atrial fibrillation in geriatric patients. Z Gerontol Geriatr. 2012;45(1):55–66; quiz 7-8
42. Mertz KJ, Lee DC, Sui X, Powell KE, Blair SN. Falls among adults: the association of cardiorespiratory fitness and physical activity with walking-related falls. Am J Prev Med. 2010;39(1):15–24.
43. Laszlo R, Lesevic H, Enders K, Steinacker JM. Atrial fibrillation: sports and oral anticoagulation. Deutsche Zeitschrift für Sportmedizin. 2017;68(6):142–7.
44. Shendre A, Beasley TM, Brown TM, Hill CE, Arnett DK, Limdi NA. Influence of regular physical activity on warfarin dose and risk of hemorrhagic complications. Pharmacotherapy. 2014;34(6):545–54.
45. Kirchhof P, Benussi S, Kotecha D, Ahlsson A, Atar D, Casadei B, et al. 2016 ESC guidelines for the management of atrial fibrillation developed in collaboration with EACTS: the Task Force for the management of atrial fibrillation of the European Society of Cardiology (ESC) Developed with the special contribution of the European Heart Rhythm Association (EHRA) of the ESCEndorsed by the European Stroke Organisation (ESO). Eur Heart J. 2016;37(38).
46. Piepoli MF, Hoes AW, Agewall S, Albus C, Brotons C, Catapano AL, et al. 2016 European Guidelines on cardiovascular disease prevention in clinical practice: the Sixth Joint Task Force of the European Society of Cardiology and Other Societies on Cardiovascular Disease Prevention in Clinical Practice (constituted by representatives of 10 societies and by invited experts)Developed with the special contribution of the European Association for Cardiovascular Prevention & Rehabilitation (EACPR). Eur Heart J. 2016;37(29):2315–81.
47. Mezzani A, Hamm LF, Jones AM, McBride PE, Moholdt T, Stone JA, et al. Aerobic exercise intensity assessment and prescription in cardiac rehabilitation: a joint position statement of the European Association for Cardiovascular Prevention and Rehabilitation, the American Association of Cardiovascular and Pulmonary Rehabilitation and the Canadian Association of Cardiac Rehabilitation. Eur J Prev Cardiol. 2013;20(3):442–67.
48. Zipes DP, Link MS, Ackerman MJ, Kovacs RJ, Myerburg RJ, Estes NA 3rd, et al. Eligibility and disqualification recommendations for competitive athletes with cardiovascular abnormalities: task force 9: arrhythmias and conduction defects: a scientific statement from the American Heart Association and American College of Cardiology. Circulation. 2015;132(22):e315–25.
49. Piepoli MF, Corra U, Benzer W, Bjarnason-Wehrens B, Dendale P, Gaita D, et al. Secondary prevention through cardiac rehabilitation: from knowledge to implementation. A position paper from the Cardiac Rehabilitation Section of the European Association of Cardiovascular Prevention and Rehabilitation. Eur J Cardiovasc Prev Rehabil. 2010;17(1):1–17.
50. Corra U, Piepoli MF, Carre F, Heuschmann P, Hoffmann U, Verschuren M, et al. Secondary prevention through cardiac rehabilitation: physical activity counselling and exercise training: key components of the position paper from the cardiac rehabilitation section of the European Association of Cardiovascular Prevention and Rehabilitation. Eur Heart J. 2010;31(16):1967–74.
51. Van Gelder IC, Hagens VE, Bosker HA, Kingma JH, Kamp O, Kingma T, et al. A comparison of rate control and rhythm control in patients with recurrent persistent atrial fibrillation. N Engl J Med. 2002;347(23):1834–40.
52. Wyse DG, Waldo AL, DiMarco JP, Domanski MJ, Rosenberg Y, Schron EB, et al. A comparison of rate control and rhythm control in patients with atrial fibrillation. N Engl J Med. 2002;347(23):1825–33.
53. Younis A, Shaviv E, Nof E, Israel A, Berkovitch A, Goldenberg I, et al. The role and outcome of cardiac rehabilitation program in patients with atrial fibrillation. Clin Cardiol. 2018;41(9):1170–6.

54. Proietti M, Boriani G, Laroche C, Diemberger I, Popescu MI, Rasmussen LH, et al. Self-reported physical activity and major adverse events in patients with atrial fibrillation: a report from the EURObservational Research Programme Pilot Survey on Atrial Fibrillation (EORP-AF) General Registry. Europace. 2017;19(4):535–43.
55. Gorenek B, Pelliccia A, Benjamin EJ, Boriani G, Crijns HJ, Fogel RI, et al. European Heart Rhythm Association (EHRA)/European Association of Cardiovascular Prevention and Rehabilitation (EACPR) position paper on how to prevent atrial fibrillation endorsed by the Heart Rhythm Society (HRS) and Asia Pacific Heart Rhythm Society (APHRS). Europace. 2017;19(2):190–225.
56. Reed JL, Terada T, Chirico D, Prince SA, Pipe AL. The effects of cardiac rehabilitation in patients with atrial fibrillation: a systematic review. Can J Cardiol. 2018;34(10S2):S284–S95.
57. Risom SS, Zwisler AD, Johansen PP, Sibilitz KL, Lindschou J, Gluud C, et al. Exercise-based cardiac rehabilitation for adults with atrial fibrillation. Cochrane Database Syst Rev. 2017;2:CD011197.
58. Diehl K, Thiel A, Zipfel S, Mayer J, Litaker DG, Schneider S. How healthy is the behavior of young athletes? A systematic literature review and meta-analyses. J Sports Sci Med. 2012;11(2):201–20.
59. Lisha NE, Sussman S, Fapa F, Leventhal AM. Physical activity and alcohol use disorders. Am J Drug Alcohol Abuse. 2013;39(2):115–20.
60. Tamminen KA, Holt NL, Crocker PR. Adolescent athletes: psychosocial challenges and clinical concerns. Curr Opin Psychiatry. 2012;25(4):293–300.
61. Myrstad M, Lochen ML, Graff-Iversen S, Gulsvik AK, Thelle DS, Stigum H, et al. Increased risk of atrial fibrillation among elderly Norwegian men with a history of long-term endurance sport practice. Scand J Med Sci Sports. 2014;24(4):e238–44.

# Exercise in Specific Diseases: Pacemakers and Implantable Cardioverter Defibrillators

# 50

Kumar Narayanan and Eloi Marijon

**Learning Objectives**

Understand the pathophysiology, clinical issues and risks-benefits involved with regard to exercise and sports participation in individuals with pacemakers and ICDs.

1. Summarize the current evidence available on this topic.
2. Discuss the recommendations from current guidelines on physical activity and exercise in this special population.
3. Develop a practical approach, based on current knowledge, for clinical decision-making for the individual patient.

## 50.1 Scope of the Problem

Cardiac Implantable Electronic Devices (CIEDs), including

(a) pacemakers,
(b) Implantable Cardioverter Defibrillators (ICDs) and
(c) Cardiac Resynchronization Therapy (CRT)

are now an integral part of heart disease management, with large trials [1–3] demonstrating their utility, and international guidelines [4, 5] giving specific

K. Narayanan, MD, FHRS
Paris Cardiovascular Research Center, Inserm U970, Paris, France

Cardiology Department, Medicover Hospitals, Hyderabad, India
e-mail: kumar.narayanan@inserm.fr

E. Marijon, MD, PhD (✉)
Paris Cardiovascular Research Center, Inserm U970, Paris, France

Cardiology Department, European Georges Pompidou Hospital, Paris, France



A. Pressler, J. Niebauer (eds.), *Textbook of Sports and Exercise Cardiology*,
https://doi.org/10.1007/978-3-030-35374-2_50

recommendations for their use. CIEDs may be implanted for structural heart disease (various cardiomyopathies) or non-structural, purely arrhythmic disorders such as conduction system diseases and channelopathies. The range of conditions therefore encompass a wide spectrum of patient types, both young and old, many of whom may be having active lifestyles. This is more so, as improved diagnostic techniques, family screening, genetic testing [6] and pre-sports screening [7, 8] have led to an expanding pool of potentially younger patients implanted with devices. Both the diagnosis of a cardiac condition and the implantation of a CIED invariably represent a significant upheaval in the patient's life, forcing a reassessment of their overall situation, work and activities. One of the important, but incompletely understood aspects is the appropriateness and extent of physical activity in these subjects [9]. While regular exercise and cardiac rehabilitation have been found to be beneficial overall and therefore recommended [10, 11], relatively lesser attention has been paid to the subgroup with CIEDs. Questions about whether it is safe to exercise, the intensity of activity, playing recreational sports etc. all deserve careful attention and it is incumbent upon the treating cardiologist to try and give as clear a guidance as possible to patients in this often-confusing scenario.

## 50.2 Potential Concerns Related to Physical Activity in CIED Patients

### 50.2.1 Implantable Cardioverter Defibrillators (ICDs)

ICDs are implanted in a variety of cardiac conditions in order to diagnose and treat (by anti-tachycardia pacing or shock) potentially lethal cardiac arrhythmias. Hence an obvious concern in these patients is the risk of arrhythmia and attendant ICD shock during exercise.

- Studies suggest a transiently elevated risk for arrhythmias and cardiac arrest during exercise [12, 13], likely related to increased sympathetic drive, and other possible mechanisms such as dehydration and electrolyte imbalance.
- Additionally, the possibility of inappropriate shocks may also be higher in view of sinus tachycardia and a greater likelihood of other supraventricular arrhythmias during exercise [14].
- A greater chance of arrhythmia occurrence in turn, raises the possibility of syncope and resultant bodily injury.
- There is also the fear that ICD shocks may be less effective in terminating arrhythmias secondary to increased catecholamine levels during exertion [15, 16].

- Malfunction of the pulse generator as well as the lead, such as insulation defect, lead fracture etc., may occur as a result of mechanical trauma to the device due to bodily impact or stretching of the leads due to vigorous arm movements [6].

Occurrence of either appropriate or inappropriate shocks during exercise can also result in a negative psychological impact, with some subjects becoming permanently discouraged from carrying out further exercise or sports [17]. Lastly there is the concern that physical activity may lead to progression of the underlying substrate, especially in certain situations such as arrhythmogenic right ventricular cardiomyopathy (ARVC) [18].

### 50.2.2 Pacemakers and CRT

Patients exercising with routine or CRT pacemakers may be susceptible to other types of problems:

- Lack of adequate rate responsiveness may result in inadequate heart rate rise to cope with the demands of exercise.
- Excessive increases in sinus rate may result in undesirable upper rate behavior such as occurrence of 2:1 AV block causing sudden symptoms.
- Despite rate adaptive AV delays, AV synchrony may be adversely affected at higher rates, compromising exercise tolerance.
- In CRT recipients, frequent ectopics during exercise or spontaneous conduction with short AV interval can lead to loss of biventricular pacing [19, 20].
- Similarly, AV and VV optimizations done at rest may not be ideal during exercise, resulting in suboptimal CRT function and symptoms [21].
- Additionally, susceptibility to pacemaker malfunction, related to issues such as T wave oversensing, exaggerated myopotentials etc. can all increase with exercise.
- Pacemaker dependent subjects, such as those with complete AV block may suffer syncope or falls if there is device or lead malfunction during exercise.

## 50.3 Disadvantages of Restricting Exercise in CIED Recipients

Although logical concerns exist with regard to exercise in a patient with pacemaker or ICD, on the other hand one needs to consider the potential harm in restricting physical activity. The cardiovascular benefits of regular exercise are well established [22, 23]. Improvements in exercise capacity and health related quality of life have been well documented across all heart failure subgroups [24] and this applies to patients with CIEDs as well.

- For example, post CRT implantation, both cardiac function and exercise tolerance improve, but these gains may be lost in the absence of a proper cardiac rehabilitation program.

Guided exercise training can further improve exercise capacity (peak oxygen uptake, $VO_2$peak) and skeletal muscle function [25]. In both CRT and ICD recipients, exercise-based rehabilitation leads to

(a) better quality of life,
(b) improved endothelial function, and
(c) reductions in anxiety and depression [26, 27].

Improved physical activity levels have also been directly linked to survival [28]. Conversely, exercise and sports restriction may have adverse physical and psychological consequences especially in younger subjects [29]. Therefore there is a clear need for proper assessment and guidance in such patients, with studies suggesting that this population, especially ICD recipients, are often inadequately referred for rehabilitation programs [30].

## 50.4 Safety and Efficacy of Exercise in Pacemaker-/ICD-Recipients

Several studies have now demonstrated the safety and benefits of especially moderate intensity exercise among device recipients:

- The COPE-ICD trial, which randomized 196 patients with ICD to 12 weeks of exercise training versus usual care, demonstrated significant improvements in fitness and general health, without an increase in ICD shocks [31].
- The larger HF-ACTION trial randomized more than 1000 patients with an ICD to receive exercise training or regular care and found that randomization to exercise was not a predictor of increased ICD shocks [32]. Training resulted in an improvement in exercise capacity, although reduction in hospitalization or all-cause mortality was not demonstrated [33].
- Dougherty et al. prospectively studied the impact of moderately strenuous aerobic exercise after ICD implantation and reported improvements in peak oxygen consumption with no impact on ICD shocks or hospitalization compared to usual care [34].
- A prospective assessment of symptom limited treadmill exercise testing in a large ICD cohort showed no adverse events in the form of death, sustained ventricular arrhythmias or inappropriate shocks [35].
- A 2012 systematic review by Isaksen et al., confined to ICD patients, demonstrated that shocks during actual exercise were rare and exercise training improved aerobic fitness significantly; in fact, the overall frequency of shocks was greater in sedentary compared to active individuals [36].

- A more recent and larger review, encompassing all device types (pacemakers, ICDs and ventricular assist devices) confirmed both the very low adverse event rates associated with moderate to high intensity exercise training and the benefit of improved aerobic fitness [37].

Similar information is available from observational and registry data:

- In a 2006 Heart Rhythm Society survey, most member physicians reported their ICD patients participating in fairly vigorous activity such as basketball, running and skiing. Although ICD shocks occurred by report in up to 40% of such patients, serious adverse events including physical injury, damage to device and failed shocks were uncommon [38].
- A prospective, multinational sports registry, though involving only athletes with implanted ICDs, nevertheless conveyed reassuring data on the safety of participation in vigorous sports, both competitive as well as recreational, with no instances of physical injury or failure to terminate arrhythmias [17, 39].
  - The overall incidence of shocks in this registry also did not appear to significantly differ from unselected young ICD populations [40], although, as expected, shocks were more frequent during activity compared to rest.

Thus it seems that fairly vigorous exercise and rehabilitative activity is feasible in device patients, with anecdotal reports raising the possibility of meaningful return to work in even high intensity occupations such as firefighters [41].

## 50.5 Specific Considerations

While assessing the overall issue of exercise for patients with pacemakers or ICDs, some specific issues warrant consideration:

- The individual underlying pathology is important, with diseases such as catecholaminergic polymorphic VT (CPVT) and arrhythmogenic right ventricular cardiomyopathy (ARVC) more frequently associated with exercise-related shocks [39, 42].
- Also, in patients with structural cardiomyopathy, the possibility of vigorous exercise worsening the underlying substrate is another potential concern:
  - In ARVC-patients with genetically defective desmosomes, increased ventricular wall stress during physical exercise can further disrupt cell-cell junctions and accelerate fibrofatty myocardial replacement, thereby contributing to disease progression [43] and a potentially worse long term arrhythmia risk as well.
  - In fact, even in asymptomatic mutation carriers of ARVC, exercise has been linked to development and progression of disease [18].
  - Similarly, in hypertrophic cardiomyopathy (HCM), intense activity may predispose to repeated bouts of small vessel myocardial ischemia and damage, promoting more fibrosis [44].

- The type of exercise proposed is also important, with certain activities and sports such as bowling, golf and brisk walking being traditionally considered to be at low cardiovascular demand, whereas others may entail higher cardiovascular stress.

## 50.6 What Do the Guidelines Say?

Guidelines for physical activity or sports in patients with CIEDs have mainly focused on competitive athletes, from which recommendations can in turn be inferred for ordinary subjects, as the level of exercise intensity is expected to be lower:

- The 2015 ACC/AHA guidelines for athletes with pacemakers [45] suggest that athletic participation can be allowed provided the underlying substrate does not pose a high risk.
  - For pacemaker dependent patients, activities with a risk of collision and potential device damage should be avoided; protective padding to the device should be considered for all patients.
  - As far as ICDs are concerned, generally low intensity sports (Level IA; see Chap. 1) are recommended, and higher intensity can also be considered in the absence of recent active arrhythmia.
  - An arrhythmia/shock free period of at least 3 months is advised, especially if considering high intensity physical activity [45].
- Similarly, current European guidelines do not prohibit either leisure sports or even potentially competitive sports in patients with ICDs, but do stress the importance of a full discussion of the relevant risks-benefits with the individual, as well as the necessity of considering the underlying condition so as to exercise caution in high risk subsets, particularly ARVC [46].
  - Earlier European recommendations for individuals with pacemakers reiterate the issue of avoiding activities with risk of collision or device damage.
  - In addition, gathering information from a Holter or submaximal exercise test is recommended to program appropriate rate responsiveness.
  - Judicious utilization of device stored data such as atrial or ventricular high rate episodes is also advisable to ensure ongoing surveillance and appropriate management in exercising individuals [47].

Overall, guidelines have evolved over time and become more permissive in terms of even allowing vigorous exercise in patients with devices. Given the multitude of benefits associated with recreational sports and exercise training, it is evident that all CIED patients should not only be allowed but, in fact encouraged to engage in moderate intensity exercise, with appropriate precautions depending on device type and underlying pathology.

## 50.7 Clinical Approach to the Individual Patient

A planned exercise rehabilitation program is essential for all cardiac patients including those with CIEDs and should be implemented whenever possible. Generally, regular physical activity can be planned starting about 4–6 weeks after device implantation to allow for basic healing and lead fixation [48]. However, it is important to individualize the exercise prescription for each patient for which a number of variables need to be taken into account (Fig. 50.1). These can be broadly thought of as patient-/device-related factors and exercise-related factors.

### 50.7.1 Patient-/Device-Related Factors

This category includes

(a) the indication for ICD (primary vs. secondary with accordingly differing arrhythmia risk),
(b) time since last arrhythmia or shock,
(c) nature of the underlying cardiac disease (risk of arrhythmia or disease progression),
(d) the type of device (CRTD vs. ICD vs. pacemaker),
(e) number of leads, and
(f) the extent of pacemaker dependence.

One needs to carefully consider all measures which can be potentially undertaken to optimize patient-/device-related factors with respect to safely undertaking exercise. This planning should ideally begin right from the time of device implantation.

- For instance, given the lack of evidence for better discrimination with a dual chamber ICD [49, 50], two leads should not be implanted unless a compelling need exists. Reducing unnecessary leads will decrease the potential for activity related damage.
- Device programming is another important aspect.
  - In line with current thinking, especially for primary prevention, a high rate cut off or long detection times would also help minimize inappropriate shocks for sinus or supraventricular tachycardia associated with exercise [51, 52].
  - Setting a monitor zone in ICDs should always be considered as it can yield a wealth of diagnostic information including heart rates achieved during

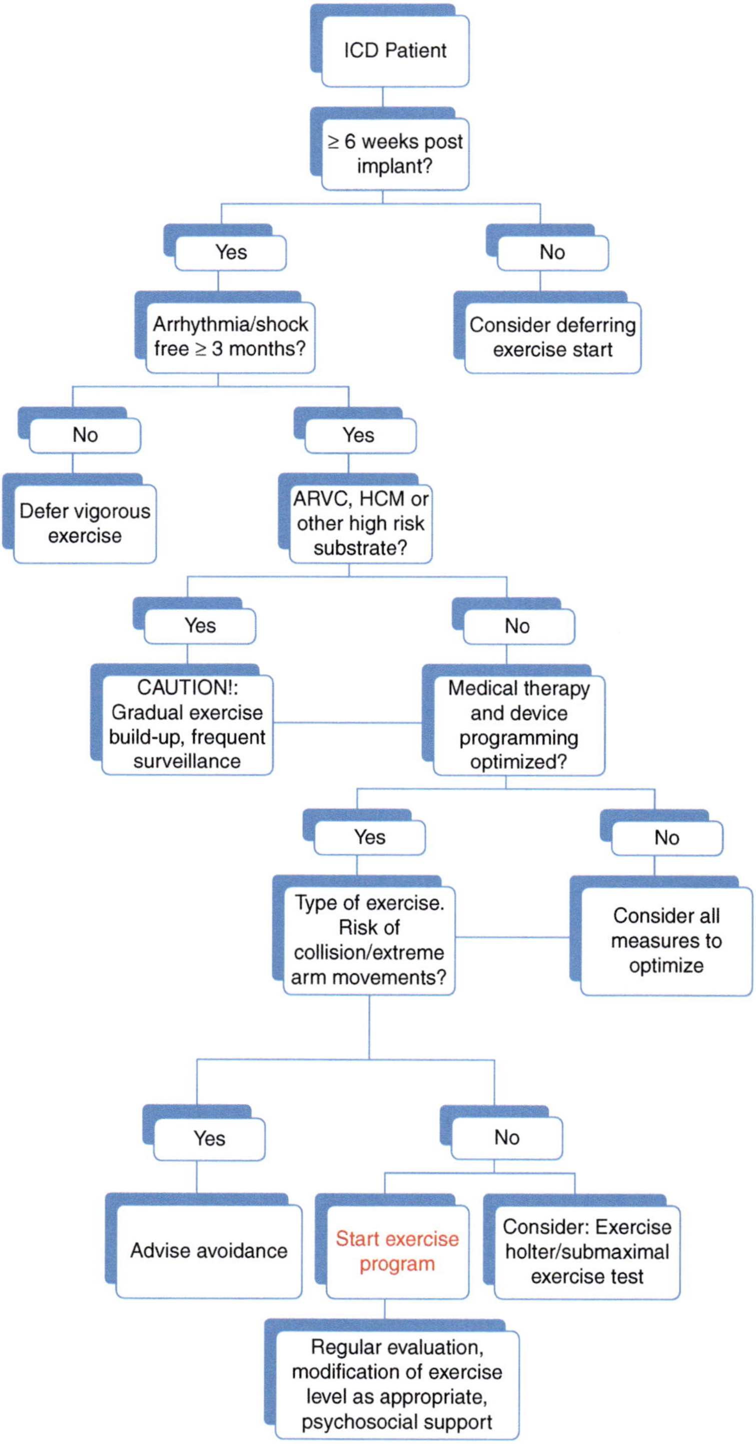


**Fig. 50.1** Suggested approach to exercise and leisure sports in a patient implanted with an ICD

exercise as well as the occurrence of exercise related arrhythmias which can help adjust medical therapy and titrate exercise levels [48].
  - Similarly for pacemakers and CRTs, the dynamic fluctuations of heart rate during exercise should be considered and appropriate programming done for ensuring adequate rate responsiveness, AV synchrony and continued biventricular pacing during exercise.
  - Upper tracking rates should be kept sufficiently high to avoid undesirable upper rate behavior and inappropriate triggering of PMT response during exercise [20].
- As already mentioned, an extended Holter or an exercise test can help assess heart rate patterns during exercise and improve programming decisions.
- Careful attention should be paid to stored diagnostic data in modern pacemakers such as atrial/ventricular high rate episodes or occurrence of myopotential oversensing with certain types of exercise [47].

In addition to ensuring device optimization, the risk of the underlying condition has to be considered, with for instance, a more cautious, gradual "build up" of activity levels in high risk variants such as ARVC with more frequent surveillance. Optimizing medical therapy for the specific pathology is obviously crucial to reduce activity related arrhythmia risk. A specific aspect concerns the use of beta blockers which are often part of medical therapy but may be associated with fatigue or perceived low energy, potentially interfering in some with exercise capacity. Although a recent registry in athletes did not show an association between beta blocker use and shocks [17], given the theoretical benefits for arrhythmia prevention, beta blockers should be continued in most situations. Additionally, the profound psychological impact of shocks is important to recognize, with several studies showing an adverse impact on quality of life [53, 54] and discontinuation of exercise driven by a fear of shocks. Hence a comprehensive exercise rehabilitation in CIED patients should combine supervised training with ongoing psychological counselling and education to help patients cope [31].

### 50.7.2 Exercise-Related Factors

The type of exercise proposed to be undertaken should be carefully considered.

- As already mentioned, activities with risk of collision and extreme repetitive ipsilateral (to device side) arm movements, should be avoided.
- While most patients can safely participate in low intensity (Class IA) sports such as billiards, golf, bowling etc., exercise testing under supervision as well as ambulatory heart rate monitoring during exercise, with, for instance a wrist device, can help provide additional guidance with regard to the intensity of exercise which may be undertaken [55].
- In ICD patients, it may be prudent to aim for a target heart rate during exercise that is at least 20–30 bpm lower than the lowest VT zone to minimize risk of inappropriate shocks [48].

- Lastly it is important to emphasize that risk is a dynamic phenomenon and periodic reassessments of the underlying condition are important to ensure appropriateness of the exercise level on an ongoing basis.

## 50.8 Future Directions and Conclusion

Although it is clear that the benefits of planned exercise and cardiac rehabilitation outweigh the risks in CIED patients, further studies should focus on addressing knowledge gaps in this field. A variety of different exercise testing protocols depending on patient condition and lifestyle would probably be more useful compared to a single one in fine-tuning recommendations. Further research is needed on the best way to respond to shocks encountered during exercise. More data are also needed on women and whether differences exist by ethnicities. Furthermore, follow up data in the patients' usual or home setting would be useful. The increasing diffusion of home monitoring holds promise in this regard and data obtained by remote transmission can help guide home-based training on an ongoing basis after an initial center-based rehabilitation program [56]. This can also improve motivation and long-term adherence to an exercise program.

Newer techniques and developments in the device field have the potential to improve outcomes. The fully subcutaneous ICD, eliminating intravascular leads, could be advantageous in reducing lead-related issues during activity [57], and studies evaluating this technique are needed. Physiologic pacing methods such as His Bundle-pacing, which is even being proposed as an alternative to CRT, also hold promise in improving outcomes in the near future [58].

In conclusion, it is imperative that the multiple benefits of physical exercise should not be denied to patients with cardiac implanted devices. Hence, it is important that treating cardiologists be familiar with all issues related to exercise in this setting. An individualized approach, based on the underlying condition, activity level, optimal device programing and a thorough discussion, respecting patient autonomy should form the basis of care for these patients.

**Clinical Pearls**

- Expanding indications and improved screening have led to an increasing pool of physically active patients receiving cardiac implantable electronic devices (CIED).
- An exercise-based cardiac rehabilitation program has several physical and psychological benefits which holds true for CIED patients as well, and every effort must be made to implement this in all cases.
- Concerns related to exercise in CIED-patients include increased arrhythmia risk, appropriate and inappropriate shocks, undesirable pacemaker responses during exercise and damage to the device or leads.
- Data from both randomized and observational studies suggest that moderate to vigorous exercise is safe in patients with pacemakers and ICDs without an undue

risk of arrhythmias, shocks or major adverse events. Accordingly, both American and European guidelines suggest that even medium to intense exercise can be undertaken in device patients with ongoing supervision and specific precautions related to device type and underlying pathology.

- The exercise prescription for patients with devices needs to be individualized, taking into account several factors such as the cardiac condition, device type, arrhythmia history etc. Optimal medication, device programming and a thorough discussion with the patient are key elements in the decision process.

## Review

### Questions

1. A 20-year-old college student implanted with an ICD seeks advice on participating in leisure time sports. Which of the following conditions would be most concerning for disease progression due to exercise?
   (a) Long QT Syndrome
   (b) Brugada Syndrome
   (c) Arrhythmogenic Right Ventricular Cardiomyopathy
   (d) Repaired Tetralogy of Fallot
2. Guidelines on exercise in patients with ICDs recommend which of the following:
   (a) Participation in impact sports.
   (b) Waiting for an arrhythmia-free period of at least 3 months before vigorous exercise.
   (c) Strictly no exercise for all secondary prevention ICD recipients.
   (d) Psychological evaluation before starting exercise.

### Answers

1. (**c**) Studies have shown that patients with ARVC have a particularly high risk of disease progression due to exercise, with resultant increase in likelihood of malignant arrhythmic events. Even in asymptomatic genetic mutation carriers, exercise has been shown to promote conversion to overt disease with an increased rate of clinical events. Hence in ARVC, greater caution is warranted with respect to vigorous exercise and sports. The other listed conditions do not have a risk of underlying disease progression due to exercise as such.
2. (**b**) As per guidelines for patients with ICDs, it is recommended to wait for an arrhythmia/shock free period of at least 3 months before participating in vigorous exercise. This potentially reduces the likelihood of arrhythmia or shocks during renewed exercise and also gives an opportunity to optimize anti-arrhythmic drugs and overall management to minimize the risk of future events. Participation in sports with risk of impact or collision is not advisable in CIED

patients. Although, ongoing psychosocial support can be useful as part of an exercise rehabilitation program for CIED patients, formal psychological evaluation is not mandatory before allowing exercise. Lastly, there is no recommendation disallowing exercise for secondary prevention ICD recipients.

## References

1. Bardy GH, Lee KL, Mark DB, Poole JE, Packer DL, Boineau R, et al. Amiodarone or an implantable cardioverter-defibrillator for congestive heart failure. N Engl J Med. 2005;352(3):225–37.
2. Bristow MR, Saxon LA, Boehmer J, Krueger S, Kass DA, De Marco T, et al. Cardiac-resynchronization therapy with or without an implantable defibrillator in advanced chronic heart failure. N Engl J Med. 2004;350(21):2140–50.
3. Moss AJ, Zareba W, Hall WJ, Klein H, Wilber DJ, Cannom DS, et al. Prophylactic implantation of a defibrillator in patients with myocardial infarction and reduced ejection fraction. N Engl J Med. 2002;346(12):877–83.
4. Brignole M, Auricchio A, Baron-Esquivias G, Bordachar P, Boriani G, Breithardt OA, et al. 2013 ESC Guidelines on cardiac pacing and cardiac resynchronization therapy: the Task Force on cardiac pacing and resynchronization therapy of the European Society of Cardiology (ESC). Developed in collaboration with the European Heart Rhythm Association (EHRA). Eur Heart J. 2013;34(29):2281–329.
5. Epstein AE, DiMarco JP, Ellenbogen KA, Estes NA 3rd, Freedman RA, Gettes LS, et al. 2012 ACCF/AHA/HRS focused update incorporated into the ACCF/AHA/HRS 2008 guidelines for device-based therapy of cardiac rhythm abnormalities: a report of the American College of Cardiology Foundation/American Heart Association Task Force on Practice Guidelines and the Heart Rhythm Society. Circulation. 2013;127(3):e283–352.
6. Heidbuchel H. Implantable cardioverter defibrillator therapy in athletes. Cardiol Clin. 2007;25(3):467–82. vii
7. Corrado D, Pelliccia A, Bjornstad HH, Vanhees L, Biffi A, Borjesson M, et al. Cardiovascular pre-participation screening of young competitive athletes for prevention of sudden death: proposal for a common European protocol. Consensus statement of the study Group of Sport Cardiology of the working group of cardiac rehabilitation and exercise physiology and the working group of myocardial and pericardial diseases of the European Society of Cardiology. Eur Heart J. 2005;26(5):516–24.
8. Corrado D, Pelliccia A, Heidbuchel H, Sharma S, Link M, Basso C, et al. Recommendations for interpretation of 12-lead electrocardiogram in the athlete. Eur Heart J. 2010;31(2):243–59.
9. Hansen D, Dendale P, Berger J, Meeusen R. Rehabilitation in cardiac patients:what do we know about training modalities? Sports Med. 2005;35(12):1063–84.
10. Fletcher GF, Ades PA, Kligfield P, Arena R, Balady GJ, Bittner VA, et al. Exercise standards for testing and training: a scientific statement from the American Heart Association. Circulation. 2013;128(8):873–934.
11. Piepoli MF, Corra U, Adamopoulos S, Benzer W, Bjarnason-Wehrens B, Cupples M, et al. Secondary prevention in the clinical management of patients with cardiovascular diseases. Core components, standards and outcome measures for referral and delivery: a policy statement from the cardiac rehabilitation section of the European Association for Cardiovascular Prevention & Rehabilitation. Endorsed by the Committee for Practice Guidelines of the European Society of Cardiology. Eur J Prev Cardiol. 2014;21(6):664–81.
12. Albert CM, Mittleman MA, Chae CU, Lee IM, Hennekens CH, Manson JE. Triggering of sudden death from cardiac causes by vigorous exertion. N Engl J Med. 2000;343(19):1355–61.
13. Siscovick DS, Weiss NS, Fletcher RH, Lasky T. The incidence of primary cardiac arrest during vigorous exercise. N Engl J Med. 1984;311(14):874–7.

14. Anselme F, Mletzko R, Bowes R, Mabo P, Sadoul N, Schoels W, et al. Prevention of inappropriate shocks in ICD recipients: a review of 10,000 tachycardia episodes. Pacing Clin Electrophysiol. 2007;30(Suppl 1):S128–33.
15. Sousa J, Kou W, Calkins H, Rosenheck S, Kadish A, Morady F. Effect of epinephrine on the efficacy of the internal cardioverter-defibrillator. Am J Cardiol. 1992;69(5):509–12.
16. Venditti FJ Jr, John RM, Hull M, Tofler GH, Shahian DM, Martin DT. Circadian variation in defibrillation energy requirements. Circulation. 1996;94(7):1607–12.
17. Heidbuchel H, Willems R, Jordaens L, Olshansky B, Carre F, Lozano IF, et al. Intensive recreational athletes in the prospective multinational ICD sports safety registry: results from the European cohort. Eur J Prev Cardiol. 2019;26(7):764–75.
18. James CA, Bhonsale A, Tichnell C, Murray B, Russell SD, Tandri H, et al. Exercise increases age-related penetrance and arrhythmic risk in arrhythmogenic right ventricular dysplasia/cardiomyopathy-associated desmosomal mutation carriers. J Am Coll Cardiol. 2013;62(14):1290–7.
19. Iliou MC, Blanchard JC, Lamar-Tanguy A, Cristofini P, Ledru F. Cardiac rehabilitation in patients with pacemakers and implantable cardioverter defibrillators. Monaldi Arch Chest Dis. 2016;86(1–2):756.
20. Strik M, Socie P, Ploux S, Bordachar P. Unexpected and undesired side-effects of pacing algorithms during exercise. J Electrocardiol. 2018;51(6):1023–8.
21. Kim CH, Cha YM, Shen WK, Maccarter DJ, Taylor BJ, Johnson BD. Effects of atrioventricular and interventricular delays on gas exchange during exercise in patients with heart failure. J Heart Lung Transplant. 2014;33(4):397–403.
22. Blair SN, Kohl HW 3rd, Paffenbarger RS Jr, Clark DG, Cooper KH, Gibbons LW. Physical fitness and all-cause mortality. A prospective study of healthy men and women. JAMA. 1989;262(17):2395–401.
23. Kodama S, Saito K, Tanaka S, Maki M, Yachi Y, Asumi M, et al. Cardiorespiratory fitness as a quantitative predictor of all-cause mortality and cardiovascular events in healthy men and women: a meta-analysis. JAMA. 2009;301(19):2024–35.
24. Taylor RS, Walker S, Smart NA, Piepoli MF, Warren FC, Ciani O, et al. Impact of exercise rehabilitation on exercise capacity and quality-of-life in heart failure: individual participant meta-analysis. J Am Coll Cardiol. 2019;73(12):1430–43.
25. Patwala AY, Woods PR, Sharp L, Goldspink DF, Tan LB, Wright DJ. Maximizing patient benefit from cardiac resynchronization therapy with the addition of structured exercise training: a randomized controlled study. J Am Coll Cardiol. 2009;53(25):2332–9.
26. Belardinelli R, Capestro F, Misiani A, Scipione P, Georgiou D. Moderate exercise training improves functional capacity, quality of life, and endothelium-dependent vasodilation in chronic heart failure patients with implantable cardioverter defibrillators and cardiac resynchronization therapy. Eur J Cardiovasc Prev Rehabil. 2006;13(5):818–25.
27. Isaksen K, Munk PS, Giske R, Larsen AI. Effects of aerobic interval training on measures of anxiety, depression and quality of life in patients with ischaemic heart failure and an implantable cardioverter defibrillator: a prospective non-randomized trial. J Rehabil Med. 2016;48(3):300–6.
28. Kramer DB, Jones PW, Rogers T, Mitchell SL, Reynolds MR. Patterns of physical activity and survival following cardiac resynchronization therapy implantation: the ALTITUDE activity study. Europace. 2017;19(11):1841–7.
29. Rahman B, Macciocca I, Sahhar M, Kamberi S, Connell V, Duncan RE. Adolescents with implantable cardioverter defibrillators: a patient and parent perspective. Pacing Clin Electrophysiol. 2012;35(1):62–72.
30. Berg SK, Thygesen LC, Svendsen JH, Christensen AV, Zwisler AD. Physical activity in primary versus secondary prevention indication implantable cardioverter defibrillator recipients 6-12 months after implantation - a cross-sectional study with register follow up. Arch Phys Med Rehabil. 2015;96(3):426–31.

31. Berg SK, Pedersen PU, Zwisler AD, Winkel P, Gluud C, Pedersen BD, et al. Comprehensive cardiac rehabilitation improves outcome for patients with implantable cardioverter defibrillator. Findings from the COPE-ICD randomised clinical trial. Eur J Cardiovasc Nurs. 2015;14(1):34–44.
32. Piccini JP, Hellkamp AS, Whellan DJ, Ellis SJ, Keteyian SJ, Kraus WE, et al. Exercise training and implantable cardioverter-defibrillator shocks in patients with heart failure: results from HF-ACTION (heart failure and a controlled trial investigating outcomes of exercise TraiNing). JACC Heart Fail. 2013;1(2):142–8.
33. Zeitler EP, Piccini JP, Hellkamp AS, Whellan DJ, Jackson KP, Ellis SJ, et al. Exercise training and pacing status in patients with heart failure: results from HF-ACTION. J Card Fail. 2015;21(1):60–7.
34. Dougherty CM, Glenny RW, Burr RL, Flo GL, Kudenchuk PJ. Prospective randomized trial of moderately strenuous aerobic exercise after an implantable cardioverter defibrillator. Circulation. 2015;131(21):1835–42.
35. Voss F, Schueler M, Lauterbach M, Bauer A, Katus HA, Becker R. Safety of symptom-limited exercise testing in a big cohort of a modern ICD population. Clin Res Cardiol. 2016;105(1):53–8.
36. Isaksen K, Morken IM, Munk PS, Larsen AI. Exercise training and cardiac rehabilitation in patients with implantable cardioverter defibrillators: a review of current literature focusing on safety, effects of exercise training, and the psychological impact of programme participation. Eur J Prev Cardiol. 2012;19(4):804–12.
37. Alswyan AH, Liberato ACS, Dougherty CM. A systematic review of exercise training in patients with cardiac implantable devices. J Cardiopulm Rehabil Prev. 2018;38(2):70–84.
38. Lampert R, Cannom D, Olshansky B. Safety of sports participation in patients with implantable cardioverter defibrillators: a survey of heart rhythm society members. J Cardiovasc Electrophysiol. 2006;17(1):11–5.
39. Lampert R, Olshansky B, Heidbuchel H, Lawless C, Saarel E, Ackerman M, et al. Safety of sports for athletes with implantable Cardioverter-defibrillators: long-term results of a prospective multinational registry. Circulation. 2017;135(23):2310–2.
40. Berul CI, Van Hare GF, Kertesz NJ, Dubin AM, Cecchin F, Collins KK, et al. Results of a multicenter retrospective implantable cardioverter-defibrillator registry of pediatric and congenital heart disease patients. J Am Coll Cardiol. 2008;51(17):1685–91.
41. Adams J, DeJong S, Arnett JK, Kennedy K, Franklin JO, Berbarie RF. High-intensity cardiac rehabilitation training of a firefighter after placement of an implantable cardioverter-defibrillator. Proc (Bayl Univ Med Cent). 2014;27(3):226–8.
42. Ostby SA, Bos JM, Owen HJ, Wackel PL, Cannon BC, Ackerman MJ. Competitive sports participation in patients with catecholaminergic polymorphic ventricular tachycardia: a single center's early experience. JACC Clin Electrophysiol. 2016;2(3):253–62.
43. Saberniak J, Hasselberg NE, Borgquist R, Platonov PG, Sarvari SI, Smith HJ, et al. Vigorous physical activity impairs myocardial function in patients with arrhythmogenic right ventricular cardiomyopathy and in mutation positive family members. Eur J Heart Fail. 2014;16(12):1337–44.
44. Hindieh W, Adler A, Weissler-Snir A, Fourey D, Harris S, Rakowski H. Exercise in patients with hypertrophic cardiomyopathy: a review of current evidence, national guideline recommendations and a proposal for a new direction to fitness. J Sci Med Sport. 2017;20(4):333–8.
45. Zipes DP, Link MS, Ackerman MJ, Kovacs RJ, Myerburg RJ, Estes NAM 3rd. Eligibility and disqualification recommendations for competitive athletes with cardiovascular abnormalities: task force 9: arrhythmias and conduction defects: a scientific statement from the American Heart Association and American College of Cardiology. J Am Coll Cardiol. 2015;66(21):2412–23.
46. Pelliccia A, Solberg EE, Papadakis M, Adami PE, Biffi A, Caselli S, et al. Recommendations for participation in competitive and leisure time sport in athletes with cardiomyopathies, myocarditis, and pericarditis: position statement of the sport cardiology section of the European Association of Preventive Cardiology (EAPC). Eur Heart J. 2019;40(1):19–33.

47. Heidbuchel H, Panhuyzen-Goedkoop N, Corrado D, Hoffmann E, Biffi A, Delise P, et al. Recommendations for participation in leisure-time physical activity and competitive sports in patients with arrhythmias and potentially arrhythmogenic conditions part I: supraventricular arrhythmias and pacemakers. Eur J Cardiovasc Prev Rehabil. 2006;13(4):475–84.
48. Heidbuchel H, Carre F. Exercise and competitive sports in patients with an implantable cardioverter-defibrillator. Eur Heart J. 2014;35(44):3097–102.
49. Defaye P, Boveda S, Klug D, Beganton F, Piot O, Narayanan K, et al. Dual- vs. single-chamber defibrillators for primary prevention of sudden cardiac death: long-term follow-up of the Defibrillateur Automatique Implantable-Prevention Primaire registry. Europace. 2017;19(9):1478–84.
50. Hu ZY, Zhang J, Xu ZT, Gao XF, Zhang H, Pan C, et al. Efficiencies and complications of dual chamber versus single chamber implantable cardioverter defibrillators in secondary sudden cardiac death prevention: a meta-analysis. Heart Lung Circ. 2016;25(2):148–54.
51. Moss AJ, Schuger C, Beck CA, Brown MW, Cannom DS, Daubert JP, et al. Reduction in inappropriate therapy and mortality through ICD programming. N Engl J Med. 2012;367(24):2275–83.
52. Tan VH, Wilton SB, Kuriachan V, Sumner GL, Exner DV. Impact of programming strategies aimed at reducing nonessential implantable cardioverter defibrillator therapies on mortality: a systematic review and meta-analysis. Circ Arrhythm Electrophysiol. 2014;7(1):164–70.
53. Schron EB, Exner DV, Yao Q, Jenkins LS, Steinberg JS, Cook JR, et al. Quality of life in the antiarrhythmics versus implantable defibrillators trial: impact of therapy and influence of adverse symptoms and defibrillator shocks. Circulation. 2002;105(5):589–94.
54. Schulz SM, Massa C, Grzbiela A, Dengler W, Wiedemann G, Pauli P. Implantable cardioverter defibrillator shocks are prospective predictors of anxiety. Heart Lung. 2013;42(2):105–11.
55. Stove MP, Haucke E, Nymann ML, Sigurdsson T, Larsen BT. Accuracy of the wearable activity tracker Garmin forerunner 235 for the assessment of heart rate during rest and activity. J Sports Sci. 2019;37(8):895–901.
56. Parahuleva MS, Soydan N, Divchev D, Lusebrink U, Schieffer B, Erdogan A. Home monitoring after ambulatory implanted primary cardiac implantable electronic devices: the home ambulance pilot study. Clin Cardiol. 2017;40(11):1068–75.
57. Bardy GH, Smith WM, Hood MA, Crozier IG, Melton IC, Jordaens L, et al. An entirely subcutaneous implantable cardioverter-defibrillator. N Engl J Med. 2010;363(1):36–44.
58. Upadhyay GA, Vijayaraman P, Nayak HM, Verma N, Dandamudi G, Sharma PS, et al. On-treatment comparison between corrective His bundle pacing and biventricular pacing for cardiac resynchronization: a secondary analysis of His-SYNC Trial. Heart Rhythm. 2019;16:1797–807.

# Exercise in Specific Diseases: Abdominal Aortic Aneurysm

51

Jonathan Myers and Josef Niebauer

**Learning Objectives**

1. Recognize the definition of abdominal aortic aneurysms (AAA), understand the growth in their prevalence and the impact of AAA as a leading cause of sudden death.
2. Recognize risk factors for AAA.
3. Understand the safety of exercise testing in AAA.
4. Understand the hemodynamic influences of exercise on the aneurysm area.
5. Appreciate the potential benefits of rehabilitation in AAA.
6. Recognize the effects of regular exercise on AAA growth.

## 51.1 Introduction

An abdominal aortic aneurysm (AAA) is a localized dilation caused by weakening of the vessel wall, most often in the infrarenal area. It is usually defined as an outer aortic diameter >3.0 cm (normal diameter of the aorta is <2.0 cm) (Fig. 51.1). AAAs are usually asymptomatic and are often not discovered until they rupture or cause symptoms due to localized pressure on adjacent tissues. The major complication is rupture of the aneurysm; this is a life-threatening event, as large amounts of blood spill into the abdominal cavity and can lead to death within minutes. In the past, few data were available on the effects of physical activity in AAA, and these patients

J. Myers (✉)
Cardiology Division, Veterans Affairs Palo Alto Health Care System and Stanford University, Stanford, CA, USA

J. Niebauer
Institute of Sports Medicine, Prevention and Rehabilitation, Paracelsus Medical University Salzburg, Salzburg, Austria
e-mail: j.niebauer@salk.at



A. Pressler, J. Niebauer (eds.), *Textbook of Sports and Exercise Cardiology*,
https://doi.org/10.1007/978-3-030-35374-2_51

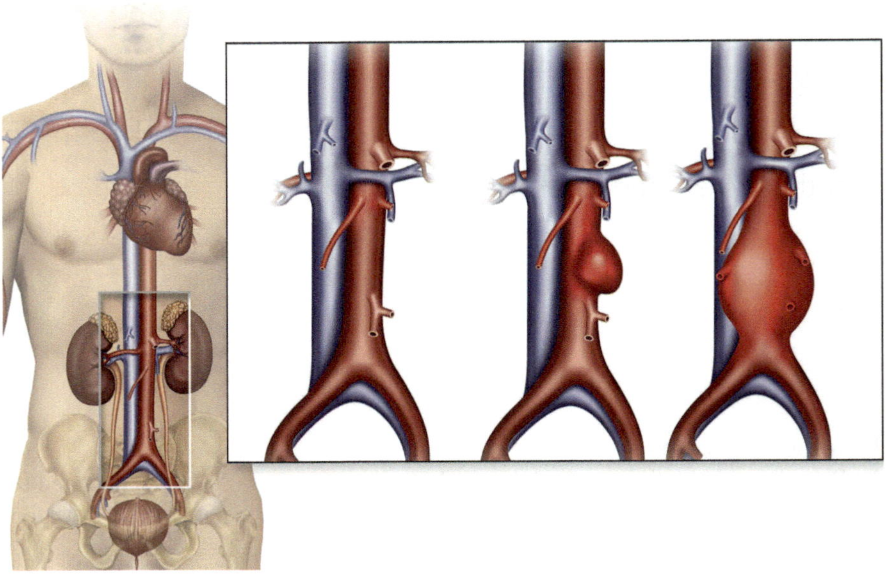

**Fig. 51.1** Illustration of a normal abdominal aorta (left) and an abdominal aorta with a moderate (center) and large (right) aneurysm

were generally discouraged from participating in exercise programs. However, this has begun to change with the recent publication of some notable randomized trials of exercise training in patients with AAA. The purpose of this chapter is to review the available data on exercise testing and training in AAA and discuss the potential for exercise therapy to reduce AAA risk and limit AAA progression.

## 51.2 Definition of Abdominal Aortic Aneurysm

AAA is defined by a localized dilation caused by weakening of the vessel wall, most often in the infrarenal area.

- AAA is usually defined as an outer aortic diameter >3.0 cm (normal diameter of the aorta is <2.0 cm).
  - If the outer diameter exceeds 5.5 cm, the aneurysm is considered to be *large* and such patients are considered candidates for surgical repair [1, 2].

AAAs are usually asymptomatic and are often not discovered until they rupture or cause symptoms due to localized pressure on adjacent tissues. The major complication is rupture of the aneurysm, which is a life-threatening event. Many factors can contribute to an AAA, including each of the major risk factors for cardiovascular disease. AAAs occur most commonly among individuals between the ages of 65 and 75 years and are more common among men (4–5 times higher incidence) and among smokers [1–7].

## 51.3 Detection of AAA

Detection of AAA has improved considerably in recent years through greater media attention, public outreach programs [8], and the addition of AAA ultrasound screening to guideline recommendation in the US and Europe, including the adoption of AAA screening to the US Medicare program:

- In 2005 (updated in 2014), a US Preventive Services Task Force (USPSTF) report recommended that men aged 65–75 years who had ever smoked be screened for AAA on one occasion by abdominal ultrasound [9, 10].
  - However, the USPSTF found that there is little benefit to repeat screening in men who have a negative ultrasound and that men over age 75 are unlikely to benefit from screening.

While the USPSTF recommended against screening for women, a 2008 budget amendment termed "screening abdominal aortic aneurysms very efficiently" (SAAAVE) authorized the Centers for Medicare and Medicaid Services to cover screening for men in the 65 to 75 year age range who had smoked more than 100 cigarettes in their lifetime, in addition to men *and* women in this age range with a family history of AAA disease [11]. While there are slight differences between professional organizations, screening criteria are generally similar to the USPSTF recommendations, including those from the Canadian Society for Vascular Surgery [12] and the European Society for Vascular Surgery [13].

- Abdominal ultrasonography has been used as the screening modality in the large randomized trials of screening for AAA, because of its high sensitivity and specificity and low cost.
  - With a sensitivity >95% and a specificity nearly 100%, ultrasonography has excellent test characteristics for diagnosing and following patients with AAA [1, 9, 10].

## 51.4 Epidemiology of AAA

Abdominal aortic aneurysms account for an increasing burden on health care costs in the Western world:

- AAA is the 13th leading cause of death in the US, and is the third leading cause of sudden death in men >60 years of age, accounting for roughly 4–5% of sudden deaths [14, 15].
- AAA is directly related to age, with a prevalence of approximately 6% in men >60 years, increasing to roughly 11% in men >80 years [3, 16].
- The prevalence of AAA varies considerably depending on the presence of other risk factors.
- The most important modifiable risk factor is cigarette smoking; smokers are 2 to 9 times more likely to develop AAA than non-smokers [6, 16–19].

- Other major risk factors for AAA include
  - Hypertension,
  - obesity,
  - inflammation, and
  - white race [5–7, 16–21].

## 51.5 Physical Inactivity as a Risk Factor

While data are relatively limited, patients with AAA represent a population that could potentially benefit from exercise therapy and secondary prevention, since associated risk factors such as hypertension, obesity and inflammation are amenable to exercise training.

- Physical inactivity is associated with microvascular dysfunction, inflammation, and other factors related to AAA, including obesity [22–24].
- Regular exercise has been shown to favorably alter epicardial and peripheral flow dynamics, resulting in improved blood flow to ischemic areas in patients with vascular diseases [23–30].
- The luminal diameter of epicardial and other vessels change rapidly in response to mechanical (flow-related) and endogenous or pharmacological stimuli, and endothelial health is enhanced by exercise training [23, 27–30].
- Studies have shown that acute exercise favorably alters adverse hemodynamic conditions in the abdominal aorta in patients with AAA, including lessening peripheral resistance and oscillatory sheer stress which may attenuate AAA growth [31–33].

## 51.6 Safety of Exercise Testing in AAA

Guidelines on exercise testing have generally not addressed patients with AAA. A 1997 recommendation suggested that individuals with AAA should not undergo *maximal* exercise testing, that heart rate should not exceed 100 beats/min, and that excessive rises in double-product (systolic blood pressure x heart rate) be avoided due to concerns about the potential for rupture [34].

Pre-operative risk assessments in patients with AAA have largely employed pharmacologic stress with dobutamine, ostensibly to avoid an excessive rise in systolic blood pressure [35]. However, these limitations have been based on intuition rather than known risks associated with exercise in AAA.

The ACC/AHA Practice Guidelines for the Management of Patients with Peripheral Vascular Disease [36] suggest that AAA patients should not be fearful of moderate activity, and that efforts should be made to improve fitness in the event that surgery is required.

Limited data are available regarding maximal exercise test responses in patients with AAA. Undoubtedly this is because of limited awareness of AAA until recent years, and the tendency to refer these patients to pharmacologic stress testing because of concerns about safety. While the American Heart Association (AHA) Guidelines on Exercise Testing reviewed the applications of the test in a wide variety of cardiovascular and related conditions, AAA is not mentioned [37]. Likewise, exercise testing is not mentioned in the AHA/American College of Cardiology Guidelines for the Management of Peripheral Arterial Disease [35].

Three recent studies have assessed the safety of maximal exercise testing in patients with AAA.

1. Best and colleagues [38] retrospectively evaluated 262 patients with AAA diameters >4.0 cm who had undergone exercise testing at the Mayo Clinic. One patient with a large (6.1 cm diameter) aneurysm was reported to have had a rupture 12 h after the exercise test. While this event may or may not have been related to the exercise test, this yielded a rupture rate of 0.4%.
2. In a case report, Puls and Thadani described a patient with a 7.0 cm aneurysm who underwent supine exercise nuclear ventriculography [39]. Six minutes into the test, at a work rate of 450 kpm (approximately 65 W) and a blood pressure of 200/100 mmHg, the patient complained of excruciating low back pain. The test was stopped, an ultrasound was performed revealing a rupture, and the patient underwent surgical repair. Two days following surgery, the patient died of myocardial infarction. It is notable that these two exercise test-related events occurred in patients with very large aneurysms (6.1 and 7.0 cm), which represent obvious contraindications to exercise.
3. In the Abdominal Aortic Aneurysm: Simple Treatment and Prevention (AAA STOP) trial, more than 500 maximal exercise tests were conducted in patients with small AAA, (i.e. 2.5–5.0 cm) [40].
   (a) No exercise test responses occurred that were serious enough to be considered an "event" by conventional definitions.
   (b) A comparison of exercise test responses between patients with AAA and subjects of similar age referred for exercise testing for clinical reasons is presented in Table 51.1.
   (c) While the occurrence of hyper- and hypotensive responses were slightly higher in AAA subjects than those among age-matched referrals, the incidence of these responses was similar to other studies in subjects referred for exercise testing for clinical reasons.
   (d) Notably, there were no instances of sustained or non-sustained ventricular tachycardia in the AAA subjects; this contrasts the incidence rate of 1.5% in age-matched subjects referred for exercise testing for clinical reasons; an incidence rate of 1.0% previously reported in the same exercise lab [43]; and rates ranging from 0.08% to 1.1% reported elsewhere [44].

**Table 51.1** Comparison of exercise test responses between patients with abdominal aortic aneurysm (AAA) and subjects referred for exercise testing for clinical reasons (adapted from [40])

| Variables | AAA subjects (n = 306) | VA referrals (n = 2155) | p-value |
|---|---|---|---|
| **Rest** | | | |
| Heart rate (beats/min) | 63 ± 11 | 70 ± 13 | <0.001 |
| Systolic blood pressure (mmHg) | 132 ± 15 | 138 ± 20 | <0.001 |
| Diastolic blood pressure (mmHg) | 75 ± 9 | 79 ± 20 | <0.01 |
| **Maximal exercise** | | | |
| Heart rate (beats/min) | 127 ± 23 | 129 ± 22 | 0.13 |
| Systolic blood pressure (mmHg) | 184 ± 30 | 176 ± 27 | <0.001 |
| Diastolic blood pressure (mmHg) | 80 ± 13 | 84 ± 26 | <0.01 |
| Perceived exertion | 18.6 ± 1.4 | 16.7 ± 2.3 | <0.001 |
| Respiratory exchange ratio | 1.10 ± 0.11 | 1.09 ± 0.15 | 0.38 |
| Oxygen uptake (ml/kg/min) | 20.0 ± 6.3 | 20.3 ± 7.3 | <0.54 |
| Estimated oxygen uptake (METs) | 7.0 ± 2.6 | 6.4 ± 2.7 | <0.001 |
| Percent age-predicted VO2[a] | 77.4 ± 24 | 79.5 ± 29 | 0.47 |
| Percent age-predicted estimated METs[b] | 96 ± 36 | 90 ± 37 | 0.002 |
| **Reasons for stopping** | | | |
| Hypotensive response (%) | 2.9 | 0.19 | <0.001 |
| Hypertensive response (%) | 3.6 | 0.65 | <0.001 |
| Ventricular tachycardia (≥3 beat run, %) | 0 | 1.5 | – |
| Claudication (%) | 8.4 | 3.7 | <0.001 |
| **Ischemic changes** | | | |
| ST depression ≥1.0 mm (%) | 11.1 | 36.6 | <0.001 |
| Angina (%) | 1.6 | 10.7 | <0.001 |
| **Prognostic scores** | | | |
| Duke score (annual mortality) | 4.7 ± 5 (3.1%) | 1.6 ± 6 (3.5%) | <0.001 |
| VA score (annual mortality) | −5.6 ± 3 (2.5%) | −4.1 ± 4 (2.5%) | <0.001 |

*METs* metabolic equivalent of tasks, *VA* Veterans Affairs
[a]Using equation from Ref. [41]
[b]Using equation from Ref. [42]

## 51.7 Safety of Exercise Training in AAA

Undoubtedly there have been many post-MI, post PCI, or heart failure patients with occult small AAA who have participated in rehabilitation programs in the years prior to the wider screening programs and awareness of the condition that exists today. Numerous studies have reported on event rates associated with cardiac rehabilitation programs, and these studies have been summarized in various sources, including national guidelines [45].

- There are no specific incidences of AAA rupture reported in these studies, although the possibility that an AAA event was attributed to acute MI or another cause cannot be discounted.

## 51.8 Role of Fitness and Physical Activity Patterns in Predicting Outcomes

There are limited data in the literature regarding the applications of fitness and physical activity patterns in the context of risk for AAA.

- Peak $VO_2$ has been used to estimate pre- and post-operative risk among patients undergoing vascular surgery in recent years, and AAA subjects with preserved exercise capacity have been demonstrated to have better post-surgical outcomes vs. those with lower exercise capacity [46–49].
- In the UK Small Aneurysm Trial (UKSAT) [50], patients with small AAA (4.0–5.5 cm) who were poorly fit (based on a global pre-operative score) benefited particularly from early surgery, with a 44% higher survival when expressed as aneurysm-related mortality.
- In a Swedish cohort of >33,000 men and women, physically inactive subjects classified crudely as "not walking or cycling to work" had a nearly threefold higher risk of developing AAA [51].
- In a 6-year follow-up of Finnish smokers, subjects categorized as "no exercise in leisure time" had a 29% higher risk of developing AAA [19].
- In a cross-sectional study of 6386 subjects in Norway, the odds ratios for AAA presence among active vs. inactive men and women (defined as < or >3 h low intensity activity in the last year) were 0.80 and 0.79, respectively [51].
- A major conclusion from the Endovascular Aneurysm Repair II (EVAR II) trial was that improving patient fitness, particularly cardiovascular, pulmonary, and renal function, should be the focus of treatment prior to considering repair [52].
- In a follow-up analysis in which EVAR I and EVAR II data were combined, the benefit of endovascular repair was demonstrated to be most convincing in the fittest patients [53].

These studies suggest that in addition to modifying conventional risk markers for vascular disease, efforts to improve fitness by increasing activity should be included in the prevention and treatment paradigm for AAA.

## 51.9 Effects of Rehabilitation in AAA

A summary of studies addressing exercise training in AAA are outlined in Table 51.2 [54–59]. All studies have been performed in pre-surgical AAA (<5.5 cm). The studies generally show that training responses and safety are similar to post-MI patients and other groups referred for cardiac rehabilitation. Some studies tested patients only to the ventilatory threshold (VT) due to safety concerns; thus, the effects of training on *maximal* exercise capacity are unknown from

**Table 51.2** Summary of studies of exercise training in abdominal aortic aneurysm (AAA)

| Author (ref #) | Year | # Subjects | AAA | Intervention | Main findings |
|---|---|---|---|---|---|
| Kothmann et al. [54] | 2009 | 30 | Small AAA under surveillance (<5.5 cm) | 6 weeks supervised training (30 min moderate intensity cycle ergometry, twice weekly) at VT | $VO_2$ at VT increased by 10% in the exercise group compared with controls |
| Myers et al. [55] | 2010 | 108 | Small AAA (3.0–5.5 cm) | 1 year exercise training (at home/in house combination) | Exercise group increased exercise capacity (42% increase in treadmill time, 24% increase in estimated METs), reduced C-reactive protein, reduced W/H ratio |
| Tew et al. [56] | 2012 | 28 | Small AAA (3.0–5.0 cm) | 12 weeks of supervised training, 3 days/week | Increase in $VO_2$ at the VT; no change in AAA size |
| Myers et al. [57] | 2014 | 140 | Small AAA (3.0–5.5 cm) | Up to 3 years exercise training (at home/in house combination) | Increases in peak $VO_2$ and $VO_2$ at VT; reduced submaximal heart rate in exercise group; no change in AAA growth rate |
| Barakat et al. [58] | 2013 | 20 | AAA awaiting aneurysm repair | 6 weeks supervised exercise program, 3 sessions/week, 1 h/session cardio/strength combination | Increased peak $VO_2$ and $VO_2$ at VT, increased exercise time |
| Nakayama et al. [59] | 2018 | 212 | Small AAA (3.0–5.5 cm) | Moderate aerobic training, 30 min sessions, 1–3 days/week for 3 months | Slower AAA growth rate in the exercise group vs. usual care |

*VT* ventilatory anaerobic threshold, *METs* metabolic equivalent of tasks, *W/H* waist-to-hip

these studies. The conservative approach using exercise testing only to the level of the VT underscores the fact that little is known about exercise in this population and highlights the perception that a high level of exertion in AAA may adversely affect the aneurysm or lead to rupture.

The largest randomized trial to date was AAA STOP [57]:

- 140 subjects 50–85 years of age were included with aortic diameters ≥3.0 and < 5.5 cm.
- They followed a standard regimen using a combination of in-house and home exercise aerobic and resistance training.
- Regardless of where training occurred, subjects were interviewed weekly by telephone to obtain estimates of recreational energy expenditure using a 7-day activity recall tool.
- The overall goal of training was to achieve a relatively ambitious mean energy expenditure of 2000 kcals/week, or the equivalent of roughly 1 h of moderate exercise/day.

- Maximal exercise tests were performed. Exercise capacity results at 3, 12, and 24 months are presented in Fig. 51.2.
  - Significant training responses were observed, including improvements in peak $VO_2$, maximal exercise time, and $VO_2$ at the ventilatory threshold.
  - No participants in the training group experienced AAA-related symptoms, exercise-related clinical events or excessive growth rates.

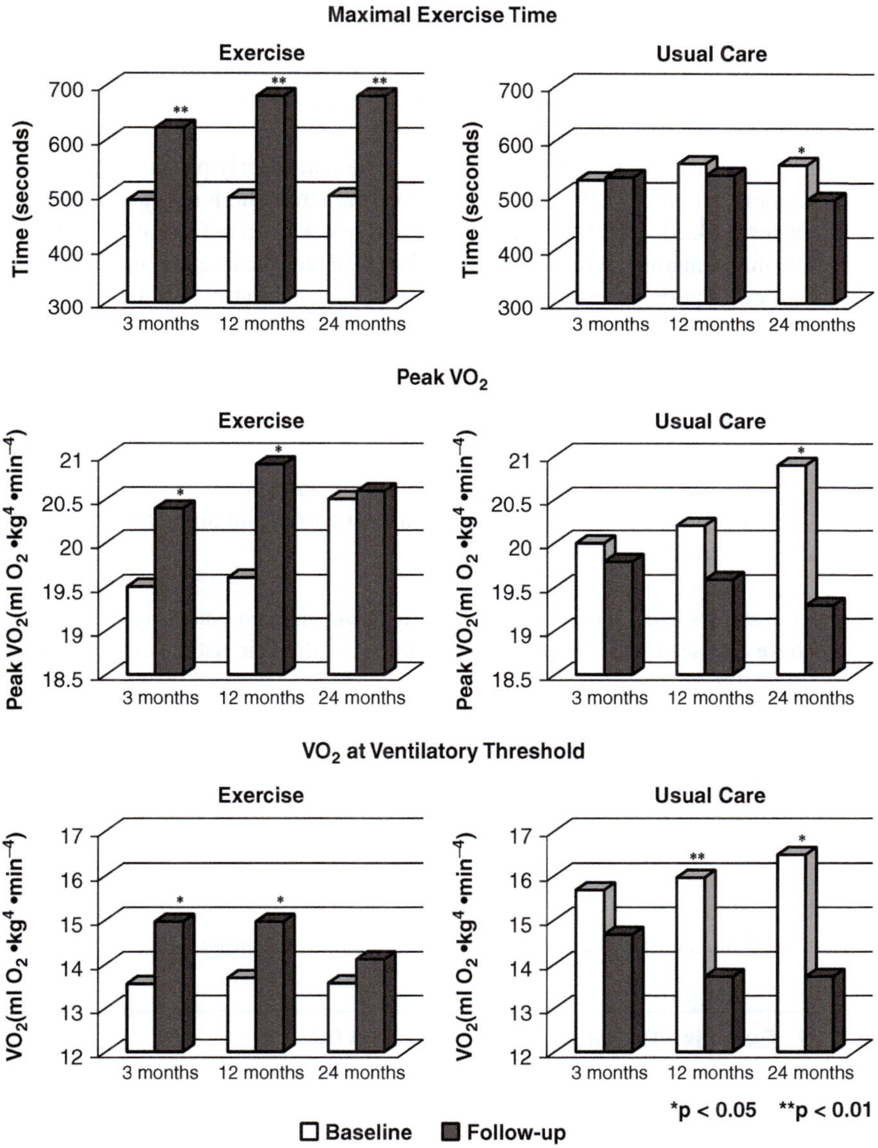


**Fig. 51.2** Comparisons of maximal exercise time, peak $VO_2$, and $VO_2$ at the ventilatory threshold in the exercise and usual care groups at 3 months, 1 year, and 2 years (reprinted with permission from [55])

- The mean recreational energy expenditure of 1999 kcals/week is roughly double the minimum amount widely recommended in guidelines on physical activity and health.
- Training did not influence AAA growth rates.

## 51.10 Hemodynamic Effects of Exercise in AAA

Hemodynamic factors, including sheer stress, cyclic strain, and various other pressure forces play an important role in the normal adaptive response of the vasculature to changes in physiologic demands as well as maladaptive responses that lead to cardiovascular disease [29, 30].

The abdominal aorta has been suggested to be particularly prone to unfavorable hemodynamic conditions due low mean wall shear stress, high retrograde flow, and other factors [24, 31–33, 60, 61]. Exercise training is known to favorably modify the systemic inflammatory state, and the vascular shear stress caused by moderate exercise has been demonstrated to improve endothelial function in radial, femoral, and coronary arteries [27, 29, 30, 62].

It has therefore been suggested that regular exercise may also provide localized benefits to the abdominal aortic vasculature by triggering biologic processes that lead to protection from the progression of atherosclerosis. These processes include hemodynamic conditions that inhibit atherosclerosis such as unidirectional laminar flow, increased wall shear stress, upregulation of endothelial vasodilator mechanisms, and downregulation of vasoconstrictor properties, inflammatory molecules, and adhesion proteins [24, 30, 32, 60–65].

- Recent studies using magnetic resonance imaging and computational fluid dynamics have characterized abdominal aortic flow conditions in patients with AAA.
- Acute bouts of submaximal exercise have been demonstrated to counteract these abnormal hemodynamic conditions by attenuating retrograde flow and increasing wall shear stress in the abdominal aorta [24, 31–33, 60, 61].
- These studies have consistently observed that unfavorable hemodynamic conditions at rest in AAA are improved with even modest levels of acute exercise.

While the association between regular exercise and AAA progression has yet to be fully explored, these studies suggest that regular exercise may modify disease progression in AAA by altering local hemodynamic conditions.

## 51.11 Exercise Recommendations in AAA

Although data are limited on the physiologic effects of exercise training in patients with AAA, it seems reasonable to expect that moderate exercise typical of standard outpatient rehabilitation programs is safe and beneficial in these patients.

- The ACC/AHA Practice Guidelines for the Management of Patients with Peripheral Vascular Disease [36] recommend modest activity in AAA patients, in part to counteract the reductions in fitness that have been shown to be associated with poor outcomes among patients who eventually require surgery [46–49, 52, 53].
- The Society for Vascular Surgery Practice Guidelines for AAA recommend that during surveillance for patients with small AAA, management should include counseling that moderate activity does not precipitate rupture and may limit AAA growth rate [66].
- For patients with aneurysms in general, the American College of Sports Medicine (ACSM) recommends moderate aerobic exercise, 20–40 min per session, 3–4 days/week, with an emphasis on exercise duration over intensity [67].
- The recommendations for small AAA also include low resistance strength training as a complement to the aerobic component.

It would be appropriate to perform a treadmill test, particularly for patients wishing to engage in more vigorous activities, both to assess the physiologic response to exercise and to ascertain that the patient does not have a hypertensive response [67]. The test should be performed while on their standard medication, e.g. beta blockers and/or other antihypertensive medications, and recommendations for activity should be targeted below a systolic blood pressure rise of 180 mmHg on the treadmill test [67].

## 51.12 Summary

Rehabilitation programs have been broadening their referral base in recent years to include non-traditional patients such as post-cardiac transplant, implantable cardioverter-defibrillators (ICDs), heart failure, and post-PCI patients, and stable patients with small AAA would appear to be good candidates for rehabilitation programs as well. Given that cardiac rehabilitation has evolved from traditional exercise-based programs to comprehensive secondary prevention and chronic disease management centers [68], AAA patients would be ideal candidates for intervention since AAA is a disease strongly associated with cardiometabolic risk [5, 17, 20, 21, 24]. Concerns about risks associated with moderate levels of exercise appear to be unfounded [36, 40, 49, 57, 58, 67]. While the effects of training in patients with AAA appear to be similar to other groups, available data remain limited, and more studies are needed to explore the role of rehabilitation in the prevention and treatment of AAA.

**Clinical Pearls**

- AAA commonly is an asymptomatic weakening of the aortic wall and unfortunately often the first symptoms are caused by rupture, an often lethal event.
- AAA of <5.5 cm are considered small; patients with large AAA, i.e. >5.5 cm, are considered candidates for repair.

- Risk factors for AAA are identical with those of other cardiovascular diseases, i.e. smoking, physical inactivity, hypercholesterolemia, hyperglycemia, obesity, arterial hypertension.
- AAA is directly related to age and occurs most commonly between 65 and 75 years of age; it is more common among men (4–5 times higher incidence) and among smokers.
- Detection of AAA has improved thanks to greater media attention, public outreach programs, and addition of ultrasound screening to guideline recommendations in the US and Europe.
- Given that cardiac rehabilitation has evolved from traditional exercise-based programs to comprehensive secondary prevention and chronic disease management centers [68], AAA patients are ideal candidates not only for exercise-based rehabilitation programs but also for comprehensive secondary prevention since it is a disease strongly associated with cardiometabolic risk.
- Concerns about risks associated with moderate levels of exercise in patients with stable, small AAAs appear to be unfounded.

## Review

### Questions

1. The incidence of abdominal aortic aneurysm has increased markedly in recent years. Which factors account for this increase?
2. AAAs occur most commonly in whom?
3. Do patients with AAA respond to exercise training like other cardiac patients or differently?

### Answers

1. This increase is owed—among others—to the aging of the population, better detection methods, public outreach programs, and guideline-directed inclusion of AAA ultrasound screening for particular at-risk populations.
2. It occurs most commonly in men between the ages of 65 and 75 years with a history of smoking.
3. Responses to exercise programs are similar in AAA patients to those observed in post-MI patients and other groups referred for cardiac rehabilitation.

## References

1. Erbel R, Aboyans V, Boileau C, Bossone E, Bartolomeo RD, Eggebrecht H, et al. 2014 ESC Guidelines on the diagnosis and treatment of aortic diseases: Document covering acute and chronic aortic diseases of the thoracic and abdominal aorta of the adult. The Task Force for the diagnosis and treatment of aortic diseases of the European Society of Cardiology (ESC). Eur Heart J. 2014;35(41):2873–926.

2. Brewster DC, Cronenwett JL, Hallett JW Jr, Johnston KW, Krupski WC, Matsumura JS, et al. Guidelines for the treatment of abdominal aortic aneurysms. Report of a subcommittee of the Joint Council of the American Association for Vascular Surgery and Society for Vascular Surgery. J Vasc Surg. 2003;37(5):1106–17.
3. Nordon IM, Hinchliffe RJ, Loftus IM, Thompson MM. Pathophysiology and epidemiology of abdominal aortic aneurysms. Nat Rev Cardiol. 2011;8(2):92–102.
4. Derubertis BG, Trocciola SM, Ryer EJ, Pieracci FM, McKinsey JF, Faries PL, et al. Abdominal aortic aneurysm in women: prevalence, risk factors, and implications for screening. J Vasc Surg. 2007;46(4):630–5.
5. Iribarren C, Darbinian JA, Go AS, Fireman BH, Lee CD, Grey DP. Traditional and novel risk factors for clinically diagnosed abdominal aortic aneurysm: the Kaiser multiphasic health checkup cohort study. Ann Epidemiol. 2007;17(9):669–78.
6. Golledge J, Muller J, Daugherty A, Norman P. Abdominal aortic aneurysm: pathogenesis and implications for management. Arterioscler Thromb Vasc Biol. 2006;26(12):2605–13.
7. Kent KC. Clinical practice. Abdominal aortic aneurysms. N Engl J Med. 2014;371(22):2101–8.
8. Aneurysm Outreach Inc. 2018. https://www.crowdrise.com/aaaneurysmoutreach.
9. U. S. Preventive Services Task Force. Screening for abdominal aortic aneurysm: recommendation statement. Ann Intern Med. 2005;142(3):198–202.
10. LeFevre ML, U. S. Preventive Services Task Force. Screening for abdominal aortic aneurysm: U.S. Preventive Services Task Force recommendation statement. Ann Intern Med. 2014;161(4):281–90.
11. Preventive services: abdominal aortic aneurysm screening. 2008. http://www.medicare.gov/Health/AAA.asp.
12. Mastracci TM, Cina CS, Canadian Society for Vascular Surgery. Screening for abdominal aortic aneurysm in Canada: review and position statement of the Canadian Society for Vascular Surgery. J Vasc Surg. 2007;45(6):1268–76.
13. Moll FL, Powell JT, Fraedrich G, Verzini F, Haulon S, Waltham M, et al. Management of abdominal aortic aneurysms clinical practice guidelines of the European society for vascular surgery. Eur J Vasc Endovasc Surg. 2011;41(Suppl 1):S1–S58.
14. Cowan JA Jr, Dimick JB, Henke PK, Rectenwald J, Stanley JC, Upchurch GR Jr. Epidemiology of aortic aneurysm repair in the United States from 1993 to 2003. Ann N Y Acad Sci. 2006;1085:1–10.
15. Aggarwal S, Qamar A, Sharma V, Sharma A. Abdominal aortic aneurysm: a comprehensive review. Exp Clin Cardiol. 2011;16(1):11–5.
16. Sidloff D, Stather P, Dattani N, Bown M, Thompson J, Sayers R, et al. Aneurysm global epidemiology study: public health measures can further reduce abdominal aortic aneurysm mortality. Circulation. 2014;129(7):747–53.
17. Blanchard JF, Armenian HK, Friesen PP. Risk factors for abdominal aortic aneurysm: results of a case-control study. Am J Epidemiol. 2000;151(6):575–83.
18. Lee AJ, Fowkes FG, Carson MN, Leng GC, Allan PL. Smoking, atherosclerosis and risk of abdominal aortic aneurysm. Eur Heart J. 1997;18(4):671–6.
19. Tornwall ME, Virtamo J, Haukka JK, Albanes D, Huttunen JK. Life-style factors and risk for abdominal aortic aneurysm in a cohort of Finnish male smokers. Epidemiology. 2001;12(1):94–100.
20. Golledge J, Clancy P, Jamrozik K, Norman PE. Obesity, adipokines, and abdominal aortic aneurysm: health in men study. Circulation. 2007;116(20):2275–9.
21. Lindblad B, Borner G, Gottsater A. Factors associated with development of large abdominal aortic aneurysm in middle-aged men. Eur J Vasc Endovasc Surg. 2005;30(4):346–52.
22. Hamburg NM, McMackin CJ, Huang AL, Shenouda SM, Widlansky ME, Schulz E, et al. Physical inactivity rapidly induces insulin resistance and microvascular dysfunction in healthy volunteers. Arterioscler Thromb Vasc Biol. 2007;27(12):2650–6.
23. Mobius-Winkler S, Linke A, Adams V, Schuler G, Erbs S. How to improve endothelial repair mechanisms: the lifestyle approach. Expert Rev Cardiovasc Ther. 2010;8(4):573–80.
24. Dalman RL, Tedesco MM, Myers J, Taylor CA. AAA disease: mechanism, stratification, and treatment. Ann N Y Acad Sci. 2006;1085:92–109.

25. Myers JN. Exercise and fitness. In: Perk J, Mathes P, editors. Cardiovascular prevention and rehabilitation. London: Springer; 2007. p. 77–87.
26. Gielen S, Schuler G, Hambrecht R. Exercise training in coronary artery disease and coronary vasomotion. Circulation. 2001;103(1):E1–6.
27. Sixt S, Beer S, Bluher M, Korff N, Peschel T, Sonnabend M, et al. Long- but not short-term multifactorial intervention with focus on exercise training improves coronary endothelial dysfunction in diabetes mellitus type 2 and coronary artery disease. Eur Heart J. 2010;31(1):112–9.
28. Niebauer J, Hambrecht R, Velich T, Hauer K, Marburger C, Kalberer B, et al. Attenuated progression of coronary artery disease after 6 years of multifactorial risk intervention: role of physical exercise. Circulation. 1997;96(8):2534–41.
29. Adams V, Reich B, Uhlemann M, Niebauer J. Molecular effects of exercise training in patients with cardiovascular disease: focus on skeletal muscle, endothelium, and myocardium. Am J Physiol Heart Circ Physiol. 2017;313(1):H72–88.
30. Niebauer J, Cooke JP. Cardiovascular effects of exercise: role of endothelial shear stress. J Am Coll Cardiol. 1996;28(7):1652–60.
31. Tang BT, Cheng CP, Draney MT, Wilson NM, Tsao PS, Herfkens RJ, et al. Abdominal aortic hemodynamics in young healthy adults at rest and during lower limb exercise: quantification using image-based computer modeling. Am J Physiol Heart Circ Physiol. 2006;291(2):H668–76.
32. Taylor CA, Hughes TJ, Zarins CK. Effect of exercise on hemodynamic conditions in the abdominal aorta. J Vasc Surg. 1999;29(6):1077–89.
33. Les AS, Shadden SC, Figueroa CA, Park JM, Tedesco MM, Herfkens RJ, et al. Quantification of hemodynamics in abdominal aortic aneurysms during rest and exercise using magnetic resonance imaging and computational fluid dynamics. Ann Biomed Eng. 2010;38(4):1288–313.
34. Pyeritz RE. Aneurysms and Marfan syndrome. In: Durstine JL, Moore G, editors. ACSM's exercise management for persons with chronic diseases and disabilities. 1st ed. Champaign, IL: Human Kinetics; 1997.
35. Kertai MD, Bax JJ, Boersma E, Van Urk H, Poldermans D. The prognostic value of dobutamine stress echocardiography in patients with abdominal aortic aneurysm and concomitant coronary artery disease. J Cardiovasc Surg. 2003;44(3):423–30.
36. Hirsch AT, Haskal ZJ, Hertzer NR, Bakal CW, Creager MA, Halperin JL, et al. ACC/AHA guidelines for the management of patients with peripheral arterial disease (lower extremity, renal, mesenteric, and abdominal aortic): a collaborative report from the American Associations for Vascular Surgery/Society for Vascular Surgery, Society for Cardiovascular Angiography and Interventions, Society for Vascular Medicine and Biology, Society of Interventional Radiology, and the ACC/AHA Task Force on Practice Guidelines (writing committee to develop guidelines for the management of patients with peripheral arterial disease)—summary of recommendations. J Vasc Interv Radiol. 2006;17(9):1383–97; quiz 98.
37. Fletcher GF, Ades PA, Kligfield P, Arena R, Balady GJ, Bittner VA, et al. Exercise standards for testing and training: a scientific statement from the American Heart Association. Circulation. 2013;128(8):873–934.
38. Best PJ, Tajik AJ, Gibbons RJ, Pellikka PA. The safety of treadmill exercise stress testing in patients with abdominal aortic aneurysms. Ann Intern Med. 1998;129(8):628–31.
39. Puls A, Thadani U. Rupture of abdominal aortic aneurysm during exercise. Gated blood pool studies. Am J Med. 1986;81(5):887–9.
40. Myers J, Powell A, Smith K, Fonda H, Dalman RL, Stanford AAA SCCOR Investigators. Cardiopulmonary exercise testing in small abdominal aortic aneurysm: profile, safety, and mortality estimates. Eur J Cardiovasc Prev Rehabil. 2011;18(3):459–66.
41. Wasserman Hansen JE, Sue DY, Stringer WW, Whipp BJ. Principles of exercise testing and interpretation. 5th ed. Philadelphia: Lippincott, Williams and Wilkins; 2012.
42. Morris CK, Myers J, Kawaguchi T, Ueshima K, Hideg A, Froelicher VF. Nomogram based on metabolic equivalents and age for assessing aerobic capacity in men. J Am Coll Cardiol. 1993;22:175–82.

43. Yang JC, Wesley RC Jr, Froelicher VF. Ventricular tachycardia during routine treadmill testing. Risk and prognosis. Arch Intern Med. 1991;151(2):349–53.
44. Beckerman J, Wu T, Jones S, Froelicher VF. Exercise test-induced arrhythmias. Prog Cardiovasc Dis. 2005;47(4):285–305.
45. Thompson PD, Franklin BA, Balady GJ, Blair SN, Corrado D, Estes NA 3rd, et al. Exercise and acute cardiovascular events placing the risks into perspective: a scientific statement from the American Heart Association Council on Nutrition, Physical Activity, and Metabolism and the Council on Clinical Cardiology. Circulation. 2007;115(17):2358–68.
46. Carlisle J, Swart M. Mid-term survival after abdominal aortic aneurysm surgery predicted by cardiopulmonary exercise testing. Br J Surg. 2007;94(8):966–9.
47. Smith TB, Stonell C, Purkayastha S, Paraskevas P. Cardiopulmonary exercise testing as a risk assessment method in non cardio-pulmonary surgery: a systematic review. Anaesthesia. 2009;64(8):883–93.
48. Lee JT, Chaloner EJ, Hollingsworth SJ. The role of cardiopulmonary fitness and its genetic influences on surgical outcomes. Br J Surg. 2006;93(2):147–57.
49. Rose GA, Davies RG, Appadurai IR, Lewis WG, Cho JS, Lewis MH, et al. Cardiorespiratory fitness is impaired and predicts mid-term postoperative survival in patients with abdominal aortic aneurysm disease. Exp Physiol. 2018;103(11):1505–12.
50. Brown LC, Thompson SG, Greenhalgh RM, Powell JT, UK Small Aneurysm Trial Participants. Fit patients with small abdominal aortic aneurysms (AAAs) do not benefit from early intervention. J Vasc Surg. 2008;48(6):1375–81.
51. Singh K, Bonaa KH, Jacobsen BK, Bjork L, Solberg S. Prevalence of and risk factors for abdominal aortic aneurysms in a population-based study: the Tromso study. Am J Epidemiol. 2001;154(3):236–44.
52. EVAR trial participants. Endovascular aneurysm repair and outcome in patients unfit for open repair of abdominal aortic aneurysm (EVAR trial 2): randomised controlled trial. Lancet. 2005;365(9478):2187–92.
53. Brown LC, Greenhalgh RM, Howell S, Powell JT, Thompson SG. Patient fitness and survival after abdominal aortic aneurysm repair in patients from the UK EVAR trials. Br J Surg. 2007;94(6):709–16.
54. Kothmann E, Batterham AM, Owen SJ, Turley AJ, Cheesman M, Parry A, Danjoux G. Effect of short-term exercise training on aerobic fitness in patients with abdominal aortic aneurysms: a pilot study. Br J Anaesth. 2009;103:505–10.
55. Myers JN, White JJ, Narasimhan B, Dalman RL. Effects of exercise training in patients with abdominal aortic aneurysm: preliminary results from a randomized trial. J Cardiopulm Rehabil Prev. 2010;30(6):374–83.
56. Tew GA, Moss J, Crank H, Mitchell PA, Nawaz S. Endurance exercise training in patients with small abdominal aortic anuerysm: a randomized controlled pilot study. Arch Phys Med Rehabil. 2012;93:2148–53.
57. Myers J, McElrath M, Jaffe A, Smith K, Fonda H, Vu A, et al. A randomized trial of exercise training in abdominal aortic aneurysm disease. Med Sci Sports Exerc. 2014;46(1):2–9.
58. Barakat HM, Shahin Y, Barnes R, Gohil R, Souroullas P, Khan J, McCollum PT, Chetter IC. Supervised exercise program improves aerobic fitness in patients awaiting abdominal aortic aneurysm repair. Ann Vasc Surg. 2014;28:74–9.
59. Nakayama A, Morita H, Nagayama M, Hoshina K, Uemura Y, Tomoike H, Komuro I. Cardiac rehabilitation protects against the expansion of abdominal aortic aneurysm. J Am Heart Assoc. 2018;7(5). https://doi.org/10.1161/JAHA.117.007959; pii: e007959.
60. Taylor CA, Cheng CP, Espinosa LA, Tang BT, Parker D, Herfkens RJ. In vivo quantification of blood flow and wall shear stress in the human abdominal aorta during lower limb exercise. Ann Biomed Eng. 2002;30(3):402–8.
61. Suh GY, Les AS, Tenforde AS, Shadden SC, Spilker RL, Yeung JJ, et al. Quantification of particle residence time in abdominal aortic aneurysms using magnetic resonance imaging and computational fluid dynamics. Ann Biomed Eng. 2011;39(2):864–83.

62. Gielen S, Schuler G, Adams V. Cardiovascular effects of exercise training: molecular mechanisms. Circulation. 2010;122(12):1221–38.
63. Malek AM, Alper SL, Izumo S. Hemodynamic shear stress and its role in atherosclerosis. JAMA. 1999;282(21):2035–42.
64. Topper JN, Cai J, Falb D, Gimbrone MA Jr. Identification of vascular endothelial genes differentially responsive to fluid mechanical stimuli: cyclooxygenase-2, manganese superoxide dismutase, and endothelial cell nitric oxide synthase are selectively up-regulated by steady laminar shear stress. Proc Natl Acad Sci U S A. 1996;93(19):10417–22.
65. Topper JN, Gimbrone MA Jr. Blood flow and vascular gene expression: fluid shear stress as a modulator of endothelial phenotype. Mol Med Today. 1999;5(1):40–6.
66. Chaikof EL, Brewster DC, Dalman RL, Makaroun MS, Illig KA, Sicard GA, et al. The care of patients with an abdominal aortic aneurysm: the Society for Vascular Surgery practice guidelines. J Vasc Surg. 2009;50(4 Suppl):S2–49.
67. Fonda H, Myers J. Aneurysms. In: Durstine JL, Moore G, editors. ACSM's Exercise Management for Persons with chronic diseases and disabilities. 4th ed. Champaign: Human Kinetics; 2016.
68. Ades PA, Balady GJ, Berra K. Transforming exercise-based cardiac rehabilitation programs into secondary prevention centers: a national imperative. J Cardpulm Rehabil. 2001;21(5):263–72.

# Correction to: Textbook of Sports and Exercise Cardiology

Axel Pressler and Josef Niebauer

## Correction to: A. Pressler, J. Niebauer (eds.), Textbook of Sports and Exercise Cardiology, https://doi.org/10.1007/978-3-030-35374-2

The original version of the chapter 5 and chapter 26 is revised as follows,

In Chapter 5, Figure 5.1 data has been corrected.

Initially the chapter 26 was published with the co-author name as Eric Solberg.

Now chapter 26 and List of contributors, Table of contents in the Front matter was updated with the Author's full name as Erik Ekker Solberg.

The updated online version of this book can be found at
https://doi.org/10.1007/978-3-030-35374-2
https://doi.org/10.1007/978-3-030-35374-2_5
https://doi.org/10.1007/978-3-030-35374-2_26



A. Pressler, J. Niebauer (eds.), *Textbook of Sports and Exercise Cardiology*,
https://doi.org/10.1007/978-3-030-35374-2_52

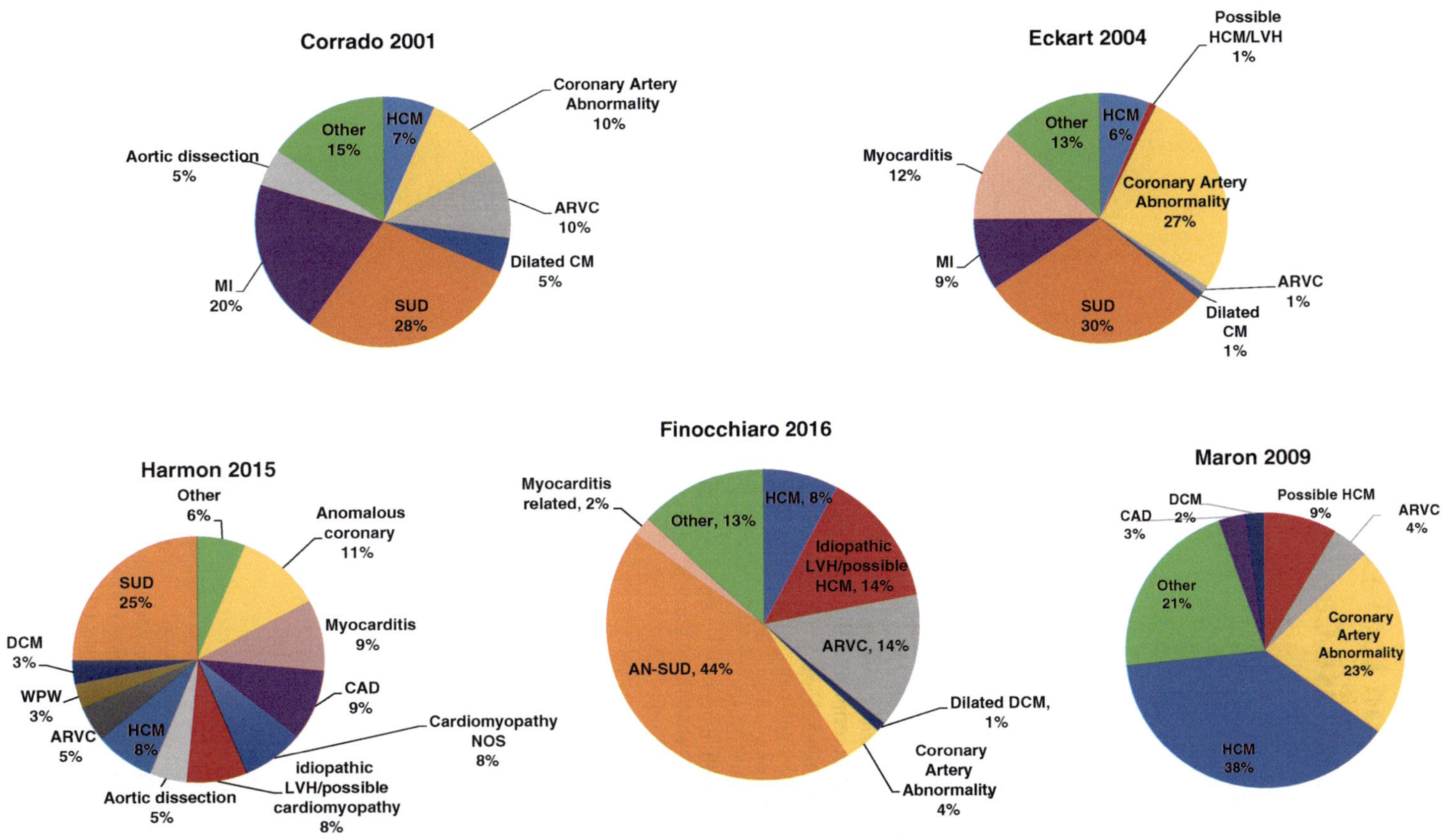


**Fig. 5.1** Graphic comparison of etiology of SCD in athletes. (Created from data reported in [7, 17, 18, 20])

# Index




A. Pressler, J. Niebauer (eds.), *Textbook of Sports and Exercise Cardiology*,
https://doi.org/10.1007/978-3-030-35374-2

**M**

## T

GPSR Compliance

*The European Union's (EU) General Product Safety Regulation (GPSR) is a set of rules that requires consumer products to be safe and our obligations to ensure this.*

*If you have any concerns about our products, you can contact us on ProductSafety@springernature.com*

In case Publisher is established outside the EU, the EU authorized representative is:

Springer Nature Customer Service Center GmbH
Europaplatz 3
69115 Heidelberg, Germany

**Batch number: 10732051**

Printed by Printforce, the Netherlands